Sophia Lahusen Bair
541 968 8199
P 314 294 9263

MANUAL OF CARDIOVASCULAR MEDICINE

Third Edition

MANUAL OF CARDIOVASCULAR MEDICINE

Third Edition

Editors

Brian P. Griffin, MD, FACC
Director, Cardiovascular Disease Training Program
The John and Rosemary Brown Endowed Chair in Cardiovascular Medicine
Cleveland Clinic
Cleveland, Ohio

Eric J. Topol, MD, FACC
Director, Scripps Translational Science Institute
Chief Academic Officer, Scripps Health
Professor of Translational Genomics, TSRI
Senior Consultant, Division of Cardiovascular Diseases
Scripps Clinic
La Jolla, California

Guest Editors

Deepu Nair, MD
Kellan Ashley, MD
Chief Fellows, Cardiovascular Medicine
Cleveland Clinic
Cleveland, Ohio

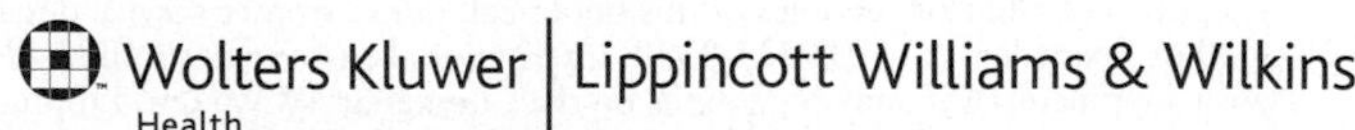

Philadelphia • Baltimore • New York • London
Buenos Aires • Hong Kong • Sydney • Tokyo

Acquisitions Editor: Frances DeStefano
Managing Editor: Chris Potash and Leanne McMillan
Project Manager: Rosanne Hallowell
Manufacturing Manager: Benjamin Rivera
Marketing Manager: Angela Panetta
Art Director: Risa Clow
Production Services: Aptara, Inc.

Third Edition

530 Walnut Street
Philadelphia, PA 19106
LWW.com

Printed in China

Library of Congress Cataloging-in-Publication Data

Manual of cardiovascular medicine / editors, Brian P. Griffin, Eric J. Topol ; guest editors, Deepu Nair, Kellan Ashley.—3rd ed.
p. ; cm.
Includes bibliographical references and index.
ISBN 978-0-7817-7854-1 (alk. paper)
1. Cardiology—Handbooks, manuals, etc. 2. Heart—Diseases—Handbooks, manuals, etc. I. Griffin, Brian P., 1956- II. Topol, Eric J., 1954-.
[DNLM: 1. Heart Diseases—diagnosis. 2. Heart Diseases—therapy.
WG 210 M294 2009]
RC669.15.M35 2009
616.1′2—dc22

2008034724

To purchase additional copies of this book, call our customer service department at (800) 638-3030 or fax orders to (301) 223-2320. International customers should call (301) 223-2300.

Visit Lippincott Williams & Wilkins on the Internet at LWW.com. Lippincott Williams & Wilkins customer service representatives are available from 8:30 am to 6 pm, EST.

10 9 8 7 6 5 4

RRC0910

To our families
—BG, EJT, DN, KA

CONTENTS

SECTION III: VALVULAR HEART DISEASE

SECTION IV: ARRYTHMIAS

SECTION V: VASCULAR AND PERICARDIAL DISEASES

SECTION VI: ADULT CONGENITAL HEART DISEASE

SECTION VII: CLINICAL CARDIOLOGY

SECTION VIII: PREVENTIVE CARDIOLOGY

SECTION IX: NONINVASIVE ASSESSMENT

SECTION XII: COMMON GENETIC ISSUES IN CARDIOLOVASCULAR DISEASE

SECTION XIII: CARDIOVASCULAR DRUGS

CONTRIBUTORS

Unless otherwise noted, the following contributors are affiliated with the Cleveland Clinic Foundation, Cleveland, Ohio.

Zuheir Abrahams, MD
Advanced Fellow in Heart Failure/Transplantation

Mateen Akhtar, MD
Fellow in Cardiovascular Medicine

Carlos Alves, MD
Fellow in Cardiac Electrophysiology

Saif Anwaruddin, MD
Fellow in Interventional Cardiology

Kellan E. Ashley, MD
Chief Cardiovascular Fellow

Arman T. Askari, MD
Associate Program Director
Cardiovascular Disease Training Program

Bethany A. Austin, MD
Fellow in Cardiovascular Medicine

Christopher T. Bajzer, MD
Staff Interventional Cardiologist

Bryan Barandowski, MD
Chief Cardiac Electrophysiology Fellow

Nitin Barman, MD
Interventional Cardiology
Department of Cardiovascular Medicine
Mt. Sinai Hospital
New York, New York

John R. Bartholomew, MD
Chief, Section of Vascular Medicine

Gregory G. Bashian, MD
Fellow in Cardiovascular Medicine

Anthony A. Bavry, MD
Fellow in Interventional Cardiology

Matthew C. Becker, MD
Fellow in Interventional Cardiology

Mandeep Bhargava, MD
Staff Cardiac Electrophysiologist

P. Peter Borek, MD
Felllow in Cardiac Electrophysiology

Andrew Boyle, MD
Assistant Professor of Medicine
University of Minnesota
Minneapolis, Minnesota

Thomas D. Callahan, MD
Staff Cardiac Electrophysiologist

Daniel J. Cantillon, MD
Fellow in Cardiovascular Medicine

Adnan K. Chhatriwalla
Fellow in Interventional Cardiology

Leslie Cho, MD
Director, Women's Heart Center

Arti Choure, MD
Fellow in Cardiovascular Medicine

Ryan D. Christofferson, MD
Interventional Fellow

Ronan J. Curtin, MD
Staff Cardiologist

Ryan P. Daly, MD
Fellow in Cardiovascular Medicine

Ross A. Downey, MD
Fellow in Cardiac Electrophysiology

John M. Galla, MD
Fellow in Cardiovascular Medicine

Stephen Gimple, MD
Fellow in Cardiovascular Medicine

Gonzalo Gonzalez-Stawinski, MD
Staff Cardiac Surgeon

Eiran Z. Gorodeski, MD
Fellow in Cardiovascular Medicine

Adam W. Grasso
Staff Cardiologist

Brian P. Griffin, MD
The John and Rosemary Brown Endowed Chair in Cardiovascular Medicine
Director, Cardiovascular Medicine Fellowship Program

Christian Gring, MD
Staff Cardiologist
Wake Heart & Vascular Associates
Raleigh, North Carolina

Carmel M. Halley, MD
Advanced Fellow in Cardiovascular Medicine

Mazen Hanna, MD
Staff Cardiologist

Brian Hardaway, MD
Fellow in Cardiovascular Medicine

Thomas J. Helton, DO
Fellow in Cardiovascular Medicine

Ron Jacob, MD
Advanced Fellow in Cardiac Imaging

Apur R. Kamdar, MD
Fellow in Cardiovascular Medicine

Matthew A. Kaminski, MD
Fellow in Cardiovascular Medicine

Anne Kanderian, MD
Advanced Fellow in Cardiovascular Medicine

Samir R. Kapadia, MD
Director, Interventional Cardiology Fellowship

Esther S. H. Kim, MD
Vascular Fellow

Yuli Y. Kim, MD
Fellow in Cardiovascular Medicine

Amar Krishnaswamy
Fellow in Cardiovascular Medicine

Deborah H. Kwon, MD
Fellow in Cardiovascular Imaging

Timothy H. Mahoney, MD
Fellow in Cardiovascular Medicine

Anjli Maroo, MD
Staff Cardiologist
Department of Cardiology
Fairview Hospital
Cleveland, Ohio

A. Thomas McRae III, MD
Staff Cardiologist
Department of Cardiology
Centennial Hospital
Nashville, Tennessee

Telly A. Meadows, MD
Fellow in Cardiovascular Medicine

Kamran I. Muhammed, MD
Fellow in Cardiovascular Medicine

Debabrata Mukherjee, MD
Director, Cardiac Catheterization Laboratory
Gill Heart Institute
University of Kentucky
Lexington, Kentucky

Wilfried Mullens, MD
Fellow in Heart Failure and Cardiovascular Transplantation

Deepu Nair, MD
Chief Cardiovascular Medicine Fellow

Marc S. Penn, MD, PhD
Associate Program Director
Department of Cardiovascular Medicine

Athar M. Qureshi, MD
Associate Staff
Department of Pediatric Cardiology

Russell Raymond, MD
Staff Interventional Cardiologist

Mark Robbins, MD
Assistant Professor of Medicine
Department of Medicine
Vanderbilt University
Nashville, Tennessee

Robert A. Schweikert, MD
Chief of Cardiology
Akron General Hospital
Akron, Ohio

Shaun Senter, MD
Fellow in Cardiovascular Medicine

Medhi H. Shishehbor, MD
Interventional Cardiology Fellow

W. H. Wilson Tang, MD
Staff Cardiologist

Khaldoun G. Tarakji, MD
Fellow in Cardiovascular Medicine

Patrick Tchou, MD
Staff Cardiac Electrophysiologist

Maran Thamilarasan, MD
Staff Cardiologist

George Thomas, MD
Fellow in Cardiac Electrophysiology

Eric J. Topol, MD
Director, Scripps Translational Science Institute
Chief Academic Officer, Scripps Health
Professor of Translational Genomics, TSRI
Senior Consultant, Division of Cardiovascular Diseases
Scripps Clinic
La Jolla, California

Richard Troughton, MB, BCh, PhD
Associate Professor
Department of Medicine
University of Otago, Christ Church
Christ Church, New Zealand

Samuel Unzek, MD
Fellow in Cardiovascular Medicine

Oussama Wazni, MD
Staff Cardiologist

Tim Williams, MD
Cardiovascular Associates of Charlottesville
Charlottesville, South Carolina

PREFACE

The aims of the *Manual of Cardiovascular Medicine* remain the same in its third edition: to provide a concise but thorough overview of current diagnosis and practice in cardiovascular medicine. It has been written predominantly by staff and fellows in cardiovascular medicine and related fields at Cleveland Clinic. This edition has been extensively revised and updated to reflect significant changes in diagnosis and management of cardiovascular disease since the last edition 4 years ago. A chapter on genetics in cardiovascular disease has been added and, where appropriate, current ACC/AHA or other important guidelines have been added.

I wish to thank all who contributed to this and previous editions. Specifically, I wish to recognize the Guest Editors, Deepu Nair and Kellan Ashley, who did a phenomenal job of maintaining the timeline and the quality of the contributions. I am very grateful also to the section editors for their exceptional work in ensuring that the various chapters are topical and accurate. I am particularly thankful to Drs. Marc Penn, Arman Askari, and Venu Menon for their mentorship of the fellows over the years. I wish to thank Lois Adamski, the educational coordinator of the Cardiovascular Disease Training Program at Cleveland Clinic, and Barbara Robinson, my personal assistant, without whose help this edition would not have been possible. Fran DeStefano and all at Wolters Kluwer have been excellent colleagues in ensuring a reader-friendly text. I am deeply indebted to John and Rosemary Brown, for endowing a Chair in Cardiovascular Medicine that helps support my academic activity, and for their wonderful friendship over the years. Finally, I wish to express my immense gratitude to my family: to my parents for instilling in me a thirst for knowledge, and to my wife Mary without whose support, patience, and fortitude, this and all other endeavors would be impossible.

Brian P. Griffin, MD

MANUAL OF CARDIOVASCULAR MEDICINE

Third Edition

Ischemic Heart Disease I

ACUTE MYOCARDIAL INFARCTION 1

Ryan D. Christofferson

I. EPIDEMIOLOGY. Acute myocardial infarction (MI) is the leading cause of death in North America and Europe. In the United States, the annual death toll from coronary heart disease is higher than 800,000 (1). More than 1 million people each year in the United States sustain an acute MI. An additional 300,000 or more are estimated to die of acute MI before hospitalization. An American has an acute MI every 25 seconds, and someone dies of cardiovascular disease every 36 seconds. Including patients who die before hospital admission, the overall mortality rate of acute MI is >30%, although the incidence and mortality have declined over the last 30 years with the advent of the coronary care unit, fibrinolytic therapy, and catheter-based reperfusion. Although primary percutaneous coronary intervention (PCI) has been shown to lower mortality, a substantial number of patients with acute MI are not eligible for this therapy. Many patients do not have ready access to hospitals that perform 24-hour PCI for acute MI. With the elderly representing an increasing proportion of the population who have a high incidence of and mortality from acute MI and decreased eligibility for fibrinolytic therapy, it probably will remain the leading cause of death over the next several decades. Moreover, the increased incidence of diabetes and obesity stemming from a global shift to a Western diet and lifestyle will increase the sequelae of coronary artery disease in the future.

II. PATHOPHYSIOLOGY. Coronary **plaque fissuring or rupture** is the initiating event of acute MI. Rupture of the fibrous cap of a coronary atheroma exposes the underlying subendothelial matrix to formed elements of circulating blood, leading to activation of platelets, thrombin generation, and thrombus formation. This is a dynamic process that involves cyclical transitioning between complete vessel occlusion, partial vessel occlusion, and reperfusion. Occlusive thrombus in the absence of significant collateral vessels most often results in acute ST-segment-elevation MI (STEMI). The pathophysiology of STEMI and non–ST-segment elevation MI (NSTEMI) is similar, and this explains the substantial overlap in acute coronary syndromes with regard to ultimate outcome, extent of necrosis, and mortality rates. However, the recognition of ST-segment elevation remains important because it generally mandates the need for emergent reperfusion therapy.

III. DEFINITION. A recent expert consensus document (2) redefined acute MI as the detection of a rise and/or fall in cardiac biomarkers with at least one value above the 99th percentile of the upper reference limit (URL), together with evidence of ischemia. Ischemia was defined as any symptoms of ischemia, electrocardiographic changes suggestive of new ischemia, development of pathologic Q waves on electrocardiogram (EKG) or imaging evidence of infarction. Included in the definition was sudden cardiac death with evidence of myocardial ischemia (new ST-elevation, left bundle-branch block, or coronary thrombus), biomarker elevation >3× URL for post-PCI patients, or >5× URL for post coronary artery bypass grafting (post-CABG) patients.

TABLE 1.1 Clinical Classification of Different Types of Myocardial Infarction

Type 1	Spontaneous MI related to ischemia from a coronary plaque rupture or dissection
Type 2	MI due to ischemia resulting from increased oxygen demand or decreased supply
Type 3	Sudden cardiac death with symptoms of ischemia, new ST-elevation, or LBBB or coronary thrombus
Type 4a	MI associated with PCI
Type 4b	MI associated with stent thrombosis
Type 5	MI associated with CABG

CABG, Coronary artery bypass grafting; LBBB, left bundle-branch block; MI, myocardial infarction; PCI, percutaneous coronary intervention.
Adapted from Thygesen K, Alpert JS, White HD. Universal definition of myocardial infarction. *J Am Coll Cardiol* 2007;50:2173–2175.

Documented stent thrombosis was recognized in this new definition as well (Table 1.1). Established MI was defined as any one criterion that satisfies the following: development of new pathologic Q waves on serial ECGs, imaging evidence of MI, or pathologic findings of healed or healing MI.

IV. CLINICAL DIAGNOSIS. In any patient with a clinical history of chest pain suspected to be of cardiac origin, an ECG should be obtained within 5 minutes of presentation and interpreted promptly to determine eligibility for reperfusion therapy. If the **ECG demonstrates acute ST-segment elevation or new left bundle-branch block (LBBB), emergent reperfusion treatment with fibrinolysis or primary PCI is indicated.** During this evaluation period, a targeted medical history and physical examination should be performed. If the patient's history is compatible with cardiac ischemia and the ECG does not meet the criteria for reperfusion therapy, the patient may have unstable angina or NSTEMI. These syndromes are discussed in Chapter 2.

A. Signs and symptoms

1. The classic symptoms are severe, **crushing substernal chest pain** described as a squeezing or constricting sensation with frequent radiation to the left arm, often associated with an impending sense of doom. The discomfort is similar to that of angina pectoris, but it is typically more severe, of longer duration (usually more than 20 minutes), and is not relieved with rest or nitroglycerin. Peak intensity usually is not instantaneous, as it would be with pulmonary embolus or aortic dissection.
   a. The chest discomfort may radiate to the neck, jaw, back, shoulder, right arm, and epigastrium. Pain in any of these locations without chest pain is possible. Myocardial ischemic pain localized to the epigastrium is often misdiagnosed as indigestion. Acute MI can occur without chest pain, especially among postoperative patients, the elderly, and those with diabetes mellitus.
   b. If the pain radiates to the back and is described as tearing or knifelike, aortic dissection should be considered.
2. Associated symptoms may include diaphoresis, dyspnea, fatigue, lightheadedness, palpitations, acute confusion, indigestion, nausea, or vomiting. Gastrointestinal symptoms are especially common with inferior infarction.

B. Physical examination. In general, the physical examination does not add much to the diagnosis of acute MI. However, the examination is extremely important in excluding other diagnoses that may mimic acute MI, in risk stratification, in the diagnosis of impending heart failure, and in serving as a baseline examination to monitor for mechanical complications of acute MI that may develop.

1. **Risk stratification,** which aids in treatment decisions and counseling patients and families, is based in part on age, heart rate, blood pressure, and on the presence or absence of pulmonary edema and a third heart sound.

2. The **mechanical complications** of mitral regurgitation and ventricular septal defect often are heralded by a new systolic murmur (see Chapter 3). Early diagnosis of these complications relies on well-documented examination findings at baseline and during the hospital course.

V. DIFFERENTIAL DIAGNOSIS. The differential diagnosis of ST-elevation includes conditions with comorbid ischemia such as acute aortic dissection, conditions with ST elevation but no ischemia, such as left ventricular (LV) hypertrophy, and conditions with chest pain but no ischemia such as myopericarditis (Table 1.2). The most common differential diagnostic considerations are discussed in the following text.

A. Pericarditis. Chest pain that is worse when the person is supine and improves when the person is sitting upright or slightly forward is typical of pericarditis. Care must be taken in excluding acute MI, however, because pericarditis can complicate acute MI. The electrocardiographic abnormalities of acute pericarditis may also be confused with acute MI. Diffuse ST-segment elevation is the hallmark of acute pericarditis, but this finding may be seen in acute MI that involves the left main coronary artery or a large "wrap-around" left anterior descending artery. PR-segment depression, peaked T waves, or electrocardiographic abnormalities out of proportion to the clinical scenario may favor the diagnosis of pericarditis. The ST-segment elevations in pericarditis are often concave, whereas the ST-segment elevations in acute MI are usually convex. Reciprocal ST depression does not occur in pericarditis, except in leads aVR and V_1. Echocardiography may be useful, not in evaluating pericardial effusion, which may occur in either condition, but in documenting the lack of wall-motion abnormalities in the setting of ongoing pain and ST elevation.

B. Myocarditis. As with pericarditis, the symptoms and electrocardiographic findings of myocarditis may be similar to those of acute MI. Echocardiography is less useful in differentiating this syndrome from acute MI, because diffuse LV dysfunction may be encountered in either condition. A complete history often reveals a more insidious onset and associated viral syndrome with myocarditis.

C. Acute aortic dissection. Sharp, tearing chest pain that radiates through the chest to the back is typical of aortic dissection (see Chapter 25). This type of radiation pattern should be investigated thoroughly before administration of antithrombotic, antiplatelet, or fibrinolytic therapy. Proximal extension of the dissection into either coronary ostium can account for acute MI. A chest radiograph may reveal a widened mediastinum. Transthoracic echocardiography may reveal a dissection flap in the proximal ascending aorta. If it does not, a more definitive diagnosis should be obtained with transesophageal echocardiography, computerized tomography (CT), or magnetic resonance imaging (MRI).

D. Pulmonary embolism. Shortness of breath associated with pleuritic chest pain but without evidence of pulmonary edema suggests pulmonary embolism. Echocardiography helps to rule out wall-motion abnormalities and may identify right

TABLE 1.2 Differential Diagnostic Considerations for STEMI

Comorbid ischemia	ST elevation but no ischemia	Chest pain but no ischemia
Aortic dissection	Early repolarization	Aortic dissection
Systemic arterial embolism	Left ventricular hypertrophy	Myopericarditis
Hypertensive crisis	Left bundle-branch block	Pleuritis
Aortic stenosis	Hyperkalemia	Pulmonary embolism
Cocaine use	Brugada syndrome	Costochondritis
Arteritis		GI disorders

Adapted from Christofferson RD. Acute ST-elevation myocardial infarction. In: Shishehbor MH, Wang TH, Askari AT, et al., eds. *Management of the patient in the coronary care unit.* New York: Lippincott Williams & Wilkins, 2008.

ventricular (RV) strain, which is an indication for fibrinolytic therapy in the setting of pulmonary embolism.

E. Esophageal disorders. Gastroesophageal reflux disease, esophageal motility disorders, and esophageal hyperalgesia can cause chest pain, the character of which is very similar to cardiac ischemic pain. These disorders can often coexist in patients with coronary disease, thereby complicating the diagnosis. A workup for coronary disease should precede evaluation of esophageal disorders. Symptoms that may be suggestive but not diagnostic of chest pain of an esophageal origin include postprandial symptoms, relief with antacids, and lack of radiation of pain.

F. Acute cholecystitis can mimic the symptoms and ECG findings of inferior acute MI, although the two can coexist. Tenderness in the right upper quadrant, fever, and an elevated leukocyte count favor cholecystitis, which can be diagnosed by means of hepatobiliary iminodiacetic acid (HIDA) scanning.

VI. LABORATORY EXAMINATION

A. Creatinine kinase. An elevated level of creatinine kinase (CK) is rarely helpful in making the diagnosis of acute MI for a patient with ST-segment elevation. Because it usually takes 4 to 6 hours to see an appreciable rise in CK levels, a normal value may signify recent complete occlusion. CK and CK-MB (myocardial band) levels can be elevated in the presence of pericarditis and myocarditis, which may cause diffuse ST-segment elevation. CK levels are more helpful in gauging the size and timing of acute MI than in making the diagnosis. CK levels peak at 24 hours, but the peak CK level is believed to occur earlier among patients who undergo successful reperfusion. False-positive results of CK elevation occur in a variety of settings, including skeletal muscle disease or trauma (e.g., rhabdomyolysis).

B. Troponins. Troponin T and troponin I assays are particularly useful in the diagnosis and management of unstable angina and NSTEMI because of their high sensitivity, ability to be used and interpreted rapidly at bedside, and nearly universal availability. However, the lag time (3 to 6 hours) between occlusion and detectable elevations in serum levels limits their usefulness in the diagnosis of acute STEMI. Data have suggested that a single troponin T concentration measured 72 hours after acute MI may be predictive of MI size, independent of reperfusion (3). Troponin elevation in the absence of ischemic heart disease can be found in congestive heart failure (CHF), aortic dissection, hypertrophic cardiomyopathy, pulmonary embolism, acute neurologic disease, cardiac contusion, or drug toxicity.

C. Myoglobin. Damaged cardiac myocytes rapidly release this protein into the bloodstream. Peak levels occur between 1 and 4 hours, allowing for early diagnosis of acute MI. However, myoglobin lacks cardiac specificity, thereby limiting its clinical utility. Studies have indicated that it might play a role in risk stratification after reperfusion therapy (4).

VII. DIAGNOSTIC TESTING

A. Electrocardiography

1. **Definitive electrocardiographic diagnosis** of acute MI requires ST elevation of 1 mm or more in two or more contiguous leads, often with reciprocal ST depression in the contralateral leads. In leads V_2-V_3, 2 mm of ST elevation in men and 1.5 mm in women is required for accurate diagnosis.
2. **ECG subsets.** ST-segment elevations can be divided into subgroups that may be correlated with the infarction-related artery and risk for death. These five subgroups are listed in Table 1.3 and illustrated in Figure 1.1.
3. **Left Bundle-Branch Block (LBBB)**
   a. **New LBBB in the setting of symptoms consistent with acute MI** may indicate a large, anterior wall acute MI involving the proximal left anterior descending coronary artery and should be managed as acute STEMI.
   b. **In the absence of an old ECG or in the presence of LBBB at baseline** the diagnosis of acute STEMI can be made in the presence of LBBB with greater than 90% specificity on the basis of the criteria listed in Table 1.4 and illustrated in Figure 1.2.

TABLE 1.3 Acute Myocardial Infarction: ECG Subsets and Correlated Infarct-Related Artery and Mortality

Category	Anatomy of occlusion	ECG findings	30-Day mortality rate (%)[a]	1-Year mortality rate (%)
1. Proximal LAD	Proximal to first septal perforator	ST ↑ V_{1-6}, I, aVL and fasicular or bundle-branch block	19.6	25.6
2. Mid-LAD	Proximal to large diagonal but distal to first septal perforator	ST ↑ V_{1-6}, I, aVL	9.2	12.4
3. Distal LAD or diagonal	Distal to large diagonal or diagonal itself	ST ↑ V_{1-4}, or I, aVL, V_{5-6}	6.8	10.2
4. Moderate to large inferior (posterior, lateral, right ventricular)	Proximal RCA or left circumflex	ST ↑ II, III, aVF, and any of the following: a. V_1, V_3R, V_4R b. V_{5-6} c. R > S in V_1, V_2	6.4	8.4
5. Small inferior	Distal RCA or left circumflex branch	ST ↑ II, III, aVF only	4.5	6.7

LAD, Left anterior descending (coronary artery); ↑, increased; RCA, right coronary artery.
[a]Mortality rate based on GUSTO I cohort population in each of the 5-year categories, all receiving reperfusion therapy.
From Topol EJ, Van de Werf FJ. Acute myocardial infarction: early diagnosis and management. In: Topol EJ, ed. *Textbook of cardiovascular medicine.* New York: Lippincott-Raven, 1998, with permission.

c. Right bundle-branch block (RBBB) complicates interpretation of ST elevation in leads V_1 through V_3. The diagnosis of anterior acute MI is possible when the normal secondary T-wave changes (i.e., opposite the terminal deflection of the QRS complex) in a patient with RBBB in leads V_1 through V_3 or V_4 are replaced with T waves of concordant polarity with the QRS (i.e., pseudonormalization). RBBB does not obscure ST-segment elevation in other leads.

B. Echocardiography may be helpful in the evaluation of LBBB of undetermined duration in that the lack of regional wall-motion abnormality in the presence of continuing symptoms makes the diagnosis of acute MI unlikely.

VIII. RISK STRATIFICATION. It is possible and useful to estimate the risk of death of a patient with acute MI. The estimate can aid in making treatment decisions and recommendations and in counseling patients and families. Five simple baseline parameters have been reported to account for more than 90% of the prognostic information for 30-day mortality. These characteristics are given in descending order of importance: age, systolic blood pressure, Killip classification (Table 1.5), heart rate, and location of MI (Table 1.3, Fig. 1.1) (5).

IX. THERAPY

A. Immediate management and stabilization

1. Aspirin. Immediate administration of aspirin is indicated for all patients with acute MI, unless there is a clear history of true aspirin allergy (not intolerance). Aspirin therapy conveys as much mortality benefit as streptokinase, and the combination provides additive benefit (6). The dose should be four, chewable 81-mg tablets (for more rapid absorption) or one 325-mg nonchewable tablet. If oral administration is not possible, a rectal suppository can be given. If true aspirin allergy is present, clopidogrel monotherapy is the best alternative.

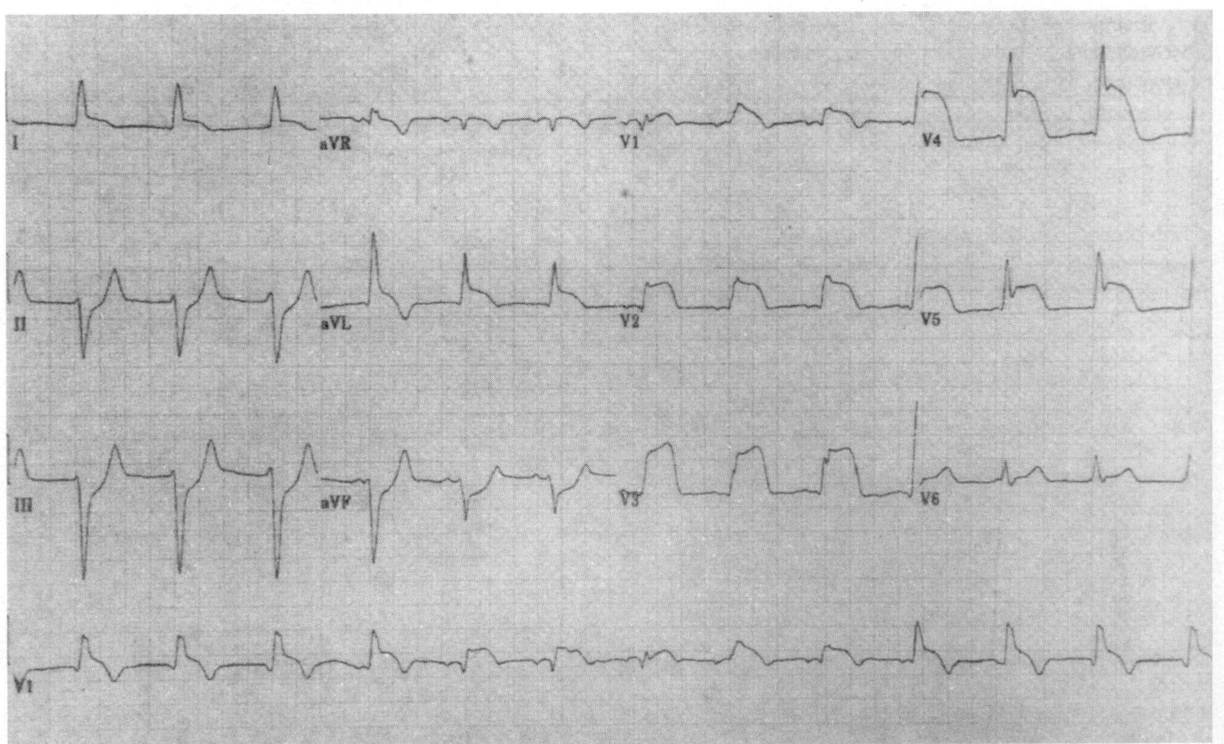

Figure 1.1. Electrocardiographic subsets of acute myocardial infarction (MI). **A:** Large anterior MI with conduction disturbance [proximal left anterior descending coronary artery (LAD)]. (*Continued*)

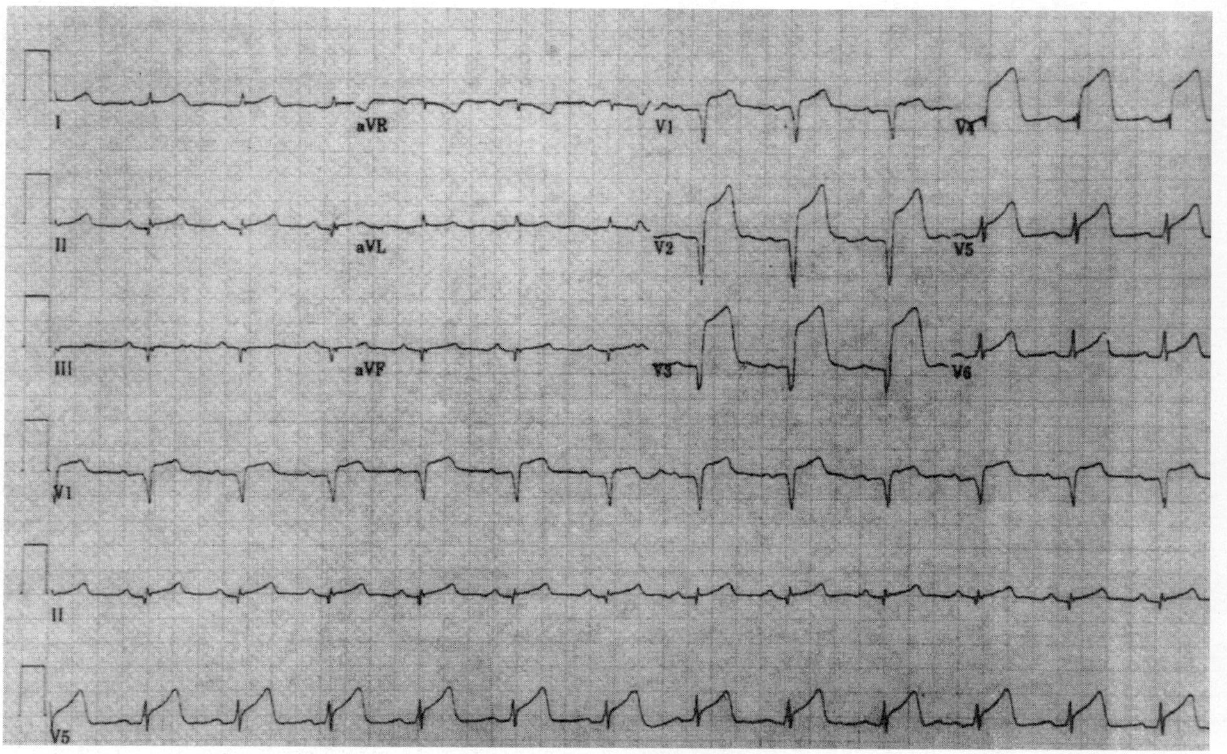

Figure 1.1. B: Anterior MI without conduction disturbance (mid-LAD). (*Continued*)

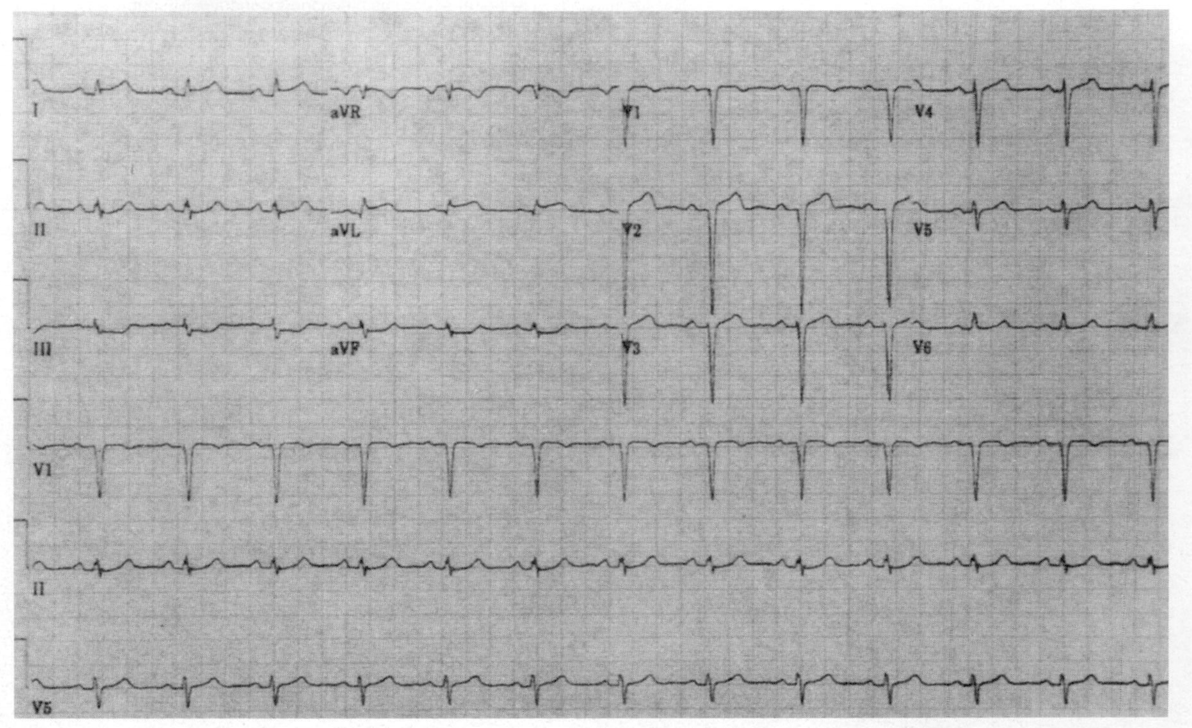

Figure 1.1. **C:** Lateral MI (distal LAD, diagonal branch, or left circumflex branch). (*Continued*)

D

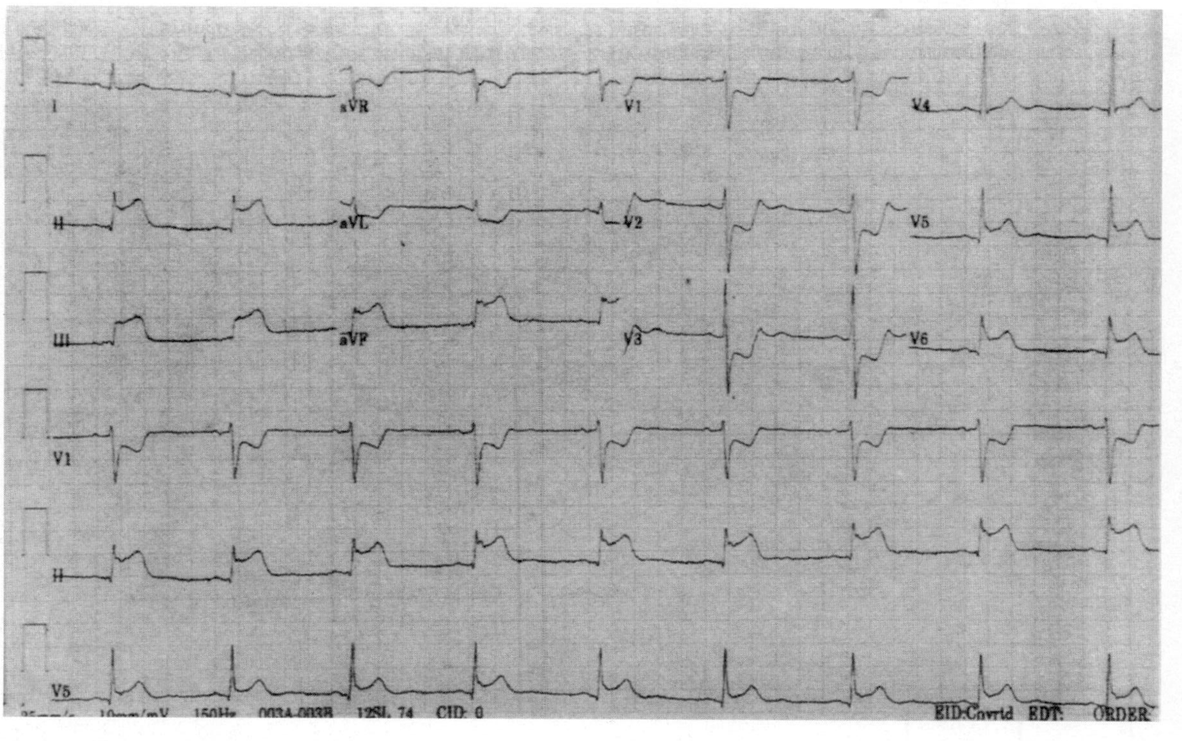

Figure 1.1. D: Large inferior MI with reciprocal changes [proximal right coronary artery (RCA)]. (*Continued*)

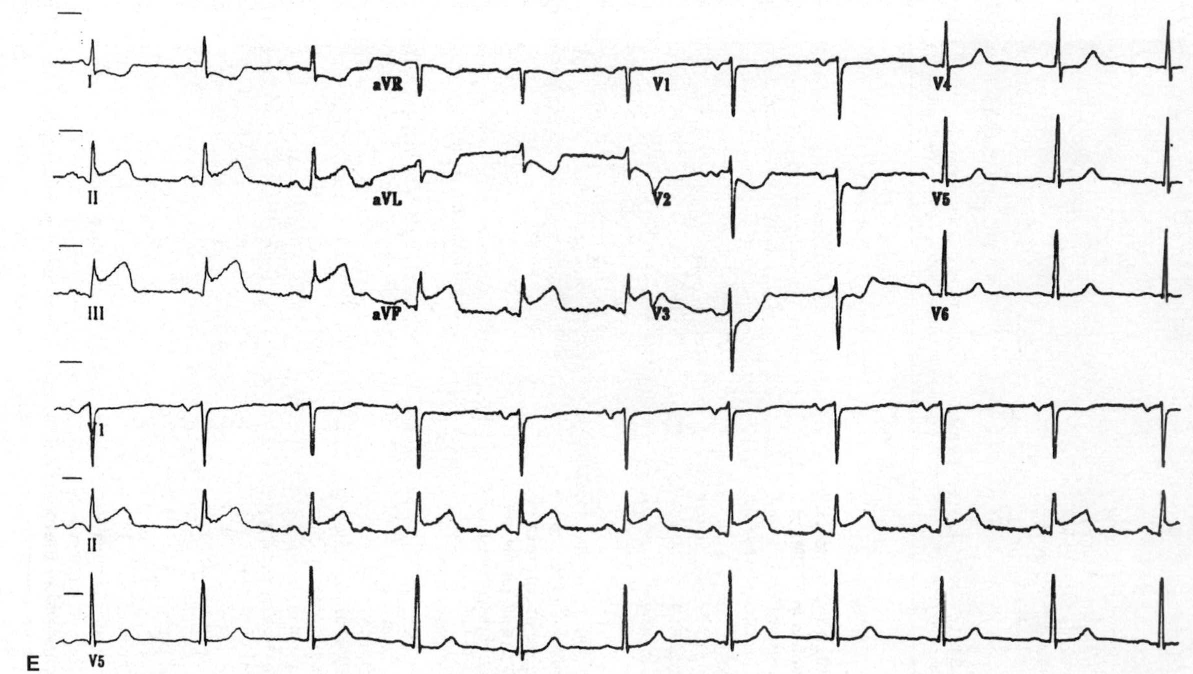

Figure 1.1. E: Small inferior MI (distal RCA). (From Topol EJ, Van de Werf FJ. Acute myocardial infarction: early diagnosis and management. In: Topol EJ, ed. *Textbook of cardiovascular medicine.* New York: Lippincott-Raven, 2002, with permission.)

TABLE 1.4 Electrocardiographic Criteria for the Diagnosis of Acute Myocardial Infarction in the Presence of Left Bundle-Branch Block

Criterion	Score[a]
ST-segment elevation $\geq$1 mm concordant with QRS	5
ST-segment depression $\geq$1 mm in lead V_1, V_2, or V_3	3
ST-segment elevation $\geq$5 mm discordant with QRS	2

[a]Point scores for each criterion met are added. Total point score of 3 yields $\geq$90% specificity and an 88% positive predictive value.
Adapted from Sgarbossa EB, Pinski SL, Barbagelata A, et al. Electrocardiographic diagnosis of evolving acute myocardial infarction in the presence of left bundle branch block. *N Engl J Med* 1996;334:481–487.

2. **Thienopyridines.** Recent data indicate that **clopidogrel should be added to aspirin in STEMI patients regardless of whether they undergo primary PCI or fibrinolysis**. The CLARITY-TIMI 28 trial showed pretreatment with clopidogrel to be safe and effective without increased bleeding among patients treated with fibrinolytic therapy, with many receiving subsequent PCI (~57%) (7). The composite endpoint of cardiovascular death, re-infarction or revascularization was reduced from 14.1% to 11.6% ($p = 0.03$) by clopidogrel pretreatment. A subsequent large randomized double-blind placebo-controlled trial ($N = 22{,}891$) called COMMIT/CCS-2 found a significant reduction in all-cause mortality (8.1% vs. 7.5%) but no difference in major bleeding (8). An oral loading dose of 300 mg is given, followed by 75 mg daily. Where CABG is planned it is recommended to wait 5 to 7 days after clopidogrel administration before surgery unless urgent revascularization is needed (9).
3. **Oxygen.** Supplemental oxygen by means of nasal cannula should be given to all patients with suspected MI. Administration through a face mask or endotracheal tube may be necessary for patients with severe pulmonary edema or cardiogenic shock.
4. **Nitroglycerin.** It is worthwhile to give sublingual nitroglycerin (0.4 mg) to determine whether the ST-segment elevation represents coronary artery spasm while arrangements for reperfusion therapy are being initiated. Patients should be questioned about recent use of sildenafil (Viagra) because administration of nitroglycerin within 24 hours of sildenafil may cause life-threatening hypotension. A meta-analysis performed before the age of routine reperfusion suggested a mortality benefit with intravenous nitroglycerin (10), although routine use of oral nitrates after MI had no benefit in two large randomized trials in the modern era. Nitroglycerin can be useful in the management of acute MI complicated by CHF, ongoing symptoms, or hypertension. A 30% reduction in systolic blood pressure can be expected with appropriately aggressive dosing (10 to 20 μg/min with 5 to 10 μg/min increases every 5 to 10 min). Intravenous therapy can be continued for 24 to 48 hours, after which time patients with heart failure or residual ischemia can convert to oral or topical therapy with an appropriate nitrate-free interval to avoid tachyphylaxis.
5. **Reperfusion therapy.** The primary goal in the management of acute MI is to institute reperfusion therapy as quickly as possible. All patients with ST-segment elevation or new LBBB MI who seek treatment within 12 to 24 hours from onset of continuous symptoms should be considered for immediate reperfusion therapy. Persistent ischemic symptoms after 12 hours may indicate a stuttering course of occlusion, spontaneous reperfusion, and reocclusion, and may indicate potential continued benefit for early therapy.
   a. **Benefit.** The benefit of reperfusion therapy has been well documented in the management of acute MI, regardless of age, gender, and most baseline

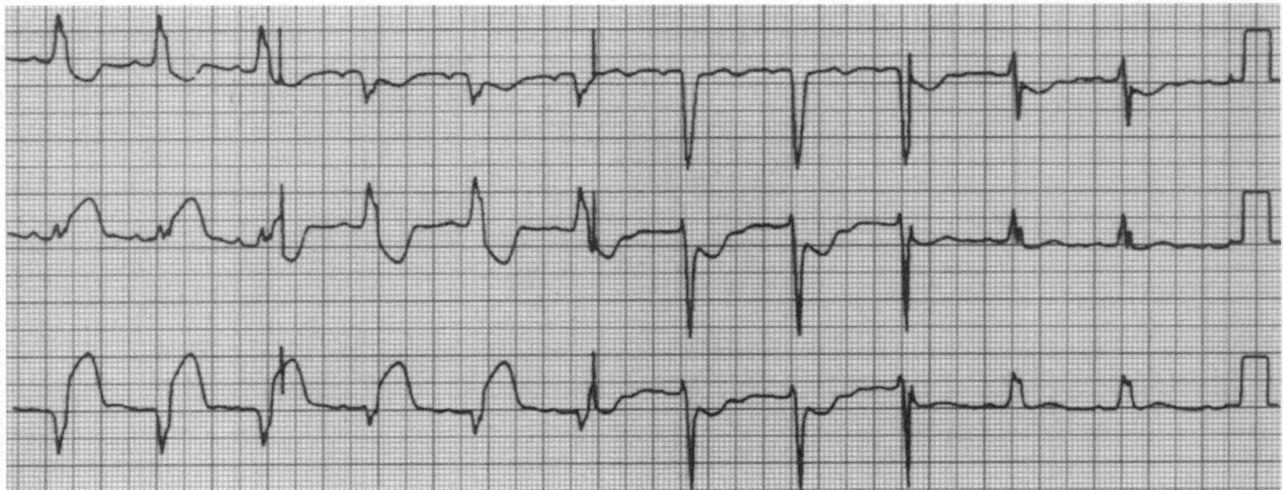

Figure 1.2. Electrocardiogram displays all of the criteria for the diagnosis of acute myocardial infarction (MI) in the setting of left bundle-branch block (LBBB): ST-segment elevation greater than 1 mm, concordant with QRS in lead II (5 points); ST-segment depression greater than 1 mm in leads V_2 and V_3 (3 points); and ST-segment elevation greater than 5 mm, discordant with QRS in leads III and VF (2 points). A score of 10 points indicates an extremely high likelihood of inferior MI. (From Sgarbossa EB, Wagner G, 1997, with permission.)

TABLE 1.5 30-Day Mortality Based on Hemodynamic (Killip) Class

Killip class	Characteristics	Patients (%)	Mortality rate (%)
I	No evidence of CHF	85	5.1
II	Rales, ↑ JVD, or S_3	13	13.6
III	Pulmonary edema	1	32.2
IV	Cardiogenic shock	1	57.8

CHF, Congestive heart failure; ↑, increased; JVD, jugular venous distention; S_3, third heart sound. Adapted from Lee KL, Woodlief LH, Topol EJ, et al. Predictors of 30-day mortality in the era of reperfusion for acute myocardial infarction. Results from an international trial of 41,021 patients. GUSTO-I Investigators. *Circulation* 1995;91:1659–1668.

characteristics. However, the patients who derive the most benefit are those treated earliest and those at highest risk, such as those with anterior MI.

b. Time to treatment is paramount. Patients treated in the first hour have the highest morality benefit. It is unclear whether this results entirely from the prevention of myocardial damage or whether those who seek treatment early have a larger infarction and are preselected to derive pronounced benefit. Regardless, **numerous trials support an inverse relation between time to treatment and survival benefit.** This relationship appears more consistent with fibrinolytic therapy than for direct PCI. After 12 hours of continuous symptoms, there is little net benefit to pharmacologic reperfusion with fibrinolytics, although recent data indicate that the benefit of primary PCI in terms of infarct-size reduction may extend even beyond 12 to 24 hours (BRAVE-2 study), even among patients without persistent chest pain (11).

c. Fibrinolysis versus direct PCI. After it has been determined that a patient is a candidate for reperfusion therapy, the decision to use fibrinolytic or direct PCI therapy must be made quickly.

(1) If facilities for immediate coronary angiography and PCI are available within 90 minutes of first medical contact, this is the preferred therapy. Pooled data from several large trials show a significant (22%) reduction in short-term mortality for patients treated with primary angioplasty (12). This benefit was durable because there were significant reductions in the incidence of death, nonfatal MI, and recurrent ischemia at long-term follow-up. PCI is also associated with a reduction in the incidence of intracerebral hemorrhage compared to fibrinolytic therapy.

(2) If facilities for immediate coronary angiography and direct PCI are not available, fibrinolytic therapy, unless contraindicated, should be instituted within 30 minutes of first medical contact. Anticipated prolonged transfer time to a primary PCI facility (medical contact-to-balloon time >90 minutes) is also an indication for fibrinolytic therapy (9). There is some controversy regarding the use of primary PCI with prolonged transfer times. Several trials, including the DANAMI-2 (Danish Multicenter Randomized Study on Thrombolytic Therapy Versus Acute Coronary Angioplasty in Acute Myocardial Infarction) (13), AIR-PAMI (Air-Primary Angioplasty in Myocardial Infarction) (14), and the PRAGUE (Primary Angioplasty in Patients Transferred from a General Community Hospital to Specialized PTCA Units) (15), have investigated the benefit of on-site fibrinolysis compared with transfer to tertiary centers for direct PCI. These studies have found improved outcomes in patients randomized to a transfer strategy and direct PCI even after taking into account the increased time for patient transfer. For example, patients in DANAMI 2 randomized to transfer PCI had a significantly lower 30-day incidence of death, MI, or stroke (8.5% vs. 14.3%, $p = 0.002$) despite a median time from randomization to balloon inflation of 112 minutes. However, **current guidelines are designed to emphasize early reperfusion, whether this is with primary PCI or thrombolytic therapy** (9).

(3) If a contraindication to fibrinolytic therapy exists or there is some question of the diagnosis, arrangements should be made for transfer to a PCI facility.

(4) Because of the relative lack of efficacy of lytic therapy among patients with cardiogenic shock or prior bypass operations, such patients are especially well suited for primary PCI. However, if a long delay (>3 hours) is anticipated, fibrinolytic therapy may still be considered while arrangements for coronary angiography are made.

d. Primary PCI. Once the decision has been made to perform reperfusion with primary PCI, the patient should be moved to the cardiac catheterization laboratory and undergo angiography as rapidly as possible. After the culprit lesion has been identified, reperfusion should be achieved with standard PCI techniques (see Chapter 59).

(1) Platelet glycoprotein IIb/IIIa inhibitors (GP IIb/IIIa). Several clinical trials have documented the benefits of abciximab in improving clinical outcomes after primary PCI with or without stenting in patients with STEMI. Results from the RAPPORT (ReoPro and Primary PTCA Organization and Trial) showed a nearly 50% reduction in death, MI, or urgent total vascular resistance (TVR) at 30 days in patients treated with abciximab compared with placebo at the time of PCI (11.2% vs. 5.8%, $p = 0.03$) (16). The ADMIRAL (Abciximab before Direct Angioplasty and Stenting in Myocardial Infarction Regarding Acute and Long-Term Follow-up) study found a significant reduction in the composite endpoint of death, MI, urgent TVR at 30-days in patients randomized to abciximab before direct PCI or stenting (6.0% vs. 14.6%, $p = 0.01$) (17). The finding of favorable outcomes with abciximab and stenting was replicated by the ACE trial, which compared stenting alone to stenting with abciximab, showing a reduction of >50% in a similar composite endpoint with abciximab and stenting (18). As a result, abciximab (0.25 mg/kg by intravenous [IV] bolus, followed by 0.125 mcg/kg/min infusion over 12 hours) should be considered in the care of all patients undergoing primary PCI for acute MI. Although a point of some debate, it appears that tirofiban may be equivalent to abciximab in terms of infarct size and bleeding events (19). In addition, early (emergency department) administration of eptifibatide or tirofiban may increase primary patency rates, although hard outcomes data are lacking with these alternative therapies.

(2) Aspiration devices and distal embolic protection. Although aspiration catheters have been shown to improve ST-segment resolution and myocardial blush, they have not been shown to improve clinical outcomes. Similarly, distal embolic protection has failed to show any benefit in multiple trials and may in fact increase infarct size. The major criticism of these trials is the exclusion of patients with large thrombus burden. Regardless of this caveat, these devices are not routinely recommended for acute PCI.

(3) Coronary stenting. The early benefit of angioplasty over thrombolytic therapy is attenuated with more extended follow-up. In the GUSTO IIb (Global Use of Strategies to Open Occluded Coronary Arteries) trial in which use of accelerated tissue plasminogen activator (tPA) was compared with angioplasty alone (percutaneous transluminal coronary angioplasty, PTCA), the reduction in rates of death and nonfatal MI at 30 days (13.7% tPA vs. 9.6% PTCA) dwindled, and by 6 months, the difference (16.1% for tPA vs.14.1% for PTCA) had lost statistical significance (20). This loss of effect may be at least partially caused by restenosis of the target lesion that was managed directly with angioplasty. Although coronary stents are known to reduce rates of restenosis during elective PCI, it was once believed that stents should not be placed in thrombus-laden lesions, such as those associated with acute MI, because of risk for in-stent thrombosis. However, clinical trials with adequate antiplatelet therapy have shown stenting to be safe. The STENT-PAMI (STENT-Primary Angioplasty in Myocardial Infarction) (21) study found coronary stenting significantly reduced the need for target vessel revascularization at 6 months (7.7% vs. 17.0%, $p < 0.001$). These findings were confirmed in the CADILLAC (Controlled Abciximab and Device Investigation to Lower Late Angioplasty Complications) (22) trial, which found that coronary stenting significantly reduced the incidence of restenosis at 6 months (40.8% vs. 22.2%, $p < 0.0001$), independent of abciximab use. The introduction of the drug-eluting stent (DES) has led to the application of these stents in acute MI patients, with uncertain clinical benefit. Although early registry data and several small randomized trials have shown potential safety and efficacy for DES in this setting, early indication of possible increased risk of late stent thrombosis with DES in acute MI has limited their use.

e. **Fibrinolytic therapy.** The lifesaving capability of early fibrinolytic therapy has been well established, beginning with the Gruppo Italiano per lo Studio della Sopravivenza nell'Infarto Miocardico (GISSI I) trial (23) in 1986. Pooled data show a relative reduction in mortality of 18% and an absolute reduction of nearly 2%. Even more dramatic long-term mortality benefit may be the result of preservation of normal LV function.

(1) **Contraindications.** The only **absolute contraindications to fibrinolytic therapies are recent cerebrovascular accident (CVA), hemorrhagic CVA, intracranial neoplasm, active internal bleeding, and suspected aortic dissection.** The presence of one of these, or one or more of the relative contraindications listed in Table 1.6, would favor PCI, even if it meant delaying reperfusion.

(2) **Choice of agent**

(a) **Alteplase (tPA).** The GUSTO I (Global Utilization of Streptokinase and Tissue Plasminogen Activator for Occluded Coronary Arteries) trial showed that use of accelerated alteplase significantly reduced the 30-day mortality rate by 15% relative to streptokinase (SK) with subcutaneous or intravenous heparin (24). This mortality reduction correlated with significantly higher rates of TIMI (thrombolysis in myocardial infarction) 3 flow at 90 minutes compared with SK (54% vs. 31%, $p < 0.001$). The benefit was initially challenged because of the high cost of alteplase (approximately US $2200 per episode of MI) compared with streptokinase (approximately US $300). For alteplase, this corresponds to a cost of US $32,678 per year of life saved, less than that of the well-accepted standard of hemodialysis for end-stage renal disease (25). The benefit was seen across all subgroups, although the patients at highest risk derived the most benefit. The accelerated protocol consisted of an intravenous bolus dose of 15 mg followed by 0.75 mg/kg (up to 50 mg) over 30 minutes and then 0.5 mg/kg over 60 minutes. Alteplase is considered a fibrin-specific agent because of its relative selectivity for clot-bound fibrin.

(b) **Reteplase.** The first of the third-generation fibrinolytic agents approved for use in the United States, reteplase is a less fibrin-specific mutation of alteplase. Reteplase has a longer half-life than alteplase and can be administered in a double bolus (10 mg each, 30 minutes apart). The GUSTO III trial (26) showed no mortality benefit of reteplase over alteplase, but its ease of use may help to reduce time to administration.

(c) **Tenecteplase (TNK),** another third-generation fibrinolytic, is characterized by its improved fibrin specificity, enhanced resistance to plasminogen activator inhibitor (PAI-1), and decreased plasma clearance.

TABLE 1.6 Contraindications and Cautions for Use of Thrombolytic Agents to Manage Myocardial Infarction

Absolute contraindications
Previous hemorrhagic stroke at any time; ischemic stroke within 3 months
Known intracranial neoplasm, structural cerebral vascular lesion, or closed-head injury within 3 months
Active bleeding or bleeding diathesis (excluding menses)
Suspected aortic dissection
Relative contraindications
Severe, uncontrolled hypertension at presentation (blood pressure >180/110 mm Hg) or history of chronic severe hypertension
History of ischemic stroke >3 months, dementia, or known intracerebral pathologic condition not covered in contraindications
Current use of anticoagulants, the risk increases with increasing INR
Traumatic or prolonged (>10 min) CPR or major surgery (<3 wk)
Noncompressible vascular punctures
Recent (within 2–4 wk) internal bleeding
For streptokinase or anistrepeplase: prior exposure (more than 5 days prior) or prior allergic reaction
Pregnancy
Active peptic ulcer

CPR, Cardiopulmonary resuscitation; INR, international normalized ratio.
Adapted from Antman EM, Anbe DT, Armstrong PW, et al. ACC/AHA guidelines for the management of patients with ST-elevation myocardial infarction: A report of the American College of Cardiology/American Heart Association Task Force on Practice Guidelines (Committee to Revise the 1999 Guidelines for the Management of Patients with Acute Myocardial Infarction). *J Am Coll Cardiol* 2004;44:E1–E211.

These properties allow it be administered as a single bolus. The ASSENT 2 (Assessment of the Safety and Efficacy of a New Thrombolytic) trial found no mortality difference between TNK and tPA at 30 days (27). However, TNK was associated with significantly less noncerebral bleeding and improved mortality in patients treated more than 4 hours after symptom onset. The weight-adjusted dose of TNK is 30 to 40 mg (ASSENT 1).

(d) Streptokinase (SK). This first-generation nonfibrin specific lytic is a reasonable alternative to second- or third-generation agents if newer agents are not available or cannot be used because of limited financial resources. Because of the possible development of antibodies, SK should not be administered to a patient who has received it in the past. Because overall rate of intracerebral hemorrhage is lower with SK (0.5%) than with tPA (0.7%), some cardiologists advocate its use in the care of high-risk patients, such as elderly patients with a history of a cerebrovascular event or severe hypertension. SK is a nonfibrin specific agent capable of lysing circulating and clot-bound plasminogen to plasmin. This process results in substantial systemic fibrinogenolysis, fibrinogenemia, and elevation in fibrin degradation products.

(3) Bleeding complications after fibrinolysis. The most serious **complication** of fibrinolytic therapy is **intracerebral hemorrhage, which occurs in approximately 0.5% to 0.7% of patients receiving such therapy. The major risk factors for intracranial hemorrhage include age (>75 years), hypertension, low body weight, female gender, and coagulopathy** (e.g., prior Coumadin use). The diagnosis must be considered if a patient has severe headache, visual disturbances, new neurologic deficit, acute confusional state, or seizure. If the clinical suspicion is high, fibrinolytic, antithrombin, and antiplatelet therapy should be interrupted while emergency CT or MRI is performed and neurosurgical consultation is obtained. Surgical evacuation may be lifesaving. Even with prompt recognition and treatment, the mortality rate is higher than 60%; elderly patients (>75 years) have a mortality rate higher than 90%. There is some controversy regarding the risk of fibrinolytic therapy in these patients as the literature reports are conflicting. An observational study (28) from the Medicare database found patients older than 75 years had an increased risk of death at 30 days with fibrinolytic therapy [relative risk (RR) = 1.38, 95% confidence interval (CI): 1.12 to 1.71, $p = 0.003$]. However, an updated meta-analysis of nine randomized trials (29,30) found the risk reduction with fibrinolysis in patients older than 75 years was 16% [odds ratio (OR) = 0.84, 95% CI: 0.72 to 0.98, $p < 0.05$]. There appears to be a decreasing relative benefit with fibrinolysis in the elderly, but an absolute gain in lives saved. The only randomized trial to specifically study management of STEMI in the elderly found patients treated with PCI had significantly lower 30-day and 1-year mortality rates than patients treated with fibrinolysis (30). However, the TIMI-Extract 25 study more recently indicates that fibrinolytic therapy may be safe in the elderly if a reduced dose of enoxaparin is used (31). Gastrointestinal, retroperitoneal, and access-site bleeding may complicate fibrinolytic therapy but are usually not life threatening if promptly recognized and managed. In any case, the best treatment of acute STEMI in elderly patients appears to be primary PCI.

(4) Prehospital fibrinolysis. Early administration of fibrinolytic therapy by emergency services has been shown to potentially reduce infarct size but lacks solid randomized trial data advocating its routine use. It has also been found to reduce time to treatment (32,33), but this did not translate into a reduction in mortality. Although a meta-analysis (34) of prehospital fibrinolytic trials did find a 17% reduction of in-hospital mortality, it remains to be seen whether this strategy can improve long-term outcomes in clinical practice.

f. Combination fibrinolytic therapy with GP IIb/IIIa inhibitors (without PCI)

(1) Rationale. Sustained tissue-level reperfusion occurs in only 25% of patients treated with fibrinolytic therapy. Platelets have paradoxically increased activity after fibrinolysis and are important mediators in the tendency for vessel reocclusion. Aspirin is pathway specific and, therefore, a relatively weak antiplatelet agent. Glycoprotein (GP) IIb/IIIa inhibitors, however, are potent antiplatelet agents that block the final common pathway of platelet aggregation, and for this reason, they have been studied in combination with half-dose fibrinolysis.

(2) Clinical trials. GUSTO V found the addition of abciximab to half-dose reteplase did not reduce mortality at 30 days or 1 year compared with full-dose reteplase, but it did reduce reinfarctions and complications after MI (35). ASSENT 3 also found comparable reductions in reinfarction with the combination of half-dose tenecteplase and abciximab (36).

(3) Contraindications. GUSTO V found the rate of intracranial hemorrhage in elderly patients (>75) treated with combination therapy was almost twice that of standard lytic therapy (2.1% vs. 1.1%, $p = 0.07$). ASSENT 3 confirmed this finding. Age older than 75 years is, therefore, an additional contraindication for combination lytic therapy. No increase in intracranial hemorrhage was seen in younger patients.

g. Rescue percutaneous revascularization is defined as the use of PCI when fibrinolytic therapy has proved unsuccessful. Despite the proven mortality benefit, more than 30% of patients who received lytic therapy have TIMI 0 to 1 flow at 90 minutes, whereas patency at 90 minutes has been shown to correlate with long-term survival (37). If reperfusion is not clearly evident 90 minutes after initiation of lytic therapy, particularly among patients with large acute MI, the decision to perform emergency angiography and mechanical reperfusion should be made promptly. Patients in cardiogenic shock, with severe CHF, or compromising arrhythmias after lytic therapy should undergo immediate coronary angiography and should not await clinical assessment of reperfusion.

(1) Clinical determination of successful reperfusion. It can be difficult to determine clinically whether a patient has successfully reperfused with fibrinolytic therapy. Resolution of chest pain is an inaccurate measure of reperfusion, because the pain may be blunted by narcotic analgesia or the partial denervation that is known to occur among some patients with MI. Serial assessment of 12-lead ECGs is a more reliable indicator of reperfusion, although it also is suboptimal. An accelerated idioventricular rhythm (AIVR) is fairly specific for reperfusion, but arrhythmias other than AIVRs are not reliable indicators because a variety of ventricular and supraventricular arrhythmias may be observed in patients with nonreperfused infarction-related artery. The complete resolution of chest pain and electrocardiographic changes (defined as more than 70% resolution of ST-segment elevation), accompanied by a run of AIVR, is highly specific for successful reperfusion, but it occurs in less than 10% of patients receiving lytic therapy. Resolution of ST-segment elevation by more than 70% is correlated with effective tissue level reperfusion, and this finding has been correlated with better clinical outcomes and angiographic reperfusion.

(2) Benefit. It has been shown in the RESCUE (Randomized Evaluation of Salvage Angioplasty with Combined Utilization of Endpoints) trial (38) that patients with anterior MI who have unsuccessful thrombolysis (TIMI 0 or 1 flow) have a significant benefit from rescue angioplasty. In addition, the REACT trial demonstrated that among patients with failed reperfusion with lytics, treatment with rescue angioplasty with or without PCI is associated with an ~50% reduction in death, re-infarction, stroke, and severe heart failure (39). GRACIA I evaluated an early invasive strategy (within 24 hours) versus an ischemia-guided approach among patients with STEMI treated with fibrinolytic therapy. This trial primarily demonstrated a reduction in revascularization events with the early invasive approach, although a trend was seen toward fewer deaths and re-infarcts. Based on the above data, an early angiography strategy (within 24 hours) may also be considered a reasonable approach in all patients who receive lytic therapy. However, this approach should be differentiated from the facilitated PCI strategy described later.

(3) Routine late angiography is discussed in Chapter 4.

(4) Recurrent ischemia after MI is an indication for coronary angiography and revascularization (see Chapter 4).

h. Facilitated PCI refers to the use of an initial pharmacologic regimen to improve vessel patency rates prior to planned PCI. This method has been proposed as a way to manage patients with acute MI who present to hospitals without 24-hour catheterization laboratory facilities. Various facilitated PCI strategies have been proposed, including high-dose heparin, early GP IIb/IIIa inhibitors, full-dose or reduced-dose fibrinolytics, and combination fibrinolytics and GP IIb/IIIa inhibitors. Theoretical advantages include earlier time to reperfusion, improved hemodynamic stability, smaller infarct size, greater procedural success and improved survival, albeit at increased risk of bleeding complications. The ASSENT-4 PCI (Assessment of Safety and Efficacy of a New Treatment Strategy with PCI) trial was the largest study to evaluate full-dose fibrinolytic therapy (tenecteplase) plus PCI versus primary PCI alone. The trial was terminated prematurely because of higher in-hospital mortality rates (6% vs. 3%; $p = 0.01$) and higher primary composite endpoints (death, shock, and heart failure within 90 days) with full-dose fibrinolytics plus PCI versus PCI alone (18.6% vs. 13.4%; $p = 0.0045$) (40). The FINESSE (Facilitated Intervention with Enhanced

Speed to Stop Events) trial, reported preliminarily at the European Society of Cardiology in September 2007, compared half-dose reteplase with abciximab versus abciximab alone versus placebo in patients undergoing primary PCI for STEMI. Although more patients with fibrinolytic plus GP IIB/IIIA inhibitor had an open artery on arrival to the catheterization laboratory, the composite primary endpoint of death or complications of MI at 90 days was no different among the various strategies (9.8% half-dose fibrinolytic + GP IIB/IIIA inhibitor, 10.5% GP IIb/IIIa inhibitor alone and 10.7% placebo; p = NS) the bleeding rates were higher with the half-dose fibrinolytic + IIB/IIIA inhibitor. Finally, a large meta-analysis of multiple smaller trials recently confirmed that primary PCI is superior to facilitated PCI (41). Current guidelines recommend the use of facilitated PCI only with regimens other than full-dose lytics when patients are at high risk, but PCI is not immediately available within 90 minutes and bleeding risk is low (9). In addition, more recent data (CARESS-in-AMI) would indicate that patients treated with half-dose fibrinolytics and abciximab benefit from immediate transfer for PCI as opposed to rescue PCI (42).

i. **The late open artery hypothesis** postulates that benefit in terms of improved ventricular function, increased electrical stability, and provision of collaterals can be gained by late patency of occluded infarct arteries. However, OAT (Occluded Artery Trial) failed to show benefit of angioplasty for late total occlusion within 3 to 28 days after MI (43). Criticism of this trial includes exclusion of high-risk patients with New York Heart Association (NYHA) class III or IV heart failure, rest angina, clinical instability, multivessel disease (left main or three-vessel disease), or severe inducible ischemia on stress testing. Regardless of these concerns, this study has led to a new **class III recommendation against PCI of a totally occluded artery >24 hours after STEMI in asymptomatic patients without the previously noted high-risk criteria** (9).

j. **Emergency coronary bypass surgery** may be the treatment of choice for patients in whom the intent is to perform direct or rescue percutaneous mechanical reperfusion but are found to have a critical left main-stem lesion or severe three-vessel disease unapproachable with percutaneous revascularization. Studies of this strategy are fairly encouraging, especially when patients can be taken to the operating room early in the course of infarction, before severe myocardial necrosis has occurred. Right ventricular infarction is a relative contraindication to bypass surgery because it complicates the discontinuation of cardiopulmonary support.

k. **PCI in small hospitals or without surgical backup.** The C-PORT (Atlantic Cardiovascular Patient Outcomes Research Team) trial (44) found a reduced 6-month composite outcome of death, MI, and stroke in patients with acute MI randomized to primary PCI versus fibrinolytic therapy (12.4% vs. 19.9%, $p = 0.03$), even when PCI was performed at hospitals without surgical backup. All the community hospitals involved in this study underwent a formal "PCI development program." With adequate training, primary PCI may be a safe and efficacious treatment, even in smaller hospitals. However, in cases where surgical backup is not available, primary PCI is still not recommended.

B. Adjuvant Therapy

1. Antithrombins

a. **Heparin without fibrinolysis.** Although heparin was never shown to reduce mortality in the era before reperfusion, the trials that examined this issue were underpowered. A meta-analysis of three large trials (45) suggested a mortality benefit with intravenous heparin. Reductions in the incidence of LV thrombus and stroke have been especially evident among patients with large anterior MI or documented thrombus.

b. **Heparin with fibrinolysis.**

(1) tPA. As an adjunct to tPA, heparin has been shown to improve late patency. Most cardiologists consider heparin to be an essential adjunct to tPA to overcome the thrombogenic state induced by systemic fibrinolytic therapy. Although it has not been shown to improve mortality compared with placebo, intravenous heparin was used in conjunction with accelerated tPA in the GUSTO I trial. The dose of heparin recommended in the American Heart Association (AHA)/American College of Cardiology (ACC) guidelines is 60 U/kg bolus (maximum, 4000 units), followed by 12 U/kg per hour (maximum, 1000 U/hour). The goal activated partial thromboplastin time (aPTT) should be adjusted to 1.5 to 2.0 times control (50 to 70 seconds).

(2) Streptokinase. There are no data to support the use of intravenous heparin with streptokinase, unless the patient has recurrent ischemia or has another indication for heparin therapy. In the GUSTO I trial, intravenous heparin was equivalent to subcutaneous heparin when used with streptokinase, which has considerably more fibrinogenolytic action than alteplase.

(3) Third-generation agents. The use of unfractionated heparin as adjunctive therapy with reteplase and tenecteplase has been validated in GUSTO III and ASSENT 2, respectively.

c. Heparin with direct angioplasty. When direct angioplasty is planned, patients should receive a GP IIb/IIIa inhibitor such as abciximab. An initial low-dose, weight-adjusted bolus of heparin also should be given (50 to 70 U/kg up to 7000 U). This combination resulted in the lowest rate of death and ischemic complications in the EPILOG (Evaluation in PTCA to Improve Long-Term Outcome with Abciximab Glycoprotein IIb/IIIa Blockade) trial (46). If abciximab is not given, standard procedural doses of heparin (100 U/kg, up to 10,000 U) may be administered before the procedure.

d. Low–molecular-weight heparins and direct thrombin inhibitors have recently received attention to improve upon outcomes obtained with adjunctive unfractionated heparin (UFH) use. Table 1.7 summarizes the observations from trials of anticoagulants in STEMI.

(1) Rationale for use. Unfractionated heparin is neutralized by activated platelets and cannot inhibit clot-bound thrombin. Because thrombin is a key component of a coronary thrombus and has paradoxically increased activity after fibrinolysis, its inhibition is essential to sustain vessel patency after fibrinolysis. Enoxaparin, a low–molecular-weight heparin, is advantageous because of its consistent bioavailability, diminished inhibition by platelet factor 4, and a reduced incidence of heparin-induced

TABLE 1.7 Summary of Findings from Trials of Low–Molecular-Weight Heparins for STEMI

Pharmacologic agent	30-day efficacy	Safety	Use during PCI
Enoxaparin	Appears superior to UFH with fibrinolysis	Increased risk of serious bleeds	Can be used to support PCI after fibrinolysis
Fondaparinux	Appears superior to placebo/UFH in fibrinolysis. Trend toward worse outcomes with primary PCI	Trend toward decreased risk of serious bleeds	Increased risk of catheter thrombosis when used alone

PCI, percutaneous coronary intervention; UFH, unfractionated heparin.
Adapted from Antman EM, Hand M, Armstrong PW, et al. 2007 focused update of the ACC/AHA 2004 guidelines for the management of patients with ST-elevation myocardial infarction: a report of the American College of Cardiology/American Heart Association Task Force on Practice Guidelines. *J Am Coll Cardiol* 2008;51:210–247.

thrombocytopenia. Direct thrombin inhibitors such as hirudin and bivalirudin can inhibit fibrin-bound thrombin in addition to fluid-phase thrombin. Unlike UFH, they have more reproducible pharmacokinetics and are unaffected by circulating inhibitors.

(2) Clinical trials data

(a) Enoxaparin plus fibrinolytics. ASSENT 3 found patients treated with full-dose TNK and enoxaparin (30 mg IV, followed by 1 mg/kg twice daily) had a lower 30-day risk of death or MI compared with full-dose TNK and UFH (6.8% vs. 9.1%, $p = 0.020$). The Enoxaparin as Adjunctive Antithrombin Therapy for ST-Elevation Myocardial Infarction (ENTIRE–TIMI 23) trial (47) found patients treated with full-dose TNK and enoxaparin had reduced rates of death or MI at 30 days compared with full-dose TNK and UFH (15.9% vs. 4.4%, $p = 0.005$). The rate of major hemorrhage was also slightly lower in the full-dose TNK plus enoxaparin group. It appears that full-dose TNK plus enoxaparin results in salutary effects on ischemic endpoints similar to that of combination therapy (half-dose TNK plus abciximab) with a better safety profile in patients older than 75 years (36). The HART II (Heparin and Aspirin Reperfusion) study (48) found enoxaparin not to be inferior to UFH after fibrinolysis, with trends toward reduced vessel reocclusion and improved rates of TIMI 3 flow in the enoxaparin-treated arm. These findings were confirmed in the phase III trial entitled EXTRACT-TIMI 25, comparing enoxaparin to UFH in fibrinolysis (31). Despite finding a reduction in composite endpoints of death and re-infarction, the primary benefit was in re-infarction, not MI. The result is that both UFH and enoxaparin are considered reasonable treatment strategies with fibrinolytic therapy. The EXTRACT-TIMI 25 trial did not have a primary PCI subset, however, among patients who underwent subsequent PCI after fibrinolysis, enoxaparin appeared to be superior to UFH without increased bleeding events (31). Fondaparinux is an additional low-molecular weight heparin that has been studied in acute MI. The OASIS-6 trial evaluated fondaparinux with fibrinolytics and appeared to demonstrate benefit versus placebo/UFH in terms of death and re-infarction at 30 days (9.7% vs. 11.2%; HR = 0.86) without an increased risk in bleeding (49). However, in the primary PCI subset, there was no benefit and a significant increase in guiding-catheter thrombosis, which has limited its widespread use.

(b) Direct thrombin inhibitors. Several large trials failed to show a significant benefit of hirudin over heparin during fibrinolysis in acute MI. Newer agents have been studied in recent trials. The HERO-2 (Hirulog and Early Reperfusion or Occlusion) trial (50) found no mortality difference at 30 days in patients with acute STEMI treated with SK and adjunctive bivalirudin in comparison to SK and UFH. The bivalirudin arm had significantly fewer re-infarctions but significantly higher rates of bleeding. Additional study is needed before direct thrombin inhibitors can be routinely recommended in acute MI, although ongoing trials will soon be reported on this topic. A clear indication for these agents is heparin-induced thrombocytopenia. A form of hirudin, lepirudin (0.4 mg/kg bolus up to 44 mg, followed by an infusion of 0.15 mg/kg for 2 to 10 days) has been approved. Argatroban (2 μg/kg/min infusion) is also approved for this indication.

(3) β-Blockers. Extensive data from the era before reperfusion established the usefulness of β-blockers in reducing recurrent ischemia, arrhythmias, and mortality. Several small randomized trials performed in the fibrinolytic reperfusion era confirmed the anti-ischemic and antiarrhythmic benefits, although short-term mortality was not affected. As a result, prior recommendations have stated that β- blockers should be administered to all patients within the first 24 hours of acute MI, unless contraindicated by severe reactive airways disease, hypotension, bradycardia, or cardiogenic shock. However, more recent data from the PCI era have shown no difference in mortality and no difference in the composite endpoint of death, re-infarction, or ventricular fibrillation arrest (51). The COMMIT/CCS-2 metoprolol trial, a large ($N = 22{,}929$) randomized controlled trial found that the metoprolol group had more ventricular fibrillation arrest (2.5% vs. 3.0%; $p = 0.001$) and shock (5.0% vs. 3.9%; $p < 0.001$). The incidence of shock was most notable in patients with Killip class II and III. This has led to a change in guidelines recommending more judicious use of early (<24 hours) β-blockers, avoiding use in patients with significant signs of heart failure, low cardiac output, risk of cardiogenic shock, or other relative contraindications to their use (9).

(a) **For ongoing ischemia with tachycardia or hypertension,** after rapid evaluation of ventricular function, intravenous metoprolol can be given (5 mg every 5 minutes until desired blood pressure and pulse achieved). Patients who tolerated the intravenous loading can begin moderate oral doses (12.5 to 50 mg of metoprolol, two to four times daily). The dose should be subsequently titrated upward to the maximally tolerated dose (200 mg of sustained-release metoprolol, once daily). Use of β-blockers should be avoided in patients with tachycardia of unclear origin, as these agents can decompensate heart failure in patients with compensatory tachycardia.

(4) **Angiotensin-converting enzyme (ACE) inhibitors** can be started orally in the first 24 hours for all patients without hypotension, acute renal failure, or other contraindications. These medications were shown to reduce mortality in the GISSI 3 (51) and ISIS 4 (International Study of Infarct Survival) (52) trials. ACE inhibitors should be continued indefinitely for patients with LV dysfunction or clinical CHF, because these patients have been shown to derive a mortality benefit. The Heart Outcomes Prevention Evaluation (HOPE) study (53) found that high-risk patients, including those with prior MI but normal LV function, still had long-term benefit from ramipril. Intravenous formulations of these agents should not be used because they have not demonstrated benefit and may increase mortality. Rather, a graded oral regimen is advised. Angiotensin-receptor blockers (ARBs) remain a viable option for ACE inhibitor–intolerant patients.

(5) **Calcium channel blockers.** Evidence for a potential increase in mortality has limited the use of calcium channel blockers in the care of patients with acute MI. They are indicated for the management of supraventricular tachyarrhythmia, cocaine-induced MI, or relief of postinfarction angina unresponsive to β-blockade. Otherwise, these agents should be avoided. Short-acting agents, such as nifedipine, are contraindicated because of their reflex sympathetic activation. Verapamil and diltiazem should be avoided in patients with LV dysfunction or CHF. Amlodipine is an effective antianginal and appears safe to use for this indication in patients with CHF.

(6) **Magnesium.** There was once considerable enthusiasm for the routine use of intravenous magnesium in patients with MI, based on the findings of LIMIT 2, which observed a 24% reduction in mortality compared with placebo. The larger ISIS 4 and MAGIC trials failed to duplicate this benefit, however, and enthusiasm has waned. Some speculated that the lack of effect in ISIS 4 was because of delayed administration or low control-group mortality. In the modern era, magnesium is not routinely used other than to replete serum magnesium levels that are lower than 2.0 μg/dL or for the management of *torsade de pointes* (1 to 2 g over 5 minutes).

(7) **Aldosterone antagonists.** The use of aldosterone-blocking agents has been shown to be beneficial in post-MI patients. The RALES

(Randomized Aldactone Evaluation Study) found a reduction in all-cause mortality with use of aldactone in patients with ischemic cardiomyopathy and NYHA class III or IV heart failure. However, the only randomized trial to address the use of such agents among patients with ventricular dysfunction after STEMI is the EPHESUS (Eplerenone Post-Acute Myocardial Infarction Heart Failure Efficacy and Survival Study), where eplerenone was found to be beneficial.

(8) Diabetes control. The DIGAMI (Diabetes Mellitus, Insulin Glucose Infusion in Acute Myocardial Infarction) study found a significantly lower mortality rate at 1 year compared with standard therapy (8.6% vs. 18.0%, $p = 0.020$) in diabetic patients treated with aggressive blood glucose reduction with an insulin infusion during hospitalization, followed by multidose subcutaneous insulin injections. However, a small trial (OASIS-6 GIK) and a large (>20,000 patients) randomized trial (CREATE-ELCA) failed to show any benefit to glucose–insulin–potassium (GIK) infusions. As a result, it appears prudent to institute sound glucose control, but it is not necessary to aggressively pursue glucose control with GIK infusions.

(9) Antiarrhythmics. The use of lidocaine or other antiarrhythmic agents is not warranted for the prophylactic suppression of ventricular tachycardia and fibrillation. Although lidocaine may decrease tachyarrhythmias, there is no survival benefit. There also is evidence to suggest an increase in mortality related to an increased incidence of bradycardia and asystole. In addition, there is evidence that "high-dose" amiodarone may actually increase mortality. Antiarrhythmic therapies are discussed in greater detail in Chapter 20.

(10) Intraaortic balloon pump (IABP). In the treatment of patients with cardiogenic shock, IABP counterpulsation is the preferred means of augmenting systolic pressure because use of an IABP decreases afterload and oxygen requirements while increasing diastolic coronary flow. IABP is contraindicated in the care of patients with marked aortic regurgitation, because it may worsen the regurgitation and cause rapid hemodynamic deterioration (see Chapter 57).

(11) Inotropic agents. In general, these agents should be avoided whenever possible because of their tendency to increase myocardial oxygen demand and their associated risk of tachycardia and arrhythmias. If IABP counterpulsation proves insufficient, intravenous inotropic support may be warranted, but its use should be guided by means of pulmonary arterial catheter monitoring whenever possible.

(a) Patients with hypotension accompanied by a pulmonary capillary wedge pressure (PCWP) less than 15 mm Hg should be managed with rapid infusion of boluses of normal saline solution, as should patients with inferior MI who have concomitant RV infarction.

(b) After intravascular volume has been repleted and the PCWP is greater than 15 mm Hg, dopamine may be indicated at doses up to 20 μg/kg per minute if hypotension or signs of heart failure persist. Norepinephrine may be used as second-line therapy. The benefits of improved cerebral and systemic perfusion pressure by an increase in inotropy usually come at the cost of increased afterload and myocardial oxygen demand from vasoconstriction.

(c) Dobutamine can be useful when PCWP is greater than 18 mm Hg in the setting of mild to moderate hypotension (70 to 90 mm Hg), or when nitroglycerin or nitroprusside are contraindicated because of risk for inducing hypotension. Use of phosphodiesterase inhibitors such as milrinone, which have combined vasodilating and inotropic actions, is problematic because of their arrhythmogenicity and tendency to increase myocardial oxygen consumption. Use of these drugs to maintain adequate systemic pressure and forward output is acceptable if the other therapies have failed. The main goal, however, should be to avoid these agents or reduce the need for them in terms of absolute dose and duration.

(12) Implantable cardioverter–defibrillators (ICDs). Posited to reduce the risk of sudden death following acute MI, ICDs were routinely implanted an average of 18 days following the index MI event in patients with reduced ventricular function and autonomic dysfunction (DINAMIT trial) (55). Although there was a decrease in cardiovascular death, this study failed to demonstrate any reduction in all-cause mortality, leading to the recommendation to wait 6 months following revascularization before defibrillator evaluation.

(13) Anticoagulation for large anterior wall MIs. Historical teaching (not based on randomized data) has advocated anticoagulating patients for 6 weeks after a large anterior wall MI with the goal of prevention of LV thrombus development. However, in the era of primary PCI with coronary stenting, this recommendation would necessitate treatment with aspirin, clopidogrel, and coumadin, placing patients at fairly high risk for bleeding. Some clinicians recommend anticoagulation only if there is objective evidence of LV thrombus by echocardiography. Others still recommend empiric anticoagulation, but with a slightly lower target international normalized ratio (INR, 1.5 to 2.0).

X. ACUTE MI ASSOCIATED WITH COCAINE ABUSE.

The pathophysiologic process and management of acute MI associated with cocaine use differ from those of classic MI.

A. Pathophysiology

1. **The underlying pathophysiologic factor** in acute MI associated with cocaine abuse is believed to be coronary spasm or thrombus formation caused by α-adrenergic stimulation. This can occur in a normal segment of artery or be superimposed on mild to moderate atherosclerosis. Atherosclerosis is accelerated by chronic cocaine use.
2. **Increased oxygen demand** caused by β-adrenergic stimulation of heart rate and contractility also contributes to the onset of ischemia.

B. Clinical presentation.

Chest pain caused by infarction after cocaine ingestion typically occurs within 3 hours, although it can vary from minutes to days, and depends on the route of administration (median of 30 minutes with intravenous cocaine, 90 minutes with crack smoking, and 135 minutes with nasal inhalation). More than 80% of persons with infarction are also cigarette smokers. Studies with animals have demonstrated a synergistic effect between cigarette smoking and cocaine use.

C. Therapy

1. **Initial management** of ST-segment elevation associated with cocaine use includes the routine administration of aspirin, oxygen, and heparin. Aggressive use of sublingual and intravenous nitroglycerin or intravenous calcium channel blockers is advised in an effort to relieve coronary spasm.
2. **β-Blockers are contraindicated in patients with cocaine-induced acute MI.** Although they block undesirable β-adrenergic effects, these agents allow unopposed α-adrenergic stimulation and have been associated with increased mortality in nonrandomized analyses.
3. **Reperfusion therapy must be considered if vasodilator therapy is unsuccessful** in relieving symptoms and ST-segment changes.
4. **Immediate angiography and mechanical revascularization as appropriate** may be even more beneficial in cocaine-induced MI patients. Many patients who use cocaine have contraindications to thrombolysis, such as severe hypertension or persistent vasospasm without thrombosis, which is not amenable to thrombolytic therapy.

XI. POSTOPERATIVE ACUTE MI

A. Etiology and pathophysiology.

Acute MI following noncardiac operations most commonly occurs on the third or fourth postoperative day Conventional theory was that MI was caused by a combination of increased oxygen demand and arterial shear stress associated with the increased adrenergic drive that accompanies pain and ambulation in the postoperative period. Intravascular volume shifts caused by redistribution of fluids, intravenous administration of fluids, and decreased enteral intake all contribute to the risk of postoperative MI. It is apparent that there is a postoperative inflammatory state associated with hypercoagulability, marked by an increase in fibrinogen and other acute-phase reactants. Recent data would indicate that perioperative management of patients with DESs may be problematic, as risk for stent thrombosis may be speculated to be increased in this mileu, whereas antiplatelet therapies are discontinued to reduce bleeding risks.

B. Therapy. Management is complicated by limitations on the use of fibrinolytic agents and anticoagulant therapies. Therapy relies more heavily on the intravenous use of β-blockers and urgent angiography and mechanical revascularization. The optimal antiplatelet or anticoagulation regimen for recent (<1 year) DES patients undergoing noncardiac surgery is not known.

XII. SIMPLIFIED REPERFUSION STRATEGY. The wealth of data regarding reperfusion strategies and adjunctive therapies in acute MI detailed previously may lead to confusion regarding the optimal approach. Based on guideline recommendations, a simplification of the STEMI management strategy can be achieved.

A. For patients presenting with acute MI where primary PCI is available, a reasonable strategy would involve pre-hospital administration of aspirin, emergency department initiation of UFH or enoxaparin and clopidogrel, as well as nitrates and β-blocker therapy if not contraindicated, and immediate transfer to the catheterization laboratory with abciximab infusion begun at the time of PCI. Coronary stenting with bare metal stents and subsequent assessment of ventricular function is performed, allowing risk stratification and initiation of additional adjunctive therapies such as statins, ACE inhibitor, and aldosterone antagonists. The early administration of any GP IIb/IIIa inhibitor in the emergency department remains a reasonable option in patients undergoing primary PCI.

B. For patients presenting to a hospital where primary PCI is not available, but immediate transfer (medical contact to balloon time <90 minutes) to a PCI facility is available, a similar strategy is employed, with initiation of aspirin, clopidogrel, heparin, nitrates, and β-blockers prior to transfer, although patients at high risk with potentially longer transfer times may benefit from the addition of GP IIb/IIIa inhibitor or half-dose fibrinolytics plus GP IIb/IIIa inhibitor prior to transfer.

C. If anticipated transfer times will exceed the medical contact-to-PCI time of 90 minutes, then fibrinolytic therapy should be instituted in eligible patients within 30 minutes of medical contact. The choice of UFH or enoxaparin remains operator dependent, with either option reasonable. Among patients receiving fibrinolytics, immediate transfer to a PCI facility is preferable, and an early angiography (<24 hours) strategy may be useful, although assessment for persistent ischemia prior to angiography is reasonable in low-risk patients. Full-dose fibrinolytics followed by immediate planned PCI should not be undertaken, however, as this strategy has shown increased mortality.

ACKNOWLEDGMENTS

The author thanks Drs. Deepak P. Vivekananthan and Michael A. Lauer for their contributions to earlier editions of this chapter.

References

1. Rosamond W, Flegal K, Friday G, et al. Heart disease and stroke statistics—2007 update: a report from the American Heart Association Statistics Committee and Stroke Statistics Subcommittee. *Circulation* 2007;115:e69–171.
2. Thygesen K, Alpert JS, White HD. Universal definition of myocardial infarction. *J Am Coll Cardiol* 2007;50:2173–2195.
3. Licka M, Zimmermann R, Zehelein J, et al. Troponin T concentrations 72 hours after myocardial infarction as a serological estimate of infarct size. *Heart* 2002;87:520–524.
4. Srinivas VS, Cannon CP, Gibson CM, et al. Myoglobin levels at 12 hours identify patients at low risk for 30-day mortality after thrombolysis in acute myocardial infarction: a Thrombolysis In Myocardial Infarction 10B substudy. *Am Heart J* 2001;142:29–36.

5. Lee KL, Woodlief LH, Topol EJ, et al. Predictors of 30-day mortality in the era of reperfusion for acute myocardial infarction. Results from an international trial of 41,021 patients. GUSTO-I Investigators. *Circulation* 1995;91:1659–1668.
6. Randomised trial of intravenous streptokinase, oral aspirin, both, or neither among 17,187 cases of suspected acute myocardial infarction: ISIS-2. ISIS-2 (Second International Study of Infarct Survival) Collaborative Group. *Lancet* 1988;2:349–360.
7. Sabatine MS, Cannon CP, Gibson CM, et al. Addition of clopidogrel to aspirin and fibrinolytic therapy for myocardial infarction with ST-segment elevation. *N Engl J Med* 2005;352:1179–1189.
8. Chen ZM, Jiang LX, Chen YP, et al. Addition of clopidogrel to aspirin in 45,852 patients with acute myocardial infarction: randomised placebo-controlled trial. *Lancet* 2005;366:1607–1621.
9. Antman EM, Hand M, Armstrong PW, et al. 2007 focused update of the ACC/AHA 2004 guidelines for the management of patients with ST-elevation myocardial infarction: a report of the American College of Cardiology/American Heart Association Task Force on Practice Guidelines. *J Am Coll Cardiol* 2008;51:210–247.
10. Yusuf S, Collins R, MacMahon S, et al. Effect of intravenous nitrates on mortality in acute myocardial infarction: an overview of the randomised trials. *Lancet* 1988;1:1088–1092.
11. Schomig A, Mehilli J, Antoniucci D, et al. Mechanical reperfusion in patients with acute myocardial infarction presenting more than 12 hours from symptom onset: a randomized controlled trial. *JAMA* 2005;293:2865–2872.
12. Keeley EC, Boura JA, Grines CL. Primary angioplasty versus intravenous thrombolytic therapy for acute myocardial infarction: a quantitative review of 23 randomised trials. *Lancet* 2003;361:13–20.
13. Andersen HR, Nielsen TT, Rasmussen K, et al. A comparison of coronary angioplasty with fibrinolytic therapy in acute myocardial infarction. *N Engl J Med* 2003;349:733–742.
14. Grines CL, Westerhausen DR, Jr., Grines LL, et al. A randomized trial of transfer for primary angioplasty versus on-site thrombolysis in patients with high-risk myocardial infarction: the Air Primary Angioplasty in Myocardial Infarction study. *J Am Coll Cardiol* 2002;39:1713–1719.
15. Widimsky P, Groch L, Zelizko M, et al. Multicentre randomized trial comparing transport to primary angioplasty vs immediate thrombolysis vs combined strategy for patients with acute myocardial infarction presenting to a community hospital without a catheterization laboratory. The PRAGUE study. *Eur Heart J* 2000;21:823–831.
16. Brener SJ, Barr LA, Burchenal JE, et al. Randomized, placebo-controlled trial of platelet glycoprotein IIb/IIIa blockade with primary angioplasty for acute myocardial infarction. ReoPro and Primary PTCA Organization and Randomized Trial (RAPPORT) Investigators. *Circulation* 1998;98:734–741.
17. Montalescot G, Barragan P, Wittenberg O, et al. Platelet glycoprotein IIb/IIIa inhibition with coronary stenting for acute myocardial infarction. *N Engl J Med* 2001;344:1895–1903.
18. Antoniucci D, Rodriguez A, Hempel A, et al. A randomized trial comparing primary infarct artery stenting with or without abciximab in acute myocardial infarction. *J Am Coll Cardiol* 2003;42:1879–1885.
19. Danzi GB, Sesana M, Capuano C, et al. Comparison in patients having primary coronary angioplasty of abciximab versus tirofiban on recovery of left ventricular function. Am J Cardiol 2004;94:35–39.
20. A clinical trial comparing primary coronary angioplasty with tissue plasminogen activator for acute myocardial infarction. The Global Use of Strategies to Open Occluded Coronary Arteries in Acute Coronary Syndromes (GUSTO IIb) Angioplasty Substudy Investigators. *N Engl J Med* 1997;336:1621–1628.
21. Grines CL, Cox DA, Stone GW, et al. Coronary angioplasty with or without stent implantation for acute myocardial infarction. Stent Primary Angioplasty in Myocardial Infarction Study Group. *N Engl J Med* 1999;341:1949–1956.
22. Stone GW, Grines CL, Cox DA, et al. Comparison of angioplasty with stenting, with or without abciximab, in acute myocardial infarction. *N Engl J Med* 2002;346:957–966.
23. Long-term effects of intravenous thrombolysis in acute myocardial infarction: final report of the GISSI study. Gruppo Italiano per lo Studio della Streptochi-nasi nell'Infarto Miocardico (GISSI). *Lancet* 1987;2:871–874.
24. An international randomized trial comparing four thrombolytic strategies for acute myocardial infarction. The GUSTO investigators. *N Engl J Med* 1993;329:673–682.
25. Mark DB, Hlatky MA, Califf RM, et al. Cost effectiveness of thrombolytic therapy with tissue plasminogen activator as compared with streptokinase for acute myocardial infarction. *N Engl J Med* 1995;332:1418–1424.
26. A comparison of reteplase with alteplase for acute myocardial infarction. The Global Use of Strategies to Open Occluded Coronary Arteries (GUSTO III) Investigators. *N Engl J Med* 1997;337:1118–1123.
27. Van De Werf F, Adgey J, Ardissino D, et al. Single-bolus tenecteplase compared with front-loaded alteplase in acute myocardial infarction: the ASSENT-2 double-blind randomised trial. *Lancet* 1999;354:716–722.
28. Thiemann D. Primary angioplasty vs thrombolysis in elderly patients. JAMA 2000;283:601–602.
29. Indications for fibrinolytic therapy in suspected acute myocardial infarction: collaborative overview of early mortality and major morbidity results from all randomised trials of more than 1000 patients. Fibrinolytic Therapy Trialists' (FTT) Collaborative Group. *Lancet* 1994;343:311–322.
30. de Boer MJ, Ottervanger JP, van't Hof AW, et al. Reperfusion therapy in elderly patients with acute myocardial infarction: a randomized comparison of primary angioplasty and thrombolytic therapy. *J Am Coll Cardiol* 2002;39:1723–1728.
31. Antman EM, Morrow DA, McCabe CH, et al. Enoxaparin versus unfractionated heparin with fibrinolysis for ST-elevation myocardial infarction. *N Engl J Med* 2006;354:1477–1488.
32. Morrow DA, Antman EM, Sayah A, et al. Evaluation of the time saved by prehospital initiation of reteplase for ST-elevation myocardial infarction: results of The Early Retavase-Thrombolysis in Myocardial Infarction (ER-TIMI) 19 trial. *J Am Coll Cardiol* 2002;40:71–77.
33. Weaver WD, Cerqueira M, Hallstrom AP, et al. Prehospital-initiated vs hospital-initiated thrombolytic therapy. The Myocardial Infarction Triage and Intervention Trial. *JAMA* 1993;270:1211–1216.
34. Morrison LJ, Verbeek PR, McDonald AC, et al. Mortality and prehospital thrombolysis for acute myocardial infarction: A meta-analysis. *JAMA* 2000;283:2686–2692.
35. Topol EJ. Reperfusion therapy for acute myocardial infarction with fibrinolytic therapy or combination reduced fibrinolytic therapy and platelet glycoprotein IIb/IIIa inhibition: the GUSTO V randomised trial. *Lancet* 2001;357:1905–1914.

36. Efficacy and safety of tenecteplase in combination with enoxaparin, abciximab, or unfractionated heparin: the ASSENT-3 randomised trial in acute myocardial infarction. *Lancet* 2001;358:605–613.
37. The effects of tissue plasminogen activator, streptokinase, or both on coronary-artery patency, ventricular function, and survival after acute myocardial infarction. The GUSTO Angiographic Investigators. *N Engl J Med* 1993;329:1615–1622.
38. Ellis SG, da Silva ER, Heyndrickx G, et al. Randomized comparison of rescue angioplasty with conservative management of patients with early failure of thrombolysis for acute anterior myocardial infarction. *Circulation* 1994;90:2280–2284.
39. Gershlick AH, Stephens-Lloyd A, Hughes S, et al. Rescue angioplasty after failed thrombolytic therapy for acute myocardial infarction. *N Engl J Med* 2005;353:2758–2768.
40. Primary versus tenecteplase-facilitated percutaneous coronary intervention in patients with ST-segment elevation acute myocardial infarction (ASSENT-4 PCI): randomised trial. *Lancet* 2006;367:569–578.
41. Keeley EC, Boura JA, Grines CL. Comparison of primary and facilitated percutaneous coronary interventions for ST-elevation myocardial infarction: quantitative review of randomised trials. *Lancet* 2006;367:579–588.
42. Di Mario C, Dudek D, Piscione F, et al. Immediate angioplasty versus standard therapy with rescue angioplasty after thrombolysis in the Combined Abciximab REteplase Stent Study in Acute Myocardial Infarction (CARESS-in-AMI): an open, prospective, randomised, multicentre trial. *Lancet* 2008;371:559–568.
43. Hochman JS, Lamas GA, Buller CE, et al. Coronary intervention for persistent occlusion after myocardial infarction. *N Engl J Med* 2006;355:2395–2407.
44. Aversano T, Aversano LT, Passamani E, et al. Thrombolytic therapy vs primary percutaneous coronary intervention for myocardial infarction in patients presenting to hospitals without on-site cardiac surgery: a randomized controlled trial. *JAMA* 2002;287:1943–1951.
45. Mitchell JR. Anticoagulants in coronary heart disease—retrospect and prospect. *Lancet* 1981;1:257–262.
46. Platelet glycoprotein IIb/IIIa receptor blockade and low-dose heparin during percutaneous coronary revascularization. The EPILOG Investigators. *N Engl J Med* 1997;336:1689–1696.
47. Antman EM, Louwerenburg HW, Baars HF, et al. Enoxaparin as adjunctive antithrombin therapy for ST-elevation myocardial infarction: results of the ENTIRE-Thrombolysis in Myocardial Infarction (TIMI) 23 Trial. *Circulation* 2002;105:1642–1649.
48. Ross AM, Molhoek P, Lundergan C, et al. Randomized comparison of enoxaparin, a low-molecular-weight heparin, with unfractionated heparin adjunctive to recombinant tissue plasminogen activator thrombolysis and aspirin: second trial of Heparin and Aspirin Reperfusion Therapy (HART II). *Circulation* 2001;104:648–652.
49. Yusuf S, Mehta SR, Chrolavicius S, et al. Effects of fondaparinux on mortality and reinfarction in patients with acute ST-segment elevation myocardial infarction: the OASIS-6 randomized trial. *JAMA* 2006;295:1519–1530.
50. White H. Thrombin-specific anticoagulation with bivalirudin versus heparin in patients receiving fibrinolytic therapy for acute myocardial infarction: the HERO-2 randomised trial. *Lancet* 2001;358:1855–1863.
51. Chen ZM, Pan HC, Chen YP, et al. Early intravenous then oral metoprolol in 45,852 patients with acute myocardial infarction: randomised placebo-controlled trial. *Lancet* 2005;366:1622–1632.
52. GISSI-3: effects of lisinopril and transdermal glyceryl trinitrate singly and together on 6-week mortality and ventricular function after acute myocardial infarction. Gruppo Italiano per lo Studio della Sopravvivenza nell'infarto Miocardico. *Lancet* 1994;343:1115–1122.
53. ISIS-4: a randomised factorial trial assessing early oral captopril, oral mononitrate, and intravenous magnesium sulphate in 58,050 patients with suspected acute myocardial infarction. ISIS-4 (Fourth International Study of Infarct Survival) Collaborative Group. *Lancet* 1995;345:669–685.
54. Yusuf S, Sleight P, Pogue J, et al. Effects of an angiotensin-converting-enzyme inhibitor, ramipril, on cardiovascular events in high-risk patients. The Heart Outcomes Prevention Evaluation Study Investigators. *N Engl J Med* 2000;342:145–153.
55. Hohnloser SH, Kuck KH, Dorian P, et al. Prophylactic use of an implantable cardioverter-defibrillator after acute myocardial infarction. *N Engl J Med* 2004;351:2481–2488.

Landmark Trials

Gruppo Italiano per lo Studio dell Streptochi-nasi nell'Inrarto Miocardico. Long-term effects of intravenous thrombolysis in acute myocardial infarction: final report of the GISSI study. *Lancet* 1987;2:871–874.

Gruppo Italiano per lo Studio dell Streptochi-nasi nell'Inrarto Miocardico. GISSI-3: effects of lisinopril and transdermal glyceryl trinitrate singly and together on 6-week mortality and ventricular function after acute myocardial infarction. *Lancet* 1994;343:1115–1122.

The GUSTO Investigators. An international randomized trial comparing four thrombolytic strategies for acute myocardial infarction. *N Engl J Med* 1993;329:673–682.

GUSTO IIb Angioplasty Substudy Investigators. A clinical trial comparing primary coronary angioplasty with tissue plasminogen activator for acute myocardial infarction. *N Engl J Med* 1997;336:1621–1628.

The GUSTO III Investigators. A comparison of reteplase with alteplase for acute myocardial infarction. *N Engl J Med* 1997;337:1118–1123.

ISIS-2 (Second international study of infarct survival) Collaborative Group. Randomised trial of intravenous streptokinase, oral aspirin, both, or neither among 17,187 cases of suspected acute myocardial infarction. *Lancet* 1988;2:349–360.

The GUSTO V Investigators. Reperfusion therapy for acute myocardial infarction with fibrinolytic therapy or combination reduced fibrinolytic therapy and platelet glycoprotein IIb/IIIa inhibition: the GUSTO V randomised trial. *Lancet* 2001;357:1905–1914.

The ASSENT-3 Investigators. Efficacy and safety of tenecteplase in combination with enoxaparin, abciximab, or unfractionated heparin: the ASSENT-3 randomised trial in acute myocardial infarction. *Lancet* 2001;358:605–613.

CLARITY-TIMI 28. Sabatine MS, Cannon CP, Gibson CM, et al. Addition of clopidogrel to aspirin and fibrinolytic therapy for myocardial infarction with ST-segment elevation. *N Engl J Med* 2005;352:1179–1189.

COMMIT/CCS-2. Chen ZM, Jiang LX, Chen YP, et al. Addition of clopidogrel to aspirin in 45,852 patients with acute myocardial infarction: randomised placebo-controlled trial. *Lancet* 2005;366:1607–1621.

The ASSENT-4 PCI Investigators. Primary versus tenecteplase-facilitated percutaneous coronary intervention in patients with ST-segment elevation acute myocardial infarction (ASSENT-4 PCI): randomised trial. *Lancet* 2006;367:569–578.

OAT. Primary versus tenecteplase-facilitated percutaneous coronary intervention in patients with ST-segment elevation acute myocardial infarction (ASSENT-4 PCI): randomised trial. *Lancet* 2006;367:569–578.

EXTRACT-TIMI 25. Antman EM, Morrow DA, McCabe CH, et al. Enoxaparin versus unfractionated heparin with fibrinolysis for ST-elevation myocardial infarction. *N Engl J Med* 2006;354:1477–1488.

Key Reviews

Antman EM, Anbe DT, Armstrong PW, et al. ACC/AHA guidelines for the management of patients with ST-elevation myocardial infarction: A report of the American College of Cardiology/American Heart Association Task Force on Practice Guidelines (Committee to Revise the 1999 Guidelines for the Management of Patients with Acute Myocardial Infarction). *J Am Coll Cardiol* 2004;44:E1–E211.

Antman EM, Hand M, Armstrong PW, et al. 2007 focused update of the ACC/AHA 2004 guidelines for the management of patients with ST-elevation myocardial infarction: a report of the American College of Cardiology/American Heart Association Task Force on Practice Guidelines. J Am Coll Cardiol 2008;51:210–247. New MI definitions.

Falk E, Shah PK, Fuster V. Coronary plaque disruption. *Circulation* 1995;92:657–671.

Thygesen K, Alpert JS, White HD. Universal definition of myocardial infarction. *J Am Coll Cardiol* 2007;50:2173–2195.

White HD, Van de Werf FJ. Thrombolysis for acute myocardial infarction. *Circulation* 1998;97:1632–1646.

Relevant Book Chapters

Bavry AA, Bhatt DL. Revascularization and reperfusion therapy. In: *Managing acute coronary syndromes in clinical practice*. London: Current Medical Group, 2008.

Christofferson RD. Acute ST-elevation myocardial infarction. In: Shishehbor MH, Wang TH, Askari AT, et al., eds. *Management of the patient in the coronary care unit*. New York: Lippincott Williams & Wilkins, 2008.

Topol EJ, Van de Werf FJ. Acute myocardial infarction: early diagnosis and management. In: Topol EJ, ed. *Textbook of cardiovascular medicine*. New York: Lippincott Williams & Wilkins, 2007.

2 UNSTABLE ANGINA AND NON–ST-SEGMENT-ELEVATION MYOCARDIAL INFARCTION

Telly A. Meadows

I. INTRODUCTION. **Unstable angina (UA)** and **non–ST-segment-elevation myocardial infarction (NSTEMI)** remain leading causes of morbidity and mortality in the United States, accounting for more than 1.5 million hospital admissions in the year 2004 alone. These conditions are part of a continuum of acute coronary syndromes (ACS) that ranges from UA and NSTEMI to ST-segment-elevation MI (STEMI). **The clinical presentation of non–ST-elevation acute coronary syndromes (NSTE-ACS) can be insidious,** ranging from **progressive exertional angina** to **postinfarction angina.** Because **NSTEMI is distinguished from UA by the presence of elevated serum levels of cardiac biomarkers**, serial measurements in patients presenting with ACS should be performed. With improvements in the diagnosis and risk stratification of patients with UA and NSTEMI, therapeutic approaches to NSTE-ACS have continued to evolve.

II. CLINICAL PRESENTATION

A. Risk factors

1. **Clinical characteristics indicative of high-risk.** Symptoms may include an **acceleration of ischemic symptoms within the preceding 48 hours, angina at rest (>20 minutes), congestive heart failure (S_3 gallop, pulmonary edema, rales), known reduced left ventricular (LV) function, hypotension, new or worsening mitral regurgitation murmur, age >75 years, diffuse ST-segment changes on an electrocardiogram (ECG, ≥0.5 to 1 mm), and the presence of elevated serum cardiac biomarkers (typically creatine kinase MB [CK-MB], troponin T, or troponin I).** Patients at intermediate or low risk have angina of short duration, no ischemic ST-segment changes on ECG, are negative for cardiac biomarkers, and are hemodynamically stable (Table 2.1).

TABLE 2.1 Risk Stratification of Patients with Unstable Angina

High risk[a]	Intermediate risk	Low risk
One of the following must be present:	No high-risk feature but must have one of the following:	No high- or intermediate-risk features present
Accelerating tempo of ischemic symptoms in preceding 48 h	Prior MI, peripheral or cerebrovascular disease	
Prolonged ongoing rest pain (>20 min): moderate or high likelihood of CAD	Prolonged rest pain (>20 min) that resolves	Increased frequency or duration of angina
Pulmonary edema: most likely caused by ischemia	Rest angina (>20 min or relieved with rest or sublingual NTG)	Angina provoked by less exertion
Rest angina with dynamic ST changes ≥0.5 mm	Nocturnal angina	New-onset angina (within 2 wk to 2 mo)
New or worsening rales, S_3, or MR murmur	New-onset, severe angina within 2 wk with moderate or high likelihood of CAD	
Hypotension, bradycardia, tachycardia		
Bundle-branch block, new or presumed new	T-Wave changes	Normal or unchanged ECG
Sustained ventricular tachycardia	Pathologic Q waves or resting ST-depression (<1 mm) in multiple lead groups	
Positive serum cardiac biomarkers	Slightly elevated CK-MB, troponin T, troponin I (e.g., TnT 0.01 but <0.1 ng/mL)	Normal cardiac markers
	Age older than 70 years	

CAD, Coronary artery disease; ECG, electrocardiogram; MR, mitral regurgitation; NTG, nitroglycerin.
[a]Risk stratification involves considering clinical characteristics and ECG findings to make early triage decisions.

2. **Electrocardiogram.** The initial electrocardiogram can help risk-stratify patients with UA. Ideally, this should be performed within 10 minutes of arrival to the emergency department. Patients with ST-segment deviation (i.e., ST depression or transient ST elevation) ≥0.5 mm or with pre-existing left bundle-branch block (LBBB) are at increased risk for death or MI at 1 year after presentation. ST-segment elevation ≥0.5 mm in lead aVR raises the possibility of left main or three-vessel coronary artery disease (CAD). **T-wave inversions alone generally are not predictive of adverse ischemic events.**
3. **NSTEMI.** NSTEMI predicts a poorer prognosis among patients with UA. Multivariate predictors of NSTEMI in patients with ACS include **prolonged chest pain** (>60 minutes), **ST-segment deviations** (depression or transient elevation), and **new or recent onset of angina** (in the past month). Elevations in the levels of troponin I or troponin T, contractile proteins released from necrotic cardiac myocytes, are independently predictive of morbidity and mortality among patients with UA (discussed later) (1,2). According to the European Society of Cardiology/American College of Cardiology (ESC/ACC), troponin elevations in this clinical setting are, by definition, NSTEMI.
4. **Clinical risk classification systems.** Numerous scores have been derived to facilitate risk assessment and guide medical therapy in patients with NSTE-ACS. It is important to note that these scores can be used to determine which patients may benefit most from early invasive therapy as opposed to a more conservative approach. The **Braunwald classification system** risk-stratifies patients with UA at

TABLE 2.2 Braunwald Classification of Unstable Angina

Class	Characteristics[a]
I	**Exertional angina**
	New onset, severe, or accelerated
	Angina of <2 mo duration
	More frequent angina
	Angina precipitated by less exertion
	No rest angina in the last 2 mo
II	**Rest angina, subacute**
	Rest angina within the last month but none within 48 h of presentation
III	**Rest angina, acute**
	Rest angina within 48 h of presentation
	CLINICAL CIRCUMSTANCES
A	**Secondary unstable angina**
	Caused by a noncardiac condition, such as anemia, infection, thyrotoxicosis, or hypoxemia
B	**Primary unstable angina**
C	**Postinfarction unstable angina**
	Within 2 wk of documented myocardial infarction

[a]This classification can be used for risk stratification. Clinical characteristics at presentation and severity of angina are considered.

presentation (Table 2.2). Braunwald defined UA according to the **characteristics of anginal pain** and the **underlying cause.** Patients with increasing Braunwald class have been shown to have increasing risk of recurrent ischemia and death at 6 months. Vital clinical characteristics not included in this classification were age, the presence of comorbid conditions (e.g., diabetes mellitus, renal insufficiency), electrocardiographic criteria, and the presence of positive cardiac markers.

The thrombolysis in myocardial infarction (TIMI) unstable angina risk score, based on the TIMI 11B and ESSENCE trials, incorporates **the combination of age, clinical characteristics, ECG changes, and cardiac markers for risk stratification** (Table 2.3). A higher risk score correlated with an increase in the incidence of death, new or recurrent MI, and recurrent ischemia requiring revascularization (3). The GRACE prediction score, which incorporates nine clinical variables derived from the medical history and clinical findings on initial presentation and during hospitalization, can be used to estimate the in-hospital and 6-month outcomes for patients hospitalized with any form of ACS (4,5). Other risk stratification scores based on the PURSUIT trial and the GUSTO IV-ACS trial (Table 2.4) have also been described. Together, these various clinical risk-stratification systems help to identify high-risk patients likely to benefit most from more aggressive therapy.

B. Demographics. Compared with STEMI, patients with **UA/NSTEMI** are **older,** have a higher incidence of **cardiac risk factors or comorbid conditions (e.g., diabetes, hypertension, hypercholesterolemia)** and a greater likelihood of **prior MI and revascularization procedures** (i.e., percutaneous coronary intervention [PCI] and coronary artery bypass grafting [CABG]).

C. Signs and symptoms. Chest pain due to UA may be rest pain or may be triggered with minimal exertion and can be new onset or increased in severity, frequency, or precipitated with less effort than prior angina. Compared with stable angina, **chest pain in UA** is usually more **severe and protracted,** often requiring several doses of sublingual nitroglycerin or extended periods of rest for relief. UA or NSTEMI cannot be differentiated on the basis of chest pain characteristics or ECG abnormalities

TABLE 2.3 TIMI Risk Score

Score	Incidence of death, new or recurrent MI, recurrent ischemia requiring revascularization
0/1	4.7%
2	8.3%
3	13.2%
4	19.9%
5	26.2%
6/7	40.9%
	SCORING SYSTEM
One point when risk factor is present, zero points if absent (total of 7 points are possible):	
Age >65 y	
Presence of more than three risk factors for coronary artery disease	
Prior coronary stenosis ≥50%	
Presence of ST-segment deviation on admission electrocardiogram	
More than two episodes of angina within past 24 h	
Prior use of aspirin in past 7 d	
Elevated cardiac markers	

TABLE 2.4 GUSTO Risk Score

Risk score	30-Day mortality rate
0–5	0.4%
6–10	2.8%
11–15	8.7%
16–19	25.0%
20–22	41.7%
SCORING SYSTEM	
Points are assigned based on the following crlteria:	
Age (y)	Points
50–59	2
60–69	4
70–79	6
80+	8
Clinical history	
Prior heart failure	2
Prior stroke/TIA	2
Prior MI/revasc./chronic angina	1
Vitals & Lab. Values	
Heart Rate ≥90	3
Elevated troponin and CK-MB	3
Cr >1.4 mg/dL	2
CRP (μ/L) >20	2
10–20	1
Anemia	1

CRP, C-Reactive protein; MI, myocardial infarction; Revasc., revascularization; TIA, transient ischemic attack.

alone. **The only way this determination can be made is with evidence of myocardial necrosis by measurement of cardiac biomarkers.**

D. Differential diagnosis. It is vitally important to determine the probability that the chest pain or presenting symptom(s) are caused by ACS resulting from obstructive CAD. The exclusion of other diagnoses that mimic angina such as costochondritis, pneumonia, or pericarditis, as well as other life-threatening conditions such as aortic dissection, pneumothorax, and pulmonary embolus, is essential. Hypertensive urgency or emergency, thyrotoxicosis, systemic infection, and other precipitating causes of myocardial ischemia and secondary unstable angina should also be sought.

E. Physical findings. Physical examination alone is insufficient for the diagnosis of UA. **Signs of heart failure** (elevated jugular venous pressure [JVP], S_3), impaired myocardial performance (S_4) or peripheral vascular disease (PVD) (i.e., bruits over major vessels) may be present. These findings predict a higher likelihood of significant CAD.

III. LABORATORY EVALUATION

A. Electrocardiogram. Common ECG findings in UA/NSTEMI include **ST-segment depression, transient ST-segment elevation, and T-wave inversion.** However, **approximately 20% of patients with an NSTEMI confirmed by cardiac enzymes have no ischemic ECG changes. Moreover, a "normal" ECG pattern is not sufficient to rule out ACS in patients with chest pain** (>4% of patients presenting with chest pain and normal ECG patterns are diagnosed with UA) (6). Persistent ST-segment elevation of ≥1 mm in two or more contiguous leads or new LBBB suggests acute STEMI and should be urgently treated with reperfusion therapy (see Chapter 1). As previously mentioned, ST-segment elevation ≥0.5 mm in lead aVR raises the possibility of left main or three-vessel CAD. **T-wave inversions are the least specific of ECG changes in ACS.** However, new, deep, **symmetric T-wave inversions of ≥2 mm** across the precordium in patients presenting with UA often correspond to acute ischemia, usually related to a severe proximal left anterior descending (LAD) artery stenosis. In this setting, revascularization often results in improved ventricular function and normalization of the electrocardiogram.

1. Older classification systems recognized NSTEMI as **non–Q-wave MI** because myocardial necrosis occurs without ECG evidence of transmural injury. Because of the inability to determine the transmural extent of myocardial injury based on the presence or absence of ST-segment elevation, **NSTEMI** has become the preferred terminology.
2. Analysis of 1473 UA or NSTEMI patients in the **TIMI III trial** revealed transient ST-segment elevation in 10%, ST-segment depression in 33%, T-wave inversion in 46%, and no ischemic ECG changes in 9% (7).

B. Cardiac enzymes

1. **Creatine kinase (CK).** Among the most commonly used biochemical markers for the evaluation of patients with suspected ACS are CK and the MB isoenzyme of CK, measured serially every 6 to 8 hours for the first 24 hours. Total CK levels **peak at 12 to 24 hours** after the onset of symptoms, and **CK-MB levels peak at 10 to 18 hours** after the onset of symptoms. The CK-MB isoenzyme is more specific and more sensitive than the total CK measurement for documenting myocardial necrosis. Although a low level of CK and CK-MB is usually found in normal patients, values above the upper limit of normal for a given laboratory suggest the presence of myocardial necrosis. **Many nonischemic conditions, such as pericarditis, skeletal muscle injury, and renal failure** can cause elevations of total CK levels or, and less likely, an increase in CK-MB.
2. **Troponins.** Cardiac troponins are contractile proteins found only in cardiac myocytes. Many clinical trials have used troponin levels for diagnosis and prognosis in ACS. Serum levels of **troponins I and T typically rise within 3 to 12 hours** after myocardial necrosis, remain elevated afterward for much longer than CK (10 to 14 days), and do not correlate well with the extent of myocardial damage. Although troponins are more sensitive and specific for myocardial injury than CK and CK-MB, elevated troponin levels can be seen in other nonischemic cardiac conditions (advanced heart failure, acute pericarditis) and in the setting of

renal insufficiency. In the setting of NSTE-ACS, troponins have important prognostic significance beyond that specified by clinical criteria, with elevated levels portending a worse prognosis.

In the **GUSTO IIb** trial of patients with UA, the 30-day mortality rate for patients with an elevated troponin T level (>0.1 ng/mL) was 11.8%, compared with 3.9% for patients with normal troponin levels. Elevated troponin levels in the setting of NSTE-ACS have also been associated with increased likelihood of multivessel disease, high-risk culprit lesions, and intracoronary thrombus visible at the time of angiography.

3. **Recommendations.** Because of the increased sensitivity and specificity of troponin measurements as well as their correlation with future prognosis, troponin levels are the preferred biomarker and should be drawn in all patients presenting with ACS. Serial CK and CK-MB levels should also be measured, as they can give a better indication of infarct size and temporal course.

C. Other biochemical markers

1. **C-Reactive protein (CRP).** In the TIMI 11A trial, patients with UA/NSTEMI with an elevated quantitative CRP (levels ≥1.55 mg/dL) had a higher mortality rate, even those patients with negative troponin T level (5.80% vs. 0.36%, $p = 0.006$). Patients with an elevated CRP and a positive troponin T level had the highest mortality rates. Patients with either an elevated CRP concentration or a positive troponin level had an intermediate mortality rate, and patients without an elevated CRP or a positive troponin had the lowest mortality (9.10% vs. 4.65% vs. 0.36%, respectively, $p = 0.0003$) (8).
2. **Other markers.** Research aimed at identifying additional novel biochemical markers that may help to further risk-stratify and tailor therapy in ACS continues to rapidly evolve. Novel markers being developed generally fall into one of the following categories: markers of necrosis (troponin), inflammation (hs-CRP, myeloperoxidase, pregnancy-associated plasma protein A, soluble CD-40 ligand, interleukin-6), hemodynamic stress or neurohormonal activation (brain natriuretic peptide [BNP], N-terminal fragment of pro-**brain natriuretic peptide** [NT-proBNP]), coagulation, platelet activation, vascular damage (creatinine clearance, cystatin C), accelerated atherosclerosis (hemoglobin A1c, HbA1c), and proteogenomics. Many of these biomarkers have been shown to be independent predictors of risk in NSTE-ACS. As the number of available biomakers continues to grow, further studies evaluating the utility of a multimarker approach (combination of individual markers, possibly from various classes) continue to be performed.

IV. PATHOPHYSIOLOGY. The pathophysiology of ACS encompasses a complex interplay of plaque rupture, platelet activation and aggregation leading to thrombus formation, endothelial dysfunction, vasospasm, and vascular remodeling.

A. Plaque rupture. UA, NSTEMI, and STEMI share a common initiating event: atheromatous plaque fissure or rupture. Plaque rupture stimulates platelet deposition, activation, and aggregation at the site of injury, followed by activation of the coagulation cascade and thrombus formation. Factors contributing to plaque instability include lymphocyte and macrophage activation and increased inflammation. Infection with *Chlamydia pneumoniae* also may be involved. Ruptured plaques or culprit lesions in patients, even when medically stabilized, tend to progress in comparison to stable lesions. Follow-up angiography of 85 patients with UA who were medically stabilized 8 months after initial presentation revealed that 25% of culprit lesions progressed in disease severity (usually to complete occlusion), compared with 7% of nonculprit lesions. This progression of disease correlated with future cardiac events (9).

B. Thrombus formation. Exposure of circulating platelets to subendothelial contents results in platelet adhesion, aggregation, and, ultimately, thrombus formation. With platelet activation, the glycoprotein (GP) IIb/IIIa receptor on the platelet surface undergoes a conformational change, facilitating further platelet activation and aggregation. This markedly increases thrombin production, further expanding and stabilizing the thrombus.

C. **Vasospasm** can be induced by the local production of vasoactive substances released from the subendothelial matrix or propagating thrombus, or it can occur as a primary phenomenon. Severe localized spasm of a coronary artery segment (i.e., Prinzmetal's angina) may also result in ACS. This vasospasm frequently occurs at sites of unstable plaque and is thought to contribute to thrombus formation. Even angiographically normal coronary arteries with underlying endothelial dysfunction may be subject to vasospasm.

D. **Multiple lesions.** Although a single culprit lesion is often found at angiography, multiple culprit lesions are not uncommon in patients presenting with UA/NSTEMI, attesting to the global nature of the disease. In a substudy of patients with NSTEMI, **multiple apparent culprit lesions were found in 14% of patients**, whereas a single culprit lesion was found in 49%. An intravascular ultrasound study of patients with NSTEMI undergoing angiography and possible PCI revealed an average of 2.1 plaque ruptures per patient, with 79% of patients having a lesion in a different location than that of the culprit lesion.

E. **Secondary causes.** UA can also result from a supply–demand mismatch of oxygen delivery to the myocardium. With stable obstructive coronary lesions, precipitants of UA include **increased myocardial oxygen demand** (i.e., tachycardia, severe hypertension, cocaine use, hyperthyroidism, fever, or sepsis) and **decreased oxygen supply** (i.e., anemia or hypoxemia).

V. DIAGNOSTIC TESTING.

UA remains predominantly a clinical diagnosis. Diagnostic testing can confirm or refute the initial clinical suspicion of UA through documentation of myocardial ischemia, myocardial damage manifested as elevated cardiac biomarker levels, or new LV wall-motion abnormalities, and substantial coronary arterial plaque burden. Noninvasive testing is generally used in low-risk patients with UA.

A. **Echocardiography.** In patients presenting with ACS, echocardiography may be helpful to demonstrate wall-motion abnormalities correlating with acute ischemia. However, small amounts of ischemic myocardium may be insufficient to produce wall-motion abnormalities that are evident echocardiographically. Moreover, these wall-motion abnormalities may be transient and seen only at the time of acute ischemia. New wall-motion abnormalities cannot be differentiated from pre-existing ones. In the presence of existing CAD or known LV dysfunction, echocardiography may be limited in its ability to definitively diagnose acute ischemia. Poor acoustic windows and limited availability of trained sonographers also limit its universal availability and applicability. The utility of echocardiography in patients with UA primarily resides in the evaluation of **resting LV function,** especially in patients with signs or symptoms of congestive heart failure (CHF).

B. **Noninvasive stress testing.** Stress testing has been thought to be contraindicated in the evaluation of patients with UA because of the concern for acute occlusion with increased cardiac workloads in the presence of unstable plaques. However, patients at low or even intermediate risk who remain pain free for at least 12 to 24 hours and without any symptoms of heart failure can safely undergo functional testing. Intermediate-risk patients include those with an age >70 years; slightly elevated cardiac biomarkers (e.g., troponin T >0.01 ng/mL but <0.1 ng/mL), T-wave changes; pathologic QS; or minimal resting ST-depressions (<1 mm) on ECG; rest angina or present with atypical symptoms; or prior history of MI, CABG, peripheral or cerebrovascular disease, or aspirin use.

1. **Cardiac catheterization** should be considered for patients found to have an **abnormal thallium scan** on stress testing, because they are at increased risk for adverse ischemic events. Patients who have **normal thallium scan** without fixed or reversible perfusion defects can be **discharged** from the hospital and followed up on an outpatient basis.
2. If patients are unable to exercise, **pharmacologic stress testing** can be done instead with dobutamine or dipyridamole. However, no large-scale studies using these modalities for stress testing have been performed in this patient population.

C. **Diagnostic cardiac catheterization.** In patients with UA, cardiac catheterization reveals angiographically normal coronary arteries or mild disease (all lesions <50%) in 10% to 20% of patients, single-vessel disease in 30% to 35%, two-vessel disease in 25% to 30%, three-vessel disease in 20% to 25%, and left main artery disease in 5% to 10%.

D. Key suggestions

1. Patients who do not undergo cardiac catheterization should undergo **stress testing. Patients found to have a reversible perfusion defect or wall-motion abnormality on stress testing should undergo cardiac catheterization.**
2. An early invasive approach, performing a **cardiac catheterization** with plans for revascularization, is only of clear benefit in high-risk patients (Table 2.1). In other patients, an early conservative approach with selective invasive therapy is the preferred approach (see Section P. Early invasive versus conservative strategies).

E. Other imaging modalities. Coronary CT angiography and cardiac magnetic resonance imaging are currently being evaluated in clinical studies for use as alternative imaging methods for assessment of patients with low pre-test probability of CAD presenting with possible unstable angina.

VI. THERAPY. In patients with UA, the immediate goals of medical therapy are the **treatment of platelet activation/aggregation and thrombus formation** in conjunction **with antianginal therapy.** Based on patient's risk, it is important to decide early between an early invasive approach to therapy versus an initial conservative strategy. Patients with recurrent symptoms despite maximal medical therapy, high-risk scores (e.g., TIMI, GRACE, PURSUIT), elevated cardiac biomarkers, hemodynamic instability, reduced left ventricular function, prior CABG, or prior PCI within 6 months should undergo urgent cardiac catheterization and percutaneous intervention. Patients at low risk who can be stabilized may warrant only medical therapy with selective use of angiography. In most cases of UA/NSTEMI, occlusive thrombus is not found at the time of cardiac catheterization. **The primary goal of revascularization is not acute reperfusion as it is in STEMI, but rather minimization of subsequent morbidity and mortality (i.e., death, nonfatal MI, and refractory angina).**

A. Priority of medical therapy

1. Antiplatelet agents with aspirin and clopidogrel
2. Antianginal therapy with nitrates and β-blockers
3. Anticoagulant therapy with unfractionated heparin, low–molecular-weight heparin (LMWH), direct thrombin inhibitors, or factor Xa inhibitor
4. Glycoprotein IIb/IIIa inhibitors in high-risk patients or those undergoing early PCI

B. Antiplatelet agents

1. **Aspirin.** Despite being a relatively weak inhibitor of platelet aggregation, aspirin has a significant effect on mortality in UA. There are several pathways that lead to platelet activation, of which aspirin blocks only the cyclooxygenase-derived thromboxane A_2 pathway. Aspirin therapy for UA/NSTEMI has been studied in five major clinical trials at doses ranging from 75 to 325 mg/day. Overall, treatment with aspirin reduced the combined endpoint of death or nonfatal MI by 50%.
   a. **Pharmacokinetics.** The onset of aspirin's antiplatelet effect is quite rapid, with substantial inhibition of thromboxane A_2 production within 15 minutes, translating into measurable platelet inhibition within 60 minutes. It should be given **as soon as patients present with ACS.** Because aspirin's inhibition of cyclooxygenase is irreversible, its antiplatelet effect is durable, lasting 7 to 10 days.
   b. **Dosing.** Unless contraindicated (e.g., active bleeding, documented hypersensitivity to aspirin), an intial dose of 162 to 325 mg of nonenteric coated aspirin (chewed and swallowed) should be given to all patients with suspected UA. **Those patients allergic or intolerant to aspirin should receive clopidogrel as soon as possible.** Subsequent daily aspirin doses can be reduced, with the preferred dose for secondary prevention being 81 to 162 mg daily. For patients who undergo PCI, aspirin at 162 to 325 mg/day is recommended for at least 1 month after bare metal stenting, 3 months after sirolimus-eluting stent implantation, and 6 months after paclitaxel-eluting stent implantation followed by 81 to 162 mg/day indefinitely thereafter.

2. **Thienopyridines (ticlopidine and clopidogrel).** Ticlopidine and clopidogrel inhibit adenosine diphosphate (ADP)–induced platelet aggregation. Compared with placebo, ticlopidine reduced rates of death or MI at 6 months among patients with UA to a degree similar to that of aspirin.

   In the **CURE** trial, patients with UA or NSTEMI had a lower rate of cardiovascular death, nonfatal MI, or stroke when treated with aspirin and clopidogrel versus aspirin alone (9.3% vs. 11.4%, p <0.001). Patients treated with this combination experienced lower rates of refractory ischemia, heart failure, or revascularization. However, an increased rate of major bleeding (3.7% vs. 2.7% for aspirin) was seen in patients receiving clopidogrel, predominantly in those undergoing CABG.

   In a substudy of the CURE trial, **PCI-CURE**, pretreatment with clopidogrel resulted in lower rates of cardiovascular death, nonfatal MI, or urgent target-vessel revascularization at 30 days (4.5% vs. 6.4%) in patients with UA/NSTEMI undergoing PCI. Long-term treatment with clopidogrel resulted in lower rates of cardiovascular death, nonfatal MI, or revascularization, without a significant increase in major bleeding (10). The benefit of clopidogrel pretreatment in PCI was further confirmed in the **CREDO** trial in which patients receiving a 300-mg loading dose plus 1 year of 75 mg daily maintenance therapy of clopidogrel had a 26.9% relative reduction in death, nonfatal MI, or stroke at 1 year compared to those receiving only 1 month of maintenance therapy without any loading dose of clopidogrel (11).

   a. **Pharmacokinetics.** Ticlopidine's onset of action is delayed, usually taking 2 to 3 days for maximum antiplatelet effect. Clopidogrel has a shorter onset of action when 300 mg is given, with antiplatelet activity being detected within 2 hours after administration.
   b. **Side effects.** Ticlopidine can cause neutropenia (1% to 5% of patients) and is rarely associated with thrombotic thrombocytopenic purpura (TTP). There have also been case reports of TTP with clopidogrel therapy.
   c. **Dosing.** Ticlopidine is given as a loading dose of 500 mg followed by 250 mg twice daily. The conventional loading dose for clopidogrel has been 300 mg; however, there is evidence demonstrating a more rapid and heightened platelet inhibitory response, resulting in decreased ischemic events after PCI with use of a 600-mg loading dose of clopidogrel. The optimal loading dose—300 mg versus 600 mg—for clopidogrel is still being evaluated in clinical studies. Clopidogrel maintence therapy is 75 mg daily.
   d. **Recommendations.** Clopidogrel is preferred over ticlopidine because of a more rapid onset of action, less frequent dosing, and fewer serious side effects. Clopidogrel therapy (loading dose plus maintenance therapy) is recommended for all patients diagnosed with NSTE-ACS. The benefit of treatment must be balanced against the significant bleeding risk in the minority that will undergo CABG. For patients unlikely to undergo revascularization by CABG, clopidogrel should be initiated at the time aspirin is started. If patients undergo CABG, at least 5 days without clopidogrel is recommended to decrease the risk of perioperative complications, including reoperation for bleeding. For inpatients treated with an early invasive approach, some centers delay initiation of clopidogrel until coronary anatomy is defined at diagnostic angiography and decisions are made about revascularization (percutaneous versus surgical). Clopidogrel maintenance therapy should be provided for at least 1 month, although ideally 1 year, in patients treated medically or with PCI and bare metal stenting. Given the small but increased risk of stent thrombosis in patients who undergo PCI with drug-eluting stents, clopidogrel maintenance therapy should continue for a minimum of 1 year, and even longer if no contraindication exists.
   e. Another oral thienopyridine currently undergoing clinical evaluation is prasugrel. In preclinical studies, prasugrel has been shown to have a more potent antiplatlelet effect than clopidogrel. The **TRITON-TIMI 38** trial evaluated the efficacy of prasugrel versus clopidogrel in patients presenting with ACSs with

planned PCI. In this study of 13,608 patients, use of prasugrel as compared to clopidogrel resulted in a significant reduction in the primary efficacy endpoint of death from cardiovascular causes, nonfatal MI, or nonfatal stroke (9.9% vs. 12.1%, $p < 0.001$). However, the salutory benefits in reduction of ischemic events with prasugrel came at the expense of an increase in late bleeding events, including a significant increase in rates of both major bleeding (2.4% vs. 1.1%, $p = 0.03$) and fatal bleeding (0.4% vs. 0.1%, $p = 0.002$) (12). There are also two other nonthienopyridine ADP receptor antagonists, cangrelor and AZD6140, being evaluated in phase 3 clinincal studies.

C. Anticoagulants. There are an increasing number of anticoagulant therapies available for use in NSTE-ACS including unfractionated heparin, LMWH, direct thrombin inhibitors, and a factor Xa inhibitor. All patients with UA/NSTEMI should have some form of anticoagulant thearapy added to the antiplatelet therapy. The decision of which therapy to choose will ultimately depend on the patient's risk and initial management strategy (invasive vs. conservative).

1. Heparin. Unfractionated heparin (UH) in combination with aspirin reduces the incidence of ischemic events in patients with UA. A meta-analysis of six trials in patients with UA demonstrated that treatment with aspirin plus UH reduced the incidence of death or nonfatal MI by 33% compared with treatment with aspirin alone, although this difference did not quite reach statistical significance (13). The treatment effect of heparin may also wane after therapy is discontinued.

a. Duration of therapy. Although the optimal length for therapy with unfractionated heparin is unknown, studies have suggested that therapy must be continued for at least 3 to 7 days to achieve clinical benefit.

b. Rebound ischemia. Rebound ischemia is thought to result from the accumulation of thrombin during UH administration and the ensuing platelet aggregation. Studies have shown that this rebound ischemia can be attenuated with the concomitant use of aspirin.

c. Recommendations. Intravenous UH can be used for anticoagulant therapy in patients with NSTE-ACS undergoing either an invasive or conservative treatment strategy unless contraindicated (e.g., active bleeding, known hypersensitivity, history of heparin-associated thrombocytopenia).

d. Dosing. Initially, heparin should be given as a weight-adjusted bolus (60 U/kg), followed with an infusion (15 U/kg/hour). The activated partial thromboplastin time (aPTT) should be monitored every 6 hours until it stabilizes between 50 and 70 seconds, and monitored subsequently every 12 to 24 hours thereafter. Standardized heparin nomograms have simplified and streamlined the initial orders for UH and the subsequent adjustment of dosing based on aPTT levels.

2. Low-molecular-weight heparin. The advantages of LMWH compared with UH include increased bioavailability, a fixed dosing regimen, more effective thrombin inhibition, lower rates of heparin-induced thrombocytopenia, and cost savings because serial aPTT levels do not have to be monitored.

a. Comparison with heparin. A meta-analysis of 12 trials involving 17,157 patients with UA/NSTEMI that compared the use of several different LMWHs with UH found no significant benefit with LMWHs compared with UH (odds ratio [OR] = 0.88, 95% confident interval [CI] 0.69 to 1.12, $p = 0.34$).

In the **ESSENCE** trial, however, patients with UA/NSTEMI had a lower rate of death, MI, or recurrent angina at 30 days when treated with the LMWH, enoxaparin, than with UH (19.8% vs. 23.3%, $p = 0.016$). Patients treated with enoxaparin also underwent fewer revascularization procedures and experienced similar rates of major bleeding. Similarly, in the **TIMI 11B** study, patients with UA/NSTEMI treated with enoxaparin had a lower rate of death, MI, or urgent revascularization at 43 days compared with UH (17.3% vs. 19.7%, $p = 0.048$). Enoxaparin has been shown to be superior to UH in this patient population and may be used instead of UH, unless CABG is anticipated within 24 hours.

In the **SYNERGY** trial of 9978 high-risk patients with NSTE-ACS treated with an invasive therapeutic approach, enoxaparin was found to be noninferior but not superior to unfractionated heparin. The rate of death or MI at 30 days was 14% in the enoxaparin group and 14.5% in the UH group ($p = 0.396$). There was an increase in major bleeding per the TIMI criteria in those patients randomized to enoxaparin as compared to UH (9.1% vs. 7.6%, $p = 0.008$). Post hoc analysis suggested that crossover from enoxaparin to UH may have partly been the reason for this excess bleeding risk associated with enoxaparin (14).

b. Dosing. **Enoxaparin** is administered as 1 mg/kg given subcutaneously every 12 hours. No routine laboratory values have to be followed. However, in certain clinical settings (e.g., renal insufficiency, severe obesity), an anti-Xa level can be measured. The therapeutic anti-Xa level has yet to be determined in patients with UA/NSTEMI or in patients undergoing PCI, but the commonly accepted therapeutic range is 0.5 to 1.0 anti-Xa units per mL.

c. Recommendations. In patients with NSTE-ACS who may undergo either a conservative or early invasive therapy, enoxaparin is an acceptable agent for anticoagulation. In low-risk patients selected to be managed conservatively, enoxaparin may be preferred over UH.

3. Direct thrombin inhibitors. Direct thrombin inhibitors (DTIs) inhibit clot-bound thrombin more effectively than UH and are not inactivated by plasma proteins or platelet factor 4. Hirudin is an older generation DTI that is no longer used clinically and has been supplanated by its synthetic derivative, bivalirudin.

a. Bivalirudin (previously, Hirulog). Bivalirudin is a synthetic derivative of hirudin, with a shorter half-life, that reversibly inhibits thrombin. In the **ACUITY** trial of 13,819 patients with UA/NSTEMI, the clinical efficacy of bivalirudin plus GP IIb/IIIa inhibition was noninferior to heparin with GP IIb/IIIa inhibition with 30-day rates of ischemia of 7.7% versus 7.3%, respectively. In those patients receiving thienopyridine therapy prior to PCI, bivalirudin alone had similar efficacy along with lower bleeding rates as compared to heparin plus GP IIb/IIIa inhibition. However, bivalirudin alone was inferior to heparin plus GP IIb/IIIa inhibition in those patients who did not receive a thienopyridine prior to PCI (15).

b. Recommendations. Current guidelines recommend bivalirudin as a possible choice for anticoagulant therapy in conjunction with GP IIb/IIIa inhibition or a thienopyridine prior to angiography in patients presenting with NSTE-ACS with a planned invasive therapeutic approach. Bivalirudin is not recommended in those patients determined to undergo an initial conservative approach with medical therapy.

4. Factor Xa inhibitors. Fondaparinux is a heparin pentasaccharide analog that selectively inhibits factor Xa in the coagulation cascade. In comparison to unfractionated heparin, fondaparinux has decreased binding to plasma proteins along with dose-independent clearance with a longer half-life. These properties translate into more predictable and sustained anticoagulation, which permits fixed-dose, once daily administration.

a. Comparison with enoxaparin. The **OASIS-5** trial evaluated the efficacy of fondaparinux versus enoxaparin in 20,078 patients with UA/NSTEMI. Patients receiving fondaparinux (2.5 mg subcutaneously [SQ] once daily) had a similar rate of the combined endpoint of death, MI, or refractory ischemia at 9 days as those randomized to enoxaparin (1.0 mg/kg SQ twice daily). The use of fondaparinux was associated with a lower rate of major bleeding at 9 days as compared to enoxaparin (2.2% vs. 4.1%, $p < 0.001$). However, in this trial there was an increased incidence of catheter-associated thrombus noted, and the trial protocol was changed to allow for use of open-label unfractionated heparin, which initially was not allowed during PCI (16).

b. Dosing. The dosing of fondaparinux for UA/NSTEMI is 2.5 mg SQ once daily. Fondaparinux is renally cleared and its use is contraindicated in those patients with a creatinine clearance (CrCl) <30 mL/min.

c. **Recommendation.** Fondaparinux can be used for anticoagulant therapy in those patients selected to undergo a conservative medical approach. It is the preferred therapy in patients with increased risk of bleeding being managed with medical therapy. For patients who undergo angiography and PCI, adjuvant UH is recommended, given the increased rates of catheter-associated thrombus with fondaparinux in the **OASIS-5** trial.

D. Platelet glycoprotein IIb/IIIa antagonists

1. **Background.** Platelet aggregation requires the activation of glycoprotein (GP) IIb/IIIa receptors on the platelet surface. The GP IIb/IIIa receptors of adjacent platelets bind fibrinogen molecules that allow cross-linking of the platelets, which subsequently initiates thrombus formation. Blocking the GP IIb/IIIa receptor inhibits platelet aggregation and reduces thrombus formation.
2. **Intravenous glycoprotein IIb/IIIa inhibitors. Abciximab,** the Fab fragment of a murine monoclonal antibody to the human GP IIb/IIIa receptor, binds this receptor tightly and inhibits platelet aggregation for days after the drug infusion is discontinued. In addition to its affinity for the GP IIb/IIIa receptor, abciximab inhibits other receptors, including the vitronectin receptor on endothelial cells and the MAC-1 receptor on leukocytes. **Eptifibatide** is a cyclic peptide inhibitor derived from snake venom with rapid onset and a short half-life. Because of its short half-life, continuous drug infusion is required to sustain maximal inhibition of platelet aggregation. **Tirofiban** and **lamifiban**, nonpeptide antagonists of the GP IIb/IIIa receptor, have half-lives between 4 and 6 hours.

a. **Use in UA during PCI.** Abciximab and eptifibatide have been approved by the FDA for use as adjunctive therapy during PCI. Tirofiban has been approved for the treatment of UA, with continuation of its use into the catheterization laboratory.

(1) **Abciximab** was studied in patients with UA undergoing high-risk percutaneous transluminal coronary angioplasty (PTCA) in the Evaluation of 7E3 for the Prevention of Ischemic Complications **(EPIC)** trial. In 489 patients, abciximab lowered major ischemic event rates (12.8% for placebo vs. 4.8% for abciximab, $p = 0.012$) at 30 days, primarily because of a reduced rate of death or MI (17). This benefit was maintained at long-term follow-up (3 years). In the Evaluation in PTCA to Improve Long-term Outcome with abciximab Glycoprotein IIb/IIIa blockade **(EPILOG)** trial, treatment with abciximab in addition to heparin was associated with a significant reduction in the rate of death, MI, or urgent revascularization at 30 days (11.7% vs. 5.2% in the low-dose heparin group, $p < 0.001$) expanding the benefit to low- and intermediate-risk patients undergoing PCI (18). In the EPILOG trial, a lower, weight-adjusted dosing algorithm of heparin resulted in similar major and minor bleeding rates between abciximab and placebo. In the c7E3 Fab Antiplatelet Therapy for Unstable Refractory Angina **(CAPTURE)** study, abciximab given 18 to 24 hours before PCI reduced the rate of death, MI, and urgent intervention (10.8% vs. 15.4%, $p = 0.017$). Patients treated with abciximab also had a higher rate of thrombus resolution and improved procedural success (19). Results from the Evaluation of Platelet IIb/IIIa Inhibitor for Stenting (**EPISTENT**) trial demonstrated that when **stents and abciximab** are used together, the rate of adverse ischemic events and long-term (1-year) mortality is lower than that with stents alone. Abciximab (bolus of 0.25 mg/kg abciximab is followed by 12-hour infusion at10 μg/min) is commonly used during PCI in patients with ACS.

(2) **Tirofiban.** In the Randomized Efficacy Study of Tirofiban for Outcomes and Restenosis **(RESTORE)** trial, patients presenting with ACS who underwent PCI within 72 hours of presentation were treated with heparin and aspirin with the addition of tirofiban or placebo. Treatment with tirofiban resulted in a reduction in the short-term rate of death, MI, or revascularization for failed PTCA or recurrent ischemia without an increase in major bleeding. In the Platelet Receptor Inhibition for Ischemic

Syndrome Management **(PRISM)** trial, treatment with tirofiban (the dose used was a 0.6 μg/kg/min bolus for 30 minutes, followed by an infusion of 0.15 μg/kg/min) in patients with UA resulted in a 32% decrease in the rate of death, MI, or refractory ischemia at 48 hours (3.8% vs. 5.6%, $p = 0.01$). The composite endpoint, however, was not significantly different at 30 days, although the mortality was reduced (3.6% vs. 2.3%). Notably, very few patients underwent PCI during the treatment period (1.9%). In the Platelet Receptor Inhibition for Ischemic Syndrome Management in Patients Limited to Very Unstable Signs and Symptoms **(PRISM-PLUS)** trial, tirofiban in addition to heparin was associated with a decreased rate of death, MI, or refractory ischemia compared with heparin alone at 7 days (12.9% vs. 17.9%, $p = 0.004$), at 30 days (18.5% vs. 22.3%, $p = 0.03$), and at 6 months (27.7% vs. 32.1%, $p = 0.02$).

(3) Eptifibatide was evaluated in the Platelet Glycoprotein IIb/IIIa in Unstable Angina: Receptor Suppression Using Integrilin Therapy **(PURSUIT)** trial. Eptifibatide treatment (180 μg/kg bolus followed by an infusion of 1.3 or 2.0 μg/kg/min) in patients with UA/NSTEMI was associated with a decreased rate of death or nonfatal MI at 30 days compared with placebo (14.2% vs. 15.7%, $p = 0.04$), although with an increased rate of bleeding.

b. Use independently of PCI. Eptifibatide and tirofiban have been approved for use in the care of patients with UA as a primary medical therapy whether PCI is performed or not. A pooled analysis of the **CAPTURE, PURSUIT,** and **PRISM-PLUS** trials revealed that during the study medication infusion, treatment with a GP IIb/IIIa inhibitor resulted in a reduction of death or nonfatal MI of 34% in patients with UA/NSTEMI, suggesting an early benefit during medical treatment that may be independent of its effect during PCI. However, in the **GUSTO IV–ACS** trial, patients with UA/NSTEMI treated with abciximab bolus and infusion for 24 or 48 hours received no benefit in addition to conventional therapy with aspirin and heparin, with the 30-day incidence of death or MI being similar across groups (8.0% placebo, 8.2% for 24-hour infusion, 9.1% for 48-hour infusion). Medical management was encouraged during the first 48 hours, and only 1.6% of patients underwent PCI while on the study drug. In patients not likely to be treated with an early invasive strategy, abciximab has shown no benefit using the dosing protocol described in that trial.

c. Recommendations. The benefit of GP IIb/IIIa inhibitors is predominantly in patients who subsequently undergo PCI. However, in the contempory era with newer anticoagulant therapies and use of higher loading doses of clopidogrel (600 mg) there is less clarity regarding the utility of adjuvant GP IIb/IIIa inhibition with PCI. The **ISAR-REACT 2** trial randomized 2022 patients with NSTE-ACS undergoing PCI to abciximab or placebo in addition to pretreatment with a 600-mg loading dose of clopidogrel. Overall, there was a 25% reduction in death, MI, or urgent target-vessel revascularization noted in those patients who received abciximab. However, this benefit was observed solely in those patients with elevated troponin levels (20). Also, the **ACUITY** trial suggests that GP IIb/IIIa inhibition is unnecessary in those patients who have received bivalirudin plus clopidogrel pretreatment with a loading dose of at least 300 mg at least 6 hours prior to angiography.

For patients with UA/NSTEMI undergoing an **early invasive strategy**, the American College of Cardiology/American Heart Association (ACC/AHA) guidelines state that either a GP IIb/IIIa inhibitor or clopidogrel can be used upstream in lower-risk patients, whereas combination therapy with both is favorable in those patients with high-risk features, early recurrent ischemic discomfort, or those having a delay to angiography. If PCI is likely to be performed and there is no expectable delay to angiography, then abciximab can be used upstream for GP IIb/IIIa inhibition. Otherwise, eptifibatide or tirofiban is the preferred GP IIb/IIIa inhibitor of choice.

3. **Subgroups that benefit from glycoprotein IIb/IIIa inhibitors**
   a. **Troponin-positive status.** Several studies have shown that the benefit of these agents resides primarily with patients presenting with elevated cardiac troponins. In the **CAPTURE** trial, patients with UA with an elevated troponin T level had a greater reduction in the rate of death or nonfatal MI with abciximab therapy than patients with a normal troponin T level. This continues to be true in the contemporary era of dual antiplatlet therapy with aspirin and clopidogrel as discussed earlier with the results of the **ISAR-REACT 2** trial. Therefore, elevated troponin levels continue to identify patients at higher risk for adverse cardiac events who may benefit particularly from therapy with glycoprotein IIb/IIIa inhibitors.
   b. **Diabetics.** In a meta-analysis of diabetic patients with ACS, the use of GP IIb/IIIa inhibitors was associated with decreased mortality at 30 days (6.2% vs. 4.6%, $p = 0.007$). In diabetic patients with ACS undergoing PCI, treatment with GP IIb/IIIa inhibitors was associated with a more marked benefit (mortality rate: 4.0% vs. 1.2%, $p = 0.002$). In this same analysis, GP IIb/IIIa inhibitors did not confer the same improvement in mortality to nondiabetic patients (3.0% vs. 3.0%). These data suggest that diabetic patients, in particular, benefit from the use of these agents, particularly when undergoing PCI during the initial hospitalization (21).
4. **Summary.** In a meta-analysis of six trials totaling 31,402 patients with ACS, treatment with GP IIb/IIIa inhibitors was associated with a 9% reduction in the rate of death and MI at 30 days (10.8% vs. 11.8%, $p = 0.015$). This treatment benefit was primarily in patients who subsequently underwent revascularization with PCI or CABG within 30 days (OR for death or MI = 0.89, 95% CI: 0.80 to 0.98) and in patients with elevated troponin levels (OR = 0.85, 95% CI: 0.71 to 1.03). Treatment with GP IIb/IIIa inhibitors, however, was associated with an elevated risk of major (not intracranial hemorrhage [ICH]) bleeding (2.4% vs. 1.4%, $p < 0.0001$).
5. **Oral glycoprotein IIb/IIIa inhibitors.** Oral GP IIb/IIIa inhibitors have not been shown to be beneficial and may increase mortality. The reason for this dichotomy between the benefit seen with intravenous GP IIb/IIIa inhibitors and the detriment seen with oral inhibitors is not entirely clear. One possible explanation is that the oral agents, in contrast to the intravenous GP IIb/IIIa inhibitors, have partial agonist activity, which actually leads to an increase in fibrinogen binding and platelet aggregation on administration.

E. **Nitrates.** Despite a lack of randomized clinical trial data, nitrates remain a mainstay of treatment for patients with UA with chest pain.
1. **Dosing.** Sublingual nitroglycerin or nitroglycerin spray (0.4 mg) should be administered immediately and repeated every 5 minutes (three times) to relieve anginal discomfort. If angina persists, intravenous nitroglycerin may be started (at 10 to 20 μg/min). Intravenous nitroglycerin can be quickly titrated (5 to 10 μg/min increases every 5 to 10 minutes) to relieve angina. Caution must be exercised as it may cause profound hypotension. Topical (nitroglycerin transdermal patch, 0.2 to 0.6 mg/hour, or nitro-paste, 1 to 2 inches, replaced every 6 hours), or oral nitrates (isosorbide dinitrate, 10 to 40 mg orally three times daily, or isosorbide mononitrate, 30 to 120 mg orally each day) can also be used in patients to prevent recurrent anginal symptoms. Tolerance to nitrates is dose- and interval-dependent and can occur within 24 hours of initiation, requiring higher doses of nitrates. After symptoms are controlled, changing from intravenous to topical or oral formulations with nitrate-free intervals can limit this phenomenon.
2. **Contraindications.** Known **hypersensitivity to nitrates, hypotension. Sildenafil (Viagra) use** within the prior 24 hours has been associated with hypotension, MI, and death.

F. **β-Blockers.** β-Blockers may relieve myocardial ischemia by lowering myocardial oxygen demand through its effects on blood pressure, heart rate, and contractility. A meta-analysis of 4700 patients with UA and impending MI showed that β-blockers reduced the risk for MI, but no clear effect on mortality was seen.

1. **Indications.** Patients with UA with angina should be started on β-blocker therapy to relieve ischemia. The goals of therapy are a resting heart rate of usually 50 to 60 beats/min and relief of angina. Cardioselective β-blockers (e.g., metoprolol, atenolol) are typically used to minimize side effects.
2. **Contraindications.** Contraindications to β-blocker therapy include **advanced atrioventricular block, active bronchospasm, cardiogenic shock, hypotension, baseline bradycardia,** and **congestive heart failure.**
3. **Dosing.** Patients with ongoing anginal pain or persistent hypertension can initially be treated with intravenous β-blockers. Intravenous metoprolol can be given in 5-mg increments every 5 to10 minutes until the desired heart rate and blood pressure response is achieved. Oral metoprolol therapy can then be started at a dose of 25 to 50 mg every 6 to 12 hours, and can be subsequently titrated as necessary.

G. Calcium channel blockers. Calcium channel blockers have diverse physiologic effects, including vasodilation, decreased or slowed atrioventricular conduction, and negative inotropy and chronotropy. A meta-analysis of calcium channel blocker trials in the management of UA showed no effect on death or nonfatal MI. However, short-acting nifedipine increased the risk for MI or recurrent angina compared with metoprolol. Diltiazem may reduce adverse events among patients with UA, except in patients with LV dysfunction or pulmonary congestion on physical examination, who experienced worse outcomes with diltiazem.

1. **Indications.** Calcium channel blockers are recommended for patients with UA, **only in patients with contraindications to** β-blockers or when **β-blockers and nitrates fail** to fully relieve symptoms of ischemia. Calcium channel blockers are preferred in patients with variant angina or cocaine-induced vasospasm.
2. **Contraindications.** Contraindications to calcium channel blockers include LV dysfunction or signs and symptoms of congestive heart failure, hypotension, or atrioventricular conduction abnormalities.

H. Angiotensin-converting enzyme (ACE) inhibitors. In patients with STEMI or in patients with LV dysfunction, ACE inhibitors improve survival and ventricular remodeling. The effects of ACE inhibitors in the care of patients with UA or NSTEMI are less well defined. However, **if patients have LV dysfunction, ACE inhibitors should be added to existing medical therapy.** Moreover, in the long term, ACE inhibitors should be considered in every patient with UA/NSTEMI, especially given the overall favorable data for their use in patients with CAD.

I. Lipid-lowering therapy. 3-Hydroxy-3-methylglutaryl coenzyme A **(HMG-CoA)** reductase inhibitors **(i.e., statins)** have been shown to be integral in primary and secondary prevention of CAD. Early initiation of statin therapy has beneficial effects in patients with NSTE-ACS as well. In the **MIRACL** study involving 3086 patients with UA/NSTEMI, treatment with atorvastatin 24 to 96 hours after presentation was associated with a decreased rate of death, nonfatal MI, cardiac arrest, or recurrent ischemia at 16 weeks [14.8% vs. 17.4%, relative risk (RR) = 0.84, 95% CI: 0.70 to 1.00, $p = 0.048$], primarily because of reduced recurrent symptomatic ischemia requiring hospitalization. The **PROVE IT-TIMI 22** trial demonstrated the salutory effects of aggressive lipid-lowering therapy in patients with ACS. In this study, 4162 patients with ACS were randomized to pravastatin 40 mg daily (standard therapy) or atorvastatin 80 mg daily (intensive therapy) and followed for a mean of 24 months. There was a significant 16% reduction in the rate of death, MI, unstable angina requiring rehospitalization, revascularization, and stroke at 2 years in those randomized to more intensive lipid-lowering therapy compared to standard lipid therapy (22.4% vs. 26.3%, $p = 0.005$) (22). Further analysis from this trial demonstrated an early clinical benefit, which correlated with concomitant reductions in CRP levels, at 30 days with use of intensive lipid-lowering therapy. These early benefits from statin therapy are likely caused by the "pleiotropic" or nonlipid-lowering effects of statins such as their anti-inflammatory, antioxidant, and antithrombotic properties. Statin's anti-inflammatory effects are likely responsible for beneficial effects in the periprocedural MI reduction seen in patients with NSTE-ACS treated with PCI. In the **ARMYDA-ACS** study, patients with NSTE-ACS undergoing PCI, pretreatment (12 hours prior to PCI) with atorvastatin 80 mg as compared to placebo resulted in a significant reduction in death, MI, or unplanned revascularization at 30 days (5% vs. 17%, $p = 0.01$) that was driven entirely by the reduction in periprocedural MI rates (5% vs. 15%, $p = 0.04$) (23).

J. Aldosterone receptor antagonists. The use of the aldosterone receptor antagonist, eplerenone, has been shown to have salutory effects on morbidity and mortality in the early management of patients with post acute myocardial infarction complicated by decreased LV function with symptomatic heart failure. In the **EPHESUS** trial, 6642 patients post-MI (3 to 14 days) with LV ejection fraction $\leq$40% along with either symptomatic heart failure or diabetes mellitus were randomized to oral eplerenone (starting dose of 25 mg, titrated to maximum of 50 mg/day) versus placebo in addition to optimal medical therapy. In those individuals randomized to eplerenone as compared to placebo there was a significant reduction in overall mortality (14.4% vs. 16.7%, $p = 0.008$), cardiovascular mortality (12.3% vs. 14.6%, $p = 0.005$), and cardiovascular mortality or hospitalization for cardiovascular events (26.7% vs. 30%, $p = 0.002$) at mean follow-up of 16 months (24). There is an increased risk for hyperkalemia with use of this agent, particularly in those patients with abnormal renal function. In the **EPHESUS** study, there was a significant increase in the risk of serious hyperkalemia (serum potassium $\geq$6.0 mmol/L) associated with the use of eplerenone as compared to those in the placebo group (5.5% vs. 3.9%, $p = 0.002$). Eplerenone should not be used in those patients with severe renal insufficiency.

K. Antiarrhythmic agents. The presence of hemodynamically significant ventricular arrhythmias should be treated with appropriate medications such as amiodarone or lidocaine. In a pooled analysis of 26,416 patients with UA/NSTEMI, the incidence of ventricular fibrillation or tachycardia was 2.1%. Patients with ventricular arrhythmias had an increased mortality rate at 30 days and 6 months (25). However, prophylactic use of antiarrhythmic agents (i.e., flecainide and encainide) for increased ventricular ectopy has been associated with increased mortality.

L. Fibrinolytic agents. Although fibrinolytic therapy has decreased mortality and improved LV function among patients with STEMI, use of these agents is associated with worse outcomes in patients with UA and NSTEMI. A meta-analysis of fibrinolytic therapy in the management of UA demonstrated an increase in death or nonfatal MI in patients receiving fibrinolytics (9.8% for fibrinolytics vs. 6.9% for placebo). The lack of efficacy of fibrinolytic agents in these patients may result from the prothrombotic milieu induced by exposure of clot-bound thrombin after fibrin cleavage. Plasmin generation increases, and platelets are activated, perpetuating this prothrombotic state. Fibrinolytic agents would not be expected to dramatically improve coronary blood flow in UA because of the nonocclusive nature of thrombi in these patients.

M. PCI. The goals of PCI in patients with UA/NSTEMI are to relieve symptoms (e.g., angina) and to improve prognosis (e.g., prevent death, MI, and recurrent ischemia).

Studies done in the 1980s suggest that patients with UA had worse outcomes with PTCA than patients with stable angina. In the **TIMI IIIb** trial of UA patients treated with PTCA, the incidence of periprocedural MI was 2.7%, emergency CABG was 1.4%, and death was 0.5%. Although the initial technical success rate of PTCA was very high at 96%, 28% of these patients needed repeat revascularization within 1 year after the intervention.

Coronary stents **reduce the rate of abrupt vessel closure and restenosis** after PCI and are considered standard therapy during contemporary percutaneous revascularization procedures. Drug-eluting stents (DESs) have reduced rates of restenosis beyond that achieved with bare metal stents at the expense of a moderate increase in risk of late coronary thrombosis. In several retrospective analyses of patients with stable and UA treated with intracoronary stenting, no significant differences in complication rates or restenosis were seen in patients with stable compared with those with unstable symptoms. Adjunctive pharmacologic agents (e.g., GP IIb/IIIa receptor inhibitors) reduce periprocedural ischemic complications and improve long-term outcomes after percutaneous revascularization (discussed earlier).

N. Surgical revascularization. The decision to refer a patient for CABG involves multiple factors including age, comorbidities, severity of coronary atherosclerotic disease, prior revascularization procedures (i.e., CABG or PCI), and the technical feasibility and durability of percutaneous revascularization. Recent studies comparing CABG to PCI, some of which included patients with unstable angina, have found no significant difference in hard outcomes including death, MI, or stroke. However, none of these studies utilized contemporary practices in interventional cardiology (dual- and triple-antiplatelet therapy and DES).

Decisions about percutaneous versus surgical revascularization should not be significantly influenced because patients present with UA/NSTEMI. In patients with diabetes mellitus, LV dysfunction, or significant burden of disease (i.e., left main disease, three-vessel disease, or two-vessel disease with proximal LAD involvement, LV dysfunction), CABG still may be the preferred revascularization strategy, although PCI is increasingly evolving into a legitimate alternative in this setting as well.

O. Intraaortic balloon counterpulsation. In patients presenting with UA who have medically refractory angina, placement of an intraaortic balloon pump (IABP) should be considered. By reducing myocardial oxygen demand and increasing coronary perfusion pressure, the IABP may produce almost immediate relief of angina and ischemic ECG changes. In a consecutive series of patients with UA, 1% of patients required an IABP to relieve ischemia. Placement of an IABP is a short-term strategy, serving only as a bridge to revascularization in patients with medically refractory UA.

P. Early invasive versus conservative strategies. Two approaches to managing patients with NSTE-ACS have evolved. Based on a host of factors, including an overall assessment of patient risk, a decision to pursue either an early invasive or an initial conservative strategy needs to be decided early in the management of NSTE-ACS (Table 2.5). Overall, patients selected to have early invasive therapy will have coronary angiography performed within 24 hours of admission, or sooner, depending on the clinical situation. Those patients elected to a conservative strategy are managed with optimal medical therapy and undergo angiography only in select circumstances such as development of recurrent symptoms or objective evidence of ischemia while on appropriate medical therapy. There have been several studies comparing these two strategies. Bavry et al. (26) performed a contemporary meta-analysis on seven randomized trials evaluating an early invasive versus a conservative approach in the management of patients with NSTE-ACS. In this pooled analysis of 8375 patients, there was a 25% reduction in all cause mortality at 2 years

TABLE 2.5 Initial Management Strategy in NSTE-ACS: Early Invasive Versus Conservative (Selective Invasive) Approach

Early invasive	Conservative
Hemodynamic instability Arrhythmia instability High risk score (e.g., TIMI, GRACE, PURSUIT) Elevated troponin T or I Refractory angina despite aggressive medical therapy Prior PCI within 6 months or prior CABG Signs or symptoms of congestive heart failure New or worsening mitral regurgitation Left ventricular function <40%	Low risk score (e.g., TIMI, GRACE, PURSUIT) Physician or patient preference in low- to intermediate-risk patient

with use of early invasive as compared to conservative therapy (4.9% vs. 6.5%, $p = 0.001$) (26). Early invasive therapy also reduced the incidence of nonfatal MI and rehospitalization for unstable angina by 17% and 31%, respectively.

1. **Randomized trials**
   a. Two earlier trials performed prior to the current era of antiplatelet therapy and coronary stenting were the **TIMI IIIb** and **VANQWISH** trials. Both of theses trials showed similar long-term outcomes (death or MI) between early invasive and conservative treatment strategies; however, there was an increase in early mortality associated with invasive therapy in the VANQWISH study (27), and these two trials were excluded from the recent meta-analysis, since both are noncontemporary.
   b. In the **FRISC II** trial, patients with UA/NSTEMI were randomized in a factorial design to an early invasive or conservative strategy and to dalteparin or placebo. An early invasive strategy was associated with a reduction in the rate of death or MI at 6 months (9.4% vs. 12.1%, $p = 0.031$) and reduced symptoms of angina and rehospitalization, regardless of treatment with dalteparin.
   c. In the **TACTICS-TIMI 18** trial, patients with UA/NSTEMI treated with aspirin, heparin, and tirofiban were randomized to an early invasive or a conservative strategy. Patients assigned to an **early invasive approach underwent catheterization within 4 to 48 hours** with revascularization as appropriate. Patients assigned to the conservative arm underwent cardiac catheterization only if there was objective evidence of recurrent ischemia or abnormal stress test. An early invasive strategy was associated with a reduction in the composite of death, nonfatal MI, or rehospitalization for ACS at 6 months (15.9% vs. 19.4%, $p = 0.025$), as well as a reduction in the incidence of death or nonfatal MI at 6 months (7.3% vs. 9.5%, $p < 0.05$).
   d. In the **RITA 3** trial, an early invasive strategy for moderate-risk patients with UA/NSTEMI was associated with a decreased rate of death, MI, or refractory angina compared with conservative therapy at 4 months (9.6% vs. 14.5%, $p = 0.001$). This was caused primarily by a reduction in refractory angina (28). These results suggest that even in moderate-risk patients, an early invasive strategy may be preferred. The RITA 3 investigators also reported a meta-analysis of trials comparing an early invasive versus a conservative approach, with an association between the early invasive approach and a decreased incidence of death or nonfatal MI at 1 year (RR = 0.88, 95% CI: 0.78 to 0.99).
   e. In the **ISAR-COOL** trial, patients with UA/NSTEMI treated with intensive medical therapy (aspirin, heparin, clopidogrel [600-mg loading dose], and tirofiban) were randomized to immediate invasive therapy (median time of 2.4 hours) versus delayed invasive therapy after a "cooling off" period (median time of 86 hours). Those who had early intervention had a significant reduction in death or MI at 30 days compared to those who had a "cooling off" period (5.9% vs. 11.6%, $p = 0.04$) (29).
   f. In the **ICTUS** trial, 1200 patients with NSTE-ACS with elevated troponins were randomized to either early invasive therapy (angiography within 24 to 48 hours) or initial conservative strategy with selective invasive therapy. There was no difference in the primary composite endpoint of death, MI, or rehospitalization for ACS at 1 year between the two groups (22.7% vs. 21.2%, $p = 0.33$). The aggressive medical therapies and high rates of revascularization (47%) in the initial conservative strategy group are two among many potential explanations for the findings in this trial (30).
2. **Recommendations.** Overall, recent ACC/AHA guidelines **recommend management with an early invasive strategy in patients with refractory angina despite medical therapy, hemodynamic or electrical instability, or patients at high risk for adverse events. However, an initial conservative strategy with selective invasive therapy can also be considered in stabilized patients with an elevated risk for clinical events, including those with positive troponins.** Notably, the

preferred approach in women with low-risk features is a conservative strategy, however, those at high-risk have recommendations similar to those for men.

VII. FOLLOW-UP. Patients with UA usually receive definitive therapy during hospitalization, but close follow-up care after hospital discharge is imperative. There are no guidelines regarding noninvasive stress testing of patients without symptoms who have undergone percutaneous or surgical revascularization for UA. If anginal symptoms recur after hospital discharge, stress testing or cardiac catheterization can be performed, depending on the clinical presentation.

Follow-up must also include lifestyle alteration, risk-factor modification, and secondary prevention. An exercise regimen in stable patients, smoking cessation efforts, and dietary changes are helpful. **The long-term use of aspirin, clopidogrel, β-blockers, statins/cholesterol-lowering regimens, and/or ACE inhibitors should not be neglected.** Statin therapy should be given to all patients status post NSTE-ACS, regardless of baseline low-density lipoprotein cholesterol (LDL-C) levels. LDL-C levels should be lowered to $\leq$100 mg/dL with strong consideration for levels $\leq$70 mg/dL. Hypertension, dyslipidemia, and diabetes mellitus must be diagnosed and aggressively treated. Antianginals (i.e., nitrates, β-blockers, and possibly calcium antagonists) should be used for symptom relief. Patients must be reassured and educated about their acceptable level of activity.

ACKNOWLEDGMENTS

The authors thank Drs. David S. Lee and Matthew T. Roe for their contributions to this chapter.

References

1. Antman EM, Tanasijevic MJ, Thompson B, et al. Cardiac-specific troponin I levels to predict the risk of mortality in patients with acute coronary syndromes. *N Engl J Med* 1996;335:1342–1349.
2. Hamm CW, Goldmann BU, Heeschen C, et al. Emergency room triage of patients with acute chest pain by means of rapid testing for cardiac troponin T or troponin I. *N Engl J Med* 1997;337:1648–1653.
3. Antman EM, Cohen M, Bernink PJ, et al. The TIMI risk score for unstable angina/non-ST elevation MI: a method for prognostication and therapeutic decision making. *JAMA* 2000;284:835–842.
4. Granger CB, Goldberg RJ, Dabbous O, et al. Predictors of hospital mortality in the global registry of acute coronary events. *Arch Intern Med* 2003;163:2345–2353.
5. Eagle KA, Lim MJ, Dabbous OH, et al. A validated prediction model for all forms of acute coronary syndrome: estimating the risk of 6-month postdischarge death in an international registry. *JAMA* 2004;291:2727–2733.
6. Slater DK, Hlatky MA, Mark DB, et al. Outcome in suspected acute myocardial infarction with normal or minimally abnormal admission electrocardiographic findings. *Am J Cardiol* 1987;60:766–770.
7. Effects of tissue plasminogen activator and a comparison of early invasive and conservative strategies in unstable angina and non-Q-wave myocardial infarction. Results of the TIMI IIIB Trial. Thrombolysis in Myocardial Ischemia. *Circulation* 1994;89:1545–1556.
8. Morrow DA, Rifai N, Antman EM, et al. C-Reactive protein is a potent predictor of mortality independently of and in combination with troponin T in acute coronary syndromes: a TIMI 11A substudy. Thrombolysis in Myocardial Infarction. *J Am Coll Cardiol* 1998;31:1460–1465.
9. Chen L, Chester MR, Redwood S, et al. Angiographic stenosis progression and coronary events in patients with "stabilized" unstable angina. *Circulation* 1995;91:2319–2324.
10. Mehta SR, Yusuf S, Peters RJ, et al. Effects of pretreatment with clopidogrel and aspirin followed by long-term therapy in patients undergoing percutaneous coronary intervention: the PCI-CURE study. *Lancet* 2001;358:527–533.
11. Steinhubl SR, Berger PB, Mann JT 3rd, et al. Early and sustained dual oral antiplatelet therapy following percutaneous coronary intervention: a randomized controlled trial. *JAMA* 2002;288:2411–2420.
12. Wiviott SD, Braunwald E, McCabe CH, et al. Prasugrel versus clopidogrel in patients with acute coronary syndromes. *N Engl J Med* 2007;357:2001–2015.
13. Oler A, Whooley MA, Oler J, Grady D. Adding heparin to aspirin reduces the incidence of myocardial infarction and death in patients with unstable angina. A meta-analysis. *JAMA* 1996;276:811–815.
14. Ferguson JJ, Califf RM, Antman EM, et al. Enoxaparin vs unfractionated heparin in high-risk patients with non-ST-segment elevation acute coronary syndromes managed with an intended early invasive strategy: primary results of the SYNERGY randomized trial. *JAMA* 2004;292:45–54.
15. Stone GW, McLaurin BT, Cox DA, et al. Bivalirudin for patients with acute coronary syndromes. *N Engl J Med* 2006;355:2203–2216.
16. Yusuf S, Mehta SR, Chrolavicius S, et al. Comparison of fondaparinux and enoxaparin in acute coronary syndromes. *N Engl J Med* 2006;354:1464–1476.
17. Lincoff AM, Califf RM, Anderson KM, et al. Evidence for prevention of death and myocardial infarction with platelet membrane glycoprotein IIb/IIIa receptor blockade by abciximab (c7E3 Fab) among patients with unstable angina undergoing percutaneous coronary revascularization. EPIC Investigators. Evaluation of 7E3 in Preventing Ischemic Complications. *J Am Coll Cardiol* 1997;30:149–156.
18. Platelet glycoprotein IIb/IIIa receptor blockade and low-dose heparin during percutaneous coronary revascularization. The EPILOG Investigators. *N Engl J Med* 1997;336:1689–1696.

19. Randomised placebo-controlled trial of abciximab before and during coronary intervention in refractory unstable angina: the CAPTURE Study. *Lancet* 1997;349:1429–1435.
20. Kastrati A, Mehilli J, Neumann FJ, et al. Abciximab in patients with acute coronary syndromes undergoing percutaneous coronary intervention after clopidogrel pretreatment: the ISAR-REACT 2 randomized trial. *JAMA* 2006;295:1531–1538.
21. Roffi M, Chew DP, Mukherjee D, et al. Platelet glycoprotein IIb/IIIa inhibitors reduce mortality in diabetic patients with non-ST-segment-elevation acute coronary syndromes. *Circulation* 2001;104:2767–2771.
22. Cannon CP, Braunwald E, McCabe CH, et al. Intensive versus moderate lipid lowering with statins after acute coronary syndromes. *N Engl J Med* 2004;350:1495–1504.
23. Patti G, Pasceri V, Colonna G, et al. Atorvastatin pretreatment improves outcomes in patients with acute coronary syndromes undergoing early percutaneous coronary intervention: results of the ARMYDA-ACS randomized trial. *J Am Coll Cardiol* 2007;49:1272–1278.
24. Pitt B, Remme W, Zannad F, et al. Eplerenone, a selective aldosterone blocker, in patients with left ventricular dysfunction after myocardial infarction. *N Engl J Med* 2003;348:1309–1321.
25. Al-Khatib SM, Granger CB, Huang Y, et al. Sustained ventricular arrhythmias among patients with acute coronary syndromes with no ST-segment elevation: incidence, predictors, and outcomes. *Circulation* 2002;106:309–312.
26. Bavry AA, Kumbhani DJ, Rassi AN, et al. Benefit of early invasive therapy in acute coronary syndromes: a meta-analysis of contemporary randomized clinical trials. *J Am Coll Cardiol* 2006;48:1319–1325.
27. Boden WE, O'Rourke RA, Crawford MH, et al. Outcomes in patients with acute non-Q-wave myocardial infarction randomly assigned to an invasive as compared with a conservative management strategy. Veterans Affairs Non-Q-Wave Infarction Strategies in Hospital (VANQWISH) Trial Investigators. *N Engl J Med* 1998;338:1785–1792.
28. Fox KA, Poole-Wilson PA, Henderson RA, et al. Interventional versus conservative treatment for patients with unstable angina or non-ST-elevation myocardial infarction: the British Heart Foundation RITA 3 randomised trial. Randomized Intervention Trial of unstable Angina. *Lancet* 2002;360:743–751.
29. Neuman FJ, Kastrati A, Pogatsa-Murray G, et al. Evaluation of prolonged antithrombotic pretreatment ("cooling-off" strategy) before intervention in patients with unstable coronary syndromes: a randomized controlled trial. *JAMA* 2003;290:1593–1599.
30. de Winter RJ, Windhausen F, Cornel JH, et al. Early invasive versus selectively invasive management for acute coronary syndromes. *N Engl J Med* 2005;353:1095–1104.

Landmark Articles

ACC/AHA 2007 Guidelines for the Management of Patients With Unstable Angina/Non ST-Elevation Myocardial Infarction: A Report of the American College of Cardiology/American Heart Association Task Force on Practice Guidelines (Writing Committee to Revise the 2002 Guidelines for the Management of Patients With Unstable Angina/Non ST-Elevation Myocardial Infarction): Developed in Collaboration with the American College of Emergency Physicians, the Society for Cardiovascular Angiography and Interventions, and the Society of Thoracic Surgeons: Endorsed by the American Association of Cardiovascular and Pulmonary Rehabilitation and the Society for Academic Emergency Medicine. *Circulation* 2007;116:e148–304.

A comparison of aspirin plus tirofiban with aspirin plus heparin for unstable angina. Platelet Receptor Inhibition in Ischemic Syndrome Management (PRISM) Study Investigators. *N Engl J Med* 1998;338:1498–1505.

Antman EM, Cohen M, Bernink PJ, et al. The TIMI risk score for unstable angina/non-ST elevation MI: A method for prognostication and therapeutic decision making. *JAMA* 2000;284:835–842.

Cannon CP, Braunwald E, McCabe CH, et al. Intensive versus moderate lipid lowering with statins after acute coronary syndromes. *N Engl J Med* 2004;350:1495–1504.

Cohen M, Demers C, Gurfinkel EP, et al. A comparison of low-molecular-weight heparin with unfractionated heparin for unstable coronary artery disease. Efficacy and Safety of Subcutaneous Enoxaparin in Non-Q-Wave Coronary Events Study Group. *N Engl J Med* 1997;337:447–452.

Fuster V, Badimon L, Badimon JJ, et. al. The pathogenesis of coronary artery disease and the acute coronary syndromes. *N Engl J Med* 1992;326:242–250.

Hamm CW, Heeschen C, Goldmann B, et al. Benefit of abciximab in patients with refractory unstable angina in relation to serum troponin T levels. c7E3 Fab Antiplatelet Therapy in Unstable Refractory Angina (CAPTURE) Study Investigators. *N Engl J Med* 1999;340:1623–1629.

Inhibition of the platelet glycoprotein IIb/IIIa receptor with tirofiban in unstable angina and non-Q-wave myocardial infarction. Platelet Receptor Inhibition in Ischemic Syndrome Management in Patients Limited by Unstable Signs and Symptoms (PRISM-PLUS) Study Investigators. *N Engl J Med* 1998;338:1488–1497.

Invasive compared with non-invasive treatment in unstable coronary-artery disease: FRISC II prospective randomised multicentre study. FRagmin and Fast Revascularisation during Instability in Coronary artery disease Investigators. *Lancet* 1999;354:708–715.

Schwartz GG, Olsson AG, Ezekowitz MD, et al. Effects of atorvastatin on early recurrent ischemic events in acute coronary syndromes: the MIRACL study: a randomized controlled trial. *JAMA* 2001;285:1711–1718.

Stone GW, McLaurin BT, Cox DA, et al. Bivalirudin for patients with acute coronary syndromes. *N Engl J Med* 2006;355:2203–2216.

Theroux P, Ouimet H, McCans J, et. al. Aspirin, heparin, or both to treat acute UA. *N Engl J Med* 1988;319:1105–1111.

Yusuf S, Zhao F, Mehta SR, et al. Effects of clopidogrel in addition to aspirin in patients with acute coronary syndromes without ST-segment elevation. *N Engl J Med* 2001;345:494–502.

Key Meta-analyses

Bavry AA, Kumbhani DJ, Rassi AN, et al. Benefit of early invasive therapy in acute coronary syndromes: a meta-analysis of contemporary randomized clinical trials. *J Am Coll Cardiol* 2006;48:1319–1325.

Boersma E, Harrington RA, Moliterno DJ, et al. Platelet glycoprotein IIb/IIIa inhibitors in acute coronary syndromes: a meta-analysis of all major randomized clinical trials. *Lancet* 2002;359:189–198.

Direct thrombin inhibitors in acute coronary syndromes: principal results of a meta-analysis based on individual patients data. *Lancet* 2002;359:294–302.

Eikelboom JW, Anand SS, Malmberg K, et al. Unfractionated heparin and low-molecular-weight heparin in acute coronary syndrome without ST elevation: a meta-analysis. *Lancet* 2000;355:1936–1942.

Relevant Book Chapters

Gersh BJ, Braunwald EG, Rutherford JD. Chronic coronary artery disease: unstable angina. In: Braunwald EG, ed. *Heart disease: a textbook of cardiovascular medicine,* 5th ed. Philadelphia: WB Saunders, 1997:1331–1339.

Granger CB, Califf RM. Stabilizing the unstable artery. In: Califf RM, Mark DB, Wagner GS, eds. *Acute coronary care,* 2nd ed. St. Louis: Mosby, 1995:525–541.

Moliterno DJ, Granger CB. Differences between unstable angina and acute myocardial infarction: the pathophysiological and clinical spectrum. In: Topol EJ, ed. *Acute coronary syndromes.* New York: Marcel Dekker, 1998:67–104.

White HD. Unstable angina: ischemic syndromes. In: Topol EJ, ed. *Textbook of cardiovascular medicine.* Philadelphia: Lippincott-Raven, 1998:365–393.

3 COMPLICATIONS OF MYOCARDIAL INFARCTION

John M. Galla and Debabrata Mukherjee

I. INTRODUCTION. In-hospital mortality among patients with acute myocardial infarction (MI) is primarily caused by circulatory failure from severe left ventricular (LV) dysfunction or from one of the complications of MI. These complications may be broadly classified as mechanical, electrical or arrhythmic, ischemic, embolic, or inflammatory **(e.g., pericarditis).**

II. MECHANICAL COMPLICATIONS. Serious and life-threatening mechanical complications of acute MI include ventricular septal defect (VSD), papillary muscle rupture, cardiac free-wall rupture, large ventricular aneurysms, LV pump failure, cardiogenic shock, dynamic LV outflow tract (LVOT) obstruction, and right ventricular (RV) failure.

A. Ventricular septal rupture (VSR)

1. Clinical presentation. VSR occurred in 1% to 2% of patients after acute MI in the prethrombolytic era (1) and accounted for 5% of the periinfarction mortality. The incidence has dramatically decreased in the post thrombolytic era. In the Global Utilization of Streptokinase and Tissue Plasminogen Activator for Occluded Coronary Arteries (GUSTO I) trial, the incidence of VSR was approximately 0.2% (2), occurring with equal frequency in anterior and nonanterior sites. VSR is more likely to occur in patients who are **older, female, and hypertensive; have no history of smoking; and have anterior infarction, an increased heart rate, and a worse Killip class designation on admission.** VSR may develop as early as 24 hours after MI but is usually seen 2 to 5 days after MI (2). Fibrinolytic therapy is not associated with increased risk of VSR (3).

a. Signs and symptoms. Patients with post-MI VSR may appear relatively comfortable early in the disease course and have no clinically significant orthopnea or pulmonary edema. Recurrence of angina, pulmonary edema, hypotension, and shock may develop abruptly later in the course. Alternatively, precipitous onset of hemodynamic compromise characterized by hypotension, biventricular failure, and a new murmur may be the initial manifestation.

b. Physical findings. The diagnosis should be suspected when a new **pansystolic murmur** develops, especially in the setting of worsening hemodynamic profile and biventricular failure. For this reason, it is important that **all patients with**

MI have a well-documented cardiac examination at presentation and frequent evaluations thereafter.

(1) The murmur is usually best heard in the **lower left sternal border**; it is accompanied by a **thrill in 50% of cases.** In patients with a large VSR and severe heart failure or shock, the murmur may be of low intensity or inaudible, but **the absence of a murmur does not rule out VSD.**

(2) Several features differentiate the murmur of VSR from that of mitral regurgitation (MR) caused by rupture of the papillary muscle (Table 3.1). The murmur may radiate to the base and the apex of the heart. A third heart sound (S_3), loud P_2, and signs of tricuspid regurgitation may be present.

2. Histopathology. The defect usually occurs at the myocardial infarct border zone, located in the **apical septum with anterior MI** and in the **basal posterior septum with inferior MI.** A VSR almost always occurs in the setting of a transmural MI. The defect may not always be a single large defect; a meshwork of serpiginous channels can be identified in 30% to 40% of patients. Multiple fenestrations are especially common with inferior MIs.

3. Laboratory examination and diagnostic testing

a. An electrocardiogram (ECG) may show atrioventricular (AV) node or infranodal conduction abnormalities in approximately 40% of patients.

b. Echocardiography

(1) Echocardiography with color flow imaging is **the test of choice** for diagnosis of VSR.

(a) Basal VSR is best visualized in the parasternal long axis with medial angulation, the apical long axis, and the subcostal long axis.

(b) Apical VSR is best visualized in the apical four-chamber view.

(2) In some cases, transesophageal echocardiography may help in determining the extent of the defect and assessing suitability for potential off-label percutaneous closure.

(3) Echocardiography may help determine the size of the defect and the magnitude of the left-to-right shunt by comparing flow across the pulmonary valve with flow across the aortic valve.

(4) Echocardiography also is useful in defining LV and RV function, two important determinants of mortality.

c. Right heart catheterization. Pulmonary artery catheterization with oximetry is helpful in diagnosing a VSR by demonstrating stepped-up oxygen saturation in the right ventricle and pulmonary artery. **Location of the increase is significant** because there have been case reports of enhanced oxygen saturation in the peripheral pulmonary artery due to acute MR. Diagnosis involves fluoroscopically guided measurement of oxygen saturation in the superior and inferior vena cavae; high, mid, and low right atrium; base, mid, and apical levels of the right ventricle; and the pulmonary artery.

TABLE 3.1 Differential Diagnosis of New Systolic Murmur After Acute Myocardial Infarction

Differentiating features	Ventricular septal rupture	Papillary muscle rupture
Location of MI	Anterior > nonanterior	Inferoposterior > anterior
Location of murmur	Lower left sternal area	Cardiac apex
Intensity	Loud	Variable; may be faint
Thrill	50% of patients	Rare
V waves in PCWP	Present or absent	Almost always present
V waves in PA tracing	Absent	Present
O_2 step-up in PA	Almost always present	Present or absent

MI, myocardial infarction; PA, pulmonary artery; PCWP, pulmonary capillary wedge pressure.

(1) Normal saturations for these chambers are 64% to 66% in the superior vena cava (SVC), 69% to 71% in the inferior vena cava (IVC), 64% to 67% in the right atrium, 64% to 67% in the right ventricle, and 64% to 67% in the pulmonary artery.

(2) A left-to-right shunt across the ventricular septum typically results in a **7% or greater** increase in oxygen saturation between the SVC or IVC and the right atrium or a **5% or greater** increase in oxygen saturation between the right atrium and the right ventricle or pulmonary artery.

(3) Shunt fraction is calculated as follows:

$$Q_p/Q_s = Sao_2 - Mvo_2/Pvo_2 - Pao_2$$

In this equation, Q_p is pulmonary flow; Q_s is systemic flow; Sao_2 is arterial oxygen saturation; Mvo_2 is mixed venous oxygen saturation; Pvo_2 is pulmonary venous oxygen saturation; and Pao_2 is pulmonary arterial oxygen saturation. $Q_p/Q_s \geq 2$ suggests a considerable shunt, **and is more likely to necessitate surgical correction. In the acute MI setting, any VSD or shunt should be considered for surgical repair, regardless of the shunt fraction.**

(4) For a patient with an intracardiac shunt, cardiac output measured by means of the thermodilution technique is inaccurate; **the Fick method should be used.** The **key to measurement of accurate systemic flow** in the presence of a shunt is that the mixed venous oxygen content measured in the pulmonary artery will be abnormally elevated and must be measured in the chamber immediately **proximal** to the shunt (i.e., the right atrium or superior and inferior vena cavae in the case of VSD). When using IVC and SVC saturations to estimate cardiac output, the mixed venous oxygen saturation (Svo_2) may be estimated as (3(SVC)+IVC)/4. The Fick equation is calculated as follows:

$$\text{Cardiac output} = O_2\ \text{consumption}/(Sao_2 - Svo_2) \times \text{Hgb} \times 1.34 \times 10$$

4. Therapy

a. Priority of therapy. Early surgical closure is the treatment of choice, even if the patient's condition is stable.

b. Medical therapy

(1) Although initial reports suggested that delaying surgery to allow healing of friable tissue improved surgical mortality, it was likely that lower mortality was as a result of selection bias (4). The mortality rate for patients with VSD treated medically is 24% at 72 hours and 75% at 3 weeks (5). Patients should be considered for urgent surgical repair.

(2) Vasodilators can decrease left-to-right shunt and increase systemic flow by means of reducing systemic vascular resistance (SVR); however, a greater decrease in pulmonary vascular resistance may actually increase shunting. The vasodilator of choice is intravenous nitroprusside, which is started at 5 to 10 μg/kg/min and titrated to a mean arterial pressure (MAP) of 70 to 80 mm Hg.

c. Percutaneous therapy. An intraaortic balloon pump (IABP) should be inserted as early as possible as a bridge to a surgical procedure, unless there is marked aortic regurgitation. IABP counterpulsation decreases SVR, decreases shunt fraction, increases coronary perfusion, and maintains blood pressure. After insertion of an IABP, vasodilators can be tailored with hemodynamic monitoring.

d. Surgical therapy. Surgical closure is **the treatment of choice** even if the patient's condition is stable.

(1) Cardiogenic shock and multisystem failure are associated with high surgical mortality, further supporting earlier operations on these patients before complications develop (6).

(2) Surgical mortality is high among patients with **basal septal rupture associated with inferior MI** (70% compared with 30% in patients with anterior infarcts) because of the greater technical difficulty and the need for concomitant mitral valve repair in these patients, who often have coexisting MR (7).

(3) Early surgical intervention in the care of patients in hemodynamically stable condition **is associated with lower mortality** than watchful waiting and delayed surgical treatment (8).

(4) Although surgical closure remains the treatment of choice for these defects, emerging data suggest that percutaneous closure may be a viable treatment for high-risk surgical patients and patients from whom surgical closure has failed. Use of a pediatric VSD occluder device has been approved on a compassionate basis for patients who are deemed at too high-risk for surgery.

B. Mitral regurgitation. The GUSTO I trial revealed MR to be a **predictor of poor prognosis.** MR of mild to moderate severity is common among patients with acute MI, occurring in 13% to 45% of patients (9,10). Even mild or moderate MR is associated with increased mortality (10). Multiple mechanisms may account for MR. These include dilation of the mitral valve annulus as a result of LV dilation; papillary muscle dysfunction with a concomitant ischemic regional wall-motion abnormality near the insertion of the posterior papillary muscle; and partial or complete rupture of the chordae or papillary muscle (11). Most MR is transient, asymptomatic, and benign. However, severe MR caused by papillary muscle rupture is a life-threatening and manageable complication of acute MI. Historical reports indicate that papillary muscle rupture occurs between days 2 and 7. However, the SHOCK (SHould we emergently revascularize Occluded coronaries for Cardiogenic shocK?) Trial Registry demonstrated a median time to papillary muscle rupture of 13 hours (12). Papillary muscle rupture accounts for 7% of the cases of cardiogenic shock and 5% of mortality after acute MI (13). The overall incidence is 1%.

1. Clinical presentation. Papillary muscle rupture is more likely to occur with inferior MI. Fibrinolytic agents decrease the overall incidence, but rupture may occur earlier in the post-MI period. In some instances, the hemodynamic stress imposed by acute MI causes rupture of a chordae in patients who are predisposed to this problem.

a. Signs and symptoms. Complete transection of the papillary muscles is rare and usually results in immediate shock and death. Patients with rupture of one or more heads of papillary muscle typically have sudden, severe respiratory distress from the development of pulmonary edema and impending cardiogenic shock.

b. Physical findings. A new **pansystolic murmur that is audible at the cardiac apex with radiation to the axilla or the base of the heart suggests acute MR.** In posterior papillary muscle rupture, the murmur radiates to the left sternal border and may be confused with the murmur of VSD or aortic stenosis (intensity of the murmur does not predict the severity of MR). The **murmur may often be quiet, soft, or absent** in patients with poor cardiac output or in persons with elevated left atrial pressures due to the rapid equilibration of pressures.

2. Pathophysiology. Papillary muscle rupture is **more common with an inferior MI.** It involves the posteromedial papillary muscle because of its single blood supply through the posterior descending coronary artery (14). The anterolateral papillary muscle is perfused through the left anterior descending (LAD) and left circumflex coronary arteries. **In 50% of patients, the infarct is relatively small.**

3. Laboratory examination

a. An ECG usually shows evidence of recent inferior or posterior MI.

b. A chest radiograph may demonstrate pulmonary edema. In some patients, focal pulmonary edema may be seen in the right upper lobe because of flow directed at the right pulmonary veins.

4. Diagnostic testing

a. Two-dimensional echocardiography with Doppler and color flow imaging is the diagnostic modality of choice.

(1) The **mitral valve leaflet is usually flail** with severe MR.
(2) Color flow imaging is useful in differentiating papillary muscle rupture with severe MR from VSD after MI.
(3) In some patients with posteriorly directed jets, the amount of MR may not be fully appreciated with transthoracic echocardiography. In these patients, **transesophageal echocardiography** may be particularly helpful in quantifying the severity and elucidating the mechanism of MR.

b. Pulmonary artery catheterization. Hemodynamic monitoring with a pulmonary artery catheter may reveal large V waves in the pulmonary capillary wedge pressure (PCWP) tracing. However, patients with VSD also may have large V waves because of increased pulmonary venous return in a normal-sized and normally compliant left atrium. Among patients with severe MR and reflected V waves in the pulmonary artery tracing, **oxygen saturation in the pulmonary artery may be higher** than that in the right atrial blood, complicating differentiation from VSD (15). There are two means for differentiating MR from VSD:

(1) Prominent V waves in the pulmonary artery tracing before the incisura almost always are associated with acute severe MR (Fig. 3.1).
(2) Blood for oximetry is obtained with fluoroscopy to ensure sampling from the main pulmonary artery rather than distal branches.

5. Therapy

a. Priority of therapy. Papillary muscle rupture should be identified early. Patients should receive **aggressive medical therapy** and be considered for **emergency surgical repair.**

b. Medical therapy

(1) **Vasodilator therapy** is very useful in the treatment of patients with acute MR. Nitroprusside decreases SVR, reduces regurgitant fraction, and increases stroke volume and cardiac output. Nitroprusside is started at 5 to 10 μg/kg/min and is titrated to a MAP of 70 to 80 mm Hg.
(2) **Vasodilators cannot be used** as first-line treatment in patients with **hypotension**, and an IABP should be inserted promptly. An IABP decreases

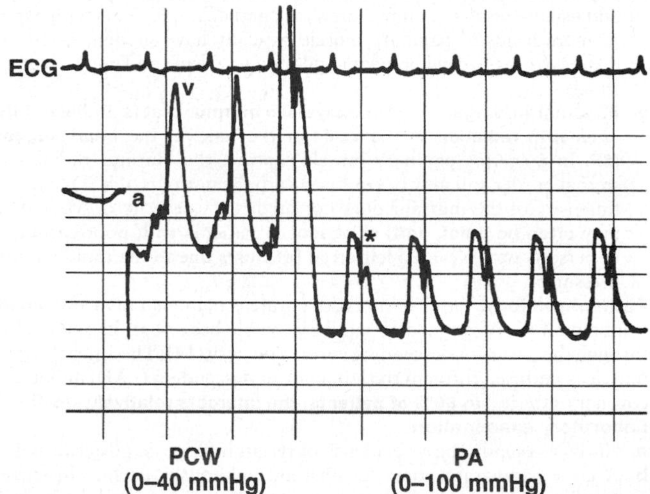

Figure 3.1. Giant V waves on the pulmonary capillary wedge (PCW) tracing can be transmitted to the pulmonary artery (PA) pressure, producing a notch *(asterisk)* on the pulmonary artery downslope. (Adapted from Kern M. *The cardiac catheterization handbook,* 2nd ed. St. Louis: Mosby–Year Book, 1991.)

LV afterload, improves coronary perfusion, and increases forward cardiac output. Patients with hypotension can be given vasodilators after insertion of an IABP to improve hemodynamic values. Patients with moderate MR after MI benefit from vasodilators.

c. **Percutaneous therapy.** Improvement in hemodynamic values and reduction in MR has been reported after percutaneous intervention in the care of patients with severe MR caused by papillary muscle ischemia rather than rupture. **Percutaneous interventions have no role in true papillary muscle rupture.**

d. **Surgical therapy** should be **considered immediately** for patients with papillary muscle rupture.

(1) The prognosis is very poor among patients treated medically. Even though perioperative mortality (20% to 25%) is higher than it is for elective surgical treatment, surgical repair should be considered for every patient.

(2) **Coronary angiography** should be performed before surgical correction, because revascularization during mitral valve replacement (MVR) is associated with improved short- and long-term mortality (16).

(3) Patients with moderate MR who do not improve with afterload reduction may benefit from mitral valve repair. Many of these valves can be repaired and may not require replacement.

C. Cardiac rupture

1. **Clinical presentation.** Cardiac free-wall rupture occurs in 3% of post-MI patients. It accounts for approximately **10% of mortality after MI.** Rupture occurs in the first 5 days in 50% of patients and within 2 weeks in 90% of patients. Free-wall rupture occurs only after transmural MI. Risk factors include advanced age, female sex, hypertension, first MI, and poor coronary collateral vessels.

a. **Signs and symptoms**

(1) **Acute course.** With acute rupture, patients have electromechanical dissociation and sudden death. Sudden onset of chest pain with straining or coughing may suggest the onset of myocardial rupture.

(2) **Subacute course.** Some patients may have a subacute course as a result of contained rupture, with pain suggestive of pericarditis, nausea, and hypotension. In a large retrospective analysis of post-MI patients, 6.2% of patients sustained free-wall rupture. Approximately one-third presented with subacute disease (17). Immediate bedside echocardiography may reveal localized pericardial effusion or pseudoaneurysm.

b. **Physical findings.** Jugular venous distention, pulsus paradoxus, diminished heart sounds, and a pericardial rub suggest subacute rupture. New to-and-fro murmurs may be heard in patients with subacute rupture or pseudoaneurysm.

2. **Pathophysiology.** Free-wall rupture constitutes part of the early hazard function among patients treated with thrombolytic agents. (Mortality among patients who receive thrombolytic agents is higher for the first 24 hours and is partially attributable to cardiac rupture.) Nevertheless, the overall incidence of free-wall rupture is not greater in patients treated with thrombolytics (18). Rupture most commonly occurs at the lateral wall, although any wall may be involved.

There are three distinct types of free-wall rupture. **Type I** occurs within the first 24 hours and is a full-thickness rupture (this rupture type increases with thrombolytics), **type II** ruptures occur as a result of erosion of the myocardium at the site of infarction, and **type III** ruptures occur late and are located at the border zone of the infarction and normal myocardium. **Type III ruptures occur less frequently in patients treated with thrombolytics.** It has been postulated that type III ruptures occur as a result of dynamic LVOT obstruction and resultant increased wall stress (19).

3. **Laboratory examination.** In addition to evidence for new MI, an ECG may show junctional or idioventricular rhythm, low-voltage complexes, and tall precordial T waves. A large proportion of patients have transient bradycardia immediately preceding rupture.

4. **Diagnostic testing.** There may not be time for diagnostic testing in the treatment of patients with acute rupture.

a. **Echocardiography** reveals findings of **cardiac tamponade** in patients with a subacute course: right atrial systolic collapse of more than one third of cardiac systole, RV diastolic collapse, dilated inferior vena cava (i.e., inferior vena cava plethora), and marked respiratory variation in mitral (>25%) and tricuspid (>40%) inflow.

b. **Cardiac catheterization.** Hemodynamic evaluation with a pulmonary artery catheter may reveal equalization of pressures in the right atrium, RV diastolic pressure, and PCWP consistent with pericardial tamponade. During left heart catheterization, there may be significant respiratory variation in the systolic blood pressure (pulsus paradoxus) present on arterial tracings.

5. **Therapy.** Reperfusion therapy has reduced the overall incidence of cardiac rupture and shifted its occurrence to earlier after acute MI.

a. **Priority of therapy.** The goal is to rapidly identify the problem and perform emergency surgical treatment.

b. **Medical therapy** has little role in the treatment of these patients, except for aggressive supportive care in anticipation of surgical correction.

c. **Percutaneous therapy**

(1) **Immediate pericardiocentesis** should be performed on patients with tamponade as soon as the diagnosis is made and while arrangements are being made for transport to the operating room.

(2) If the index of suspicion is high and the patient's condition is unstable, pericardiocentesis should be attempted without waiting for diagnostic test results.

(3) An indwelling catheter should be clamped and left in the pericardial cavity and connected to a drainage bag during transfer to the operating room so that continued decompression of the pericardial cavity with recurrent hemodynamic compromise can be achieved.

d. **Surgical therapy.** Emergency thoracotomy with surgical repair is the definitive therapy and is the **only chance for survival among patients with cardiac rupture.**

D. **Pseudoaneurysm** (i.e., contained rupture)

1. **Clinical presentation**

a. **Signs and symptoms.** Pseudoaneurysms may remain clinically silent and be discovered during routine investigations. However, some patients may have recurrent tachyarrhythmia and heart failure.

b. **Physical findings.** Some patients may have systolic, diastolic, or to-and-fro murmurs related to flow of blood across the narrow neck of the pseudoaneurysm during LV systole and diastole.

2. **Pathophysiology.** Pseudoaneurysm is caused by contained rupture of the LV free wall.

a. The pseudoaneurysm may remain small or undergo progressive enlargement. The outer walls are formed by the pericardium and mural thrombus.

b. Pseudoaneurysms communicate with the body of the left ventricle through a narrow neck, the diameter of which is <**50% of the diameter of the fundus.**

3. **Laboratory examination and diagnostic testing**

a. A **chest radiograph** may show cardiomegaly with an abnormal bulge on the cardiac border.

b. An **ECG** may have a persistent ST elevation, as with true aneurysms.

c. **Echocardiography, magnetic resonance imaging,** or **computed tomography** is used to **confirm the diagnosis.**

4. **Therapy.** Spontaneous rupture may occur without warning in approximately one third of patients with a pseudoaneurysm. **Surgical resection is recommended for patients with or without symptoms, regardless of the size of the pseudoaneurysm, to minimize the risk of death.**

E. **LV pump failure and cardiogenic shock.** LV dysfunction is common after acute MI, and the severity of dysfunction correlates with the extent of myocardial injury. Patients with small infarcts may have regional wall-motion abnormalities with overall normal LV function because of compensatory hyperkinesia of the unaffected

TABLE 3.2 30-Day Mortality Based on Hemodynamic (Killip) Class in the GUSTO I Trial

Killip class	Characteristics	Patients (%)	Mortality rate (%)
I	No evidence of CHF	85	5.1
II	Rales, ↑ JVD, or S_3	13	13.6
III	Pulmonary edema	1	32.2
IV	Cardiogenic shock	1	57.8

CHF, congestive heart failure; ↑, increased; JVD, jugular venous distention.
(Adapted from Fox AC, Glassman E, Isom OW. Surgically remediable complications of myocardial infarction. *Prog Cardiovasc Dis* 1979;107:852–855.)

segments. **Prior MI, older age, female sex, diabetes, and anterior infarction** are risk factors for development of cardiogenic shock.

1. Classification

a. Killip and Kimball (20) classified four subsets of patients on the basis of clinical presentation and physical findings at the onset of MI (Table 3.2). They reported an 81% mortality rate with cardiogenic shock (Killip class IV). The 30-day mortality rate for the 0.8% of GUSTO I patients with cardiogenic shock treated with thrombolytic agents was 58% (21).

b. Four hemodynamic subsets (4) are based on PCWP and cardiac index (Table 3.3). The hemodynamic subsets correlate well with mortality rate. Subset II represents congestive heart failure (CHF) without shock. Patients in subset III may be hypovolemic and respond to fluid replacement. Subset IV satisfies criteria for true cardiogenic shock. There is an approximately 50% mortality in subset IV; however, data are largely compiled from the era before reperfusion (22).

2. Clinical presentation

a. Signs and symptoms. Patients may develop respiratory distress, diaphoresis, and cool, clammy extremities in addition to the typical signs and symptoms of acute MI. Patients in cardiogenic shock may have severe orthopnea, dyspnea, and oliguria in addition to altered mental status from cerebral hypoperfusion.

b. Physical findings. A dyskinetic segment of the ventricle may be apparent during inspection or may be felt during palpation. An S_3 gallop may be heard in patients with poor ventricular function.

3. Etiology. Table 3.4 lists the causes of cardiogenic shock. Patients with acute MI and cardiogenic shock typically have **severe three-vessel disease** and commonly have substantial involvement of the LAD (23). Autopsy studies have revealed that at least 40% of the left ventricle is affected in patients with cardiogenic shock (24). Forty percent of patients have prior MI. If the previous MI was large, even a small, acute MI may cause shock.

4. Laboratory examination

a. Lactic acidosis, elevated creatinine levels, and arterial hypoxemia are common.

TABLE 3.3 Forrester Classification

Subset	PCWP	Cardiac index	Mortality rate
I	<18	>2.2	3
II	>18	>2.2	9
III	<18	<2.2	23
IV	>18	<2.2	51

PCWP, pulmonary capillary wedge pressure.

TABLE 3.4 Causes of Cardiogenic Shock
COMPLICATIONS OF ACUTE MYOCARDIAL INFARCTION
Extensive left ventricular infarction
Extensive right ventricular infarction
Ventricular septal rupture
Acute severe mitral regurgitation
Cardiac tamponade with or without free-wall rupture
OTHER CONDITIONS
Aortic dissection
Myocarditis
Massive pulmonary embolism
Critical valvular stenosis
Acute mitral or aortic regurgitation
Calcium channel blocker or β-blocker overdose

b. A chest radiograph reveals pulmonary congestion.

c. Patients with cardiogenic shock resulting from LV failure usually have extensive electrocardiographic abnormalities consistent with massive infarction, severe diffuse ischemia, or evidence of a large, prior MI.

d. Extensive ST-segment depressions are common.

e. An unremarkable ECG in the presence of shock suggests another cause of shock, such as aortic dissection or mechanical complications of acute MI (e.g., free-wall rupture, VSR, papillary muscle rupture, dynamic LVOT obstruction).

5. Diagnostic testing

a. Cardiac catheterization. Hemodynamic monitoring with an arterial line and pulmonary artery catheter helps influence minute-to-minute care. Hemodynamic data help identify RV infarction, acute MR, and VSR that contribute to the shock state.

b. Echocardiography helps determine the extent of myocardial necrosis and identify complications of MI that contribute to cardiogenic shock.

6. Therapy

a. Priority of therapy. An **IABP** should be inserted as soon as possible in a patient with cardiogenic shock without the contraindications of aortic dissection or more than moderate aortic insufficiency.

b. Medical therapy

(1) Vasodilators play an important role in the management of post-MI heart failure by means of afterload reduction. The main determinants of myocardial oxygen consumption are heart rate, contractility, and wall stress. Wall stress depends on peak LV pressure, volume, and wall thickness. Vasodilators reduce wall stress and decrease oxygen requirements; they also improve cardiac output by decreasing SVR. Vasodilators are indicated **only to treat patients with adequate arterial pressure.**

(a) Nitroglycerin. Intravenous nitroglycerin is the drug of choice among vasodilators because it is less likely to produce coronary steal and is antiischemic. The starting dose is 10 to 20 μg/min, and it is increased by 10 μg/min every few minutes. Nitroglycerin is titrated to achieve a MAP of approximately 70 mm Hg.

(b) Nitroprusside. Intravenous nitroprusside may be added if further reduction in afterload is warranted because nitroglycerin is predominantly a venodilator. Nitroprusside is started at 5 to 10 μg/kg/min, and it is titrated to a MAP of approximately 70 mm Hg. Caution should be exercised in the acute MI setting given the suggestion of increased mortality with nitroprusside.

(2) Angiotensin-converting enzyme (ACE) inhibitors improve LV performance by reducing cardiac preload and afterload in patients with heart failure or acute MI. ACE inhibitors should be instituted early in the care of patients with pulmonary congestion, particularly in those with hypertension. On the basis of the beneficial effects on infarct expansion in the International Study of Infarct Survival (ISIS 4) and Gruppo Italiano per lo Studio della Sopravvivenza nell'Infarto Miocardio (GISSI 3) trials, early (<12 hours) initiation of captopril at 6.25 mg three times daily is recommended. The amount may be doubled with each subsequent dose as tolerated, up to 50 mg every 8 hours. **ACE inhibitors should not be given to patients with cardiogenic shock.**

(3) Diuretics. Patients with mild pulmonary edema MI can be treated with diuretics such as furosemide. Furosemide (20 mg IV) is administered initially for patients with normal creatinine levels. This can be followed with higher and repeated doses as needed.

(4) Cardiac glycosides. The use of digitalis glycosides in the setting of an acute MI should be restricted to treatment of patients with atrial fibrillation or atrial flutter, or to treatment of patients with heart failure that persists after appropriate therapy.

(5) β-Adrenergic agonists. Patients with severe heart failure and cardiogenic shock (i.e., PCWP >18 with persistent cardiac index <2.2 and MAP <65) may need dopamine and dobutamine. β-Blockers are contraindicated in this population, because they exacerbate the already life-threatening low cardiac function.

- **(a) Dopamine** is started at a dose of 3 μg/kg/min and increased gradually to a maximal dose of 20 μg/kg/min.
- **(b) Dobutamine** has positive inotropic action comparable to that of dopamine but is less chronotropic and may **decrease afterload.** Dobutamine is started at a dose of 2.5 μg/kg/min and increased to a maximum dose of 30 μg/kg/min.

(6) Phosphodiesterase inhibitors. Milrinone, a phosphodiesterase inhibitor with inotropic and vasodilator action, may be beneficial in some patients, especially those with right ventricular dysfunction. Milrinone is given as a 50-μg/kg bolus over 10 minutes, followed by an infusion of 0.375 to 0.75 μg/kg/min. The bolus may be omitted in the care of patients with marginal blood pressures. Table 3.5 lists the hemodynamic effects of medications used to manage heart failure. Patients without adequate MAP may not tolerate milrinone.

TABLE 3.5 Hemodynamic Effects of Medications Used to Manage Heart Failure

Medication	Preload ↓	Afterload ↓	Contractility	Vasoconstriction
Dopamine (medium dose)	–	–	++	–
Dopamine (high dose)	–	–	++	++
Dobutamine	+	++	+++	–
Milrinone	++	++	+++	–
Nitroglycerin	+++	+	–	–
Nitroprusside	+++	+++	–	–

–, No effect; +, little effect; ++, moderate effect; +++, great effect.

(7) **Vasopressors.** Some patients may need norepinephrine to maintain arterial pressure. Norepinephrine is started at 2 μg/min and titrated to 20 μg/min to maintain a MAP of 70 to 75 mm Hg. Pure α-adrenergic agonists like phenylephrine should be avoided, as they act primarily by increasing afterload, which may acutely worsen patients already in cardiogenic shock

c. **Percutaneous therapy**

(1) **IABP.** An IABP should be inserted as soon as possible in a patient with cardiogenic shock. It reduces afterload, improves cardiac output, and decreases the myocardial oxygen requirement by means of reduction in wall stress.

(2) **Percutaneous ventricular assist device.** Traditional mechanical circulatory support from an IABP may prove insufficient in certain patients, and consideration may be given to more aggressive support with a percutaneous left ventricular assist device. These systems provide left atrial to femoral artery bypass flow at rates up to 4.0 L/min and can serve as a bridge to recovery or more definitive therapy.

(3) **Percutaneous coronary intervention (PCI).** Percutaneous coronary intervention of the infarction-related artery has been associated with a good prognosis among patients with cardiogenic shock attributed to depressed LV function; **the approximate reduction in the mortality rate is from 50% to 60%.** In most studies, investigators performed percutaneous transluminal coronary angioplasty (PTCA) on the infarct-related artery only. Some investigators, however, reported multivessel PCI with more complete revascularization. Considering the dismal prognosis for patients with acute MI and cardiogenic shock, immediate percutaneous revascularization should be considered.

d. **Surgical therapy**

(1) Emergency surgical revascularization is indicated in the care of patients with severe multivessel disease or substantial left main coronary artery stenosis.

(2) Other surgical modalities that may be used in extreme cases include the use of LV or biventricular assist devices or extracorporeal membrane oxygenation as a bridge to heart transplantation. Some patients may gradually discontinue the use of assist devices after recovery of the stunned portion of myocardium.

F. **RV failure.** Mild RV dysfunction is common after MI of the inferior or inferior posterior wall; however, hemodynamically significant RV impairment occurs in only 10% of patients with inferior or inferoposterior wall MI and commonly involves the proximal right coronary artery. Because the right ventricle has lower oxygen requirements, is thin walled, is perfused during systole and diastole, and often has collateral blood flow from the LAD and thebesian veins, it is unusual to have extensive, irreversible damage (25).

1. **Clinical presentation**

a. **Signs and symptoms.** The triad of hypotension, jugular venous distention (JVD) with clear lungs, and absence of dyspnea is highly specific (but has poor sensitivity) for RV infarction (26). Patients with severe RV failure have symptoms of a low cardiac output state, including diaphoresis; cool, clammy extremities; and altered mental status. Patients often are hypotensive and oliguric. Use of nitrates or β-blockers as standard MI treatment may precipitate profound hypotension and provide the first clue of RV involvement. Table 3.6 lists the causes of hypotension among patients with inferior wall MI.

b. **Physical findings.** Patients with RV failure without concomitant LV failure have elevated jugular venous pressure (JVP) and RV S_3 with clear lungs. The combination of JVP >8 cm H_2O and **Kussmaul's sign** (i.e., failure of JVP to decrease with inspiration) is sensitive and specific for severe RV failure. Rarely, elevated right-sided pressures can result in right-to-left shunting. This should

TABLE 3.6	Causes of Hypotension Among Patients With Inferior Myocardial Infarction
Severe right ventricular infarction	
Bradyarrythmia	
Acute severe mitral regurgitation	
Prior myocardial infarction	
Left ventricular septal rupture	
Bezold-Jarisch reflex	

be considered in patients with RV infarction and hypoxia. Table 3.7 lists the clinical findings associated with a RV infarction.

2. **Pathophysiology.** RV involvement depends on the location of the right coronary artery occlusion. Marked dysfunction occurs only if occlusion is proximal to the acute marginal branch. The degree of RV involvement also depends on whether collateral flow from the LAD is present and the extent of blood flow through the thebesian veins. The right ventricle is a thin-walled chamber that has low oxygen demand with coronary perfusion during the entire cardiac cycle; extensive and irreversible infarction is, therefore, rare. Most patients with RV infarction who survive the acute phase spontaneously improve after 48 to 72 hours.
3. **Laboratory examination**
   a. An **ECG** usually shows inferior MI. ST elevation in V_4R in the setting of suspected RV infarction has a positive predictive value of 80%. ST-segment elevation exceeding 1 mm may be seen in V_1 and occasionally in V_2 and V_3 (Fig. 3.2).
   b. A chest radiograph usually is normal; there is no evidence of pulmonary congestion.
4. **Diagnostic testing**
   a. **Two-dimensional echocardiography** is the diagnostic **study of choice** for RV infarction. It may demonstrate RV dilation, severe RV dysfunction, and usually shows LV inferior wall dysfunction. It is also useful in differentiating RV infarction from other syndromes that can mimic it, such as cardiac tamponade.
   b. **Pulmonary artery catheterization.** Hemodynamic monitoring with a pulmonary artery catheter usually reveals **high right atrial pressures with low PCWP.** Acute RV failure results in underfilling of the left ventricle and a low cardiac output state. The PCWP usually is low unless concomitant, severe LV dysfunction is present. In some patients, RV dilation can cause decreased LV performance resulting from ventricular interdependence. As the right ventricle dilates, the septum flattens or bows into the left ventricle and restricts ventricular filling. A right arterial pressure >10 mm Hg and right arterial pressure-to-PCWP ratio ≥0.8 strongly suggests RV infarction (27,28).

TABLE 3.7	Clinical Findings Associated with Right Ventricular Infarction
Hypotension	
Elevated jugular venous pressure	
Kussmaul's sign	
Abnormal jugular venous pressure pattern (Y ≥ X descent)	
Tricuspid regurgitation	
Right-sided S_3 and S_4	
Pulsus paradoxus	
High-grade atrioventricular block	

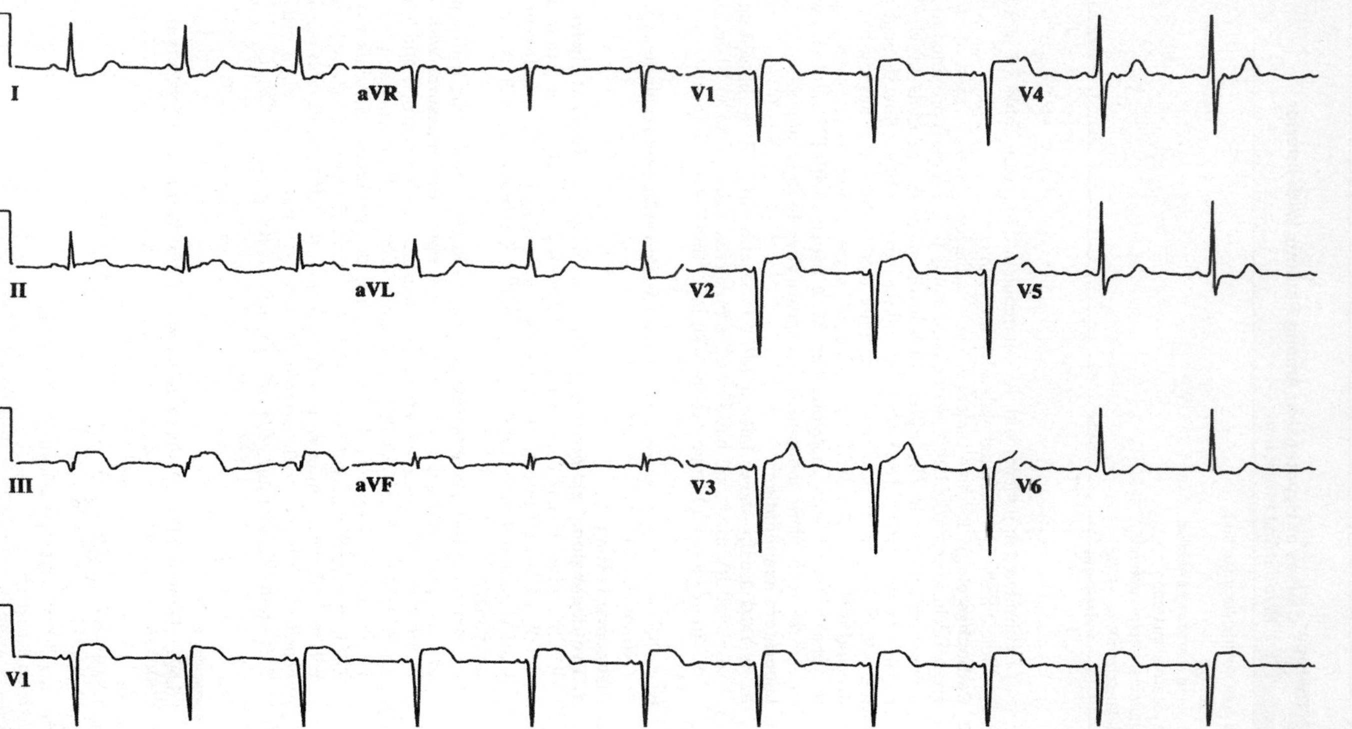

Figure 3.2. Electrocardiogram shows acute inferior myocardial infarction with right ventricular involvement.

5. **Therapy**
   a. **Medical therapy**
      (1) **Fluid administration.** Management of RV infarction involves volume loading to increase preload and cardiac output. Some patients may require several liters in 1 hour. **Hemodynamic monitoring is crucial** because overzealous fluid administration to a patient with severe RV dilation can further decrease LV preload and cardiac output. (The septum shifts toward the left ventricle, and intrapericardial pressure shifts substantially.) The target central venous pressure is approximately 15 mm Hg.
      (2) **Inotropes.** When volume loading fails to increase cardiac output, use of inotropes is indicated. Administration of dobutamine markedly increases cardiac index and RV ejection fraction and is superior to afterload reduction with nitroprusside (29).
   b. **Percutaneous therapy**
      (1) Patients who undergo successful reperfusion of RV branches have improved RV function and decreased 30-day mortality rates (30).
      (2) AV sequential pacing may markedly improve the condition of a patient with RV infarction, bradyarrhythmias, or loss of sinus rhythm. **A longer AV delay of approximately 200 ms and a heart rate of 80 to 90 beats/min are usually optimal for these patients.**
      (3) An IABP may be useful, especially in cases of concomittant LV dysfunction.
   c. **Surgical therapy**
      (1) **Pericardiectomy** may be considered in the care of patients with refractory shock as it reverses the septal impingement on LV filling.
      (2) An **RV assist device** is indicated in the care of patients who remain in cardiogenic shock despite the foregoing measures.

G. **Ventricular aneurysm**
1. **Clinical presentation**
   a. **Signs and symptoms**
      (1) **Acute aneurysms.** Acute development of a large LV aneurysm can result in severe CHF and even cardiogenic shock. Patients with an acute MI that involves the apex of the left ventricle, particularly those with transmural anteroapical infarcts, are at greatest risk. Acute aneurysms expand during systole. This expansion wastes contractile energy generated by normal myocardium and puts the entire ventricle at a mechanical disadvantage.
      (2) **Chronic aneurysms** which persist >6 weeks after MI, are less compliant than acute aneurysms and rarely expand during systole. They occur in 10% to 30% of patients after MI, especially MI involving the anterior wall. Patients with chronic aneurysms may have heart failure, ventricular arrhythmias, and systemic embolism, but they frequently have no symptoms.
   b. **Physical findings.** A dyskinetic segment of the ventricle may be apparent during inspection or may be felt during palpation. S_3 gallop may be heard in patients with poor ventricular function.
2. **Pathophysiology.** Expansion of infarction and progressive LV dilation are associated with occlusion of an infarct-related artery, and inhibition of LV dilation is associated with an open infarct-related artery. The early open artery hypothesis contends that early reperfusion results in myocardial salvage and inhibits infarct expansion. Late reperfusion limits infarct expansion through multiple mechanisms, including immediate change in infarction characteristics, preservation of small amounts of residual myofibrils and interstitial collagen, accelerated healing, the scaffold effect of a blood-filled vasculature, and elimination of ischemia in viable but dysfunctional myocardium.
3. **Diagnostic testing**
   a. **ECG**
      (1) **Acute aneurysms.** The ECG reveals evidence of ST-elevation MI, which may persist despite evidence of reperfusion.
      (2) **Chronic aneurysms.** ST elevation that persists >6 weeks occurs among patients with chronic ventricular aneurysms.

b. **A chest radiograph** may reveal a localized bulge in the cardiac silhouette.
c. **Echocardiography** is the diagnostic **test of choice** and accurately depicts the aneurysmal segment. It also may reveal the presence of a mural thrombus. Echocardiography is useful in differentiating a true aneurysm from a pseudoaneurysm. True aneurysms have a wide neck, whereas pseudoaneurysms have a narrow neck in relation to the diameter of the aneurysm.
d. Cardiac **magnetic resonance imaging** also depicts the aneurysm.

4. **Therapy**
   a. **Medical therapy**
      (1) **Acute aneurysm.** Heart failure with acute aneurysms is managed with intravenous vasodilators and an IABP. ACE inhibitors have been shown to reduce infarct expansion and progressive LV remodeling. Because infarct expansion starts early, ACE inhibitors should be started within the first 24 hours of the onset of acute MI if blood pressure allows.
      (2) **Chronic aneurysm.** Heart failure with chronic aneurysms is managed with ACE inhibitors, digoxin, and diuretics.
      (3) **Anticoagulation**
         (a) Anticoagulation with **warfarin sodium** is indicated for patients with a mural thrombus. Patients are initially treated with intravenous heparin with a target partial thromboplastin time (PTT) of 50 to 65 seconds. Warfarin is started simultaneously. Patients should be treated with warfarin with a target international normalized ratio (INR) of 2 to 3 for 3 to 6 months.
         (b) It is **controversial whether patients with large aneurysms without thrombus should receive anticoagulants.** Many clinicians prescribe anticoagulants for 6 to 12 weeks after the acute phase in patients with large anterior MIs.
         (c) Patients with LV aneurysms and a low global ejection fraction (<40%) have a higher stroke rate and should take anticoagulants for at least 3 months after the acute event. They may be subsequently observed with echocardiography. Anticoagulation is reinitiated if a thrombus develops.
   b. **Percutaneous therapy**
      (1) A patent infarction-related artery has beneficial effects on LV remodeling that are independent of myocardial salvage (i.e., decreased 1-year mortality, decreased LV dilation, and expansion). These patients may be candidates **for late reperfusion with percutaneous intervention** (>12 hours but <24 hours). There are no data to suggest benefit with percutaneous intervention after 24 hours.
      (2) Implantation of an implantable cardioverter–defibrillator (ICD) is indicated in the care of patients with chronic aneurysms and in those with normal LV function and intractable ventricular arrhythmias refractory to medications. Patients with depressed ejection fractions (<30%) after an MI are candidates for prophylactic ICD placement.
   c. **Surgical therapy.** Patients with refractory heart failure and refractory ventricular arrhythmias should be considered for surgical resection. Surgical resection may be followed by conventional closure or newer techniques (e.g., inverted T closure, endocardial patch) to maintain LV geometry. Revascularization is beneficial to patients with a large amount of viable myocardium in the aneurysmal segment.

H. **Dynamic LVOT obstruction.** Dynamic LVOT obstruction is an **uncommon complication** of acute anterior MI. Although this complication has been cited only in case reports, it may be an underappreciated and underreported complication.

1. **Clinical presentation**
   a. **Signs and symptoms.** Patients may have respiratory distress, diaphoresis, and cool, clammy extremities in addition to the typical signs and symptoms of acute MI. Patients with severe obstruction may appear to be in cardiogenic

shock with severe orthopnea, dyspnea, and oliguria in addition to altered mental status from cerebral hypoperfusion.

b. **Physical findings** frequently include a new systolic ejection murmur heard best at the left upper sternal border with radiation to the neck. A new systolic murmur can be heard at the apex with radiation to the axilla as a result of systolic anterior motion of the mitral leaflet. An S_3 gallop, pulmonary rales, hypotension, and tachycardia also may occur.

2. **Pathophysiology.** The development of LVOT obstruction depends on hyperkinesis of basal and mid segments of the left ventricle. The increased contractile force of these regions decreases the cross-sectional area of the LVOT. The resulting increased velocity of blood through the outflow tract can produce decreased pressure below the mitral valve and result in the leaflet being drawn anteriorly toward the septum (i.e., Venturi effect). This results in further outflow tract obstruction and in MR. It has been postulated that this complication can play a role in free-wall rupture. LVOT obstruction leads to increased end-systolic intraventricular pressure, which leads to increased stress of the weakened, necrotic infarcted zone.

3. **Diagnostic testing. Echocardiography** is the diagnostic test of choice and helps evaluate the hyperkinetic segments, the LVOT obstruction, and the presence of systolic anterior motion (SAM) of the mitral leaflet.

4. **Medical therapy** centers on decreasing myocardial contractility and heart rate while expanding intravascular volume and increasing afterload (modestly).

   a. **β-Blockers** should be added slowly and with careful monitoring of heart rate, blood pressure, and pulmonary venous oxygen saturation (SvO_2).

   b. **Intravenous hydration** should be initiated with several small (250-mL) boluses of normal saline to increase preload and decrease LVOT obstruction and SAM. The patient's hemodynamic and respiratory status should be monitored closely during this therapeutic intervention.

III. COMPLICATIONS OF ARRHYTHMIA.

Arrhythmias are the most common complications after acute MI. They affect approximately 90% of patients who have had an MI (see Chapters 19 through 24).

IV. ISCHEMIC COMPLICATIONS

A. Clinical presentation

1. **Infarct extension** is a progressive increase in the amount of myocardial necrosis within the same arterial territory as the original MI. This may manifest as subendocardial MI that extends to transmural MI or as MI that extends and involves the adjacent myocardium.

   a. Patients usually have continuous or recurrent **chest pain**, new **electrocardiographic changes**, and prolonged elevations in creatine kinase (CK) level.

   b. **Echocardiography** or **nuclear imaging** helps confirm the diagnosis by showing a larger infarct than was seen immediately after the MI.

   c. **Reinfarction** occurs more frequently when the infarction-related artery reoccludes then when it remains patent; however, reocclusion of the infarction-related artery does not always cause reinfarction. After thrombolytic therapy, reocclusion is found on angiograms of 5% to 30% of patients and is associated with a poor outcome.

2. **Postinfarction angina**

   a. **Recurrent angina** within a few hours to 30 days after acute MI is defined as postinfarction angina. The incidence is between 23% and 60%. The frequency of postinfarction angina is higher after non–Q-wave MI and after administration of thrombolytic agents.

   b. Patients with postinfarction angina have a worse prognosis in regard to sudden death, reinfarction, and acute cardiac events.

   c. The pathophysiologic mechanism of postinfarction angina is similar to that of unstable angina and should be managed as such.

3. **In-hospital reinfarction.** Infarction in a separate territory (i.e., recurrent infarction) may be difficult to diagnose in the first 24 to 48 hours after the initial event. Infarct extension and infarction in a separate territory may be difficult to differentiate. Reinfarction occurs in approximately 4.7% of patients with acute MI and is more common in patients older than 70 years, women patients with diabetes mellitus, and those with prior MI.
   a. It may be very difficult to delineate the electrocardiographic changes of reinfarction from the evolving electrocardiographic changes of the index MI.
   b. CK isoforms are more useful in diagnosing reinfarction than are the troponins. Recurrent elevations in CK-MB after normalization or a rise to >50% of the prior value is regarded as the standard for reinfarction
   c. Echocardiography reveals a wall motion abnormality in a new area.

B. Therapy

1. **Medical therapy.** Aggressive medical therapy with aspirin, heparin, nitrates, and β-blockers is indicated in the care of patients who have had MI and have ongoing ischemia.
2. **Percutaneous therapy**
   a. An **IABP** should be promptly inserted in patients with hypotension and those with severe LV systolic dysfunction.
   b. Urgent **coronary angiography** with percutaneous intervention is indicated after stabilization with medical therapy or as an emergency if the patient's condition is unstable or the patient has refractory chest pain. Percutaneous or surgical revascularization improves the prognosis of these patients.

V. EMBOLIC COMPLICATIONS. The incidence of clinically evident systemic embolism after MI is approximately 2%. The incidence is higher among patients with **anterior wall MI.** The overall incidence of mural thrombus after MI is approximately 20%. Large anterior MI may be accompanied by mural thrombus in 60% of patients.

A. Clinical presentation

1. **Signs and symptoms.** The most common clinical presentation of embolic complications is stroke, although patients may have limb ischemia, renal infarction, and intestinal ischemia. Most episodes of systemic emboli occur in the first 10 days after acute MI.
2. **Physical findings.** The physical findings depend on the site of embolism.
   a. Patients with stroke have a neurologic deficit.
   b. Embolism to the peripheral circulation causes limb ischemia, which makes the extremity cold, pulseless, and painful.
   c. Renal infarctions may cause hematuria and flank pain.
   d. Mesenteric ischemia causes abdominal pain and bloody diarrhea.

B. Therapy

1. **Intravenous heparin** is administered for 3 or 4 days to a target PTT of 50 to 65 seconds to patients with large anterior MI or mural thrombi.
2. **Oral warfarin sodium therapy** should be continued for 3 to 6 months for patients with mural thrombi and those with large akinetic areas detected by echocardiography.
3. In one study, patients with a large MI treated with heparin followed by oral anticoagulation (INR of 2 to 3) for 1 month had a decrease from 3% to 1% in the incidence of cerebral emboli.

VI. PERICARDITIS

A. Early pericarditis. The incidence of early pericarditis after acute MI is approximately 10%. The inflammation usually develops 24 to 96 hours after MI (31).

1. **Clinical presentation.** Early pericarditis occurs among patients with transmural MI. Most of these patients have no symptoms, although transient pericardial friction rubs may be audible in some patients.
   a. **Signs and symptoms**
      (1) Patients report progressive, severe chest pain that lasts for hours. The **pain is postural**: worse when the patient is supine and alleviated if the patient sits up and leans forward. The pain usually is pleuritic in nature and is worsened with deep inspiration, coughing, and swallowing.

(2) Radiation of pain to the trapezius ridge is nearly pathognomonic for acute pericarditis and does not occur in patients with ischemic pain. The pain also may radiate to the neck and less frequently to the arm or back.

b. Physical findings. The presence of a pericardial friction rub is pathognomonic for acute pericarditis; however, it can be evanescent.

(1) The rub is best heard at the left lower sternal edge with the diaphragm of the stethoscope.

(2) The rub has three components—one component each in atrial systole, ventricular systole, and ventricular diastole. In about 30% of patients, the rub is biphasic, and in 10% it is uniphasic.

(3) The development of pericardial effusion may cause fluctuation in the intensity of the rub, although the rub may still be heard despite substantial pericardial effusion.

2. Etiology and pathophysiology. Pericarditis typically results from an area of localized pericardial inflammation overlying the infarcted myocardium. The inflammation is fibrinous in nature. The development of an evanescent pericardial rub correlates with a larger infarct and hemodynamic derangements.

3. Laboratory examination and diagnostic testing

a. An **ECG** is the most useful test in the diagnosis of pericarditis; however, evolving electrocardiographic changes may make the diagnosis difficult for patients who have had MI. Unlike ischemia, in which the changes are limited to a particular territory, pericarditis produces generalized electrocardiographic changes.

(1) The ST-segment elevation seen with pericarditis is a concave upward or saddle-shaped curve.

(2) In pericarditis, T waves become inverted after the ST segment becomes isoelectric, whereas in acute MI, T waves may become inverted when the ST segment is still elevated.

(3) Four phases of electrocardiographic abnormality have been described in association with pericarditis (Table 3.8).

b. Chest radiography is of limited value in the diagnosis of pericarditis.

c. Echocardiography may reveal pericardial effusion, which strongly suggests pericarditis, although the absence of effusion does not rule out the diagnosis.

4. Therapy

a. Aspirin is used to manage post-MI pericarditis in doses of 650 mg every 4 to 6 hours.

b. Nonsteroidal antiinflammatory agents and corticosteroids should not be used to treat these patients. These agents may interfere with myocardial healing and contribute to infarct expansion (32).

c. Colchicine may be beneficial to patients with recurrent pericarditis.

B. Late pericarditis (i.e., Dressler's syndrome). The incidence of Dressler's syndrome is between 1% and 3%. The syndrome occurs 1 to 8 weeks after MI. The pathogenesis is unknown, but an autoimmune mechanism has been suggested.

1. Clinical presentation. Patients have chest discomfort that suggests pericarditis, pleuritic chest pain, fever, arthralgia, malaise, an elevated leukocyte count, and an elevated sedimentation rate. Echocardiography may reveal pericardial effusion.

TABLE 3.8 Electrocardiographic Changes of Pericarditis

Stage I	ST elevation, upright T waves
Stage II	ST elevation resolves, upright to flat T waves
Stage III	ST isoelectric, inverted T waves
Stage IV	ST isolelectric, upright T waves

2. **Therapy** is similar to that for early post-MI pericarditis: aspirin and avoidance of nonsteroidal antiinflammatory drugs and corticosteroids. However, if >4 weeks have elapsed since the MI, nonsteroidal agents and even steroids may be indicated for severe symptoms.

ACKNOWLEDGMENT

The authors would like to thank Dr. David Tschopp for his contributions to this chapter.

References

1. Topaz O, Taylor AL. Interventricular septal rupture complicating acute myocardial infarction: from pathophysiologic features to the role of invasive and noninvasive diagnostic modalities in current management. *Am J Med* 1992;93:683–688.
2. Gershaw BS, Granger CB, Bunbaum Y, et al. Risk factors, angiographic patterns and outcomes in patients with ventricular septal defect complicating acute myocardial infarction. GUSTO I Investigators. *Circulation* 2000;101:27–32.
3. Chatterjee K. Complications of acute myocardial infarction. *Curr Probl Cardiol* 1993;18:1–79.
4. Giuliana ER, Danielson GK, Pluth JR, et al. Postinfarction ventricular septal rupture. Surgical considerations and results. *Circulation* 1974;49:455–459.
5. Fox AC, Glassman E, Isom OW. Surgically remediable complications of myocardial infarction. *Prog Cardiovasc Dis* 1979;107:852–855.
6. Menon V, White H, LeJemtel T, et al. The clinical profile of patients with suspected cardiogenic shock due to predominant left ventricular failure. *J Am Coll Cardiol* 2000;36:1071–1076.
7. Moore CA, Nygard TW, Kaser DI, et al. Postinfarction ventricular septal rupture: the importance of location of infarction and right ventricular function in determining survival. *Circulation* 1986;74:45–55.
8. Ryan TJ, for the American College of Cardiology/American Heart Association. Guidelines for the management of patients with acute myocardial infarction. *J Am Coll Cardiol* 1999;34:890–911.
9. Barzilai B, Gessler C, Perez JE, et al. Significance of Doppler-detected mitral regurgitation in acute myocardial infarction. *Am J Cardiol* 1988;61:220–223.
10. Lehmann KG, Francis CK, Dodge HT, et al. Mitral regurgitation in early myocardial infarction: incidence, clinical detection, and prognostic implications. TIMI Study Group. *Ann Intern Med* 1992;117:10–17.
11. Wei JY, Hutchins GM, Bulkley BH. Papillary muscle rupture in fatal acute myocardial infarction: a potentially treatable form of cardiogenic shock. *Ann Intern Med* 1979;90:149–152.
12. Thompson CR, Christopher BE, Sleeper LA, et al. Cardiogenic shock due to acute severe mitral regurgitation complicating acute myocardial infarction: a report for the SHOCK Trial Registry. *J Am Coll Cardiol* 2000;36;1104–1109.
13. Hochman JS, Buller CE, Sleeper LA, et al. Cardiogenic shock complicating acute myocardial infarction—etiologies, management and outcome: overall findings of the SHOCK Trial Registry. *J Am Coll Cardiol* 2000;36:1063–1070.
14. Voci P, Bilotta F, Caretta Q, et al. Papillary muscle perfusion pattern: a hypothesis for ischemic papillary muscle dysfunction. *Circulation*. 1995;91:1714–1718.
15. Fuchs RM, Heuser RR, Yin FCP, et al. Limitations of pulmonary wedge V waves in diagnosing mitral regurgitation *Am J Cardiol* 1982;49:849–854.
16. Kishon Y, Oh J, Schaff H, et al. Mitral valve operation in postinfarction rupture of a Papillary muscle: immediate results and long term follow-up of 22 patients. *Mayo Clin Proc* 1992;67:1023–1030.
17. Lopez-Sendon J, Gonzales A, Lopez de Sa E, et al. Diagnosis of subacute ventricular wall rupture after acute myocardial infarction: sensitivity and specificity of clinical, hemodynamic, and echocardiographic criteria. *J Am Coll Cardiol* 1992;19:1145–1153.
18. Becker R, Charlesworth A, Wilcox R, et al. Cardiac rupture associated with thrombolytic therapy: impact of time to treatment in the Late Assessment of Thrombolytic Efficacy (LATE) study. *J Am Coll Cardiol* 1995;25:1063–1068.
19. Bartunek J, Vanderheyden M, de Bruyne B. Dynamic left ventricular outflow tract obstruction after anterior myocardial infarction: a potential mechanism of myocardial rupture. *Eur Heart J* 1995;16:1439–1442.
20. Killip T, Kimball JT. Treatment of myocardial infarction in a coronary care unit: a two year experience with 250 patients. *Am J Cardiol* 1967;20:457–461.
21. Holmes DR, Bates ER, Kleiman NS, et al, for the GUSTO I investigators. Contemporary reperfusion therapy for cardiogenic shock: the GUSTO I trial experience *J Am Coll Cardiol* 1995;26:668–674.
22. Forrester JS, Diamond GA, Chatterjee K. Medical therapy of acute myocardial infarction by application of hemodynamic subsets. *N Engl J Med* 1976;295:1356–1361.
23. Wong SC, Antonelli T, Sleeper LA, et al. Angiographic findings and clinical correlates in patients with cardiogenic shock complicating acute myocardial infarction in the SHOCK Registry. *J Am Coll Cardiol* 2000;36:1077–1083.
24. Alonso DR, Scheidt S, Post M, et al. Pathophysiology of cardiogenic shock: quantification of myocardial necrosis, clinical pathological and electrocardiographic correlation. *Circulation* 1973;48:588–596.
25. Dell'Italia LJ, Lembo NJ, Starling MR, et al. Hemodynamically important right ventricular infarction: follow-up evaluation of right ventricular systolic function at rest and during exercise with radionuclide ventriculography and respiratory gas exchange. *Circulation* 1987;75:996.
26. Dell'Italia LJ, Starling MR, O'Rourke RA. Physical examination for exclusion of hemodynamically important right ventricular infarction. *Ann Intern Med* 1983;99:608–611.
27. Dell'Italia LJ, Starling MR, Crawford MH, et al. Right ventricular infarction: identification by hemodynamic measurements before and after volume loading and correlation with noninvasive techniques. *J Am Coll Cardiol* 1984;4:931–939.
28. Dell'Italia LJ, Starling MR. Right ventricular infarction: an important clinical entity. *Curr Probl Cardiol* 1984;9:1–58.
29. Dell'Italia LJ, Starling MR, Blumhardt R, et al. Comparative effects of volume loading, dobutamine, and nitroprusside in patients with predominant right ventricular infarction. *Circulation* 1985;72:1327–1335.

30. Bowers TR. Effect of reperfusion on biventricular function and survival after right ventricular infarction. *N Engl J Med* 1998;338:933–940.
31. Lichstein E. Early post-myocardial infarction pericarditis. *Pract Cardiol* 1982;8:60–66.
32. Berman J, Haffajee CA, Alpert JS. Therapy of symptomatic pericarditis after myocardial infarction: retrospective and prospective studies of aspirin, indomethacin, prednisone, and spontaneous resolution. *Am Heart J* 1981;101:750–753.

4 POST–MYOCARDIAL INFARCTION RISK STRATIFICATION AND MANAGEMENT

Shaun Senter and Mehdi H. Shishehbor

I. INTRODUCTION. More than 1.5 million patients will have an acute coronary syndrome (ACS) in the United States each year. At least 1 million will have evidence of myocardial infarction (MI), for which mortality and morbidity remain considerable. Although patient outcomes have improved, well-documented therapies are widely underprescribed. After identifying patients with MI, the goal of the physician must be to successfully stratify patients according to risk, implement medical interventions, and initiate risk-factor modification during the initial hospitalization.

II. RISK STRATIFICATION. Post-MI risk stratification identifies patients at high risk for subsequent cardiovascular events who will benefit from revascularization.

A. Age is the most important predictor of mortality after MI. The average age of patients with first MI is 65 years. Although older patients are at greatest risk and may benefit most, they receive less-aggressive treatment compared to younger patients, who have the lowest overall mortality.

B. Assessment of left ventricular (LV) function

1. **LV function** is the second most important predictor of mortality after MI. An inverse relation exists between LV ejection fraction (LVEF) and mortality. Mortality is greatest for patients with an LVEF less than 40%.
2. Assessment of LV function is indicated for all patients diagnosed with MI. Echocardiography, left ventriculography during diagnostic catheterization, or radionuclide angiography are useful in evaluating LV function. Although no imaging modality is proven to be superior, availability, expertise, and cost are important considerations when deciding which procedure to use.

C. Other indicators. Biomarkers are useful in further risk stratifying patients after MI. Elevated serum **troponin, C-reactive protein**, and **B-type natriuretic peptide** are associated with increased risk for recurrent cardiac events. The level of creatinine kinase-myocardial band (**CK-MB**) elevation is directly associated with mortality. New **ST-segment changes**, both elevationa and depression, portend higher risk of death, heart failure, recurrent ischemia, and severe coronary artery disease (CAD). **Electrical instability** such as ventricular fibrillation, ventricular tachycardia, and atrial fibrillation is associated with increased risk. Anterior MI, renal insufficiency, poor glycemic control, and anemia are also associated with worse outcomes.

D. Risk models. Various models utilize a combination of the aforementioned risk factors to quantitate a predictive score of patient risk for subsequent cardiac events and mortality. Examples included Thrombolysis In Myocardial Infarction (TIMI), Gruppo Italiano per lo Studio della Sopravvivenza nell'Infarto Miocardio (GISSI), and the Global Registry of Acute Coronary Events (GRACE) (1–3).

E. Assessment of residual ischemia (Fig. 4.1). The extent of CAD and the presence of residual ischemia are two strong predictors of mortality among patients who have

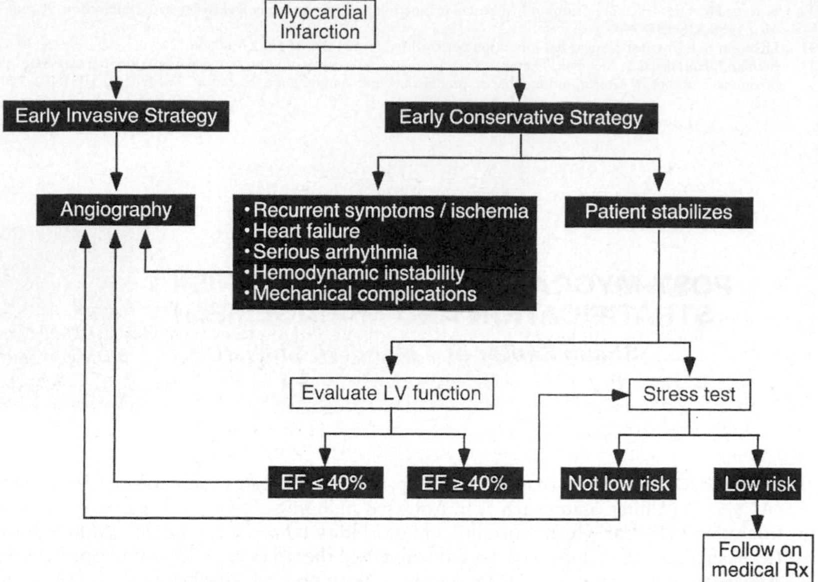

Figure 4.1. Post–myocardial infarction risk stratification.

had an MI. For this reason, low- and intermediate-risk patients who do not have ongoing ischemia or heart failure for at least 12 to 24 hours are candidates for submaximal stress testing.

1. **Submaximal exercise stress test is optimal for noninvasive risk stratification.** This test provides considerable prognostic information, assesses functional capacity, and can guide cardiac rehabilitation after discharge.
2. **Echocardiography** or **radionuclide imaging is** recommended in patients who have uninterpretable electrocardiograms (e.g., baseline ST-T changes, LV hypertrophy, intraventricular conduction delays, paced rhythm, or digoxin-related effects). Addition of either imaging modality increases both the sensitivity and specificity of detecting CAD.
3. **Dobutamine, adenosine, and dipyridamole** are pharmacologic agents safely used in conjunction with imaging for post-MI stress testing if a patient cannot exercise (see Chapter 5).
4. **American College of Cardiology and American Heart Association (ACC/AHA) guidelines** recommend a submaximal exercise stress test within 72 hours of discharge for all patients with uncomplicated MI who have not undergone coronary angiography or inpatient stress test. Patients who achieve at least three metabolic equivalents of the task (METs) have a good prognosis. Inability to achieve three METs, hypotension during exercise, or marked ST-segment depression or elevation is an indication for coronary angiography.

III. THERAPY AFTER MI

A. Coronary angiography

1. Indications

a. Coronary angiography is indicated in patients with recurrent angina or ischemia on medical therapy or higher risk findings on noninvasive stress testing. These include reduced ejection fraction, wall-motion abnormalities, perfusion defects, and evidence of ischemia.

b. An **"invasive strategy" utilizing early coronary angiography** is indicated for patients with elevated troponin, congestive heart failure, failed thrombolysis, mechanical complications, and electrical or hemodynamic instability.

c. **Patients with a history of prior revascularization,** either percutaneous coronary intervention (PCI) or coronary artery bypass grafting (CABG), should generally be referred for angiography.

d. Mechanical complications of MI include ventricular septal defect, LV aneurysm, and acute mitral regurgitation due to papillary muscle rupture. Coronary angiography is generally preferred before surgical intervention to identify potential bypass targets and to further assess the mechanical problem. In rare instances when hemodynamic instability precludes angiography, the surgeon may bypass all or selected coronary arteries.

e. **Open-artery hypothesis.** Nonrandomized studies have demonstrated that coronary patency after MI is an important predictor of subsequent mortality. Patients who have had an MI with an occluded artery have increased LV dilation, more spontaneous and induced arrhythmias, and a worse prognosis than patients who have patent infarction-related arteries. All these factors may be related to adverse LV remodeling after MI.

2. **Contraindications.** Catheterization should not be performed on patients who are ineligible for surgical or percutaneous revascularization because of severe comorbid conditions or who do not consent to angiography because of personal preference.

3. **Controversy.** Low-risk, asymptomatic patients who have sustained an uncomplicated MI generally have a good long-term prognosis and may not need to undergo angiography. These patients presumably are those without high-risk features on noninvasive stress testing who will receive aggressive medical therapy and risk factor modification. Still many cardiologists advocate catheterization for all patients after MI.

4. **PCI.** A new era of PCI therapy that includes glycoprotein IIb/IIIa inhibitors, thienopyridines, and drug-eluting stents continues to significantly affect the options and outcomes for patients undergoing revascularization. Currently in the United States, stents are utilized in more than 85% of lesions deemed appropriate for PCI. New devices and techniques continue to be developed and employed to improve patient outcomes after MI.

B. **CABG after MI** can be divided into two categories: emergency and elective.

1. **Emergency CABG.** The indications and management considerations for emergency CABG are discussed in Chapter 1.

2. **Elective CABG.** CABG has been shown to provide a survival benefit for patients with left main (>50% stenosis) or extensive three-vessel CAD. Surgical revascularization remains preferable for patients with severe LV dysfunction, diabetes, or two-vessel disease with proximal left anterior descending involvement and either high-risk noninvasive stress test results or LV dysfunction. However, the Arterial Revascularization Therapies Study (ARTS) demonstrated no significant difference in mortality, MI, or stroke among patients with multivessel disease and normal-to-moderately decreased LV function randomized to CABG versus PCI (4). Target-vessel revascularization was higher in the PCI group. The mortality benefit that patients with diabetes may derive from CABG must be weighed against an increased risk of stroke.

3. **Operative risk.** No prospective, randomized trials have been performed to determine the optimal timing of elective CABG after MI. Most data suggest that CABG 3 to 7 days after MI is associated with a low operative mortality similar to that of elective bypass in patients without recent infarction. **Operative risk increases** among patients with LV dysfunction, advanced age, and multiple comorbid conditions (e.g., diabetes mellitus, chronic obstructive pulmonary disease, chronic renal insufficiency). Emergency CABG and reoperations on patients with prior bypass surgery are associated with a higher operative mortality.

IV. SECONDARY PREVENTION

A. **Smoking cessation is mandatory.** Smoking doubles the rate of re-infarction and death after MI, causes coronary artery spasm, and reduces the effectiveness of

β-blocker therapy. The risk reduction attributed to smoking cessation is rapid, and nearly equals that of post-MI patients who never smoked in only 3 years. Half of all patients who stop smoking after MI will begin smoking again within 6 to 12 months. Many approaches to smoking cessation have been attempted, including pharmacologic therapy, formal smoking cessation programs, hypnosis, and abstinence.

1. **Nicotine substitutes** can be delivered by a variety of vehicles, including transdermal patches, chewing gum, nasal spray, and inhalers. These systems can deliver 30% to 60% of the nicotine of cigarettes. Although nicotine substitutes are not recommended for the acute phase of MI, use of these agents is safe in later phases. Patients who start smoking again should discontinue the use of nicotine substitutes.
2. **Pharmacotherapy. Bupropion** appears to be an effective aid in smoking cessation. The dose is doubled after 3 days and then taken twice daily for 7 to 12 weeks. Patients set a goal to stop smoking 1 to 2 weeks into therapy. **Varenicline**, a partial agonist of nicotine receptors, provides nicotine stimulation while blocking cigarette nicotine effects. In head-to-head trials, varenicline was more effective than buproprion. Like buproprion, therapy is for 12 weeks.
3. **Recommendations.** Physicians can aid patients in their effort to stop smoking by using a stepped approach with education and a firm recommendation to quit smoking, devising a plan, and reinforcement of effort to quit. Patients who are likely to relapse are older, less educated, or heavy smokers. Formal smoking cessation programs have been shown to have high rates of patient abstinence. Coinhabitants should also stop smoking to increase the likelihood of success.

B. Lipid management

1. **Low-density lipoprotein (LDL).** Most patients with acute MI have abnormal lipid profiles. Several large, secondary prevention trials have demonstrated that lowering of lipids can reduce the incidence of future mortality and reinfarction (5–8).
   a. **Diagnostic testing.** All patients who have had an MI should have a complete lipid panel [e.g., total cholesterol, LDL cholesterol, high-density lipoprotein (HDL) cholesterol, and triglycerides] determined within 24 hours of admission. If this is not possible, a random cholesterol level can be measured immediately and a complete lipid profile determined 4 weeks after MI.
   b. **Diet.** Current ACC/AHA guidelines recommend that all patients should start the AHA step II diet (less than 7% of total calories as saturated fat and less than 200 mg/day cholesterol). However, adherence to the step II diet is low (9).
   c. **Therapy.** The National Cholesterol Education Program III **(NCEP III)** recommends a target LDL cholesterol level less than 100 mg/dL, with a goal of less than 70 mg/dL in very-high risk patients (e.g., post-MI) (10–11). The Lipid Treatment Assessment Project found that only 38% of patients with dyslipidemia achieve the NCEP LDL goals, with an even lower rate (18%) among patients with known CAD. Given the results of the Heart Protection Study (HPS), a 3-hydroxy-3-methylglutaryl coenzyme A (HMG-CoA) reductase inhibitor, or **statin, should be initiated in all patients irrespective of LDL levels,** owing to potential benefits in addition to lipid lowering, including anti-inflammatory and antithrombotic effects (12). The Myocardial Ischemia Reduction with Aggressive Cholesterol-Lowering (MIRACL) and Pravastatin or Atorvastatin Evaluation and Infection Therapy (PROVE-IT) trials demonstrate that **early initiation of aggressive lipid-lowering statin therapy** during an ACS is associated with a **reduction in major cardiovascular events, including death** (13–14.) Long-term compliance with statins is improved by in-hospital initiation of therapy (77% vs. 40%) (15). Other therapies include bile-acid sequestrants, niacin, gemfibrozil, moderate alcohol consumption (particularly red wine), and exercise. These may be used in conjunction with statin therapy.
2. **HDL.** Low HDL cholesterol level is an independent risk factor for MI. The NCEP III recommends an HDL level of at least 40 mg/dL. Consideration can be given to therapy with exercise, niacin, or gemfibrozil.

3. **Triglycerides.** Hypertriglyceridemia may be an independent risk factor for CAD, commonly accompanied by low HDL levels or diabetes. Fenofibrate, niacin, or gemfibrozil can be added when triglyceride levels exceed 200 mg/dL, particularly if a low HDL level is concurrent.

C. **Diabetes management.** Aggressive glycemic control in diabetic patients during and after MI results in a reduction in mortality (16). Lifestyle modification and pharmacotherapy with rigorous follow-up are essential for glycemic control and prevention of futre events.

D. **Antiplatelet therapy**

1. All patients who have had an ACS should take **aspirin** upon presentation and continue indefinitely unless there are absolute contraindications. Aspirin therapy after MI results in a mortaliy reduction of 25 lives per 1000 patients treated. Aspirin reduces the rates of vascular mortality, nonfatal stroke, and nonfatal MI. Doses of 75 to 162 mg daily are recommended for all patients presenting with ACS. Patients receiving dual antiplatelet therapy (e.g., aspirin plus thienopyridines) have fewer side effects such as bleeding at lower aspirin doses.
2. **Thienopyridines** (i.e., clopidogrel and ticlopidine) inhibit platelets via adenosine diphosphate antagonissm. Only in patients with true aspirin allergy should thienopyridines be used as an aspirin-alternative therapy. The Clopidogrel versus Aspirin in Patients at Risk of Ischaemic Events (CAPRIE) trial demonstrated significant reduction in ischemic stroke, MI, or vascular death with clopidogrel over aspirin (17). Clopidogrel is favored over ticlopidine because of a greater incidence of hematologic dyscrasia associated with ticlopidine. In the Clopidogrel in Unstable Angina to Prevent Recurrent Events (CURE) trial, the combination of clopidogrel and aspirin was given early for ACS without ST-segment elevation, thereby reducing cardiovascular death, MI, stroke, in-hospital ischemia, and revascularization with benefit seen at 1 year of therapy. The Clopidogrel as Adjunctive Reperfusion Therapy (CLARITY) and Clopidogrel and Metoprolol in Myocardial Infarction Trial (COMMIT) trials demonstrated the benefit of clopidogrel in patients with ST-elevation MI with repurfusion via lytics or PCI (18–19). Opinions vary as to whether to withhold clopidogrel in patients who are likely to proceed to CABG, because of an increased risk of bleeding with surgery. However, in our institution, eligible patients usually receive a 600-mg loading dose of clopidogrel on admission to the emergency room.
3. **Adding other medications,** such as sulfinpyrazone and dipyridamole, has not been shown to be more efficacious than aspirin alone and is not recommended for patients who have had an MI.

E. **Warfarin sodium**

1. **Patients** with a large anterior MI and LV thrombus treated with warfarin are at decreased risk for embolic stroke. Randomized trials do not exist, but many physicians recommend 6 weeks of warfarin therapy for this group of patients. This may assist in stabilization and endothelialization of the thrombus.
2. Data for the routine use of warfarin in conjunction with aspirin for secondary prevention of reinfarction are conflicting. The Combination Hemotherapy and Mortality Prevention (CHAMP) study and the Coumadin Aspirin Reinfarction Study (CARS) trial found no benefit for the addition of warfarin to standard aspirin therapy (23–24). However, combination therapy with aspirin and warfarin decreased infarct-related artery reocclusion and recurrent events in the Antithrombotics in the Prevention of Reocclusion in Coronary Thrombolysis (APRICOT 2) trial (25). The routine use of warfarin after MI is currently not recommended except for other established indications for anticoagulation, such as atrial fibrillation or prosthetic heart valves.

F. **β-Blockers**

1. **Indications.** β-Blockers are anti-ischemic, antihypertensive, antiarrhythmics, and reduce LV wall stress. Mortality reduction results from decreased risk of sudden death, non–sudden cardiac death, and nonfatal infarction. Overall, the use of β-blockers reduces post-MI events by approximately 20%.

a. **The beneficial effects of β-blockers are greatest among patients who are at high risk,** such as patients with anterior infarction, complex ventricular ectopy, advanced age, and LV dysfunction. In the Clopidogrel and Metoprolol in Myocardial Infarction Trial (COMMIT) trial, metoprolol given at presentation significantly reduced re-infarction and ventricular fibrillation in patients with acute MI who were hemodynamically stable; mortality benefit was not significant and probably the result of a net hazard during days 0 to 1 for patients presenting with New York Heart Association (NYHA) class III or IV heart failure (26). Several studies have found that only 50% of patients who sustain an MI actually receive β-blockers. **β-Blockers should be started as soon as possible in hemodynamically stable patients with MI,** and should be continued indefinitely. Moderate LV dysfunction and compensated congested heart failure are not contraindications to β-blocker treatment.

b. **β-Blockers** without intrinsic sympathomimetic activity, such as carvedilol, metoprolol, propranolol, timolol, and atenolol, appear to have the greatest benefit. Reduction in heart rate seems to be important in achieving a mortality benefit.

2. **Contraindications.** Relative contraindications include second- or third-degree heart block, severe asthma, severe chronic obstructive pulmonary disease, severe or decompensated congestive heart failure, heart rate less than 60 beats/min, and severe peripheral vascular disease. In patients with heart rate greater than 100 beats/min, cardiogenic shock should be ruled out by history and examination before administering β-blockers. Diabetes is not an absolute contraindication; however, the dose of the β-blocker may have to be reduced or discontinued if hypoglycemic episodes are frequent or severe

G. **Angiotensin-converting enzyme (ACE) inhibitors**

1. **Indications.** Ventricular remodeling can be attenuated by ACE inhibitors, reducing ventricular dilation and development of congestive heart failure. During infarction, the expression of ACE increases within the myocardium. Several large randomized clinical trials have demonstrated that ACE inhibitors reduce mortality. These trials include Survival and Ventricular Enlargement (SAVE), Acute Infarction Ramipril Efficacy (AIRE), and Trandolapril Cardiac Evaluation (TRACE) (27–29). The greatest benefit was found among patients with large areas of infarction, anterior infarction, and infarction that impaired LV function. **ACE inhibitor therapy should be started in all patients after an acute MI** in the absence of contraindications. ACE inhibitor therapy should be continued for 6 weeks in patients with preserved LV function. Therapy should be continued indefinitely in the setting of LV dysfunction (ejection fraction less than 40%), heart failure, hypertension, or diabetes, although the ACC/AHA guidelines give class IIa recommendation for indefinite therapy in all patients after MI regardless of LV function or comorbities. Angiotensin receptor blocker (ARB) may be substituted if ACE inhibitors are not tolerated. Dual therapy may be considered in the context of persistent symptomatic heart failure with LVEF less than 40% despite single therapy with ACE inhibitor or ARB.

2. **Side effects** include cough, worsening renal function, hypotension, and angioedema.

H. **Calcium channel blockers.** The preferred agent after ACS is a β-blocker unless truely contraindicated. Calcium channel blockers are reserved for patients with **refractory angina** and not recommended for routine use after MI by the ACC/AHA guidelines.. Longer-acting preparations should be used if necessary, whereas short-acting dihydropyridine antagonists should be avoided.

1. **Indications.** The use of calcium channel blockers should be limited to patients with refractory angina or rapid atrial arrhythmias, or to patients with clear contraindications to the use of β-blockers.

2. **Contraindications.** Calcium channel blockers should be avoided in patients with congestive heart failure or high-degree atrioventricular block after an MI. Short-acting dihydropyridine antagonists, such as nifedipine, may increase the risk of death or infarction after MI. Short-acting nifedipine may be especially harmful to

patients with hypotension or tachycardia, and can induce coronary steal or reflex sympathetic activation, which increases myocardial oxygen demand. Verapamil and diltiazem are contraindicated in the care of patients with LV dysfunction or congestive heart failure after MI. These agents may be useful in patients with contraindications to β-blockers who do not have LV dysfunction or congestive heart failure. Few data are available for the effect of the second-generation agents, amlodipine and felodipine, on survival after MI.

I. Estrogen replacement therapy. The Heart and Estrogen/progestin Replacement Study (HERS) found no benefit to hormone replacement therapy as secondary prevention for coronary disease, as therapy was associated with an early increase in death and MI (30). The Women's Health Initiative (WHI) also observed an increased risk of cardiovascular events and breast cancer with hormone replacement therapy (31). Initiation of estrogen for primary and secondary prevention of cardiovascular disease is not recommended and should be discontinued at the time of MI.

J. Antioxidants. Previous epidemiologic studies suggested vitamin E, vitamin C, and beta-carotene were associated with a lower incidence of CAD. The HPS did not demonstrate a mortality or cardiovascular benefit from antioxidant therapy. Several other large randomized trials have failed to show either primary or secondary benefit for other similar vitamin supplementation strategies. The ACC/AHA guidelines, therefore, do not support the use of vitamin C or vitamin E, beta-carotene, or folate with or without B_6 and B_{12}, for primary or secondary prevention.

V. PREVENTION OF SUDDEN CARDIAC DEATH AFTER MI

A. Risk Stratification for Sudden Cardiac Death (SCD)

1. **All patients are at risk** for sudden cardiac death after MI, with the greatest risk encountered during the first year (3% to 5%), most commonly due to ventricular arrhythmias.
2. **Reduced LV function (<40%) remains the best predictor of mortality.** Measurement of LV function soon after MI may reflect myocardial stunning, so echocardiography should be remeasured again at the time of possible implantable cardioverter–defibrillator (ICD) implantation, usually 40 days after MI for primary prevention or 3 months if reperfused after MI, via either PCI or CABG.
3. Several studies have suggested that patients with an occluded infarct-related artery have a markedly worse mortality than patients with a patent artery. In the reperfusion era, this may be less often the case.
4. Many studies have found that patients who have more than six premature ventricular contractions per hour have a 60% increased risk for sudden cardiac death. Patients with ventricular fibrillation or sustained ventricular tachycardia more than 48 hours after MI also are at increased risk. Monomorphic ventricular tachycardia is less likely to be related to the current MI suggesting a preexisting increased risk for SCD.
5. Various techniques have been tested to identify patients at increased risk for sudden cardiac death, but none is sensitive enough to be recommended for routine use. Signal-averaged ECG, heart rate variability, QT-interval dispersion, and baroreflex sensitivity are noninvasive tests, with each test having a low (<30%) positive predictive value. Repolarization alternans (T-wave alternans) appears to have a higher sensitivity and specificity for inducible ventricular arrhythmia during electrophysiologic testing. Still invasive electrophysiologic testing has a low predictive value for future cardiac events. Consequently, **these modalities are not recommended for routine post-MI risk stratification.**

B. Therapy

1. The only medications proven to reduce risk for sudden cardiac death are **β-blockers.** All patients should receive β-blockers after an MI unless absolutely contraindicated.
2. **Other medications. Amiodarone** has multiple antiarrhythmic effects, but is primarily classified as a class III agent. Trials of amiodarone in the care of patients who have had an MI with LVEF less than 40% have shown conflicting results, although a significant reduction in mortality has not been demonstrated. Amiodarone is still the preferred antiarrhythmic therapy for symptomatic or

sustained ventricular arrhythmias in post-MI patients. The prophylactic use of sotalol after MI has been associated with increased mortality (33). The use of type IC antiarrhythmic agents (i.e., encainide, flecainide, and propafenone) after MI is contraindicated (34).

3. The Defibrillator IN Acute Myocardial Infarction Trial (DINAMIT) found no mortality benefit despite a reduction in arrhythmogenic death when ICDs were implanted within 40 days after MI despite LVEF <35%. (35) The Multicenter Automatic Defibrillator Implantation Trial II (MADIT II) investigators and others demonstrated a survival benefit in patients with LV dysfunction and *previous* MI receiving a prophylactic ICD (see Chapter 22) (36). Therefore, at the present time LV function should be evaluated 3 months after ACS to determine whether ICD is indicated. An LVEF <35%, 3 months after ACS is considered class I indication.

VI. THERAPY AND PREVENTION AFTER HOSPITAL TREATMENT

A. **Cardiac rehabilitation programs** seek to achieve treatment goals of exercise, weight loss, proper diet, and smoking cessation.

1. Formal rehabilitation programs use **exercise and patient education** to help patients modify their lifestyles. The benefits of cardiac rehabilitation include improvement in a patient's commitment to treatment, increased functional capacity, and reduced likelihood of readmission for recurrent ischemia. The **social support** offered is associated with a 25% reduction in both cardiac and all-cause mortality. Depression after MI is common, and patients must be screened during follow-up. Depression is also an independent risk factor for mortality, possibly by decreasing commitment to therapy and exercise. There are limited data regarding the safety and efficacy of antidepressant medications in the post-MI setting. In a small study, sertraline was safe and efficacious for the treatment of major depressive disorder after ACS (37).
2. **Home programs and family care.** Although cardiac rehabilitation has been shown to have many benefits, less than one half of patients who have had an MI participate in formal programs. Home programs may be helpful, but they do not provide the social network found in group rehabilitation programs. Because most cardiac arrests after MI occur within 18 months after discharge, family members should be encouraged to learn basic cardiopulmonary resuscitation.

B. Soon after receiving the diagnosis of MI, patients should be counseled regarding **lifestyle modification** to improve weight control, diet, exercise, lipid control, blood pressure, and smoking cessation.

1. Optimal control of hypertension and diabetes should be achieved. The Diabetes Control and Complication Trial (DCCT) and the United Kingdom Prospective Diabetes Study (UKPDS) determined the need for strict glucose control of insulin and non–insulin-dependent diabetes (38–39). Improvement in serum glucose levels decreases the progression of microvascular complications. In both trials, a trend toward decreased microvascular events among the groups that received aggressive treatment was observed.
2. **Weight reduction.** Among adults in the United States, approximately two-thirds of the population, or nearly 130 million persons, are overweight [i.e., body mass index (BMI) >25 kg/m^2). Patients should be encouraged to achieve (or maintain) an ideal body weight. All patients should begin an AHA step II diet to achieve lipid goals. As fewer than 50% of patients comply with the step II diet, many patients will need additional pharmacologic therapy to manage hyperlipidemia.
3. **Resumption of daily activities**
   a. At discharge, all patients who have had an MI should receive information regarding resumption of sexual activity, driving, return to work, and exercise.
   b. **Sexual activity** can be resumed within a week for most patients. **Sildenafil is absolutely contraindicated in patients on concomitant nitrate therapy** and should not be used within 24 hours of nitrate use. **Driving** can also be resumed within a week. Most patients who have had an MI who do not have symptoms can **return to work** within 2 weeks.
   c. A patient's performance on an **exercise test** can be used to generate an activity prescription. Patients who can perform at least 5 METs on a submaximal

exercise test without marked ST-segment depression or development of angina have a good long-term prognosis.

d. Because of the lowered oxygen tension in most commercial aircraft (pressurized to 7500 to 8000 feet), only patients in stable condition should **travel by plane** within the first 2 weeks after MI. They should carry sublingual nitroglycerin and request a wheelchair for transportation.

ACKNOWLEDGMENTS

The authors thank Drs. John H. Chiu and Elaine K. Moen for their contributions to earlier editions of this chapter.

References

1. Morrow DA, Antman EM, Charlesworth A, et al. TIMI risk score for ST-elevation myocardial infarction: a convenient, bedside, clinical score for risk assessment at presentation: an intravenous nPA for treatment of infarcting myocardium early II trial substudy. *Circulation* 2000;102:2031–2037.
2. Marchioli R, Avanzini F, Barzi F, et al. Assessment of absolute risk of death after myocardial infarction by use of multiple-risk-factor assessment equations: GISSI-Prevenzione mortality risk chart. *Eur Heart J* 2001;22:2085–2103.
3. Granger CB, Goldberg RJ, Dabbous O, et al. Predictors of hospital mortality in the Global Registry of Acute Coronary Events. *Arch Intern Med* 2003;63: 2345–2353.
4. Serruys PW, Unger F, Souse JE, et al. Comparison of coronary-artery bypass surgery and stenting for the treatment of multivessel disease. *N Engl J Med* 2001;344:1117–1124.
5. Randomised trial of cholesterol lowering in 4444 patients with coronary heart disease: the Scandinavian Simvastatin Survival Study (4S). *Lancet* 1994;344:1383–1389.
6. Sacks FM, Pfeffer MA, Moye LA, et al. The effect of pravastatin on coronary events after myocardial infarction in patients with average cholesterol levels. Cholesterol and Recurrent Events Trial investigators. *N Engl J Med* 1996;335:1001–1009.
7. Tonkin AM. Management of the Long-Term Intervention with Pravastatin in Ischaemic Disease (LIPID) study after the Scandinavian Simvastatin Survival Study (4S). *Am J Cardiol* 1995;76:107C–112C.
8. Cannon CP, Braunwald E, McCabe CH, et al. Intensive versus moderate lipid lowering with statins after acute coronary syndromes. *N Engl J Med* 2004;350:1495–1504.
9. Pearson TA, Laurora I, Chu H, Kafonek S. The Lipid Treatment Assessment Project (L-TAP): a multicenter survey to evaluate the percentages of dyslipidemic patients receiving lipid-lowering therapy and achieving low-density lipoprotein cholesterol goals. *Arch Intern Med* 2000;160:459–467.
10. Third Report of the National Cholesterol Education Program (NCEP) Expert Panel on Detection, Evaluation, and Treatment of High Blood Cholesterol in Adults (Adult Treatment Panel III) final report. *Circulation* 2002;106:3143–1421.
11. Grundy SM, Cleeman JI, Merz CN, et al. Implications of recent clinical trials for the National Cholesterol Education Program Adult Treatment Panel III guidelines. *Circulation* 2004;110:227–239.
12. MRC/BHF Heart Protection Study of cholesterol lowering with simvastatin in 20,536 high-risk individuals: a randomised placebo-controlled trial. *Lancet* 2002;360:7–22.
13. Schwartz GG, Olsson AG, Ezekowitz MD, et al. Effects of atorvastatin on early recurrent ischemic events in acute coronary syndromes: the MIRACL study: a randomized controlled trial. *JAMA* 2001;285:1711–1718.
14. Cannon CP, Braunwald E, McCabe CH, et al. Intensive versus moderate lipid lowering with statins after acute coronary syndromes. *N Engl J Med* 2004;350:1495–1504.
15. Muhlestein JB, Horne BD, Blair TL, et al. Usefulness of in-hospital prescription of statin agents after angiographic diagnosis of coronary artery disease in improving continued compliance and reduced mortality. *Am J Cardiol* 2001;87:257–261.
16. Malmberg K, Ryden L, Efendic S, et al. Randomized trial of insulin-glucose infusion followed by subcutaneous insulin treatment in diabetic patients with acute myocardial infarction (DIGAMI study): effects on mortality at 1 year. *J Am Coll Cardiol* 1995;26:57–65.
17. A randomised, blinded, trial of Clopidogrel versus Aspirin in Patients at Risk of Ischaemic Events (CAPRIE). CAPRIE Steering Committee. *Lancet* 1996;348:1329–1339.
18. Yusuf S, Zhao F, Mehta SR, et al. Effects of clopidogrel in addition to aspirin in patients with acute coronary syndromes without ST-segment elevation. *N Engl J Med* 2001;345:494–502.
19. Peters RJ, Mehta SR, Fox KA, et al. Effects of aspirin dose when used alone or in combination with clopidogrel in patients with acute coronary syndromes: observations from the Clopidogrel in Unstable angina to prevent Recurrent Events (CURE) study. *Circulation* 2003;108:1682–1687.
20. Sabatine MS, Cannon CP, Gibson CM, et al, for the CLARITY-TIMI 28 investigators. Addition of clopidogrel to aspirin and fibrinolytic therapy for myocardial infarction with ST-segment elevation. *N Engl J Med* 2005;352:1179–1189.
21. COMMIT (ClOpidogrel and Metoprolol in Myocardial Infarction Trial) collaborative group. Addition of clopidogrel to aspirin in 45,852 patients with acute myocardial infarction: Randomised placebo-controlled trial. *Lancet* 2005;366:1607–1621.
22. Sabatine MS, Cannon CP, Gibson CM, et al. Effect of clopidogrel pretreatment before percutaneous coronary intervention in patients with ST-elevation myocardial infarction treated with fibrinolytics. The PCI-CLARITY study. *JAMA* 2005;294:1224–1232.
23. Fiore LD, Ezekowitz MD, Brophy MT, et al, for the Combination Hemotherapy and Mortality Prevention (CHAMP) Study Group. Department of Veterans Affairs Cooperative Studies Program Clinical Trial comparing combined warfarin and aspirin with aspirin alone in survivors of acute myocardial infarction: primary results of the CHAMP study. *Circulation* 2002;105:557–563.

24. Randomised double-blind trial of fixed low-dose warfarin with aspirin after myocardial infarction. Coumadin Aspirin Reinfarction Study (CARS) Investigators. *Lancet* 1997;350:389–396.
25. Brouwer MA, van den Bergh PJ, Aengevaeren WR, et al. Aspirin plus coumarin versus aspirin alone in the prevention of reocclusion after fibrinolysis for acute myocardial infarction: results of the Antithrombotics in the Prevention of Reocclusion in Coronary Thrombolysis (APRICOT)-2 trial. *Circulation* 2002;106:659–665.
26. COMMIT (ClOpidogrel and Metoprolol in Myocardial Infarction Trial) collaborative group. Early intravenous then oral metoprolol in 45,852 patients with acute myocardial infarction: randomised placebo-controlled trial. *Lancet* 2005;366:1622–1632.
27. Pfeffer MA, Braunwald E, Moye LA, et al. Effect of captopril on mortality and morbidity in patients with left ventricular dysfunction after myocardial infarction: results of the Survival and Ventricular Enlargement trial. The SAVE Investigators. *N Engl J Med* 1992;327:669–677.
28. Effect of ramipril on mortality and morbidity of survivors of acute myocardial infarction with clinical evidence of heart failure. The Acute Infarction Ramipril Efficacy (AIRE) Study Investigators. *Lancet* 1993;342:821–828.
29. Kober L, Torpe-Pederson C, Carlsen JE, et al. A clinical trial of the angiotensin-converting-enzyme inhibitor trandolapril in patients with left ventricular dysfunction after myocardial infarction. Trandolapril Cardiac Evaluation (TRACE) Study Group. *N Engl J Med* 1995;333:1670–1676.
30. Hulley S, Grady E, Bush T, et al. Randomized trial of estrogen plus progestin for secondary prevention of coronary heart disease in postmenopausal women. Heart and Estrogen/progestin Replacement Study (HERS) Research Group. *JAMA* 1998;280:605–613.
31. Risks and benefits of estrogen plus progestin in healthy postmenopausal women: principal results from the Women's Health Initiative randomized controlled trial. Women's Health Initiative Investigators. *JAMA* 2002;288:321–333.
32. MRC/BHF Heart Protection Study of antioxidant vitamin supplementation in 20,536 high-risk individuals: a randomised placebo-controlled trial. *Lancet* 2002;360:23–33.
33. Waldo AL, Camm AJ, deRuyter H, et al. Effect of D-sotalol on mortality in patients with left ventricular dysfunction after recent and remote myocardial infarction. The SWORD Investigators: Survival with Oral D-Sotalol. *Lancet* 1996;348:7–12.
34. Hohnloser SH, Kuck KH, Dorian P, et al. Prophylactic use of an implantable cardioverter-defibrillator after acute myocardial infarction. *N Engl J Med* 2004;351:2481–2488.
35. Preliminary report: effect of encainide and flecainide on mortality in a randomized trial of arrhythmia suppression after myocardial infarction. The Cardiac Arrhythmia Suppression Trial (CAST) Investigators. *N Engl J Med* 1989;321:406–412.
36. Moss AJ, Zareba W, Hall WJ, et al, for the Multicenter Automatic Defibrillator Implantation Trial II. Prophylactic implantation of a defibrillator in patients with myocardial infarction and reduced ejection fraction. *N Engl J Med* 2002;346:877–883.
37. Glassman AH, O'Connor CM, Califf RM, et al. Sertraline treatment of major depression in patients with acute MI or unstable angina. *JAMA* 2002;288:701–709.
38. The effect of intensive treatment of diabetes on the development and progression of long-term complications in insulin-dependent diabetes mellitus. The Diabetes Control and Complications Trial Research Group. *N Engl J Med* 1993;329:977–986.
39. Intensive blood-glucose control with sulphonylureas or insulin compared with conventional treatment and risk of complications in patients with type 2 diabetes (UKPDS 33). UK Prospective Diabetes Study (UKPDS) Group. *Lancet* 1998;352:837–853.

Landmark Articles

Bates ER, Califf RM, Stack RS, et al. Thrombolysis and Angioplasty in Myocardial Infarction (TAMI-1) trial: influence of infarct location on arterial patency, left ventricular function and mortality. *J Am Coll Cardiol* 1989;13:12–18.

Randomised trial of intravenous atenolol among 16,027 cases of suspected acute myocardial infarction: ISIS-1. First International Study of Infarct Survival Collaborative Group. *Lancet* 1986;2:57–66.

Key Reviews

Anderson JL, Adams CD, Antman EM, et al. ACC/AHA 2007 guidelines for the management of patients with unstable angina/non-ST-Elevation myocardial infarction: a report of the American College of Cardiology/American Heart Association Task Force on Practice Guidelines. *J Am Coll Cardiol* 2007;50:1–157.

Executive Summary of the Third Report of The National Cholesterol Education Program (NCEP) Expert Panel on Detection, Evaluation, and Treatment of High Blood Cholesterol in Adults (Adult Treatment Panel III). *JAMA* 2001;285:2486–2497.

Relevant Book Chapters

Antman JL. Unstable angina and non-ST elevation MI. In: Zipes DP, et al., eds. *Braunwald's heart disease: a textbook of cardiovascular medicine*, 7th ed. Philadelphia: WB Saunders, 2005.

Anwaruddin S. Mechanical complications of acute myocardial infarction. In: Shishehbor MH, et al., eds. *Management of the patient in the coronary care unit*.

Bhatt DL, Newby LK. Post-myocardial infarction management. In: Topol EJ, ed. *Textbook of cardiovascular medicine*, 3rd ed. Philadelphia: Lippincott Williams & Wilkins, 2006:327–345.

STABLE ANGINA

Amar Krishnaswamy and Samir R. Kapadia

5

I. INTRODUCTION. Angina pectoris, derived from the Greek "ankhon" (strangling) and the Latin "pectus" (chest), is the term used to describe the syndrome of chest discomfort resulting from myocardial ischemia. Angina is characterized as stable or unstable on the basis of symptom pattern.

A. Anginal symptoms are defined as stable if there is no substantial change in symptoms over several weeks. Symptoms of stable angina can fluctuate from time to time, depending on myocardial oxygen consumption, emotional stress, or change in ambient temperature. In general, the clinical definition of stable angina pectoris closely correlates with the stability or quiescence of an atherosclerotic plaque.

B. Angina is said to be unstable when the symptom pattern worsens abruptly (increase in frequency and duration) without an obvious cause of increased myocardial oxygen consumption.

C. For some patients with new-onset angina that has been stable over a few weeks, clear distinction between stable and unstable angina is not possible. These patients can be considered to be in an intermediate stage between unstable and stable angina.

II. CLINICAL PRESENTATION. For most patients with chest pain, the diagnosis of angina pectoris can be made with careful history taking. The presence of risk factors for coronary artery disease (CAD), such as hypertension, diabetes mellitus, smoking, family history, hyperlipidemia, and advanced age increases the likelihood that the chest pain is being caused by myocardial ischemia.

A. Signs and symptoms. The constellation of symptoms characteristic of angina pectoris include the following four cardinal features.

1. Location. Discomfort is commonly located in the retrosternal area with radiation to the neck, shoulders, arms, jaws, epigastrium, or back. In some instances, it involves these areas without affecting the retrosternal area.

2. Relation to a trigger. Symptoms typically are triggered by physical activity, emotional stress, exposure to cold, consuming a heavy meal, or smoking.

a. Some patients will experience the resolution of angina despite continued exertion, which is known as the walk through phenomenon. Others may experience the warm-up phenomenon, in which an initial exertion produces angina, but a similar second exertion does not reproduce anginal symptoms. These circumstances probably result from the recruitment of collateral coronary flow during the initial episode of ischemia.

b. Decubitus angina, which is a less common manifestation, occurs with a change in posture and is believed to be caused by a shift in blood volume. Nocturnal angina, which occurs at night, frequently is associated with nightmares and tachyarrhythmias.

3. Character. Most patients describe angina as vague chest discomfort. They describe squeezing, burning, tightness, choking, heaviness, and occasionally a hot or cold sensation. Many patients do not perceive angina as pain *per se*. Some patients have dyspnea, profound fatigue, weakness, lightheadedness, nausea, diaphoresis, altered mental status, or syncope in the absence of any chest discomfort. These symptoms are often referred to as anginal equivalents.

4. Duration. The chest pain associated with ischemia typically lasts 3 to 5 minutes. Ischemic pain usually does not last more than 30 minutes without causing myocardial infarction (MI). Chest pain triggered by emotional distress tends to last longer than that triggered by exercise. Chest pain that lasts less than 1 minute is unlikely to be of cardiac origin, especially when it is not associated with other typical symptoms or findings.

5. It should be stressed that women may present with symptom constellations that may be atypical in location or quality in comparison to the symptoms described by men, or manifest as anginal equivalents such as nausea or dyspnea.
6. Chest pain is defined as "typical angina" if it consists of characteristic substernal discomfort, is provoked by stress, and is relieved by rest or nitroglycerin. It is considered "atypical" if it involves two or less of the previously mentioned critera.
7. **Classification.** Various classifications are available to assess severity and to predict outcome among patients with angina. The Canadian Cardiovascular Society classification is the most popular (Table 5.1). Other classification systems include the Specific Activity Scale, the Duke Activity Status Index and the Braunwald classification.

B. Physical findings. For patients with a history of chest pain, physical examination helps to identify risk factors for CAD and occult cardiac abnormalities.

1. **The signs associated with a high risk for CAD** include elevated blood pressure or manifestations of hypertensive vascular disease such as retinal arteriopathy, signs of hyperlipidemic conditions including corneal arcus or xanthelasma, and evidence of carotid or other peripheral vascular disease.
2. **Physical examination** performed during an episode of chest pain may reveal rales, an S_3 or S_4 gallop, or a systolic murmur from ischemic mitral regurgitation, all of which generally disappear with resolution of symptoms.

C. Baseline electrocardiogram (ECG)

1. A baseline ECG is **useful for the initial screening** for CAD, although about 60% of patients with chest pain have a normal ECG. Presence of a Q wave or persistent ST depression is associated with an unfavorable outcome. The ECG can also demonstrate other abnormalities, such as left ventricular (LV) hypertrophy, bundle-branch block, and preexcitation syndromes.
2. Information obtained from the ECG is **useful in the assessment of chest pain** and helps to stratify patients who are at risk for an adverse event.
3. ECG at the time of chest pain can also **help to identify the cause of the chest pain.** Transient changes in the T-wave, ST-segment, or conduction patterns point toward a cardiac source of the chest pain. A normal ECG does not exclude ischemia as being the cause of chest pain.

III. DIAGNOSTIC TESTING.

For a patient with stable CAD, investigations are aimed at risk stratification and management of symptoms and unfavorable outcomes.

A. Stress testing. The basic principle of stress testing is to provoke ischemia or produce coronary vasodilation, followed by functional assessment with different

TABLE 5.1 Classification of Angina

Canadian cardiovascular society (CCS) class	Definition	Comment
I	Ordinary physical activity does not cause angina	Angina only with extraordinary exertion at work or recreation
II	Slight limitation of ordinary activity	Angina with walking more than 2 blocks on a level surface or climbing more than 1 flight of stairs at a normal pace
III	Marked limitation of ordinary physical activity	Walking 1 to 2 blocks on a level surface or climbing 1 flight of stairs at a normal pace
IV	Inability to carry on any activity without discomfort	Angina at rest or with minimal activity or stress

systems to detect ischemia. Stress tests can be categorized according to the methods used to provoke and detect myocardial ischemia. The sensitivity and specificity of each test to identify coronary stenosis vary according to the study population, definition of disease, definition of a positive test result, protocol used for the stress testing, and experience of the interpreter. The following parameters provide important prognostic information regarding exercise stress testing.

1. **Methods to induce ischemia.** Exercise is the most physiologically sound and useful method for inducing ischemia. Pharmacologic testing can be used for patients who cannot exercise adequately.
   a. **Exercise**
      (1) **Mechanism.** Exercise increases myocardial contractility, preload, and afterload, causing an increase in myocardial oxygen demand. The increase in oxygen demand is proportional to the rate-pressure product (i.e., heart rate and systolic blood pressure). Because the increased heart rate is primarily responsible for the increased oxygen demand, adequacy of exercise response is judged on the basis of heart rate achieved during exercise. An exercise test is considered adequate if 85% or more of age-predicted maximum heart rate (220 – age) is achieved.
      (2) **Strengths.** Exercise testing provides an objective assessment of functional capacity, which provides useful prognostic information. The prognosis of a patient with stable angina largely depends on the exercise capacity and the stage at which ischemia is induced.
      (3) **Chronotropic incompetence** is defined as an inability to attain 85% of maximum predicted heart rate with maximum effort among patients who have not been treated with negative chronotropic agents; it is a marker for poor prognosis. β-Blockers specifically render the chronotropic incompetence measurement uninterpretable.
      (4) **Heart rate recovery** is defined as the difference between heart rate at peak exercise and 1 minute later, is also a predictor of outcome. A value of 12 beats per minute or less is considered abnormal and is associated with a decrease in survival.
      (5) **The Duke Treadmill Score** (DTS) uses the duration of exercise, the amount of ST-segment deviation during or after exercise, and the amount of angina provoked to predict outcome. The DTS is calculated using the following formula: DTS = exercise time (minutes) – (5 × maximum net ST deviation) – (4 × angina index). (The angina index score is as follows: 0 = no angina, 1 = non-limiting angina, 2 = angina limiting further testing). A DTS of –11 or lower is considered high risk, –10 to 4 is considered moderate risk, and 5 or greater is considered low risk.
      (6) **Limitations.** Exercise testing is not useful for patients with claudication, severe lung problems, arthritis, poor physical fitness, or other conditions that limit the ability to adequately exercise.
   b. **Pharmacologic testing** with adenosine and dipyridamole. Adenosine acts through a specific adenosine receptor to cause coronary microvascular vasodilation, and helps to detect coronary stenosis by causing a discrepancy in myocardial blood flow. The stenosed artery is not able to increase blood flow in the same way as a normal artery. With severe epicardial stenosis, this leads to coronary steal, in which blood is diverted to normal vessels from the stenosed vessel, causing ischemia. Dipyridamole acts by inhibiting cellular uptake of adenosine and leads to similar biologic effects as adenosine but with slower onset, longer duration of action, and higher patient-to-patient variability. Dipyridamole is the most widely used agent because its duration of action is 20 to 30 minutes, which allows for vasodilation that is sufficiently sustained for radionuclide deposition. Dipyridamole is less frequently associated with complete heart block than adenosine.
      (1) **Strengths.** Pharmacologic testing, which depends on coronary flow reserve rather than increasing myocardial oxygen demand, may be a better way of assessing coronary perfusion because changes in flow reserve may

precede development of ischemia. Because discrepancy in flow pattern is easily detected with radionuclide tracers, adenosine and dipyridamole are ideal for use in a nuclear stress laboratory.

(2) Limitations. Heart block (first and second degree) commonly develops with infusion of adenosine. Hemodynamically significant heart block, however, is rare. Because of the short half-life of adenosine, reversal with aminophylline is rarely needed. Both adenosine and dipyridamole can cause bronchospasm, hypotension, chest pain, flushing, dizziness, and dyspnea. Because of its longer duration of action, side effects associated with the use of dipyridamole may necessitate reversal with aminophylline.

Because electrocardiographic changes and wall-motion abnormalities are less likely to occur with these agents, they are not ideal for stress echocardiography. The significance of increased lung uptake of the radionuclide tracer with dipyridamole is unclear. Results of tests involving use of these agents have lower negative predictive value compared with results of exercise stress tests.

c. Pharmacologic testing with dobutamine

(1) Mechanism. Dobutamine and the less commonly used arbutamine (β_1-agonists) increase the rate-pressure product, causing an increase in myocardial oxygen demand. For adequate stress, patients should achieve 85% or more of maximum predicted heart rate. Atropine and handgrip can be used as adjuncts to achieve an adequate heart rate response.

(2) Strengths. This pharmacologic stress mimics physiologic changes during exercise, but the rate-pressure product usually is lower than that from exercise testing. There is evidence that chronotropic incompetence with dobutamine infusion is associated with poor outcome. Electrocardiographic changes with dobutamine infusion have a predictive value similar to that of electrocardiographic changes associated with exercise.

(3) Limitations. Atrial fibrillation, ventricular tachycardia, and hypotension can be precipitated in some patients, leading to premature termination of the test. Patients with aortic stenosis, hypertrophic cardiomyopathy, severe LV dysfunction, and mitral stenosis are at the greatest risk, and dobutamine is typically not used in these settings. β-Adrenergic blockers may interfere with use of this method of stress testing.

2. Methods to assess ischemia

a. Stress ECG

(1) Strengths. Exercise ECG provides useful information about the patients with normal baseline ECGs who are at high risk for CAD. It is less useful when the pretest probability of CAD is low. Stress ECG helps to ascertain whether a patient is at high risk for future adverse events. Patients with results indicative of high risk (Table 5.2) have an annual mortality rate exceeding 5%. Stress ECG is used to identify a safe limit for exercise in patients with stable angina. For some patients, exercise testing is used to

TABLE 5.2 High Risk Predicted with Exercise Electrocardiogram
Inability to complete 6 minutes of Bruce protocol
Early positive test result ($\leq$3 min)
Strongly positive test result ($\geq$2 min ST depression)
Sustained ST depression $\geq$3 minutes after cessation of exercise
Down-sloping ST depression
Ischemia at low ($\leq$120 beats/min) heart rate
Flat or lowered blood pressure response
Serious ventricular arrhythmia at heart rate $\leq$120 beats/min

evaluate the response to antianginal therapy. These patients continue to receive medications, and a maximum capacity stress test is performed to determine the functional benefit of the therapy.

(2) Limitations. The sensitivity and specificity of stress ECG are poor among patients with an abnormal baseline ECG, LV hypertrophy, ventricular pacing, left bundle-branch block (LBBB), or intraventricular conduction disturbance, and among patients taking digitalis or other medications that affect conduction and depolarization. Stress ECG is not indicated for judging the functional significance of a specific stenosis because it does not localize ischemia (except in the presence of ST-segment elevation). The viability of myocardium cannot be determined with stress ECG.

(3) Sensitivity and specificity. For exercise ECG testing, sensitivity ranges from 48% to 94% (mean, 65%), and specificity ranges from 58% to 98% (mean, 70%). Specificity of the test is poor for assessing restenosis. Electrocardiographic changes during dipyridamole or adenosine infusion have high specificity but poor sensitivity. Electrocardiographic changes during dobutamine and arbutamine infusion have sensitivity and specificity similar to those of exercise ECG.

b. Echocardiographic imaging

(1) Strengths. Stress echocardiography is an economical test with good specificity for identifying ischemic territories. This is assessed by the induction of regional wall-motion abnormalities with stress, or dilation of the left LV cavity with stress (which may indicate global ischemia). Stress echocardiography also can be used to assess the severity and significance of valvular heart dysfunction, certain structural heart diseases (i.e., hypertrophic cardiomyopathy), or pulmonary hypertension.

Exercise stress echocardiography should be performed for patients who can exercise. There has been increasing interest in a supine bicycle test, because it allows imaging at peak exercise rather than immediately after peak exercise, thereby increasing the likelihood of detecting ischemia. Exercise-induced wall-motion abnormalities help to identify and localize ischemic myocardium.

If the patient is unable to exercise, a dobutamine stress test can be performed. A biphasic response with dobutamine, in which contractility initially increases with lower doses of dobutamine and then decreases with higher doses, is diagnostic of ischemia. Dobutamine stress testing also is useful for assessing the viability of the myocardium.

At some medical centers, dipyridamole and adenosine stress tests are performed with echocardiographic imaging. Compared with stress echocardiography with exercise or dobutamine or arbutamine, this method is less sensitive in detecting underlying CAD.

(2) Limitations. Results of stress echocardiography are difficult to interpret in some patients with a hypertensive response to exercise and in some patients with severe mitral or aortic regurgitation. Preexisting wall-motion abnormalities further complicate image interpretation. In addition, image quality and experience of the interpreter greatly influence the accuracy of this test. Patients with hypertrophic cardiomyopathy (HCM) and a high resting gradient should not be referred for dobutamine stress echocardiography owing to the risk of hemodynamic compromise and ventricular arrhythmias.

(3) Sensitivity and specificity. Sensitivity to identify flow-limiting coronary stenosis with exercise echocardiography varies from 70% to 90% (mean, about 75%) and specificity ranges from 85% to 95% (mean, about 85%). Dobutamine echocardiography has similar sensitivity and specificity. The sensitivity and specificity of stress echocardiography decrease with poor image quality and among patients with LBBB, small LV cavity, substantial valvular heart disease, hypertensive response to exercise, and dilated cardiomyopathy. The decline in sensitivity and specificity is caused by inadequate visualization of the myocardial walls, wall-motion abnormalities not directly related to ischemia, and premature test termination.

c. Radionuclide imaging

(1) Radiopharmaceuticals. Single positron emission computed tomography (SPECT) can be performed after injection with thallium-201 or technetium (Tc)-99m–labeled radiopharmaceuticals. Positron emission tomography (PET) can be performed after injection of rubidium-82.

(a) The initial distribution of thallium is directly proportional to coronary blood flow, but because thallium quickly redistributes, images must be acquired soon after peak exercise. With Tc-labeled isotopes, repeat injection is necessary to visualize blood flow at rest, but the images do not have to be acquired immediately after exercise.

(b) The Tc-labeled isotopes have a shorter half-life and higher energy than thallium. Five to ten times higher doses can be safely given to patients. This higher dosage improves images for obese patients and women with large breast tissue.

(c) Rubidium has an even shorter half-life and a higher energy than technetium. This results in much less scattering and unwanted attenuation. Furthermore, there is a suggestion that PET imaging provides greater spatial resolution and diagnostic accuracy in comparison to SPECT imaging.

(2) Strengths. Radionuclide vasodilator stress testing provides useful information regarding prognosis for patients with stable angina. It is most useful in patients who cannot exercise, have a pacemaker, have baseline electrocardiographic or echocardiographic abnormalities, or have intermediate exercise stress test results.

(a) An abnormal perfusion scan is associated with 15-fold higher cardiovascular mortality than patients with a normal scan. The mortality rate is higher with an increasing number of segments with abnormal perfusion. The most important segment that determines prognosis is the proximal septum, which corresponds to the proximal left anterior descending (LAD) artery distribution.

(b) Exercise-induced dilation of the left ventricle and increased lung thallium uptake also are predictive of poor outcome. If the scan is normal, there is less than a 1% risk for nonfatal MI or death in the subsequent year.

(3) Limitations. The sensitivity of radionuclide imaging is higher than that of stress echocardiography, but the specificity is lower. Attenuation or artifact from adjoining tissue [i.e., gastrointestinal (GI) tract, breast] can decrease the sensitivity and specificity of radionuclide imaging.

(4) Sensitivity and specificity. The sensitivity to identify flow-limiting coronary stenosis varies from 75% to 90% (mean, about 80%); specificity ranges from 65% to 90% (mean, about 70%). The sensitivity and specificity are decreased among patients with severe obesity, three-vessel disease, and LBBB.

B. Echocardiography is a noninvasive method for analyzing the anatomic structure and function of the heart. It provides useful information in the overall assessment of suspected stable angina.

1. Regional wall-motion abnormalities involving the left ventricle are commonly caused by CAD. Moderate impairment in LV systolic function, LV hypertrophy, and presence of substantial mitral regurgitation are associated with poor outcome. LV systolic function frequently guides the choice of medical therapy.
2. Echocardiography is the test of choice to rule out aortic stenosis or hypertrophic cardiomyopathy. Dobutamine stress echocardiography and PET can be used to assess myocardial viability for patients with angina and considerable LV dysfunction.

C. Magnetic resonance imaging (MRI)

1. MRI has many cardiac applications in addition to ischemia evaluation. It offers information on the aorta, pericardium, thrombi and cardiac masses, congenital heart disease, valvular heart disease, pulmonary artery disease, and myocardial disease. MRI uses gadolinium to evaluate regional wall-motion abnormalities and ejection fraction, which appear to correlate well with radionuclide images. The MRI also can provide direct visualization of the coronary arteries, although CT angiography is much better for this application.
2. MRI is typically used as an adjunct to echocardiography. Its weaknesses include increased cost, lack of portability, and the inability to be used in the growing population of patients with pacemakers and defibrillators.

D. Positron emission tomography (PET)

1. PET imaging allows for the metabolic evaluation of myocardium after injection of fluorine-18 labeled deoxyglucose (FDG). PET detects ischemic myocardium and can differentiate hibernating myocardium from myocardial scarring. Small studies have suggested an improved diagnostic accuracy for PET over SPECT imaging in the assessment of CAD.
2. PET is not able to provide significant anatomic information on structures such as the aorta, pericardium, or cardiac masses.

E. Electron beam computed tomography (EBCT)

1. EBCT is a noninvasive method of obtaining cross-sectional images of the heart in fractions of a second. This decreases motion artifact and allows quantification of small coronary artery calcification. The test is rapid (lasting less than a few minutes), does not require any pharmacologic agents, and provides a "calcium score." For detecting obstructive CAD defined as greater than 50% diameter stenosis, the sensitivity is approximately 90%, and the specificity is 54%.
2. EBCT is not able to provide explicit information on the degree of arterial stenosis. Although the technology allows for a decrease in motion artifact, there is not sufficient detail to accurately quantify and localize atherosclerotic lesions. EBCT is useful as a screening tool for CAD with abnormal findings leading to further risk factor modification and cardiovascular risk assessment.

F. Multidetector computed tomography (MDCT)

1. **Strengths.** The acquistion of multiple slices simultaneously with coronary CT angiography (CCTA) allows for evaluation of the epicardial coronary tree using a noninvasive approach. The sensitivity of CCTA for assessing coronary stenosis approaches 97% with a specificity of 86% when using 64-slice machines. With technologic advances allowing a greater number of slices to be acquired simultaneously, the accuracy of this study is expected to increase. Importantly, the negative predictive value of CCTA is 99%, with an optimal study and appropriate patient selection.
2. **Limitations.** For optimal image quality, the heart rate must be between 60 and 70 beats per minute, which may be achieved through the use of β-blockers at the time of imaging if tolerated by the patient. The patient must sustain a breath-hold for 15 to 20 seconds during imaging. Severe coronary artery calcification or previous coronary stent placement may significantly detract from image quality, rendering the study uninterpretable. Larger stents may be grossly evaluated for patency, but accurate quantification for in-stent restenosis in positions distal to the left main coronary artery is not always feasible.

G. Coronary angiography

1. **Strengths.** Coronary angiography is the standard for anatomic assessment of coronary arterial stenosis and provides important prognostic information.
   a. Risk for MI increases with incremental stenosis. Patients with more than 75% stenosis involving at least one coronary artery have a lower survival rate than patients with 25% to 50% or less than 25% stenosis. Even for mild stenosis, risk for MI is markedly higher than for no stenosis.
   b. The severity of lesions demonstrated with angiography is not predictive of plaque stability; two-thirds of patients with acute MI have stenosis of less than

50% diameter at the site of plaque rupture before MI. It is possible, however, to assess plaque instability on the basis of angiographic characteristics or morphologic features of the lesion.

(1) Eccentric lesions with narrow necks, overhanging edges, or scalloped borders (type II plaques) are more unstable than concentric lesions with smooth borders (type I lesions).

(2) Lesion roughness (i.e., irregular borders) is predictive of future infarction.

(3) The morphologic characteristics of the plaque help to judge the feasibility and risk of percutaneous or surgical intervention.

c. Ventriculography performed at the time of selective coronary angiography adds an important dimension to risk stratification by providing an index of LV systolic function and regional wall-motion characteristics.

2. Indications. In the management of stable angina, use of angiography is variable. An American College of Cardiology and American Heart Association (ACC/AHA) task force classified the indications for coronary angiography into three categories. The relevant indications in the context of stable angina are presented in Table 5.3.

3. Limitations. Coronary angiography underestimates plaque burden, possibly because of vascular remodeling and the diffuse nature of the disease. Coronary angiography does not depict intraluminal plaque burden and does not show coronary flow reserve. Adjunctive use of intravascular ultrasonography greatly facilitates investigation of hazy areas on coronary angiograms, which may be caused by calcium, thrombus, severe eccentric lesion, or dissection. Intravascular ultrasonography (IVUS) can also assess positive and negative remodeling, which has been shown to correlate with stable and unstable syndromes.

H. Intravascular ultrasonography allows visualization of the cross-sectional image of coronary arteries. This modality helps to quantitate plaque area, artery size, and

TABLE 5.3 Indications for Coronary Angiography in Stable Angina

Class I (general agreement among cardiologists)
Severe anginal symptoms (CCS class III or IV) with optimal medical therapy
Stress testing indicators of high-risk coronary disease
Survivors of sudden cardiac arrest
Symptoms of congestive heart failure with angina
Clinical predictors of severe coronary artery disease
Class II (frequently used but controversial)
Symptoms of angina and positive stress test
Inadequate information from noninvasive testing
Severe angina that improves to mild/moderate angina with medical therapy
Anginal symptoms and intolerance of medical therapy
Asymptomatic patients with positive stress test
Patients who are unable to be evaluated noninvasively
Patients with an occupation that involves an unusual degree of risk
Patients suspected of ischemic symptoms caused by nonatherosclerotic coronary disease (i.e., vasculitis, radiation coronary disease)
Suspicion of coronary vasospasm with the need for provocative testing
Suspicion of left main or three-vessel coronary disease
Recurrent hospitalization for chest pain and need for definitive coronary evaluation
Patients with intermediate or high probability of CAD and a desire for definitive diagnosis
Class III (unjustified use of angiography)
Mild symptoms that resolve with medical therapy
Patients who would not undergo revascularization
Patients with low probability of CAD and a desire for definitive diagnosis

CAD, coronary artery disease; CCS, Canadian Cardiovascular Society.

luminal stenosis; assess hazy areas on coronary angiograms, questionable areas of stenosis, and extent of stenosis; and sometimes determine the calcium content of a plaque. Hypodense areas in a plaque may correlate with high lipid content, which may indicate fast-growing or potentially unstable plaque. This information can help to assess the need and options for therapy. This modality does not, however, have a role in routine evaluation of patients with stable angina, due to the invasive nature of the test.

I. Invasive functional assessment. Invasive assessment of the functional significance of stenosis can be made by means of coronary blood flow measurement with intracoronary Doppler ultrasound and direct measurement of a pressure gradient across a stenosis.

1. With the help of a small transducer mounted on a guidewire, coronary blood flow can be measured by means of a fixed sample volume and pulsed Doppler.
   a. In the left coronary artery, most coronary flow occurs during diastole. In normal arteries, a ratio of proximal-to-distal flow velocity approaching 1 is considered normal. In the presence of coronary stenosis, coronary blood flow becomes mainly systolic because the diastolic component of the flow is jeopardized first.
   b. Three indices can help identify physiologically important stenoses:
      (1) Diastolic-to-systolic average peak coronary flow velocity in a ratio of less than 1.8 distal to the obstruction
      (2) A proximal-to-distal average peak coronary flow velocity ratio more than 1.7
      (3) Coronary flow reserve (i.e., increase in coronary flow with adenosine, which is administered after intracoronary nitroglycerin) with a less than twofold increase in peak velocity
2. **Direct measurement of pressure gradients** can be accomplished with a transducer mounted on a catheter. Ratio of mean pressure distal and proximal to the lesion after maximum vasodilation (fraction flow reserve, or FFR) of less than 0.75 indicates a hemodynamically significant lesion. These techniques supplement angiography in determining the functional significant of an angiographic stenosis. The importance of this invasive assessment in predicting the patient's overall risk for future cardiac events is similar to that of a positive stress test.

J. Holter monitoring

1. After MI, increased ventricular ectopy is predictive of increased cardiovascular morbidity and mortality. This association is less important among patients with stable angina without prior MI, and routine Holter testing for risk stratification is not indicated. However, no medical treatment aimed at suppressing ventricular ectopy has been shown to improve outcome.
2. When silent ischemia is suspected, there is probably a role for Holter monitoring to identify these clinically asymptomatic events. Silent ischemia detected by Holter monitoring has been correlated indirectly with outcome. Ischemia detected by this method should call for more aggressive treatment and evaluation.

IV. THERAPY.

The goals of therapy are to prevent cardiovascular morbidity and mortality and to improve quality of life.

A. Priority of therapy. Medical therapy, percutaneous coronary intervention (PCI), and coronary artery bypass grafting (CABG) have been shown to control symptoms and improve exercise time to ischemia, but effectiveness varies. Medical therapy and CABG improve cardiovascular mortality, morbidity, and quality of life. PCI has been shown to improve anginal symptoms but has not yet been shown to decrease mortality.

B. Pharmacologic therapy

1. **Platelet inhibitors**
   a. The Antiplatelet Trialists' Collaboration was a meta-analysis that included approximately 100,000 patients from 174 trials involving antiplatelet therapy. This trial showed that aspirin (acetylsalicylic acid, ASA) reduced the rate

of stoke, MI, and death among high-risk patients, including those with stable angina without previous MI. A recent systematic review confirms that, while optimal dosing is controversial, there is general support in the literature for limiting the dose of ASA to 75 to 81 mg daily. Approximately 5% to 10% of patients with CAD have aspirin resistance, defined as a lack of decrease in platelet function associated with aspirin use. Aspirin resistance has been shown to result in higher thrombotic events in people with peripheral vascular disease. Patients who demonstrate increased platelet reactivity despite aspirin therapy have been found to have increased risks for stroke, MI, and vascular death compared with aspirin responders.

b. Among patients with true allergy or intolerance to aspirin, ticlopidine and clopidogrel have been shown to decrease the frequency of fatal and nonfatal vascular events in peripheral, cerebral, and coronary vessel disease.

(1) Clopidogrel is second-line therapy in patients unable to tolerate aspirin. In high-risk patients with prior cardiac surgery or ischemic events, the use of clopidogrel as monotherapy, or in addition to aspirin, is beneficial. The use and duration of dual antiplatelet therapy with clopidogrel and aspirin in the setting of drug-eluting stent (DES) implantation is currently under intense review, although general consensus at this time is to continue therapy for at least 12 to 24 months, and potentially indefinitely. Clopidogrel is usually well tolerated and has few side effects.

(2) In the initial analysis of the CHARISMA trial, performed on a large group of patients included with either prior cardiovascular events or multiple cardiovascular risk factors, there was no benefit to the use of dual-antiplatelet therapy over aspirin alone in preventing myocardial infarction or death. More recent analysis of pre-specified subgroups, which included higher-risk patients only (such as those with prior MI), did show a decrease in cardiovascular events for the group receiving clopidogrel in addition to aspirin. This suggests that in an appropriate group of patients who require a more intense antiplatelet regimen, the addition of thienopyridine therapy to aspirin, may be beneficial.

(3) Ticlopidine has been associated with side effects such as neutropenia, thrombocytopenia, and pancytopenia, and with the development of thrombotic thrombocytopenic purpura. Blood count monitoring is necessary. Ticlopidine is rarely used because of its side-effect profile.

2. Lipid-lowering agents. Among patients with established CAD, lipid-lowering therapy has demonstrated marked reduction in disease progression and risk for subsequent cardiovascular events. Statins are potent inhibitors of 3-hydroxy-3-methylglutaryl coenzyme reductase (HMG-CoA reductase), and have proven themselves as indispensable therapeutic agents in both primary and secondary prevention of cardiovascular events and death. They are the most effective medical therapy for lowering levels of low-density lipoprotein (LDL), and have also been shown to upregulate nitric oxide (NO) synthase, decrease expression of endothelin-1 mRNA, improve platelet function, and decrease production of detrimental free radicals; all of which promote normal endothelial function.

a. Indications. The Scandinavian Simvastatin Survival Study (4S), Cholesterol and Recurrent Events (CARE), Long-Term Intervention with Pravastatin in Ischemic Disease (LIPID), and Heart Protection Study (HPS) trials have provided convincing evidence that in patients with evidence of vascular disease with normal or elevated cholesterol levels, statins decrease mortality, the rate of MI, and the need for CABG.

b. Effectiveness. Recent studies have shown that in patients with stable CAD (TNT) or post-ACS (PROVE IT-TIMI-22), aggressive lipid lowering to an LDL goal of 70 mg/dL decreases the risks of cardiovascular death, MI, and stroke compared to patients treated to an LDL goal of 100 mg/dL. There is also a suggestion that aggressive statin use results in a mild degree of plaque regression as measured by IVUS.

c. Choice of agents. Because the benefits of lipid-lowering medication appear to be caused by a class effect of HMG-CoA reductase inhibitors, any statin that is effective and economical can be used. The quantification of lipoprotein(a) [Lp(a)], fibrinogen, apolipoprotein (apo A), and apo B100 is investigational. Bile acid sequestrants primarily reduce LDL cholesterol and should not be used in patients with triglyceride levels higher than 300 mg/dL, because these agents may exacerbate hypertriglyceridemia. Nicotinic acid reduces LDL and triglyceride levels, and is the most effective of the available lipid-lowering medications at increasing high-density lipoprotein (HDL) level. It is also the only agent that lowers Lp(a). Fibric acid derivatives are most effective against hypertriglyceridemia; they raise HDL level modestly and have little effect on LDL. They are the first line of treatment in patients with triglyceride levels higher than 400 mg/dL. Omega-3 fatty acids are used to treat hypertriglyceridemia that is refractory to niacin and fibric acid therapy.

(1) Current evidence supports aggressive lowering of LDL cholesterol levels in patients with established coronary disease, or CAD equivalents, to a goal of 70 mg/dL (class IIa). A level of HDL cholesterol >45 mg/dL, and triglycerides <150 mg/dL are secondary goals of dietary, lifestyle, and pharmacologic therapy.

(2) The side effects of statin therapy, including myositis and hepatitis are quite rare. Blood tests are not necessary for routine follow-up of patients on these medications, and should only be measured based upon clinical suspicion of an untoward effect.

3. Nitrates (Table 5.4)

a. Mechanism of action. Nitrates decrease cardiac workload and oxygen demand by means of reducing preload and afterload of the left ventricle. They also redistribute blood flow to the ischemic subendocardium by means of decreasing LV end-diastolic pressure and vasodilation of epicardial vessels. Nitrates may even inhibit platelet aggregation.

b. Evidence for effectiveness. Nitrates can decrease exercise-induced myocardial ischemia, alleviate symptoms, and increase exercise tolerance in patients with stable angina.

TABLE 5.4 Nitrates

Medication	Route of administration	Each dose	Frequency
Nitroglycerin (glyceryl trinitrate, Nitro-Bid, Nitrostat, Nitro-Dur)	Sublingual tablet	0.15–0.6 mg	As needed
	Sublingual spray	0.4 mg	As needed
	Sustained-release capsule	2.5–9.0 mg	Every 6–12 h
	Ointment (topical)	0.5–2 inches (1.25–5 cm)	Every 4–8 h
	Disk (patch)	1 disk (2.5–15 mg)	Every 24 h
	Intravenous	5–400 μg/min	Continuous
	Buccal tablet	1 mg	Every 3–5 h
Isosorbide dinitrate (Isordil, Sorbitrate, Dilatrate-SR)	Sublingual tablet	2.5–10 mg	Every 2–3 h
	Chewable tablet	5–10 mg	Every 2–3 h
	Oral tablet	10–40 mg	Every 6 h
	Sustained-release tablet	40–80 mg	Every 8–12 h
Isosorbide-5-mononitrate (Imdur, Ismo)	Sublingual tablet	10–40 mg	Every 12 h
	Sustained release	60 mg	Every 24 h
Erythrityl tetranitrate (Cardilate)	Sublingual tablet	5–10 mg	As needed
	Tablet	10 mg	Every 8 h

(1) Adding nitrates to an optimal β-blocker regimen does not improve frequency of anginal episodes, glycerol trinitrate consumption, exercise duration, or duration of silent ischemia.

(2) In some small studies, the efficacy of nitrates in reducing anginal episodes was increased with concomitant use of angiotensin-converting enzyme (ACE) inhibitors.

(3) No study has shown survival benefit with the use of nitrates to treat patients with chronic stable angina.

c. Selection of preparations. Because nitrates have a fast onset of action, a sublingual tablet or oral spray offers immediate relief of an anginal episode.

(1) For short-term prophylaxis (up to 30 minutes), nitroglycerin tablets can be used when activities known to precipitate angina are anticipated. Timing and frequency of the doses can be individualized according to the diurnal rhythm of anginal episodes. A nitrate-free interval of about 8 hours is adequate for preventing tolerance.

(2) Use of long-acting medications and transcutaneous delivery systems improve compliance but still necessitate a nitrate-free interval.

d. Side effects. Oral nitrates should be taken with meals to prevent heartburn.

(1) Headache is common and can be severe. Severity usually decreases with continued use and often can be controlled by decreasing the dose.

(2) Transient episodes of flushing, dizziness, weakness, and postural hypotension can occur, but these effects usually are abrogated by positioning and other procedures that facilitate venous return.

(3) Glaucoma is not precipitated by the use of nitrates.

e. Drug interactions

(1) Hypotension can occur with the use of other vasodilators, such as ACE inhibitors, hydralazine, or calcium channel blockers. Concurrent use of sildenafil (Viagra) and nitrates can lead to severe hypotension and, therefore, is absolutely contraindicated.

(2) Extremely high intravenous doses ($>$200 μg/min) of nitrates can displace heparin from antithrombin III and cause relative heparin resistance. Frequent measurement of partial thromboplastin time (PTT) is necessary when the nitroglycerin infusion rate is high and frequently changed.

f. Controversies

(1) **Tolerance.** Sustained therapy attenuates the vascular and antiplatelet effects of nitrates. Although the basis for this phenomenon of nitrate tolerance is not completely understood, sulfhydryl depletion, neurohormonal activation, and increased plasma volume are likely involved. Administration of *N*-acetylcysteine, ACE inhibitors, or diuretics does not consistently prevent nitrate tolerance. Intermittent nitrate therapy is the only way to avoid nitrate tolerance.

(2) **Rebound.** Intermittent use of nitrates is not associated with serious rebound of angina among patients taking maintenance therapy with β-blockers. Dosing to allow for a longer nitrate-free interval also is not associated with rebound.

4. β-Blockers (Table 5.5)

a. Mechanism of action. Blocking the β_1-adrenergic receptors in the heart decreases the rate-pressure product and oxygen demand. Decreased tension in the LV wall allows favorable redistribution of blood flow from the epicardium to endocardium.

(1) Coronary vasospasm is rare from the β_2-receptor blocking effect, but use of β-blockers should be avoided among patients with known, active vasospasm.

(2) β-Blockers have a variable degree of membrane-stabilizing effect.

TABLE 5.5 β-Blockers

Compound	Daily dose (mg)	Frequency	Excretion	Lipid solubility	Intrinsic sympathomimetic activity	Membrane stabilization
			Selective β_1-blockers			
Metoprolol						
Short-acting	50–400	Every 12 h	Liver	Moderate		
Long-acting		Every 24 h			None	Possible
Atenolol	25–200	Every 24 h	Kidney	None	None	None
Acebutolol	200–600	Every 12 h	Kidney	Moderate	Low	Low
Betaxolol	20–40	Every 24 h	Kidney		Low	
			Nonselective β ($\beta_1+\beta_2$) blockers			
Propranolol	80–320	Every 4–6 h	Liver			
Long-acting		Every 12 h		High	None	Moderate
Nadolol	80–240	Every 24 h	Kidney	Low	None	None
Timolol	15–45	Every 12 h	Liver	Moderate	None	None
Pindolol	15–45	Every 8–12 h	Kidney	Moderate	Moderate	Possible
Labetalol[a]	600–2400	Every 6–8	Liver	None	None	Possible
Carvedilol[a]						
Short-acting	25–50	Every 12 h	Liver	Moderate	None	Possible
Long-acting	10–80	Every 24 h				

[a]Also a potent α_1-antagonist.

b. Evidence for effectiveness. β-Blockers decrease mortality after MI. The mortality benefit is not proved among patients with stable angina without prior MI, although symptomatic improvement is well documented.

c. Side effects. The most important side effects are related to blockade of β_2-receptors. However, data show that some of the side effects may occur less frequently than previously believed, and potentially lifesaving therapy should be offered to those at greatest risk for adverse events.

(1) Bronchoconstriction, masking of symptoms caused by hypoglycemic reaction among patients with diabetes, exacerbation of symptoms of peripheral vascular disease, and central nervous system (CNS) side effects such as somnolence, lethargy, depression, and vivid dreaming are well documented. The CNS side effects are thought to be related to the lipid solubility of these compounds.

(2) Symptomatic bradycardia and precipitation of heart failure are concerns for patients with a diseased conduction system or preexisting heart failure, respectively.

(3) Decreased libido, impotence, and reversible alopecia can be a problem for some patients.

(4) β-Blockers adversely alter lipid profile by increasing LDL cholesterol and decreasing HDL cholesterol.

d. Drug interactions. Severe bradycardia and hypotension can occur with concomitant use of some calcium channel blockers.

e. Selection of preparations. Cardioselectivity, lipid solubility, mode of excretion, and frequency of dosing are the main consideration when selecting a particular agent. Intrinsic sympathomimetic activity is not a clinically important factor in the choice of a medication, although benefits in patients with CAD have been decreased with agents having intrinsic sympathomimetic activity.

f. Effect on lipids. The clinical significance of lipid abnormalities associated with β-blockers is unclear. β-Blockers have been associated with a decline in HDL level and a rise in triglycerides level. β-Blockers can improve survival among patients in New York Heart Association (NYHA) class I or II heart failure and angina. The condition of a patient with NYHA class III or IV disease should be stabilized before β-blocker therapy is instituted.

5. Calcium channel blockers (Table 5.6)

a. Mechanism of action. These agents block calcium entry into vascular smooth muscle cells and cardiac cells by inhibiting calcium channels, but they do not affect the regulation of intracellular calcium release. The result is decreased contractions of muscle cells.

(1) The four types of calcium channels are L, T, N, and P.

(2) The T-type calcium channels are located in the atria and sinoatrial node and affect the phase I of depolarization.

(3) L-Type channels contribute to entrance of calcium into the cell during phase III of the action potential.

(4) The N and P types of channels are present mainly in the nervous system.

(5) The three main groups of calcium channel blockers are dihydropyridines (e.g., nifedipine), benzothiazipines (e.g., diltiazem), and phenylalkylamines (e.g., verapamil).

(6) The dihydropyridines bind to the extracellular portion of the L channels at a specific site. They do not bind to the T channels and do not have a negative chronotropic effect. Because of their extracellular site of action, dihydropyridines do not inhibit receptor-induced intracellular calcium release.

(7) Verapamil binds to the intracellular part of the L channel and inhibits the T channel. Intracellular calcium release is inhibited by verapamil because of its intracellular binding site, and reflex sympathetic activation is less effective. Use dependence occurs with verapamil because open channels are needed for transport of the drug into the intracellular binding site.

TABLE 5.6 Calcium Channel Blockers

Compound	Each dose (mg)	Frequency	Vasodilation	Sinoatrial node inhibition	Atrioventricular node inhibition	Negative inotrope
Nifedipine	30–120	Every 8 h	5	1	0	1
Nifedipine XL (Procardia)	30–180	Every 24 h				
Diltiazem	30–90	Every 6–8 h	3	5	4	2
Diltiazem CD (Cardizem)	120–300	Every 24 h				
Verapamil	40–120	Every 6–8 h	4	5	5	4
Verapamil SR (Calan, Isoptin)	120–240	Every 12 h				
Amlodipine (Norvasc)	2.5–10	Every 24 h	4	1	0	1
Felodipine (Plendil)	5–20	Every 24 h	5	1	0	0
Bepridil (Vascor)	200–400	Every 24 h	4	4	4	5
Isradipine (DynaCirc)	2.5–10	Every 24 h	4	4	0	0
Nicardipine (Cardene)	10–20	Every 8 h	5	1	0	0

0, No activity; 5, most potent effect. Intermediate numbers suggest intermediate potency of effects.

In stable angina, verapamil helps by improving rate pressure product and increasing oxygen delivery from coronary vasodilation.

b. Evidence of effectiveness. Numerous placebo-controlled, double-blind trials have shown that calcium channel blockers decrease the number of anginal attacks and attenuate exercise-induced depression of ST segments.

(1) Studies comparing the efficacy of β-blockers and calcium channel blockers in the management of stable angina in which death, infarction, and unstable angina were used as endpoints showed calcium channel blockers to be as effective as β-blockers.

(2) Increased mortality caused by short-acting nifedipine among patients with CAD was demonstrated in a retrospective study and meta-analysis. If the use of nifedipine is contemplated, a long-acting preparation in conjunction with β-blocker therapy is the safer approach. The mechanism of increased mortality is unclear, but reflex tachycardia and coronary steal phenomenon are potential explanations.

c. Side effects. The most common side effects are hypotension, flushing, dizziness, and headache. Because a negative inotropic effect can precipitate heart failure, the use of calcium channel blockers to treat patients with impaired LV function is relatively contraindicated. Conduction disturbances and symptomatic bradycardia occur with the use of compounds that have a marked inhibitory effect on the sinoatrial and atrioventricular nodes. Bepridil is known to prolong QTc, and QT monitoring is necessary when this medication is used.

d. Drug interactions. Digitalis levels are increased by calcium channel blockers. The use of these drugs is contraindicated in the presence of digitalis toxicity.

e. Selection of preparations. Calcium channel blockers have a variable negative inotropic effect.

(1) Amlodipine is most likely to be tolerated by patients with compensated heart failure. In decompensated heart failure, all calcium channel blockers should be avoided. Amlodipine is the only calcium channel blocker approved for angina by the U.S. Food and Drug Administration (FDA).

(2) Patients with conduction disturbances should take agents with minimal effects on the conduction system. Longer-acting preparations minimize the risk for precipitation of angina caused by reflex tachycardia.

6. ACE inhibitors. The rationale for using ACE inhibitors to manage chronic stable angina comes from post-MI and heart failure trials that demonstrated a significant reduction in ischemic events with the use of ACE inhibitors.

a. It is possible that ACE inhibitors, by decreasing mainly the preload and, to some extent, afterload, decrease myocardial oxygen demand and help in the management of chronic stable angina. The Heart Outcomes Prevention Evaluation (HOPE) trial in high-risk patients with CAD, stroke, diabetes, and peripheral vascular disease showed that ramipril was associated with a significant reduction in death, MI, and stroke in this high-risk population. A recent meta-analysis found that ACE inhibitors reduce the risk of these outcomes even in patients with atherosclerosis who do not have evidence of systolic dysfunction.

b. The relative efficacy of different ACE inhibitors for relieving ischemia has not been well studied.

c. Serious side effects of ACE inhibitors include cough, hyperkalemia, and decreased glomerular filtration rate. They are contraindicated in the care of patients with hereditary angioedema or patients with bilateral renal artery stenosis.

7. Hormone replacement therapy (HRT). The lipid profiles of women change unfavorably after menopause. LDL, total cholesterol, and triglyceride levels increase, and HDL level decreases. All these changes have an adverse effect on cardiovascular morbidity and mortality. Several large case-controlled and prospective cohort studies suggested that the postmenopausal use of estrogen alone or in combination with medroxyprogesterone acetate has a favorable effect on lipid profile and cardiovascular events. However, the Women's Health Initiative (WHI) showed an increased risk of cardiovascular and cerebrovascular events in postmenopausal women receiving HRT. Another randomized trial quantifying coronary atherosclerosis angiographically showed negative results with respect to estrogen use. As a result, it has been postulated that the previously shown benefits might have been caused by the "healthy user" effect, and the use of HRT for primary prophylaxis against cardiovascular events is not recommended.

a. **Benefits of use.** Although the use of estrogen has shown an increase in cardiovascular events, it is associated with some specific favorable findings. The positive effects of estrogen use include maintenance of normal endothelial function, reduction in levels of oxidized LDL, alteration in vascular tone, maintenance of normal hemostatic profile, a favorable effect on plasma glucose levels, reduction of osteoporotic fractures, and a reduction in menopausal symptoms.
b. **Side effects** include bleeding, nausea, and water retention. Because doses of estrogen are small, these side effects are uncommon. For patients with an intact uterus, routine gynecologic examination is mandatory for cancer surveillance. The risk of breast cancer is also increased with the use of HRT, and routine screening is beneficial.

8. **Antioxidants.** The role of vitamins A, C, and E is unclear in patients with CAD.
   a. The initial observational studies involving daily vitamin E supplementation reducing the risk for cardiovascular events among patients with proven atherosclerotic heart disease appeared promising. However, when vitamin E was tested in a randomized fashion, no benefit to its use was proved. There are also data suggesting that vitamin E may attenuate the effect of statins. Vitamins A, C, and E are not recommended for the secondary prevention of cardiovascular events.
   b. Data are lacking about vitamins A and C. Most of the available information suggests no benefit of taking supranormal doses of these vitamins. Vitamin A does not prevent LDL oxidation, even though it binds to LDL molecules. Because it is water soluble, vitamin C does not bind to the LDL molecule. These two vitamins are not recommended for prevention of progression of atherosclerosis.
   c. The role of probucol, a lipid-lowering medication with antioxidant properties, is under investigation.
9. **Ranolazine**
   a. Ranolazine has recently been shown to work by inhibiting the late sodium channel in myocytes, which can otherwise remain open in pathologic states such as ischemia and heart failure. By reducing late sodium entry into myocytes, ranolazine causes reduced sodium-dependent calcium entry into the cytosol. This downstream reduction in intracellular calcium levels is thought to reduce diastolic stiffness, thereby improving diastolic blood flow and reducing ischemia and angina. Earlier studies had suggested that ranolazine's effects were primarily through its impact on fatty acid metabolism; however, the weight of evidence now suggests that late sodium-channel inhibition is its primary mechanism.
   b. Numerous randomized studies of ranolazine, with or without background antianginal therapy, have shown a benefit in patients with stable angina with respect to frequency of anginal attacks, exercise duration, time to ST-segment depression on treadmill testing, and use of sublingual nitroglycerin.
   c. **Side effects.** Dizziness, headache, and GI intolerance are the most common side effects noted. Prolongation of the QT interval has been reported, especially in patients with hepatic or liver dysfunction due to decreased metabolism. Prolonged QT interval at baseline or during treatment follow-up is a contraindication to its use.

d. **Drug interactions.** Inhibitors of CYP 3A4, such as azole antifungals, nondihydropyridine calcium-channel blockers, macrolide antibiotics, protease inhibitors, and grapefruit juice should not be used concommitantly due to inhibition of ranolazine metabolism.

10. **Newer pharmacologic approaches**

a. Therapy with direct infusion of vascular endothelial growth factor (VEGF) and basic fibroblast growth factor (bFGF) proteins have been shown to increase collateral blood flow in animal models. Studies are underway to investigate the role of these agents in improving collateral blood flow to the ischemic myocardium of patients with angina. Although early results are encouraging, long-term risks and benefits of such therapy remain largely unknown.

b. Approaches involving the use of gene therapy to cause overexpression of these endogenous growth factors to control the development of collateral blood vessels have been proposed. These approaches are under investigation.

11. **Enhanced external counterpulsation (EECP)** has become a treatment option for patients with stable angina.

a. EECP involves the intermittent compression of the lower extremities in an effort to increase diastolic pressure and augment coronary blood flow. Three sets of balloons are wrapped around the lower legs, lower thighs, and upper thighs, with precise cuff inflation and deflation gated with the ECG. The lower cuffs are inflated at the start of diastole as represented by the beginning of the T wave, and simultaneous deflation of all three chambers is triggered just before systole at the onset of the P wave.

b. In patients with refractory angina, clinical trials have demonstrated improvements in exercise tolerance, reduction in anginal symptoms, decreased use of nitroglycerin, and improvements in objective measures of ischemia as measured by thallium scintigraphy. These benefits are maintained at 2 years of follow-up.

C. **Percutaneous Coronary Intervention.** The effectiveness of PCI to control symptoms in chronic stable angina and to prevent death or MI has been compared with medical management and CABG.

1. **Compared with medical treatment**

a. The Angioplasty Compared with Medicine (ACME) trial compared PCI with medical therapy in approximately 200 patients with single-vessel and multivessel CAD. Patients with single-vessel CAD showed better symptomatic relief at 6 months with PCI but no difference in mortality or MI. Patients with two-vessel CAD had no significant differences in symptoms, mortality, or MI.

b. The Medicine, Angioplasty or Surgery Study (MASS) randomized approximately 200 patients with proximal LAD artery disease to medical therapy, PCI, or CABG. This study demonstrated no difference in the primary endpoint (i.e., death, MI, or refractory angina necessitating revascularization). Patients randomized to CABG had a lower incidence of events compared with the other two groups, driven by a decrease in repeat revascularization procedures.

c. The Randomized Intervention Treatment of Angina trial (RITA-2) randomized more than 1000 patients with stable angina to medical therapy or PCI. After 2.7 years of follow-up, the primary endpoint (i.e., death or MI) was lower in the medically treated group. There was an improvement in angina, exercise capacity, and perceived quality of life in patients who underwent PCI. There was also a higher incidence of revascularization in the medically treated group.

d. The study on Optimal Medical Therapy with or without PCI for Stable Coronary Disease (by the COURAGE Trial Research group) was recently reported and received extensive coverage in the press and medical community. In patients with severe angiographic disease of one or more vessel, and either classic symptoms or documented ischemia on provocative testing, PCI with bare-metal stenting did not reduce the risk of death or major adverse cardiovascular events compared with optimal medical therapy alone. The aggressive degree to which optimal medical therapy was pursued, however, may not be achievable in "real-world" practice. Furthermore, it should be stressed that all of the patients were enrolled after angiography had been performed, and, therefore, excluded any patients for whom the cardiologist preferred PCI as definitive treatment.

e. The recent Occluded Artery Trial (OAT) tested the hypothesis that routine PCI of totally occluded arteries 3 to 28 days after MI in high-risk but asymptomatic patients would improve outcomes. In the 2166 patients studied, there was no statistically significant difference in long-term cardiac events between the PCI and medical therapy groups, although the PCI group had more rapid relief of angina. However, the clinical implications of this trial remain controversial, as some experts have raised questions about patient selection and PCI technique.

f. The use of the DES in comparison to bare-metal stent (BMS) has significantly decreased the risk of in-stent restenosis and the need for target-vessel revascularization, thereby improving quality of life, freedom from angina, and the risk of repeat procedures. Recently, the risk of late stent thrombosis in DES has raised the question of this stent's safety, and the appropriate duration of thienopyridine use after implantation to decrease the thrombotic risk. The absolute risk of stent thrombosis even with DES is quite low, and their use in appropriate situations is still recommended. This includes small vessels, long lesions, patients with BMS restenosis, and vein graft PCI. Dual antiplatelet therapy should be considered for at least 12 to 24 months, and potentially indefinitely.

2. Compared with CABG

a. The Emory Angioplasty versus Surgery Trial (EAST) randomized approximately 400 patients with multivessel disease to PCI or CABG. After 8 years of follow-up, there was no difference in the combined endpoint of mortality, Q-wave MI, and large thallium perfusion defect. In patients with proximal LAD disease or diabetes, there was a nonsignificant trend toward improved survival with CABG.

b. The Bypass Angioplasty Revascularization Investigators (BARI) conducted the largest trial comparing PCI with CABG in the management of multivessel disease. In this trial, there was no difference in survival between patients randomized to PCI or CABG at 7 years of follow-up, although the subgroup of patients with diabetes had a better survival rate with CABG than with PCI (76.4% vs. 55.7%).

c. The Arterial Revascularization Therapies Study (ARTS) randomized 1200 patients with multivessel disease to CABG or BMS placement. After 1 and 5 years of follow-up, there was no difference in mortality, MI, or stroke. Outcomes were similar for patients with stable and unstable angina. Among diabetic patients, however, mortality was greater for those who received PCI. There was a greater incidence of repeat revascularization in the PCI group, although the use of DES in ARTS 2 (compared to the historic CABG group from ARTS 1) shows a similar 1-year rate of revascularization between PCI and CABG.

d. The SoS (surgery or stenting) study compared almost 1000 patients with multivessel disease in the setting of ACS or non-ACS presentation. There was an increased mortality and need for repeat revascularization in the PCI group, which could not be attributed to a diabetic population. ERACI II, however, showed that in 450 patients PCI was superior to CABG with respect to death or MI at 1 year. The need for repeat revascularization was greater in the PCI group.

e. In patients with left main coronary artery (LMCA) stenosis, guidelines have long recommended CABG as the treatment of choice. However, in the era of stent placement, PCI of "unprotected" LMCA stenosis has gained favor.

Small studies have shown that the mortality difference between PCI and CABG in similarly matched groups of patients is negligible. Furthermore, recent studies comparing the experience of DES implantation in the LMCA with BMS placement has shown a marked decrease in the need for repeat revascularization.

f. At the present time, strong consideration is given to CABG in the group of patients with multivessel disease and diabetes, LV dysfunction, or LMCA who are able to undergo open-heart surgery. In the general population with multivessel or LMCA disease, however, there is a paucity of evidence showing a survival advantage to CABG over PCI. Prospective trials with modern treatment practices (including DES implantation, aggressive antiplatelet therapy, off-pump coronary artery bypass procedures, and use of arterial grafts) to compare the two revascularization modalities are currently underway.

3. Revascularization methods. Many different percutaneous methods such as balloon angioplasty, stents, atherectomy (e.g., rotablation, directional, laser), and transluminal extraction catheterization are used in conjunction with various antiplatelet and anticoagulation drug regimens. The rapidly evolving mechanical and pharmacologic approach to revascularization makes it difficult to fully apply the results of previous studies to contemporary practice. Most clinical trials include highly selected patients with lesions suitable for percutaneous intervention. This definition is in evolution because of advances in percutaneous techniques. These points should be kept in mind when recommending one therapy versus the other on the basis of evidence.

D. CABG

1. Compared with medical treatment. Compared with medical treatment, CABG improves the survival rate among patients with stable angina at high risk. Population groups at high risk include patients with three-vessel CAD, impaired LV function, or substantial LMCA stenosis.

a. This information is derived from the Coronary Artery Surgery Study (CASS), European Coronary Surgery Study (ECSS), and Veterans Administration Cooperative Study (VACS). These trials were completed before generalized awareness grew regarding the benefits of medical management with β-blockers, ACE inhibitors, antiplatelet agents, or lipid-lowering medications.

b. Surgical techniques have also changed significantly, with greater use of arterial conduits including internal mammary artery grafts, minimally invasive surgery, and improved techniques of cardiac tissue preservation and anesthesia.

2. Venous or arterial grafts. There are different techniques of CABG. The use of minimally invasive bypass surgery involving the LIMA in patients with isolated LAD artery stenosis has not shown any difference in the rate of mortality, MI, or stroke in comparison to PCI, but has shown a decrease in the need for repeat revascularization. With open sternotomy, in which the use of the left internal mammary artery (LIMA) is well studied, mammary arterial grafting has better long-term outcome compared with vein graft conduits. Given the success of the (LIMA) graft, other arterial conduits have been used, such as the right internal mammary artery (RIMA), the radial artery, and the right gastroepiploic artery.

a. Twenty percent of venous grafts are nonfunctional at 5 years, and only 60% to 70% are functional after 10 years. In contrast, greater than 90% of LIMA to LAD grafts are patent 20 years after the operation.

b. Internal mammary artery (IMA) grafts have a better patency rate at 10 years when used for LAD lesions (95%) than for circumflex (88%) or right coronary artery (76%) lesions. The patency rates are higher for LIMA compared with RIMA and for *in situ* grafts compared with free grafts.

c. Patient survival is better with an IMA graft than when only saphenous venous grafts are used. This survival benefit persists for up to 20 years.

d. The use of bilateral IMA grafts appears promising with evidence that use of the RIMA in addition to the LIMA improves survival in comparison to LIMA plus saphenous veing grafting (SVG). The use of the RIMA is technically difficult, however, and has, therefore, not been widespread. Attention has also turned to other arterial conduits.

e. The radial artery graft was introduced into clinical practice around 1970 and initially had mixed results. However, at approximately 1 year, 92% of the grafts are patent, and at 5 years 80% to 85% of grafts are open. The right gastroepiploic arterial graft has been in use for approximately 15 years, and 5-year angiographic patency rates of 92% have been reported.

3. Previous CABG. Little information is available on treatment of patients who have already undergone bypass surgery and have stable angina. Although another bypass operation may be offered to these patients, direct comparison with medical treatment in this patient population has not been made. The use of multiple arterial grafts at the time of first CABG reduces the need for reoperation.

4. Compared with PCI. This is discussed earlier in the section on PCI.

E. Other forms of revascularization

Percutaneous and intraoperative transmyocardial revascularization are potential treatments for patients with coronary disease not amenable to PCI or CABG. Some reports suggest improvement in symptoms, a decrease in perfusion defects, and improvement in contractile function after these procedures, but no survival benefit has been reported. This procedure should be reserved as palliation for patients with medically refractory angina and no other revascularization option, but it has generally fallen out of favor in recent years.

Promotion of ancillary blood vessels by means of injection of blood vessel–promoting agents such as VEGF at the time of surgical or percutaneous coronary revascularization is currently under investigation. So far the results of this form of intervention have been mixed. Smaller studies targeting improvement in perfusion and exercise tolerance suggest some benefit in the active treatment group. However, two somewhat larger studies have recently been terminated early due to lack of benefit at interim analysis.

F. Lifestyle modification

1. Exercise

a. Rationale. Exercise conditions the skeletal muscles, which decreases total body oxygen consumption for the same amount of workload. Exercise training also lowers heart rate for any level of exertion, which decreases the oxygen demand on the myocardium for any workload. Some evidence shows that higher physical activity and exercise can decrease cardiovascular morbidity and mortality.

b. Recommendation. For secondary prevention, aerobic and isotonic exercises with a goal of achieving a sustained heart rate of approximately 70% to 85% of the maximum predicted heart rate at least three or four times per week has been shown to improve survival. For beginners, a supervised exercise or rehabilitative program, in which 50% to 70% of maximal predicted heart rate is achieved, is also helpful. Isometric exercises are not recommended because they increase myocardial oxygen demand substantially.

2. Diet. A strict vegetarian diet with less than 10% fat and no dairy products has shown to be beneficial, although few patients can follow these recommendations. For all patients, individualization of approach according to personal and cultural needs helps to decrease fat and calorie intake.

3. Smoking cessation. Cigarette smoking is associated with progression of atherosclerosis, increased myocardial demand due to an α-adrenergic increase in coronary tone, and adverse effects on hemostatic values, all of which can lead to worsening of stable angina. Smoking cessation decreases cardiovascular risk among patients with established CAD, including patients who have undergone CABG. Physician counseling is the best approach to achieve this goal, and adjunctive therapies include nicotine replacement patches, gum, or sprays, or medications such as bupropion and varenicline.

4. **Psychological factors.** Anger, hostility, depression, and stress are shown to adversely affect CAD. Results of small, nonrandomized trials show that biofeedback and various relaxation techniques can help to modify these factors.

V. CONTROVERSIES IN THE APPROACH TO STABLE ANGINA.

The approach to management of stable angina remains highly controversial. Data from clinical trials evaluating the diagnostic and therapeutic strategies lag behind technical advances.

A. Controversial findings

1. Because the ideal, cost-effective methods for risk stratification are debatable, individualized approaches based on the availability of technology and expertise are commonly used.
2. The relative roles of medical therapy, PCI, and CABG are controversial, especially for patients with multivessel disease, LMCA stenosis, or silent ischemia. Heterogeneity in the response to different medications makes generalized recommendations ineffective. Drug therapy tailored according to the genetic makeup of a patient may prove to be the optimal method (e.g., platelet glycoprotein IIIa polymorphism and antiplatelet therapy) to select appropriate pharmacotherapy for an individual patient.
3. The long-term effectiveness of different surgical and percutaneous therapies in the management of stable angina also remains controversial.

B. Recommended approach.

Despite the controversies, the following approach is suggested for the treatment of patients with stable angina.

1. It is reasonable to risk-stratify patients with stable angina using stress testing with imaging, such as nuclear isotope imaging or echocardiography.
   a. LV systolic function should be assessed with echocardiography to guide therapy and to identify patients with moderate LV systolic dysfunction.
   b. Patients with small perfusion defects or small wall-motion abnormalities, high threshold for ischemia, normal LV systolic function, and clear symptoms should be treated with medication.
2. If symptoms continue after medical therapy is maximized, angiography should be planned. Coronary angiography should also be performed for patients with evidence of impaired perfusion involving multiple territories, a low threshold for ischemia, and moderate LV systolic dysfunction. For patients with vague and atypical symptoms, it may be useful to perform Holter monitoring for 24 hours to assess the contribution of silent ischemia.
3. **Single-vessel disease.** If a patient has single-vessel CAD that does not involve the LMCA or supply a large myocardial territory, medical management with risk-factor modification is the appropriate first step.
   a. If patients cannot tolerate medical treatment or have symptoms despite maximum medical therapy, revascularization therapy should be offered.
4. Among patients with **multivessel CAD**, medical treatment remains an alternative for patients who have normal LV systolic function, mild symptoms, and relatively smaller areas of myocardium at risk.
   a. At this time, surgical revascularization is indicated for patients with three-vessel disease and impaired LV systolic function, and in diabetics with multivessel disease. Ongoing studies are aimed at addressing the use of multivessel PCI in this group, in comparison to CABG, using current state-of-the-art PCI technologies.
   b. CABG or PCI is a reasonable option for the other patients with multivessel CAD, provided coronary anatomy is suitable. Because the likelihood for a repeat revascularization procedure within 1 to 3 years is higher with PCI as an initial strategy, the patient's personal preference should be a strong factor in the decision.
   c. Any doubt regarding viability of the myocardium at risk should be addressed with appropriate diagnostic studies before revascularization.
5. In patients with "unprotected" LMCA stenosis, ongoing studies are evaluating the use of PCI versus CABG. Although guideline recommendations still support CABG in this population, small studies and retrospective series have indicated that these strategies are likely to be equivalent in outcome when performed in

matched patients. Left main PCI is also useful in those patients considered to be too "high-risk" for CABG or who prefer not to undergo open-heart surgery.

6. Regardless of treatment strategy, aggressive risk-factor modification, including use of lipid-lowering agents, lifestyle modification, and aspirin therapy, is an essential component of management.

ACKNOWLEDGMENT

The authors thank Dr. Keith Ellis for his contributions to earlier editions of this chapter.

References

1. Armstrong PW. Stable ischemic syndromes. In: Topol EJ, ed. *Textbook of cardiovascular medicine*. Philadelphia: Lippincott-Raven, 2002:319–349.
2. The HOPE investigators. Effects of an ACE inhibitor, ramipril, on cardiovascular events in high risk patients. *N Engl J Med* 2000;342:145–153.
3. Holubkov R, Kennard E, Fois J. Comparison of patients undergoing enhanced external counterpulsation and percutaneous coronary intervention for stable angina pectoris. *Am J Cardiol* 2002;89:1182–1186.
4. Heart Protection Study Collaborative Group. MRC/BHF Heart protection study of cholesterol lowering with simvastatin in 20,536 high risk individuals: a randomized placebo controlled trial. *Lancet* 2002;360:7–22.
5. Ropers D, Pohle FK, Kuettner A, et al. Diagnostic accuracy of noninvasive coronary angiography in patients after bypass surgery using 64-slice spiral computed tomography with 330-ms gantry rotation. *Circulation*. 2006;114:2334–2341.
6. Cheng JWM. Ranolazine for the management of coronary artery disease. *Clin Ther* 2006;28:1996–2007.
7. Cannon CP, Steinberg BA, Murphy SA, et al. Meta-analysis of cardiovascular outcomes trials comparing intensive versus moderate statin therapy. *J Am Coll Cardiol* 2006;48:438–445.
8. Bhatt DL, Fox KAA, Hacke W, et al. for the CHARISMA investigators. Clopidogrel and Aspirin versus Aspirin Alone for the Prevention of Atherothrombotic Events. *N Engl J Med* 2006;354:1706.
9. Bhatt DL, Flather MD, Hacke W, et al. Patients with prior myocardial infarction, stroke, or symptomatic peripheral arterial disease in the CHARISMA trial. *J Am Coll Cardiol* 2007;49:1982-1988.

Landmark Articles

Alderman EL, Bourassa MG, Cohen LS, et al. Ten year follow up of survival and myocardial infarction in the randomized coronary artery surgery study. *Circulation* 1990;82:1629–1646.

Al-Mallah MH, Tleyjeh IM, Abdel-Latif AA, et al. Angiotensin-converting enzyme inhibitors in coronary artery disease and preserved left ventricular systolic function: a systematic review and meta-analysis of randomized controlled trials. *J Am Coll Cardiol* 2006;47:1576–1583.

Boden WE, O'Rourke RA, Teo KK, et al., for the COURAGE Trial Research Group. Optimal medical therapy with or without PCI for stable coronary disease. *N Engl J Med* 2007;356:1503–1516.

CAPRIE Steering Committee. A randomized, blinded trial of clopidogrel versus aspirin in patients at risk of ischemic events (CAPRIE). *Lancet* 1996;348:1329–1339.

Collaborative overview of randomised trials of antiplatelet therapy. I. Prevention of death, myocardial infarction and stroke by prolonged antiplatelet therapy in various categories of patients. *BMJ* 1994:308:81–106.

Eleven year survival in the Veterans Administration Randomized Trial of Coronary Bypass Surgery. The Veterans Administration Coronary Artery Bypass Surgery Cooperative Study Group. *N Engl J Med* 1984;311: 1333–1339.

Furberg CD, Psaty BM, Meyer JV. Nifedipine: dose related increase in mortality in patients with coronary heart disease. *Circulation* 1995;92:1326–1331.

Hulley S, Grady D, Bush T. randomized trial of estrogen plus progestin for secondary prevention of coronary heart disease in postmenopausal women. *JAMA* 1998;280:605–613.

Juul-Moller S, Edvardsson N, Jahnmatz B, et al. Double blind trial of aspirin in primary prevention of myocardial infarction in patients with stable chronic angina pectoris. *Lancet* 1992;114:1421–1425.

Mark DB, Shaw L, Harrell FE, et al. Prognostic value of a treadmill exercise score in outpatients with suspected coronary artery disease. *N Engl J Med* 1991;325:849–853.

Passamani E, Davis KB, Gilepsi MJ, et al. A randomized trial of coronary artery bypass surgery. *N Engl J Med* 1985;312:1665–1671.

Rossouw JE, Anderson GL, Prentice RL, et al., Writing Group for the Women's Health Initiative Investigators. Risks and benefits of estrogen plus progestin in healthy postmenopausal women: principal results From the Women's Health Initiative randomized controlled trial. *JAMA* 2002;288:321–333.

Sacks FM, Pfeffer MA, Moye LA, et al., for the CARE Investigators. The effect of pravastatin on coronary events after myocardial infarction in patients with average cholesterol levels. Cholesterol and Recurrent Events Trial Investigators. *N Engl J Med* 1996:335:1001–1009.

Silvestri M, Barragan P, Sainsous J, et al. Unprotected left main coronary artery stenting: immediate and medium-term outcomes of 140 elective procedures. *J Am Coll Cardiol* 2000;35:1543–1550.

The Bypass Angioplasty Revascularization (BARI) Investigators. Comparison of coronary bypass surgery with angioplasty in patients with multivessel disease. *N Engl J Med* 1996;335:217–225.

The LIPID Study Group. Prevention of cardiovascular events and death with pravastatin in patients with coronary heart disease and a broad range of initial cholesterol levels. *N Engl J Med* 1998;339:1349–1357.

The Scandinavian Simvastatin Survival Study Group. Randomized trial of cholesterol lowering in 4444 patients with coronary artery disease: The Scandinavian Simvastatin Survival Study (4S). *Lancet* 1994;344:1383–1389.

Varmauskas E. Twelve year follow up of survival in the Randomized European Coronary Artery Surgery Study. *N Engl J Med* 1988;319:332–337.

Key Reviews

Campbell CL, Smyth S, Montalescot G, Steinhubl SR. Aspirin dose for the prevention of cardiovascular disease. *JAMA* 2007;297:2018–2024.

Diaz MN, Frei B, Vita JA, Keaney JF Jr. Mechanism of disease: antioxidant and atherosclerotic heart disease. *N Engl J Med* 1997;337:408–416.

Ferrari R. Major differences among the three classes of calcium antagonists. *Eur Heart J* 1997;18:A56–A70.

Fihn SD, Williams SV, Daley J. Guidelines for the management of patients with chronic stable angina: treatment. *Ann Intern Med* 2001;135:616–632.

Mark DB, Nelson CL, Califf RM, et al. Continuing evolution of therapy for coronary artery disease. *Circulation* 1994;89:2015–2125.

Parker JD, Parker JO. Drug therapy: nitrate therapy for stable angina pectoris. *N Engl J Med* 1998;338:520–531.

Wilson RF. Assessing the severity of coronary stenosis [Editorial]. *N Engl J Med* 1996;334:1735–1737.

Yla-Herttuala S. Rissanen TT. Vajanto I. Hartikainen J. Vascular endothelial growth factors: biology and current status of clinical applications in cardiovascular medicine. *J Am Coll Cardiol* 2007;49:1015–1026.

6 OTHER ISCHEMIC SYNDROMES: SILENT ISCHEMIA AND SYNDROME X

Apur R. Kamdar, Tim Williams, and Marc S. Penn

SILENT ISCHEMIA

I. INTRODUCTION. Silent ischemia represents an underappreciated manifestation of coronary artery disease (CAD), occurring in up to 20% to 40% of patients with stable and unstable coronary syndromes. By definition, patients are asymptomatic, lacking typical or atypical anginal symptoms. Silent ischemia may be documented by a variety of diagnostic modalities, including resting electrocardiogram (ECG), ambulatory ECG (AECG), nuclear scintigraphy, and echocardiography.

II. CLINICAL PRESENTATION. Patients may be loosely categorized into three groups, collectively representing a continuum of silent ischemia.

A. Type I have **asymptomatic** ischemia with no known CAD history with **asymptomatic** myocardial infarction patterns. Clinicians may discover evidence of subclinical myocardial infarction (MI) from a resting ECG or a preoperative stress test. In the Framingham Study, 12.5% of patients with MI had an unrecognized "silent" infarction. Patients may also present with arrhythmias or sudden death from subsequent scar. These patients are considered to have an ineffective "anginal warning system" (1).

In addition, a subset of this group includes patients with **asymptomatic** ischemia without a history of infarction. Silent ischemia is often discovered by stress tests after referral for aggressive primary screening. This type of screening may occur in patients with diabetes, strong family histories, or a high-risk electron beam computed tomography (EBCT) result. Given the increasingly technological nature of medical culture, the prevalence of these patients is likely to rise. AECG is rarely used as a primary screening modality. The American College of Cardiology and American Heart Association (ACC/AHA) guidelines consider the use of AECG for ischemia monitoring in asymptomatic individuals a class III recommendation.

B. Type II have **symptomatic** MIs but subsequent **asymptomatic** ischemic syndromes. Ischemia is often missed because of a lack of symptoms. Patients in this category are most often encountered after a positive stress test or the rarely ordered AECG. Type II patients may have an abnormal **pain threshold.**

C. **Type III** encompasses the largest patient population with silent ischemia. These patients with known CAD have both **symptomatic** and **asymptomatic** ischemia. Between 20% and 40% of patients with chronic anginal symptoms have silent ischemia. About 75% of ischemic episodes are silent, and only 25% are symptomatic.

III. DIAGNOSTIC TESTING.

Most patients with silent ischemia are either never identified or identified retrospectively. In the Asymptomatic Cardiac Ischemic Pilot (ACIP) study, patients with frequent silent ischemic events were at increased risk for advanced coronary disease, including high-risk coronary anatomy such as three-vessel disease. Currently, testing to detect ischemia in asymptomatic patients is controversial. The ACC/AHA guidelines considers the use of exercise ECG testing (without imaging) in asymptomatic patients with possible myocardial ischemia on AECG or severe coronary calcification on EBCT a *class IIb recommendation*. The use of exercise plus imaging stress testing (echo, nuclear) in asymptomatic patients with a low-risk Duke treadmill score on exercise ECG testing is a *class III recommendation*. In patients with an intermediate or high-risk Duke treadmill score, it is a *class IIb recommendation*.

IV. MECHANISMS

A. **The exact explanation** for a lack of symptoms in the face of unequivocal ischemia remains **unknown.** It likely represents abnormal modulation of cardiac **pain perception at different levels in the afferent pathway of the heart.**

B. **The association between diabetes and silent ischemia and painless infarction** has been attributed to **autonomic neuropathy** (3,4). A higher threshold for pain has been related to increased baseline plasma β-endorphin levels and increased age. A potential connection exists between baroreceptor function and pain perception. This may explain the relationships among increased systolic blood pressure, reduced sensitivity to ischemic pain, and the demonstration of anginal relief with carotid sinus stimulation. Results of one study (4) suggested that the gating of afferent signals at the thalamic level is a potential mechanism for silent ischemia. Patients with symptoms had activation of basal frontal, anterior, and ventral cingulate cortices and the left temporal pole. **Cortical activation was limited to the right frontal region in patients with silent ischemia.** It also has been proposed that, among type III patients, asymptomatic ischemia may represent shorter and less severe episodes compared with symptomatic episodes (5,6).

V. MANAGEMENT

A. **Medications** effective in preventing symptomatic ischemia (i.e., nitrates, calcium antagonists, and β-blockers) and in decreasing myocardial O_2 demand are also effective in reducing or eliminating episodes of silent ischemia. In one randomized study (7), metoprolol was better than diltiazem in reducing the mean number and duration of ischemic episodes. However, the combination of calcium antagonists and β-blockers was more effective than either agent alone. Lipid-lowering therapy has also shown a reduction of ischemia on AECG. The ACC/AHA guidelines currently regard the use of ASA (aspirin), β-blockers, ACE inhibitors, and statins as class I recommendations in asymptomatic patients with evidence of previous MI and class IIa recommendations in patients without history of previous MI (2).

B. The **goal of therapy remains controversial.** It is not clear whether therapy should be guided by ischemia or angina. The ACIP study revealed no difference in benefit from either of these approaches. However, 2-year follow-up data from this study demonstrated improved prognosis with initial revascularization compared with angina- or ischemia-guided medical therapy (7). The SWISSI I (Swiss Interventional Study on Silent Ischaemia type I) study randomized 54 type I subset patients to treatment with antianginal medications and aspirin vs. risk factor modification only. Their findings showed that treatment with the combination of antianginal drug therapy and aspirin appeared to significantly reduce cardiac events, including cardiac death, nonfatal myocardial infarction, or acute coronary syndrome. In addition, these patients had consistently lower rates of exercise-induced ischemia during follow-up (8). The SWISSI II study randomized 201 type II silent ischemia patients to PCI versus ongoing anti-ischemic medical therapy. The results showed a significant decrease in rates of cardiac death, nonfatal myocardial infarction, and subsequent need for revascularization in patients in the PCI group over a 10-year follow-up period (9). Similarly, in type I silent ischemia patients, with an ineffective "anginal warning system" it has been suggested that it may be reasonable to treat silent ischemia in a manner equivalent to that for symptomatic ischemia in the general population in terms of revascularization and medical therapy (1).

VI. PROGNOSIS. Myocardial ischemia, whether symptomatic or asymptomatic, is associated with poorer outcomes among patients with CAD. Patients with frequent and accelerating episodes of ST-segment depression on ambulatory ECG monitoring are at higher risk for subsequent cardiac events than patients with few or no such episodes. The Copenhagen Holter study examined the significance of ischemic changes on AECG in asymptomatic, healthy individuals between the ages of 55 and 75 years (type I subset). They found that patients with silent ischemia had a threefold higher risk of subsequent cardiac events over a 5-year follow-up period (10). Circadian effects of asymptomatic ST depression on AECG have been noted with changes being more common in the morning hours; however, nocturnal ST-segment changes have been associated with multivessel CAD or left-main narrowing (1). It has not been proven conclusively, however, that detection of silent ischemia is an independent risk factor for future cardiac events (11–14).

VII. CONTROVERSIES

A. Patients with silent ischemia on AECG monitoring represent heterogeneous populations. This may be a marker of unstable, complex coronary plaque or microvascular dysfunction. Results of the angiographic substudy of the ACIP study suggested that most patients with silent ischemia have proximal coronary lesions or complex coronary plaques (15). This hypothesis has not been tested in a larger population and continues to be investigated.

B. The potential role of **AECG monitoring** for ischemia still needs to be determined to assess its utility compared with more commonly used tests, such as exercise testing with thallium imaging. Different populations at specific times after their events should be carefully examined to answer these questions. Currently, the exercise ECG test remains the most useful and validated screening test for significant CAD.

C. Medical therapy should be used to decrease or eliminate ischemia; however, the relative role of medical therapy compared with revascularization still remains unclear.

SYNDROME X

I. INTRODUCTION. Syndrome X is defined as the constellation of effort induced **angina-like discomfort** in the setting of **angiographically normal coronary arteries** (without inducible spasm on ergonovine provocation testing). This chest pain is usually indistinguishable from traditional ischemic angina caused by obstructive coronary disease and is, therefore, considered a diagnosis of exclusion.

II. PRESENTATION. In the clinical setting, syndrome X is a diagnosis given to patients with persistent **anginal symptoms,** often with abnormal stress testing despite a **normal angiogram** and **negative workup** for noncardiac chest pain. Up to 25% of all coronary angiograms performed in the United States for symptoms of chest pain are normal, yet, most cardiologists do not routinely use ergonovine provocation or intravascular ultrasound to evaluate for variant angina or angiographically silent coronary atherosclerosis in this subset of patients (1). When intravascular ultrasonography (IVUS) studies have been performed in these patients a spectrum of findings ranging from normal vessels to intimal thickening to nonobstructive atheromatous plaque has been reported (2). Syndrome X has an increased occurrence in women (3:1 preponderance), both pre- and postmenopausal (3). Of note, abnormal cardiac physical examination findings and LV dysfunction on stress testing are both uncommon in syndrome X.

III. ETIOLOGY AND PATHOPHYSIOLOGY. Syndrome X represents a heterogeneous population and may represent multiple processes with varying causes. **Endothelial dysfunction, microvascular ischemia, and abnormal pain perception have all been implicated in the genesis of this disorder.** Endothelial dysfunction as demonstrated by abnormal coronary flow reserve (CFR), single positron emission computed tomography (SPECT) stress, and positron emission tomography (PET) stress testing is common in these patients. In addition, behavioral and psychiatric conditions often coexist. Specific treatment aimed at managing behavioral issues may lead to symptomatic improvement in chest pain in some patients.

IV. DIAGNOSTIC TESTING. Because syndrome X is a **diagnosis of exclusion**, both traditional obstructive coronary atherosclerosis and causes of noncardiac chest pain must be ruled out before a final diagnosis can be made. Multislice CT angiography may play an increasingly important role in avoiding invasive angiography in some of these patients. Laboratory testing for endothelial dysfunction is not widely utilized in the clinical setting. Abnormal CFR in the catheterization laboratory can help confirm abnormalities in microcirculatory control, often accompanied by endothelial dysfunction in patients with syndrome X. C-Reactive protein (hsCRP) has been shown to correlate with the severity of symptoms and ECG changes in this population (4).

V. THERAPY. The **primary goal** of therapy should be **aggressive cardiac risk factor modification** including lifestyle changes and lipid treatment, although the **ideal treatment regimen is unknown.** β-Blockers have been shown to be very effective in controlling anginal symptoms in this population and are considered superior to calcium channel blockers and nitrates (5). Other treatments that have provided benefit include tricyclic antidepressants (imipramine) (6), oral aminophylline, (7) and estrogen in postmenopausal women (8). Given the recent data on estrogens, caution should be exercised when considering estrogen therapy in patients with suspected syndrome X.

VI. PROGNOSIS. The prognosis for patients with angina and normal coronary arteriograms is generally favorable with good long-term outcomes shown in multiple studies. However, subsets of these patients such as patients with persistent anginal symptoms and/or evidence of significant myocardial ischemia on stress testing, seem to be at higher risk and have significantly higher event rates including premature death, myocardial infarction, and stroke than the baseline population (9,10). These subsets of patients should be treated aggressively with risk-factor modification and counseled regarding lifestyle modification.

VII. OTHER. Although not clearly related to syndrome X, **Takotsubo syndrome** (aka LV apical ballooning syndrome, stress induced cardiomyopathy), is a condition which has been receiving increasing attention. Clinical features include sudden onset of chest pain, ECG changes (often ST elevation) mimicking an acute myocardial infarction, usually in the setting of severe emotional distress and catecholamine surge. The angiogram shows normal coronary arteries, and diagnosis is made on the typical appearance by LV ventriculogram or echocardiogram with basal hyperkinesis and severe apical systolic wall-motion abnormality. Most patients recover LV function and require only hemodynamic and pharmacologic support (11).

References/Silent Ischemia

1. Morrow DA, Gersh BJ. Chronic coronary artery disease: other manifestations of coronary artery disease. Libby, ed. *Braunwald's heart disease: a textbook of cardiovascular medicine*, 8th ed. Philadelphia: WB Saunders, 2008: 1396–1397.
2. Braunwald E, Antman EM, Beasley JW, et al. ACC/AHA 2002 guideline update for the management of patients with chronic stable angina: a report of the American College of Cardiology/American Heart Association Task Force on Practice Guidelines (Committee to Update the 1999 Guidelines for the Management of Patients with Chronic Stable Angina). *J Am Coll Cardiol* 2003;41:159–168.
3. Chiariello M, Indolfi C. Silent myocardial ischemia in patients with diabetes mellitus. *Circulation* 1996;93:2081–2091.
4. Ahluwalia G, Jain P, Chugh SK, et al. Silent myocardial ischemia in diabetes with normal autonomic function. *Int J Cardiol* 1995;48:147–153.
5. Nihoyannopaulos P, Marsonis A, Joshi J, et al. Magnitude of myocardial dysfunction is greater in painful than in painless myocardial ischemia: an exercise echocardiographic study. *J Am Coll Cardiol* 1995;25:1507–1512.
6. Narins CR, Zareba W, Moss AJ, et al. Clinical implications of silent versus symptomatic exercise-induced myocardial ischemia in patients with stable coronary disease. *J Am Coll Cardiol* 1997;29:756–763.
7. Davies RF, Goldberg AD, Forman S, et al. Asymptomatic Cardiac Ischemia Pilot (ACIP) study 2 year follow-up: outcomes of patients randomized to initial strategies of medical therapy versus revascularization. *Circulation* 1997;95:2037–2043.
8. Erne P, Schoenenberger AW, Zuber M, et al. Effects of anti-ischaemic drug therapy in silent myocardial ischaemia type I: the Swiss Interventional Study on Silent Ischaemia type I (SWISSI I): a randomized, controlled pilot study. *Eur Heart J* 2007;28:2110–2117. Epub 2007 July 19.

9. Erne P, Schoenenberger AW, Burckhardt D, et al. Effects of percutaneous coronary interventions in silent ischemia after myocardial infarction: the SWISSI II randomized controlled trial. *JAMA*.2007;297:1985–1991.
10. Sajadieh A, Nielsen OW, Rasmussen V, et al. Prevalence and prognostic significance of daily-life silent myocardial ischemia in middle-aged and elderly subjects with no apparent heart disease. *Eur Heart J* 2005;26:1402.
11. Leroy F, McFadden EP, Lablanche JM, et al. Prognostic significance of silent myocardial ischaemia during maximal exercise testing after a first acute myocardial infarction. *Eur Heart J* 1993;14:1471–1475.
12. Mickley H, Nielson JR, Berning J, et al. Prognostic significance of transient myocardial ischaemic after first acute myocardial infarction: five year follow-up study. *Br Heart J* 1995;73:320–326.
13. Detry JM, Robert A, Luwaert RJ, Melin JA. Prognostic significance of silent exertional myocardial ischaemia in symptomatic men without previous myocardial infarction. *Eur Heart J* 1992;13:183–187.
14. Stone PH, Chaitman BR, Forman S, et al. Prognostic significance of myocardial ischemia detected by ambulatory electrocardiography, exercise treadmill testing, and electrocardiogram at rest to predict cardiac events by one year (the Asymptomatic Cardiac Ischemia Pilot [ACIP] study). *Am J Cardiol* 1997;80:1395–1401.
15. Sharaf BL, Bourassa MG, Mcmahon RP, et al. Clinical and detailed angiographic findings in patients with ambulatory electrocardiographic ischemia without critical coronary narrowing: results from the Asymptomatic Cardiac Ischemia Pilot (ACIP) study. *Clin Cardiol* 1998;21:86–92.

Landmark Articles

Conti CR. Silent myocardial ischemia: prognostic significance and therapeutic implications. *Clin Cardiol* 1998;11:807–811.

Syndrome X

1. Bugiardini R, Bairey Merz CN. Angina with "normal" coronary arteries: A changing philosophy. *JAMA* 2005;293:477.
2. Erbel R, Ge J, Bockisch A, et al. Value of intracoronary ultrasound and Doppler in the differentiation of angiographically normal coronary arteries: a prospective study in patients with angina pectoris. *Eur Heart J* 1996;17:880–889.
3. Kaski JC, Rosano GMC, Collins P, et al. Cardiac syndrome X: clinical characteristics and left ventricular function—long-term follow-up study. *J Am Coll Cardiol* 1995;25:807–814.
4. Cosin-Sales J, Pizzi C, et al. C-Reactive protein, clinical presentation, and ischemic activity in patients with chest pain and normal coronary angiograms. *J Am Coll Cardiol* 2003;41:1468.
5. Lanza GA, Colonna G, Pasceri V, et al. Atenolol versus amlodipine versus isosorbide-5-monnitrate on anginal symptoms in syndrome X. *Am J Cardiol* 1999;84:854–856.
6. Johnson BD, Shaw LJ, Buchthal SD, et al. Prognosis in women with myocardial ischemia in the absence of obstructive coronary disease: Results from the National Institutes of Health-National Heart, Lung, and Blood Institute-Sponsored Women's Ischemia Syndrome Evaluation (WISE). *Circulation* 2004;109:2993.
7. Elliott PM, Dickinson KK, Calvino R, et al. Effect of oral aminophylline in patients with angina and normal coronary arteriograms (cardiac syndrome X). *Heart* 1997;77:523–526.
8. Kaski JC. Cardiac syndrome X in women: the role of oestrogen deficiency. *Heart* 2006;92(Suppl III):iii5–iii9.
9. Bugiardini R. Women, "non-specific" chest pain, and normal or near-normal coronary angiograms are not synonymous with favourable outcome. *Eur Heart J* 2006;27:1387.
10. Johnson BD, Shaw LJ, Pepine CJ, et al. Persistent chest pain predicts cardiovascular events in women without obstructive coronary artery disease: Results from the NIH-NHLBI-sponsored Women's Ischaemia Syndrome Evaluation (WISE) study. *Eur Heart J* 2006;27:1408.
11. Bybee KA, Kara T, Prasad A, et al. Systematic review: transient left ventricular apical ballooning: a syndrome that mimics ST-segment elevation myocardial infarction. *Ann Intern Med* 2004;141:858–865.

Relevant Book Chapters

Fox KA. Stable ischemic syndromes. In: Topol EJ, ed. *Textbook of cardiovascular medicine,* 3rd ed. Philadelphia: Lippincott Williams & Wilkins, 2007.

Morrow DA, Gersh BJ. Chronic coronary artery disease: other manifestations of coronary artery disease. Libby, ed. *Braunwald's heart disease: a textbook of cardiovascular medicine,* 8th ed. Philadelphia: WB Saunders, 2008:1395–1396.

Heart Failure and Transplantation

II

HEART FAILURE WITH SYSTOLIC DYSFUNCTION

7

Brian Hardaway and W. H. Wilson Tang

I. INTRODUCTION

A. Heart failure is a complex clinical syndrome characterized by impaired myocardial performance and progressive activation of the neuroendocrine system leading to circulatory insufficiency and congestion. With the increasing age of the population, improved survival of patients with acute myocardial infarction (MI) and reduced mortality from other diseases, the incidence of heart failure and the cost of managing patients with heart failure continue to increase. Data suggest that the lifetime risk of developing heart failure is about 20%.

B. Terminology

1. Based on the hemodynamic model, **systolic heart failure** has been defined by the presence of impaired contractility of the left ventricle, measured as ejection fraction (EF). There has been recognition that this classification is somewhat arbitrary and can vary widely with different imaging modalities, although most clinical trials have used a reduced EF as entry criterion. However, there is discordance between symptom presentation in heart failure and the degree of cardiac dysfunction. (e.g., a patient with markedly reduced EF may have minimal symptoms and can respond favorably to medical therapy).
2. The major pathophysiologic process in the progression of heart failure appears to be **cardiac remodeling,** often referred to as progressive chamber enlargement over time and obligatory reduction in EF.
3. The term **congestive heart failure (CHF)** is overused to describe heart failure, as not all patients with heart failure have signs and symptoms of congestion.
4. In some instances, the term **right heart failure** is still used to describe patients with peripheral signs and symptoms of heart failure (often from elevated right-heart filling pressures) without evidence of pulmonary congestion. This is caused by elevated venous pressures and inadequate cardiac output independent of abnormal left ventricular (LV) contractility.
5. **Acute decompensation** usually refers to episodes of acute or subacute worsening of clinical signs and symptoms of heart failure due to a wide range of precipitants (Table 7.1). The most common causes include dietary indiscretion (especially overuse of salt), medical noncompliance, and arrhythmia (especially atrial fibrillation).

C. Classification

1. The latest American College of Cardiology and American Heart Association (ACC/AHA) guidelines have classified heart failure using a new staging system that emphasizes the evolution and progression of heart failure across a continuum:
   a. Stage A: patients at high risk for developing heart failure with no structural heart disease

TABLE 7.1 Common Causes and Precipitants of Heart Failure

Causes of heart failure (WHO criteria, 1996)	Precipitants of acute heart failure
Dilated cardiomyopathy (idiopathic)	Myocardial ischemia (acute coronary syndrome, myocardial infarction and complications)
Hypertrophic cardiomyopathy	Acute valvular catastrophe
Restrictive cardiomyopathy	Hypertension (malignant, crisis)
Arrhythmogenic right ventricular cardiomyopathy	Acute myocarditis
Unclassified cardiomyopathies	Arrhythmias (rapid ventricular responses)
Fibroelastosis	Acute pulmonary embolism (right heart failure)
Systolic dysfunction without dilation	Cardiac tamponade
Mitochondrial cardiomyopathy	Toxins (alcohol, nonsteroidal anti-inflammatory agents)
Specific cardiomyopathies	Infections
Ischemic	Sodium or dietary indiscretion
Valvular obstruction or insufficiency	Medication noncompliance
Hypertensive	
Inflammatory (lymphocytic, eosinophilic, giant-cell myocarditis)	
Infectious (Chagas' disease, HIV, enterovirus, adenovirus, CMV, bacterial or fungal infections)	
Metabolic	
Endocrine (thyroid diseases, adrenal insufficiency, pheochromocytoma, acromegaly, diabetes mellitus)	
Familial storage disease (hemochromatosis, glycogen storage disease, Hurler's syndrome, Fabry-Anderson disease)	
Electrolyte deficiency syndromes (hypokalemia, hypomagnesemia)	
Nutritional disorders (kwashiorkor, anemia, beri-beri, selenium)	
Amyloid	
Familial Mediterranean fever	
General system diseases	
Connective tissue disorders (SLE, polyarteritis nodosa, rheumatoid arthritis, scleroderma, dermatomyositis, polymyositis, sarcoidosis)	
Muscular dystrophies (Duchenne's, Becker's, myotonic)	
Neuromuscular (Friedreich's ataxia, Noonan's disease)	
Toxins (alcohol, catecholamines, cocaine, anthracyclines and other chemotherapeutics, irradiation)	
Peripartum cardiomyopathy	

CMV, cytomegalovirus; HIV, human immunodeficiency virus; SLE, systemic lupus erythematosus.

b. Stage B: patients with structural heart disease who have not yet developed symptoms of heart failure

c. Stage C: patients with past or current symptoms of heart failure associated with underlying structural heart disease

d. Stage D: patients with end-stage heart failure who require specialized advanced treatment.

It is important to recognize that heart failure staging can go only in one direction, that is, once symptoms occur, patients will be considered at "stage C" even if their symptoms may resolve.

TABLE 7.2 New York Heart Association Functional Classification

Class	Description
I	Patients have cardiac disease but without resulting limitations of physical activity. Ordinary physical activity does not cause undue fatigue, palpitations, dyspnea, or anginal pain.
II	Patients have cardiac disease resulting in slight limitation of physical activity. They are comfortable at rest. Ordinary physical activity results in fatigue, palpitation, dyspnea, or anginal pain.
III	Patients have cardiac disease resulting in marked limitation of physical activity. They are comfortable at rest. Less than ordinary physical activity causes fatigue, palpitation, dyspnea, or anginal pain.
IV	Patients have cardiac disease resulting in an inability to carry on any physical activity without discomfort. Symptoms of cardiac insufficiency or of the anginal syndrome may be present even at rest. If any physical activity is undertaken, discomfort is increased.

2. In practice, heart failure is a bedside diagnosis that is defined by clinical assessment. Some patients may have cardiac dysfunction (e.g., low EF) without any symptoms, which is often referred to as having **asymptomatic heart failure or asymptomatic LV dysfunction.** Others may have preserved LV systolic function, but demonstrate typical signs and symptoms of heart failure, which is called **heart failure with preserved LV function** (see Chapter 9).
   a. The **New York Heart Association (NYHA) functional classification**, although somewhat vague, remains the most commonly used standard to describe severity of signs and symptoms (Table 7.2).
   b. The **Killip classification** is often used for patients after acute coronary syndromes.

II. SIGNS AND SYMPTOMS

A. The spectrum of signs and symptoms in heart failure varies markedly among patients. Up to one-half of all patients with LV systolic dysfunction are asymptomatic.
   1. Among patients with symptoms, the most common and earliest presenting symptom is **dyspnea**, usually with exertion. **Orthopnea** (i.e., dyspnea when lying down, usually described as number of pillows used while sleeping) is typical with more advanced cases of LV dysfunction or in decompensated heart failure. As further decompensation occurs, **paroxysmal nocturnal dyspnea** (PND) and **Cheyne-Stokes respiratory patterns** may occur.
   2. **Fatigue** and **low exercise tolerance** are common complaints in patients with heart failure.
   3. **Dizziness** may occur in the setting of impaired perfusion, but is more commonly iatrogenic (i.e., related to the use of heart failure medications). **Palpitations** and **syncope** may occur in patients with underlying arrhythmia and require prompt evaluation.
   4. **Anorexia** and **abdominal pain** are common symptoms of advanced heart failure, especially with right-heart failure. Seldom considered (but highly prevalent) symptoms include **cough, insomnia, and depressed mood.**

B. **Physical examination** of a patient with appreciable but well-compensated systolic heart failure may reveal no abnormalities. A high index of suspicion based on symptoms must be maintained. Physical signs commonly seen in the heart failure syndrome vary according to the degree of compensation, the chronicity (acute versus chronic), and chamber involvement (right-heart versus left-heart failure).
   1. Fluid or volume overload is the hallmark sign for heart failure, especially in the setting of acute decompensation and right-heart failure. Typical physical signs of volume overload in heart failure include the following:

a. **Pulmonary rales** due to accumulation of fluid in the pulmonary interstitium and alveoli from high left atrial pressures are commonly referred to as **acute cardiogenic pulmonary edema (ACPE).**
b. **Dullness** at the lung bases consistent with pleural effusion
c. **Jugular venous distention (JVD)** should be elicited at a 45-degree incline, although when JVD is very elevated, it may be apparent only with the patient sitting upright.
d. **Edema, ascites, and hepatomegaly** may occur, sometimes even with a pulsatile liver palpable during congestion.
e. systolic murmur of **mitral regurgitation (MR)** is often present in the setting of LV enlargement. Congestive heart failure caused by primary valvular heart disease will have distinctive murmurs.
f. **A third heart sound** (S_3 gallop) is best heard with the bell of the stethoscope in the left lateral position and signifies increased LV end-diastolic pressure in patients with decreased LV function.

2. Often neglected is the subtle sign of **peripheral perfusion** (e.g., color, warm or cool extremities, capillary refill), which may be important in assessing adequacy of perfusion and anemia in patients with advanced heart failure.
3. **Pulsus alternans**, or low-amplitude pulse, is also associated with advanced heart failure.
4. **Vital signs** are often important. Tachycardia, tachypnea, and narrow pulse pressures are often signs of poor prognosis or advanced disease, although body weight is often useful in monitoring the compensatory status. Blood pressure monitoring is also an important aspect in the management of heart failure.

III. LABORATORY EVALUATION

A. Blood work

1. Clinically, blood work evaluation is used to diagnose potentially reversible causes and correctable problems related to the heart failure syndrome, to identify comorbidities, to monitor and correct abnormalities before or during treatment, and to assess the disease severity to predict the prognosis of the patients with heart failure.
2. Natriuretic peptides such as **B-type natriuretic peptide (BNP) or amino-terminal pro-B-type natriuretic peptide (proBNP)** are available for clinical use as an aid to the diagnosis of heart failure. Although a normal range (BNP <100 pg/mL; proBNP <125 pg/mL if age <75 years and <450 pg/mL if age ≥75 years) is recommended to "diagnose" heart failure, there is a wide variation that is determined by the patient's age, gender, medical therapy, body mass index, renal function, perioperative status, and concomitant diseases (e.g., thyroid disease). Recent guidelines have been established with their use in the clinical setting.
   a. **Screening for heart failure.** Although cardiac dysfunction has been associated with elevated BNP or proBNP levels, the sensitivity is relatively low in asymptomatic patients and is highly dependent on the cut-off levels chosen. Strategies to screen for heart failure and cardiac dysfunction in asymptomatic patients incorporating BNP testing in several settings (e.g., patients with stage A or B heart failure, such as post-MI) are still in development.
   b. **Diagnosing heart failure.** The primary use of BNP remains in the area of diagnosing heart failure in symptomatic patients with dyspnea, fatigue, or edema. The high negative predictive value (up to 90%) in this setting allows BNP testing to be useful to rule out a cardiac cause of symptoms. However, BNP levels in the setting of acute cardiogenic pulmonary edema may not rise until a few hours later.
   c. **Monitoring heart failure therapy.** Preliminary experience has suggested that changes in BNP level parallel changes in symptoms and treatment effects, but these data are complementary to clinical assessment and should *not* replace bedside or hemodynamic assessment. A single, absolute target BNP or proBNP value should not be used. In general, diuretics and drugs inhibiting the

renin–angiotensin–aldosterone system (RAAS) lower BNP, and the response of BNP to β-adrenergic blockers may vary.

d. **Determining prognosis of heart failure.** It is generally accepted that BNP and proBNP levels correlate closely with morbidity and mortality outcome measures in many clinical settings, perhaps better than many standard prognostic tools. A higher BNP or proBNP value often stratifies the patient into a higher risk category.

3. **Blood tests to diagnose reversible causes of heart failure**
   a. **Thyroid function testing** is warranted for patients with new-onset disease.
   b. Because anemia is prevalent in patients with heart failure (up to 15% to 25% of all patients with heart failure) and can contribute to the development of high-output heart failure, a serum **hemoglobin** level should be obtained to rule out anemia as a treatable factor in the heart failure syndrome. Hemodilution from fluid retention may also cause anemia and should be treated with diuretics.
4. **Blood tests to monitor heart failure therapy**
   a. **Electrolyte abnormalities** are common among patients with heart failure and may be caused by the disease itself or by the treatment. Hypokalemia, hypomagnesemia, and metabolic alkalosis due to diuretic use, as well as hyperkalemia from drugs inhibiting the RAAS, are common and should be monitored carefully, owing to their arrhythmogenic propensity. Hyponatremia typically signifies advanced heart failure and fluid retention. Electrolyte monitoring is especially important within the first week following initiation of aldosterone receptor antagonists.
   b. **Renal function** should be closely monitored, especially when diuretics and drugs inhibiting the RAAS are administered.
   c. Elevation of **liver function test results** can occur when right-sided failure is predominant (e.g., hepatic congestion). This may be reflected in an elevation in transaminase levels or altered coagulation indices.
5. Standard preventive cardiology screening should be performed, because coronary artery disease remains the predominant cause of heart failure. In particular, routine screening for **dyslipidemia** and **glucose intolerance** or diabetes mellitus is important.

B. **The electrocardiogram (ECG)** may provide diagnostic information about the cause of heart failure.
   1. It is important to look for signs of prior MI, chamber enlargement and hypertrophy, heart block (i.e., iatrogenic or infiltrative diseases), arrhythmias, pericardial effusion (i.e., voltage <5 mm in frontal leads and <10 mm in precordial leads), and cardiac amyloidosis (i.e., low voltage and a pseudoinfarction pattern in anterior leads).
   2. Recent understanding of the role of impairment of **cardiac synchrony** in the genesis of heart failure has led to the measurement of the QRS duration and morphology to determine the potential benefits of cardiac resynchronization therapy (particularly, left bundle-branch block morphology with QRS >130 ms).
   3. **Holter monitoring** is often helpful in identifying arrhythmia (e.g., atrial fibrillation, ventricular tachycardia).

C. Examination of a **chest radiograph** should include heart size and the condition of the pulmonary parenchyma. Enlargement of the heart silhouette implies LV or biventricular failure. Patients with severe systolic dysfunction may have a normal chest radiograph if the dysfunction is compensated. A normal-sized cardiac silhouette does not exclude systolic or diastolic dysfunction. The lung field abnormalities may range from mild engorgement of the perihilar vessels to bilateral pleural effusions, Kerley B lines, and frank pulmonary edema.

D. **Echocardiography** is useful in evaluating cardiac structure and function and in identifying possible structural causes of heart failure. Although the concept of the ejection fraction is well accepted as a surrogate of pump dysfunction, structural abnormalities such as the degree of cardiac hypertrophy and dilation are related more closely to the pathophysiology and prognosis. Routine measurements of cardiac size, structure, and systolic and diastolic function are detailed in Chapter 60.

E. Right-heart catheterization (see Chapter 52). Invasive hemodynamic monitoring is often helpful in the diagnosis and inpatient management of heart failure, particularly in the titration of intravenous therapy on a minute-to-minute basis. In contrast, an elective diagnostic right-heart catheterization is indicated to better assess cardiac performance, intracardiac filling pressures, valvular area estimates, or the presence of intracardiac shunting. Right-heart catheterization can be combined with exercise testing or infusions with inotropic or vasodilatory agents to study their effects on hemodynamics.

1. **Cardiac Index** is one of the important measurements provided by right-heart catheterization. It can be calculated by means of thermodilution dilution technique or the Fick method. Some methods of right-heart catheterization allow continuous monitoring of cardiac output. Routine **determination of cardiac output** for patients with decompensated heart failure is critical to pharmacotherapy. It also provides an early indication that medication is not effective and a more aggressive approach is warranted (e.g., intraaortic balloon pump, ventricular assist device).
2. **Other key information** includes filling pressures, pulmonary arterial pressure, pulmonary capillary wedge pressure, systemic vascular resistance, pulmonary vascular resistance, pulmonary artery to pulmonary artery wedge gradient, and shunt calculation. All patients with isolated right-heart failure of unknown causation should be evaluated for intracardiac shunting by means of echocardiography. They also should undergo an oxygen saturation study at the time of right-heart catheterization.

F. Left-heart catheterization (see Chapter 58). In the care of patients with a history of coronary artery disease, evaluation of the coronary anatomy may be warranted to identify the cause of decompensation and to guide therapy, to identify whether decompensation is caused by ischemia, and to determine whether revascularization (percutaneous or surgical) is indicated.

G. Endomyocardial biopsy (see Chapter 56) is indicated only when primary myocardial disease is suspected and other causes of decompensation have been ruled out. Biopsy seldom yields information to change the treatment plan, although important prognostic information may be obtained (e.g., in cases of cardiac amyloidosis).

H. Viability assessment is important in the assessment of patients with heart failure and coronary artery disease to detect and quantify the amount of ischemia and hibernation (see Chapter 45). This is possible with dobutamine echocardiography, [^{18}F] fluorodeoxyglucose positron emission tomography, or thallium-201 single-photon emission computed tomography. Magnetic resonance imaging is used increasingly in the evaluation of scar and hibernating myocardium. Revascularization is appropriate in those patients with significant ischemia or viability, whereas medical therapy and cardiac transplantation may be required when scar predominates.

I. Metabolic stress testing. Patients being considered for heart transplantation undergo risk stratification with a metabolic stress test. Patients with a peak oxygen consumption $<$14 mL/kg per minute or exercise tolerance $<$50% predicted for age have a poor prognosis and should be considered for transplantation. This examination also is beneficial in differentiating the effects of respiratory from those of cardiac dysfunction on patients with dyspnea during exertion.

J. Arrhythmia workup with Holter monitoring (see Chapters 20 and 21)

K. Other considerations. The choice of test usually is based on the availability and accuracy of the test equipment within the local medical community. For patients who need very accurate measurements of systolic function (e.g., patients undergoing chemotherapy), radionuclide ventriculography (MUGA scan) is the preferred imaging modality. For patients believed to have valvular or congenital heart disease, transthoracic and transesophageal echocardiography or cardiac magnetic resonance imaging are preferred.

IV. ETIOLOGY. It is important to identify the cause of heart failure if possible to tailor therapy. Identification of a causative agent or reversible course is important (Table 7.1).

A. Dilated cardiomyopathy is a condition in which cardiac mass increases (i.e., **cardiac remodeling**), leading to dilation and impaired systolic function in the absence of epicardial coronary artery disease. Nonischemic dilated cardiomyopathy often responds to medical therapy and has a better prognosis than when the cause of heart failure is coronary artery disease.

1. Dilated cardiomyopathy is the most common cardiomyopathy among young people (about 25% of cases). Signs and symptoms of heart failure may be absent.
2. Although viral infection (i.e., viral cardiomyopathy) has been implicated as an etiologic factor in some cases, the underlying cause is not well understood in most cases (i.e., **idiopathic dilated cardiomyopathy**).

B. Ischemic cardiomyopathy is a condition caused by disease of the coronary arteries with resultant wall-motion abnormalities and impaired LV function. It is the most common cardiomyopathy in the United States (up to two-thirds of all cases).

1. The degree of atherosclerosis may involve the epicardial coronary arteries or smaller subendocardial vessels, as occurs among persons with diabetes and hypertension. However, **the presence of coronary artery stenosis does not equal ischemic cardiomyopathy.** In some cases, discrepancies between the location and severity of coronary artery stenoses and dysfunctional myocardium may suggest the existence of underlying dilated cardiomyopathy.
2. Ischemic cardiomyopathy may be associated with ventricular aneurysm, MR from papillary muscle dysfunction, or arrhythmia.
3. Percutaneous and surgical revascularization and reconstructive surgery (see Chapter 11) should be carefully considered in all patients with ischemic cardiomyopathy to slow or even reverse the progression of heart failure. This includes careful definition of coronary anatomy and accurate assessment of myocardial viability in some cases, even with multiple modalities (see Chapter 45).

C. Hypertensive and diabetic cardiomyopathy are seldom considered as stand-alone diagnoses. Progression from LV hypertrophy to dysfunction in hypertensive patients (so-called burnt-out hypertensive heart) most likely results from microvascular ischemia, is common, and can be delayed or reversed with medical therapy. Hypertension and diabetes also contribute significantly to the development of coronary artery disease and ischemic cardiomyopathy.

D. Cardiotoxic agents. The list of toxins that can produce cardiomyopathy is extensive (Table 7.1). Identification of the toxin and removal of the offending agent may halt progression of heart failure and in some instances lead to improvement.

1. **Chemotherapeutic agents. Anthracycline** toxicity can cause myocyte destruction and cardiomyopathy. Patients who receive a cumulative dose of doxorubicin hydrochloride of <400 mg/m^2 are at low risk for this syndrome, whereas those who receive a cumulative dose exposure >700 mg/m^2 have nearly a 20% likelihood of development of cardiomyopathy. Other cardiotoxic drugs that require careful cardiac monitoring include cyclophosphamide and trastuzumab.
2. **Alcohol** consumption is a common cause of toxin-mediated cardiomyopathy. It accounts for up to 30% of all cases of nonischemic cardiomyopathy and may not necessarily correlate with the amount of alcohol consumed. Total abstinence from alcohol may completely reverse this disease in its early stages. The continued use of alcohol is associated with high mortality (50% at 3 to 6 years).

E. Inflammatory cardiomyopathy (or, myocarditis) is discussed in Chapter 11.

F. Valvular disorders that produce chronic volume overload, such as MR and aortic regurgitation, are most commonly responsible for valve-related systolic heart failure. Differentiating primary MR (i.e., mitral valve abnormalities such as prolapse) from secondary MR (due to annular dilation) can be difficult. A long-standing history of cardiac murmur favors the diagnosis of primary MR, whereas a centrally directed MR jet without apparent leaflet abnormalities favors secondary MR. Severe aortic stenosis and outflow tract obstruction commonly lead to progressive LV dysfunction (see Chapters 14 and 15).

G. Metabolic disorders

1. Thyroid disorders

a. Hypothyroidism is common in patients with heart failure. Severe hypothyroidism (i.e., myxedema) may cause decreased cardiac output and heart failure. Bradycardia and pericardial effusion can develop in extreme cases of hypothyroidism. Treatment consists of thyroid replacement, beginning at 25 to 50 μg of levothyroxine per day for elderly patients or 100 μg each day for young, otherwise healthy patients.

b. Severe manifestations of **hyperthyroidism** may include heart failure, especially among the elderly and patients with low ventricular reserve. Atrial fibrillation is a common accompanying arrhythmia, occurring in 9% to 22% of patients with thyrotoxicosis. Angina pectoris that had previously been stable may become unstable. Nonspecific symptoms such as fatigue, weight loss, and insomnia predominate. A high index of suspicion also is necessary in the care of patients with inappropriate tachycardia or atrial fibrillation, especially if atrial fibrillation is resistant to digoxin. Patients treated with amiodarone are at increased risk for hyperthyroidism.

2. Thiamine deficiency (beriberi). Although rare in Western countries, thiamine deficiency is still common in developing countries. It also occurs in persons who observe fad diets for long periods and in those with alcoholism. Wet beriberi includes the features of high-output cardiac failure such as marked edema, peripheral vasodilatation, and pulmonary congestion. The signs and symptoms of dry beriberi include glossitis, hyperkeratosis, and peripheral neuropathy. Laboratory evaluation may show metabolic acidosis caused by lactic acid and depressed ketolase levels in red blood cells. Intravenous therapy with 100 mg of thiamine followed by daily oral dietary replacement can lead to dramatic improvement in clinical symptoms. Some patients may develop thiamine deficiency with chronic diuretics.

3. High-output heart failure from anemia. Acute anemia caused by rapid blood loss is associated with depressed cardiac output caused by hypovolemia. Chronic anemia, however, causes symptoms of CHF due to compensatory mechanisms. Most healthy persons tolerate moderate degrees of chronic anemia (hemoglobin <9 g/dL) without symptoms of CHF, but persons with baseline heart disease have symptoms early. However, even normal hearts experience CHF with chronic anemia of severe proportions (hemoglobin <4 g/dL). The main compensatory mechanisms are decreased vascular resistance, increased 2,3-diphosphoglycerate (DPG), which shifts the hemoglobin–oxygen dissociation curve to the right, fluid retention, and increased cardiac output caused by resting tachycardia. Management of the cause of anemia and blood transfusion with diuresis improve clinical symptoms. Patients with CHF should be given transfusions slowly (1 to 2 units over 24 hours) and undergo diuresis.

4. Other metabolic causes of high-output heart failure include Paget's disease, Albright's syndrome, and pregnancy. The treatment is individualized on the basis of the underlying disorder.

H. Inherited cardiomyopathies

1. Familial dilated cardiomyopathy. Approximately 20% to 30% of the cases of dilated cardiomyopathy are thought to be familial and may have a worse prognosis.

2. Inherited myopathies such as Duchenne's muscular dystrophy, limb girdle dystrophy, and myotonic dystrophy are genetic diseases associated with dilated cardiomyopathy. Friedreich's ataxia is associated with hypertrophic cardiomyopathy but in rare instances can cause dilated cardiomyopathy. Mitochrondrial cardiomyopathies may also present with dilated cardiomyopathy.

3. Fabry's disease (α-galactosidase A deficiency) is a rare metabolic disorder that leads to LV hypertrophy because of progressive accumulation of globotriaosylceramide in the vascular endothelium leading to ischemia. Fabry's disease can be diagnosed by measuring α-galactosidase A activity, and enzyme replacement therapy is available. Fabry's disease may manifest in a manner similar to that of hypertrophic cardiomyopathy.

4. **Arrhythmogenic right ventricular dysplasia (ARVD)** usually manifests in young persons as syncope, sudden death from ventricular arrhythmias, or, less commonly, right-sided heart failure. There is a male predominance, and the condition often is diagnosed after syncope or sudden death occurs during exercise. The diagnosis of ARVD is difficult to make with endomyocardial biopsy because of the patchy nature of the disease. Magnetic resonance imaging helps in identifying fatty infiltration of the right ventricle. Long-standing right-heart failure produces evidence of RV hypertrophy and strain pattern. Management of ARVD includes antiarrhythmic drugs and devices, diuretics, digoxin, and sodium restriction. **Uhl's anomaly** is also known as parchment heart because of the paper-thin right-ventricular wall characteristic of this disease. This disease more often manifests in early childhood with signs of right-heart failure. The disease involves death of myocytes throughout the right ventricle. Uhl's anomaly is more refractory to treatment than ARVD and may be an indication for heart transplantation.

V. TREATMENT. Understanding the distinction between acute and chronic therapies is important. For example, short-term inotropic therapy is sometimes needed to bridge patients from their acute decompensation, even though long-term inotropic therapy is associated with an increased risk of mortality from arrhythmia. In contrast, administration of spironolactone in the acutely decompensated patient (and, therefore, volume-depleted from recent diuresis) may pose an increased risk of developing hyperkalemia and renal failure.

A. Acute medical therapies are used in patients with decompensated heart failure, for which short-term hemodynamic stabilization and optimization of tissue perfusion are the main goals to normalize cardiac filling pressures. Rapid diagnosis and treatment of the underlying cause should be aggressively pursued and managed. In the setting of acute heart failure, hemodynamic monitoring should be considered in guiding therapy (see Chapter 23).

1. Maximizing oxygenation capacity is vital. All patients should be positioned upright and receive supplemental oxygen as needed to ensure adequate ventilation. Mechanical ventilation should be considered if indicated, and anemia should be corrected.

2. **Vasodilators.** ACPE is often a result of impaired diastolic filling and elevated blood pressure. Vasodilators are the first-line drug therapy for the management of ACPE among patients who are not in cardiogenic shock.

   a. The most common errors in using vasodilators in the acute setting are the following:

   (1) The inability to closely monitor patient status, allowing undertreatment because of the failure to up-titrate therapy

   (2) Overreacting toward changes in blood pressure (most often due to erroneous or insufficient data), causing unnecessary changes in dosage

   (3) The lack of concomitant up-titration of an oral vasodilator regimen

   b. Nitroglycerin may be given rapidly in the emergency setting (0.4 to 0.8 mg, given sublingually every 3 to 5 minutes) and by means of intravenous infusion in the subacute setting (starting dosage of 0.2 to 0.4 μg/kg/min) and titration every 5 minutes on the basis of symptoms or mean arterial pressure (MAP). The sublingual dose can be considered as a large-dose bolus equivalent of nitroglycerin infusion (400 μg), even though it may be only partially absorbed. Contrary to general belief, there is no maximal limit to the dose of nitroglycerin until hypotension ensues. However, increasing the dose to more than 300 to 400 μg/min probably will not provide additional benefit, and another vasodilating agent usually is needed. Headache is the most common side effect.

   c. Sodium nitroprusside is a potent vasodilator that requires careful hemodynamic monitoring (usually by an arterial line). A starting dosage of 0.1 to 0.2 μ/kg per minute is used and titrated every 5 minutes to achieve a clinical response or until hypotension develops. Thiocyanate toxicity, although widely publicized, is rare in management of acute heart failure. However, nitroprusside should be used with caution in the care of patients with severe renal dysfunction. Long-term, high-dose infusion of nitroprusside should be avoided. In patients with myocardial ischemia, nitroglycerin is often preferred over sodium nitroprusside because of the potential for coronary steal.

d. **Nesiritide** is a novel intravenous vasodilator that has gained popularity in the acute care setting because of its ease of use. Nesiritide is indicated for decompensated heart failure and can be infused in the telemetry unit without invasive hemodynamic monitoring. Nesiritide infusion reduces plasma BNP levels (but not NT-proBNP). An optional starting dose of 2 mg/kg delivered by intravenous bolus followed by an infusion at a rate of 0.01 mg/kg per minute for up to 48 hours has been shown to be effective. In select cases, it has been shown to produce large-volume diuresis without significant renal compromise, and urinary output should be monitored carefully. Nesiritide should be avoided in patients with renal failure, hypotension, and other contraindications of vasodilator therapy (e.g., severe aortic stenosis with preserved systolic LV function).

3. **Diuretics.** In addition to the ability to gradually reduce intravascular volume, diuretics have an immediate vasodilator effect, which may be responsible for the immediate beneficial effect in patients with ACPE. Because many patients with ACPE do not have whole-body salt and water excess, the **judicious use of diuretics** is recommended. Patients without chronic exposure to loop diuretics usually respond to 20 to 40 mg of intravenous furosemide. Patients undergoing long-term furosemide therapy usually need an intravenous bolus dose at least equivalent to their oral dose, and in some cases continuous infusions may provide more effective diuresis without cardiorenal compromise. When using intravenous diuretics, a therapeutic goal (with net fluid balance or estimated dry weight) should be established, so that conversion to an oral regimen can be instituted at the appropriate time. Adverse effects that should be closely monitored include hypotension, hypokalemia, hypomagnesemia, hypocalcemia, and renal azotemia (estimates of fractional excretion of sodium is inaccurate in this setting because of alterations in urinary electrolyte excretion by diuretics).

4. **Inotropic therapy.** When signs and symptoms of decompensated heart failure persists despite administration of vasodilators and diuretics, aggressive hemodynamic monitoring is needed to determine the need for inotropic therapy. **Inotropic therapy is used for temporary hemodynamic support and has not been shown to improve survival.** For patients without significant hypotension, intravenous dobutamine or milrinone can be used to augment cardiac output. Both drugs are associated with increased oxygen demand and cardiac arrhythmias and should be used with extreme caution to treat patients with ischemia and preexisting arrhythmias. Both drugs may cause hypotension, although this is more common with loading doses of milrinone. **There is no evidence to support the use of chronic or intermittent infusion of inotropic agents.** In cases of severe hypotension (especially as a result of drug administration of vasodilators or β-blockers), temporary use of vasopressors such as dopamine, norepinephrine, and phenylephrine may be necessary en route to mechanical assist support.

a. **Dobutamine** has a shorter half-life than milrinone and usually is the drug of choice in the acute setting. Dobutamine infusions act rapidly and are usually begun at 2.5 to 5.0 μg/kg per minute. On the basis of hemodynamic response, it may be titrated by 1 to 2 μg/kg per minute every 30 minutes until the desired effect is reached or until dosage reaches 15 to 20 μg/kg per minute.

b. **Milrinone** is a vasodilator and an inotropic agent and should be used cautiously to treat patients with borderline hypotension. For patients who need an immediate inotropic response, a loading dose of 50 μg/kg is followed by an infusion of 0.375 to 0.75 μg/kg per minute.

5. **Positive airway pressure ventilation** has been used for hypoxic patients with ACPE. It has demonstrated clinical improvement and success in avoiding

impending intubations only in small clinical studies and primarily in the acute setting to avoid intubations.

6. **Ultrafiltration** has been used as an alternative to pharmacologic diuresis in acute decompensated heart failure with significant cardiorenal compromise or overtly fluid overloaded states. Recent studies have demonstrated its safety and potential benefits, although its invasiveness and appropriate usage remains to be determined.

B. Chronic medical therapies. The goals of medical therapy are to prolong survival and to improve symptoms and functional status. Our strategy for medical management of chronic heart failure is illustrated in Table 7.3.

1. **Angiotensin-converting enzyme (ACE) inhibitors** have been established to reduce morbidity and mortality among patients with systolic heart failure. The mechanism of long-term benefit is most likely related to attenuation of the neurohormonal response by the RAAS in the syndrome of heart failure.
   a. **Use of an ACE inhibitor is the first-line therapy for asymptomatic LV dysfunction and symptomatic heart failure.** The dose of the ACE inhibitor should be increased to the target dose (Table 7.4). Although there are theoretical benefits of using "tissue" ACE inhibitors (e.g., quinapril, ramipril), there are no data to support their preferential use. Relative contraindications include hyperkalemia (potassium >5.5 mEq/day), renal insufficiency (creatine >3.0 mg/dL), and hypotension (systolic blood pressure <90 mm Hg) and should be gauged on a case-by-case basis. It is not advisable to stop ACE inhibitors in patients with systolic heart failure, even when there is complete resolution of symptoms.
   b. After initiation, close monitoring is warranted to look for **hyperkalemia** and **renal insufficiency.**
      (1) **Hypotension** is common, especially with first dose in a volume-depleted patients (e.g., after aggressive diuresis). This may require down-titration of diuretic doses and other vasodilator therapy. Captopril is usually used in the acute setting (e.g., after infarction) for this reason, because the half-life is relatively short.
      (2) **Renal insufficiency** and **hyperkalemia** are common and usually occur when ACE inhibitors are given in the setting of depleted intravascular volume (e.g., after aggressive diuresis). ***It is crucial to discontinue other nephrotoxic agents (e.g., nonsteroidal anti-inflammatory agents)*** and ensure adequate kidney perfusion (i.e., not hypotensive). ***If blood urea nitrogen or creatine levels increase by less than 50%, ACE inhibitors can be continued safely; if they increase by more than 50%, the ACE inhibitor dose should be halved; if they increase by more than 100%, the ACE inhibitor should be held and switched to hydralazine or isosorbide dinitrate.*** In the case of hyperkalemia, discontinuation of potassium supplementation and reducing the ACE inhibitor dose constitute the best strategy.
   c. Unique side effects of ACE inhibitors are cough and angioedema.
      (1) The **cough** associated with use of ACE inhibitors is related to increased levels of bradykinin. The cough tends to be dry, nonproductive, and involuntary. A true ACE-inhibitor cough rarely resolves with changing the dose or the type of ACE inhibitor. All attempts should be made to identify an alternative cause of the cough before discontinuing ACE inhibitors.
      (2) **Angioedema** is a rare complication of use of ACE inhibitors (0.4%). It involves soft tissue edema of the lips, face, tongue, and, occasionally, the oropharynx and epiglottis. Angioedema usually begins within 2 weeks of initiation of ACE-inhibitor therapy, but some patients present with this complication months to years after starting therapy. **Angioedema is an absolute contraindication to the use of any type of ACE inhibitor or angiotensin II receptor blocker (ARB).**
2. **ARBs** are specific receptor antagonists to the angiotensin II type 1 receptors that are commonly used as antihypertensive agents. Although they theoretically provide more complete inhibition of the deleterious effects of angiotensin II than

TABLE 7.3 The Cleveland Clinic Foundation Heart Failure Management Standards of Care

Initial evaluation

Determine systolic versus diastolic dysfunction
Determine cause beyond LV function (complete metabolic profile and blood count, thyroid function, electrocardiogram, chest radiography)
Consider determining plasma B-type natriuretic peptide level as an aid to diagnosis and management of HF
Determine heart failure staging and NYHA functional class
Adjunctive studies: metabolic stress testing (peak V_{O_2}, PET scan)

Nonpharmacologic therapies

Patient education regarding diet, medications, fluid management (including daily weights, "ideal weight," and how to treat weight increases), activity and signs or symptoms of worsening conditions. Advise daily weight monitoring.
Fluid restriction: <2 L/d, increase to <1.5 L/d when serum sodium <130 mg/dL
Sodium restriction: ≤3 g sodium diet for mild HF (NYHA I–II), ≤2 g sodium diet for advanced HF (NYHA III–IV); dietary consult recommended
Cardiac rehabilitation, home health consult recommended

Pharmacologic therapies

Diuretics: for volume overload, titrate to euvolemia
- Maintenance dosing versus aggressive dosing with symptoms
- Add thiazide drugs 30 minutes before loop diuretics for synergistic response if necessary

ACE inhibitors and other RAAS drugs: titrate to target dose, as tolerated
- Do not use if serum creatinine >3.0 mg/dL or potassium >5.5 mg/dL
- Begin therapy if SBP >90 mm Hg without vasodilator therapy or >80 mm Hg and asymptomatic with other vasodilator therapy (do not hold vasodilator unless SBP <80 mm Hg or signs or symptoms of orthostasis, mental obtundation or reduced urine output)
- Begin therapy if serum sodium >134 mg/dL, may need further diagnostic evaluation of fluid status and decompensation if ≤134 mg/dL
- Add spironolactone for NYHA III–IV or post-MI without hyperkalemia or renal dysfunction
- Alternative to ACE inhibitors: ARBs or hydralazine plus isosorbide dinitrate combination
  ARBs show equivalency with ACE inhibitors, and add-on ARBs have shown to reduce cardiovascular morbidity and mortality in chronic heart failure
  Hydralazine and isosorbide dinitrate fixed combination should be considered in African American patients with advanced heart failure.

β-Adrenergic Blockers: titrate to target dose, as tolerated
- Use in NYHA II–III (may use NYHA I patients with history of MI or hypertension or NYHA IV patients who are euvolemic and no signs/symptoms of volume overload)
- Contraindicated in patients with history of severe hepatic failure, bronchospasm, bradycardia (<50 beats/min without symptoms or <60 beats/min with symptoms), heart block, sick sinus syndrome without permanent pacemaker, overt congestion, or symptomatic hypotension
- Should take with food and stagger dose with vasodilator therapy and adjust diuretics; titrate up every 2–4 weeks as tolerated until target dose is reached
- Reduce β-blocker dose if dizziness or lightheadedness, worsening heart failure (edema, weight gain, dyspnea), significant bradycardia; reinstate β-blocker
  - If off <72 hours and no cardiogenic shock—restart with same dose
  - If off >72 hours and <7 days and no cardiogenic shock—restart at half dose
  - If off >7 days or episode of cardiogenic shock—restart at lowest dose and retitrate

Digoxin: generally give low dose of 0.125 mg/d, may reduce dose if low body mass index or renal insufficiency is present
- Usually indicated after hospitalization
- Watch for signs of digoxin toxicity, bradycardia
- No indication for monitoring digoxin levels, but if known should maintain <1.2 mg/dL

ACE, angiotensin-converting enzyme; ARB, angiotensin II receptor blocker; HF, heart failure; MI, myocardial infarction; NYHA, New York Heart Association; RAAS, renin–angiotensin–aldosterone system; SPB, systolic blood pressure.

TABLE 7.4 Drug Dosing for Common Medical Therapies for Chronic Heart Failure

Drug	Start (mg)	Target (mg)	Max (mg)
Ace inhibitiors			
Captopril (Capoten)	6.25–12.5 tid	50 tid	100 tid
Enalapril (Vasotec)	2.5–5 bid	10 bid	20 bid
Lisinopril (Prinivil, Zestril)	2.5–5 qd	20 qd	40 qd
Ramipril (Altace)	1.25–2.5 bid	5 bid	10 bid
Quinapril (Accupril)	5 bid	20 bid	20 bid
Fosinopril (Monopril)	2.5 or 5 bid	20 bid	20 bid
Benazepril (Lotensin)[a]	2.5 or 5 bid	20 bid	20 bid
Moexipril (Univasc)[a]	7.5 qd	30 qd	30 qd
Trandolapril (Mavik)	1 qd	4 qd	4 qd
Angiotensin receptor blockers			
Candesartan (Atacand)	16 qd	32 qd	32 qd
Valsartan (Diovan)	80 qd	160 qd	320 qd
Losartan (Cozaar)[a]	12.5–25 qd	50 qd	100 qd
Irbesartan (Avapro)[a]	150 qd	300 qd	300 qd
Telmisartan (Micardis)[a]	40 qd	80 qd	80 qd
Hydralazine isosorbide dinitrate			
Hydralazine	25 qid	50–75 qid	100 qid
Isosorbide dinitrate	10–20 tid	20–80 tid	80 tid
BiDil (fixed-dose hydralazine-isosorbide dinitrate)	25/37.5 mg tid	50/75 mg tid	50/75 mg tid
Aldosterone antagonist			
Spironolactone (Aldactone)	12.5–25 qd	25 qd	50 bid
Eplerenone (Inspra)	50 qd	100 qd	100 qd
Diuretics			
Furosemide (Lasix)	10 qd (IV) 20 qd (PO)	As required	1,000 qd (IV) 240 bid (PO)
Bumetanide (Bumex)	1 qd	As required	10 qd
Torsemide (Demadex)	10 qd	As required	200 qd
Ethacrynic acid (Edecrin)	50 qd	As required	200 bid
Hydrochlorothiazide (HCTZ)	25 qd	As required	50 qd
Triamterene (Maxzide)	50 qd	As required	100 bid
Metolazone (Zaroxolyn)	2.5 qd	As required	10 qd
β-blockers			
Carvedilol (Coreg)	3.125 bid	6.25–25 bid	50 bid
Metoprolol succinate (Toprol XL)	25 qd	150–200 qd	200 qd
Bisoprolol (Zebeta)[a]	1.25 qd	10 qd	20 qd

[a] Not yet approved by the FDA for management of heart failure.

do ACE inhibitors, clinical trials have not shown any superiority in patients with heart failure. In general, ARBs are used and monitored in the same manner as ACE inhibitors. These drugs are reserved for patients who are ACE-inhibitor intolerant, although in practice, these drugs are extensively used. ARBs have a similar side-effect profile (e.g., hypotension, renal insufficiency, hyperkalemia), although they are better tolerated clinically. Whether they can produce extra benefit when used in addition to ACE inhibitors is still being debated in light of conflicting results from CHARM and VALIANT.

3. The combination of **hydralazine** and **isosorbide dinitrate** is the original vasodilator combination therapy. Recently, a fixed-dose combination (Bidil) has shown to confer both a morbidity and mortality benefit in African Americans with

NYHA class III–IV heart failure despite standard medications with preserved blood pressure and evidence of cardiac remodeling. Hydraazine and isosorbide dinitrate are also indicated when patients are unable to tolerate ACE inhibitors or ARBs because of severe renal insufficiency or angioedema. Rare side effects of hydralazine may include reflex tachycardia and a lupus-like syndrome. Nitrates can cause headaches and tolerance if used continuously.

4. β-Adrenergic blockers (i.e., **β-blockers).** Once considered to be contraindicated for patients with heart failure, β-blockers are now considered **first-line therapy for symptomatic patients with heart failure (NYHA class II or III)** because of the consistent mortality benefits. The exact mechanism of action is not well understood, even though it is presumed to act on the neurohormonal axis.

a. It is often customary to start ACE inhibitors before using β-blockers. This is particularly true in patients with advanced heart failure, when there is a narrow margin of error. The rationale of titrating one drug before the other is to better monitor potential side effects, and the exact sequence is somewhat historical. In some patients (e.g., those who are post-MI or with tachycardia), β-blockers may be of particular benefit and should be started promptly, before or concurrently with ACE inhibitors.

b. Only carvedilol, bisoprolol, and metoprolol succinate have been approved for the medical treatment of chronic heart failure. Although atenolol and metoprolol tartrate are widely available and relatively inexpensive, there is no evidence to support their use in this population.

c. Current recommendations are to start β-blockers in those who are deemed euvolemic by clinical assessment (not decompensated). The general principle is to "start low and go slow." The initial dose is **slowly up-titrated every 2 to 4 weeks over 3 to 4 months to the target dose**, provided that the patient can tolerate the adverse effects. It is imperative to maintain contact with the patient and to adjust vasodilator or diuretic therapy during drug titration. **There is a potential risk of worsening clinical status with drug withdrawal.** It is not advisable to stop β-blockers in patients with a history of heart failure, even if there is complete resolution of symptoms and LV dysfunction.

d. Side effects are common when using β-blockers. Patients should understand that these drugs are used to prolong survival and usually do not improve symptoms.

(1) Dizziness and **lightheadedness** are common and related to hypotension or heart block. **Significant bradycardia** mandates dose reduction of β-blockers and other heart rate–lowering agents such as digoxin and amiodarone. **Advanced heart block** is a contraindication to β-blockers unless a permanent pacemaker is available. **Hypotension** can be managed by lowering diuretics and ACE-inhibitor doses and by staggering the timing of drug administration (e.g., β-blockers taken 2 hours after vasodilator therapy or ACE inhibitors taken in the evening and β-blockers in the morning). In practice, carvedilol (with its nonselective, α_1-blocking, vasodilating effects) may have greater blood pressure–lowering effects than selective β_1-agents such as metoprolol succinate (Toprol XL), although both drugs are well tolerated (up to 70% of heart failure patients in our clinics).

(2) Worsening heart failure is still an important adverse effect of β-blockers because of its known negative inotropic effects. This is particularly common during the early titration phase, when patients may present with worsening congestion, fluid retention, and fatigue. Intensification of salt restriction and diuretic regimen and reductions or slower increase in β-blocker dose may be necessary.

5. Aldosterone receptor antagonists such as spironolactone have long been used as a weak, potassium-sparing diuretic in patients with heart failure. The concept of incomplete blockade of the RAAS by ACE inhibitors led to studies that demonstrated significant benefits of aldosterone antagonism in patients with advanced heart failure.

a. Spironolactone is indicated in **patients with advanced systolic heart failure (recent or current NYHA class III or IV, left ventricular ejection fraction (LVEF ≤35%) already treated with ACE inhibitors and β-blockers and without significant renal dysfunction (creatinine >2.5 mg/dL) or hyperkalemia (potassium >5 mEq/L).** Eplerenone is indicated for patients with postinfarction heart failure (LVEF ≤40%).

b. Spironolactone is prescribed in **low dose** (25 mg/day if creatine <2.0 mg/dL and potassium <4.5 mEq/L), and there usually is no need to up-titrate the dose. In most cases, the dose of potassium supplementation should be reduced or held.

c. Chemistry panel should be monitored in 1 to 2 weeks after initiation and monitored at regular intervals. Some patients may require a lower dose (12.5 mg/day or 25 mg every other day) at initiation or during follow-up (if creatine = 2 to 2.5 mg/dL or potassium = 4.5 to 5 mEq/L). One trial demonstrated significant mortality benefits in using eplerenone (25 to 50 mg/day) in patients with post-MI heart failure.

d. The most common side effect for aldosterone antagonists is **hyperkalemia,** particularly in patients with concomitant **renal insufficiency** and diabetes mellitus (with renal tubular acidosis), which usually requires dose reduction or discontinuation. **Painful gynecomastia** and **galactorrhea** may occur when using spironolactone, but these side effects are rare in patients on eplerenone.

6. **Diuretics** are used to maintain euvolemia and to improve symptoms. Overuse of diuretics, however, may cause worsening organ perfusion (e.g., acute renal failure), weakness, and electrolyte abnormalities.

a. The **lowest possible dose of diuretic needed to prevent substantial volume overload** should be used. A patient often must tolerate some degree of peripheral edema if right-sided heart failure exists. In some patients, a moderate degree of renal insufficiency is tolerated to maintain relative euvolemia. Some patients who are relatively asymptomatic and demonstrate no signs of fluid retention (i.e., supported by a relatively low plasma BNP level) may not need any diuretic therapy.

b. An effective and inexpensive initial regimen includes 20 to 120 mg of furosemide taken orally each day. If furosemide doses higher than 120 mg/day are needed, a second evening dose usually is prescribed. If this regimen fails, a daily dose of a thiazide diuretic, such as metolazone (Zaroxolyn) or hydrochlorothiazide (HCTZ), often is added.

c. More expensive loop diuretics (e.g., torsemide, bumetanide) may have better bioavailability. In select cases, they may be more effective in diuretic-resistant patients. Unlike furosemide (which has a 1:2 intravenous-to-oral dose conversion), the intravenous and oral doses are equivalent.

d. The concept of **diuretic resistance** is evolving. Although there is an entity with recurrent exacerbation of decompensated heart failure despite maximal diuretic therapy, most cases involve dietary (sodium) indiscretion and medication noncompliance.

7. **Digoxin** is a positive inotropic and negative chronotropic drug. It is commonly used to treat **patients with heart failure and concomitant atrial fibrillation.**

a. Digoxin is safe and significantly reduces hospitalization for heart failure. The use of 0.125 mg of digoxin each day to treat patients with normal renal function is recommended.

b. Serum digoxin levels probably have no correlation with clinical response, and monitoring is, therefore, unnecessary unless toxicity is suspected or in the setting of worsening renal insufficiency. Usually levels less than 1.2 nmol/L are desirable. The side effects of digoxin may be more pronounced in the setting of hypokalemia.

c. It is still unclear whether digoxin is beneficial in all patients with heart failure, although it is generally advisable to start patients on digoxin after an index hospitalization for heart-failure exacerbation to reduce subsequent morbidity.

Studies have shown that withdrawal of digoxin is often associated with worsening clinical status.

8. **Electrolyte supplementation** is perhaps the most important and least emphasized area of monitoring of ongoing drug therapy for heart failure. Potassium depletion is common with diuretic therapy, whereas hyperkalemia can be caused by ACE inhibitors, spironolactone, or worsening renal insufficiency. In general, oral potassium supplementation is necessary to maintain serum potassium level in the ideal range of 4.0 to 5.0 mEq/L. Magnesium, thiamine, and calcium depletion are also common with long-standing diuretic therapy.

C. **Chronic nonmedical therapies.** The goals of device therapy are to ameliorate symptoms and improve functional status in advanced heart failure.

1. **Patient education and disease management programs** remain the most effective treatment strategy for patients with systolic heart failure. Sodium restriction and medication compliance are the key to preventing disease progression and exacerbations. Drugs such as nonsteroidal anti-inflammatory agents should be avoided. Control of blood pressure, glucose levels, and lipid concentrations should be emphasized. Many patients can perform self-monitoring (i.e., daily weights and examinations) and care (i.e., titration of diuretics) similar to that in diabetes care.
2. **Cardiac resynchronization therapy (CRT).** The development of biventricular pacing technology has identified a subgroup of patients with heart failure and dyssynchrony (particularly those with the left bundle branch block morphology) that may gain substantial morbidity benefits from CRT. Patients with significant LV dysfunction (EF <30%), advanced heart failure (i.e., symptomatic despite maximal standard therapy), and with a QRS duration of more than 130 ms on the ECG may be considered for CRT.
3. **Exercise training.** There is clear evidence from the literature that exercise training improves endothelial function and functional capacity in patients with chronic heart failure. A supervised cardiac rehabilitation program should be advised if available. Patients should be advised to maintain all activities of daily living as tolerated.

IV. CONTROVERSIES IN THE TREATMENT OF SYSTOLIC HEART FAILURE

A. **Anticoagulation** in the setting of systolic heart failure is controversial, and the benefits of using warfarin to prevent cerebrovascular events is unclear.

1. The general rule in regard to anticoagulation of patients with heart failure is to use **warfarin sodium** in the following settings:
   a. Ventricular thrombi documented by echocardiography
   b. Any history of atrial fibrillation
   c. Pulmonary embolism or chronic deep venous thrombosis
   d. After a large, transmural, anterior wall MI with a large akinetic or dyskinetic wall.
2. Most patients with heart failure are on an extensive regimen of medications, and care should be used when adding any medication because of the possible side effect and drug-interaction profile of the new medication. Whether use of warfarin sodium lowers mortality rates among patients with decreased LVEF (<35%) without other indications for anticoagulants is unknown. Use of warfarin certainly complicates the medical regimen and increases the risk for bleeding complications.

B. **Antiarrhythmic therapy in systolic heart failure.** Sudden cardiac death is unpredictable and accounts for nearly one-half of deaths among patients with systolic heart failure. Although frequent premature ventricular contractions (PVCs) are a marker of increased mortality in these patients, studies involving patients who have had an MI revealed that the use of conventional antiarrhythmic agents to suppress PVCs leads to higher mortality.

1. **Amiodarone** has been extensively studied in the care of patients with systolic heart failure because of its low incidence of proarrhythmia and its favorable hemodynamic effects. Data from four large, randomized trials involving

TABLE 7.5 Common Clinical Predictors of Poor Survival in Systolic Heart Failure

- Increased age
- Functional capacity—high New York Heart Association functional class
- Severely reduced LV ejection fraction (Left venticular end-diastolic dimension [LVEF] <25%), extensive cardiac remodeling (LVIDd >65 mm) or reduced cardiac index (CI <2.5)
- Concomitant diastolic dysfunction (especially restrictive mitral inflow and dilated left atrium) and increase in pulse pressure
- Reduced right ventricular function
- Atrial fibrillation, tachycardia, and reduced heart rate variability
- Low peak V_{O_2} with maximal exercise (14 mL/min/kg), low heart rate response to exercise, increased peripheral chemosensitivity (ventilatory response to hypoxia) and low V_E/V_{CO_2}
- High plasma B-type natriuretic peptide (BNP) and N-terminal proBNP levels
- Anemia of heart failure
- Markers of reduced tissue perfusion:
  - Low mean arterial pressure
  - Renal insufficiency (creatinine clearance <60 mL/min)
  - Attenuated response to diuretics and lack of hemodynamic and structural improvement (reverse remodeling) with medical therapy
  - Persistent signs of congestion and fluid retention, including hepatic insufficiency
  - Serum sodium <135 mg/dL
- Cardiac and neurohormonal biomarkers (cardiac troponin, norepinephrine, cytokines, endothelin-1, urotensin-II, cardiotropin-I)
- Cardiac dyssynchrony (QRS >130 ms, left bundle-branch block)
- Depression
- Nocturnal Cheyne-Stokes respiration, and obstructive sleep apnea

patients with systolic heart failure but without previous sustained ventricular tachyarrhythmia suggested the following:

a. Amiodarone appears not to be harmful to patients with systolic heart failure and frequent PVCs, and it demonstrated a trend toward reducing overall mortality.

b. Amiodarone reduces the incidence of arrhythmic death among these patients.

2. **Implantable cardioverter–defibrillators (ICDs)** (see Chapter 22) are increasingly used to prevent sudden cardiac death, particularly in patients with a history of MI and systolic heart failure (EF <35%) following the MADIT-II and SCD-HeFT studies. There is little doubt that this strategy improves survival, but the logistics and the huge cost to society remain controversial because many patients with systolic heart failure are likely to qualify for this expensive therapy. Careful discussion regarding risks and benefits are warranted, preferably with an electrophysiologist.

V. PROGNOSIS. Heart failure, when caused by systolic or diastolic dysfunction, is associated with a high mortality rate. In the Framingham study, patients with heart failure had mortality rates four to eight times higher than that of the general population of the same age. A patient with NYHA class IV disease has a 1-year survival rate of between 30% and 50%—a mortality rate that is as high as that for some malignancies (Table 7.5). Recently, the Seattle Heart Failure Model provides reliable prediction based on clinically available variables.

Landmark Articles

The BEST Investigators. A trial of the beta-blocker bucindolol in patients with advanced chronic heart failure. *N Engl J Med* 2001;344:1659–1667.

The CIBIS-II Investigators. The Cardiac Insufficiency Bisoprolol Study II (CIBIS II): a randomized trial. *Lancet* 1999;353:9–13.

Cohn JN, Archibald DG, Ziesche S, et al. Effect of vasodilator therapy on mortality in chronic congestive heart failure: results of a Veterans Administration Cooperative Study (V-Heft I). *N Engl J Med* 1986;314:1547–1552.

Cohn JN, Tognoni G, for the Valsartan Heart Failure Trial Investigators. A randomized trial of the angiotensin-recepto blocker valsartan in chronic heart failure. *N Engl J Med* 2001;345:1667–1675.
CONSENSUS Trial Study Group. Effects of enalapril on mortality in severe congestive heart failure: results of the Cooperative North Scandinavian Enalapril Survival Study (CONSENSUS). *N Engl J Med* 1987;316:1429–1435.
The Digitalis Investigation Group: The effect of digoxin on morbidity and mortality in patients with heart failure. *N Engl J Med* 1997;336:525–533.
MERIT-HF Study Group. Effect of metoprolol CR/XL in chronic heart failure: Metoprolol CR/XL Randomized Intervention Trial in Congestive Heart Failure (MERIT-HF). *Lancet* 1999;353:2001–2007.
Packer M, Bristow MR, Cohn JN, et al. The effect of carvedilol on morbidity and mortality in patients with chronic heart failure. *N Engl J Med* 1996;334:1349–1355.
Packer M, Coats ACS, Fowler MB, et al. Effect of carvedilol on survival in severe chronic heart failure. *N Engl J Med* 2001;344:1651–1658.
Packer M, Poole-Wilson PA, Armstrong PW, et al. Comparative effects of low and high dose of the ACE inhibitor, lisinopril, on morbidity and mortality in chronic heart failure. *Circulation* 1999;100:2312–2318.
Pfeffer MA, McMurray JJ, Velazquez EJ, et al. Valsartan, Captopril, or both in myocardial infarction complicated by heart failure, left ventricular dysfunction, or both. *N Engl J Med* 2003;1349:1893–1906.
Pfeffer MA, Swedberg K, Granger CB, et al. Effects of candesartan on mortality and morbidity in patients with chronic heart failure: the CHARM overall programme. *Lancet* 2003;362:759–766.
Pitt B, Poole-Wilson PA, Segal R, et al. Effect of losartan compared with captopril on mortality in patients with symptomatic heart failure (Evaluation of Losartan in the Elderly survival study [ELITE II]). *Lancet* 2000;355:1582–1587.
SOLVD Investigators. Effect of enalapril on survival in patients with reduced left ventricular ejection fractions and congestive heart failure. *N Engl J Med* 1991;325:293–302.
Taylor A, Ziesche S, Yancy C, et al. Combination of isosorbide dinitrate and hydralizine in blacks with heart failure. *N Engl J Med* 2004;351:2049–2057.

Key Reviews

Adams KF, Lindenfeld J, Arnold JMO, et al. Executive Summary: HFSA 2006 comprehensive heart failure practice guideline. *J Card Fail* 2006;12:10–38.
Hunt SA, Abraham WT, Chin MH, et al. ACC/AHA 2005 guideline update for diagnosis and management of chronic heart failure in the adult: Executive summary. A Report of the American College of Cardiology/American Heart Association Task Force on Practice Guidelines (Writing Committee to Review the 2001 Guidelines for the Evaluation and Management of Heart Failure): Developed in Collaboration with the American College of Chest Physicians and the International Society for Heart and Lung Transplantation, Endorsed by the Heart Rhythm Society. *J Am Coll Cardiol* 2005;46:1116–1143.
Tang WH, Francis GS, Morrow DA, et al. National Academy of Clinical Biochemistry Laboratory Medicine Practice Guidelines: clinical utilization of cardiac biomarker testing in heart failure. *Circulation* 2007;116:e99–e109.

Relevant Book Chapters

Systolic heart failure. In: Libby P, Bonow RO eds. *Braunwald's heart disease: a textbook of cardiovascular medicine,* 8th ed. Philadelphia: WB Saunders, 2007.
Heart failure with preserved systolic function. In: Libby P, Bonow RO, eds. *Braunwald's heart disease: a textbook of cardiovascular medicine,* 8th ed. Philadelphia: WB Saunders, 2007.
Francis GS, Sonnenblick E, Tang WH. Pathophysiology of heart failure. In: Valentin F, ed. *Hurst's the heart,* 13th ed. New York: McGraw-Hill, 2007.
Tang WH, Young JB. Chronic heart failure. In: Topol EJ, ed. *Textbook of cardiovascular medicine,* 3rd ed. Philadelphia: Lippincott Williams & Wilkins, 2006.

Useful Websites

Seattle Heart Failure Model: http://depts.washington.edu/shfm/
HFSA Heart failure guidelines: http://www.heartfailureguidelines.org/

8 HEART FAILURE WITH PRESERVED LEFT VENTRICULAR EJECTION FRACTION

Ryan P. Daly

I. INTRODUCTION

A. Epidemiologic population studies suggest that nearly one-half of patients with heart failure have a preserved ejection fraction; the proportion in those hospitalized has been reported to range from 24% to 55%. The survival of patients with heart failure and preserved ejection fraction was once thought to be better than those with a decreased ejection fraction, but recent evidence suggests similar mortality rates.

Heart failure with preserved left ventricular ejection fraction (HFpEF) is the preferred term over diastolic heart failure, as the physiologic abnormalities are not solely restricted to either diastole or systole. Many patients with signs or symptoms of heart failure and preserved ejection fraction may have causes other than diastolic dysfunction. Furthermore systolic indices other than ejection fraction, (e.g., myocardial velocities or ventricular–arterial coupling) are usually abnormal. Diastolic heart failure more properly represents a subset of patients with heart failure and preserved left ventricular (LV) ejection fraction.

To date there have been no large randomized, controlled clinical outcome trials of therapies that demonstrate a mortality benefit, although the results of a number of ongoing trials are eagerly awaited.

B. A consensus definition of diastolic heart failure is lacking. Diastolic heart failure may be defined as **(1) signs *or* symptoms of congestive heart failure; (2) normal or mildly abnormal systolic LV function; (3) evidence of diastolic dysfunction.** It arises from a disturbance in ventricular relaxation or distensibility, necessitating elevated left atrial (LA) filling pressures to achieve adequate cardiac output. Diastole is defined as the part of the cardiac cycle that begins with aortic valve closure and ends with equalization of LA and LV pressures (just preceding mitral valve closure). It is divided into two phases: isovolumic relaxation time and the auxotonic phase. The latter is subdivided into rapid filling, slow filling, and atrial contraction phases (Fig. 8.1).

C. Early diastole depends on active relaxation of the ventricle, as well as passive properties of the ventricle that include wall thickness, chamber geometry, and myocardial stiffness. Relaxation is an energy-dependent process and is influenced by load (pre- or afterload), inactivation, and nonuniformity. High afterload, as in the case of severe hypertension, will delay the rate of ventricular pressure fall and may lead to elevation of filling pressures. Myocardial inactivation is determined by calcium homeostatis, mediated in part by Sarco/Endoplasmic Reticulum Ca^{2+}-ATPase (SERCA) and the calcium ATPase and its inhibitory protein phospholamban as well as by myofilament regulators of cross-bridge cycling (calcium detachment). These processess are dependent upon myocardial energetics (ADP/ATP ratio and Pi concentration), and consequently are impaired by hypoxia and ischemia, and as well as by increased LV mass. Lastly, nonuniformity refers to how in some patients regional ventricular relaxation may occur asynchronously and lead to a slower rate of ventricular pressure fall. **The time constant of isovolumic relxation, tau (τ), is used to describe this rate of fall in LV pressure. This is the hemodynamic measure of myocardial relaxation, as tau increases, active relaxation occurs more slowly.** A tau greater than 48 ms is considered abnormal.

Active relaxation produces negative intraventricular pressures and creates a suction effect that is maximum at the cardiac apex. Meanwhile, LA pressure rises

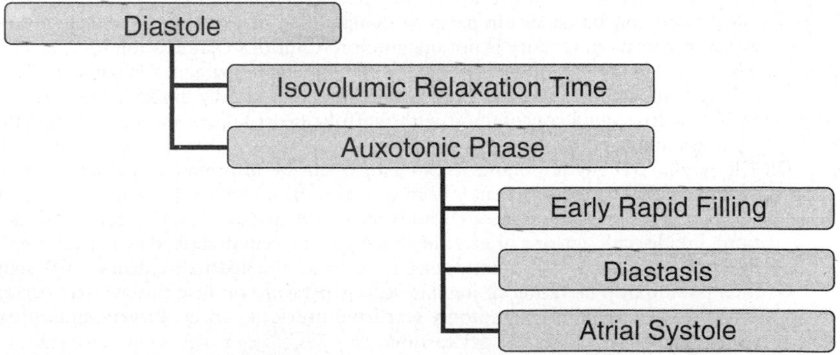

Figure 8.1. Phases of diastole.

as blood returns through the pulmonary veins. When LA pressure exceeds LV pressure, the mitral valve opens, and rapid diastolic filling occurs. **Passive filling of the LV depends on many factors: the viscoelastic properties of the myocardium (myocardial stiffness), chamber size and shape, wall thickness, intrathoracic pressure, and pericardial constraint.**

D. The viscoelastic properties or compliance of the LV can be expressed as dP/dV (i.e., change in pressure over volume), and is determined by the myocardial cytoskeleton and the composition of the extracellular matrix (ECM). The cytosketal protein titin provides most of the elastic force of cardiac myocytes. Pertubations in the composition of the ECM, primarily the amount and quality of the fibrillar collagen in terms of the degree of cross-linking and glycosylation, play an important role in determining myocardial stiffness. Perturbation of the matrix of the ventricle may occur with ischemia (i.e., from epicardial coronary disease or subendocardial ischemia) and with pressure-induced myocyte hypertrophy (i.e., adverse remodeling), which causes increased collagen content and a stiffer chamber. Infiltrative cardiomyopathies (e.g., amyloid, sarcoid, mucopolysaccharidoses) reduce the elastic recoil of the ventricle. Myocardial stiffness generally increases with age owing to a decrease in the elastic properties of the myocardium.

E. As rapid ventricular filling occurs, LV relaxation and recoil continues at a lesser rate. LA pressure falls, and the phase of slow, passive filling occurs. **LA contraction occurs, contributing 25%** to LV filling in the normal heart but significantly more in patients with impaired filling.

F. Diastolic function depends on five important parameters:

1. Heart rate (i.e., diastole is disproportionately shortened with faster heart rates)
2. Circulating fluid volume
3. Anatomic considerations (e.g., LA, mitral valve, pulmonary veins, LV mass, pericardium)
4. Active myocardial relaxation (i.e., myoenergetics)
5. Passive pressure-volume relationship (e.g., collagen composition, infiltration)

II. CLINICAL PRESENTATION

A. Analogous to systolic dysfunction, diastolic dysfunction may be asymptomatic in a compensated patient. Heart failure is predominantly a disease of the elderly. Older patients are more likely to be female and have a preserved ejection function. The symptoms of diastolic heart failure are indistinguishable from those of systolic heart failure. Fatigue, impaired effort tolerance, dyspnea, wheeze, abdominal bloating, early satiety, and peripheral edema may occur in isolation or in any combination. Dyspnea is usually the earliest symptom. Palpitations may herald the onset of (poorly tolerated) atrial fibrillation. Syncope or sudden death may occur because of tachyarrhythmias or bradyarrhythmias. Some patients may have predominantly right-sided signs and symptoms, typically those with pericardial constriction or restriction.

B. The signs of diastolic heart failure are neither sensitive nor specific. **Signs of congestion may be absent in patients complaining of dyspnea, especially in the outpatient setting.** Obesity is not uncommon. Cautious examination for systemic disorders that may result in diastolic dysfunction, including hemochromatosis, sarcoidosis, amyloidosis, and diabetes, is warranted but usually unrewarding. Hypertension is frequently concomitant with diastolic heart failure and may precipitate acute decompensation.

C. The jugular venous pulse and its waveform can be informative. Jugular venous distention (JVD) has consistently been shown to be a very specific sign of elevated cardiac filling pressures (although not specific for diastolic over systolic dysfunction). Freidriech's sign or a brief *y* duration/rapid descent described as a "flickering" in otherwise distended JVD may suggest pericardial constriction. Kussmaul's sign (i.e., paradoxical elevation of jugular venous pressure on inspiration) may occur. There may be a midline sternotomy scar from previous cardiac surgery, indicating the substrate for constrictive pericarditis.

D. Overall, none of the following clinical signs can reliably distinguish systolic from diastolic heart failure: JVD, rales, displaced apical impulse, third heart sound (S_3), fourth heart sound (S_4,) hepatomegaly, and edema. Abdominal distention and frank ascites may occur. A hepatojugular relex may also be present The liver may be engorged and palpably enlarged. Sacral edema may predominate over pedal edema in bed-bound patients.

III. LABORATORY EXAMINATION

A. Electrocardiogram (ECG). A normal resting ECG does not rule out diastolic dysfunction. **The most common abnormality seen is LV hypertrophy caused by systemic hypertension**, but voltage and axis changes are neither sensitive nor specific. Previous myocardial infarction may be indicated by a Q wave or, more frequently, a non–Q wave with diffuse ST-segment changes. Abnormal P waves reflect overload of left, right, or both atria. A pseudoinfarction pattern or dramatic voltage changes can occur with hypertrophic cardiomyopathy. Atrioventricular block can occur in infiltrative cardiomyopathies, classically expressed in sarcoid. Low-voltage QRS complexes occur in tamponade and obesity. Small QRS complexes, in the presence of myocardial thickening on echocardiography, should raise the suspicion of cardiac amyloid. Atrial fibrillation is a common finding in diastolic dysfunction.

B. Chest radiograph. In the compensated state, the chest radiograph may be normal. In decompensated states, pulmonary edema or pulmonary venous hypertension is frequently observed. Cardiomegaly and pulmonary venous hypertension occur with almost the same frequency in isolated diastolic heart failure as in systolic heart failure. LA enlargement is occasionally seen on plain films. Pericardial or mitral valvular calcification is sometimes visible on chest radiographs. Other clues about possible causes include sternal wires (i.e., constriction), globular heart (i.e., pericardial effusion), and primary pulmonary tuberculosis (i.e., pericardial constriction).

C. Specific laboratory investigations. These studies may be prompted by the history and physical examination and include determinations of serum glucose (i.e., diabetes), ferritin (i.e., hemochromatosis), serum calcium, angiotensin-converting enzyme (sercoidosis), autoantibodies (i.e., amyloid), and protein electrophoresis (i.e., amyloid). B-type natriuritic peptide (BNP) may be used to exclude HFpEF as a cause of dyspnea but not to establish the diagnosis of HFpEF.

IV. ETIOLOGY.

Any factor that affects the diastolic-filling properties discussed previously can result in diastolic heart failure, and many occur in combination. Diastolic heart failure is associated with older age, hypertension, diabetes, female gender, and LV hypertrophy. Pericardial disease and hypertrophic cardiomyopathy are discussed elsewhere in this book.

A. Myocardial ischemia. Myocyte relaxation is an intensely energy-dependent phenomenon. Acute and chronic ischemia can result in impaired active relaxation and acute diastolic heart failure (in addition to systolic heart failure). Chronic ischemia, established myocardial infarction (i.e., scar), or adverse remodeling in myocardium remote from sites of infarction may increase collagen formation and impair passive filling by altered passive chamber compliance. Ischemia can also cause atrial fibrillation (with loss of atrial kick) and other tachyarrhythmias, shortening diastolic filling time. Heart failure with preserved ejection fraction has been found to be common among patients with non–ST-segment-elevation myocardial infarction (NSTEMI) and confers an increased mortality over acute coronary syndrome (ACS) alone.

B. LV hypertrophy may be a result of hypertrophic cardiomyopathy, systemic hypertension, or LV outflow obstruction (e.g., aortic valvular stenosis, subvalvular stenosis). Increased wall thickness reduces passive filling. Subendocardial ischemia, common in left ventricular hypertrophy (LVH), may impair active myocyte relaxation. Atrial fibrillation, which may occur with hypertensive heart disease, contributes to diastolic dysfunction.

C. Restrictive cardiomyopathies are defined as diseases of the myocardium that are characterized by restrictive filling and reduced diastolic volume of either or both ventricles with normal or near-normal systolic function. Atrioventricular block and symptomatic bradycardias requiring pacemaker insertion commonly coexist. Atrial fibrillation is poorly tolerated and common. Restrictive cardiomyopathies can be classified as primary or secondary.

1. **Primary restrictive cardiomyopathies.** Causes include endomyocardial fibrosis, Loeffler's endocarditis, and idiopathic restrictive cardiomyopathy.
   a. **Endomyocardial fibrosis** occurs in tropical areas and affects children and young adults. Histologically it is characterized by granulation tissue, collagen, and extensive connective tissue lining the endocardium. It affects both (50%), left (40%), or isolated right (10%) ventricles and is associated with a 2-year mortality rate of up to 50%. Atrial fibrillation, mitral regurgitation, and thromboembolism are common. The response to medical treatment is poor. Endocardial decortication may be beneficial for those with NYHA class III or IV symptoms. This technique has high operative mortality, (15 to 20%), but when successful, reduced symptoms and may favorably affect survival.
   b. **Loeffler's endocarditis** is more commonly seen in temperate climates and generally occurs as part of the idiopathic hypereosinophilic syndrome. It typically manifests in middle age. Features include eosinophilia, restrictive cardiac disease, and nervous system and marrow involvement. Mural thrombus frequently occurs. Aside from conventional heart failure medications (including anticoagulation), corticosteroids and hydroxyurea are useful in treatment. Surgery may be required for advanced fibrotic disease.
   c. **Idiopathic restrictive cardiomyopathy** is a disease of exclusion. It usually occurs sporadically, but may be inherited with an autosomal dominant pattern in association with distal skeletal myopathy and occasionally heart block. Echocardiography reveals near-normal LV dimensions and function, biatrial enlargement, and variable hypertrophy. Endomyocardial biopsy is unremarkable or shows nonspecific changes. The condition may manifest at any age throughout childhood or adult life. Survival time varies, with a mean of 9 years. Cardiac transplantation may be indicated in selected patients.
2. **Secondary restrictive cardiomyopathies.** Causes include infiltrative (e.g., amyloidosis, sarcoidosis, radiation carditis) and storage diseases (e.g., hemochromatosis, glycogen storage disorders, Fabry's disease).
   a. **Amyloid heart disease** is classified as primary, secondary, familial, or senile (Table 8.1). Primary amyloid is caused by light-chain immunoglobulin overproduction from a monoclonal population of plasma cells, usually associated with multiple myeloma. Secondary amyloid is associated with chronic inflammatory conditions such as Crohn's disease, rheumatoid arthritis, tuberculosis, and familial Mediterranean fever. Familial and senile amyloid heart diseases are related to overproduction of transthyretin. Suspected amyloid disease of the heart is usually diagnosed by endomyocardial biopsy. The prognosis is generally poor, with a median survival of 2 years. Treatment is directed toward relief of symptoms of congestion. Liver transplantation has been used in cases of familial amyloidosis. Amyloidosis in the presence of systemic manifestations is a contraindication to cardiac transplantation.
   b. **Sarcoidosis** is a systemic disease of unknown origin that results in the deposition of noncaseating granulomas in the lungs (i.e., bihilar lymphadenopathy), spleen, lymph nodes, skin, liver, parotid glands, and the heart. At autopsy, cardiac involvement is seen in 25% of patients, although it is clinically recognized in only 5%. Clinically cardiac sarcoidosis may be clinically evident as asymptomatic conduction abnormalites to fatal ventricular arrhythmias. Complete heart block is present in 20% to 30% of patients. First-degree heart block and bundle-branch blocks may also be seen. Sarcoid granuloma in the ventricular myocardium become substrate for ventricular arrhythmias. Ventricular tachycardia is the most common arrhythmia. Sudden cardiac death caused by arrhythmia is the leading cause of death in patients with sarcoid (67%). Congestive heart failure may occur, owing to infiltration of the myocardium, presenting early like a restrictive cardiomyopathy with a preserved ejection fraction. In later stages the ventricle may become dilated with regional wall-motion abnormalites. Diagnosis of cardiac involvement can be difficult to confirm; endomyocardial biopsy has specific features of

TABLE 8.1 Amyloid Heart Disease

Type of amyloid	Pathophysiology	Systemic features	Specific therapy
Primary (AL)	Monoclonal gammopathy—myeloma	Nephrotic syndrome, hepatomegaly, hypo-splenism, macroglossia (20%), sensory and autonomic neuropathy	Melphalan, prednisone (both of debated value)
Secondary	Excess immunoglobulin production from chronic inflammatory conditions—Crohn's disease, rheumatoid arthritis, tuberculosis, familial Mediterranean fever	Related to underlying condition in addition to systemic deposition features amyloid	Directed at underlying disease process, antiproliferative agents as for primary
Familial	Abnormal transthyretin (protein produced in liver that is deposited in cardiac tissue)	Fewer systemic manifestations; macroglossia is rare; more likely to cause conduction disturbance than other types	Liver transplantation
Senile	Excess transthyretin	Uncommon production	None

giant cells and noncaseating granulomas, but because of the patchy nature of the condition, it has a sensitivity of only 20% to 30%. Echocardiography is not sensitive in detecting early cardiac sarcoid; however, it may demonstrate increased ventricular septal thickness, mimicking hypertrophic cardiomyopathy, pericardial effusions, abnormal wall motion, regional wall thinning, or left ventricluar dilation. Contrast-enhanced magnetic resonance imaging (MRI) and 18F-fluorodeoxyglucose (18F-FDG) have been shown to be highly sensitive modalites for detecting myocardial involvement; they may be useful in detecting early cardaic sarcoid and evaluating the response to treatment. Corticosteroid treatment may slow progression of cardiac disease and prolong survival. Steroids do not prevent sudden death. ICD placement is recommended in patients with cardiac sarcoidosis and a history of non-sustained ventricular tachycardia, or low ejection fraction (EF). Pacemaker placement may be indicated in patients demonstrating conduction-system involvement. Cardiac transplantation for cardiac sarcoidosis may be necessary in selected patients.

c. **Radiation carditis** can manifest decades after exposure to thoracic radiotherapy. It can involve most cardiac structures, including coronary arteries (with ostial stenoses occurring classically), valves (with resultant calcification and stenosis or regurgitation), myocardium, and pericardium. Myocardial and pericardial involvement can cause constrictive pericarditis, a restrictive myocarditis, or both. Treatment depends on the degree of constriction; overall these patients tend to do poorly even with surgery.

d. **Metabolic storage diseases** are characterized by intracellular deposition of substances within the myocyte and resultant impaired viscoelastic properties.

(1) Hemochromatosis is a state of iron overload, caused by increased absorption from the gastrointestinal tract (i.e., primary) or by repeated blood transfusions necessitated by chronic anemia or hemoglobinopathy (i.e., secondary). Primary hemochromatosis is an autosomal recessive condition linked to chromosome 6 and is associated with iron deposition in multiple organs including the liver, skin, pancreas (so-called bronze-diabetes), gonads, and joints. It manifests as a restrictive cardiomyopathy, and treatment is by phlebotomy.

(2) **Glycogen storage diseases** are genetically transmitted inborn errors of metabolism and include Gaucher's, Hurler's, and Fabry's diseases. Fabry's disease is worthy of special mention because a specific therapy exists (recombinant α-galactosidase) that can cause regression of restrictive pathology. Cardiac involvement may be seen as increased LV wall thickness simulating a hypertrophic cardiomyopathy. The heart may be involved with other organ systems or may be the only organ involved, an atypical "cardiac" variant. **This atypical variant may represent up to 4% or more of patients with nonobstructive hypertrophic cardiomyopathy (HCM), and even higher proportions of late onset HCM.**

V. DIAGNOSTIC TESTING

A. **Echocardiography** is the best modality to assess diastolic function. It is pivotal in making the diagnosis of diastolic heart failure by documenting systolic function; eliminating valvular pathologies; and assessing ventricular mass, pericardium, and pericardial fluid collections. Diastolic heart failure is unlikely when no structural abnormalities are found by echocardiography. There are multiple echo-derived indices of diastolic function that have been well validated. Interpretation of echo indices requires an understanding of the normal effects of aging and the interplay of concomitant valvular pathophysiology and loading conditions. The following parameters are useful in determining diastolic function:

1. **Isovolumic relaxation time (IVRT)** is defined as the interval from the closure of the aortic valve to the opening of the mitral valve. It is measured between the end of ejection and the onset of mitral flow, by orienting the transducer using continuous wave (CW) between the inflow and outflow velocities in the long axis or apical five-chamber views. Alternatively, place a pulsed-wave (PW) sample in the left ventricular outflow tract (LVOT), but close enough to the anterior mitral valve leaflet to record both velocities. CW recordings provide a more reliable measure of IVRT than PW Doppler. Three to five cycles should be averaged when measuring IVRT. This value is prolonged when ventricular relaxation is delayed. See Table 8.2 for values associated with each diastolic pattern.

2. **Transmitral flow pattern.** In sinus rhythm, using PW Doppler across the mitral inflow tract, two waves are seen: the early E wave, corresponding to rapid ventricular filling as the mitral valve opens, and the A wave, which reflects atrial contraction. In healthy people younger than 50 years, E is larger than A (i.e., E/A ratio >1). The E-wave deceleration time is the time from peak E inflow velocity to decay to zero. With age, hypertension, or ischemia, the viscoelastic properties of the ventricle decrease, and the E wave decreases in amplitude, has a gentler slope, and has a longer deceleration time. The atrial kick is proportionately greater, and E–A reversal occurs, with an E/A ratio less than 1. With progression of diastolic dysfunction, LA pressure rises further to compensate, and the E wave becomes more prominent than the A wave (i.e., pseudonormalization). Repeating mitral valve inflow measurements during a Valsalva maneuver or after administration of nitroglycerin to decrease preload often reverts a pseudonormal pattern to one of impaired relaxation ($E < A$). A patient with a truly normal pattern has a reduction in both E and A velocities, but the E/A ratio should not change.

It is typically measured by placing a 2-mm sample volume at the mitral leaflet tips in the four-chamber apical view. The early E wave is driven by flow and the instantaenous transvalvular gradient and is influenced by the LA compliance and the rate of LV relaxation. The transmitral inflow pattern is affected by a multitude of techinical and physiologic factors not limited to sample volume

TABLE 8.2 Stages of Diastolic Dysfunction and Echocardiographic Characteristics

Characteristic	Normal adult	Delayed relaxation	Pseudonormal	Restrictive (Reversible)	Restrictive (irreversible)
Diastolic dysfunction grade	0	1	2	3	4
Clinical scenario	Normal	Age, ischemia, HCM, LVH, hypovolemia	Progression of hypertrophy and/or ischemia, changed loading conditions, systolic dysfunction	Advanced heart failure, severely reduced LV compliance and elevated filling pressures	As for stage 3, but fails to revert to stage 2 with treatment
E/A ratio					
Mitral deceleration time (ms)	150–220	>220	150–200	<150	<150
IVRT (ms)	<100	>100	60–100	<60	<60
S/D Ratio	>1	>1	< or >1	<1	<1
Ar wave (cm/s)	<35	< or >35, depending on LAP	>35	>35	>35
Vp (cm/s)	>45	<45	<45	<45	<45
TDIE′ (cm/s)	>8	<8	<8	<8	<8
Mean LAP	Normal	N/↑	↑↑	↑↑↑	↑↑↑
Tau (τ)	Normal	↑	↑	↑↑	↑↑
NYHA class	Normal	I–II	II–III	III–IV	IV

AR, Atrial reversal (pulmonary veins); CMM, color M-mode echocardiography; E/A, E/A wave; HCM, hypertrophic cardiomyopathy; IVRT, isovolume relaxation time; LAP, left atrial pressure; LV, left ventricular; LVH, left ventricular hypertrophy; NYHA, New York Heart Association; S/D Ratio, systolic to diastolic flow velocity ratio in pulmonary veins; TDIE′, tissue Doppler imaging early diastolic velocity; V_p(cm/s), flow propagation velocity.

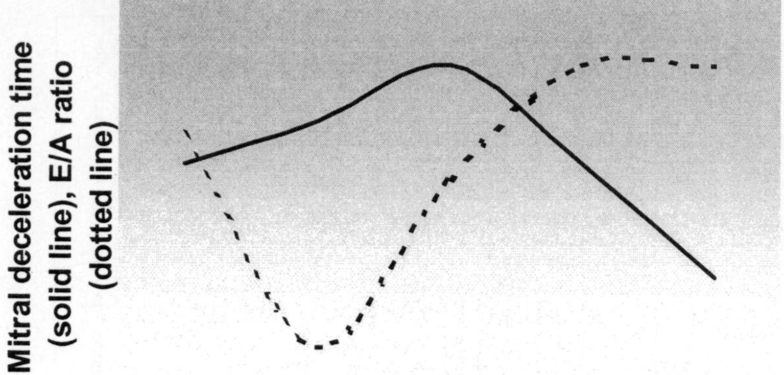

Figure 8.2. Progression of mitral deceleration and the E/A ratio in diastolic dysfunction.

(size and location), transducer angle, respiration, heart rate, PR interval, age, loading conditions, and ventricular compliance. Many different combinations of LV relaxation and LA filling pressures may result in the same transmitral inflow pattern.

3. **Transmitral deceleration time.** As diastolic dysfunction progresses, the elasticity of the ventricle is further impaired, and deceleration time is shortened. This index is a potent predictor of functional capacity and prognosis. Deceleration times can predict pulmonary capillary wedge pressure (PCWP), with DTs less than 130 ms associated with a PCWP of 20 mm Hg or greater. The E/A ratio generates a U-shaped curve, and deceleration time follows an inverted U-shaped curve (Fig. 8.2).
4. **Pulmonary venous flow** is usually measured in the right upper pulmonary vein with PW Doppler in the apical four-chamber view. Flow can be visualized first with color Doppler using a low velocity scale (40 cm/s). Wall filters should be kept at low levels; use a sample volume of 4 mm and place it in the pulmonary vein. Common mistakes include placing the sample volume near the pulmonary vein but still in the LA or measuring posterior atrial wall motion.
   a. S wave. Represents the forward flow into the LA from the pulmonary veins (toward the transducer), causing a positive S wave; this wave is often biphasic, with S1 occuring in response to atrial relaxation and S2 related to mitral annular descent. S1 is reduced in atrial fibrillation (AF). S2 is increased by LV contractility and decreased by elevated LA pressure (LAP) and mitral regurgitation.This corresponds to the *x* descent on the pulmonary capillary wedge tracings.
   b. D wave. As the mitral valve opens, the left atrium empties into the LV, allowing further flow of blood toward the transducer and a positive D wave, this is largely determined by the transmitral E wave, and corresponds to *y* descent on pulmonary capillary wedge tracings. It is decreased by impaired LV relaxation.
   c. A wave. With atrial contraction, some blood inevitably leaks back into the pulmonary veins from the transducer, causing a small negative A wave (.i.e, atrial reversal). The peak A-wave velocity increases with resistance to atrial forward flow from increased left ventricular end-diastolic pressure (LVEDP) of ventricular stiffness, with peak velocities >35 cm/s associated with elevated filling pressures. When the LVEDP is elevated, with atrial contraction, the LV

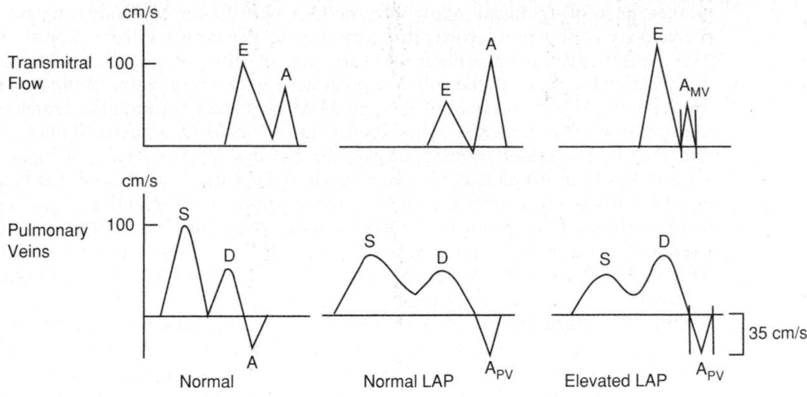

Figure 8.3. Changes in pulmonary venous flow.

pressure may become larger than the LAP, shortening the duration of the transmitral A wave relative to the pulmonary venous (PV) A-wave duration. This difference between the transmitral and PV atrial wave durations, when it exceeds 20 to 30 ms has been found to correlate with an LVEDP greater than 20 mm Hg (Fig. 8.3).

d. In the early stages of diastolic dysfunction, the S wave is greater than D. With the development of pseudonormal or restrictive physiology, D is greater than S, as the D wave correlates with transmitral E (low E/A ratio). With development of increasing LA pressure, the S wave becomes "blunted," reducing the S/D ration to less than 1, this ratio is a less sensitive measure of elevated LAP in patients with preserved ejection fractions, however.

5. Tissue Doppler imaging mitral annular velocity. This novel ultrasound technology is now used routinely in assessment of diatolic function. It is used to image the myocardial tissue, which has high amplitude, but (relative to blood) lower velocity (1–20 cm/s). Velocities are obtained by placing a 5-mm sample volume (gate) over the lateral or septal mitral annulus, and the aliasing velocity should be lowered to 20 to 30 cm/s to optimize the signal. The lateral annulus tends to have higher velocities than the septal mitral annulus. Sweep speed should be set to 50 to 100 mm/s to optimize the spectral display. The myocardial velocities have three main components: Systolic S′ (Sa), early diastolic E (Ea), and the late diastolic velocities A′ (Aa). The early diastolic velocity (E′) reflects the rate of myocardial relaxation. The ratio of transmitral flow E to E′ can be used to predict filling pressures. An E/E′ greater than 10 using the lateral mitral annulus predicts a PCWP greater than 12 mm Hg. A PCWP is likely normal if the E/E′ is less than 8. Late diastolic filling A′ correlates inversely with LAP and has been correlated with LA function. Normal diastolic function is evidenced by an E′ value greater than 8 cm/s. The advantage of using E′ over mitral Doppler indices in the assessment of LV relaxation is that E′ is less affected by preload or LA pressures. In the differentiation between restrictive and constrictive cardiomyopathy, although the mitral inflow pattern may be the same in both, E′ is normal in constriction but markedly diminished in restrictive cardiomyopathy.

6. Flow propagation velocity (Vp) by Color M Mode. This index is related to the base to apex diastolic intracavitary pressure gradients that occur as the ventricle relaxes, promoting mitral inflow into the LV cavity. Color M Mode can assess the velocity of this flow propagation, producing a color wave front. The slope of the outer edge of this wave front represents Vp (flow propagation velocity). It is obtained by placing the color Doppler across the mitral valve in the apical four-chamber view, and then placing an M Mode cursor through the center of the brightest inflow velocity. The Nyquist limit should be adjusted (lower) so that the central highest velocity jet is blue. Normal Vp is 45 cm/s or higher; a value less than 40 cm/s is consistent with impaired relaxation and can help in differentiating a normal transmitral inlow pattern from pseudonormal. Vp is relatively load-independent and has been shown to correlate well with invasive measures of LV relaxation. It may be inaccurate in concentric hypertrophy with small LV cavities. However, it cannot be used in the presence of inflow obstruction such as mitral stenosis.

7. **Strain rate imaging.** Strain is a dimensionless index, obtained through integrating strain rate over time, and represents the force required to produce a deformation of the myocardium, expressed as the percent change from the original dimension. Measurements in the long axis represent regional shortening fraction (longitudinal strain) and regional thickening in the short axis. Systolic strain represents the change in length of the myocardium between end diastole and end systole. It provides a relatively load insensitive measure of regional rather than global contractility. Strain and strain rate may be derived through tissue Doppler or feature tracking. Tissue Doppler Imaging (TDI)-derived strain still demonstrates significant Doppler angle dependency. Speckle tracking overcomes the limitation of angle dependence through the frame-by-frame tracking of characteristic speckle patterns. These patterns are created by natural acoustic markers that cause interference to the ultrasound beam in the myocardium. Tracking these speckles and how they move over time yields strain and strain rate data. The role of these modalities in assessing diastolic function remains investigational. Strain and strain rate have been found to correlate with myocardial fibrosis, and have been used to assess the response of the ventricle to treatment in hypertension, HCM, aortic stenosis, and Fabry's disease. The prognostic significance of these changes remains undefined.

B. Invasive hemodynamic assessment. Left- and right-sided catheterization can be employed to assess diastolic function and provide the most accurate clinical assessment of LV relaxation; however, this modality is invasive and requires the use of expensive catheters. It is not used in the routine evaluation of diastology. Invasive hemodynamic monitoring may be very useful in helping differentiate between restrictive and constrictive physiologies when noninvasive modalities fail to do so.

C. Radionuclide techniques. Normalized peak filling rate (NPFR) is a noninvasive index of LV relaxation; however, it is limited by loading conditions and does not provide filling pressures. It is rarely used clinically.

D. Magnetic resonance imaging (MRI) and computed tomography (CT). MRI can provide gold standard measurements of LA and LV volume and mass as well as LV filling parameters similar to those obtained by echocardiography. It is an acceptable alternative to echo if image quality from transthoracic echocardiography (TTE) is poor. However, given its cost, the technical expertise required for its optimal employment, and limited availability, it is not used routinely in the clinical evaluation of diastolic function. MRI is useful in the assessment of constriction versus restriction and in differentiating hypertrophic cardiomyopathy from other types of hypertrophy, for example, restrictive cardiomyopathies.

E. Endomyocardial biopsy (see Chapter 57). Endomyocardial biopsy is an invasive technique that may be used if there is strong suspicion of infiltrative myocardial diseases. However, many of the infiltrative diseases, especially sarcoidosis, are patchy in distribution, and safe endomyocardial biopsy has a relatively low sensitivity in this situation.

VI. STAGING OF DIASTOLIC HEART FAILURE. By using echocardiographically derived criteria, it is possible for diastolic dysfunction to be graded as stage I through IV

(Table 8.2). Many patients with suspected diastolic dysfunction have atrial fibrillation, and the E/A ratio and Ar wave velocities cannot be obtained. The beat-to-beat variation in diastolic filling times necessitates the averaging of several cycles. Mitral deceleration time and color M-mode flow propagation can provide accurate staging of atrial fibrillation.

VII. THERAPY. NO TREATMENT HAS BEEN SHOWN TO BE EFFECTIVE FOR DIASTOLIC HEART FAILURE. There is a significant lack of data from large randomized, placebo-controlled clinical trials in this population. None to date has demonstrated a mortality benefit. Therapy currently is directed toward relief of congestion, treatment of ischemia, and heart rate and blood pressure control. Nonpharmacologic therapies such as sodium and fluid restriction are important to help prevent volume overload. Moderate aerobic exercise may improve cardiopulmonary conditioning. Current therapeutic approaches use interventions that have been developed to treat systolic heart failure or the underlying pathophysiologic processes (e.g., hypertension, ischemic heart disease). The current ACC/AHA 2005 guidelines are listed in Table 8.3.

A. Symptomatic treatment. Diuretics should be used to reduce pulmonary congestion and peripheral edema. Caution must be taken not to over-diurese, because many patients require elevated filling pressures to ensure adequate stroke volume. Pre-renal diuretic-induced azotemia is common in patietns with diastolic heart failure. Absorption of orally administered diuretics is impaired in decompensated states, necessitating intravenous administration. Invasive monitoring with Swan-Ganz catheterization may be required. Patients should be educated about salt and

TABLE 8.3 Guidelines Adapted from ACC/AHA/ASE 2005 Update

Class I guidelines	
Control systolic and diastolic hypertension	1. Physicians should control hypertension in accordance with published guidelines. (Level of Evidence: A)
Diuretics	1. Physicians should use diuretics to control pulmonary congestion and peripheral edema. (Level of Evidence: C)
Ventricular rate should be controlled in presence of atrial fibrillation.	1. Physicians should control ventricular rate in AF. (Level of Evidence: C)
Class IIa guidelines	
Coronary revascularization	1. In patients with CAD in whom ischemia is having an adverse effect on cardiac function. (Level of Evidence: C)
Class IIb guidelines	
Restoration and maintenance of sinus rhythm	1. May be useful in improving symptoms. (Level of Evidence: C)
Digoxin	1. Usefulness in reducing symptoms is not well established. (Level of Evidence: C)
β-Blockers, angiotensin-converting enzymes inhibitors, angiotensin II receptor blockers, or calcium antagonists and controlled hypertension	1. Might be effective in minimizing symptoms. (Level of Evidence: C)

AF, Atrial fibrillation; CAD, coronary artery disease.

fluid restriction and the importance of daily weights. Nitrates provide symptomatic relief but should be used cautiously to avoid precipitating hypotension. Cautiously administered intravenous nitrates (with invasive hemodynamic monitoring) can effectively treat acute decompensation and acute pulmonary edema related to diastolic dysfunction.

B. Systolic and diastolic blood pressure should be treated in accordance with JNC VII guidelines (The Seventh Report of the Joint National Committee on Prevention, Detection, Evaluation, and Treatment of High Blood Pressure).

C. Coronary revascularization should be considered in patients with coronary artery disease, in whom ischemia is thought to be having an adverse effect on cardiac function.

D. Ventricular rate should be controlled in the presence of atrial fibrillation. Heart rate is a primary determinant in diastolic filling, and tachycardia is poorly tolerated. β-Blockers and calcium channel blockers allow improved diastolic filling by slowing the heart, and may be beneficial through their negative inotropic effect. However, neither has been proven to do more than reduce symptoms. The use of β-blockers and calcium channel blockers to treat patients with moderate to severe diastolic dysfunction should be undertaken with extreme caution.

E. Atrial fibrillation is poorly tolerated in patients with diastolic dysfunction, and precipitates decompensation in many patients. Restoration and maintenance of sinus rhythm seems of logical benefit, but few data supporting this approach are available.

F. Angiotensin receptor blockers (ARBs) are known to reduce LV hypertrophy and lead to improved diastolic filling through afterload reduction. In CHARM-Preserved, candesartan demonstrated a trend toward reduction in cardiovascular death, and had a modest impact in reducing heart failure hospitalization.

G. Angiotensin-converting enzyme (ACE) inhibitors theoretically should be of benefit in HFpEF, as hypertension, LV hypertrophy, diabetes, and coronary artery disease (CAD) are common in this population. Perindopril for Elderly People with Chronic Heart Failure (PEP-CHF) study failed to demonstrate a mortality benefit with perindopril, but this study was hindered by high rates of drug discontinuation. I-PRESERVE is ongoing, and it may clarify the role of ACE inhibitors in this population.

H. Digoxin has been shown to reduce symptoms and hospitalizations in both systolic and diastolic heart failure, although it had no effect on mortality.

I. Spironolactone is useful as a potassium-sparing diuretic; its role in diastolic heart failure remains unclear. The National Heart, Lung, and Blood Institute (NHLBI)–funded TOPCAT study is ongoing and may provide answers about the value of spironolactone in this population.

J. Nitrates may provide symptomatic relief but should be used cautiously so as to not precipitate hypotension. Cautiously administering intravenous nitrates (with invasive hemodynamic monitoring) can effectively treat acute decompensation and acute pulmonary edema related to diastolic dysfunction.

K. Positive inotropic agents should be used with extereme caution, and are rarely employed. Dobutamine or milrinone may be used for their lusitropic (enhanced relaxation) effects, but only with invasive hemodynamic monitoring.

L. Dialysis is occasionally used to unload the ventricle in severe cases when diuresis cannot be achieved because of the cardiorenal, avid salt- and water-retaining state that occurs in many such patients. Patients with end-stage renal disease have regression of hypertrophy and reduced diastolic heart failure after hemodialysis.

Practical Approach to HFpEF

1. Treat the underling condition. Diastolic heart failure usually occurs in the setting of other cardiovascular conditions, most commonly CAD and hypertension. Treatment of coronary artery disease should include antiplatelet agents, β-blockade, lipid-lowering therapy, and revascularization, when appropriate.

2. Most patients with diastolic heart failure have hypertension that warrants aggressive treatment. Therapy may induce regression of hypertrophy, thereby improving the myocardial energetics and viscoelastic properties of the myocardium.
3. Surgical options should be explored for specific disease states, such as valve replacement for aortic stenosis and pericardiectomy for constrictive pericarditis. Cardiac transplantation has been successful in patients with idiopathic restrictive cardiomyopathy.

VIII. PROGNOSIS. Heart failure with preserved ejection fraction was once thought to confer a better prognosis than systolic dysfunction. Recent evidence demonstrates their survival is similar. Twenty-two percent to 29% of patients with HFpEF die within 1 year of being discharged from their first hospitalization; 65% die within 5 years. Unlike patients with systolic dysfunction, no effective treatment has been found to improve this dismal outcome. The two groups have also been found to have similar rates of readmission for heart failure.

IX. CLINICAL CONTROVERSIES: CONSTRICTION VERSUS RESTRICTION. Constrictive pericarditis is caused by fibrosis and/or calcification of the pericardium, causing it to become rigid and thus inhibit the diastolic filling of the heart. In restrictive cardiomyopathy there is inherent myocardial disease, where infiltration of the myocardium creates decreased compliance.

Historically constrictive pericarditis was characterized by extensive calcification and thickening of the pericardium, usually as a consequence of tuberculosis. In the current era, constrictive disease is frequently secondary to mantle chest radiation or open heart surgery. These patients often have less diffuse calcification, and the thickness of the pericardium may even be normal. Furthermore, radiation therapy or open heart surgery may be complicated by constrictive pericarditis, restrictive cardiomyopathy, or both.

Differentiation between these two conditions is important, but may be challenging. Constrictive pericarditis can be cured frequently through pericardial stripping. Restrictive cardiomyopathies unfortunately are usually only treated by medical therapy. Significant overlap between these two conditions can cause diagnostic dilemmas. Table 8.4 outlines the principal differences between these two conditions. A distinction must be made between anatomic findings (e.g., calcification of the pericardium) and constrictive physiology.

Two-dimensional echocardiography with Doppler is useful in distinguishing constriction from constriction (Table 8.4). The use of transmitral inflow velocity to assess for respiratory variation remains a cornerstone of evaluation. In constriction, the heart is encased and behaves as a rigid box, and there is ventricular interdependence. The cardiac chambers are shielded from the effects of respiration. The pulmonary veins lie outside the pericardium. On inspiration, the pulmonary veins have greater capacity, and blood is less inclined to enter the left atrium. Mitral inflow is, therefore, considerably reduced (>25%) on inspiration in constriction. A reduced diastolic hepatic vein flow reversal is also seen in constrictive pericarditis. In restriction and in normal pericardium, there is less than 10% variability in mitral-valve inflow with respiration. However a significant number ~12% of patients with constrictive pericarditis do not demonstrate respiratory variation.

On cardiac catheterization the most valuable information in the diagnosis of constrictive pericarditis remains the demonstration of dynamic respiratory ventricular discordance, whereby the LVEDP decreases with inspiration and the right ventricular end-diastolic pressure RVEDP rises. In constrictive pericarditis, the severity of constriction is proportional to the degree of ventricular interaction. This is useful in cases where patients demonstrate both restrictive and constrictive physiologies, for example, post radiation therapy. Patients with a large degree of ventricular discordance with respiration benefit the most from a pericardial stripping. Those with little ventricular discordance, but with severely elevated diastolic pressures out of proportion to the discordance, have primarily restrictive myocardial disease, and the signs and symptoms of right-sided heart failure will remain or become worse if the pericardium is removed.

TABLE 8.4 Constrictive Versus Restrictive Physiology

Evaluation	Constrictive pericarditis	Restrictive cardiomyopathy
History	Open heart surgery Tuberculosis Radiotherapy	Chronic inflammatory disease Tuberculosis Multisystem involvement Renal disease (amyloid)
Physical examination	Chest scars Tattoos (previous radiotherapy) Kussmaul's sign Apex impalpable Pericardial knock Friedreich's sign	Mitral and tricuspid regurgitant murmurs common Kussmaul's sign rare Apical pulse prominent S3+
Electrocardiogram	Low voltage (<50%)	Low voltage (classically in amyloidosis) Left axis deviation Pseudoinfarction Atrial fibrillation Conduction disturbance or delay
2D Echocardiogram	Pericardial thickening Normal chamber wall thickness "Septal bounce" due to rapid early diastolic filling with abrupt displacement of the interventricular septum	Increased wall thickness "Speckling" of interventricular septum Thickened valves Giant atrial enlargement
Doppler echocardiography	>25% reduction in mitral inflow E′ wave velocity with inspiration Increased flow across tricuspid valve with inspiration Augmentation of hepatic vein diastolic flow reversal with inspiration	Mitral and tricuspid valvular regurgitation Concordant reduction (<10%) in mitral and tricuspid inflow velocities with inspiration Augmentation of hepatic vein diastolic flow reversal with expiration
Tissue Doppler imaging E′	>8 cm (cm/s)	<8 (cm/s)
Color M-mode flow propagation velocity (Vp)	>100 cm/s	<45 cm/s
Cardiac catheterization	RVEDP = LVEDP (<5 mm Hg difference) RVSP <50 mm Hg RAP >15 mm Hg RVEDP <1/3 RVSP Significant changes with respiration	VEDP often >5 mm Hg greater than RVEDP, but RVEPD may equal LVEPD
Endomyocardial biopsy	Usually normal	May reveal specific histology (e.g., amyloid)
MRI/CT of chest	Pericardium thickened	Pericardium usually normal

CT, Computerized tomography; LVEDP, left ventricular end-diastolic pressure; RAP, right atrial pressure; MRI, magnetic resonance imaging; RVEDP, right ventricular end-diastolic pressure; RVSP, right ventricular systolic pressure.

ACKNOWLEDGMENTS

The author thanks Drs. John G. Peterson and W.H. Wilson Tang for their contributions to earlier editions of this chapter.

Landmark Articles

Bennett KM, Hernandez AF, et al. Heart failure with preserved left ventricular systolic function among patients with non-ST segment elevation acute coronary syndromes. *Am J Cardiol* 2007;99:1351–1356.

Bhatia RS, Tu JV, Lee DS, et al. Outcome of heart failure with preserved ejection fraction in a population-based study. *N Engl J Med* 2006;355:260–269.

Bonow RO, Udelson JE. Left ventricular diastolic dysfunction as a cause of congestive heart failure. *Ann Intern Med* 1992;117:502–510.

Garcia MJ, Thomas JD, Klein AL. New Doppler echocardiographic applications for the study of diastolic function. *J Am Coll Cardiol* 1998;32:865–875.

Hurrell DG, Nishamura RA, Higano ST, et al. Value of dynamic respiratory changes in left and right ventricular pressures for the diagnosis of constrictive pericarditis. *Circulation* 1996;93:2007–2013.

Persson H, Lonn E, Edner M, et al. Diastolic dysfunction in heart failure with preserved systolic function: need for objective evidence. *J Am Coll Cardiol* 2007;49:687–694.

Yancy CW, Lopatin M, Stevensons LW, et al. Clinical presentation, management, and in-hospital outcomes of patients admitted with acute decompensated heart failure with preserved systolic function. *J Am Coll Cardiol* 2006;47:76–84.

Guidelines

Hunt SA, Abraham WT, Chin M, et al. ACC/AHA 2005 Guideline update for the diagnosis and management of chronic heart failure in the adult. Circulation 2005;112:e154–e235.

Paulus WJ, Tschope C, Sanderson JE, et al. How to diagnose diastolic heart failure: a consensus statement on the diagnosis of heart failure with normal left ventricular ejection fraction by the Heart failure and Echocardiography Assoications of the European Society of Cardiology. *Eur Heart J* 2007;28:2539–2550.

Key Reviews

Doughan AR, Williams BR. Cardiac sarcoidosis. *Heart* 2006;92:282–288.

Hogg K, McMurray J. Treatment of heart failure with preserved systolic function: a review of the evidence. *Eur Heart J Suppl* 2004;6[Suppl H]:H61–H66.

Hogg K, Swedberg K, McMurray J. Heart failure with preserved left ventricular systolic function: epidemiology, clinical characteristics, and prognosis. *J Am Coll Cardiol* 2004;43:317–327.

Kushwaha SS, Fallon JT, Fuster V, Restrictive cardiomyopathy. *N Engl J Med* 1997;336:267–276.

Leite-Moreira AF. Current perspectives in diastolic dysfunction and diastolic heart failure. *Heart* 2006;92:712–718.

Mottram PM, Marwick TH. Assessment of diastolic function: what the general cardiologist needs to know. *Heart* 2005;91:681–695.

Nishimura RA, Jaber W. Understanding diastolic heart failure. *J Am Coll Cardiol* 2007;49:695–697.

Quinones, MA. Assessment of diastolic function. *Prog Cardiovasc Dis* 2005;45:340–355.

Stoylen A, Slordahl S, Skjelvan GK, et al. Strain rate imaging in normal and reduced diastolic function: comparison with pulsed Doppler tissue imaging of the mitral annulus. *J Am Soc Echocardiogr* 2001;14:264–274.

Waggoner AD, Bierig SM. Tissue Doppler imaging: a useful echocardiographic method for the cardiac sonographer to assess systolic and diastolic ventricular function. *J Am Soc Echocardiogr* 2001;14:1143–1152.

Zile MR, Brutsaert DL. New concepts in diastolic dysfunction and diastolic heart failure. Part I. Diagnosis, prognosis, and measurements of diastolic function. *Circulation* 2002;105:1387–1393.

Zile MR, Brutsaert DL. New concepts in diastolic dysfunction and diastolic heart failure. Part II. Causal mechanisms and treatment. *Circulation* 2002;105:1503–1508.

9 HYPERTROPHIC CARDIOMYOPATHY

Eiran Z. Gorodeski, Mark Robbins, and A. Thomas McRae III

I. INTRODUCTION. Hypertrophic cardiomyopathy (HCM) is most commonly defined as significant myocardial hypertrophy in the absence of an identifiable cause. It is the preferred term because it does not connote that obstruction (present in only approximately 25% of cases) is an invariable component of the disease, as did *idiopathic hypertrophic subaortic stenosis, hypertrophic obstructive cardiomyopathy, and muscular subaortic stenosis.*

II. CLINICAL PRESENTATION

A. Natural history

1. The **histologic features** of HCM are disarray of cell-to-cell arrangement, disorganization of cellular architecture, and fibrosis. The most common sites of ventricular involvement are, in decreasing order, the septum, apex, and midventricle. One-third of patients have wall thickening limited to one segment. These morphologic and histologic features, which vary in phenotypic and clinical expression, give rise to the characteristically unpredictable natural history of HCM.
2. The **prevalence** of HCM is approximately 1 in 500, and the condition appears to be familial in origin. This makes HCM one of the most common genetically transmitted cardiovascular diseases. It is found among 0.5% of unselected patients referred for echocardiographic examination, and is a leading cause of sudden death among athletes younger than 35 years.

B. Signs and symptoms

1. **Heart failure.** Symptoms, which include dyspnea, dyspnea on exertion, paroxysmal nocturnal dyspnea, and fatigue, are largely a consequence of two processes: elevated left ventricular (LV) diastolic pressure caused by diastolic dysfunction, and dynamic LV outflow obstruction.
   a. Events that accelerate heart rate, decrease preload, shorten diastolic filling time, increase LV outflow obstruction (i.e., exercise and tachyarrhythmias), or worsen compliance (i.e., ischemia) exacerbate these symptoms.
   b. Between 5% and 10% of patients with HCM progress to severe LV systolic dysfunction, characterized by progressive LV wall thinning and cavity enlargement.
2. **Myocardial ischemia.** Myocardial ischemia occurs in obstructive and nonobstructive HCM.
   a. The **clinical** and **electrocardiographic** presentation is similar to that of ischemic syndromes in persons without HCM. Ischemia has been demonstrated with thallium perfusion studies, elevated myocardial lactate levels during rapid atrial pacing, and positron emission tomography (PET).
   b. Although the exact mechanism of ischemia is in question, the physiologic process probably is a **mismatch of supply and demand.** Contributing factors include the following:
      (1) Small-vessel coronary disease with decreased vasodilator capacity
      (2) Elevated myocardial wall tension as a consequence of delayed diastolic relaxation time and obstruction to LV outflow
      (3) Decreased capillary–to–myocardial fiber ratio
      (4) Decreased coronary perfusion pressure
3. **Syncope and presyncope** usually are a consequence of diminished cerebral perfusion caused by inadequate cardiac output. These episodes are commonly associated with exertion or cardiac arrhythmia.
4. **Sudden death.** The annual mortality rate for HCM is 1% to 6%. Most deaths are sudden or unexpected.
   a. Not all patients with HCM are at equal **risk for sudden death.** Twenty-two percent of patients with sudden death have no symptoms. Sudden death appears to be most common among older children and young adults; it is rare in the first decade of life. Approximately 60% of deaths occur during periods of inactivity; the remaining deaths occur after vigorous physical exertion.
   b. **Arrhythmogenic and ischemic mechanisms** can initiate a clinical spiral of hypotension, decreased diastolic filling time, and increased outflow obstruction that often culminates in death.

III. PHYSICAL EXAMINATION

A. Inspection of the jugular venous system may reveal a prominent *a* wave that indicates hypertrophy and lack of compliance of the right ventricle. A precordial heave, representing right ventricular (RV) strain, can be found in persons with concomitant pulmonary hypertension.

TABLE 9.1 Effects of Maneuvers or Pharmacologic Intervention to Differentiate Hypertrophic Cardiomyopathy from Aortic Stenosis

Maneuver	Physiologic effect	HCM	AS	MR
Valsalva and standing	Decreases VR, SVR, CO	↑	↓	↓
Squat and handgrip	Increases VR, SVR, CO	↓	↑	↑
Amyl nitrite	Increases VR Decreases SVR, LV volume	↑	↑	↓
Phenylephrine	Increases SVR, VR	↓	↑	↑
Extrasystole	Decreased LV volume	↑	↓	No change
Post-Valsalva release	Increased LV volume	↓	↑	No change

AS, aortic stenosis; CO, cardiac output; HCM, hypertrophic cardiomyopathy; LV, left ventricular; MR, mitral regurgitation; SVR, systemic vascular resistance; VR, venous return; ↓, decrease; ↑, increase.

B. Palpation

1. The **apical precordial pulse usually is laterally displaced and diffuse.** LV hypertrophy may cause a presystolic apical impulse or palpable fourth heart sound (S_4). A three-component apical impulse may occur, with the third impulse resulting from a late systolic bulge of the left ventricle.
2. The carotid pulse has been classically described as bifid. This **rapid carotid upstroke followed by a second peak** is caused by a hyperdynamic left ventricle.

C. Auscultation

1. S_1 (first heart sound) usually is normal and is preceded by S_4.
2. S_2 (second heart sound) can be normal or paradoxically split as the result of the prolonged ejection time of patients with severe outflow obstruction.
3. The **harsh, crescendo–decrescendo systolic murmur** associated with HCM is heard best at the left sternal border. It radiates to the lower sternal border but not to the neck vessels or axilla.
   - **a.** An important aspect of the murmur is its **variation in intensity and duration** with ventricular loading conditions. During periods of increased venous return, the murmur is of shorter duration and is less intense. In the underfilled ventricle and during periods of increased contractility, the murmur is harsh and of longer duration.
   - **b. Maneuvers that affect preload and afterload** can be helpful in diagnosing HCM and differentiating it from other systolic murmurs (Table 9.1).
     - **(1)** The **concomitant murmur of mitral insufficiency** can be differentiated because of its holosystolic, blowing quality that radiates to the axilla.
     - **(2)** A soft, early, decrescendo, **diastolic murmur of aortic insufficiency** is found in approximately 10% of patients with HCM.
     - **(3)** (3) Dynamic auscultation maneuvers (Table 9.1)

IV. GENETIC ASPECTS OF HCM. Familial HCM is inherited as an autosomal dominant trait and is caused by missense mutations involving a single amino acid substitution. To date, more than 200 individual mutations causing HCM have been identified. Currently there is only one commercially available HCM genetic test (Laboratory for Molecular Medicine, Harvard Medical School, www.hpcgg.org/lmm), which tests for the eight most common HCM-associated myofilament-encoding genes (Table 9.2). Multiple analyses suggest that these common genetic subtypes are essentially phenotypically indistinguishable. A study by Binder, et al., from the Mayo Clinic, suggested that septal morphology as detected by echocardiography can guide genetic testing choice, with a septum with a reverse curve being most highly correlated with a genetic mutation (Fig. 9.1).

The genetic alterations that encompass familial HCM should be differentiated from those of other diseases with similar phenotypic expression, such as apical HCM and HCM of the elderly, and from the myocyte disarray and systolic dysfunction that occurs in a family without hypertrophy.

TABLE 9.2 Eight Genes Included in Panel of Only Commercially Available Familial Hypertrophic Cardiomyopathy Gene Test

Gene	Name	Locus
MYH7	Myosin, heavy chain 7	14q12
MYBPC3	Myosin-binding protein c	11p11.2
TNNT2	Troponin T2	1q32
TNNI3	Troponin I	19q13.4
TPM1	Topomyosin 1	15q22.1
ACTC	Actin, alpha	15q14
MYL2	Myosin regulatory light chain	12q23-q24.3
MYL3	Myosln essential light chain	3p

Gene test available through Laboratory for Molecular Medicine, Harvard Medical School (www.hpcgg.org/lmm). Detection rate in patients with clinical symptoms of HCM is ~55% to 70%. Approximate cost $4150.

A **poor prognosis and a higher risk for sudden death** are associated with certain mutations within the β-myosin heavy chain. Troponin T mutations are associated with higher mortality even in the absence of characteristic hypertrophy. As genetic testing is further refined and made more affordable it will become more commonplace in the diagnosis and management of patients with HCM.

V. DIAGNOSTIC TESTING

A. Electrocardiogram (ECG). Although most patients have electrocardiographic evidence of disease, no changes are pathognomonic for HCM. Common electrocardiographic findings in HCM are listed in Table 9.3.

B. Echocardiography is the preferred diagnostic method because of its high sensitivity and low risk profile.

1. **M-Mode and two-dimensional** echocardiographic criteria for the diagnosis of HCM are listed in Table 9.4. Some cardiologists have used two-dimensional imaging to include all patterns of RV and LV hypertrophy in establishing the diagnosis of HCM (Table 9.5).
2. **Doppler echocardiography** enables recognition and quantification of the consequences of **systolic anterior motion (SAM) of the mitral valve.**
   a. Approximately one-fourth of patients with HCM have a resting pressure gradient between the body and outflow tract of the left ventricle; others have only provocable gradients.
   b. The **diagnosis of HCM with obstruction** is based on resting gradients greater than 30 mm Hg or provocable gradients greater than 50 mm Hg. These

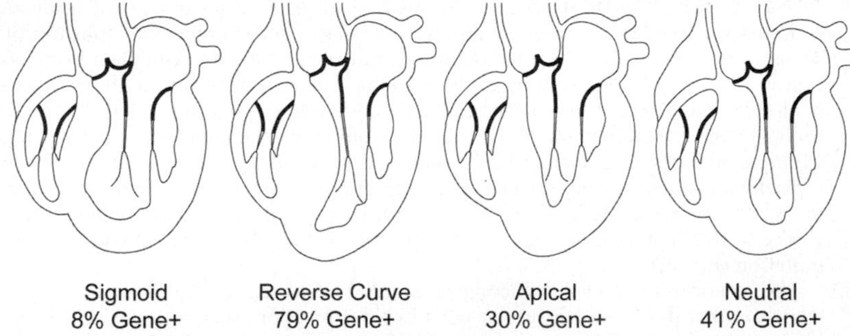

Figure 9.1. Correlation between septal morphology and known genetic mutations.

TABLE 9.3	Electrocardiographic Findings in Hypertrophic Cardiomyopathy
Evidence of right and left atrial enlargement	
Q waves in the inferolateral leads	
Voltage criteria for large negative precordial T waves (associated with Japanese variant)	
Left-axis deviation	
Short PR interval with slurred upstroke	

gradients correlate directly with the time of onset and duration of contact between the mitral leaflet and the septum. The earlier and longer the contact, the higher the pressure gradient.

(1) Inducing obstruction and, therefore, gradients, in patients believed to have latent obstruction, can be accomplished with substances (e.g., amyl nitrite, isoproterenol, dobutamine) or maneuvers (e.g., Valsalva maneuver, exercise) that decrease LV preload or increase contractility.

(2) The most accepted explanation for SAM is that the high-flow velocity caused by the narrowed outflow tract draws the mitral valve anteriorly toward the septum, resulting in subaortic obstruction and flow gradients **(i.e., Venturi effect).**

(3) Although the clinical relevance of outflow obstruction has been debated, relief by means of surgical or pharmacologic technique is associated with clinical improvement among many patients. Echocardiographic recognition of HCM and of HCM with outflow obstruction is, therefore, important.

c. Recognition of mitral regurgitation (MR) Echocardiographic evaluation of MR and the detection of valve anomalies may have a considerable effect on medical and surgical strategies in the care of patients with HCM.

(1) Approximately 60% of patients with HCM have structural abnormalities of the mitral valve, including increased leaflet area, elongation of leaflets, and anomalous insertion of papillary muscles directly into the anterior mitral leaflet.

(2) When there is no leaflet abnormality, the degree of MR is directly related to the severity of obstruction and lack of leaflet coaptation.

C. Magnetic resonance imaging (MRI). Advantages of MRI in the evaluation of HCM include excellent resolution, lack of radiation, inherent contrast, three-dimensional imaging, and tissue characterization. Disadvantages are cost, length of study, and exclusion of patients with contraindications to exposure to

TABLE 9.4	Two-dimensional, M-mode, and Doppler Echocardiographic Criteria for Diagnosis of Hypertrophic Cardiomyopathy
Asymmetric septal hypertrophy (>13 mm)	
Systolic anterior motion of the mitral valve	
Small left-ventricular cavity	
Septal immobility	
Premature closure of the aortic valve	
Resting gradients >30 mm Hg	
Provacable gradients >50 mm Hg	
Normal or increased motion of the posterior wall	
Reduced rate of closure of the mitral valve in mid-diastole	
Mitral valve prolapse with regurgitation	
Maximal left ventricular diastolic wall thickness >15 mm	

TABLE 9.5 Echocardiographic Classification of Left Ventricular Hypertrophy in Hypertrophic Cardiomyopathy

Type	Location	Frequency (%)
1	Anterior septum	10
2	Anterior and posterior septum	20
3	Anterior and posterior septum including the lateral free wall	52
4	Regions other than the anterior septum and posterior free wall	18

magnetism, such as patients with implantable cardioverter–defibrillators (ICDs) or pacemakers.

1. MRI can detect **LV hypertrophy** missed by echocardiography, specifically in the anterolateral and basal left ventricular free walls.
2. **Myocardial scar**, often found in patients with HCM, can be detected as **delayed hyperenhancement with gadolinium-contrast MRI**. Some small studies have suggested that the amount of hyperenhancement may be a predictor of sudden cardiac death (SCD) in this patient population.
3. Evaluation of regional myocardial function with use of **cine MRI**.
4. Improved identification of MR, SAM, abnormal papillary muscles, and diastolic dysfunction.

D. **Cardiac catheterization** has a role in the evaluation of coronary anatomic features before myectomy or a mitral valve operation and evaluation of ischemic symptoms. Characteristic findings of HCM during hemodynamic assessment are listed in Table 9.6 and illustrated in Figure 9.2.

1. Patients with normal coronary arteries may have **typical ischemic symptoms.** These symptoms may indicate myocardial bridges, phasic narrowing during systole, reduced coronary flow reserve, or systolic reversal of flow in the epicardial vessels.
2. **Left ventriculography** usually reveals a hypertrophied ventricle, prominent septal bulge, nearly complete obliteration of the ventricular cavity during systole, SAM, and MR. The spade-like appearance of the ventricular cavity is confined to ventricles with apical involvement.

E. **Radionuclide scanning and PET.** With some distinctions, the role of **radionuclide scanning** for assessment of ischemia is similar for patients with or without HCM. **Fixed defects** that represent scar and presumed myocardial infarction usually are associated with reduced ventricular function and exercise capacity. **Reversible defects** may reflect ischemia caused by atherosclerotic disease or reduced coronary reserve in disease-free arteries. Although often clinically silent, these reversible defects are likely to be associated with increased risk for sudden death, especially among younger patients with HCM.

TABLE 9.6 Hemodynamic Findings During Cardiac Catheterization

Subaortic or mid-ventricular outflow gradient on catheter pullback
Spike-and-dome pattern of aortic pressure tracing[a]
Elevated right and left ventricular end-diastolic pressures
Elevated pulmonary capillary wedge pressure
Increased V wave on wedge tracing[b]
Elevated pulmonary arterial pressure

[a]A consequence of outlet obstruction.
[b]May result from either mitral regurgitation or elevated left atrial pressure.

1. The characteristic **radionuclide ventriculographic findings** of HCM include abnormal diastolic filling, delayed peak filling, and prolonged isovolumic relaxation.
2. **PET** has higher sensitivity than conventional radionuclide scanning, and attenuation can be corrected during PET. [^{18}F] Fluorodeoxyglucose (FDG) PET studies have corroborated the clinical features of ischemia with pronounced impairment of coronary vasodilator reserve and resultant subendocardial underperfusion.

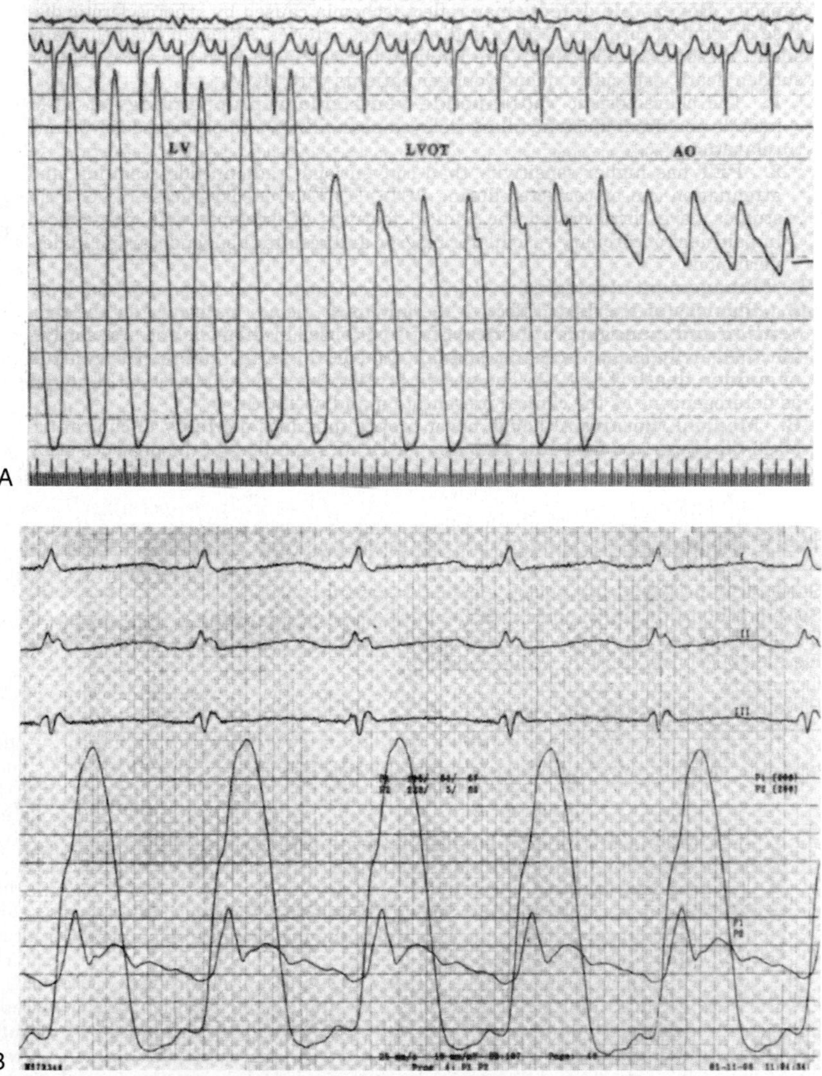

Figure 9.2. Hemodynamic tracings. **A:** Pressure difference in left ventricular outflow tract (LVOT) and left ventricle. **B:** Spike and dome of LV pressure. (*Continued*)

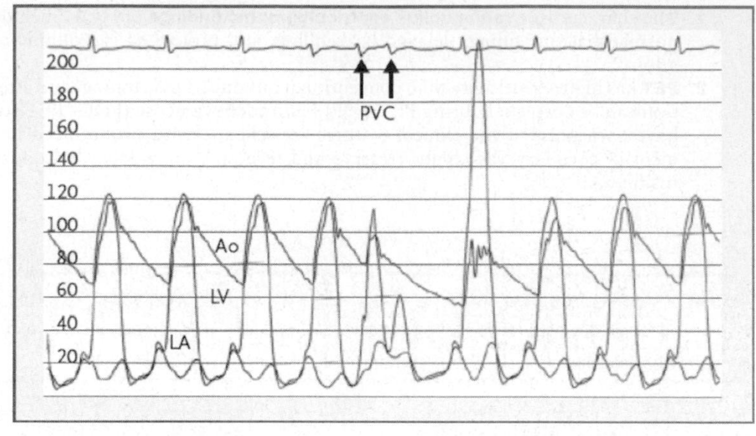

Figure 9.2. (*Continued*) **C:** Severe increase in the LV-Ao gradient in the beat after a premature ventricular contraction (PVC) (Brockenbrough-Braunwald-Morrow sign) due to an increase in contractility and decrease in afterload during the post-PVC beat.

VI. MANAGEMENT STRATEGIES

A. Priority of therapy. Effective therapy must include pathways for the **prevention and management of heart failure** caused by diastolic and systolic dysfunction, arrhythmias, ischemia, and failed medical therapy and the **prevention of sudden death** (Fig. 9.3). The specific strategies for patients with HCM can be as heterogeneous as the clinical presentation and evolution.

B. Medical therapy. Although never proved to reduce mortality in clinical trials, **β-blockers are first-line therapy** for HCM, regardless of the presence of LV outflow obstruction.

1. **β-Blockers** are effective in relieving angina, dyspnea, and syncope in as many as 70% of patients in some studies. β-Blockers with additional α-blocking properties, such as carvedilol and labetalol, should probably not be used as first-line agents because of their additional vasodilating properties.
   a. The mechanism of action of β-blockers is inhibition of sympathetic stimulation brought about by the negative inotropic and chronotropic properties of the drugs. β-Blockers diminish myocardial oxygen requirements and augment diastolic filling, which mitigate angina and the detrimental effects of LV outflow obstruction, respectively.
   b. **Contraindications** to the use of β-blockers are the presence of bronchospastic lung disease, a high-degree heart block in the absence of cardiac pacing, and decompensated LV systolic dysfunction.
2. **Calcium channel blockers** are considered to be second-line agents that are also effective in reducing the common symptoms of HCM in patients who are intolerant of or have undergone unsuccessful treatment with β-blockers.
   a. **Calcium channel blockers** have a negative inotropic effect and reduce the heart rate and blood pressure. They may also have beneficial effects on diastolic function by improving rapid diastolic filling, although possibly at the expense of higher LV end-diastolic pressures. The beneficial effects seem to be limited to the nondihydropyridines **verapamil** and **diltiazem** (Table 9.7).
   b. Because of the unpredictable hemodynamic effects of their vasodilator properties, calcium channel blockers should be administered cautiously to patients with considerable outlet obstruction and elevated pulmonary pressures. **Contraindications** to the use of calcium channel blockers include evidence of conduction system abnormalities in the absence of a pacer or in the presence of systolic dysfunction.

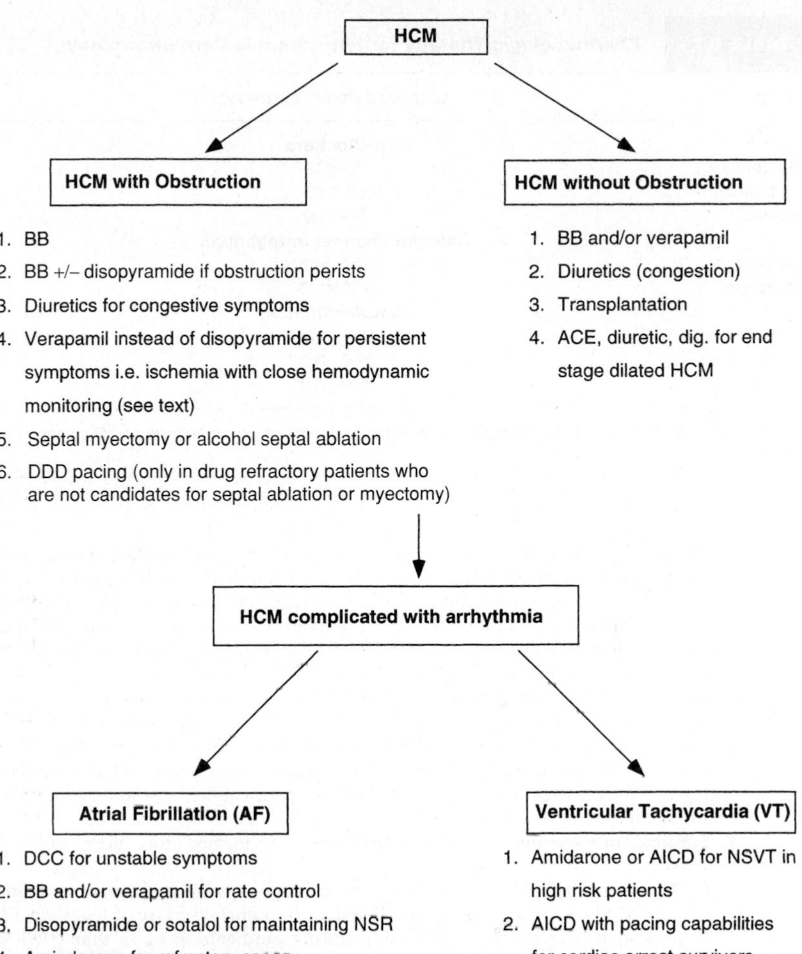

Figure 9.3. Management algorithm for hypertrophy cardiomyopathy. ACE, angiotensin-converting enzyme inhibitor; AF, atrial fibrillation; AICD, automatic implantable cardioverter–defibrillator; BB, β-blocker; DCC, direct current cardioversion; DDD, dual chamber; Dig, digoxin; HCM, hypertrophic cardiomyopathy; NSVT, nonsustained ventricular tachycardia; VT, ventricular tachycardia.

3. **Disopyramide**, a class 1A antiarrhythmic agent, may be an effective alternative or adjunct to β-blocker and calcium channel blocker therapy. Its strong negative inotropic qualities coupled with its ability to suppress ventricular and supraventricular arrhythmias make it an effective treatment when marked outflow obstruction or arrhythmias are manifested. Potential disadvantages are anticholinergic properties, accumulation in patients with hepatic or renal

TABLE 9.7 Pharmacologic Therapy for Hypertrophic Cardiomyopathy

Drug	Standard dose[a] (mg/day)
	β-Blockers
Propanolol	80–240
Metoprolol	50–200
Atenolol	50–100
	Calcium channel antagonists
Verapamil	120–360
Diltiazem	120–360
	Antiarrythmics
DIsopyramide	400–1200
Amiodarone	200–400
Sotalol	160–320

[a]Doses can be increased to treat patients with persistent symptoms who have no evidence of an adverse response.

dysfunction, the possibility of augmenting atrioventricular nodal conduction in the presence of atrial fibrillation, and waning hemodynamic effects with time. It is because of these significant side effects that disopyramide is typically used in a very symptomatic patient when a more definitive procedure is being planned, such as surgical myectomy or alcohol septal ablation. It is not considered to be a long-term treatment for HCM.

C. Nonpharmacologic treatment. Transplantation is the only option for patients with severely symptomatic, nonobstructive HCM. However, persons with obstruction who continue to have symptoms despite optimal medical treatment are candidates for septal myotomy–myectomy with or without mitral valve replacement (best option in hands of experienced surgeon), alcohol septal ablation, and dual-chamber pacing (generally poor option).

1. **Surgical management** of HCM has been performed for more than 40 years.
   a. When performed by an experienced surgeon, **septal myotomy-myectomy** (i.e., Morrow procedure) is associated with a mortality rate of less than 1% to 2%. It is effective in abolishing resting gradients in more than 90% of patients, and most patients have long-lasting symptomatic relief. Enlargement of the LV outflow tract has been found to reduce SAM, MR, LV systolic and end-diastolic pressures, left atrial pressure, and resting gradients. A retrospective study by Ommen et al. from the Mayo Clinic published in 2005, demonstrated that patients who underwent myectomy had significantly longer survival and less incidence of sudden cardiac death (SCD) as compared to patients with obstruction who did not get surgery. In fact, after myectomy survival was no different as compared to HCM patients who did not have obstruction at baseline.
   b. **Mitral valve replacement** with a low-profile prosthesis abrogates outflow obstruction, but it is considered mainly for patients with mild septal thickening, failed myotomy-myectomy, or intrinsic abnormalities of the mitral apparatus.
2. **Alcohol septal ablation**—essentially a controlled infarction of the septum—is an alternative to myotomy-myectomy. Because it has a high rate of complications including complete heart block (CHB) and extensive myocardial infarction, it is generally used in patients who are not candidates for surgical myectomy. There are no randomized trials comparing myectomy and septal ablation.
   a. **Technique.** In the cardiac catheterization laboratory, a guidewire is advanced through the left main trunk to probe the first or second septal

perforator, or both. An angioplasty catheter is placed in the proximal portion of the septal branch for vessel isolation. Ultrasonic contrast agents are infused in the cannulated perforator to define the area at risk for infarction. Infusion of 1 to 4 mL of absolute alcohol causes infarction in the zone of septal myocardium served by the cannulated septal branch. In most centers, a temporary ventricular pacing catheter is placed into the right ventricular apex before performing the ablation, in order to manage any transient conduction abnormalities.

b. Results. In the majority of patients there is a marked immediate decrease in the LV outflow tract (LVOT) gradient. This gradient response is thought to be triphasic: immediate reduction (due to stunning), early reappearance, and sustained fall by 3 months after the procedure (due to remodeling). Within this initial period, most patients attain good symptomatic relief. Risks of the procedure include high-grade atrioventricular block, coronary dissection, large anterior-wall myocardial infarction, and electrical instability of the scar that forms as a result of the infarction. Long-term results of this technique are not available.

3. Dual-chamber pacing. Initial reports of symptom relief and decreased LVOT obstruction with dual-chamber pacing have been questioned. Pacing may have deleterious effects on ventricular filling and cardiac output. Randomized, crossover trials demonstrated that much of the symptomatic benefit from pacing could be attributed to the placebo effect. The latest pacing guidelines (ESC, 2007) indicate that pacing should only be considered in patients with drug refractory HCM with resting or provoked LVOT gradient and contraindications for septal ablation or myectomy (class IIb). In persistently symptomatic patients with LVOT obstruction who have previously had a pacemaker implanted, our practice is to lengthen their atrioventricular (AV) delay in an effort to maximize diastolic filling, which may lessen the LVOT obstruction.

4. Special management considerations

a. Atrial fibrillation, which occurs in approximately 10% of patients with HCM, can have devastating consequences. Atrial fibrillation decreases diastolic filling time, and loss of atrial systole can lead to acute hemodynamic decompensation and pulmonary edema. Because of the increased risk for thromboembolism, all patients with HCM-associated atrial fibrillation should receive anticoagulation therapy. Atrial fibrillation should be treated with aggressive; efforts to restore and maintain sinus rhythm are indicated.

(1) Acute paroxysms of atrial fibrillation are best managed with cardioversion. The treatment of choice for the prevention of recurrence is disopyramide or sotalol; low-dose amiodarone is reserved for refractory cases. When considerable obstruction is present, the combination of a β-blocker and disopyramide or sotalol is an alternative.

(2) Chronic atrial fibrillation may be well tolerated if the heart rate is controlled with β-blockers or calcium-channel antagonists. For patients who do not tolerate atrial fibrillation and cannot be maintained in sinus rhythm, AV nodal ablation and implantation of a dual-chamber pacemaker may be an option.

b. Risk stratification for sudden death. Ascertaining whether a patient is at high risk for sudden death requires establishing risk factors with sufficient sensitivity, specificity, and positive predictive value to prompt implementation of preventive therapy, such as placement of an ICD or permanent pacemaker and administration of amiodarone, the long-term efficacy of which has not been established.

(1) Although no conclusive data exist on the relative value of the markers associated with sudden death, accepted **risk factors** include the following:

(a) Previous cardiac arrest

(b) Sustained ventricular tachycardia

(c) Family history of sudden death
(d) Frequent nonsustained ventricular tachycardia during Holter monitoring
(e) Recurrent syncope, near syncope (especially if exertional)
(f) Abnormal decrease in exercise blood pressure
(g) Massive LV wall thickness (>30 mm)
(h) Bridging of the left anterior descending coronary artery in children
(i) Resting LVOT obstruction (>30 mm Hg)

(2) The role of **electrophysiologic testing** in the management of HCM is uncertain. Evidence that electrophysiologic testing helps to ascertain whether a patient is at increased risk for sudden death is inconclusive. Electrophysiologic studies have not consistently induced ventricular arrhythmias with standard stimulation protocols in cardiac arrest survivors. In other electrophysiologic studies, however, investigators have been able to induce nonspecific ventricular arrhythmias with unconventional stimulation protocols in patients believed to be at low risk for sudden death.

(3) Patients who survive an episode that might have ended in sudden death, have sustained ventricular arrhythmias, or have multiple risk factors for sudden death should be strongly considered for an ICD.

(4) Selection of patients to get an ICD for primary prevention is difficult. A retrospective multicenter study from the Minneapolis Heart Institute Foundation, Maron et al. (2007) evaluated the incidence of appropriate ICD interventions in patients with HCM who previously received a device for one of four SCD risk factors: history of HCM-related SCD in a relative younger than 50 years, "massive" LV hypertrophy, nonsustained ventricular tachycardia (NSVT) on Holter monitoring, and prior unexplained syncope (nonneurocardiogenic). The study concluded that one risk factor can be enough for consideration of ICD implantation. Of note there was no control group in this study.

VII. KEY SUGGESTIONS

A. Athlete's heart

1. **Differentiating HCM from hypertrophy of athletes.** Failure to diagnose HCM places an athlete at undue risk for sudden death, although incorrect labeling of HCM often leads to irrational treatments, unnecessary fears, and inappropriate recommendations concerning exercise. Diagnostic uncertainty is greatest when maximal diastolic LV wall thickness exceeds the upper limit of normal (12 mm) but is less than the defined lower limit of normal (15 mm) for HCM in the absence of SAM and LV outflow obstruction.

   a. Characteristics that **substantiate the diagnosis of HCM** include unusual patterns of hypertrophy, an LV end-diastolic diameter of less than 45 mm, septal thickening greater than 15 mm, left atrial enlargement, abnormal diastolic function, family history of HCM, and abnormal LV filling.

   b. Characteristics more consistent with the **hypertrophied heart of an athlete** are LV end-diastolic diameter greater than 45 mm, septal thickening less than 15 mm, left atrial size less than 4 cm, LV end-diastolic diameter greater than 45 mm, and a decrease in LV thickness with deconditioning.

2. **Participation in sports.** Recommendations hold true after medical or surgical intervention.

   a. Athletes with HCM with or without obstruction who are younger than 30 years should not participate in competitive, aerobically demanding sports.

   b. Individual judgment is used for athletes older than 30 years (because of the possible reduction in sudden death with age) who lack any of the following criteria that would place them at high risk: ventricular tachycardia at ambulatory monitoring, sudden death among family members with HCM, syncope, outflow gradient greater than 50 mm Hg, exercise-induced hypotension, myocardial ischemia, left atrium larger than 5 cm, severe MR, and paroxysmal atrial fibrillation.

B. Infective endocarditis (IE)

1. **Incidence and mortality.** Between 7% and 9% of patients with HCM contract bacterial endocarditis. The associated mortality rate is 39%.
2. **Predisposing factors.** Intestinal and prostate surgical procedures place patients at increased risk for bacteremia. It is unclear if dental procedures place patients with HCM at risk.
3. **Pathophysiology.** Bacterial seeding of endomyocardial lesions is caused by repeated trauma associated with hemodynamic and intrinsic valvular abnormalities.
4. **Prophylaxis.** Guidelines on the prevention of IE published by the AHA in 2007 (Table 9.8) question the practice of treating patients with HCM with antibiotics prior to dental procedures, and recommend against it. According to these guidelines only patients at high risk of IE (prior IE, prosthetic valves, repaired or unrepaired congentical heart defects) should get antibiotic prophylaxis.

C. Yamaguchi's apical HCM

1. **Clinical presentation.** Patients experience chest pain, dyspnea, fatigue, and, in rare instances, sudden death.
2. **Prevalence.** Within Japan, apical HCM constitutes 25% of all cases of HCM. Outside Japan, only 1% to 2% of cases are associated with isolated apical hypertrophy.
3. **Diagnostic testing**
   a. An **ECG** reveals giant negative T waves in the precordial leads and LV hypertrophy.

TABLE 9.8 ACC/AHA Hypertrophic Cardiomyopathy Guidelines

ACC/AHA 2006 guidelines for management of patients with ventricular arrhythmias and prevention of sudden cardiac death
(Class I, level of Evidence: B) ICD therapy should be used for treatment in patients with HCM who have sustained VT and/or VF and who are receiving chronlc optimal medical therapy and who have reasonable expectation of survival with a good functional status for more than 1 y. (Class IIa, level of Evidence: C) ICD implantation can be effective for primary prophylaxis against SCD in patients with HCM who have 1 or more major risk factor for SCD and who are receiving chronic optimal medical therapy and in patients who have reasonable expectation of survival with a good functional status for more than 1 y. Amiodarone therapy can be effective for treatment in patients with HCM with a history of sustained VT and/or VF when an ICD is not feasible. (Class IIb, level of Evidence: C) EP testing may be considered for risk assessment for SCD in patients with HCM. Amiodarone may be considered for primary prophylaxis against SCD in patients with HCM who have 1 or more major risk factor for SCD if ICD implantation is not feasible.
ACC/AHA 2007 Recommendations and Considerations Related to Preparticipation Screening for Cardiovascular Abnormalities in Competitive Athletes Competitive athletes with a family history of hypertrophic cardiomyopathy should undergo cardiovascular screening prior to participation in athletics.

b. **Echocardiographic findings include the following:**
   (1) Localized hypertrophy in the distal left ventricle beyond the origin of the chordae tendineae
   (2) Wall thickness in the apical region of at least 15 mm or a ratio of maximal apical to posterobasal thickness greater than 1.5
   (3) Exclusion of hypertrophy and other parts of the ventricular wall
   (4) No LVOT obstruction or gradient

c. **MRI** demonstrates localized hypertrophy to the cardiac apex. MRI is useful in the care of patients with poor echocardiographic windows.

d. **Cardiac catheterization** reveals a spade-like configuration of the LV cavity at end diastole and apical end-systolic LV cavity obliteration.

4. **Prognosis** is favorable compared with that associated with other forms of HCM.
5. **Therapy.** Therapeutic efforts are limited to management of diastolic dysfunction with β-blockers and calcium channel antagonists.

D. **HCM among the elderly**

1. **Clinical presentation.** In addition to the signs and symptoms of other forms of HCM, hypertension is more common with HCM in the elderly population.
2. **Incidence.** Although the incidence is unknown, HCM among the elderly probably is more common than expected.
3. **Genetic aspects.** Reports have suggested that the delayed expression of mutations in the gene for cardiac myosin-binding protein C may play an important role in HCM in the elderly.
4. **Echocardiographic findings** for elderly patients (65 years or older) are compared with findings for young patients (40 years or younger) as follows:

   a. **Common findings**
      (1) LVOT gradient, both provocable and at rest
      (2) Asymmetric hypertrophy
      (3) SAM of the mitral valve

   b. **Differences pertaining to the elderly**
      (1) Less hypertrophy
      (2) Less RV involvement
      (3) Ovoid versus crescentic left ventricle
      (4) Prominent septal bulge (i.e., sigmoid septum)
      (5) More acute angle between the aorta and septum as the aorta uncoils with age
      (6) Management of HCM in the elderly is similar to that of other forms of HCM.
      (7) The **prognosis** is favorable compared with that for forms of HCM that occur at a younger age.

Key Reviews

Fifer MA, Vlahakes GJ. Management of symptoms in hypertrophic cardiomyopathy. *Circulation* 2008;117:429–439.

Maron BJ. Hypertrophic cardiomyopathy. *Lancet* 1997;350:127–133.

Nishimura RA, Holmes DR Jr. Hypertrophic Obstructive Cardiomyopathy. *N Engl J Med* 2004;350:1320–1327.

Landmark Articles

Fananapazir L, Epstein ND. Prevalence of hypertrophic cardiomyopathy and limitations of screening methods. *Circulation* 1995;92:700–704.

Lever HM, Karam RF, Currie PS, et al. Hypertrophic cardiomyopathy in the elderly: distinctions from the young based on cardiac shape. *Circulation* 1989;79:580–589.

Maron BJ, Cerchi F, McKenna WS, et al. Risk factors and stratification for sudden death in patients with hypertrophic cardiomyopathy. *Br Heart J* 1994;72[Suppl]:S13–S18.

Maron BJ, Gardin JM, Flack JM, et al. Prevalence of hypertrophic cardiomyopathy in a general population of young adults. *Circulation* 1995;92:785–789.

Maron BJ, Isner JM, McKenna W, et al. Task force 3: hypertrophic cardiomyopathy, myocarditis, and other myopericardial diseases and mitral valve prolapse. *J Am Coll Cardiol* 1994;24:880–885.

Maron BJ, Pelliccia A, Spirito P. Cardiac disease in young trained athletes: insights methods for distinguishing athlete's heart from structural heart disease, with particular emphasis on hypertrophic cardiomyopathy. *Circulation* 1995;91:1596–1601.

Maron BJ, Spirito P, et al. Implantable cardioverter-defibrillators and prevention of sudden cardiac death in hypertrophic cardiomyopathy. *JAMA* 2007;298:405-412.
Maron MS, Olivotto I, Betocchi S. Effect of left ventricular outflow tract obstruction in clinical outcome in hypertrophic cardiomyopathy. *N Engl J Med* 2003;348:295–303.
Nishimura RA. Dual-chamber pacing for cardiomyopathies: a 1996 perspective. *Mayo Clin Proc* 1996;71:1077–1087.
Ommen SR, Maron BJ, et al. Long-term effects of surgical septal myectomy on survival in patients with obstructive hypertrophic cardiomyopathy. *J Am Coll Cardiol* 2005;46:470-476.
Spirito P, Bellone P, Harris KM. Magnitude of left ventricular hypertrophy and risk of sudden death in hypertrophic cardiomyopathy. *N Engl J Med* 2000;342:1778–1785.

10 MYOCARDITIS

Bethany A. Austin and W. H. Wilson Tang

I. INTRODUCTION. Myocarditis is defined by an inflammatory infiltration of the myocardium with associated necrosis or degeneration, or both. The disease is also known as **inflammatory cardiomyopathy** (or myocarditis with cardiac dysfunction in the World Health Organization 1995 classification for cardiomyopathy). The incidence and prevalence of myocarditis is unclear; the syndrome is underdiagnosed because of the large number of asymptomatic cases. Myocarditis usually affects younger individuals; the median age of patients with lymphocytic myocarditis is 42 years.

A. Clinicopathologic classification of myocarditis is clinically oriented but not widely used.

1. **Fulminant myocarditis** (17%) usually has a distinct onset. It can result in either complete, spontaneous resolution or rapidly progressive deterioration and death due to severe cardiac compromise. Usually there are multiple active foci of inflammatory infiltrate on histology with complete resolution.
2. **Acute myocarditis** (65% of myocarditis cases) has an indistinct onset, with moderate cardiovascular compromise and incomplete recovery, often resulting in cardiac dysfunction or subsequent death. Histologically, there are active or borderline inflammatory infiltrates that resolve completely resolve over time.
3. **Chronic active myocarditis** (11% of myocarditis cases) has a presentation similar to that of acute myocarditis, but the chronic form usually progresses to only mild or moderate cardiac dysfunction, occasionally with restrictive physiology. Histologic examination often shows ongoing fibrosis suggesting chronic inflammatory changes.
4. **Chronic persistent myocarditis** (7% of myocarditis cases) has an indistinct onset, with nonresolving active or borderline inflammatory infiltrates seen on histologic examination. Usually, there is no cardiovascular compromise.

B. Histologic classification of myocarditis, also called the Dallas classification (1986)

1. Initial biopsy
   - **a.** Myocarditis: myocardial necrosis or degeneration, or both, in the absence of significant coronary artery disease with adjacent inflammatory infiltrates or fibrosis, or both
   - **b.** Borderline myocarditis: inflammatory infiltrates too sparse or myocyte damage not apparent
   - **c.** No myocarditis: no inflammatory infiltrates or myocyte damage

2. Subsequent biopsy
   a. Ongoing (persistent) myocarditis or fibrosis, or both
   b. Resolving (healing) myocarditis or fibrosis, or both
   c. Resolved (healed) myocarditis or fibrosis, or both

C. **World Health Organization (Marburg Criteria, 1996).** A minimum of 14 infiltrating leukocytes per mm^2, preferably T lymphocytes, and up to four macrophages may be included.

II. CLINICAL PRESENTATION

A. Signs and symptoms

1. Myocarditis can be totally asymptomatic or can manifest with chest pain syndromes ranging from mild persistent chest pain of acute myopericarditis (35% of cases) to severe symptoms that mimic acute myocardial infarction.
2. About 60% of patients may have antecedent arthralgias, malaise, fevers, sweats, or chills consistent with viral infections (e.g., pharyngitis, tonsillitis, upper respiratory tract infection) 1 to 2 weeks before onset.
3. The hallmark symptoms are those of heart failure (e.g., dyspnea, fatigue, edema). The clinical history is one of acute decompensation of heart failure in a person without known cardiac dysfunction or with low cardiac risk. The diagnosis is usually presumptive, based on patient demographics and the clinical course (i.e., spontaneous recovery after supportive care).
4. In some instances, patients may present with arrhythmia in the form of syncope, palpitations caused by heart block (i.e., Stokes-Adams attack), ventricular tachyarrhythmia, or even sudden cardiac death.

B. **Physical findings.** Patients often present with signs of acute decompensated heart failure, including an S_3 (third heart sound) gallop, central and peripheral edema, jugular venous distention, and tachycardia (see Chapter 7). An audible pericardial friction rub may accompany concomitant myopericarditis. Specific findings in special cases are as follows:

1. **Sarcoid myocarditis:** lymphadenopathy, also with arrhythmias, and sarcoid involvement in other organs (up to 70%).
2. **Acute rheumatic fever** (usually affects heart in 50% to 90%): associated signs such as erythema marginatum, polyarthralgia, chorea, subcutaneous nodules **(i.e, Jones criteria)**
3. **Hypersensitive or eosinophilic myocarditis:** pruritic maculopapular rash and history of onset temporally related to initiation of potential culprit medications
4. **Giant cell myocarditis:** sustained ventricular tachycardia in rapidly progressive heart failure
5. **Peripartum cardiomyopathy:** heart failure developing in the last month of pregnancy or within 5 months after delivery (see Chapter 38)

III. LABORATORY EVALUATION

A. Inflammatory markers of myocarditis

1. **Complete blood count.** Leukocytosis is common (often lymphocytic), although the presence of eosinophilia may suggest hypersensitive (eosinophilic) myocarditis.
2. **Elevated acute phase reactants** such as erythrocyte sedimentation rates or ultrasensitive C-reactive protein are good monitors of clinical progression or response to therapy, but they have low specificity for myocarditis. Novel inflammatory markers under investigation include tumor necrosis factor-α, interleukins, interferon-γ, serum-soluble FAS and soluble FAS-ligand levels. Elevation of these markers portends a worse prognosis.
3. **Serum viral antibody titers** are usually increased fourfold or more acutely and gradually fall during convalescence. However, measurement of viral antibody titers is rarely indicated.
4. **Anticardiac antibody titers.** Because of their low specificity, measurement of anticardiac antibody titers (against sarcolemma, myosin, laminin, DP/ATP translocator, or β-adrenergic receptors) is not indicated (only 62% of myocarditis cases have titers $\geq$1:40).

B. Rheumatologic screening. Screening antinuclear antibodies (ANAs) and rheumatoid factor (RF) are often indicated. Disease-specific testing is indicated if the following conditions are suspected:

1. Systematic lupus erythematosus: anti-dsDNA (reported positive anti-Ro/SS-A and anti-La/SS-B in lupus carditis in children)
2. Polymyositis: anti-Jo_1
3. Wegner's granulomatosus: c-ANCA (antineutrophil cytoplasmic antibody)
4. Scleroderma: anti-SCL_{70}

C. Serum cardiac enzymes (markers of myonecrosis): creatinine kinase (MB subfraction) is elevated in only 7.5% of patients with biopsy-proven myocarditis, whereas the cardiac troponin I or T is elevated in at least 50% of patients with biopsy-proven myocarditis (89% to 94% specificity and 34% to 53% sensitivity).

IV. DIAGNOSTIC TESTING

A. Electrocardiogram. The electrocardiogram often reveals sinus tachycardia, although the presence of ST-segment deviation sometimes may represent focal or global ischemia. In some cases, fascicular block or atrioventricular conduction disturbances and ventricular tachyarrhythmia may be hemodynamically significant.

B. Echocardiogram. A complete echocardiogram is standard procedure for patients with suspected myocarditis to exclude alternative causes of heart failure, detect the presence of intracardiac thrombi and associated valvular disease, and quantify the degree of left ventricular (LV) dysfunction to monitor response to therapy.

1. Occasionally, focal wall-motion abnormalities and presence of pericardial fluid may prompt further workup or intervention.
2. Fulminant myocarditis is often characterized by near-normal diastolic dimensions and increased septal wall thickness, whereas acute myocarditis often has increased diastolic dimensions but normal septal wall thickness.

C. Other imaging modalities

1. **Antimyosin scintigraphy (indium III monoclonal antimyosin antibody)** provides identification of myocardial inflammation, with a high sensitivity (91% to 100%) and negative predictive value (93% to 100%) but low specificity (28% to 33%).
2. **Gallium scanning** identifies severe myocardial cellular infiltration with high specificity (98%) but low sensitivity (36%).
3. **Gadolinium-enhanced magnetic resonance imaging** is being used more frequently for diagnosis based on several small observational studies that have found up to 100% sensitivity and specificity depending on the protocol. In one study magnetic resonance imaging (MRI) was also used for guiding biopsy to areas of focal increased uptake of gadolinium in patients with clinically suspected myocarditis with significantly higher diagnostic yield than in those who did not have enhancing areas with which to guide the bioptome.

D. Coronary angiography. Cardiac angiography is often indicated to rule out coronary artery disease as the cause of new-onset heart failure as the clinical presentation of myocarditis may mimic myocardial infarction (i.e., pseudoinfarct pattern), especially if there are focal wall-motion abnormalities and localizing electrocardiographic changes.

V. ETIOLOGY.

Up to 50% of all cases may not have a clear underlying cause (i.e., idiopathic cases).

A. Infective causes (Table 10.1).

1. **Viral myocarditis.** Cardiotropic viruses such as enteroviruses (specifically the Coxsackie group B and echoviruses) may cause direct cardiotoxic injuries, cytokine activation, cytoskeletal damage, and autoimmune responses. However, data suggest that the incidence of myocarditis after infection is lower than previously projected. Viral myocarditis is often considered when accompanied with a clinical picture of recent febrile illness, often with prominent myalgias, followed by rapid onset cardiac symptoms. However, direct proof is lacking (and often unnecessary), and many cases of idiopathic dilated cardiomyopathies have been attributed to antecedent viral myocarditis. Antiviral therapies have not proved to be useful.

TABLE 10.1 Causes of Myocarditis

Cause	Examples
	Infectious causes
Viruses	Enteroviruses, coxsackievirus A and B, echovirus, influenza virus, poliovirus, herpesviruses, adenovirus, mumps, rubella, rubeola, hepatitis B or C virus, human immunodeficiency virus (HIV), Epstein-Barr virus, cytomegalovirus, parvovirus B19
Rickettsia	Rocky Mountain Spotted Fever
Fungi	Cryptococcosis, aspergillosis, coccidioidomyoosis, histoplasmosis
Protozoa	*Trypanosoma cruzi* (Chagas' disease), *Toxoplasmosis gondii*
Helminths	trichinosis, schistosomiasis
Bacteria	*Legionella, Clostridium*, streptococci, staphylococci, *Salmonella, Shigella*
Spirochetes	*Borrelia burgdorferi* (Lyme disease)
	Noninfectious causes
Hypersensitive reaction	Eosinophilic myocarditis
Cardiotoxic drugs	Catecholamines, amphetamines, cocaine, chemotherapeutic drugs (e.g., anthracyclines, fluorouracil, streptomycin, cyclophosphamide, interleukin-2, trastuzumab [Herceptin]), small pox vaccine
Collagen vascular diseases	Systemic lupus erythematosus (i.e., lupus carditis), Wegener's granulomatosis or Churg-Strauss syndrome, dermatomyositis or polymyositis, scleroderma
Systemic illnesses	Sarcoidosis, giant cell myocarditis, Kawasaki's disease, large-vessel vasculitis (e.g., polyarteritis nodosa, Takayasu's arteritis), inflammatory bowel diseases (e.g., ulcerative colitis, Crohn's disease)
Acute rheumatic fever	
Bites and stings	Venoms of scorpions, snakes, wasps, and black widow spiders
Chemicals	Hydrocarbons, carbon monoxide, thallium, lead, arsenic, cobalt
Physical injury	Irradiation, heatstroke, hypothermia
Childbirth	Peripartum cardiomyopathy
Alloantigens	Posttransplantation cellular rejection

2. Chagas' disease. Cardiomyopathy caused by *Trypanosoma cruzi* in South and Central America, particularly in persons 30 to 50 years old. It is estimated that 16 to 18 million persons are infected with *T. cruzi* in Latin America. Cardiac involvement usually appears decades after initial treatment and is the leading cause of death of persons 30 to 50 years old in the endemic areas.

a. Diagnosis

(1) Serologic test results should be positive for at least two types of test (i.e., indirect immunofluorescence, indirect hemagglutination, complement fixation, immunoenzymatic, and radioimmune assays).

(2) Cardiac lesions diagnosed by in situ polymerase chain reaction methods of analyzing biopsies.

(3) Typical electrocardiographic changes include right bundle-branch block with left anterior hemiblock, premature ventricular complexes, T-wave inversions, abnormal Q waves, variable atrioventricular blocks, low QRS voltage, and sick sinus syndrome.

(4) Echocardiographic findings include LV aneurysm with or without thrombi, posterior basal akinesis or hypokinesis with preserved septal contraction, and diastolic dysfunction.

b. Clinical presentation

(1) The acute and subacute phases (i.e., 4 to 8 weeks of acute inflammation) consist for the most part of local inflammation at the parasite entry site and flu-like symptoms. Occasionally hepatosplenomegaly and lymphadenopathy occur, but concomitant meningoencephalitis is rare. These manifestations often result from pathogen-induced cytotoxicity and inflammatory responses. More than 90% of cases resolve in 4 to 8 weeks without therapy.

(2) The chronic phase (up to 10 to 30 years after acute infection) manifests with symptoms of palpitations, syncope, chest pain, and, subsequently, heart failure. Approximately 5% to 10% of affected patients may develop direct acute-to-chronic progression.

(a) Heart failure (predominantly right sided in advanced stages) may develop in 25% to 30% of those affected.

(b) Cerebral or pulmonary thromboembolism may occur in 10% to 15% of those affected.

(c) Concomitant megaesophagus or megacolon may develop.

(d) Apical left ventricular aneurysm and apical fibrosis may develop.

(3) Chagas' disease is highly arrhythmogenic.

(a) Frequent, complex ectopic beats and ventricular tachyarrhythmia occur in 40% to 90% of affected patients, with sudden cardiac death occurring in 55% to 65%.

(b) Bundle-branch block occurs in 50% of affected patients, and bradyarrhythmia with high-grade atrioventricular block occurs in 7% to 8%.

(c) Atrial fibrillation develops in 7% to 10% of affected patients.

c. Antibiotic therapy aims to reduce parasitemia and prevent complications.

(1) Benznidazole (5 to 10 mg/kg/day q12h for 60 days) or

(2) Nifurtimox (8 to 10 mg/kg PO q24h for 90 to 120 days)

3. Human immunodeficiency virus (HIV)–related cardiomyopathy. HIV disease has been recognized as an important cause of dilated cardiomyopathy, with an estimated incidence of 1.6%. HIV type 1 (HIV-1) virions appear to infect myocardial cells in patchy distributions, leading to cytokine activation and progressive tissue damage. Cardiac autoimmunity, nutritional deficiencies, and drug toxicities (i.e., mitochondrial damage from zidovudine and vasculitis or coronary artery disease associated with highly active antiretroviral therapy [HAART] regimens) are possible contributing causes. In addition, other known viral pathogens, including cytomegalovirus (CMV), Epstein-Barr virus (EBV), and coxsackievirus B, have been isolated from endomyocardial biopsy (EMB) specimens of HIV-positive patients with myocarditis in conjunction with HIV nucleic acid sequences, suggesting that opportunistic viral infections may play an important role in the pathogenesis of this type of cardiomyopathy.

B. Peripartum cardiomyopathy (see Chapter 38)

C. Giant cell myocarditis: (i.e., pernicious myocarditis, Fiedler's myocarditis, granulomatous myocarditis, or idiopathic interstitial myocarditis). This is a rare disorder with an unclear origin. The hallmark feature is the presence of fused, multinucleated (>20 nuclei) epithelioid giant cells of histocytic origin within a diffuse, intramyocardial inflammatory infiltrate with lymphocytes.

1. Giant cell myocarditis often presents with an aggressive clinical course with progression over days to weeks. Rapidly progressive heart failure is the presentation in 75% of affected patients. Sustained ventricular tachyarrhythmia occurs in 29% of patients with giant cell myocarditis (GCM) and atrioventricular block occurs in 50%.

2. The prognosis is dismal without therapy, but the disease is often refractory to standard medical therapy, with a 1-year mortality rate of up to 80% (median survival of 3 to 5 months from symptom onset).

3. Small observational series have suggested potential benefits of immunosuppressive therapy and a randomized, prospective multicenter study is ongoing. Consideration for early cardiac transplantation is appropriate (71% 5-year survival after successful transplantation). Often, mechanical support may be required as a temporary bridge to recovery or transplantation. A 20% to 25% rate of histologic recurrence in surveillance endomyocardial biopsies has been observed after transplantation.

D. Hypersensitive reaction (i.e., eosinophilic myocarditis). Eosinophilic endomyocardial disease (i.e., Löffler's endomyocardial fibrosis, see Chapter 8) occurs as a major complication of idiopathic hypereosinophilic syndrome as a result of direct toxic damage caused by eosinophil granule proteins within the heart. Drug-induced eosinophilic myocarditis is independent of cumulative dose and duration of therapy.

The absence of peripheral eosinophilia does not rule out eosinophilic myocarditis. Although observational series suggest potential clinical benefits of corticosteroid therapy, the best strategy is to remove the causative agent when known.

1. Medications that may cause eosinophilic myocarditis include the following:
   a. Antibiotics (e.g., ampicillin, chloramphenicol, tetracycline, sulfisoxazole)
   b. Diuretics (e.g., hydrochlorothiazide, spironolactone)
   c. Anticonvulsives (e.g., phenytoin, carbamazepine)
   d. Others drugs (e.g., lithium, clozapine, indomethacin)
   e. Tetanus toxoid
2. Collagen vascular diseases such as Wegner's granulomatosus or Churg-Strauss syndrome (i.e., allergic granulomatosis and vasculitis) may also lead to eosinophilic myocarditis.
3. Other causes include parasitic infection, drug hypersensitivity, and cellular rejection after cardiac transplantation, as well as post vaccinia myocarditis after small pox vaccination.

E. Systemic autoimmune disorders with myocarditis. Although the histologic appearance of myocarditis occurring as part of sarcoidosis, systemic lupus erythematosus, or polymyositis is similar to that seen in isolated myocarditis, the natural history is different. Systemic causes of myocarditis often respond poorly to medical therapy and cardiac transplantation, and their prognoses are often unfavorable. However, small retrospective surveys and case series have identified a significant decrease in mortality and improved clinical course among cardiac sarcoid patients treated with corticosteroids.

VI. PROGNOSIS. On the basis of population studies, adults with myocarditis may present with few symptoms or with an acute toxic state of cardiogenic shock or frank heart failure (i.e., fulminant myocarditis). However, adults may present with heart failure years after the initial index event of myocarditis (up to 12.8% of patients with idiopathic dilated cardiomyopathy had presumed prior myocarditis in one case series).

A. Natural history and sequelae of myocarditis. The outlook is poor in the acute phase, regardless of clinicopathologic classification, but those surviving the acute phase have a more favorable prognosis (except for those with chronic active myocarditis).

1. Many patients may have full spontaneous clinical recovery, even after weeks of mechanical support (e.g., intraaortic balloon counterpulsation, mechanical assist devices).
2. In the Myocarditis Treatment Trial, the 1-year mortality rate was 20%, and the 4-year mortality rate was 56%.
3. In-hospital cases series point to an 11-year survival rate of 93% for patients with fulminant myocarditis and 45% for nonfulminant cases.
4. Evolution to dilated cardiomyopathy
   a. Up to one-half of patients with myocarditis develop subsequent cardiomyopathy over a range of 3 months to 13 years.
   b. Histologic evidence of myocarditis is seen in 4% to 10% of EMBs of patients with idiopathic dilated cardiomyopathy.

5. Severe heart block requiring permanent pacemaker placement occurs in 1% patients.

B. Predictors for morbidity and mortality

1. Unfavorable factors for survival include extremes of age (i.e., very old or very young), electrocardiographic abnormalities (e.g., QRS alterations, atrial fibrillation, low voltages), syncope, and specific diagnoses (e.g., peripartum cardiomyopathy, GCM).
2. Favorable factors for survival include normal ventricular function, shorter clinical history, and fulminant presentation at onset.

VII. TREATMENT

A. Heart failure management

1. Standard heart failure therapy consists of diuretics, angiotensin-converting enzyme (ACE) inhibitors, β-blockers, and aldosterone antagonists (see Chapter 8).
2. Because of its proarrhythmic properties in animal models, digoxin should be avoided.
3. Anticoagulation to prevent thromboembolic events is usually recommended in patients with apical aneurysm with thrombus (e.g., Chagas' disease, atrial fibrillation, prior embolic episodes).
4. Inotropic therapy is reserved for severe hemodynamic compromise, particularly in fulminant myocarditis.
5. Aggressive support with mechanical and surgical intervention is often indicated (see Chapters 7 and 11).
   a. Intraaortic balloon counterpulsation for hemodynamic support and afterload reduction
   b. Mechanical assistive devices (LVAD)
   c. Extracorporeal membrane oxygenation (ECMO)
6. Early consideration for cardiac transplantation should be given, especially for patients with progressive, biopsy-proven GCM or peripartum cardiomyopathy. However, patients with myocarditis have increased rates of rejection and reduced survival after heart transplantation compared to those without myocarditis, and recurrent disease may affect the allograft.

B. Exercise restriction

1. There is a theoretical increased risk of myocardial inflammation and necrosis, cardiac remodeling, and death, as shown in animal models.
2. Patients are usually advised to abstain from vigorous exercise for several months.

C. Arrhythmia management

1. Antiarrhythmics provide first-line treatment using standard therapy such as β-blockers, amiodarone, and sotalol.
2. Implantable cardioverter–defibrillators (ICDs) are used for patients stabilized in the chronic phase with persistently low ejection fraction and for those with malignant arryhythmias that are refractory to medical therapy.
3. Permanent pacemakers are used for heart block or bradyarrhythmia.

D. Follow-up

1. Clinical follow-up should be close because persistent chronic inflammation may lead to dilated cardiomyopathy. Initially, 1- to 3-month intervals are used for drug and physical activity titration.
2. Serial echocardiographic assessment of ventricular structure and function is often performed, although there is no agreement regarding the frequency of echocardiographic assessment after myocarditis.

E. Immunosuppressive therapy is reserved for refractory disease or biopsy-proven GCM. No benefits have been established for antiviral regimens or nonsteroidal anti-inflammatory agents (see VIII.B). The most recent Heart Failure Society of America (HFSA) Guidelines do not recommend routine use of immunosuppressive therapy in patients with myocarditis.

VIII. CONTROVERSIES IN MYOCARDITIS

A. Endomyocardial biopsy

1. Routine endomyocardial biopsy confirmation of myocarditis is unnecessary.

TABLE 10.2 Relevant ACC/AHA Recommendations for Role of Endomyocardial Biopsy

Scenario	Class of recommendation
New-onset heart failure of <2 weeks' duration associated with a normal-sized or dilated left ventricle and hemodynamic compromise	I
New-onset heart failure of 2 weeks' to 3 months' duration associated with a dilated left ventricle and new ventricular arrhythmias, 2nd- or 3rd-degree heart block, or failure to respond to usual care within 1 to 2 weeks	I
Heart failure of >3 months' duration associated with a dilated left ventricle and new ventricular arrhythmias, 2nd- or 3rd-degree heart block, or failure to respond to usual care within 1 to 2 weeks	IIa
Heart failure associated with a dilated cardiomyopathy of any duration associated with suspected allergic reaction and/or eosinophilia	IIa
New-onset heart failure of 2 weeks' to 3 months' duration associated with a dilated left ventricle, without new ventricular arrhythmias or 2nd- or 3rd-degree heart block that responds to usual care within 1 to 2 weeks	IIb
Heart failure of >3 months' duration associated with a dilated left ventricle, without new ventricular arrhythmias or 2nd- or 3rd-degree heart block, that responds to usual care within 1 to 2 weeks	IIb
Unexplained ventricular arrhythmias	IIb

  - **a.** The most recent HFSA recommendations are to consider biopsy in those patients with a rapid deterioration in cardiac function of unknown etiology who do not respond to standard medical therapy.
  - **b.** Incidence of biopsy-proven myocarditis in recent-onset, unexplained heart failure can be as low as 8% to 10%. Concerns have emerged that this is caused by low sensitivity of the Dallas criteria, and several recent trials of immunosuppressive therapy have utilized supplemental pathologic criteria to assess myocarditis, including upregulation of human leukocyte antigen, presence of virus, and anticardiac antibodies.
  - **c.** False-negative rates are high (50% even in four or five biopsies) because of the small number of lymphocytes and difficulties in distinguishing cell types, with wide interobserver variability.

2. However, endomyocardial biopsy may be considered in patients with the following conditions in which a diagnostic biopy may provide information on prognosis and/or therapeutic possibilities (see Table 10.2):
  - **a.** Rapidly progressive heart failure symptoms despite conventional therapy or new-onset frequent ventricular tachyarrhythmia or conduction disturbances
  - **b.** Suspected specific causes of myocarditis (e.g., GCM, eosinophilic myocarditis, cardiac sarcoidosis, vaccinia myocarditis)

3. Although specificity is high (98%), sensitivity has been found in some series to be as low as 10% to 22%. It increases with multiple biopsies, but postmortem examinations have found that more than 17 specimens were needed to make the diagnosis with 80% sensitivity in proven myocarditis cases.

4. Biopsy for staging of myocarditis
  - **a.** Cell types include lymphocytic, eosinophilic, neutrophilic, giant cell, granulomatous, and mixed.
  - **b.** Amount of cells: none (grade 0), mild (grade 1), moderate (grade 2), and severe (grade 3)

c. Distribution: focal (i.e., outside of vessel lumen), confluent, diffuse, and reparative (i.e., in fibrotic areas)

5. Other tests:
   a. Immunohistochemical staining to examine upregulation of major histocompatibility complex (MHC) antigens and quantify inflammation, although rates of correlation with biopsy-proven myocarditis have not been consistent between studies.
   b. Approximately 12% to 50% of patients with acute or chronic myocarditis have persistent viral mRNA detected in biopsy samples.

B. **Immunosuppressive therapy** in acute myocarditis

1. Routine immunosuppressive therapy is not recommended because of the neutral findings from multiple trials, including the Myocarditis Treatment Trial and the Intervention in Myocarditis and Acute Cardiomyopathy (IMAC) study. There is no Food and Drug Administration (FDA)–approved regimen for the treatment of acute or chronic myocarditis.
2. Considerations are reserved for patients with new-onset, rapidly deteriorating, advanced heart failure with suspicion of the following conditions.
   a. Giant cell myocarditis is treated with combination therapy (Table 10.3).

TABLE 10.3 Treatment Regimens for Myocarditis in Clinical Trials

Intervention in myocarditis and acute cardiomyopathy (IMAC) study[a]
Intravenous immune globulin (IVIG, Gamimune N, 10%): 1 g/kg/d IV × 2 days
Giant cell myocarditis study[b]
Cyclosporine: 25 mg PO bid, increase by 25-mg increments to target level:
Monoclonal whole-blood immunoassay: 200–300 ng/mL
High-performance liquid chromatography assay: 150–250 ng/mL
Fluorescence polarization immunoassay serum based polyclonal assay: 100–150 ng/mL
Dose reduction if renal dysfunction develops
Muromonab-CD3 (OKT-3): 5 mg IV qd × 10 days
Dose reduction if hypotension develops
Corticosteroid: methylprednisolone, 10 mg/kg IV qd × 3 days, followed by prednisone, 1–1.25 mg/kg with extended taper
Azathioprine: 200 mg PO qd
Myocarditis treatment trial[c]
Corticosteroid/cyclosporine versus corticosteroid/azathioprine versus placebo (biopsy-proven myocarditis, LVEF <45%, NYHA ≥ class II)
Oral prednisone: 1.25 mg/kg/d in divided doses × 1 week; reduce oral dose by 0.08 mg/kg/wk until dose was 0.33 mg/kg/d at week 12; maintain oral dose until week 20 and then reduce dose by 0.08 mg/kg/wk until week 24; then off.
Oral cyclosporine: 5 mg/kg bid to achieve level of 200–300 ng/mL × 1 week; adjust oral dose to achieve level of 100–200 ng/mL from weeks 2 to 4; adjust oral dose to achieve level of 60–150 ng/mL from weeks 4 to 24.
Immunosuppressive therapy for active lymphocytic myocarditis[d]
Prednisone 1 mg/kg/day for 4 weeks; reduced to 0.33 mg/kg/day for 5 months; Azathioprine 2 mg/kg/day for 6 months

LVEF, Left ventricular ejection fraction; NYHA, New York Heart Association.

[a]McNamara DM, Holubkov R, Starling RC, et al. Controlled trial of intravenous immune globulin in recent-onset dilated cardiomyopathy. *Circulation* 2001;103:2254–2259.

[b]Rosenstein ED, Zucker MJ, Kramer N. Giant cell myocarditis: most fatal of autoimmune diseases. *Semin Arthritis Rheum* 2000;30:1–16.

[c]Mason JW, O'Connell JB, Herskowitz A, et al. A clinical trial of immunosuppressive therapy for myocarditis. The Myocarditis Treatment Trial Investigators. *N Engl J Med* 1995;333:269–275.

[d] Frustaci A, Chimenti C, Calabrese F, et al. Immunosuppressive therapy for active lymphocytic myocarditis: virological and immunologic profile of responders versus nonresponders. *Circulation* 2003;107:857–863.

b. Eosinophilic or sarcoid myocarditis is treated with high-dose steroids.
c. Specific therapy is used for underlying collagen vascular diseases, if present.

3. Studies are ongoing in an attempt to identify markers to predict favorable response to immunosuppressive regimens. One recent study of 112 patients with histopathologic acute lymphocytic myocarditis who failed to improve with conventional therapy and subsequently received prednisone and azathioprine found that one-half of the treated group improved, with ejection fraction (EF) rising from 26% to 47% and improvement in biopsy findings. Of those who failed conventional therapy, those patients who responded to immunosuppression were significantly more likely to have positive cardiac antibodies (90% vs. 0%) and less likely to have viral persistence when compared with nonresponders (14% vs. 85%).

References

1. Cooper LT, Baughman KL, Feldman AM, et al. The role of endomyocardial biopsy in the management of cardiovascular disease: A scientific statement from the American Heart Association, the American College of Cardiology, and the European Society of Cardiology endorsed by the Heart Failure Society of America and the Heart Failure Association of the European Society of Cardiology. *J Am Coll Cardiol* 2007;50:1914–1931.
2. Cooper LT, Virmani R, Chapman NM, et al. National Institutes of Health-Sponsored workshop on inflammation and immunity in dilated cardiomyopathy. *Mayo Clin Proc* 2006;81:199–204.
3. Frustaci, A, Chimenti, C, Calabrese F, et al. Immunosuppressive therapy for active lymphocytic myocarditis: Virological and immunosuppressive profile of responders versus nonresponders. *Circulation* 2003;107:857–863.
4. Heart Failure Society of America. Myocarditis: Current Treatment. *J Card Fail* 2006;12:e120–122.
5. Mahrholdt H, Goedecke C, Wagner, A, et al. Cardiovascular magnetic resonance assessment of human myocarditis: A comparison to histology and molecular pathology. *Circulation* 2004;109:1250–1258.
6. McNamara DM, Holubkov R, Starling RC, et al. Controlled trial of intravenous immune globulin in recent-onset dilated cardiomyopathy. *Circulation* 2001;103:2254–2259.
7. Rosenstein ED, Zucker MJ, Kramer N. Giant cell myocarditis: most fatal of autoimmune diseases. *Semin Arthritis Rheum* 2000;30:1–16.
8. Skouri HN, Dec GW, Friedrich MG, et al. Noninvasive imaging in myocarditis. *J Am Coll Cardiol* 2006;48:2085–2093.
9. Wu, LA, Lapeyre AC, Cooper LT. Current role of endomyocardial biopsy in the management of dilated cardiomyopathy and myocarditis. *Mayo Clin Proc* 2001;76:1030–1038.

Landmark Articles

Aretz HT, Billingham ME, Edwards WD, et al. Myocarditis: a histopathologic definition and classification. *Am J Cardiovasc Pathol* 1987;1:3–14.

Cooper LT Jr, Berry GJ, Shabetai R. Idiopathic giant-cell myocarditis: natural history and treatment. Multicenter Giant Cell Myocarditis Study Group Investigators. *N Engl J Med* 1997;336:1860–1866.

Lieberman EB, Herskowitz A, Rose NR, et al. A clinicopathologic description of myocarditis. *Clin Immunol Immunopathol* 1993;68:191–196.

Mason JW, O'Connell JB, Herskowitz A, et al. A clinical trial of immunosuppressive therapy for myocarditis. The Myocarditis Treatment Trial Investigators. *N Engl J Med* 1995;333:269–275.

McCarthy RE III, Boehmer JP, Hruban RH, et al. Long-term outcome of fulminant myocarditis as compared with acute (non-fulminant) myocarditis. *N Engl J Med* 2000;342:690–695.

Parrillo JE, Cunnion RE, Epstein SE, et al. A prospective, randomized, controlled trial of prednisone for dilated cardiomyopathy. *N Engl J Med* 1989;321:1061–1068.

Key Reviews

Feldman AM, McNamara D. Myocarditis. *N Engl J Med* 2000;343:1388–1398.

Haas GJ. Etiology, evaluation, and management of acute myocarditis. *Cardiol Rev* 2001;9:88–95.

Magnani JW, Dec GW. Myocarditis: current trends in diagnosis and treatment. *Circulation* 2006;113:876–890.

Rassi A, Rassi R, Little WC. Chagas' heart disease. *Clin Cardiol* 2000;23:883–889.

Rosenstein ED, Zucker MJ, Kramer N. Giant cell myocarditis: most fatal of autoimmune diseases. *Semin Arthritis Rheum* 2000;30:1–16.

Relevant Book Chapters

Baughman KL, Hruban RH. Treatment of myocarditis. In: Smith TW, ed. *Cardiovascular therapeutics: a companion to Braunwald's heart disease.* Philadelphia: WB Saunders, 1996:243–253.

McNamara DM. Diagnosis and medical treatment of inflammatory cardiomyopathy. In: Topol EJ, ed. *Textbook of cardiovascular medicine,* 2nd ed. Philadelphia: Lippincott-Raven, 2002:1899–1914.

Relevant Websites

www.mayoclinic.com/health/myocarditis/DS0052
www.texasheartinstitute.org/HIC/Topics/Cond/myocard.cfm

NONTRANSPLANTATION SURGICAL TREATMENT FOR CHRONIC HEART FAILURE

11

Bethany A. Austin, Gonzalo Gonzalez-Stawinski, and Mazen Hanna

I. INTRODUCTION. Even with optimal medical therapy, the morbidity and mortality associated with chronic heart failure (CHF) is significant. Fortunately, there are multiple possible surgical interventions available for these patients that may help to avoid or postpone the need for transplantation. Despite the improvement in surgical techniques and an enhanced understanding of the role of reconstructing structural abnormalities of the failing heart, safety and efficacy data are still limited for many of these procedures. Elective and planned procedures for advanced heart failure [e.g., revascularization, mitral valve surgery, left ventricular (LV) reconstructive surgery, cardiomyoplasty], and urgent or bridging procedures (e.g., circulatory support devices, total artificial heart) are discussed in this chapter. Surgical approaches to the management of heart failure must be accompanied by continued aggressive pharmacologic therapy.

II. SURGICAL REVASCULARIZATION FOR ISCHEMIC CARDIOMYOPATHY

A. Pathophysiology

1. Loss of coronary flow reserve in severe coronary artery disease leads to reduction in myocardial perfusion and myofiber hypoxia, resulting in myocardial dysfunction.
2. Myocardial infarction results in necrosis and scarring, with loss of contractile function. Sites distal to infarction undergo increased mechanical stress and adverse remodeling over time, with resultant progressive ventricular dilation and impairment of systolic and diastolic function.
3. Chronic ischemic cardiomyopathy can decrease perfusion, leading to hibernation, repeated episodes of stunning, or a large infarct. The myocytes may still be viable and may subsequently recover function. Stunning and hibernation may be detected by various imaging modalities (see Chapter 45).
   a. **Stunning** is the loss of contractile function caused by a momentary total occlusion of blood flow with subsequent restoration of flow.
   b. **Hibernation** is the downregulation of myocardial function to match chronic reduced blood flow. Myocytes in hibernation manifest sustained glucose extraction, some loss of contractile material, and change in glycogen content.

B. Clinical significance

1. Heart failure, rather than angina or an acute coronary syndrome, is a common presentation of myocardial ischemia in patients with underlying cardiac dysfunction.
2. At least two-thirds of patients with cardiac dysfunction have evidence of epicardial coronary artery disease as the primary etiology. Coronary angiography is indicated when the suspicion of an ischemic cause for cardiomyopathy is high.
3. Some patients may have epicardial coronary artery disease superimposed on an underlying dilated cardiomyopathy. In this scenario, the presence of epicardial coronary artery disease may not necessarily explain the "degree" of depressed myocardial contractility. The role of revascularization remains unclear for these patients.

C. Recommendations

1. There are no randomized, controlled data regarding the outcome of coronary artery bypass grafting (CABG) in patients with severe ischemic cardiomyopathy. There are many case series and case-control studies in the literature that suggest

it imparts a significant reduction in morbidity and mortality with careful patient selection. In this regard, primary CABG should be considered for patients with a left ventricular ejection fraction (LVEF) >15%, LV end-diastolic dimensions <65 mm, distal vessels suitable for grafting, and evidence of a significant amount of ischemic or hibernating myocardium. However, these are somewhat arbitrary guidelines and many centers consider patients with more severe disease.

2. Patients with hibernating myocardium and severe LV dysfunction who undergo CABG may achieve survival comparable to those receiving cardiac transplantation (about 80% survival in 3 years).
   a. Generally, the potential for significant improvement in LV function and symptoms is assumed to be great enough to recommend revascularization when there are four or more viable segments of myocardium, representing approximately 31% of the left ventricle.
3. Surgical revascularization of the patient with severe heart failure should generally be considered part of a multifaceted holistic approach, which may include all or some of the following: valve repair, ventricular reconstructive surgery, cryoablation for ventricular arrhythmias, and maze procedure or pulmonary vein isolation procedures for atrial dysrhythmias. If therapeutic benefit is to be maximized from this approach, aggressive complimentary pharmacologic approaches are indicated postoperatively.

III. MITRAL VALVE SURGERY

A. Pathophysiology

1. As the ventricle fails, progressive dilation and abnormal geometry of the left ventricle give rise to mitral regurgitation (MR), regardless of the cause of LV dysfunction. This leads to a progressive increase in volume overload of the left ventricle, progressive LV dilation, and further worsening of MR.
2. Other alterations of the annular–ventricular apparatus and ventricular geometry contribute to the genesis of MR, including papillary muscle ischemia or infarction, myocardial thinning and dilation, blunting of the aortomitral angle, widening of the interpapillary distance, and increased leaflet-tethering leading to the loss of the zone of coaptation.

B. Clinical significance and recommendations

1. Restoration of the zone of coaptation by inserting an "undersized" annuloplasty ring may correct the MR and improve LV geometry and effective cardiac output in patients with cardiomyopathy. Unfortunately, mitral valve repair in ischemic cardiomyopathy is less successful than in degenerative MR in terms of chronic reduction of MR.
2. The subvalvular apparatus should be kept intact when possible.
3. In selected patients with heart failure, mitral valve surgery results in improved symptoms and measures of LV function and remodeling but not necessarily in improved survival.
4. In some patients, mitral valve repair with a figure-of-eight stitch (i.e., Alfieri approach) or the "edge-to-edge" technique may be used in addition to annuloplasty to secure the repair.
5. Mitral valve replacement is required in a minority of patients and may be associated with a significantly worse outcome.

IV. LEFT VENTRICLE RECONSTRUCTIVE PROCEDURES

A. Pathophysiology

1. As the failing heart dilates and the intracavity radius increases, wall stress increases (by Laplace's law). This leads to increased myocardial oxygen consumption and stimulates detrimental remodeling processes.
2. Surgical remodeling helps to decrease ventricular size and wall stress. Endoventricular circular patch plasty (EVCPP, also called the Dor procedure) is performed in patients with ischemic cardiomyopathy and significant areas of LV akinesis or dyskinesis. Partial LV resection, also called the Batista procedure, was performed in the past on patients with dilated, nonischemic cardiomyopathy and was abandoned because of poor intermediate results and increased mortality, despite promising initial short-term outcomes.

B. EVCPP

1. After an acute myocardial infarction, the necrotic muscle becomes a scar, and remodeling of the left ventricle leads to dilation and heart failure. The Dor procedure is suitable for patients with a left anterior descending artery territory scar or aneurysm with relatively preserved lateral and posterior LV wall function.
   a. It involves opening of the akinetic or dyskinetic scar and placement of a purse-string suture at the neck of the aneurysm. The residual opening may be closed with a Dacron patch, after which the ventriculotomy is closed by running sutures.
   b. This procedure is accompanied by CABG in >90% of cases. Additional valve and ablative surgical procedures are commonly performed.
2. The patients who are good candidates for EVCPP include those with a presence of LV aneurysm (or large akinetic area), an increased LV end-systolic index, absence of scar in the circumflex territory, and good target tissue and viability for concomitant CABG. Assessment of the severity of MR is needed at the time of surgery, and mitral valve repair is performed in 30% to 50% of patients undergoing EVCPP.
3. After EVCPP, the global ejection fraction is improved, end-diastolic and end-systolic volume indices for LV volumes are reduced, and there is restoration of a more normal LV geometry and improvement in New York Heart Association (NYHA) functional class.
   a. In a series of patients with advanced heart failure, the event-free survival rate was 98% at 1 year, 95.8% at 2 years, and 82.1% at 5 years.
   b. Higher preoperative NYHA class, lower LVEF (<30%), higher end-systolic volume index, and remote asynergy were independent predictors of mortality.
   c. Several ongoing trials will help to better define the role of this kind of surgical ventricular restoration (SVR) in the treatment of CHF. One of these is the Surgical Treatment of Ischemic Heart Failure (STICH) trial, a randomized controlled trial examining standard medical therapy compared to CABG plus medical therapy as well as CABG and SVR plus medical therapy.

C. Partial LV resection (i.e., **Batista procedure**) involves the resection of myocardium at the posterolateral wall between the anterolateral and posteromedial papillary muscles in nonischemic cardiomyopathy, with or without mitral annuloplasty or mitral valve replacement. For the reasons previously stated, this procedure is no longer performed.

D. Dynamic cardiomyoplasty

1. The procedure involves the mobilization of the entire latissimus dorsi muscle, which is passed into the thoracic cavity through a window created by removing the left second rib. The muscle is wrapped around the heart and anchored posteriorly, adjacent to the right atrium and pulmonary artery and anteriorly around the right ventricle.
   a. Sensing electrodes are placed epicardially on the right ventricle, and intramuscular stimulator electrodes are placed in the latissimus muscle.
   b. The muscle-conditioning process takes place 2 weeks after surgery and involves the delivery of a single pulse with every other cardiac cycle for 2 weeks. The signal is then incrementally increased every 1 to 2 weeks for 12 weeks.
2. Cardiomyoplasty is believed to work by systolic augmentation of the failing left ventricle and the girdling effect of the muscle acting as an elastic constraint. This prevents LV dilation and improves symptoms, but has no proven survival advantages. Indeed, early mortality is high, especially in those with NYHA class IV status. This procedure is rarely performed, and data are lacking on its long-term efficacy.

E. Other investigational surgical procedures

1. **Myocardial restraint device (i.e., ACORN).** The ACORN wrap is a proprietary medical textile tissue that is wrapped around the heart, and it adheres to the epicardial surface without significant fibrosis and constriction. With or without mitral valve surgery, the ACORN wrap provides diastolic support to reduce ventricular wall stress and dilatation. One recent report followed 193 patients with an average EF of 23% randomized to mitral valve surgical intervention with or without ACORN application and revealed significantly lower 30-day mortality

rates than in the original report describing the use of this device. In addition, this report noted improvement in parameters of LV remodeling and trends to improvement in clinical endpoints including need for transplantation and left ventricular assist device (LVAD) implantation. This will likely lead to larger investigations to delineate if this adjunctive intervention in those with mitral valve dysfunction and nonischemic cardiomyopathy might have a significant impact on clinical outcomes.

2. **Myosplint shape-changing device.** The Myosplint device consists of an implantable transventricular splint and two epicardial pads that are adjusted to draw the walls of the left ventricle together, thereby dividing the left ventricle into a bilobular chamber with a smaller radius. This smaller radius should translate into lower wall stress. However, the implantation may make existing MR worse, necessitating mitral valve repair.
3. **Stem cell transplantation** involves the regeneration of myocytes by replacing scarred, nonviable heart muscle with functioning contractile tissue derived from pluripotent stem cells early after a myocardial infarction. However, the feasibility of the procedure, the optimal timing and technique, the potential risks of arrhythmia, and the need for adjunctive medical support remain under investigation.

V. CIRCULATORY SUPPORT DEVICES (i.e., MECHANICAL ASSIST DEVICES)

A. Background

1. Mechanical circulatory assistance is necessary for patients who deteriorate hemodynamically and are unlikely to survive without a transplant. These devices help bridge the patients with CHF to transplantation.
2. The types of devices include the intraaortic balloon counterpulsation pump (IABP), extracorporeal membrane oxygenation (ECMO), univentricular and biventricular nonpulsatile and pulsatile ventricular assist devices (VADs), and the total artificial heart.
3. The decision about which device to use is based on duration of predicted use, reversibility of the underlying cause of cardiogenic shock, need for left-chamber versus dual-chamber support, and the patient's size.

B. Patient selection

1. Mechanical support is generally indicated in patients who have an inability to maintain hemodynamic stability despite maximal pharmacologic support, and who usually must meet criteria as candidates for cardiac transplantation.
   - **a.** Systolic blood pressure <75 to 80 mm Hg
   - **b.** Cardiac index of <1.5 to 1.8 L/min/m^2
   - **c.** Pulmonary venous saturation <50%
2. Indications for short-term circulatory support devices include the following:
   - **a.** Cardiogenic shock after cardiac surgery
   - **b.** Acute myocardial infarction with cardiogenic shock
   - **c.** Acute (fulminant) myocarditis
   - **d.** Cardiac arrest as a complication of interventional cardiac procedures (associated with high mortality and poor survival rates)
3. 2006 International Society for Heart and Lung Transplantation (ISHLT) Guidelines for Cardiac Transplant Candidates
   - **a.** The most recent ISHLT recommendations give a class I recommendation to thoroughly evaluating other clinical risk factors prior to device implantation. For instance, an inverse relationship between outcome and age >60 to 65 years has been reported. However, age by itself should not be a contraindication to implantation.
   - **b.** Patients with serum creatinine >3.0 mg/dL are at higher risk but may be considered candidates for implantation if renal failure is acute and recovery is likely (class I).
   - **c.** Pulsatile intracorporeal devices should only be implanted in patients with body surface area (BSA) >1.5 m^2.
   - **d.** In patients with abnormal liver function tests secondary to right ventricular failure, biventricular support should be considered. In addition, biventricular

support should be considered in those with irreversible pulmonary hypertension, right ventricular (RV) failure, or multiorgan dysfunction.

e. Active infection should be identified and treated before implantation.

4. If recovery is anticipated, the best option is to use the least traumatic, least complicated device for the individual patient. If recovery of ventricular function is not expected, patients should be considered for use of a long-term implantable device.

C. Short-term devices

1. Extracorporeal membrane oxygenation (ECMO)

a. ECMO is an extracorporeal system that uses a centrifugal pump to drive blood from the patient to a membrane oxygenator system for carbon dioxide and oxygen exchange.

b. Typically, the femoral artery and vein are cannulated for peripheral access, but the aorta and right atrium can be used as well. The blood is driven from the venous system to the pump and oxygenator and then back into the arterial system.

c. Once in place, the device requires systemic anticoagulation and may cause substantial trauma to blood components.

d. ECMO has the advantage of providing oxygenation in the presence of severe pulmonary dysfunction resulting in hypoxemia. It can also unload both the right and left ventricles.

e. The large number of possible complications make ECMO suitable only for short-term use and it is generally used as a bridge either to transplantation or VAD implantation if patients cannot be weaned from cardiopulmonary support.

2. **Percutaneous left ventricular support devices** (TandemHeart and Impella) are indicated only for short-term use (up to 5 days) and are similar to an IABP with respect to decreasing afterload and myocardial oxygen consumption. Unlike an IABP, these devices completely unload the ventricle rather than simply augmenting it.

a. Inserted through the femoral artery, the Impella system is based on a catheter that crosses the aortic valve into the left ventricle and aspirates blood from the left ventricle into the ascending aorta. The 12F system is mounted on a 9F catheter inserted under fluoroscopy and contains a flow pump, the output of which can reach 2.5 L/min.

b. The TandemHeart system is a left atrial-to-femoral bypass system which, although it can be inserted percutaneously, requires transseptal puncture with a 21F inflow cannula attached to a centrifugal flow pump, which can reach a maximum cardiac output of 4 L/min. This pump delivers the blood to the femoral artery.

c. These systems require anticoagulation with heparin and prolonged supervision and bed rest, and cannot support the right ventricle. They cannot be used in patients with severe peripheral vascular disease. The TandemHeart cannot be used in patients with ventricular septal defects, given the risk of hypoxia with shunt or in patients with severe aortic insufficiency, whereas the Impella cannot be used in those with mechanical or stenotic aortic valves.

d. Potential complications include hemolysis, thromboembolism, and ventricular arrhythmia caused by catheter position, as well as risk of bleeding, infection, and catheter displacement. Complications can arise from the transseptal puncture site with the TandemHeart.

e. These devices can potentially be used to support patients with acute MI with cardiogenic shock, decompensated heart failure with myocarditis, and during high-risk percutaneous coronary intervention (PCI) or valvuloplasty. The TandemHeart can be used for RV support if the catheters are placed so as to pump right atrial to pulmonary artery.

3. **Centrifugal pumps** such as the BioMedicus Biopump are extracorporeal and commonly used for biventricular support for small patients (BSA $\leq$1.5 m^2) and are commonly used with ECMO.

a. The nonpulsatile pump uses a spinning chamber to generate blood flow through rotating cones or by an impeller mechanism.

b. The cannulation site for inflow into the pump is the femoral vein, right atrium, or ventricle, and the outflow cannula is placed in the femoral artery, axillary artery, or aorta. The lines are typically left between an unclosed sternum with only skin closure. This necessitates continuous supervision by trained staff and limits the devices to short-term use only.
c. Heparin anticoagulation is needed.

4. **Pulsatile pumps** are extracorporeal, asynchronous pumps (e.g., Abiomed BVS5000) that are commonly used for right, left, or biventricular support.
   a. There are atrial and arterial cannulas. The atrial cannula is put into the right or left atrium, and the arterial cannula is in the aorta. The advantage over centrifugal systems is that subcostal lines allow sternal closure.
   b. The pump has an upper chamber and a lower chamber. The upper chamber is filled passively by continuous blood flow from the atrium. The lower chamber has two trileaflet polyurethane valves (i.e., inflow and outflow valves) and is designed to eject a stroke volume of approximately 80 mL.
   c. The pump is pneumatically driven by compressed room air and provides 4 to 5 L/min of pulsatile flow.
   d. Anticoagulation is recommended with heparin or warfarin sodium to lower the rate of thromboembolism.
   e. The disadvantages of this system are the lack of mobility and the lower flow rates achieved compared with the chronically implanted devices. A decision is made after 5 to 7 days of support, and if further mechanical support is needed, the Abiomed is removed, and a chronic device is implanted.
   f. In small retrospective studies, outcomes in terms of successful bridge to transplantation, pre- and posttransplant mortality, and hospital discharge have not been shown to be significantly different between pulsatile and nonpulsatile devices.
5. **Axial flow pumps**
   a. Nonpulsatile rotary pumps similar to centrifugal flow devices, but which generate the energy for acceleration of blood by deflecting flow in the circumferential direction with the impellers.
   b. They are smaller and less noisy than other devices, making them a good option for patients with a smaller BSA, as well as potentially decreasing risk of infection due to smaller pocket size.
   c. Major complications include an increased tendency for pump thrombus requiring significant anticoagulation and hemolysis.

D. Longer-term implantable devices

1. Several implantable devices are available for long-term use: the Novacor, the HeartMate, the Thoratec, and the CardioWest Total Artificial Heart (TAH).
   a. The Novacor is implanted within the abdominal wall. The pump receives blood from the left ventricle through an apical cannula and pumps blood through an outflow conduit to the ascending aorta. An electromagnetic converter converts electrical energy to mechanical energy that activates two pusher plates, which then squeeze the pump sac to eject the blood into the aorta. The device is synchronized to pump systole at the end of native systole. It has a maximum stroke volume of 70 mL and flows up to 10 L/min. The external controller and power packs are wearable and connected to the pump through a single percutaneous lead brought out through the right abdominal wall. The thromboembolism rate is 10%, and patients need heparin or warfarin after implantation of the device.
   b. The HeartMate device also has an implanted pump that has pneumatically or electrically actuated pusher plates to generate pump action. The cannulas are placed similar to that in the Novacor pump. It can generate volumes of 83 mL and 9 L/min. The interior surfaces of the HeartMate are designed to allow pseudointimal layering, which reduces the risk for thromboembolism. In theory, no anticoagulation is needed, but many patients receive antiplatelet agents. These devices are designed for those with a BSA >1.5 m^2.
   c. The Thoratec is a paracorporeal system that can be used for left, right, or biventricular support. Because the system is outside the body, they can be

used in patients with BSA $\leq$1.5 m^2. However, this does limit mobility and flow rates (maximum stroke volume is 65 mL and flow rates can reach to 7.2 L/min). Systemic anticoagulation is required.

d. The CardioWest TAH is implanted after removal of the native heart and provides complete support. To accommodate the sizable device, patients must have a BSA >1.7 m^2 and anteroposterior distance of the chest of >10 cm. Systemic anticoagulation is required. This device has been approved for bridge to transplantation. Another TAH, the Abiocor, is in the investigational stages of development. This device is smaller and provides more mobility.

e. Totally implantable devices such as the Arrow Lionheart LVD-2000 and the Novacor II are under development and planned for destination therapy.

2. Axial-flow pumps such as the Jarvik 2000, HeartMate II, and the MicroMed DeBakey produce continuous nonpulsatile blood flow using a small pump with rotor blades. The bearings of the rotor are in direct contact with the blood. Although the MicroMed and HeartMate II have inflow cannulas that insert in the LV apex, the Jarvik is intraventricular, eliminating the need for an inlet cannula. The intraventricular position eliminates inlet graft kinking, thrombosis, and pannus formation in the inlet graft and inlet obstruction by the septum or lateral wall of the heart. The outflow cannula is attached to the descending aorta. The small size allows the Jarvik to be surgically implanted through a left thoracotomy, with or without cardiopulmonary bypass, and it can be implanted in smaller adults or children. The MicroMed and HeartMate II require a sternotomy and are implanted into a small abdominal pocket. The axial-flow pump is a true LVAD because it augments LV function. The pump is run optimally at pump speeds of between 8000 and 12,000 rpm, and the native left ventricle is allowed to eject through the aortic valve, giving some pulsatility to the blood flow. This can generate flows up to 5 to 7 L/min. However, a big problem is that of inadequate blood flow in the ascending aorta giving rise to thrombus formation and the potential for embolic stroke. Newer generations of these devices are being made with heparin-coated surfaces in an attempt to minimize this risk. Frazier et al. reported their initial experience with the Jarvik 2000 and showed that the cardiac index increased by 43% that capillary wedge pressure decreased by 52%, and that 80% of the patients improved from NYHA class IV to I. No device thrombosis was reported.

E. Contraindications to VADs

1. Uncontrolled sepsis
2. Aortic valve incompetence needs to be corrected before implantation of the VAD because it might lead to regurgitation of blood from the outflow cannula back into the left ventricle. Severe mitral stenosis should also be treated to avoid limiting the device output due to decreased native ventricular filling.
3. Preexisting mechanical prosthetic valves may need to be changed to bioprosthetic valves to obviate the need for anticoagulation before implanting the VAD.
4. Hypercoagulable states may preclude the placement of VADs not requiring anticoagulation.
5. Aortic aneurysm or dissection may affect the optimal placement of the outflow cannula in the ascending aorta.
6. Bleeding diathesis
7. Patent foramen ovale or atrial septal defects need to be closed before implantation of VADs to prevent right to left shunting of blood and paradoxical emboli as the left side of the heart is decompressed.
8. Recent or evolving CVA
9. Multiorgan failure
10. Metastatic tumors are an absolute contraindication.

F. Predictors of poor outcomes after implantation of LVADs

1. Age
2. Right ventricular failure
3. Urine output <30 mL/hour
4. Central venous pressure >16 mm Hg
5. Receiving mechanical ventilation

6. Prothrombin time is >16 seconds; vitamin K is usually given in high doses preoperatively to patients being considered for VAD.
7. Reoperation
8. Cachexia syndrome

G. Echo-Doppler assessment of VAD dysfunction. After the implantation of the LVAD, intraoperative transesophageal echocardiography is used to assess the following factors:

1. Position of the inflow cannula at the LV apex. If the cannula is angulated toward the interventricular septum, inflow obstruction may result. The velocity of the flow across the inflow cannula is affected by multiple factors, including the flow generated by the device. However, if this velocity is >2 m/s, then obstruction of the cannula should be considered and thrombus or another mechanical cause of obstruction should be sought.
2. Whether the left ventricle has been adequately decompressed
3. The function of the aortic valve. If the flow rate through the LVAD is adequate, the aortic valve should not open. If there is significant aortic regurgitation, the aortic valve may have to be replaced.
4. Doppler interrogation of the inflow and outflow cannulas is done to exclude inflow and outflow valve dysfunction. Usually, the valves are unable to open, giving rise to increased forward flow velocities.
5. Periodic follow-up echocardiographic evaluation is performed to exclude thrombus formation, inflow cannula valve dysfunction, or endocarditis, and to evaluate LV systolic function.

H. Right ventricular assist device (RVAD)

1. Decisions for RVAD support (needed by 20% of patients) are based on hemodynamics after LVAD placement. However, implantation of long-term RVAD devices is more labor intensive and requires long bypass times for placement, which carries higher morbidity.
2. Univariate predictors of RVAD use are small body surface area, female gender, preoperative circulatory support, preoperative mechanical ventilation, and high total bilirubin and aspartate transferase values. Preoperatively, hemodynamic indices of a low mean or diastolic pulmonary artery pressure or a low right ventricular stroke work index (RVSWI <400 mm Hg · mL/m^2) may indicate the necessity for RVAD after LVAD insertion.
3. Inotropic agents, volume infusions, and vasodilators are used to optimize pulmonary pressures and LVAD flows, with right-heart hemodynamic values used as a guide. Aggressive diuresis is often necessary. If VAD flow remains <2 L/min per square meter, an RVAD system may be placed with the inflow from the right atrium and outflow to the pulmonary artery.
4. Inhaled nitric oxide has gained popularity as a potential alternative to RVAD implantation. In one center, it reduced the need for RVAD support from 7% to zero.
5. However, the RVAD use is associated with higher incidence of repeat sternotomy for bleeding, and the survival to transplantation is poor at 17%. It may be prudent for patients with risk factors for right ventricular dysfunction to receive a biventricular assist device or a total artificial heart from the start.

I. Complications

1. **Perioperative bleeding** increases with prolonged cardiopulmonary bypass times and causes excess fibrinolysis and platelet consumption. The degree of bleeding is intimately associated with right ventricular failure and RVAD support. Transfusion is associated with infection and HLA immunization, which can increase risk for hyperacute humoral rejection for a patient who goes on to transplantation. The use of LVADs, because of the need for perioperative transfusions, increases this risk from 4% to 25%. Leukocyte-poor blood products should be used to minimize this risk as much as possible.
2. **Malignant arrhythmias.** There is a high incidence of malignant cardiac arrhythmia after device implantation. Causes include cardiomyopathy, ischemia, chamber dilation, use of inotropic agents, and focal abnormalities at the sewing ring.

3. **Infection.** Antibiotic prophylaxis should be administered to prevent infection. In the long term, there is a 25% to 45% rate of infection, which temporarily removes 20% of patients from the active transplantation list. The most serious infection is VAD endocarditis, which carries a 50% mortality rate and necessitates removal or replacement of the device.
4. Embolic complications. Thromboembolism still occurs at a high rate despite appropriate anticoagulation. The Thoratec device carries a 22% risk for cerebrovascular embolic events; the Novacor, 10%; and the HeartMate, 3% to 5% over a 1-year period.

J. **Permanent VAD.** The Randomized Evaluation of Mechanical Assistance for the Treatment of Congestive Heart Failure (REMATCH) trial randomized patients with end-stage heart failure who required ionotropic therapy but were ineligible for cardiac transplantation to a vented electric LVAD or optimal medical therapy. There was a 48% relative reduction in risk of death from any cause in the group that received LVAD compared with the medically treated group. The probability of device failure was 35% at 24 months, and 10 patients had the device replaced. The LVAD group had significant improvement in quality of life over the trial, but the survival rates with permanent VAD are still far inferior to those for cardiac transplantation. This trial led to the approval of the HeartMate LVAD as destination therapy in selected patients not eligible for transplant. Follow-up of outcomes in 42 patients who were implanted with destination therapy HeartMate LVAD since REMATCH reveals improved survival rates at 1 month and 1 year, and decreased rates of infection and adverse events compared to those found in the trial patients. Occasionally patients who are implanted with the intent of destination therapy have improvement in conditions such as renal impairment or pulmonary hypertension that had precluded them from eligibility for transplantation earlier in their course and are able to be reevaluated for transplantation.

K. **Bridging to transplantation.** Patients presenting with severe, refractory low cardiac output states need mechanical support as a bridge to transplantation. However, it has been recognized that major end-organ dysfunction affects survival after transplantation. Mechanical support of the failing heart using short-term circulatory support devices can permit time to assess the reversibility of major organ dysfunction, and allow a full workup for suitability for cardiac transplantation. If the patient meets the selection criteria found in Table 11.1, full LVAD support can be implemented,

TABLE 11.1 Patient Selection Criteria for VAD Support as a Bridge to Cardiac Transplantation

1. Upper age consistent with successful cardiac transplantation, usually about age 70
2. Lower age limit determined by patient size large enough to accommodate a device
3. Suitable candidate for cardiac transplantation
4. Imminent risk of death before donor heart availability, usually with evidence of deterioration on maximal appropriate inotropic support and/or intraaortic balloon support
5. General hemodynamic guidelines:
   a. Cardiac index <1.8 L/min/m^2
   b. Systolic arterial blood pressure <90 mm Hg
   c. Pulmonary arterial capillary wedge pressure >20 mm Hg despite appropriate pharmacologic management
6. Adequate psychological criteria and external psychosocial support for transplantation and potentially prolonged LVAD support
7. Informed consent of patient or family
8. Absence of fixed pulmonary hypertension (pulmonary vascular resistance >6 Wood units)
9. Absence of irreversible renal or hepatic failure (LVAD support not expected to reverse existing renal or hepatic dysfunction)

LVAD, left ventricular assist device; VAD, ventricular assist device. Adapted from Kirklin JK, McGriffin D, Young JB. *Heart transplantation.* New York: Churchill Livingstone, 2002.

and if the major organ dysfunction normalizes, a successful bridge to transplantation can be expected. It is expected that 70% to 80% of patients with an LVAD can be successfully bridged to transplantation, compared with 36% of patients managed on inotropic agents with or without an IABP, and 80% of these transplanted patients will survive to be discharged from hospital. The percentage of transplantation patients requiring mechanical support has increased steadily from 3% in 1990 to >28% in 2004. Most LVAD implantation (75%) is for a strategy of bridge to transplantation. For those with biventricular failure that necessitates mechanical support, the options are combined RVAD and LVAD therapy or support with a total artificial heart. The CardioWest TAH has been approved for bridge to transplantation therapy.

L. Bridging to recovery. Clinical recovery sufficient to allow mechanical support device removal has been reported in small numbers at a few institutions. In theory, chronic mechanical unloading may permit reverse remodeling with downregulation of collagen production and hypertrophy and decrease in circulating inflammatory cytokines. Likelihood of successful recovery is greater in those with acute nonischemic cardiomyopathy and much less likely in those with chronic dilated cardiomyopathy. Currently, approximately 5% of LVAD implantation is peformed with a strategy of bridge to recovery.

ACKNOWLEDGMENTS

The authors thank Drs. Kenneth Ng and James O. O'Neill for their contributions to earlier editions of this chapter.

Landmark Articles

Ahuja K, Crooke GA, Grossi EA, et al. Reversing left ventricular remodeling in chronic heart failure: Surgical approaches. *Card Rev* 2007;15:184–190.

Badhwar V, Bolling SF. Mitral valve surgery in patients with left ventricular dysfunction. *Semin Thorac Cardiovasc Surg* 2002;14:133–136.

Bax JJ, Visser FC, Poldermans D, et al. Relationship between preoperative viability and postoperative improvement in LVEF and heart failure symptoms. *J Nucl Med* 2001;42:79–86.

Braile DM, Godoy MF, Thevenard GH, et al. Dynamic cardiomyoplasty: Long-term clinical results in patients with dilated cardiomyopathy. *Ann Thorac Surg* 2000;69:1445–1447.

Dakik HA, Howell JF, Lawrie GM, et al. Assessment of myocardial viability with 99mTc-sestamibi tomography before coronary artery bypass surgery. *Circulation* 1997;96:2892–2898.

DiCarli MF, Asgarzadie F, Schelbert HR, et al. Quantitation relation between myocardial viability and improvement in heart failure symptoms after revascularization in patients with ischemic cardiomyopathy. *Circulation* 1995;92:3436–3444.

DiCarli MF, Maddahi J, Rokhsar S, et al. Long-term survival of patients with coronary artery disease and left ventricular dysfunction: implications for the role of myocardial viability assessment in management decisions. *J Thorac Cardiovasc Surg* 1998;116:997.

DiDonato MD, Toso A, Maioli M, et al. Intermediate survival and predictors of death after surgical ventricular restoration. *Semin Thorac Cardiovasc Surg* 2001;13:468–475.

Feller ED, Sorensen EN, Haddad M, et al. Clinical outcomes are similar in pulsatile and nonpulsatile left ventricular assist device recipients. *Ann Thorac Surg* 2007;83:1082–1088.

Franco-Cereceda A, McCarthy PM, Blackstone EH, et al. Partial left ventriculectomy for dilated cardiomyopathy: is this an alternative to transplantation? *J Thorac Cardiovasc Surg* 2001;121:879–893.

Frazier OH, Myers TJ, Gregoric ID, et al. Initial clinical experience with the Jarvik 2000 implantable axial-flow left ventricular assist system. *Circulation* 2002;105:2855–2860.

Furnary AP, Jessup M, Moreira LF. Multicenter trial of dynamic cardiomyoplasty for chronic heart failure. *J Am Coll Cardiol* 1996;28:1175–1180.

Gronda E, Bourge RC, Costanzo MR, et al. Heart rhythm considerations in heart transplant candidates and considerations for ventricular assist devices: International Society for Heart and Lung Transplantation Guidelines for the Care of Cardiac Transplant Candidates-2006. *J Heart Lung Transplant* 2006;25:1043–1056.

Hunt SA, Baker DW, Chin MH, et al., for the American College of Cardiology/American Heart Association Task Force on Practice Guidelines (Committee to Revise the 1995 Guidelines for the Evaluation and Management of Heart Failure); International Society for Heart and Lung Transplantation; Heart Failure Society of America. ACC/AHA guidelines for the evaluation and management of chronic heart failure in the adult: executive summary, a report of the American College of Cardiology/American Heart Association Task Force on Practice Guidelines (Committee to Revise the 1995 Guidelines for the Evaluation and Management of Heart Failure): developed in collaboration with the International Society for Heart and Lung Transplantation; endorsed by the Heart Failure Society of America. *Circulation* 2001;104:2996–3007.

Kaul TK, Agnihotri AK, Fields BL, et al. Coronary bypass grafting in patients with an ejection fraction of twenty percent or less. *J Thorac Cardiovasc Surg* 1996;111:1001.

Kirklin JK, Holman WL. Mechanical circulatory support therapy as a bridge to transplant or recovery (new advances). *Curr Opin Cardiol* 2006;21:120–126.

Klotz et al. New LVAD technology and impact on outcome. *Ann Thorac Surg* 2006;82:1774–1778.

Konertz W, Dushe S, Hotz H, et al. Safety and feasibility of a cardiac support device. *J Card Surg* 2001;16:113–117.

Lee MS, Makkar RR. Percutaneous left ventricular support devices. *Cardiol Clin* 2006;24:265–275.
Long JW, Kfoury AG, Slaughter MS, et al. Long-term destination therapy with the HeartMate XVE left ventricular assist device: improved outcomes since the REMATCH study. *Congest Heart Fail* 2005;11:133–138.
McCarthy PM, Starling RC, Wong J, et al. Early results with partial left ventriculectomy. *J Thorac Cardiovasc Surg* 1997;114:755–765.
McCarthy PM, Takagaki M, Ochiai Y, et al. Device-based change in left ventricular shape: a new concept for the treatment of dilated cardiomyopathy. *J Thorac Cardiovasc Surg* 2001;122:482–490.
Pagely PR, Beller GA, Watson DD, et al. Improved outcome after coronary bypass surgery in patients with ischemic cardiomyopathy and residual myocardial viability. *Circulation* 1997;96:793–800.
Rose EA, Gelijns AC, Moskowitz AJ, et al. Long-term use of a left ventricular assist device for end-stage heart failure. *N Engl J Med* 2001;345:1435–1443.
Samady H, Elefteriades JA, Abbott BG, et al. Failure to improve left ventricular function after coronary revascularization for ischemic cardiomyopathy is not associated with worse outcome. *Circulation* 1999;100:1298–1304.
Schenk S, Reichenspurner H, Groezner JG, et al. Myosplint implantation and ventricular shape change in patients with dilated cardiomyopathy—first clinical experience. *J Heart Lung Transplant* 2001;20:217.

Suggested readings

Kirklin JK, McGriffin D, Young JB. *Heart transplantation*. New York: Churchill Livingstone, 2002.
Kumpati GS, McCarthy PM, Hoercher KJ. Surgical treatments for heart failure. *Cardiol Clin* 2001;4:669–681.
Young JB, Mills RM. *Clinical management of heart failure*. Caddo, Oklahoma: Professional Communications, 2001.

12 CARDIAC TRANSPLANTATION

Zuheir Abrahams, Wilfried Mullens, and Andrew Boyle

I. INTRODUCTION. Cardiac transplantation is now a well-established therapeutic option for a select group of patients with end-stage heart disease. It offers these patients, who have no other alternatives, a chance for extended survival and improved quality of life. Cardiac transplantation, however, should not be perceived as a curative procedure. Although the patient's primary problem of heart failure is alleviated by a successful transplantation, a new set of potential long-term complications arises primarily owing to the secondary effects of chronic immunosuppression.

In the United States, the United Network for Organ Sharing (UNOS) reports a 10% reduction in cardiac transplantations over the same time period. UNOS is a national organization which, along with local organ-procurement agencies, maintains organ transplantation waiting lists, initiates the evaluation of potential organ donors, allocates organs when a donor is identified, and compiles statistics annually on all aspects of the transplantation process, including survival. Based on data from other registries, it is estimated that >4000 cardiac transplantations are performed each year worldwide. Since 1990, the number of patients listed and waiting for a cardiac transplant in the United States has more than doubled. There is a shortage of donors, and each year 1.5 to 3 times as many patients are listed for cardiac transplantation as there are donors, so this problem is only going to escalate as the population gets older unless there is a significant increase in organ donation. The annual mortality rate while on the waiting list in 2001 was 15%, which has declined continually over the last decade, probably because of improved medical therapy for end-stage congestive heart failure and increased use of implantable cardioverter–defibrillator. As the annual number of cardiac transplantations has declined, wait times have continued to lengthen. The national median waiting time by UNOS status at listing from 2003–2004 data is as follows: 49 days for status 1A, 77 days for status 1B, and 308 days for status 2 patients. However, this can be misleading, as patients with different blood types such as blood type O, wait significantly longer than other blood types such as blood type AB on average. A blood type O status 2 patient could easily wait for >2 years for a cardiac transplantation.

The primary indication for adult cardiac transplantation over the last 5 years is fairly equally split between ischemic cardiomyopathies (42%) and nonischemic cardiomyopathies (46%) with valvular heart disease (3%), adult congenital disease (2%), re-transplantation (2%), and miscellaneous causes (5%) accounting for the rest (1). The average cardiac transplant recipient is a white (81.8%) male (77%) with an average age of 51, which reflects the demographics of the patients on the waiting list. The average donor age is 33 years, and donors >50 years of age, which were rarely reported before 1986, now account for >12% of all donors. Transplantation outcomes continue to improve despite transplanting older, sicker patients. Recent data show that 44% of recipients were on intravenous inotropic support compared to 34%, 5 years ago. Mechanical circulatory support is also more common, with 30% of patients on some form of mechanical circulatory support at time of transplantation, including 23% with a left ventricular assist device (LVAD), compared to only 15% on mechanical circulatory support (11% with an LVAD) 5 years ago (1). National survival rates post-cardiac transplantation by UNOS status at time of transplantation from 2004 data is as follows: status 1A (85.7% at 1 year, 75.2% at 3 years, and 68.8% at 5 years), status 1B (87.3% at 1 year, 80.3% at 3 years, and 72.7% at 5 years), and status 2 (90.6% at 1 year, 81.8% at 2 years, and 74% at 5 years).

Because of the scarcity of donor organs and growing transplant waiting lists, it is crucial that cardiac transplantation programs adequately screen and properly select potential transplant recipients. Effective use of this limited resource is essential to avoid "wasting" organs that become available on suboptimal recipients.

II. INDICATIONS FOR CARDIAC TRANSPLANTATION

A. Patients should be on optimal medical therapy for congestive heart failure, as recommended by the American College of Cardiology/American Heart Association guidelines, including an angiotensin-converting enzyme (ACE) inhibitor, digoxin, a diuretic, a β-blocker, and spironolactone. If a patient is intolerant to an ACE inhibitor, she or he should be on an angiotensin-receptor blocker (ARB).

B. Medically reversible causes of decompensated congestive heart failure should be excluded, including hypothyroidism, tachycardia-mediated cardiomyopathy, alcohol abuse, obstructive sleep apnea, hypertension, and medical noncompliance.

C. Surgically reversible causes of decompensated congestive heart failure should be excluded, including valvular heart disease, unrevascularized coronary artery disease with large territories of ischemia or viability, hypertrophic obstructive cardiomyopathy, and LV aneurysm for which resection would improve overall cardiac hemodynamics.

D. Patients should be too ill or not candidates for cardiac resynchronization therapy. Alternatively, cardiac resynchronization therapy might have failed to improve symptoms or to halt progression of the underlying pathology.

E. If the previous criteria are met, indications for a cardiac transplantation evaluation are as follows:

1. Cardiogenic shock requiring mechanical support (i.e., LVAD or intraaortic balloon pump counterpulsation)
2. Cardiogenic shock requiring continuous intravenous inotropic therapy for hemodynamic stabilization
3. New York Heart Association (NYHA) class III or IV congestive heart failure symptoms, particularly if progressively worsening
4. Recurrent life-threatening LV arrhythmias despite an implantable cardiac defibrillator, antiarrhythmic drug therapy (usually amiodarone), or attempted catheter-based ablation, if appropriate
5. End-stage complex congenital heart disease without pulmonary hypertension
6. Refractory angina without potential medical or surgical therapeutic options

III. COMPONENTS OF A CARDIAC TRANSPLANTATION EVALUATION AND CONTRAINDICATIONS.

The purpose of a cardiac transplant evaluation is to exclude patients with medical and psychosocial comorbidities and to quantify the severity of a patient's cardiac functional impairment. Recommended investigations prior to

TABLE 12.1 Recommended Evaluation Prior to Transplantation

Complete history and physical examination
Laboratory investigations:
- Complete blood count (CBC) with differential, complete metabolic panel
- Thyroid function studies (thyroid-stimulating hormone, TSH)
- Liver function panel, creatinine clearance
- Lipid profile, hemoglobin A1c, urinalysis

Immunologic data:
- Blood type and antibody screen
- Human leukocyte antigen (HLA) typing
- Panel of reactive antibodies (PRAs) screen

Serology for infectious diseases:
- Hepatitis HBsAg, HBsAb, HBcAb, HepCAb
- Herpes group virus
- Human immunodeficiency virus
- Cytomegalovirus (CMV) IgG antibody
- Toxoplasmosis
- Varicella and rubella titers
- Ebstein-Barr virus IgG and IgM antibodies
- Venereal Disease Research Laboratory (VDRL) or Rapid Plasma Reagin (RPR)

Cardiovascular investigations:
- Electrocardiogram (ECG), chest x-ray, echocardiogram
- Exercise test with oxygen consumption
- Right- and left-heart catheterization
- Myocardial biopsy (if indicated, for example to rule out infiltrative process such as amyloidosis)

Vascular assessment:
- Carotid Dopplers
- Peripheral vascular assessment (ankle-brachial index and/or duplex ultrasound)
- Abdominal ultrasound
- Ophthalmology examination (if indicated, for example to rule out diabetic retinopathy)

Cancer screening:
- Prostate-specific antigen (PSA) (in men if indicated)
- Papanicolaou smear (PAP smear), mammography (in women if indicated)
- Colonoscopy (if indicated)

Psychosocial evaluation:
- Support system
- Substance abuse history (alcohol, tobacco, and drug use)
- Psychiatric history

Baseline investigations:
- Dental examination
- Bone density scan
- Pulmonary function tests

transplantation are summarized in Table 12.1 and exclusion criteria for cardiac transplantation are summarized in Table 12.2.

A. Blood work. Standard blood work includes a complete blood cell count; a complete metabolic panel, including hepatic enzymes and thyroid function tests; and blood typing and antibody screening. A serologic assessment should also be performed to determine a potential recipient's presensitization to cytomegalovirus (CMV), toxoplasmosis, hepatitis B and C viruses, and human immunodeficiency virus (HIV).

1. Patients who are anemic should have a thorough evaluation, including iron studies and a colon examination. Esophagogastroduodenoscopy and a hematologic evaluation, including a bone marrow biopsy, may also be necessary. Some

TABLE 12.2 Exclusion Criteria for Cardiac Transplantation

Irreversible pulmonary parenchymal disease
Renal dysfunction with Cr >2.0–2.5 or CrCl <30–50 mL/min (unless for combined heart-kidney transplant)
Irreversible hepatic dysfunction (unless for combined heart–liver transplant)
Severe peripheral and cerebrovascular obstructive disease
Insulin-dependent diabetes with end-organ damage
Acute pulmonary embolism
Irreversible pulmonary hypertension (PVR >4.0 Wood units after vasodilators)
Psychosocial instability or substance abuse
History of malignancy with probability of recurrence
Advanced age (>70 years)
Severe obesity
Active infection
Severe osteoporosis

patients may benefit from erythropoietin treatment to increase red blood cell counts without the need for transfusions that may expose the patient to further antigens.

2. Patients found to have an elevated serum creatinine level should have further evaluation to determine its relationship to low renal perfusion. A normal urinalysis result suggests the absence of renal parenchymal disease. This should include an assessment of cardiac hemodynamics and a renal ultrasound to assess renal parenchymal size and the presence of two kidneys without evidence of obstruction.
3. Patients found to have elevated hepatic enzymes should have further evaluation to determine right-sided filling pressures, and they should have a hepatic ultrasound scan. All patients should have their hepatitis B and C virus serologies assessed.
4. The patient's serum should be screened for antibodies against HLA antigens for B and T lymphocytes, drawn from community volunteers representative of the major HLA allotypes. These antibodies are collectively referred to as panel-reactive antibodies (PRAs) and are often elevated in multiparous women and patients with multiple transfusions (often perioperatively in the past). Elevated PRA levels (>10%) necessitate a pretransplantation donor HLA crossmatch and increase the likelihood of it being positive, making waiting times longer and transplantation more difficult. If a patient has elevated PRA levels, an attempt to reduce them before transplantation with intravenous immunoglobulin, plasmapheresis, mycophenolate mofetil (MMF), or cyclophosphamide, alone or in combination, may be considered. Traditionally, each potential recipient would have a thorough HLA tissue-typing analysis, including a cytotoxicity assay for assistance in matching donor hearts. In this assay, random donor lymphocytes are incubated with recipient sera. Complement-dependent antibody-mediated cytolysis identifies potential donor-specific antibodies present in that recipient. Currently, most programs use flow cytometry to assess preformed antibodies rather than cytotoxic assays. This allows for detection of weaker interactions and provides a wider more efficient screening process.

B. Imaging

1. All patients should have coronary angiography or a functional assessment for ischemia and viability. If ischemia or viability can be demonstrated, consideration should be given to percutaneous or surgical revascularization.
2. Bilateral carotid ultrasound scans should be performed in patients with risk factors for atherosclerosis. Select patients with carotid stenoses who would otherwise be cardiac transplantation candidates may undergo pretransplantation percutaneous or surgical intervention, thereby eliminating this contraindication.

3. Occasionally an abdominal aortic ultrasound is obtained to rule out an aneurysm, particularly in patients being considered for mechanical support.

C. Functional assessment

1. Metabolic stress testing is performed to assess the severity of cardiac functional impairment. Patients with compensated congestive heart failure and a peak oxygen consumption of <14 mL/kg per minute or <50% predicted are considered sufficiently impaired for transplantation (2). Adequate patient effort during the stress test can be assessed by the respiratory exchange ratio, which should be >1.1, indicating the onset of anaerobic metabolism.
2. Generally, a right-heart catheterization is performed to assess cardiac hemodynamics and for optimization of a patient's medical therapy. Fixed, severe pulmonary hypertension, defined as a pulmonary vascular resistance (PVR) greater than 4 Woods units, is a contraindication to cardiac transplantation. In this setting, the donor right ventricle will likely immediately fail after implantation because it is not accustomed to high pulmonary pressures. An attempt should be made to medically decrease the pulmonary hypertension with inotropic agents, nitrates, or nitroprusside. Sometimes an LVAD is required to decompress the left ventricle sufficiently to reverse the pulmonary hypertension. Rarely, endomyocardial biopsy is performed, except when an infiltrative cardiomyopathy is suspected.
3. Pulmonary function tests are performed to exclude patients with significant chronic obstructive or restrictive pulmonary disease.
4. Peripheral vascular studies may be obtained to exclude patients with significant peripheral arteriosclerosis obliterans.

D. Comorbidities and implications for heart transplant listing. Advanced age, cancer, and obesity are three common comorbidities, which remain somewhat controversial with respect to their impact on whether an individual program will list a patient for heart transplantation.

1. **Age** criteria for eligibility were initially quite rigorous; however, it has become apparent that chronologic and physiologic age are often discrepant. Most centers do not have a fixed upper age limit, but generally patients >65 years of age are very carefully screened for lack of comorbidities. The International Society of Heart and Lung Transplantation (ISHLT) recommends considering patients for cardiac transplantation if they are ≤70 years of age (3). Patients >age 70 may be considered for cardiac transplantation at the discretion of the transplant program and should theoretically be in excellent health other than heart disease. An alternate-type of program for these patients has been proposed whereby older donor hearts would be utilized in this population (3).
2. Active **malignancy** other than skin cancer is an absolute contraindication to cardiac transplantation due to limited survival rates. Chronic immunosuppression is associated with a higher than average incidence of malignancy and is associated with increased recurrence of prior malignancy. Patients with cancers that have been in remission for ≥5 years and patients with low-grade cancers such as prostate cancer are generally accepted for transplant evaluation. Preexisting malignancies are heterogeneous in nature and some are readily treatable with chemotherapy, thus an individualized approach to these patients is required, and consultation with an oncologist regarding prognosis is often very helpful.
3. Traditionally, centers have been cautious when considering **obese** patients for transplantation. Most currently available data indicate that patients with a pretransplant body mass index (BMI) >30 kg/m^2 have poor outomes following cardiac transplantation, with increased rates of infection and higher mortality rates. However, this area remains controversial and some recent data presented in abstract form only demonstrate no significant mortality differences between obese (BMI, 30–34.99) transplant recipients and overweight (BMI, 25–29.99) transplant recipients. Despite this controversy, the current ISHLT recommmendations are that patients achieve a BMI <30 kg/m^2 or a percent ideal body weight <140% prior to being listed for cardiac transplantation (3). This cut-off

will vary from center to center, but generally a BMI >35 kg/ m^2 will preclude listing for cardiac transplantation.

E. Consultations

1. A **psychosocial assessment** is a crucial component of every cardiac transplantation evaluation. Accepted psychosocial contraindications for cardiac transplantations include active smoking; active substance abuse, including alcohol; medical noncompliance; and significant untreated psychological or psychiatric diagnoses. Relative psychosocial contraindications to cardiac transplantation include posttraumatic stress disorder and lack of an adequate support structure.
2. For diabetic patients, an ophthalmology consultation is obtained for an assessment of retinal end-organ damage related to the diabetes.

IV. UNOS AND THE RECIPIENT LIST. After a patient is accepted as a potential cardiac transplant recipient by a UNOS-certified transplant program, the patient's name is entered on a national list compiled by UNOS. The patient is given a status level based on predefined clinical criteria (Table 12.3), which can be adjusted as any patient's clinical situation evolves. A patient's priority on the UNOS list depends on his or her status level and the duration of time on the list. Highest priority is given to patients with status 1A and who have been waiting the longest. A critical patient initially listed as 1A immediately has a higher priority than a patient with a status 1B, regardless of the duration of time spent as status 1B. Whether a patient is hospitalized does not affect priority on the list, other than the fact that hospitalized patients are more likely to be receiving hemodynamic support (mechanical or inotropic) and have a higher status level. A hospitalized patient on continuous inotropic therapy has the same status as a similar patient on home continuous inotropic therapy. Patients on home continuous inotropic therapy awaiting cardiac transplantation are generally thought to have an increased mortality related to the proarrhythmic effect of inotropic therapy, and most

TABLE 12.3 Description of Status Levels in the United Network of Organ Sharing List

Status	Description
1A	Must be an inpatient
	Life expectancy <7 days
	LVAD and/or RVAD (maximum 30 days)
	VAD-related thromboembolism
	VAD-related infection (including the pocket and the driveline)
	Mechanical failure of VAD
	Total Artificial Heart (TAH)
	Extracorporeal membrane oxygenation (ECMO)
	Intraaortic balloon pump (IABP) with inotropic criteria
	Life-threatening refractory arrhythmias with or without a VAD
	Mechanical ventilation
	High-dose single intravenous inotrope (see doses below), or multiple intravenous inotropes, in addition to Swan-Ganz catheter
1B	Inotrope-dependent
	VAD not meeting criteria for IA status
2	Not inotrope-dependent
7	Inactive on list because of improved clinical status or short term contraindications to cardiac transplantation (e.g., active infection)
Inotrope criteria for status 1a	
1.	Two or more inotropes, regardless of dose
2.	Intravenous milrinone, at least 0.5 μg/kg/min by continuous infusion
3.	Intravenous dobutamine, at least 7.5 μg/kg/min by continuous infusion

LVAD, left-ventricular assist device; RVAD, right-ventricular assist device; VAD, ventricular assist device programs require implantation of an intracardiac defibrillator as a prerequisite for discharge.

V. WORKUP OF A POTENTIAL CARDIAC DONOR. Potential cardiac organ donors are patients who are declared brain dead but otherwise have viable internal organs. Generally, these are patients with lethal head injuries or catastrophic central nervous system events (i.e., intracranial hemorrhage, stroke, or cerebral anoxia).

A. Declaration of brain death. A neurologist or neurosurgeon usually declares the brain death of a potential organ donor. Usually, this declaration is made after a period of observation (about 12 hours) during which no neurologic improvement is seen. Physicians involved in the care of potential transplant recipients are not involved in this decision to avoid conflicts of interest. Criteria for the determination of brain death are very specific. Absence of any one of these criteria makes the patient ineligible for organ donation.

1. A known cause of death
2. Absence of hypotension, hypothermia, hypoxemia, and metabolic perturbations
3. Absence of medical or recreational drugs known to depress the central nervous system
4. Absence of cerebral cortical function
5. No response to painful stimuli
6. Absence of brainstem reflexes
   - **a.** Pupillary constriction to light
   - **b.** Corneal reflex
   - **c.** Vestibular ocular reflexes (i.e., doll's eyes or cold caloric testing)
   - **d.** Gag reflex
   - **e.** Cough reflex
7. Positive apnea test: no spontaneous respiration despite arterial PCO_2 greater than 60 mm Hg at least 10 minutes after disconnection from the ventilator.
8. An electroencephalogram (EEG) is *not* required but may be performed at the discretion of the examining physician. The EEG should demonstrate electrical silence.

B. Potential donor screening. After a patient is declared brain dead, a local organ procurement organization (OPO), under the auspices of UNOS, performs the initial evaluation of a potential donor. This evaluation includes a thorough patient and family history, focusing specifically on cardiac risk factors and potentially transmittable diseases (i.e., malignancy and infection). Preliminary blood tests are done, including determinations of cardiac enzymes; serologies for hepatitis B and C viruses, HIV, toxoplasmosis, and CMV; ABO blood group typing; and HLA antigen typing. An echocardiogram is routinely performed to assess cardiac function and to rule out congenital anomalies and valvular disease. At the request of the potential recipient's physician, a coronary angiogram may be obtained if a donor has significant cardiac risk factors, positive cardiac enzymes, or is relatively advanced in age. Cardiac donor selection criteria are summarized in Table 12.4.

If the potential recipient also has elevated **PRA levels**, a prospective complement-dependent antibody-mediated lymphocytotoxic crossmatch is usually performed, in which the recipient's serum is incubated with donor lymphocytes to identify potential donor-recipient HLA incompatibility. Many centers today perform a "virtual crossmatch" for patients with elevated PRA levels to improve donor availability. With the HLA technologies available today, the exact antigen specificity of the recipients anti-HLA antibodies are known. If the HLA-tissue typing of the potential donor does not include the antigens against which the recipient is sensitized, it is assumed that the actual crossmatch will be negative (i.e.. a "virtual" negative crossmatch). If a prospective crossmatch is not performed, a retrospective crossmatch (by lymphocytotoxic assay or by flow cytometry) is performed using donor lymphocytes obtained from donor aortic lymph nodes retrieved at the time of harvest.

C. Donor-recipient matching. UNOS maintains a computerized list of all patients listed and waiting for cardiac transplantation. A list of potential recipients with compatible blood types is generated for each potential donor organ and is made

TABLE 12.4 Cardiac Donor Selection Criteria
Must meet legal requirements for brain death
No history of chest trauma or cardiac disease
No prolonged hypotension or hypoxemia
Normal electrocardiogram (ECG)
Normal ECG
Normal cardiac angiogram, performed if indicated by donor age (male >45 years or female >50 years) and history
Negative HBsAg, hepatitis C virus (HCV), and human immunodeficiency virus (HIV) serologies
Systolic blood pressure >100 mm Hg or mean arterial pressure (MAP) >60 mm Hg
Central venous pressure (CVP) 8–12 mm Hg
Inotropic support < 10 μg/kg/min dopamine or dobutamine
Age <55 years preferred

available to the OPO. Priority on this list is given to local patients (defined as within the OPO's territory) with the highest status level who have been waiting the longest. Recent changes to the UNOS donor net criteria mean a local status 2 patient is no longer higher on the list than a status 1A patient from outside the OPO's territory.

Transplantation physicians for the potential recipient may also reject a potential organ because of a positive prospective crossmatch, donor-recipient size mismatch, or a prolonged projected ischemia time (usually related to long travel distances). Matching donor and recipient size is important, because an oversized donor organ may not allow closure of the chest without compression of the organ, and an undersized donor organ may not be able to pump a sufficient quantity of blood. Current guidelines suggest that the recipient's weight should range between 70% and 130% of a potential donor's weight.

VI. SURGICAL ISSUES RELATED TO CARDIAC TRANSPLANTATION. Most surgical issues related to cardiac transplantation are beyond the scope of this chapter and are mainly of interest to the cardiac surgeon. The main surgical issue of interest to the transplantation cardiologist is related to the anastomosis of the right atrium. The surgeon may suture the donor atrium to the recipient atrium (i.e., biatrial anastomosis) or suture the donor superior vena cava to the recipient superior vena cava and the donor inferior vena cava to the recipient inferior vena cava (i.e., bicaval anastomosis). The bicaval anastomosis approach is more time consuming but reduces the incidence of atrial arrhythmias (including sinus node dysfunction), reduces the incidence of posttransplantation tricuspid regurgitation, and improves right atrial hemodynamics. The bicaval anastomosis approach does, however, provide some potential difficulties to the cardiologist trying to perform surveillance endomyocardial biopsies because these anastomoses have a tendency to scar and narrow the central lumen over time. Currently, most centers employ the bicaval anastomosis approach, although no survival advantage has been conclusively demonstrated with the bicaval anastomosis approach.

VII. POSTOPERATIVE COMPLICATIONS AFTER CARDIAC TRANSPLANTATION

A. Surgical complications. The most common surgical complication is the development of a pericardial effusion with or without tamponade. Pericardial effusions are very common because of the large potential space left behind as the dilated and dysfunctional recipient left ventricle is replaced with a more appropriately sized donor left ventricle. Rarely, pericardial tamponade develops, necessitating percutaneous or surgical evacuation of the pericardium. Other surgical complications are much less common but can be catastrophic and usually result from a problem either at a site of anastomosis or cannulation.

B. Early graft dysfunction

1. Left ventricular systolic dysfunction. It is common for transplant recipients to require inotropic support as they come off cardiopulmonary bypass. The most commonly used inotropic agents in this setting are dobutamine, milrinone, and isoproterenol, used alone or in combination. It is also common for transplant recipients to require peripheral vasoconstrictors such as epinephrine, norepinephrine, and dopamine in the early postoperative period, because most are on large quantities of oral or intravenous vasodilators before transplantation. Most patients can be weaned from inotropic therapy and peripheral vasoconstrictors within the first 48 hours.

2. **Left ventricular diastolic dysfunction** is very common soon after cardiac transplantation. It usually results from reversible ischemia or reperfusion injury to the donor organ and usually resolves over a period of days to weeks. If the ischemia or reperfusion injury is sufficiently severe to induce significant contraction band necrosis or myocardial fibrosis, as seen on endomyocardial biopsy, chronic diastolic dysfunction can ensue. Another potential cause of diastolic dysfunction is donor–recipient mismatch, particularly with a small donor organ or acute rejection.
3. **Right ventricular dysfunction** is much more common than LV dysfunction after cardiac transplantation, especially in patients with preexisting pulmonary hypertension. The right ventricle is subjected to similar ischemic or reperfusion injury risks as the left ventricle. Right ventricular dysfunction is usually accompanied by right ventricular dilation and the failure of coaptation of the tricuspid valve leaflets, leading to severe tricuspid regurgitation. The treatment for perioperative right ventricular dysfunction is usually intravenous milrinone and nitrates to increase cardiac output and lower the PVR. In patients with refractory pulmonary hypertension, other agents to be considered include nitroprusside, nesiritide, isoproterenol, or rarely, inhaled nitric oxide. Usually, the pulmonary hypertension and right ventricular dysfunction improve over a period of days to weeks.

C. Cardiac arrhythmias. Most transplant recipients require perioperative temporary atrioventricular pacing. Sinus node dysfunction is very common, probably because of a combination of surgical trauma, ischemia or reperfusion injury, and denervation. The incidence of sinus node dysfunction is believed to be reduced by the bicaval anastomosis technique compared with the biatrial anastomosis technique. With time, the sinus node usually recovers, and a permanent pacemaker is unnecessary. Preoperative use of amiodarone increases the likelihood of bradycardia after transplantation. Other cardiac arrhythmias are rare, especially off inotropic therapy, and may signify acute rejection.

D. Renal dysfunction. Preoperatively, many transplant recipients have some degree of impaired renal function. There is a risk of worsening renal function perioperatively. This risk is compounded by the fact that the major immunosuppressive agents (i.e., cyclosporine and tacrolimus) are nephrotoxic. If renal function does worsen postoperatively, induction therapy is begun to delay initiation of cyclosporine or tacrolimus. Most centers no longer use OKT3 for induction therapy, but rather use interleukin-2 (IL-2) receptor blockers or thymoglobulin for induction therapy.

VIII. SYSTEMIC IMMUNOSUPPRESSION. Immunosuppressant protocols during and after cardiac transplantation vary greatly from program to program, and even from patient to patient within a program. Triple-therapy, which constitutes the cornerstone of modern immunosuppressive regimens in cardiac transplantation, includes a calcineurin inhibitor (such as cyclosporine or tacrolimus), an antiproliferative agent (such as MMF or azathioprine), and a corticosteroid. Controversy remains about the advisability of using cytolytic or induction therapy in the non-presensitized recipient without renal failure (Table 12.5).

A. Steroids. The mechanism by which steroids serve as immunosuppressants is complex and incompletely understood. Steroids bind to nuclear receptors, thereby preventing gene expression of various cytokines important for B- and T-cell activation and proliferation, the most important of which is IL-2. Steroids also have important anti-inflammatory properties and suppress macrophage activity. Important side effects from steroids include diabetes, hypertension, weight gain, osteoporosis, and avascular necrosis of the femoral head.

TABLE 12.5 Common Immunosuppressants

	Steroids	Calcineurin inhibitors	MMF	Azathioprine	TOR inhibitors	OKT3	Polyclonal antilymphocyte antibodies	IL-2 receptor blockers
Drugs	Prednisone (P) (PO) Solu-Medrol (S) (IV)	Neoral (N) Tacrolimus (T)			Rapamycin (R) Everolimus (E)		Atgam (A) Thymoglobulin (T)	Basiliximab (B) Daclizumab (T)
Indication	Chronic IM, acute rejection	Chronic IM	Chronic IM, skin cancer with AZA	Chronic IM	Chronic IM, vasculopathy	Induction, acute rejection	Induction, acute rejection	Induction
Dosing								
Initial	IV 125–150 mg q8h	N: 100 mg bid T: 2 mg bid	1.5 g bid	1–2 mg/kg/d	R: 2–5 mg qd E: 1.5–3 mg qd	—	—	—
Induction	—	—	—	—	—	5 mg qd × 5–15 days	A: 15 mg/kg/d T: 1.5 mg/kg/d 5–15 days	B: 20 mg days 1 and 4 D: 1 mg/kg q1–2 wk × 5 doses
Maintenance	Weaned off	Adjusted to levels	1.5 g bid	1–2 mg/kg/d	Adjusted to levels	—	—	—
Acute rejection	P: 100 mg qd × 3 S: 1g IV qd × 3	Consider change from CsA to tacrolimus	—	—	—	As above	As above	—

Target levels	—	See Tables 12.3 and 12.4	2–4 ng/mL, 12-hr trough, WBC > 4.0	WBC >3.0	R: 4–12 ng/mL 18-hr trough	CD3 count <20 cells/ mL	CD3 count <20 cells/ mL	—
Common side effects	Diabetes, osteoporosis, weight gain, hypertension, adrenal insufficiency	Nephrotoxicity, hypertension, tremors, gingival hyperplasia	Diarrhea, nausea, myelosuppression	Myelo-suppression skin cancer	Hypertriglyc-eridemia, thrombocytopenia.	Cytokine release, hypotension, capillary leak syndrome, PTLD, CMV superinfection	Thrombocytopenia fevers, chills, PTLD, CMV superinfection	—
Common drug interac-tions	—	Erythromycin, diltiazem, verapamil, rapamycin, anticonvulsants, rifampin, statins	Cholestyramine, probenecid	Allopurinol	Cyclosporine	—	—	—

AZA, Azathioprine; CMV, cytomegalovirus; CsA, cyclosporin A; IL, interleukin; IM, immunosuppression; MMF, mycophenolate mofetil; PTLD, posttransplantation lymphoproliferative disorder; TOR, target of rapamycin.

Steroid-dosing protocols vary tremendously from one institution to another. A dose of 500 to 1000 mg of intravenous Solu-Medrol is usually given before being brought to the operating room, and then 125 to 150 mg is usually repeated every 8 hours, for a total of three more doses. At that point, if the patient is extubated, oral prednisone is begun. Some centers start at a divided dose of 1 mg/kg/day and wean by 5 mg daily, whereas others start immediately at only 20 mg daily. The dose of steroid is slowly tapered, provided the patient continues to have a clean biopsy record. The trend in clinical practice is to wean most patients completely from steroids. Some centers continue to advocate the indefinite use of low-dose prednisone (2.5 to 5 mg daily). If a decision is made to withdraw steroids completely, it should be done approximately 1 month before the next scheduled biopsy to ensure continued lack of acute cellular rejection.

Steroids are also given in "pulses" to treat episodes of acute cellular rejection. If a patient has acute cellular rejection associated with hemodynamic compromise, she or he is admitted for 1 g of intravenous Solu-Medrol daily for 3 days, and may be given cytolytic therapy or plasmapheresis, or both. If no hemodynamic compromise is associated with the episode of rejection, 100 mg of oral prednisone daily for 3 days is usually sufficient, followed by repeat biopsy, at most 2 weeks later to ensure resolution.

B. Calcineurin inhibitors. Calcineurin is a phosphatase enzyme that triggers transcription of new messenger RNA after activation of the T-cell receptor by an appropriate antigen, leading to increased gene expression of IL-2 and other important cytokines. Calcineurin antagonists inhibit this phosphatase activity, thereby preventing synthesis of these cytokines, which prevents B- and T-cell proliferation.

1. **Cyclosporine (Neoral, Gengraf, Sandimmune)** is a calcineurin antagonist with a highly variable pattern of bioavailability, depending on the oral formulation taken. Bioavailability of the original soft gelatin capsule (Sandimmune) was low and depended on emulsification by bile salts. The newer microemulsion formulation (Neoral) does not depend on bile salts for emulsification and has a more consistent bioavailability. Nevertheless, there remain tremendous interpatient differences in bioavailability, and dosing of Neoral is based primarily on serum drug trough levels. Because of the narrow therapeutic range of cyclosporine, drug trough levels are also important to prevent toxicity. Nephrotoxicity is the most important side effect from cyclosporine therapy and is related to renal afferent arteriolar vasoconstriction and the resultant reduced renal perfusion. Other side effects include systemic hypertension, gingival hyperplasia, and tremors. Calcium channel blockers, particularly diltiazem, reduce hepatic metabolism of cyclosporine, thereby increasing serum drug levels. This drug interaction is frequently used clinically to reduce the oral dose of cyclosporine required to achieve a given serum drug concentration, thereby minimizing the cost of immunosuppression.

   Postoperatively, once the patient is hemodynamically stable with good urine output, cyclosporine is initiated via continuous infusion at 1 mg/hour. After the patient is able to take oral medicines, Neoral is begun at a dose of 100 mg twice daily, with adjustments in the dose based on serum trough levels (Table 12.6). The dose of Neoral is gradually reduced over a period of 1 year if the patient has a clean biopsy record.

TABLE 12.6 Target Serum Cyclosporin a Levels

Time	Target level (12-hour trough)
0–3 mo	250–350 ng/mL
3–12 mo	200–250 ng/mL
>12 mo	150–175 ng/mL

TABLE 12.7 Target Serum Tacrolimus (FK506) Levels

Time	Target level (12-hour trough)
0–30 d	12–20 ng/mL
1–6 mo	8–15 ng/mL
6–18 mo	5–15 ng/mL
>18 mo	5–10 ng/mL

2. Tacrolimus (Prograf), previously known as FK506, is another calcineurin inhibitor that has low oral bioavailability. Tacrolimus has never been prospectively shown to be superior to cyclosporine in the prevention of acute cellular rejection. However, it has become standard practice to change the cyclosporine in a patient's immunosuppressive regimen to tacrolimus in the setting of recurrent or persistent acute cellular rejection with adequate cyclosporine levels. Some programs empirically use tacrolimus for all female patients because a common side effect of cyclosporine is hirsutism. The major side effects of tacrolimus are nephrotoxicity and neurotoxicity (most commonly tremor).

Like cyclosporine, tacrolimus is initiated postoperatively once the patient is hemodynamically and renally stable. The dose of tacrolimus is 0.01 mg/kg per day administed by continuous infusion. Unfortunately, intravenous tacrolimus is seemingly more nephrotoxic than cyclosporine. Tacrolimus can be given sublingually using a 1:1 oral-to-sublingual dose ratio. After the patient is taking oral medicines, the tacrolimus is changed to 0.5 to 2 mg twice daily, with dose adjustment based on serum FK506 levels (Table 12.7).

C. Mycophenolate mofetil (CellCept). MPA inhibits DNA synthesis by inhibiting *de novo* purine synthesis. Because human lymphocytes depend on the de novo synthesis of purines for DNA replication, MPA has the unique ability to inhibit B- and T-lymphocyte proliferation without affecting DNA synthesis in other cell lines, which can obtain purines through the parallel and unaffected purine salvage pathway. MMF has become the preferred immunosuppressant over azathioprine at most transplantation centers because of a reduced mortality rate at 1 year (6.2% vs. 11.4%; $p = 0.03$), especially among patients with treated biopsy-proven rejection and severe hemodynamic compromise (32% vs. 0%). Although there is a trend toward a reduced incidence of grade 3A (now 2R) rejection in MMF-treated compared with azathioprine-treated patients, it did not reach statistical significance (45% vs. 52.9%; $p = 0.055$). The main disadvantage of MMF over azathioprine is the increased cost (almost tenfold) and the potential increased risk of opportunistic viral infections. Toxicities of MMF include gastrointestinal symptoms (nausea, vomiting, and diarrhea) and myelosuppression. Some patients on MMF develop clinically significant leukopenia, necessitating dose reduction or discontinuation of the drug. The incidence of these adverse events is higher in patients receiving >3 g/day of MMF. Most symptoms will resolve with reduction of dose.

MMF is given intravenously or orally. Because of the high bioavailability (>90%), the initial dose of MMF is 1 g taken twice daily, regardless of the route of administration. The initial dose is given within the first 12 hours after transplantation. Few centers monitor serum levels of mycophenolic acid (MPA), the active metabolite of MMF. The serum levels of MPA are higher when MMF is adminstered with tacrolimus compared to cyclosporine; therefore, it may be advisable to empirically reduce the dosage of MMF when switching from cyclosporine to tacrolimus. Although there is no consensus on dose adjustment of MMF, at the Cleveland Clinic, the dose is adjusted to maintain MPA 12-hour trough concentrations in the the range of 2 to 4 μg/mL.

D. Azathioprine (Imuran) is a purine analog that impairs DNA synthesis, thereby preventing B- and T-lymphocyte proliferation in response to antigen stimulation.

Azathioprine has largely been replaced by MMF as the antiproliferative agent of choice in the triple immunosuppressant cocktails of today. Because there is no drug-level assay available, azathioprine dosing is usually fixed between 1 and 2 mg/kg per day. The major side effect of azathioprine is myelosuppression, and the dose of azathioprine is usually adjusted to maintain a white blood cell count of more >3000/mL. Azathioprine is metabolized by xanthine oxidase, and xanthine oxidase inhibitors such as allopurinol can lead to the accumulation of toxic levels of azathioprine and profound and prolonged myelosuppression.

E. Inhibitors of the target of rapamycin (TOR) enzyme: sirolimus (Rapamune) and everolimus (Certican previously known as RAD). Immunosuppressants have been developed that inhibit the enzyme TOR. TOR is activated after IL-2 stimulation of the T-cell IL-2 receptor, and is critical for lymphocyte growth and proliferation. In contrast to calcineurin inhibitors, inhibitors of TOR do not block cytokine production (e.g., IL-2) but rather block the cellular response to these cytokines. TOR inhibitors also inhibit vascular smooth muscle cell growth and proliferation in response to various growth factors. It is hoped that this property of TOR inhibitors will help reduce the rate of progression of chronic transplant coronary vasculopathy. Unlike calcineurin inhibitors, TOR inhibitors are not nephrotoxic. When used in combination with cyclosporine, TOR inhibitors appear to act synergistically with regard to immunosuppression. However, worsening of renal function is common but can be prevented by lowering the cyclosporine dose without worsening of immunosuppression. The main side effects of this class of compounds are significant hypertriglyceridemia and thrombocytopenia.

Sirolimus and everolimus are both TOR inhibitors. They are structurally similar, but everolimus has a much higher bioavailability than sirolimus. The appropriate dosing of these agents remains unclear, but for sirolimus, it is probably 1 to 5 mg/day, and for everolimus, it is probably 1.5 to 3 mg/day. Sirolimus appears to lower the incidence of acute cellular rejection in humans (4) and to slow the progression of transplant vasculopathy (5). Preliminary human studies using intravascular coronary ultrasonography have also shown a reduction in neointimal proliferation with both sirolimus and everolimus.

It remains unclear where TOR inhibitors will fit in with current immunosuppressive protocols. The most likely scenario is use in combination with a calcineurin inhibitor and prednisone, in place of MMF or azathioprine. Alternatively, they could be used in place of calcineurin inhibitors and in combination with MMF or azathioprine and prednisone, particularly in patients with either preexisting or worsening renal dysfunction.

F. Induction therapy and therapy for steroid-resistant acute rejection. The purpose of induction therapy is to deplete T lymphocytes or to prevent lymphocyte proliferation during the most immunoreactive phase, which occurs immediately after transplantation. Induction therapy has continued to be a subject of controversy in heart transplantation for more than 20 years. Induction therapy is not routinely used in posttransplantation patients because of a lack of evidence of improved survival or less acute rejection. The two clear indications to use induction therapy are: (1) in patients who have severe renal dysfunction, which precludes the introduction of calcineurin inhibitors within the first 2 days following transplantation; and (2) in patients who have acute graft failure secondary to an immune mechanism such as with hyperacute rejection or humoral rejection. The two scenarios in which induction therapy is often used are in patients with preexisting significant renal dysfunction and in significantly presensitized patients.

The principle behind the treatment for steroid-resistant acute rejection is similar, in that the depletion of activated T lymphocytes presumably prevents further clonal expansion of the antigen-activated offending lymphocyte population.

1. **OKT3** (Muromonab-CD3) is a murine-based monoclonal anti-CD3 antibody. The CD3 antigen is part of the T-cell receptor complex present on activated, circulating T lymphocytes. OKT3 binds to the CD3 antigen and produces cell death by multiple mechanisms or T-cell receptor internalization, thereby inactivating the lymphocyte.

The dose of OKT3 is 5 mg/day, for a total of 5 to 10 days. After a course of OKT3, there is an immediate and well-recognized rebound in CD3-positive (activated) T-lymphocyte counts that can lead to acute cellular or humoral rejection. Cytokine-release syndrome frequently occurs and typically begins 30 to 60 minutes after adminstration of a dose of OKT3 and may persist for several hours. Premedication with acetaminophen, steroids, and antihistamines may help to minimize symptoms. CD3+ T cells are generally undetectable during OKT3 therapy; however, within 12 to 24 hours after cessation of OKT3, CD3+ T cells reappear in circulation, unlike after treatment with anti-thymocyte globulin (ATG) preparations, with which the lymphocyte depletion is present for weeks. Therefore, many programs prophylactically increase the steroid dose during withdrawal from OKT3. Since OKT3 is a murine-based monoclonal antibody, patients may develop antibodies toward the mouse component of the antibody that may limit the effectiveness of future courses of OKT3. Patients treated with OKT3 have had an increased incidence of posttransplantation lymphoproliferative disorder (PTLD) and lymphoma with a cumulative dose >75 mg. Opportunistic viral infections are also more common after OKT3 therapy.

2. **Polyclonal anti-lymphocyte antibodies** are produced by injecting animals with human lymphocytes or thymocytes and then collecting the animal's serum. Two commercially available formulations are anti-thymocyte globulin (Atgam), which is horse based, and Thymoglobulin, which is rabbit based. The antibodies produced in this manner are directed against a variety of targets on the surface of B and T cells and induce complement-mediated lymphocytolysis. The recommended doses of Atgam and Thymoglobulin are 15 mg/kg per day and 1.5 mg/kg per day, respectively, for a total of 7 to 10 days. Adequate lymphocyte depletion can be ensured by quantifying the CD2-positive lymphocytes, a marker present on all lymphocytes. Similar to OKT3, immunity may develop to the animal component of these antibodies, rendering them ineffective if further courses of therapy are necessary. An increased incidence of PTLD, lymphoma, and opportunistic viral infections has also been observed. Patients receiving either formulation are often prophylactically treated with ganciclovir to prevent CMV infection.

3. **IL-2 receptor blockers** are competitive fully humanized monoclonal anti-CD25 antibodies. CD25 antigen is the IL-2 receptor and is only present on the cell surface of activated T lymphocytes. In contrast to OKT3, there is no initial receptor agonist phase and no cytokine release syndrome.

   For the two commercially available IL-2 receptor blockers, basiliximab (Simulect) and daclizumab (Zenapax), there are data to support the use of daclizumab only for induction therapy after cardiac transplantation, particularly in patients with preexisting renal dysfunction in whom calcineurin inhibitor avoidance is preferable in the early postoperative period. Fewer patients treated with daclizumab, in addition to standard triple immunosuppressant therapy, developed acute rejection compared with controls (6). Patients treated with daclizumab also had a lower severity and frequency of acute rejection during the first 3 months and had a longer time to the first episode of rejection. In contrast to other agents used for induction therapy, daclizumab does not appear to increase the risk of lymphoma, PTLD, or opportunistic viral infections. The serum half-life of daclizumab is 21 days, and dosing strategies call for a dose of 1 mg/kg every 1 to 2 weeks after transplantation, for a total of five doses (including the initial dose). There is no indication for either basiliximab or daclizumab as therapy for steroid-resistant persistent acute rejection. Given the virtual absence of side effects from IL-2 receptor blockade, the critical issue that will need to be addressed for these agents to become widely used clinically is whether the reduction in early acute rejection episodes translates into improved long-term survival and a reduction in transplant coronary vasculopathy.

IX. REJECTION

A. Endomyocardial biopsy and gene expression profiling. The current gold standard of rejection surveillance after cardiac transplantation is endomyocardial biopsy. However, the endomyocardial biopsy is invasive, causes morbidity, and is subject to sampling error and interobserver variability. Alternative noninvasive monitoring therapies have been tested in the hope of overcoming these limitations, and one new technology holds particular promise: Gene expression profiling (GEP) test, which is also known as the AlloMap test.

GEP, which has been clinically available since January 2005, is a new modality for surveillance of cardiac allograft rejection. This test uses real-time polymerase chain reaction (PCR) technology to measure the expression of 20 genes (11 informative, 9 control and normalization) (8). A score ranging from 0 to 40 is generated by a multigene algorithm. The score has been shown to discriminate between quiescence and moderate/severe acute cellular rejection in the CARGO (Cardiac Allograft Rejection Gene Expression Observational) study. Scores of <34 were associated with a negative predictive value of >99% for grade ≥3A/2R rejection. Several factors influence AlloMap score, including time posttransplantation, peripheral alloimmune activity, corticosteroid dose, and cytomegalovirus. A recently published study has demonstrated that transplantation vasculopathy is associated with increased AlloMap GEP score. The one study on the cost effectiveness of this new technique has shown it to be a less expensive alternative to endomyocardial biopsy for monitoring allograft rejection in cardiac transplantation patients.

GEP or AlloMap testing can be used in clinically stable cardiac transplant recipients who are >15 years of age and 6 months or more posttransplantation. It is used to identify patients at low risk for moderate/severe (≥3A original ISHLT grade or ≥2R revised ISHLT grade) cellular rejection (8). The frequency of rejection surveillance using the GEP or AlloMap testing should be individualized to the patient's rejection history, immunosuppression regimen, time posttransplantation, and transplant center protocol. This novel technology has demonstrated great clinical promise in these early studies and may one day become the gold standard for rejection surveillance after cardiac transplantation.

B. Grading scheme. Rejection of the cardiac allograft is usually clinically silent unless it is accompanied by significant hemodynamic compromise (i.e., congestive heart failure). As a result, endomyocardial biopsies are routinely performed for rejection surveillance (see Chapter 57). Grading of endomyocardial biopsies for severity of acute cellular rejection has been standardized and updated in 2004 (Table 12.8) (7). The key changes include the simplification of the system to three categories: grade 1R (mild, low grade, formally grades 1A, 1B, and 2), grade 2R (moderate, intermediate-grade, formally grade 3A), and grade 3R (severe, high grade, formally grades 3B and 4) (9). Because the likelihood of acute rejection is highest early after transplantation, the frequency of biopsies is high during this period and then gradually tapers off, depending on the results (Table 12.9).

C. Types of rejection

1. **Hyperacute rejection** is usually fatal and is the result of allograft rejection by preformed antibodies. It can occur immediately on surgical reperfusion. The

TABLE 12.8 Grading Scale (2004) for Endomyocardial Biopsies

Grade	Severity of cellular rejection	Histologic findings
1R[a]	Mild	Interstitial and/or perivascular infiltrate with up to 1 focus of necrosis
2R	Moderate	≥2 foci of infiltrate with associated necrosis
3R	Severe	Diffuse infiltrate with multifocal necrosis ± edema ± hemorrhage ± vasculitis

[a]R = revised

TABLE 12.9 Endomyocardial Biopsy Schedule

Weeks after transplantation	Biopsy frequency
1–4	Weekly
5–12	Every 2 weeks
13–24	Monthly
25–52	Every 2 months
Year 2	Every 3–4 months
Years 3–4	Every 6 months
>4 Years	Only if clinically indicated
After biopsy with acute rejection	2 weeks after initial biopsy

incidence of hyperacute rejection is thankfully rare in the era of PRAs and prospective crossmatches.

2. **Cellular rejection** is a lymphocyte-mediated attack of the allograft characterized by lymphocytic infiltration on the endomyocardial biopsy accompanied by myocyte injury. Biopsy grades of ≥3A warrant accentuation of immunosuppression. If there is no hemodynamic compromise, patients are routinely treated as outpatients with 100 mg of prednisone taken orally for 3 days. If there is hemodynamic compromise or persistent or recurrent severe rejection (at least grade 3A), many therapeutic options are available, including 1 g of intravenous Solu-Medrol for 3 days, conversion from cyclosporine to tacrolimus, OKT3, Atgam, Thymoglobulin, plasmapheresis, photophoresis, and total lymphoid irradiation.
3. **Vascular (humoral) rejection** is an antibody-mediated phenomenon in which immunoglobulin G, immunoglobulin M, or complement deposition is demonstrated in the donor coronary microvasculature by immunofluorescence. Vascular rejection is not routinely screened for in endomyocardial biopsies unless suspected clinically because of allograft dysfunction or hemodynamic compromise. Treatment options for patients with vascular rejection include intravenous or oral steroids, plasmapheresis, or immunoadsorption.

X. INFECTIOUS DISEASE AFTER TRANSPLANTATION. As with all other immunosuppressed patients, one of the main complications experienced by cardiac transplant recipients is opportunistic infections. An infectious diseases specialist with a special interest in transplantation is an invaluable resource to any transplant program. There are several potential pathogens of particular interest in the transplanted patient.

A. CMV. Primary CMV infection occurs when a CMV-negative recipient receives a CMV-positive donor organ. Secondary CMV infection occurs when a CMV-positive recipient has a reactivation of his or her quiescent disease after immunosuppression, particularly with induction therapy or bolus immunosuppression prescribed for a rejection episode. Active CMV disease may manifest as fevers, myalgias, gastritis, colitis, pneumonitis, retinitis, or leukopenia and thrombocytopenia. The most sensitive and specific test for diagnosing CMV is by quantitative PCR. PCR detects CMV DNA in plasma and quantifies the CMV viral load. Although CMV DNA replication may be detected by PCR, most patients do not have the clinical syndrome of CMV disease. The issue of whether a detectable CMV viral load will progress to the clinical syndrome and whether to treat patients with CMV detection in the absence of symptoms remains controversial.

Prophylaxis against CMV disease is considered the standard of care for CMV-positive recipients (regardless of the CMV status of the donor) and CMV-negative patients with a CMV-positive donor. There is no consensus on the duration of ganciclovir therapy in these patients. Most patients are treated initially with intravenous ganciclovir, followed by a variable course of oral valganciclovir or acyclovir. Periodic monitoring of the CMV viral load may assist in guiding the duration of therapy in these patients.

Passive immunization with CMV immunoglobulin (CytoGam) may be considered in patients deemed at risk of CMV disease, particularly if they have low levels of serum immunoglobulins (<500 mg/dL). Patients undergoing induction therapy, polyclonal or monoclonal antibody therapy for steroid-resistant rejection, or increased immunosuppressive therapy for acute rejection therapy should be deemed at risk for reactivation of CMV disease.

The duration of therapy with valganciclovir for active CMV disease is usually 3 to 6 weeks. An undetectable CMV viral load should be demonstrated in such patients before consideration is given for antiviral therapy discontinuation.

B. *Pneumocystis carinii* pneumonia (PCP). Transplant recipients are at increased risk for the development of PCP because of their immunocompromised state. PCP is rare if appropriate prophylaxis with trimethoprim-sulfamethoxazole (TMP-SMX) is provided. Patients intolerant to TMP-SMX may be treated with inhaled pentamidine or dapsone. PCP is rarely seen at maintenance immunosuppressant doses in transplant patients. TMP-SMX may be discontinued at 6 to 12 months after transplantation in most patients.

XI. CARDIAC ALLOGRAFT VASCULOPATHY (CAV). CAV is a progressive, neointimal proliferative process in the epicardial coronary vasculature and the microcirculation. It is a significant cause of mortality beyond the first year after transplantation, accounting for 30% to 50% of deaths at 5 years. The pathophysiology of CAV is not completely understood. Initially CAV was thought to be an accelerated form of atherosclerosis; however, it is now clear that both immunologic and nonimmunologic factors are involved in the process. Chronic, subclinical, immune-mediated injury at the level of the donor coronary endothelium creates a chronic inflammatory milieu. The exact mediator of the endothelial injury remains controversial, but it is probably multifactorial, including chronic humoral and cellular rejection, ischemic and reperfusion injury at the time of transplantation, and chronic CMV infection of endothelial cells. Table 12.10 lists risk factors for the development of CAV of which older donor age and hyperlipidemia are well established risk factors, whereas the others are potential risk factors.

Because donor hearts are denervated at explantation, the transplant recipient typically will not experience cardiac angina from advanced allograft coronary vasculopathy. The clinical presentation of coronary vasculopathy previously unrecognized in a patient may include symptomatic or asymptomatic LV dysfunction, myocardial infarction, or cardiac arrhythmia, including ventricular arrhythmias, heart block, syncope, or sudden cardiac death. Owing to the usually asymptomatic nature of vasculopathy, transplant recipients have frequent surveillance studies to detect significant vasculopathy, including coronary angiography with or without intravascular ultrasound (IVUS), cardiac perfusion magnetic resonance imaging, and dobutamine echocardiography. The frequency and method of surveillance is center specific. Although coronary

TABLE 12.10 Risk Factors for the Development of Cardiac Allograft Vasculopathy

Older donor age
Hyperlipidemia
Donor brain death secondary to spontaneous intracranial hemorrhage
Cytomegalovirus infection (CMV)
Increased C-reactive protein levels (>1.66 mg/L)
Recurrent cellular rejection
Humoral (vascular) rejection
HLA antigen mismatch
Donor hepatitis B and C
Female donor
Peri-transplantation myocardial ischemia
Pretransplantation coronary atherosclerotic disease
Conventional atherosclerosis risk factors (diabetes, hypertension, and smoking)

angiography is useful for the diagnosis of nontransplantation coronary artery disease, its sensitivity is considerably less in CAV because of the diffuse nature of this disease. Coronary IVUS imaging provides useful tomographic perspective to study the development and progression of CAV and is now considered by many to be the gold standard modality for diagnosing CAV. However, not all centers have access to routine IVUS imaging and thus its use will vary greatly from center to center.

The detection of significant epicardial allograft coronary vasculopathy should prompt aggressive percutaneous or more rarely surgical revascularization. Because of its relationship to chronic rejection, advancement of the immunosuppressant regimen has also been advocated. Statins have been shown prospectively to decrease the incidence of transplantation vasculopathy and improve survival, regardless of the patient's lipid profile (9). Preliminary studies investigating the antiproliferative effects of TOR inhibitors (sirolimus and everolimus) suggest a significant reduction in coronary neointimal proliferation and, therefore, transplantation coronary vasculopathy. In the future, the development of transplantation vasculopathy may prompt a switch to a TOR inhibitor–based immunosuppressant regimen if the initial suggestion of attenuation of progression, and perhaps regression, of transplantation vasculopathy is confirmed in larger, prospective clinical trials. In severe, advanced CAV, frequently the only viable option is repeat transplantation.

XII. MALIGNANCY. Malignancy is an common and devastating complication of cardiac transplantation. In normal patients, the immune system actively defends against a variety of neoplastic processes. With the initiation of immunosuppression after transplantation, this defense mechanism is lost, and previously undeclared neoplastic foci may proliferate. Because a significant percentage of cardiac transplantation patients had ischemic cardiomyopathy and are former smokers, lung cancers can occur. Other common tumors include lymphomas, skin cancers, colon cancers, and breast cancers. Skin cancers are particularly common in patients on azathioprine, and they usually prompt a substitution of MMF for azathioprine. Posttransplantation malignancies are particularly common in patients who have received cytolytic or induction therapy with OKT3, Atgam, or Thymoglobulin, and the risk correlates with cumulative dosing of immunosuppression. The risk of developing malignancy as a result of immunosuppression is enhanced by the inability to adequately assess for overimmunosuppression. Underimmunosuppression is readily detected because of the development of acute rejection, whereas there is no clinical finding to suggest overimmunosuppression.

Post transplant lymphoproliferative disease (PTLD) is an Ebstein-Barr virus–related clonal expansion of B lymphocytes. PTLD may develop in any location but most commonly affects the gastrointestinal tract, lungs, and central nervous system. The primary treatment for PTLD is a reduction in immunosuppression (by about 50%), which can frequently be curative. Surgical debulking, systemic chemotherapy, and antiviral therapy may also be indicated in selected patients.

XIII. HYPERTENSION. Arterial hypertension commonly develops after cardiac transplantation secondary to the untoward effects of immunosuppression. Hypertension developing after cardiac transplantation occurs in most cyclosporine-treated and tacrolimus-treated patients. Three proposed mechanisms are: (1) direct sympathetic activation, (2) increased responsiveness to direct circulating neurohormones, and (3) direct vascular effects. A common endpoint of these proposed mechanisms is vasoconstriction of the renal vasculature, leading to sodium retention and an elevated plasma volume. Corticosteroids play a minor role in the pathogenesis of cardiac transplantation hypertension, which is described as a salt-sensitive type. Abnormal cardiorenal reflexes secondary to cardiac denervation may also contribute to salt-sensitive hypertension and fluid retention.

Patients with blood pressures consistently greater than 140/90 mm Hg should be treated. Titrated monotherapy with either angiotensin-converting enzyme (ACE) inhibitors or calcium channel blockers is usually effective in about 50% of the patients. Some patients will be prone to hyperkalemia secondary to the combined effect of cyclosporine and ACE inhibition on the kidney. The use of either diltiazem, verapamil, or amlodipine necessitates the use of lower doses of cyclosporine and initially more frequent cyclosporine-level monitoring because these drugs are competitive antagonists of cyclosporine at the cytochrome P450 level. Combination therapy with both an ACE inhibitor and a calcium channel blocker is a commonly employed strategy. Problematic hypertensives requiring multiple agents often require diuretics as part of their regimen. Hypertension in some patients is inadequately controlled despite maximally tolerated doses of both calcium channel blockers and ACE inhibitors. The final tier of management would be to add an α-blocker such as clonidine or doxazosin in refractory cases. β-Blockers traditionally have been avoided due to their known tendency to reduce exercise performance and because of concerns about excessive bradycardia. Some transplant cardiologists, however, routinely use β-blockers to manage hypertension in their transplant patients. Thus β-blockers are not contraindicated, but rather may be used with due caution.

XIV. OUTCOMES AFTER CARDIAC TRANSPLANTATION. Survival outcomes after cardiac transplantation continue to improve on a yearly basis despite what is generally accepted as a population of transplant recipients at greater risk primarily because of advancing recipient age and increasing severity of heart failure. The 1-year survival rate after cardiac transplantation is 84% nationwide, but it is frequently >90% at large transplantation centers. The mortality in the first year after transplantation primarily results from postoperative complications, including multi-organ failure, primary graft failure, and systemic infection. It is unlikely that any major improvements in early posttransplantation survival will occur in light of these excellent results. However, 10-year survival after cardiac transplantation is only 50%. Mortality in the long term primarily results from transplant coronary vasculopathy, malignancy, and renal failure. It is hoped that a major impact can be made on long-term survival with newer immunosuppressive drug regimens that may be less nephrotoxic and more effective at preventing transplant coronary vasculopathy.

References

1. Taylor DO, Edwards LB, Boucek MM, et al. Registry of the International Society for Heart and Lung Transplantation: Twenty-third Official Adult Heart Transplantation Report—2006. *J Heart Lung Transplant* 2006;24:869–879.
2. Hunt SA, Baker DW, Chin MH, et al. ACC/AHA guidelines for the evaluation and management of chronic heart failure in the adult. *Circulation* 2001;104:2996–3007.
3. Mehra MR, Kobashigawa JA, Starling RC, et al. Listing Criteria for Heart Transplantation: International Society for Heart and Lung Transplantation Guidelines for the Care of Cardiac Transplant Candidates—2006. *J Heart Lung Transplant* 2006;25:1024–1042.
4. Radovancevic B, El-Sabrout R, Thomas C, et al. Rapamycin reduces rejection in heart transplant recipients. *Transplant Proc* 2001;33:3221–3222.
5. Ikonen TS, Gummert JF, Hayase M, et al. Sirolimus (rapamycin) halts and reverses progression of allograft vascular disease in non-human primates. *Transplantation* 2000;70:969–975.
6. Beniaminovitz A, Itescu S, Lietz K, et al. Prevention of rejection in cardiac transplantation by blockade of the interleukin-2 receptor with a monoclonal antibody. *N Engl J Med* 2000;342:613–619.
7. Stewart S, Winters GL, Fishbein MC, et al. Revision of the 1990 working formulation for the standardization of nomenclature in the diagnosis of heart rejection. *J Heart Lung Transplant* 2005;24:1710–1720.
8. Starling RC, Pham M, Valantine H, et al. Molecular testing in the management of cardiac transplant recipients: initial clinical experience. *J Heart Lung Transplant* 2006;25:1389–1395.
9. Kobashigawa JA, Katznelson S, Laks H, et al. Effect of pravastatin on outcomes after cardiac transplantation. *N Engl J Med* 1995;333:621–627.

Landmark Articles

Hunt SA, Kouretas PC, Balsam LB, et al. Heart Transplantation. In: Zipes DP, Libby P, Bonow RO, Braunwald E, eds. *Braunwald's heart disease: a textbook of cardiovascular medicine,* 7th ed. Philadelphia: Elsevier Saunders, 2005:641–651.

Kirklin JK, Young JB, McGiffin DC, eds. *Heart transplantation*. Philadelphia: Churchill Livingstone, 2002.

Mancini DM, Eisen H, Kussmaul W, et al. Value of peak exercise oxygen consumption for optimal timing of cardiac transplantation in ambulatory patients with heart failure. *Circulation* 1991;83:778–786.

Mehra MR, Narula J, Young JB, eds. Current advances in heart transplantation. *Heart Fail Clin* 2007;1:1–105.

Norman DJ, Suki WN, eds. *Primer on transplantation*. Thorofare, NJ: American Society of Transplant Physicians, 1998:399–472.

Topol EJ, ed. *Textbook of cardiovascular medicine,* 2nd ed. Philadelphia: Lippincott Williams & Wilkins, 2002:1915–1934.

Relevant Web Sites

Scientific registry of solid-organ transplant recipients in the United States (www.ustransplants.org).

International Society for Heart and Lung Transplantation (ISHLT) (www.ishlt.org).

Valvular Heart Disease

III

AORTIC VALVE DISEASE

13

Anne Kanderian, Anjli Maroo, and Brian P. Griffin

I. AORTIC STENOSIS

A. Introduction. Aortic stenosis (AS) causes progressive obstruction of the left ventricular outflow tract (LVOT), resulting in pressure hypertrophy of the left ventricle and the classic symptoms of heart failure, syncope, and angina pectoris. Stenosis may occur at the valve, below the valve (i.e., subaortic stenosis), and above the valve (i.e., supravalvular stenosis). Valvular stenosis predominates. Untreated, AS is associated with significant morbidity and mortality. The normal aortic valve area is 3 to 4 cm^2 and is reduced to <1 cm^2 in severe valvular AS. Normally, there is little or no pressure difference across the aortic valve. In significant AS, the LV pressure may exceed that of the aorta by >50 mm Hg. However, because the pressure difference is affected by the severity of the narrowing of the aortic valve and by the flow through it, pressure measurements alone should be used with caution to characterize AS.

B. Etiology

1. **Valvular AS** has several causes, including congenital, rheumatic, bicuspid, and age-related calcific degeneration.
   a. The most common cause of AS in the United States is age-related calcific degeneration. This disorder involves calcium deposition at the fusion lines of the valve leaflets. Although normal "wear and tear" of the valve leaflets is thought to manifest as senile degeneration in the sixth or seventh decades, there is a growing body of evidence that suggests **atherosclerosis may contribute to the pathophysiology of this disease**. Aortic sclerosis is caused by calcification and thickening of the aortic valve without the increased gradients as seen in aortic stenosis. Both age-related aortic sclerosis and calcific stenosis have been associated with traditional risk factors for atherosclerosis, such as smoking, hypertension, and hyperlipidemia. Age-related aortic sclerosis is associated with an increased risk for cardiovascular death and myocardial infarction, and can progress to aortic stenosis. Other conditions associated with calcific AS include Paget's disease and end-stage renal disease.
   b. **Bicuspid valves** are present in 1% to 2% of the population, predominate in men, and occur in **9% of first-degree family members** of those afflicted. They may be stenotic or regurgitant. Occasionally, severe stenosis develops in early life, but most often, this does not happen until the fifth or sixth decade. **Bicuspid aortic valve** is associated with **coarctation, aortic root dilation, and a propensity for aortic dissection** in a minority of patients. Bicuspid aortic valves are most commonly caused by fusion of the right and left coronary cusps. Unicuspid valves open only at one commissure, are uncommon, and are usually severely stenotic at an early age. Unicuspid valve is also associated with aortopathy.

      The most recent American College of Cardiology/American Heart Association (ACC/AHA) valve guidelines (2006) highlight the importance of evaluating the aorta and valve in bicuspid aortic valve with echocardiography or, if this is inadequate, with other imaging modalities such as magnetic resonance imaging (MRI). In some instances, the aorta may require surgical intervention before the valve. The guidelines recommend that patients with an aortic diameter >4 cm and bicuspid valve should have yearly follow-up of aorta size, and should have **surgical intervention if the aorta is >5 cm or increases by >0.5 cm in a year,** irrespective of the valve lesion severity. **If the valve requires surgery, then aorta replacement is recommended if the aorta is >4.5 cm at the time of surgery**. Consideration should be given to the use of β-blockade in bicuspid valve patients without severe aortic regurgitation (AR) who have ascending aorta enlargement in order to reduce the rate of aorta dilation.

c. **Rheumatic aortic stenosis (AS)** often coexists with atrial regurgitation (AR) and mitral valve lesions. It is rare in the industrialized world as a cause of isolated severe AS. Fusion of the commissures occurs leaving a small central orifice.

2. **Subvalvular AS.** This is a congenital condition, although it may not be apparent at birth. Typically, a **fibromuscular membrane is present in the LVOT below the aortic valve.** The membrane is often circumferential and involves the anterior mitral valve leaflet. In more extreme cases, a tunnel-like obstruction may be present rather than a discrete membrane. The pathogenesis of this condition is not perfectly understood but is thought to represent a maladaptive response to abnormal flow dynamics in the LVOT. It may exist with other left-sided obstructive lesions, such as coarctation as part of Shone's syndrome. The condition may recur even after successful membrane resection. Subvalvular AS may be difficult to distinguish from hypertrophic cardiomyopathy, especially when secondary LV hypertrophy is pronounced.

3. **Supravalvular AS** is uncommon. It may occur as part of a congenital syndrome such as Williams' syndrome caused by a mutation in the elastin gene (i.e., associated hypercalcemia, elfin facies, developmental delay, small stature, and multiple stenoses in the aorta and peripheral arteries) or be caused by lipid deposits in severe forms of familial hypercholesterolemia. Obstruction occurs above the valve in the ascending aorta.

C. **Pathophysiology**

1. **Pressure overload.** All forms of AS are characterized by progressive narrowing of the LVOT. To maintain cardiac output in the face of increased afterload, the left ventricle must generate higher systolic pressures, which increases LV wall stress. In response to the pressure overload and increased wall stress, the left ventricle undergoes compensatory, concentric hypertrophy. The increase in LV wall thickness allows the wall stress to normalize according to Laplace's law: wall stress = (pressure × radius) ÷ (2 × thickness).

2. **Diastolic dysfunction.** LV diastolic function is determined by LV relaxation properties and LV compliance (i.e., change in volume with change in pressure [dV/dP]). Increased afterload and LV hypertrophy (LVH) lead to a reduction in LV compliance. Passive early diastolic filling is reduced, and maintenance of an adequate LV preload becomes more dependent on active left atrial contraction.

3. **Supply-demand mismatch.** Myocardial oxygen demand is determined by heart rate, cardiac contractility, and myocardial wall stress. Over time, LVH is unable to compensate for the increase in wall stress imposed on the left ventricle by progressive pressure overload. As the AS becomes more severe, wall stress and myocardial oxygen demand increase in parallel. Concurrently, AS is associated with a decrease in myocardial oxygen supply. Progressive LVH and diastolic dysfunction lead to an elevation in LV end-diastolic pressure (LVEDP). Elevated LVEDP leads to decreased perfusion pressure across the coronary bed and causes endocardial compression of small intramyocardial arteries, impairing coronary flow reserve. The imbalance between myocardial oxygen supply and demand can precipitate ischemia during exertion.

D. **Natural history.** The classic survival curve for patients with untreated AS, as described by Ross and Braunwald, is shown in Figure 13.1.

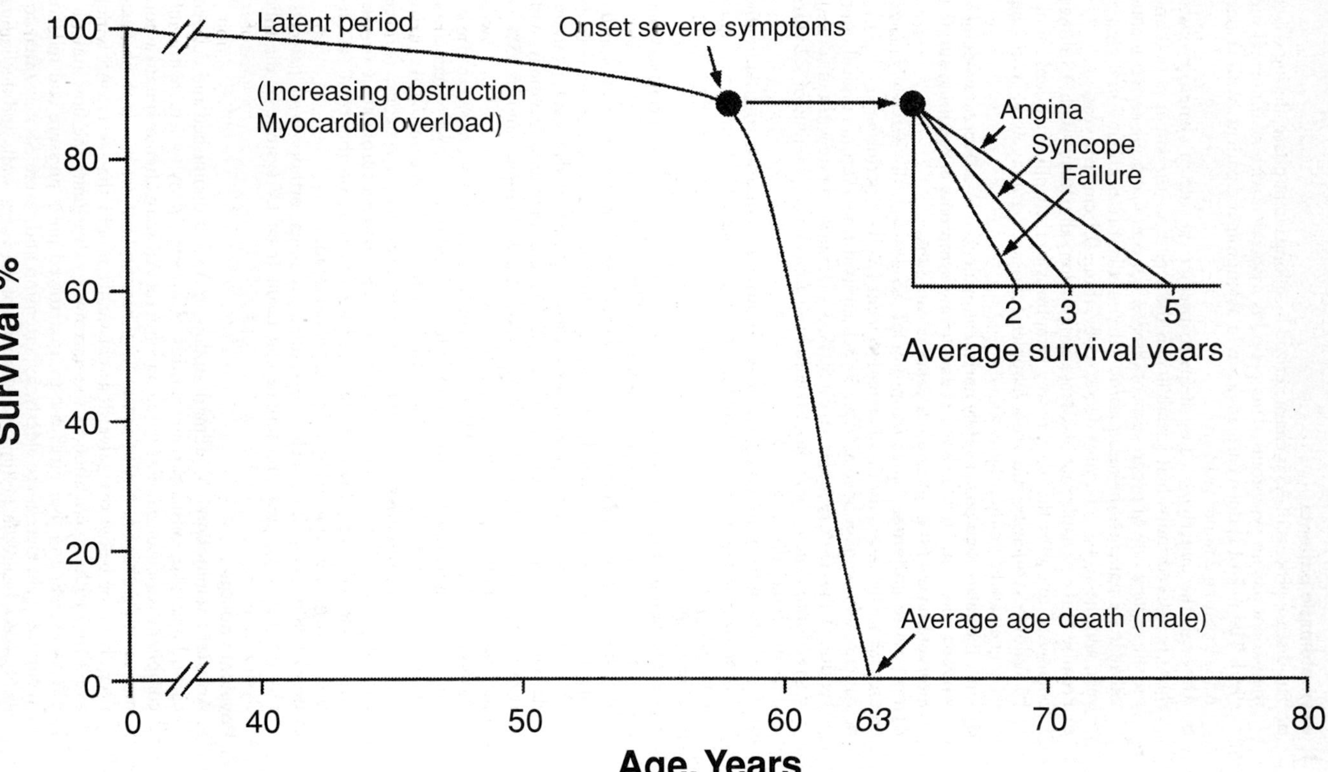

Figure 13.1. Patient survival in aortic stenosis.

1. **Asymptomatic patients**
   a. The disease process of AS is characterized by a long latent phase, during which the patient has no symptoms. This period is associated with near-normal survival. The risk of sudden cardiac death in asymptomatic patients with critical AS is less than 2% per year.
   b. Although the underlying cause helps to predict the age of symptom onset, there is marked individual variability in the length of the latent period and the subsequent rate of progression of disease. In general, among asymptomatic valvular AS patients, the mean aortic valve gradient rises about 7 mm Hg per year, and the aortic valve area decreases by about 0.1 cm^2 per year.
   c. Because of the variable rate of disease progression, all patients with AS should be advised to report the onset of any symptoms to their physician and should be followed clinically and with Doppler echocardiography with increasing frequency as the lesion progresses.
   d. Once the **valve becomes severely narrow** as evidenced by a **Doppler velocity of 4 m/sec across it, the likelihood of developing symptoms or requiring surgical intervention over the following 2 years is very high.**
2. **Symptomatic patients.** After symptoms of AS develop, the survival rate decreases markedly, unless aortic valve replacement (AVR) is performed.
   a. Patients with **angina** have a 50%, 5-year survival rate without surgical intervention. Those with **syncope** have a 50%, 3-year survival rate without surgical intervention. Patients with **heart failure** have a mean survival time of <2 years if treated medically.
   b. In patients with severe, symptomatic AS, sudden cardiac death can occur in the setting of hypotension or arrhythmia due to ischemia, LVH, or impaired LV function.

E. Clinical manifestations

1. **Signs and symptoms.** The onset of symptoms usually indicates progression to severe AS and heralds the need for surgical evaluation.
   a. **Angina.** Patients with severe AS can experience ischemia from myocardial supply—demand mismatch due to high LV diastolic pressures, decreased myocardial perfusion, and increased wall stress. Angina can also result from underlying coronary artery disease (CAD). CAD is common among patients with severe AS. It occurs in 40% to 80% of patients with angina and in 25% of patients without angina.
   b. **Syncope.** Because of fixed LVOT obstruction, patients with severe AS are unable to augment their cardiac output under conditions of low systemic vascular resistance (SVR) (i.e., induced by certain medications or vasovagal reactions). The ensuing hypotension can cause presyncope, syncope, or even cardiovascular collapse and death. Syncope can also result from atrial or ventricular arrhythmias, abnormal baroreceptor function, or abnormal vasodepressor responses induced by LV pressure overload.
   c. **Heart failure** symptoms, such as exertional dyspnea, orthopnea or paroxysmal nocturnal dyspnea, and fatigue can result from LV systolic or diastolic dysfunction.
2. **Physical findings**
   a. **Arterial examination.** A hallmark finding in AS is a diminished and delayed carotid upstroke, pulsus parvus et tardus. However, elderly patients with noncompliant vessels or patients with concomitant AR may often maintain a normal carotid pulsation, despite severe AS. These findings are rare with obstruction above or below the valve. It is classically taught that severe AS is not associated with hypertension as the narrowed valve limits the flow into the arterial system and thus gives rise to a narrowed pulse pressure and relative hypotension. In fact, in the elderly, hypertension and severe AS may often coexist, likely as a result of impaired elasticity of the aortic walls and the finding of arterial hypertension does not preclude significant associated AS.
   b. **Palpation.** With LVH and normal LV cavity dimensions, the apical impulse is usually nondisplaced, diffuse, and sustained. However, the apical impulse

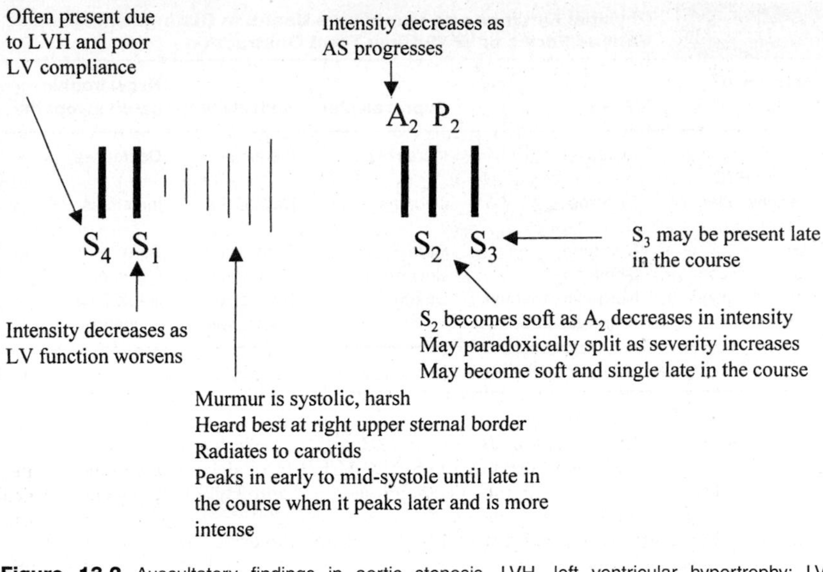

Figure 13.2. Auscultatory findings in aortic stenosis. LVH, left ventricular hypertrophy; LV, left ventricle.

may be later displaced when there is LV systolic dysfunction. A double apical impulse represents a palpable *a* wave or S_4, caused by a noncompliant left ventricle. A systolic thrill may be palpable in the second right intercostal space.

c. Auscultation. The main auscultatory findings are shown in Figure 13.2.

(1) The typical murmur of AS is a systolic ejection murmur heard at the right upper sternal border that radiates to the neck. With a mobile bicuspid valve, an aortic opening sound may precede the murmur. As the severity of stenosis increases, the murmur becomes longer and peaks later in systole. The intensity of the murmur does not necessarily correspond to the severity of AS. S_1 usually is normal in AS. As the AS becomes more severe, the aortic component of S_2 diminishes and eventually disappears, resulting in a soft, single S_2. Often, with severe AS, S_2 is paradoxically split because of the prolonged ejection duration through the severely narrowed valve. S_3 is indicative of poor LV systolic function. An S_4 is common because of reduced LV compliance.

(2) Careful examination for other murmurs should be performed. AS often is accompanied by AR. Maneuvers performed during the physical examination can help to differentiate different types of LV outflow obstruction whether this is at, below, or above the valve. These are summarized in Table 13.1.

3. Diagnostic testing

a. The typical **electrocardiogram (ECG)** of a patient with isolated severe AS usually demonstrates left atrial abnormality (80% of cases) and LVH (85% of cases).

b. Chest radiography can be entirely normal, even in patients with critical AS. The cardiac silhouette may become boot-shaped because of concentric LVH. Cardiomegaly may be identified if there is LV dysfunction or coexisting AR. Aortic valve and root calcification can be seen in adults with severe, age-related, calcific, degenerative AS. Poststenotic dilation of the ascending aorta may be evident.

TABLE 13.1 Physical Findings and Maneuvers Useful in Distinguishing Various Forms of LV Outflow Tract Obstruction

Maneuver/ finding	Valve	Supravalvular	Subvalvular	Hypertrophic cardiomyopathy
Pulse volume after PVC	Increases	Increases	Increases	Decreases
Valsalva effect on systolic murmur	Decreases	Decreases	Decreases	Increases
AR	Common	Rare	Common	Rare
S_4	Common	Uncommon	Uncommon	Common
Carotid pulse	Normal to anacrotic (parvus et tardus)	Unequal	Normal to anacrotic	Rapid jerky upstroke

AR, Atrial regurgitation; PVC, preventricular contraction.

4. Severity of aortic stenosis

The severity of AS is currently graded by ACC/AHA valve guidelines as follows:

Mild: valve area >**1.5 cm²**, mean gradient <25 mm Hg, or jet velocity <3.0 m per second

Moderate: valve area **1.0 to 1.5 cm²**, mean gradient 25 to 40 mm Hg, or jet velocity 3.0 to 4.0 m per second

Severe: valve area <**1.0 cm²**, mean gradient >40 mm Hg, or jet velocity >4.0 m per second.

5. Echocardiography

a. Transthoracic Doppler echocardiography is the method of choice as recommended by the ACC/AHA guidelines to establish the diagnosis of AS, to determine the cause and location, and to assess its severity. It should be performed when the diagnosis of AS is first suspected. Additional information may be obtained such as LV wall thickness, size, and function. After the diagnosis is established, patients should have frequent, regular clinical follow-up examinations to look for the development of symptoms. Echocardiographic follow-up can be tailored to the severity of disease: at least annually for severe AS, and more frequently as the severity increases; every 2 years for moderate AS; and every 3 to 5 years for mild AS. Development of new symptoms and signs should prompt a repeat evaluation.

(1) The parasternal long-axis, two-dimensional and M-mode views are the most helpful views to determine the precise mechanism and severity of AS and to quantitate LV chamber dimensions and wall thickness. In this view, the coaptation line of the aortic valve is normally centered within the LVOT in a trileaflet valve. The leaflets of a bicuspid valve often have an eccentric closure line, typically posterior to the midline. Systolic leaflet doming can be seen in congenital and rheumatic AS. The degree of LVH, LV chamber enlargement, or left atrial enlargement can be quantitated using two-dimensional and M-mode imaging. The LVOT diameter used in the continuity equation is measured in the two-dimensional, parasternal long-axis view. Subaortic and supravalvular AS may be detected in this view. Subaortic stenosis may be evident as a membrane below the aortic valve with normal motion of the valve. Doppler may indicate that the obstruction is occurring below the valve and often indicates AR due to the turbulent jet hitting aortic valve leaflets and causing leaflet scarring and impaired coaptation. In supravalvular AS, narrowing above the valve is evident on imaging and with Doppler.

(2) The parasternal short-axis view is the most useful view for establishing the cause of congenital AS. The number of commissures and the shape of the valve orifice should be assessed (Fig. 13.3). Trileaflet valves open

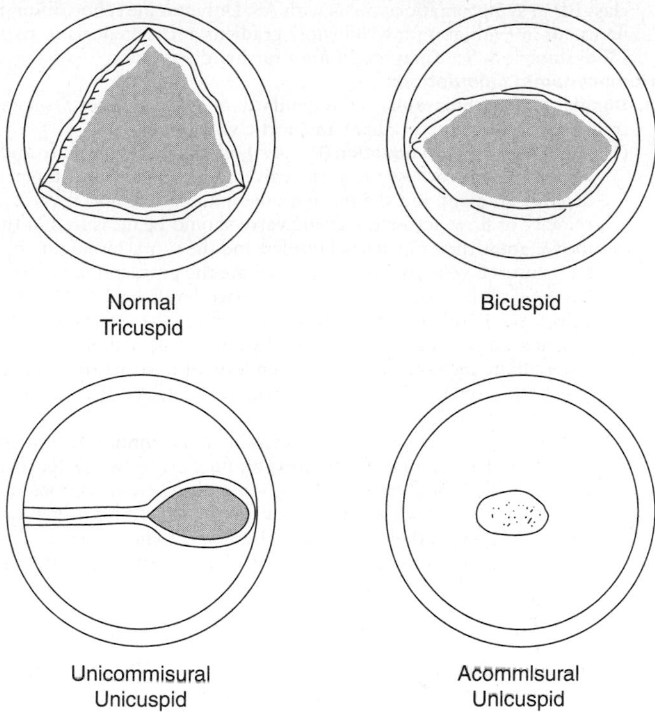

Figure 13.3. Schematic representation of parasternal short axis of a congenitally abnormal aortic valve.

as a triangle, whereas an elliptical opening suggests a bicuspid valve. In a unicuspid valve, the opening is elliptical but occurs across a radius rather than the diameter of the valve.

(3) The apical five-chamber view is well aligned with flow through the aortic valve. Continuous wave Doppler recordings across the aortic valve and pulsed-wave Doppler flow in the LVOT proximal to the aortic valve are recorded in this view for the continuity equation.

(4) Continuous-wave Doppler should be performed at multiple sites, including the suprasternal notch and the right sternal border, to ensure that the maximal velocity across the aortic valve is recorded. The dimensions of the ascending aorta should be measured, and coarctation in the descending aorta should be sought, especially in those with bicuspid aortic valves.

b. Transesophageal echocardiography (TEE). Planimetry of the aortic valve orifice is often possible with TEE and relates well to that measured by cardiac catheterization. Planimetry is difficult when the valve is extremely calcified. In bicuspid valve, the smallest area should be sought carefully, as the valve opening is not planar but rather forms a cone due to the doming of the valve as it opens. TEE is particularly useful for determining morphologic features of the valve in congenital AS. TEE is often necessary to confirm the diagnosis of subaortic membrane and to differentiate it from hypertrophic cardiomyopathy or valvular AS.

c. Dobutamine echocardiography and stress echocardiography. Exercise testing in patients with asymptomatic AS may provide useful information such as exercise-induced symptoms or abnormal blood pressure responses (ACC/AHA class IIb indication). Exercise testing is contraindicated (ACC/AHA class III) in symptomatic patients with AS. Dobutamine echocardiography may be useful in evaluating low-flow/low-gradient aortic stenosis in patients with LV dysfunction. See Chapter 46 for a further discussion.

6. Hemodynamic calculations

a. Doppler echocardiography is the standard modality used for assessment of the transvalvular pressure gradient and aortic valve area.

(1) Modified Bernoulli equation ($P = 4v^2$), in which P is pressure and v is peak velocity of flow across the aortic valve, is used to estimate the peak instantaneous gradient and the mean gradient across the aortic valve. The peak velocity of flow across the aortic valve should be measured in three areas: the LV apex, the right sternal border, and the suprasternal notch. The highest measured velocity is used to calculate the peak and mean transvalvular gradients. When stenosis is present at two levels (i.e., in LVOT and at the valve), the gradient across the LVOT reflects the integrated effects of the obstruction at both levels. It is usually impossible with Doppler to precisely differentiate the contribution of each level of obstruction to the total. This may be inferred by analysis of the images, by TEE, or by direct measurement at cardiac catheterization.

(2) Calculation of aortic valve area is based on the **continuity principle,** which states that the flow of an incompressible fluid in a closed system must remain constant. Flow in a vessel is the product of the cross-sectional area (A) of the vessel × velocity (V). Area is calculated as πR^2 or $\pi D^2/4 = 0.785D^2$, where R is the radius of the vessel and D is the diameter. A schematic representation of the variables for calculating aortic valve area is shown in Figure 13.4. The continuity equation for the aortic valve follows:

$$\text{Area}_{\text{aortic valve}} = (\text{Diameter}_{\text{LVOT}})^2 \times 0.785 \times \text{VTI}_{\text{LVOT}}/\text{VTI}_{\text{aortic valve}}$$

In the equation, VTI is the time–velocity integral. The continuity equation is valid only for valvular AS. It cannot be used to assess valve area when there are stenoses in series such as valvular and subvalvular narrowing occuring simultaneously.

(3) Care should be taken to avoid measuring post-extrasystolic beats. If the patient is in atrial fibrillation, 10 consecutive beats should be measured and averaged for both velocity measurements.

(4) During evaluation of an aortic valve prosthesis, the standard continuity equation cannot be used. Instead, the velocity ratio or **dimensionless index** is used to estimate the severity of prosthetic stenosis. It is calculated by dividing the peak velocity in the LVOT by the peak velocity through the

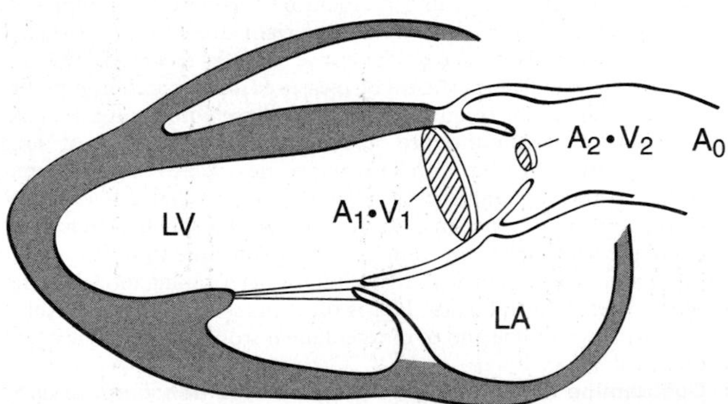

Figure 13.4. Schematic representation of parasternal long-axis view and the continuity principle. LV, left ventricle; LA, left atrium.

aortic valve. **A dimensionless index of <0.25 is generally accepted to represent severe stenosis.** This is also useful if the LVOT diameter is difficult to ascertain.

b. Cardiac catheterization was once considered the gold standard for quantification of AS but is now contraindicated (ACC/AHA class III) in the routine evaluation of a patient when echo-Doppler studies are adequate and congruent with clinical findings.

(1) Preoperative catheterization. Patients >50 years, patients with angina, and patients with significant risk factors for CAD should undergo coronary cineangiography before aortic valve operations (ACC/AHA class I).

(2) Catheter-derived hemodynamic data are indicated (ACC/AHA class I) to further evaluate the severity of AS when the clinical and echocardiographic findings diverge. Because cardiac catheterization findings often differ from those by echocardiography, it is important to understand the differences in what is being measured. The mean gradient obtained during catheterization should be equivalent to the mean gradients obtained by echocardiography. These correlate well when perfromed expertly and simultaneously. The peak gradient measured during catheterization is the peak-to-peak gradient, which is lower than the peak instantaneous gradient obtained with echocardiography (Fig. 13.5). The gradient across the aortic valve is often >50 mm Hg in severe AS with normal LV function. In the setting of reduced cardiac output of any cause, the aortic gradient may be much lower and may be <20 mm Hg in severe LV dysfunction despite critical AS.

(3) The most precise measurement of transaortic valvular gradient is made with two different catheters (one in the LV cavity and the other in the ascending aorta) or with a double-lumen pigtail catheter. Because the two-catheter technique requires cannulation of both femoral arteries, another acceptable method of measuring the peak-to-peak gradient is catheter pullback from the left ventricle to the ascending aorta. A typical pressure tracing of simultaneous LV and aortic pressures is shown in Figure 13.5.

(4) Catheterization of the patient with severe AS should be performed with low-osmolar, nonionic contrast agents. They cause less hypotension from peripheral arterial vasodilation, less bradycardia, less transient myocardial

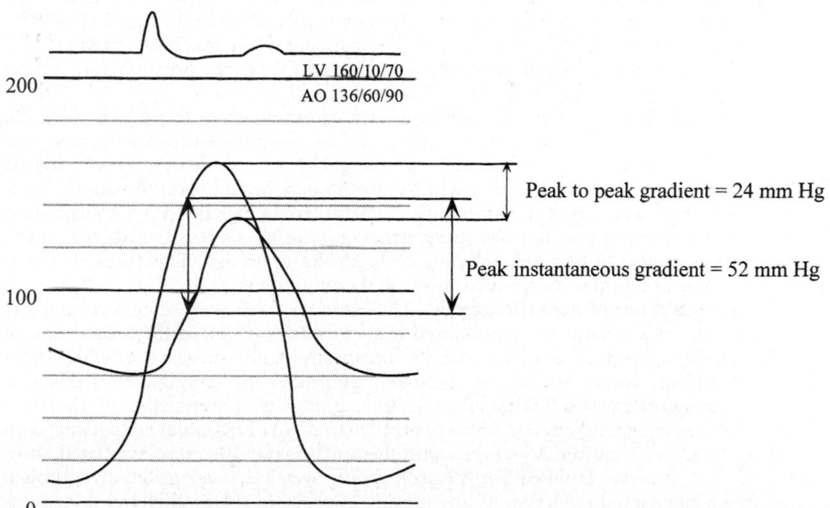

Figure 13.5. Simultaneous recording of LV and aortic pressures. LV, left ventricle; AO, aorta.

dysfunction, and less osmotic diuresis after the procedure. Left ventriculography should be avoided.

(5) The Gorlin formula is used to estimate aortic valve area (AVA):

$$AVA\ (cm^2) = \text{Stroke volume}/(44.3 \times SEP \times \text{square root of } MVG)$$

In this equation, SEP is the systolic ejection period, defined as the time from aortic valve opening to closing measured in seconds per minute. MVG is the mean valvular gradient (given in mm Hg). The **Gorlin** formula measures the **true anatomic area** of the aortic valve as it has a correction factor (the discharge coefficient) that takes into account that the flow in the area of peak narrowing (the vena contracta) is always narrower than the anatomic area. **Continuity** measures the **physiologic area** (vena contracta) and as such is smaller than that measured by Gorlin.

F. Therapy

1. Medical therapy. The mainstay of therapy for severe AS is surgical replacement of the aortic valve. Onset of symptoms in patients with severe AS is associated with a marked reduction in lifespan when treated medically rather than surgically. Medical therapy alone is ineffective treatment for severe symptomatic valvular AS.

a. Antibiotic prophylaxis. The updated 2007 American Heart Association (AHA) guideline on prevention of infective endocarditis has been extensively modified. Unless the patient has a valve prosthesis or prior history of infective endocarditis, antibiotic prophylaxis prior to dental procedures is no longer recommended in patients with valvular pathology.

b. Medical therapy in asymptomatic patients. During the asymptomatic phase, therapy is directed at primary prevention of CAD, maintenance of sinus rhythm, and blood pressure control.

c. Medical therapy in symptomatic patients. Medical therapies may be necessary in symptomatic patients with severe AS who are awaiting surgery or who are considered inoperable and require palliation. Therapy for heart failure is directed at relief of pulmonary congestion. This usually is achieved with cautious use of diuretics. Overly aggressive diuresis can cause hypotension if hypovolemia significantly impairs cardiac output. Nitrates can cause cerebral underperfusion and syncope and should be avoided or used with extreme caution. Thus the management of symptomatic patients with AS and CAD is difficult and urgent surgery is the optimal treatment where feasible. Digoxin is used for symptom relief in the setting of impaired LV systolic function and volume overload, particularly if atrial fibrillation develops.

d. Vasodilator therapy has been relatively contraindicated in patients with AS, because lowering SVR in the setting of a fixed cardiac output may cause syncope, especially in the ambulatory setting. However, patients with severe heart failure and LV dysfunction with severe AS may benefit from the careful titration of intravenous nitroprusside in the intensive care unit with concomitant invasive arterial and pulmonary artery monitoring. One study suggests an improvement in hemodynamic indices with this approach. This therapy is used only as a bridge to definitive surgical therapy.

e. Treatment of hyperlipidemia. The association between AS and risk factors for atherosclerosis has prompted trials of statins to retard the progression of AS. Retrospective studies and one prospective study suggest that when statin therapy is indicated based on current guidelines for hyperlipidemia that it is associated with a modest effect in slowing the rate of progression of AS. However, in a randomized placebo-controlled trial (SALTIRE study) of patients with significant calcific AS where statin therapy was not otherwise mandated, atorvastatin had no effect on AS progression over a 2 year period, even though a substantial reduction in low-density lipoprotein (LDL) cholesterol level ensued. Further studies are under way to try to define the role of statin therapy in AS. Meanwhile, there is no indication for statin use specific to AS, although in hyperlipidemic patients with AS, aggressive lowering of LDL level with statins appears warranted. In patients with supravalvular AS due to severe familial hyperlipidemia, improvement in the obstruction may occur after low-density lipoprotein apheresis.

2. **Percutaneous aortic balloon valvuloplasty (PABV) and percutaneous valve replacement**
   - **a.** In pediatric congenital, noncalcific AS, PABV is a safe and effective therapy, comparable to surgical repair or replacement. The goal of PABV in congenital AS is a 60% to 70% reduction in the measured peak-to-peak transvalvular gradient. Redilatation or AVR becomes necessary within 10 years of the initial PABV in >50% of children. AR is well recognized as a potential early and late complication of PABV, although moderate-to-severe AR occurs in a minority of cases.
   - **b.** In adults, PABV is not an effective long-term therapy for AS compared with surgical AVR. Although PABV initially achieves effective relief of LVOT obstruction (up to 50% improvement in aortic valve area), nearly 50% of patients have restenosis within 6 months. Moreover, PABV does not prolong survival in adults with AS. For these reasons, PABV is used mainly for palliation of symptoms or as a bridge to AVR (ACC/AHA class IIb indication). PABV is not generally recommended in asymptomatic patients with severe AS who are undergoing urgent noncardiac surgery. It is recommended that these patients undergo vigilant monitoring with careful attention to fluid balances and rapid correction of hypotension if this occurs (with phenylephrine or volume if needed).
   - **c. Percutaneous replacement of the aortic valve.** An exciting strategy currently in development is the replacement of a native aortic valve by a stented prosthetic bioprosthesis that is delivered either percutaneously from an arterial site (usually in the femoral or iliac artery) or transapically from an incision made at the LV apex on the chest wall. The delivery of the stented valve requires a highly skilled multidisciplinary team involving interventional cardiologists, cardiothoracic and vascular surgeons, cardiac anesthesiologists, and expert imaging cardiologists. The native valve is dilated with a balloon initially. The stented valve is deployed during rapid pacing to allow adequate time for successful placement. This technology has been used in both North America and Europe to treat patients who are too ill to undergo conventional aortic valve replacement and is now undergoing clinical trials. Although excellent symptomatic improvement has resulted in selected patients, the technology is still in its infancy. Paravalvular leak is still common following valve deployment, and the technique has considerable morbidity not least as it has been used up to now in very ill patients.

3. **Surgical therapy.** AVR is the surgical treatment of choice. It is preferred over repair because débridement of aortic valve calcification often results in early postoperative AR from leaflet fibrosis and retraction, a process that progresses over time.
   - **a. Recommendations for the use of AVR** in patients with AS according to the modified 2006 ACC/AHA guidelines are shown in Table 13.2. The major indications are for severe AS with symptoms or where other cardiac surgery is needed or when LV dysfunction develops as a result of severe AS.
   - **b. Surgical mortality** varies among patients with AS depending on age and other comorbidities including concomitant CAD. In an otherwise healthy individual, mortality for isolated AVR in experienced centers should be <1%. When this is the case, the 2006 ACC/AHA guidelines suggest that prophylactic surgical intervention may be warranted in severe AS, even in the absence of symptoms, especially if the valve is calcifed and therefore likely to progress rapidly (class IIb).

     Successful AVR is feasible and life enhancing, even in very elderly patients without multiple comorbidities. Outcome after surgical replacement in individuals with symptomatic AS usually is excellent, with almost normalization of expected survival. Surgical options include pulmonary valve autograft (i.e.,

TABLE 13.2 Recommendations for Aortic Valve Replacement in Patients with Aortic Stenosis (ACC/AHA Guidelines)

Class I

1. Aortic valve replacement (AVR) is indicated for symptomatic patients with severe AS.
2. AVR is indicated for patients with severe aortic stenosis (AS) undergoing coronary artery bypass grafting (CABG) or surgery on the aorta or other heart valves.
3. AVR is recommended for patients with severe AS and left ventricular (LV) systolic dysfunction (ejection fraction <0.50).

Class IIa

AVR is reasonable for patients with moderate AS undergoing CABG or surgery on the aorta or other heart valves.

Class IIb

1. AVR may be considered for asymptomatic patients with severe AS and abnormal response to exercise (e.g., development of symptoms or asymptomatic hypotension).
2. AVR may be considered for adults with severe asymptomatic AS if there is a high likelihood of rapid progression [age, calcification, and coronary artery disease (CAD)] or if surgery might be delayed at the time of symptom onset.
3. AVR may be considered in patients undergoing CABG who have mild AS when there is evidence, such as moderate to severe valve calcification, that progression may be rapid.
4. AVR may be considered for asymptomatic patients with extremely severe AS (aortic valve area <0.6 cm^2, mean gradient >60 mm Hg, and jet velocity >5.0 m per second) when the patient's expected operative mortality is 1.0% or less.

Class III

AVR is not useful for the prevention of sudden death in asymptomatic patients with AS who have none of the findings listed under the class IIa/IIb recommendations.

Ross procedure), aortic valve homograft conduit, a pericardial or porcine bioprosthesis, or a mechanical valve. The relative advantages, disadvantages, and indications for use of the different prostheses are outlined in Chapter 18.

(1) In the Ross procedure, the pulmonary valve and main pulmonary artery are removed as a unit and placed in the aortic position with reimplantation of the coronary arteries. A pulmonary homograft is placed in the pulmonic position. This procedure is best suited for pediatric and adolescent patients with growth potential, because the autograft is capable of growth, does not require anticoagulation and has an excellent hemodynamic profile. The procedure, however, is long and technically difficult and turns a single-valve problem into a double-valve problem susbsequently. Problems at the pulmonary homograft are common in adults treated with this operation.

Aortic valve homografts have been used to treat younger patients, especially those who wish to avoid anticoagulation, in the hope that greater durability of this valve might result than with a bioprosthesis. Unfortunately, more recent data suggest that any durability advantage of a homograft over a bioprosthesis in middle-aged patients is slight. Moreover, the homograft tends to calcify and is often difficult to remove at subsequent reoperations. Therefore, enthusiasm for homografts has waned, except in the setting of endocarditis of native or prosthetic valves with pyogenic complications such as abscess or fistula or when the LVOT tract is small, in which case homografts maximize the flow area and minimize the pressure gradient.

(2) **Bioprostheses** include porcine heterografts and bovine pericardial prostheses. These valves are used most often to treat patients older than 60 years because structural deterioration is much slower in this age group compared with younger patients. These valves have a low risk for thromboembolism and do not necessitate long-term anticoagulation. Because of the sewing ring and struts, all prostheses, both mechanical and biologic, have a pressure gradient across them, even with normal function. The largest possible valve should be inserted to minimize this pressure gradient. The threshold to insert bioprostheses at a younger age continues to decline given the excellent quality of life they afford.

(3) Mechanical valves. The most commonly used mechanical prostheses include the St. Jude, Medtronic-Hall, and CarboMedics prostheses. They all require anticoagulation to minimize risk for valve thrombosis and thromboembolism. These valves are durable if anticoagulation is maintained and careful antibiotic prophylaxis is used over the years. Mechanical valves are used with caution in older patients (>65 years) given the substantial increase in anticoagulation related hemorrhage and resultant mortality in this population.

c. Follow-up care. Patients without symptoms with severe AS should be observed closely and the expected symptoms of AS (shortness of breath, syncope, angina) discussed with them. They should be instructed to seek medical attention if any of these symptoms develop. Patients with severe AS should avoid competitive sports.

G. Special considerations

1. Management of asymptomatic patients with severe AS

a. High-risk patients. Most asymptomatic AS patients have low mortality and morbidity rates. A minority of asymptomatic patients, however, may die suddenly or have rapid progression of disease. These patients may benefit from AVR in the absence of symptoms. Accurate identification of such patients has been difficult. A transaortic flow velocity of >4 m per second predicted a 70% likelihood of needing an AVR within the subsequent 2 years. A flow velocity of <3 m per second corresponded to a low likelihood (<15%) of needing an AVR in the subsequent 5 years. Severe calcification of the valve and a rapid increase in the pressure gradient were predictors of poor outcome in AS in one study. Patients with highly calcified valves and a rapid increase in the pressure gradient may be considered for elective AVR after the transaortic flow velocity is >4 m per second. Other reasonable indications for AVR in patients with severe asymptomatic AS include LV dysfunction attributable to AS, exercise-induced hypotension, pulmonary hypertension (>60 mm Hg), those with a high likelihood of rapid progression, and before pregnancy.

b. Coronary artery bypass grafting (CABG) in moderate AS. Is there a need for AVR? Studies suggest a benefit of concomitant AVR in patients undergoing CABG who have an aortic valve area of <1.5 cm^2. Although concomitant AVR increases the risk of the initial surgery, the need for reoperation is significantly lower for these patients, and this may provide a survival benefit. Patients with mild AS who have evidence of moderate/severe calcification with a high likelihood of rapid progression may also undergo AVR during CABG.

2. Patients with AS and severely reduced ejection fraction. LV dysfunction in patients with AS can result from the afterload stress imposed on the left ventricle by the stenotic valve or from primary contractile dysfunction (e.g., result of other causes of cardiomyopathy). When LV dysfunction results primarily from afterload mismatch, surgical correction of AS often results in improvement or normalization of LV function. In contrast, patients with primary contractile dysfunction have an overall poor prognosis and are unlikely to benefit from AVR. It is important to determine the cause of LV dysfunction in patients with severe AS for prognostic and therapeutic purposes. These patients should be considered in three major groups: those with high transvalvular gradients (mean gradient >40 mm Hg), those with low transvalvular gradients (mean gradient <30 mm Hg), and those with aortic pseudostenosis.

a. High transvalvular gradient. A high transvalvular gradient is a surrogate measure of high-afterload mismatch. When the transvalvular gradient is substantial (e.g., mean gradient >40 mm Hg), surgical correction of AS can result in normalization of LV function.

b. Low transvalvular gradient. Patients with true anatomically severe AS (AVA <1.0 cm^2) and low transvalvular gradients (mean gradient <30 mm Hg) have a very poor prognosis without surgery. Despite a substantial operative mortality, survival appears improved in those treated surgically, especially if they demonstrate **contractile reserve** when challenged with dobutamine. Contractile reserve is defined as the ability to increase transvalvular flow by >20% from baseline. Dobutamine infusion may help to identify the subset of patients with low-gradient AS who benefit from AVR.

c. **Aortic pseudostenosis.** Patients with primary contractile dysfunction and mild AS can have a falsely small calculated valve area, mimicking severe AS. This phenomenon, called aortic pseudostenosis, occurs principally because the force generated by the weakened left ventricle is not sufficient to open a mildly stenotic valve. Differentiating low-gradient, anatomically severe AS from aortic pseudostenosis is usually accomplished by one of two methods: increasing the cardiac output with dobutamine or decreasing the total peripheral resistance with vasodilators such as nitroprusside. Patients with truly severe AS experience a parallel increase in cardiac output and in the transvalvular pressure gradient after dobutamine infusion (in the echocardiography or catheterization laboratory). The calculated valve area, therefore, does not increase. In contrast, dobutamine infusion in patients with aortic pseudostenosis results in an increase in cardiac output without a significant increase in the transvalvular pressure gradient (the mildly stenotic valve is able to accommodate the increase in blood flow). As a result, the calculated aortic valve area increases significantly ($\geq$0.3 cm^2). Nitroprusside infusion can also be used to differentiate true stenosis from pseudostenosis, albeit by a different mechanism. Vasodilators lower SVR. In true severe AS, the transvalvular gradient increases in response to vasodilators, but the fixed LV outflow obstruction does not allow cardiac output to increase concomitantly. In pseudostenosis, the valve resistance is small, and a decrease in SVR is accompanied by a significant increase in cardiac output and a decrease in the transvalvular gradient. The calculated valve area, therefore, remains the same or decreases in true stenosis and increases in pseudostenosis. The differentiation of true severe AS from aortic pseudostenosis is important because patients with aortic pseudostenosis have primary contractile dysfunction and are unlikely to benefit from AVR alone.

3. **Subaortic stenosis.** Surgical removal of the membrane in subaortic obstruction is indicated for symptoms, for asymptomatic patients with a pressure gradient larger than 50 mm Hg, and if there is evidence of concomitant moderate or greater AR as a result of damage to the aortic valve leaflets from the turbulent subvalvular jet.

II. AORTIC REGURGITATION (AR)

A. Introduction.
AR can develop from primary disease of the valve leaflets or from abnormalities of the aortic root or ascending aorta. The chronic and acute forms of AR are distinct disease entities, with different causes, clinical presentation, natural histories, and treatment strategies.

B. Etiology

1. **Chronic AR.** Disease of the valve leaflets can cause AR by inadequate leaflet coaptation, leaflet perforation, or leaflet prolapse. The most common causes of leaflet abnormalities and aortic root abnormalities that lead to the gradual development of AR are shown in Table 13.3. Subaortic stenosis can also cause AR due to a high velocity jet of blood that is a result of the outflow obstruction hitting the aortic valve, causing damage to the leaflets. Perimembranous ventricular septal defects are associated with AR as well. In addition to disease of native valve leaflets, structural deterioration of bioprosthetic valve leaflets is an important cause of chronic AR.
2. **Acute AR.** Acute AR also can result from abnormalities in the valve leaflets or in the aortic root. The causes of acute AR are limited (Table 13.4).

C. Pathophysiology

1. **Chronic AR.** AR results in diastolic regurgitation of LV stroke volume. This produces an increase in LV end-diastolic volume, thereby raising wall tension (i.e., Laplace's law). The ventricle responds to added wall tension by compensatory

TABLE 13.3 Major Causes of Chronic Aortic Regurgitation

Leaflet abnormalities	Aortic root or ascending aorta abnormalities
Rheumatic fever	Age-related aortic dilation
Infective endocarditis	Annuloaortic ectasia
Trauma	Cystic medial necrosis of the aorta (isolated biscuspid aortic valve or Marfan's syndrome)
Myxomatous degeneration	
Congenital aortic regurgitation	Systemic hypertension
Systemic lupus erythematosus	Aortitis (syphilis, giant cell arteritis)
Rheumatoid arthritis	Reiter's syndrome
Ankylosing spondylitis	Ankylosing spondylitis
Takayasu's arteritis	Behçet's syndrome
Whipple's disease	Psoriatic arthritis
Crohn's disease	Osteogenesis imperfecta
Drug induced valvulopathy	Relapsing polychondritis
	Ehlers-Danlos syndrome

eccentric hypertrophy of myocytes. As a result, during the chronic compensated phase of AR, the left ventricle is able to adapt to an increase in diastolic volume without a significant increase in end-diastolic pressure. The left ventricle produces a larger total stroke volume with each contraction, preserving normal effective forward stroke volume. Over time, however, progressive interstitial fibrosis reduces LV compliance, leading to the chronic decompensated phase. Chronic volume overload results in impaired LV emptying, an increase in LV end-systolic volume and end-diastolic pressure, further cardiac dilation, and a fall in the ejection fraction and forward cardiac output.

2. **Acute AR.** Acute AR is usually a hemodynamic emergency because the left ventricle does not have sufficient time to adapt to the rapid increase in LV volume. The effective forward stroke volume and cardiac output fall acutely, potentially resulting in hypotension and cardiogenic shock. The sudden increase in LV diastolic pressure initially causes preclosure of the mitral valve in early diastole, protecting the pulmonary vasculature from elevated diastolic pressure. However, further LV decompensation leads to diastolic MR, which allows transmission of elevated diastolic pressure to the pulmonary vascular bed, resulting in formation of pulmonary edema fluid. The tachycardia that accompanies cardiac deterioration helps shorten the diastolic-filling period during which the mitral valve is open.

D. History and clinical presentation

1. **Chronic AR** usually is asymptomatic for a long time. After LV dysfunction develops, patients gradually experience symptoms related to pulmonary congestion, including increased dyspnea with exertion, orthopnea, and paroxysmal nocturnal dyspnea. LV enlargement frequently produces an uncomfortable sensation in the chest that is exaggerated after premature ventricular contractions and in the supine

TABLE 13.4 Major Causes of Acute Aortic Regurgitation

Leaflet abnormalities	Aortic root or ascending aorta abnormalities
Traumatic rupture	Acute aortic dissection
Acute infective endocarditis	Perivalvular leak or dehiscence of prosthetic valves
Acute prosthetic valve dysfunction	
Post aortic balloon valvuloplasty	

position. Although angina is uncommon, it can be produced by latent CAD, decreased diastolic coronary perfusion pressure, nocturnal bradycardia and fall in arterial diastolic pressure, marked LV hypertrophy, and subendocardial ischemia.

2. **Acute AR.** Patients with acute, severe AR usually present with signs of sudden hemodynamic deterioration such as weakness, altered mental status, severe shortness of breath, or syncope. Untreated, these patients quickly progress to total cardiovascular collapse. When severe chest pain is part of the initial clinical presentation, aortic dissection must be strongly suspected.

E. Physical findings

1. **Chronic AR.** Patients with chronic AR can have a wide array of physical findings, especially during examination of the peripheral pulses and cardiac auscultation. The physical examination may yield clues about the cause of the AR. Patients with AR should be examined for the peripheral manifestations of infective endocarditis, signs of Marfan's syndrome, evidence of chronic aortic dissection, and signs of collagen vascular disorders.

   a. **Peripheral pulse examination.** The increased total stroke volume in chronic AR leads to an abrupt increase in arterial pressure during systole, followed by a rapid fall in arterial pressure during diastole. The widened pulse pressure accounts for a number of the physical findings associated with chronic AR (Table 13.5). Patients with chronic AR may exhibit a bisferiens pulse, characterized by double systolic peaks with increased amplitude. The signs of hyperdynamic circulation are not specific to AR, and can be seen in conditions causing high-output heart failure, including sepsis, anemia, thyrotoxicosis, beriberi, and arteriovenous fistula.

   b. **Palpation.** With severe AR, the apical impulse is typically enlarged and displaced lateral to the midclavicular line in the fifth intercostal space because of LV enlargement. The impulse may be sustained and hyperdynamic. A triple impulse typically represents a palpable, rapid, filling spike, or S_3, in addition to a palpable *a* wave. A diastolic thrill may be palpable in the second left intercostal space, as may a systolic thrill caused by increased aortic flow.

   c. **Auscultation.** The main auscultatory findings are outlined in Figure 13.6.

      (1) **Heart sounds.** S_1 may be diminished in the presence of PR-interval prolongation, LV dysfunction, or preclosure of the mitral valve. S_2 may be soft, singly split (P_2 obscured by the diastolic murmur), or paradoxically split. An S_3 may be heard with severe LV dysfunction. An S_4 often is present and represents left atrial contraction into a poorly compliant LV.

TABLE 13.5 Physical Signs Associated with Hyperdynamic Pulse in Chronic Aortic Regurgitation

Physical sign	Description
Water-hammer or Corrigan's pulse	Rapid upstroke followed by quick collapse
DeMusset's sign	Head bob with each heartbeat
Traube's sign	Pistol shot sounds heard over the femoral arteries in both systole and diastole
Müller's sign	Systolic pulsation of the uvula
Duroziez's sign	Systolic murmur over the femoral artery when compressed proximally and diastolic murmur when compressed distally or systolic-diastolic murmur with increasing compression over femoral artery
Quincke's sign	Capillary pulsations visible in the lunula of the nailbed
Hill's sign	Popliteal cuff systolic pressure exceeding brachial cuff systolic pressure by >60 mm Hg
Becker's sign	Arterial pulsations visible in the retinal arteries and pupils

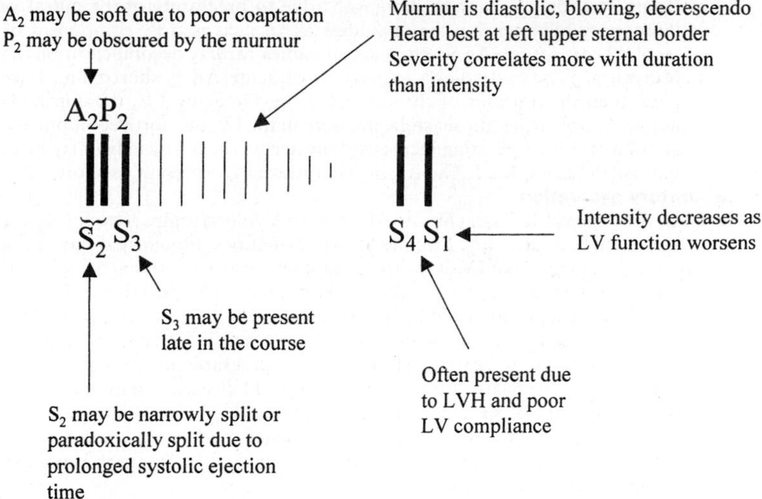

Figure 13.6. Physical findings in aortic regurgitation. LV, left ventricle; LVH, left ventricular hypertrophy.

(2) Diastolic murmur. The hallmark murmur of AR is a blowing, diastolic, decrescendo murmur that starts immediately after A_2 and is best heard in the left upper sternal border with the patient sitting up and leaning forward slightly in full expiration. In general, the severity of AR correlates with the duration of the murmur more than with its intensity. Early in the course of disease, the murmur is typically short. As the disease progresses, the murmur may become pandiastolic. In the end stages of AR, the murmur may shorten again because of rapid equilibration of pressures in the aorta and left ventricle from an elevated LVEDP. In this situation, other signs of severe AR usually are present.

(3) A **second diastolic murmur** may be audible at the apex in severe AR. The Austin Flint murmur is a middle-to-late diastolic rumble believed to be caused by vibration of the anterior mitral leaflet as it is struck by the regurgitant jet or by turbulence in the mitral inflow from partial closure of the mitral valve by the regurgitant jet. Unlike the murmur of true valvular mitral stenosis, the Austin Flint murmur is not associated with a loud S_1 or with an opening snap.

(4) A short **midsystolic ejection murmur** may be audible at the base of the heart, radiating to the neck. It reflects the increased ejection rate and large stroke volume traversing the aortic valve (i.e., functional AS).

2. Acute AR. The physical examination associated with acute AR differs considerably from the physical examination of patients with chronic AR. The physical examination may be most notable for signs of hemodynamic compromise, such as hypotension, tachycardia, pallor, cyanosis, diaphoresis, cool extremities, and pulmonary congestion.

a. Peripheral examination. The signs of hyperdynamic circulation that characterize chronic AR are often absent in acute AR. The pulse pressure may be normal or only slightly widened. The heart size is often normal, and the point of maximal intensity is not displaced laterally. When aortic dissection is suspected, blood pressures should be taken in all extremities to detect potential differences.

b. **Heart sounds.** S_1 may be diminished due to preclosure of the mitral valve. Pulmonary hypertension may manifest as an increased P_2 component of the second heart sound. An S_3 often accompanies cardiac decompensation.

c. **Murmurs.** The early diastolic murmur of acute AR is shorter and lower in pitch than the murmur of chronic AR. In severe acute AR, the murmur may not be audible when the diastolic pressure in the LV and aorta equilibrates. The systolic murmur reflecting increased flow across the aortic valve may be heard but usually is not loud. The Austin Flint murmur, if present, is short.

F. Laboratory evaluation

1. **ECG.** The typical ECG in chronic AR shows LV hypertrophy, left-axis deviation, and left atrial abnormality. Conduction abnormalities are unusual but can occur after the development of LV dysfunction. Premature atrial and ventricular beats are common. Sustained supraventricular or ventricular tachyarrhythmias are uncommon in the absence of LV dysfunction or concomitant mitral valve disease. In acute AR, the ECG usually is notable only for nonspecific ST-T-wave abnormalities.

2. **Chest radiograph.** In chronic AR, the chest radiograph may reveal marked cardiomegaly, with the heart displaced inferiorly and leftward. Dilation of the aortic knob and root may be seen. In acute AR, the LV and left atrial dimensions usually are normal. Aortic dissection can lead to a widened mediastium and/or a widened cardiac silhouette due to pericardial effusion. The chest radiograph is notable for signs of pulmonary congestion.

3. **Echocardiography.** Two-dimensional and M-mode echocardiography are useful for determining the cause of AR, evaluating the aortic root, and assessing overall LV size and function. Doppler echocardiography is useful for detecting AR and estimating severity. There are several different methods of estimating the severity of AR with color Doppler, pulsed wave Doppler, and continuous wave Doppler ultrasonography.

   a. **Two-dimensional and M-mode echocardiography.** The cause of AR can be assessed using two-dimensional echocardiography. Rheumatic AR typically causes thickening and retraction of the leaflet tips, leading to failure of cusp apposition. Bacterial endocarditis, which can cause leaflet fibrosis and retraction, leaflet perforation, or flail of the valve cusp, should be suspected if a vegetation is detected. Prolapse of the aortic valve cusps can occur in many conditions, including infective endocarditis, bicuspid aortic valve, myxomatous degeneration, and Marfan's syndrome. Aortic root abnormalities are also well visualized in the parasternal long-axis view. Aortic root dilation most often is idiopathic, although Marfan's syndrome, Ehlers-Danlos syndrome, ankylosing spondylitis, Reiter's syndrome, rheumatoid arthritis, syphilis, and giant cell arteritis are other potential causes. Symmetric dilation of the aortic root produces a central jet of AR, and focal dilation causes an eccentric jet. In the parasternal long axis, the transducer should be moved up one interspace to assess the ascending aorta. Infective destruction of the aortic wall and proximal aortic dissection flaps occasionally may be visualized on transthoracic images. M-mode echocardiography may reveal **premature closure of the mitral valve in severe, acute AR**. In acute and chronic AR, the regurgitant jet can strike the anterior mitral valve leaflet, causing it to reverberate or "flutter" in diastole. Reversed doming of the anterior mitral leaflet may be seen on two-dimensional imaging and generally indicates grade 3 to 4+ AR.

   b. **Doppler and color flow imaging.** Doppler and color flow echocardiography is used to detect AR and to assess its severity. AR is identified by Doppler imaging as high-velocity pandiastolic flow originating immediately under the aortic valve. Color flow imaging allows assessment of jet origin, size, and direction. Continuous-wave Doppler provides measurement of jet velocity and timing of flow. The maximum length of the AR jet correlates poorly with severity of regurgitation, assessed angiographically. Several other Doppler measures are used to estimate the severity of AR (Table 13.6). The ratio of the jet width to LVOT diameter is measured in the parasternal long-axis view and correlates well with the angiographic severity of AR. The pressure half-time of the aortic

TABLE 13.6 Echo-Doppler Assessment of Aortic Regurgitation Severity (modified from ACC/AHA Valve Guidelines)

	Aortic regurgitation		
	Mild	**Moderate**	**Severe**
Qualitative			
Angiographic grade	1+	2+	3–4+
Color Doppler jet width	Central jet, width <25% of LVOT	➢ mild but no signs of severe AR	Central jet, width >65% LVOT
Doppler vena contracta width (cm)	<0.3	0.3–0.6	>0.6
Quantitative (cath or echo)			
Regurgitant volume (mL per beat)	<30	30–59	≥60
Regurgitant fraction (%)	<30	30–49	≥50
Regurgitant orifice area (cm^2)	<0.10	0.10–0.29	≥0.30
Additional essential criteria			
Left ventricular size			Increased

AR, Aortic regurgitation; LVOT, left ventricular outflow tract.

regurgitant velocity is defined as the time required for the pressure gradient across the aortic valve to fall to half of its initial value. The pressure half-times of patients with mild, moderate, and severe AR have demonstrated considerable overlap. In general, shorter pressure half-times are associated with increased severity of AR, and a pressure half-time of <200 ms is nearly always associated with severe AR. Quantitation of regurgitant volume and regurgitant fraction provide the most direct correlation with quantitative angiographic estimates of AR severity. Regurgitant volume is the difference between the stroke volume across the LVOT (representing the sum of forward and regurgitant flow) and across the mitral valve inflow (representing forward flow), provided there is not significant MR. The regurgitant fraction is the ratio of the regurgitant volume divided by the LVOT stroke volume. The proximal isovelocity surface area (PISA) method also is used for estimating AR severity (see Chapter 61). The PISA method is used to calculate the effective regurgitant orifice (ERO) area. An ERO area equal to or >0.30 cm^2 is indicative of severe AR. The presence of a proximal convergence area on TTE at the aortic valve is indicative of at least moderate AR. Pulsed-wave Doppler echocardiography should be performed in the proximal descending aorta to establish the presence of diastolic flow reversal. Some degree of flow reversal is seen normally early in dastole due to reflux of blood into the coronary vasculature, but if this is >40 cm/s and continues throughout diastole, then severe AR is likely especially if this persists in the abdominal aorta. Flow reversal may also be seen with other conditions that cause blood to leak out of the arterial system such as patent ductus arteriosus (PDA) or sizeable arteriovenoou fistula.

c. TEE is used to rule out vegetation or aortic valve ring abscess in patients who may have bacterial endocarditis. In pure AR, vegetation typically occurs on the LV side of the aortic valve. TEE also is used to visualize congenital valvular abnormalities (e.g., bicuspid valve) and to exclude aortic dissection.

d. Stress echocardiography is useful for assessing the ability to exercise. However, a fall in LVEF on exercise is less predictive of occult contractile dysfunction in severe AR than it is in MR. In AR, afterload often increases substantially on exercise, precipitating a fall in ejection fraction. A fall in LVEF on stress echocardiography alone is not a primary indication for valve surgery.

TABLE 13.7 Angiographic Grading of Aortic Regurgitation

Degree of aortic regurgitation	Left ventricular opacification	Rate of clearing
Mild (1+)	Faint, incomplete	Rapid
Moderate (2+)	Faint, complete	Rapid
Moderate to severe (3+)	Equal to aortic opacification	Intermediate
Severe (4+)	Greater than aortic opacification	Slow

4. Cardiac catheterization. Cardiac catheterization is not necessary for all patients with chronic AR unless there are concerns about AR severity, hemodynamic abnormalities, or LV function, despite noninvasive testing and the physical examination. All patients older than 50 years with severe AR should undergo coronary cine angiography before any definitive surgical procedure on the valve to detect CAD. The decision to perform cardiac catheterization in younger patients should be made on an individual basis after assessment of the patient's cardiac risk profile. Catheter manipulation in patients with AR may be difficult because of dilation of the ascending aorta. Caution should be exercised when manipulating catheters in patients with Marfan's syndrome or cystic medial necrosis of the aortic wall to minimize the risk for vascular trauma. In addition to conventional coronary cine angiography, aortography should be performed to evaluate the degree of AR. The grading of AR by angiography is shown in Table 13.7. Right heart catheterization may be helpful in certain circumstances, such as new-onset heart failure or combined AR and AS.

G. Natural history. Moderate-to-severe AR may have a good prognosis for many years, provided that the patient is asymptomatic and does not exhibit signs of LV dysfunction or severe dilation. Asymptomatic patients with normal LV function require AVR at a rate of only 4% per year. Ninety percent of such patients remain asymptomatic at 3 years, 81% at 5 years, and 75% at 7 years after the diagnosis is made. Patients with mild-to-moderate AR have had 10-year survival rates of 85% to 95%. Patients with moderate-to-severe AR treated with medical therapy have 5-year survival rates of 75% and 10-year survival rates of 50%. After LV dysfunction develops, progression to symptoms is greatly accelerated, with rates approaching 25% per year. When symptoms develop, there is a rapid decline in functional status. Without surgical intervention, symptomatic patients usually die within 4 years of the onset of angina and within 2 years of the onset of heart failure. Sudden death may occur among patients with severe, symptomatic AR. Sudden cardiac death is frequently the result of ventricular arrhythmias that are primary (in the context of LV hypertrophy or dysfunction) or secondary, resulting from myocardial ischemia. It has become clear that the various dimensions used to guide surgery in AR are relative and should be interpreted in the context of patient size and gender.

H. Therapy

1. Medical therapy

a. Chronic AR

(1) Medical therapy. Vasodilators, such as hydralazine, angiotensin-converting enzyme (ACE) inhibitors, and calcium channel blockers, have been used in the treatment of chronic AR to reduce the severity of regurgitation and help delay surgical intervention. There is conflicting evidence of their value (Table 13.8). Current ACC/AHA guidelines contraindicate their use (class III) as an alternative to surgery when surgical intervention is indicated in a patient with acceptable surgical risk. Vasodilators are recommended in nonsurgical candidates with severe, chronic AR who develop symptoms or LV dysfunction. Vasodilators may also be reasonable for short-term therapy, improving the hemodynamics in patients with severe heart failure and LV systolic dysfunction prior to AVR. In asymptomatic patients, long-term

TABLE 13.8 Indications for Vasodilator Therapy in Chronic Severe Aortic Regurgitation

Indication	Class
Chronic therapy in patients with severe regurgitation who have symptoms and/or LV dysfunction when surgery is not recommended because of additional cardiac or noncardiac factors	I
Short-term therapy to improve the hemodynamic profile of patients with severe heart failure symptoms and severe LV dysfunction prior to proceeding with AVR	IIa
Long-term therapy in asymptomatic patients with severe regurgitation who have LV dilation but normal systolic function	IIb
Not indicated for long-term therapy in asymptomatic patients with mild to moderate AR and normal LV systolic function	III
Not indicated for long-term therapy in asymptomatic patients with LV systolic dysfunction who are otherwise candidates for valve replacement	III
Not indicated for long-term therapy in symptomatic patients with either normal LV function or mild to moderate LV systolic dysfunction who are otherwise candidates for valve replacement	III

AR, aortic regurgitation; AVR, aortic valve replacement; LV, left ventricular.
Bonow RO, Carabello B, Chatterjee K, et al. ACC/AHA 2006 guidelines for the management of patients with valvular heart disease: An executive summary. A report of the American College of Cardiology/American Heart Association Task Force on Practice Guidelines (Writing committee to revise the 1998 guidelines for the management of patients with valvular heart disease). *J Am Coll Cardiol* 2006;48:598–675.

vasodilator therapy may be considered for those with severe AR and normal LV systolic function who begin to demonstrate LV dilation. Long-term vasodilator therapy is not recommended for asymptomatic patients with mild-to-moderate AR and normal systolic function. These patients have a good prognosis and do not appear to benefit from vasodilator therapy. Although asymptomatic patients with LV systolic dysfunction or symptomatic patients may be treated with vasodilators in the short term, appropriate surgical candidates should be referred for AVR, and vasodilators should be continued on a long-term basis only if LV systolic dysfunction persists after AVR. The evidence for the use of specific vasodilator agents has been variable. Hydralazine was found to improve LV systolic function and to reduce LV chamber dimensions in some studies. Nifedipine was found to reduce LV volume and increase LVEF in a group of asymptomatic patients who were followed for 1 year. When compared with digoxin, nifedipine slowed the progression of LV dysfunction and delayed the time to surgical treatment in an unblinded, randomized study over a 5-year period. ACE inhibitors have been shown to decrease LV volume in some studies. However, the benefits of ACE-inhibitor therapy were seen only when blood pressure was effectively lowered.

(2) In patients with significant aortic root dilation as a result of cystic medial necrosis or related conditions, treatment with a β-blocker should be considered to slow the rate at which the aortic root enlarges. This has been proved to be beneficial in Marfan's syndrome and patients with bicuspid AV and dilated aortic roots without moderate or severe AR. After aortic root dilation is larger than 5 cm in severe AR (lower in Marfan's syndrome), aortic valve surgery and root replacement are indicated.

b. Acute AR

(1) The goal of **medical therapy** in acute AR is hemodynamic stabilization before proceeding with surgical correction. For patients presenting with cardiogenic shock, intravenous vasodilators are used to reduce the afterload stress on the LV, to lower LVEDP, and to augment forward cardiac output. In severe cases, intravenous inotropic agents may be required for temporary hemodynamic support. β-Blockers may be used with caution when acute AR is caused by an aortic dissection. β-Blockers help to reduce arterial dP/dt, which reflects the transmission of force from LV ejection to the arterial wall. Although this is an essential component of the treatment of acute aortic dissection, β-blockers increase the length of diastole by slowing the heart rate, which can exacerbate acute AR and contribute to cardiovascular collapse.

(2) A **surgical evaluation** should be performed immediately for a patient with AR caused by aortic dissection or chest trauma. The goal of medical therapy in this setting is to maximize forward cardiac output and minimize propagation of aortic dissection if present.

(3) If acute AR is associated with **endocarditis**, antibiotic therapy should be instituted as soon as all culture specimens are obtained.

2. Percutaneous therapy. Insertion of an intraaortic balloon counterpulsation device (IABP) in patients with more than moderate AR or in the presence of aortic dissection is contraindicated. Patients with combined AS and AR are poor candidates for PABV because the degree of AR is likely to increase after the procedure.

3. Surgical therapy

a. Chronic AR. The ACC/AHA guidelines on the indications for AVR in patients with chronic AR are shown in Table 13.9.

(1) Symptomatic patients. The updated ACC/AHA guidelines state that AVR is recommended for symptomatic patients with severe AR regardless of the ejection fraction.

(2) The indications for AVR in **asymptomatic patients** remain controversial. AVR is recommended when patients with chronic severe AR are undergoing CABG surgery or surgery on the aorta or other heart valves. Asymptomatic

TABLE 13.9 Indications for Aortic Valve Replacement in Severe Aortic Regurgitation

Indication	Class
Symptomatic patients with severe AR irrespective of LV systolic function	I
Asymptomatic patients with chronic severe AR and LV systolic dysfunction (EF <50%) at rest	I
Patients with chronic severe AR undergoing coronary artery bypass surgery or surgery on the aorta or other heart valves	I
Asymptomatic patients with severe AR and EF >50%, but with severe LV dilation (EDD >75 mm or ESD >55 mm[a])	IIa
Patients with moderate AS while undergoing surgery on the ascending aorta or coronary artery bypass grafting surgery.	IIb
Asymptomatic patients with severe AR and normal LV systolic function (EF >50%) when the EDD >70 mm or ESD >50 mm, when there is evidence of progressive LV dilation[a], declining exercise tolerance or abnormal hemodynamic responses to exercise.	IIb
AVR not indicated for asymptomatic patients with mild, moderate, or severe AR and normal LV systolic function at rest (EF >50%) and when degree of dilatation is not severe (EDD <70 mm, ESD <50 mm)	III

EF, ejection fraction; EDD, end-diastolic dimension; ESD, end-systolic dimension

[a]**Consider lower threshold values for patients of small stature of either gender.**

Bonow RO, Carabello B, Chatterjee K, et al. ACC/AHA 2006 guidelines for the management of patients with valvular heart disease: An executive summary. A report of the American College of Cardiology/American Heart Association Task Force on Practice Guidelines (Writing committee to revise the 1998 guidelines for the management of patients with valvular heart disease.) *J Am Coll Cardiol* 2006;48:598–675.

patients with chronic severe AR and LV systolic dysfunction (ejection fraction <50%) are at high risk for the development of symptomatic heart failure within 2 to 3 years and, therefore, should be considered for elective surgical intervention. Asymptomatic patients with normal LV systolic function at rest and evidence of severe LV dilation (LV end-diastolic dimension >75 mm, end-systolic dimension >55 mm) have an increased risk of sudden cardiac death. Their prognosis after AVR, however, is excellent, and they should be referred for valve replacement. After patients with severe LV dilation develop symptoms or LV systolic dysfunction, the perioperative mortality rate increases significantly. AVR is not recommended in asymptomatic patients with normal systolic function at rest and normal or mildly abnormal LV dimensions (end-diastolic dimension <70 mm, end-systolic dimension <50 mm).

(3) The **surgical alternatives** are discussed in section on aortic stenosis. Many patients with prolapse of bicuspid valve as the cause of AR may be candidates for surgical repair of the aortic valve. Some patients with leaflet perforation caused by infectious endocarditis may be candidates for repair in which a pericardial patch is sewn over the defect.

4. Follow-up care. Patients with chronic AR should be observed closely for the development of LV systolic dysfunction. Follow-up evaluation typically is conducted with serial echocardiography. After signs of LV systolic dysfunction manifest, consideration should be given to surgical therapy, even if the patient has no symptoms. Routine postoperative care is appropriate after AVR or repair is completed.

5. Key suggestions

a. Acute, severe AR usually is a surgical emergency. Signs of congestive heart failure and mitral valve preclosure are ominous in acute AR.

b. Valve replacement can be performed without infection of the prosthesis in active endocarditis, even when antibiotics have only recently been started. An aortic valve homograft is the preferred prosthesis in the setting of endocarditis.

c. Aortic dissection should be suspected in any patient with chest pain and AR.

d. If LV systolic dysfunction is present for <18 months, LV function is likely to improve postoperatively.

e. Heart rate usually is normal until late in the course of disease, when a low effective stroke volume is compensated with tachycardia to maintain cardiac output.

f. Rapid atrial or ventricular pacing may be used as a temporary measure to manage acute AR caused by endocarditis or trauma to improve cardiac output. The diastolic filling phase is shorter at higher heart rates; therefore, there is less time for valvular regurgitation.

Landmark Articles

Bellamy MF, Pellika PA, Klarich KW, et al. Association of cholesterol levels, hydroxymethylglutaryl coenzyme-A reductase inhibitor treatment, and progression of AS in the community. *J Am Coll Cardiol* 2002;40:1723–1730.

Bonow RO, Carabello B, Chatterjee K, et al. ACC/AHA 2006 guidelines for the management of patients with valvular heart disease: An executive summary. A report of the American College of Cardiology/American Heart Association Task Force on Practice Guidelines (Writing committee to revise the 1998 guidelines for the management of patients with valvular heart disease). *J Am Coll Cardiol* 2006;48:598–675.

Borer JS, Hochreiter C, Herrold EM, et al. Prediction of indications for valve replacement among asymptomatic or minimally symptomatic patients with chronic aortic regurgitation and normal left ventricular performance. *Circulation* 1998;97:525–534.

Brener SJ, Duffy CI, Thomas JD, et al. Progression of aortic stenosis in 394 patients: relation to changes in myocardial and mitral valve dysfunction. *J Am Coll Cardiol* 1995;25:305–310.

Connolly HM, Oh JK, Schaff HV, et al. Severe aortic stenosis with low transvalvular gradient and severe left ventricular dysfunction: result of aortic valve replacement in 52 patients. *Circulation* 2000;101:1940–1946.

Currie PJ, Sewaard JB, Chan KL, et al. Continuous wave Doppler echocardiographic assessment of severity of calcific aortic stenosis: a simultaneous Doppler-catheter correlative study in 100 consecutive patients. *Circulation* 1985;71:1162–1169.

Kelly TA, Rothbart RM, Cooper CM, et al. Comparison of outcome of asymptomatic to symptomatic patients older than 20 years of age with valvular aortic stenosis. *Am J Cardiol* 1988;61:123–130.

Khot UN, Novaro GM, Popovic ZB, et al. Nitroprusside in critically ill patients with left ventricular dysfunction and aortic stenosis. *N Engl J Med* 2003;348:1756–1763.

Novaro GM, Tiong IY, Pearce GL, et al. Effect of hydroxymethylglutaryl coenzyme a reductase inhibitors on the progression of calcific aortic stenosis. *Circulation* 2001;104:2205–2209.

Otto CM, Burwash IG, Legget ME, et al. Prospective study of asymptomatic valvular aortic stenosis: clinical, echocardiographic, and exercise predictors of outcome. *Circulation* 1997;95:2262–2270.
Otto CM, Lind BK, Kitzman DW, et al. Association of aortic-valve sclerosis with cardiovascular morbidity and mortality in the elderly. *N Engl J Med* 1999;341:142–147.
Pellikka PA, Nishimura RA, Bailey KR, et al. The natural history of adults with asymptomatic, hemodynamically significant aortic stenosis. *J Am Coll Cardiol* 1990;15:1012–1017.
Pereira JJ, Lauer MS, Bashir M, et al. Survival after aortic valve replacement for severe aortic stenosis with low transvalvular gradients and severe left ventricular dysfunction. *J Am Coll Cardiol* 2002;39:1356–1363.
Rosenhek R, Binder T, Porenta G, et al. Predictors of outcome in severe asymptomatic aortic valve stenosis. *N Engl J Med* 2000;343:611–617.
Ross J Jr, Braunwald E. Aortic stenosis. *Circulation* 1968;37[Suppl V]:V61–V67.
Wilson W, Taubert KA, Gewitz M, et al. Prevention of infective endocarditis: Guidelines from the American Heart Association. *Circulation* 2007;116:1736–1754.

Key Reviews

Braunwald E. On the natural history of severe aortic stenosis [Editorial]. *J Am Coll Cardiol* 1990;15:1018–1020.
Carabello BA. Timing of valve replacement in aortic stenosis: moving closer to perfection. *Circulation* 1997;95:2241–2243.
Carabello BA, Crawford FA. Valvular heart disease. *N Engl J Med* 1997;337:32–41.
Gaasch WH, Sundaram M, Meyer TE. Managing asymptomatic patients with chronic aortic regurgitation. *Chest* 1997;111:1702–1709.

Relevant Book Chapters

Carabello BA, Stewart WJ, Crawford FA. Aortic valve disease. In: Topol EJ, ed. *Textbook of cardiovascular medicine,* 2nd ed. Philadelphia: Lippincott-Raven, 2002:509–528.
Meier DJ, Landolfo CK, Starling MR. Role of echocardiography in the timing of surgical intervention for chronic mitral and aortic regurgitation. In: Otto CM, ed. *The practice of clinical echocardiography,* 2nd ed. Philadelphia: WB Saunders, 2002:389–416.
Shavelle DM, Otto CM. Aortic stenosis: echocardiographic evaluation of disease severity, disease progression, and the role of echocardiography in clinical decision making. In: Otto CM, ed. *The practice of clinical echocardiography,* 2nd ed. Philadelphia: WB Saunders, 2002:469–500.
Weyman AE, Griffin BP. Left ventricular outflow tract: the aortic valve, aorta, and subvalvular outflow tract. In: Weyman AE, ed. *Principles and practice of echocardiography,* 2nd ed. Philadelphia: Lea & Febiger, 1994:498–574.

14 MITRAL VALVE DISEASE

Carmel M. Halley, Maran Thamilarasan, and Brian P. Griffin

I. INTRODUCTION

A. The **mitral valvular apparatus** consists of the anterior and posterior leaflets, the mitral annulus, the chordae tendineae, and the papillary muscles.

B. Mitral regurgitation (MR) can occur as a result of malfunction of any of these components.

C. Mitral valve prolapse (MVP) exists when one or both mitral leaflets extend across the plane of the mitral valve annulus into the left atrium during systole.

D. Mitral stenosis (MS) usually is valvular, and more rarely is caused by fusion of subvalvular components.

II. MITRAL REGURGITATION

A. Clinical presentation

1. Signs and symptoms

a. With **acute, severe de novo MR,** the symptoms are caused by an abrupt rise in pulmonary capillary wedge pressure, causing pulmonary congestion. These symptoms include rest dyspnea, orthopnea, and possibly signs of diminished forward flow, including cardiogenic shock.

b. Chronic MR is usually **asymptomatic** for years. The most common presentation is an asymptomatic murmur. **When symptoms develop,** exercise intolerance and exertional dyspnea usually occur first. Orthopnea and paroxysmal nocturnal dyspnea may develop as MR progresses. Fatigue is caused by diminished forward cardiac output. With development of left ventricular (LV) dysfunction, further symptoms of congestive heart failure (CHF) are manifest. **Long-standing MR** may cause **pulmonary hypertension,** with symptoms of right ventricular (RV) failure. Atrial fibrillation may occur as a consequence of left atrial (LA) dilation.

2. Physical findings

a. Palpation. When LV function is preserved, carotid upstrokes are sharp, and the cardiac apical impulse is brisk and hyperdynamic. An early diastolic LV filling wave may be palpable because of the large volume of blood traversing from the left atrium to left ventricle. A late systolic thrust may be present in the parasternal location because of systolic expansion of the left atrium (it may be difficult to differentiate this from an RV lift). With the development of LV dilation, the apical impulse is displaced laterally. An RV heave and palpable P_2 are present if pulmonary hypertension has developed.

b. Auscultation. The main auscultatory findings are summarized in Figure 14.1. A loud S_4 (not illustrated) sometimes can be heard, particularly with acute MR. In acute, severe MR, the systolic driving pressure across the mitral valve is reduced due to a high LA pressure, and as a result, the murmur is short and relatively soft. If LA pressure is markedly elevated, the murmur of acute MR may be inaudible.

c. With advanced LV dysfunction, the typical **findings of pulmonary congestion** may be evident. If secondary RV dysfunction develops, an elevated jugular venous pulse, hepatomegaly, ascites, and peripheral edema are present.

3. The **differential diagnosis of holosystolic murmurs** includes MR, tricuspid regurgitation, and ventricular septal defect (VSD). All are high pitched, but the murmur of a VSD is often harsh in quality, unlike the blowing murmurs of MR and tricuspid regurgitation.

a. The murmur of **MR** is best heard in the apical position and often radiates to the axilla (although possibly to the base with anteriorly directed jets); those of tricuspid regurgitation and VSD typically do not. The murmur of posteriorly directed MR radiates well to the back.

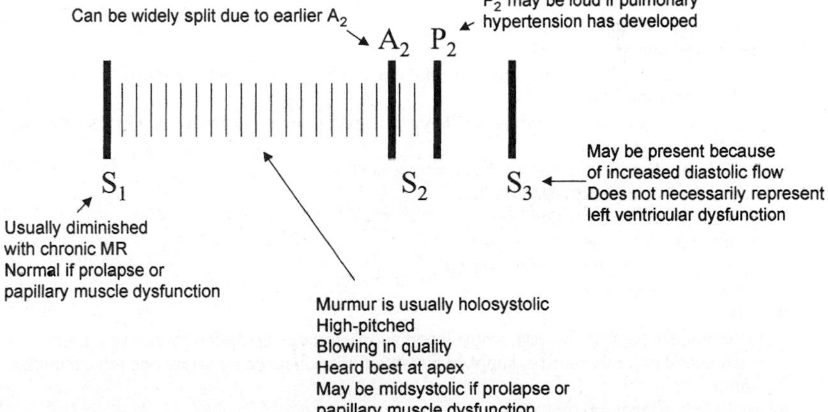

Figure 14.1. Auscultatory findings in mitral regurgitation.

b. Tricuspid regurgitation is heard best at the lower left sternal border and radiates to the right of the sternum and left midclavicular line. Like all right-sided murmurs, tricuspid regurgitation is accentuated by inspiration.

c. A **VSD** murmur also may be heard at the left sternal border and often radiates throughout the precordium.

B. Etiology and pathophysiology. MR usually has a myxomatous or ischemic rather than a rheumatic cause. Table 14.1 summarizes the causes of MR.

1. In **acute MR,** the regurgitant volume that returns from the left atrium causes a **sudden increase in LV end-diastolic volume.** The left ventricle compensates for this by means of the Frank-Starling mechanism: increased sarcomere length (preload) enhances LV contraction (inotropy). This occurs at the cost of increasing LV filling pressure and may cause symptoms of pulmonary congestion. LV wall stress (afterload) is reduced because blood is ejected into the lower-pressure left atrium as well as into the systemic circulation. Increased inotropy and reduced

TABLE 14.1 Causes of Mitral Regurgitation

LEAFLET ABNORMALITIES
Myxomatous degeneration of leaflets with excessive motion (most common)
Rheumatic disease: scarring and contraction lead to loss of leaflet tissue
Endocarditis: can cause leaflet perforations and retraction in healing phase
Aneurysms: usually from aortic valve endocarditis; aortic insufficiency produces jet lesion on mitral valve
Congenital:
Cleft mitral valve: isolated or with ostium primum atrial septal defect
Double-orifice mitral valve
Hypertrophic cardiomyopathy: systolic anterior motion of the mitral valve
MITRAL ANNULAR ABNORMALITIES
Annular dilation
From left ventricular dilation: dilated cardiomyopathy, ischemic disease, hypertension
Normal 10 cm in circumference
With sufficient dilation, loss of adequate leaflet coaptation
Tethering of leaflet and chordae can occur and produce relative restriction of leaflet motion
Mitral annular calcification
Degenerative disorder, most commonly seen in the elderly
Accelerated by hypertension or diabetes
Also seen in renal failure with dystrophic calcification
Also seen with rheumatic heart disease
Marfan's syndrome, Hurler's syndrome
Mitral regurgitation results from immobility of the annulus, loss of sphincter activity
CHORDAL ABNORMALITIES
Chordal rupture (most severe form is flail leaflet) results in loss of leaflet support usually with myxomatous degeneration
Rheumatic heart disease (chordal fibrosis and calcification)
PAPILLARY MUSCLE ABNORMALITIES
Rupture with myocardial infarction
Complete rupture typically not survived
Partial rupture more typically encountered
Dysfunctional papillary muscle
Ischemia
Posteromedial papillary muscle, single blood supply through posterior descending artery
Anterolateral papillary muscle, supplied by left anterior descending artery and left circumflex artery
Infiltrative processes: amyloid, sarcoid
Congenital: malposition, parachute mitral valve

afterload cause more complete LV emptying and hyperdynamic function. Forward cardiac output declines, however, because much of the flow is directed to the left atrium. If the acute hemodynamic insult is tolerated, the patient's condition **may progress to a chronic compensated state.**

2. In **chronic compensated MR,** there is **dilation of the left ventricle with eccentric hypertrophy.**
   a. Wall stress is normalized with the development of hypertrophy. Afterload reduction by the low-resistance left atrium is not as great as it is in the acute phase. Preload remains elevated by the same mechanism as in acute MR. LA dilation helps to accommodate the increased preload at lower filling pressures. LV function is not as hyperdynamic as in the acute state but is in the high-normal range.
   b. Patients may stay in this asymptomatic or minimally symptomatic phase for years; however, **contractile dysfunction may develop insidiously** during this phase. This is not apparent with traditional ejection phase indices (such as ejection fraction). These often appear normal because of the effect of increased preload and normal or decreased afterload.
3. In **chronic decompensated MR,** there is LV dysfunction along with progressive enlargement of the LV chamber with increased wall stress. LV dysfunction and enlargement increase the severity of MR, further contributing to the cycle of decline in LV function. Irreversible LV contractile dysfunction may be present by the time overt symptoms develop. Irreversible contractile dysfunction results in postoperative CHF and increased morbidity and mortality.

C. Laboratory examination

1. The **electrocardiographic** findings are **nonspecific.** The principal findings are LA enlargement and atrial fibrillation. LV hypertrophy and RV hypertrophy may also be seen in patients with severe MR.
2. Chest radiography. Cardiomegaly with LA and LV enlargement may be seen in chronic MR. Interstitial edema, manifest as Kerley B lines, followed by alveolar edema, may develop in acute cases or with progressive LV failure. Calcification of the mitral annulus may be visualized as a C-shaped opacity in the lateral projection.

D. Diagnostic testing

1. Echocardiography plays a pivotal role in the evaluation of MR. It is useful in **diagnosing MR and in determining its severity and cause.** MR **severity is graded as follows:** 1+ for mild, 2+ for moderate, 3+ for moderately severe, and 4+ for severe regurgitation. The American College of Cardiology/American Heart Association (ACC/AHA) Class I recommendation is for the use of Doppler echocardiography to determine the mechanism and severity of MR, to assess LA and LV size and function over time, to assess PA pressures, and to reevaluate periodically if more than mild and after mitral valve surgery. Table 14.2 summarizes the current ACC/AHA classification of MR severity by Doppler echocardiography.
   a. Color Doppler echocardiography allows diagnosis of MR by means of visualization of the regurgitant jet or jets entering the left atrium and allows assessment of severity.
      (1) Jet length and area are used in this assessment. These measurements are **reliable with central jets,** but underestimation of MR may occur with eccentric jets. Because a jet directed against the atrial wall appears smaller than a free jet of the same regurgitant volume (Coanda effect), it is common practice to upgrade the estimated severity of MR by at least one grade in this situation. The direction of the MR jet also can aid in assessing the cause of MR (Table 14.3). Regurgitation caused by prolapse or flail (excessive leaflet motion) leads to a jet away from the affected leaflet (i.e., posterior jet with anterior leaflet prolapse). MR caused by leaflet restriction (rheumatic, ischemic) is directed toward the affected leaflet.
         (a) Caveats
            i. MR assessed with **transesophageal echocardiography (TEE).** Patients often receive sedation before TEE, and the sedation may

TABLE 14.2 Assessment of Severity of Mitral Regurgitation

	Mild	Moderate	Severe[a]
Qualitative			
Angiographic grade	1+	2+	3–4+
Color Doppler jet area	Small, central jet (<4 cm^2 or <20% LA area)	Signs of MR > mild present, but no criteria for severe MR	Vena contracta width >0.7 cm with large central MR jet (area >40% of LA area) or with a wall-impinging jet of any size
Doppler vena contracta width (cm)	<0.3	0.3–0.69	≥0.70
Quantitative (cath or echo)			
Regurgitant volume (mL per beat)	<30	30–59	≥60
Regurgitant fraction (%)	<30	30–49	≥50
Regurgitant orifice area (cm^2)	<0.20	0.2–0.39	≥0.40

[a]In severe MR, evidence of LA and LV dilation is essential.
Adapted from 2006 Valve Disease ACC/AHA Guidelines.

TABLE 14.3 Mechanisms, Direction of Color Jet, and Surgical Management of Mitral Regurgitation

Jet direction	Leaflet motion	Likely cause	Surgical method
Anterior	Excessive Annuloplasty Chordal shortening Shortening of papillary muscle	Posterior leaflet prolapse	Quadrilateral resection
	Restricted	Anterior leaflet restriction	Débridement
Posterior	Excessive	Anterior leaflet prolapse	Chordal transfer or shortening
		Posterior leaflet resection to move coaptation apically	
	Restricted	Posterior leaflet restriction	Débridement, annuloplasty
	Normal	Ventricular dilatation	Annuloplasty
Central	Excessive	Bileaflet prolapse	Resection, chordal transfer
	Restricted	Bileaflet restriction	Débridement
	Normal	Ventricular dilatation	Annuloplasty
Commissural	Papillary muscle dysfunction		Reattach or fold papillary muscle
	Eccentric	Perforation or cleft	Pericardial patch

From Stewart WJ. Intraoperative echocardiography. In: Topol EJ, ed. *Textbook of cardiovascular medicine.* Philadelphia: Lippincott–Raven Publishers, 1998, with permission.

reduce systemic blood pressure (afterload). This may make the MR appear less severe than it is under normal physiologic circumstances. This effect of sedation may be mitigated to some extent by increasing afterload by handgrip or by the cautious administration of phenylephrine.

ii. In evaluation of MR in the **intraoperative setting,** there may be fluctuations in afterload and preload.

(b) Multiple factors, such as hemodynamic considerations, geometric factors (constraint imposed by LA wall), and instrumentation, may affect color Doppler measurements. This has led to the development of other measurements to quantify MR.

(2) Width of the vena contracta, which is the narrowest portion of the proximal regurgitant jet, is a **reliable indicator of the severity of MR.** The vena contracta is the narrowest portion of the MR jet downstream from the orifice. A width $\geq$**0.70 cm suggests severe MR.** High-resolution and zoom images must be used for accurate assessment of the vena contracta, or else TEE may be needed. There is some tendency for overestimation of width of the vena contracta because of limited lateral resolution.

b. Pulsed wave Doppler echocardiography of pulmonary venous flow may be useful in the assessment of the severity of MR (Fig. 14.3). Sampling of the pulmonary veins results in three distinct waves: a systolic antegrade wave, a smaller diastolic antegrade wave, and a small negative wave that represents atrial reversal during atrial contraction. With increasing MR, there is a progressive decrease in the systolic wave of pulmonary inflow with eventual reversal. **Blunting of the systolic component** of pulmonary venous flow in the presence of normal LV function suggests at least moderately severe MR. **Systolic flow reversal** suggests severe MR. Blunted pulmonary venous flow is a less reliable indicator of substantial MR in the setting of atrial fibrillation or severe LV dysfunction, since these conditions also can cause systolic blunting.

c. Pulsed-wave Doppler echocardiography of mitral inflow. Stroke volume across the regurgitant mitral valve can be estimated and compared with the stroke volume derived from pulsed-wave Doppler imaging across a competent valve (such as the aortic or pulmonary valve). The excess of flow at the mitral valve over that derived at the aortic valve is **the regurgitant volume.** These methods are both tedious and technically difficult.

d. The **proximal isovelocity surface area (PISA)** or flow convergence method provides a quantitative assessment of MR (see Fig. 14.3 and Chapter 60). Peak mitral flow rate is derived as:

$$\text{QFC} = 2\pi r^2 V$$

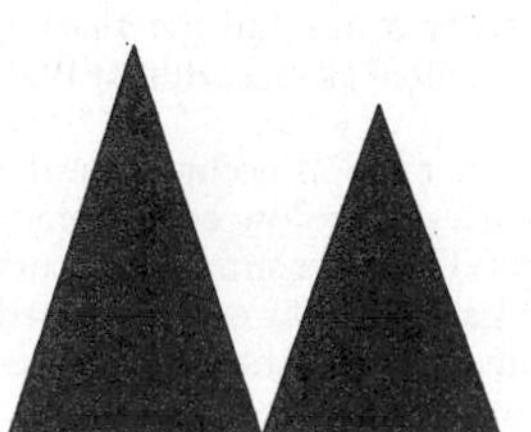

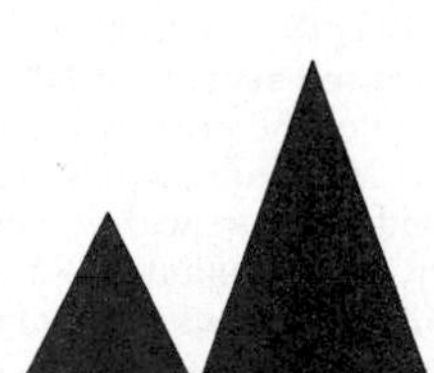

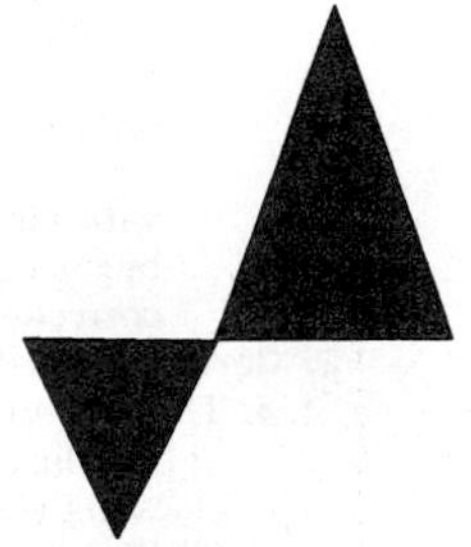

Figure 14.2. Patterns of pulmonary venous flow. *First triangle* in each panel represents flow during systole. *Second triangle* represents flow during diastole. The three potential patterns are displayed: normal flow ratio, blunted systolic flow, and reversed systolic flow.

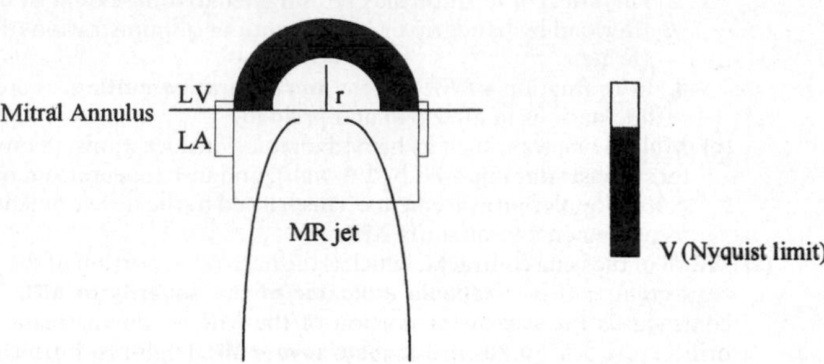

Figure 14.3. The proximal isovelocity surface area method for determining severity of mitral regurgitation.

where r is the radius of the shell and V is the aliasing velocity at that shell. **Regurgitant orifice area (ROA),** a relatively load-independent measure of regurgitation, is derived from peak flow rate by dividing by peak flow velocity [maximal MR continuous wave (CW) velocity, Vmr].

$$\text{ROA} = 2\pi\pi r^2\, V/Vmr$$

The **regurgitant volume** (RV) may be further calculated by the equation ROA × VTI*mr,* where VTI*mr* is the velocity–time integral of the regurgitant jet.

If the forward stroke volume (SV) is known, then the **regurgitant fraction** (RF%) may be derived as:

$$\text{RF} = \text{RV}/\text{RV} + \text{SV}$$

Stroke volume may be estimated in the LV outflow tract (LVOT) as area × VTI, as is performed in the continuity equation (see Chapter 13).

ROA has been shown to be prognostically powerful in MR of ischemic or degenerative origin.

(1) Simplied proximal convergence method. The preceding calculation may be simplified to allow the ROA to be estimated with only one measurement. Using this method, MR velocity is assumed to be 5 m/s and the aliasing velocity is set at 40 cm/s. The ROA may be calculated as $r^2/2$. **Higher ROA indicates an increased severity of MR.**

(2) Inaccuracies in use of the proximal convergence method occur when the orifice is nonspherical, multiple jets are present, or the flow convergence zone is constrained as occurs with eccentric jets. The latter situation occurs with a flail leaflet, as regurgitant flow and ROA are typically overestimated by use of the PISA method; accuracy may be improved by the use of angle-correction formulas.

2. Cardiac catheterization

a. The **amplitude of the v waves** on hemodynamic tracings (which are a reflection of LA filling from the pulmonary veins during ventricular systole) can provide clues to the severity of MR, particularly in acute MR.

(1) Amplitudes of v wave more than two to three times mean LA pressure suggest severe MR. However, in slowly developing MR, an abnormal v wave may not be seen. The v waves also are diminished by afterload reduction. When present (particularly with acute MR), v waves may be useful in assessing MR. **Absence of v waves does not exclude severe MR.**

(2) Other conditions that may produce prominent v waves are LV dysfunction with a dilated noncompliant left atrium, postinfarction VSD, and other situations in which there is increased pulmonary blood flow.

b. Left ventriculography allows visual assessment of the severity of MR. It is affected by multiple factors such as the adequacy of the contrast injection to fill the ventricle, the placement of the catheter, and by ventricular arrhythmia during injection. The grading system is as follows:

1. **1+ (mild):** clears with each beat; entire left atrium is never opacified.

2. **2+ (moderate):** does not clear with a single beat; may faintly opacify the entire left atrium.

3. **3+ (moderate to severe):** fills entire left atrium over two or three beats; complete opacification of the left atrium, equal in intensity to the left ventricle.

4. **4+ (severe):** complete opacification of the left atrium in one beat; contrast material refluxes into the pulmonary veins.

c. Coronary angiography is useful to detect **concomitant coronary artery disease** in these patients. Those being considered for surgery to correct MR undergo coronary angiography, even in the absence of symptoms, if they are older than 50 years or have multiple risk factors.

E. Therapy. An understanding of the pathophysiologic mechanism of MR is essential to management.

1. Acute MR

a. **Medical therapy.** If there is adequate mean arterial pressure, pharmacologic therapy with afterload-reducing agents may reduce the acute MR. Intravenous nitroprusside and nitroglycerin may reduce pulmonary pressures and maximize forward flow. If an operation is not required immediately, a change to oral agents may be made. **Afterload reducing agents**, especially angiotensin-converting enzyme (ACE) inhibitors and direct-acting vasodilators (such as hydralazine), help to maximize forward output and reduce regurgitant fraction.

b. **Percutaneous therapy.** The large sudden volume overload on a left ventricle that is not dilated or hypertrophied, causes symptoms of pulmonary congestion and even cardiogenic shock. For such patients with acute hemodynamically significant MR, especially from postinfarction papillary muscle rupture, placement of an intraaortic balloon pump (IABP) may serve as a temporary stabilizing measure until surgical repair can be undertaken.

c. **Surgical therapy.** Patients with acute, severe MR usually require urgent surgical intervention.

2. Chronic MR

a. Choosing the appropriate therapy (see Table 14.4 for a summary of the current ACC/AHA guidelines)

(1) Most patients who have **moderately severe to severe MR** and are **symptomatic** should be considered for elective surgical treatment. Decisions need to be individualized based on the age of the patient, the likelihood of valve repair, comorbidities, LV function, and the likelihood that surgical intervention will improve symptoms and/or survival.

(2) Generally, **intervention for symptoms is indicated for severe MR if the cause of the MR is primary to the valve** (i.e., prolapse, rheumatic or congenital in origin). When the **valve lesion is secondary to ventricular dysfunction,** either from ischemic heart disease or from dilated cardiomyopathy, **aggressive medical management with afterload reduction** (see subsequent text) is indicated first, and surgical intervention considered for refractory symptoms. In ischemic MR, if revascularization is indicated anyway, then valve repair should also be performed where possible. The success rate and long-term durability of operative management for ischemic MR is significantly lower than that associated with repair of primary MV disease.

(3) In **severe MR due to dilated cardiomyopathy associated with severe symptoms** and refractory to medical management and cardiac resynchronization therapy (CRT) (if indicated), mitral valve repair may lead

TABLE 14.4 Indications for Mitral Valve Surgery in Mitral Regurgitation

Class I

(a) Mitral valve (MV) surgery is recommended for the symptomatic patient with acute severe mitral regurgitation (MR).

(b) MV surgery is of benefit for patients with chronic severe MR and New York Heart Association (NYHA) functional class II, III, or IV symptoms in the absence of severe left ventricular (LV) dysfunction (severe LV dysfunction is defined as ejection fraction <0.30) and/or end-systolic dimension >55 mm.

(c) MV surgery is of benefit for asymptomatic patients with chronic severe MR and mild to moderate LV dysfunction, ejection fraction 0.30 to 0.60, and/or end-systolic dimension ≥40 mm.

(d) MV repair is indicated over MV replacement in most patients with severe chronic MR who require surgery, and patients should be referred to surgical centers experienced in MV repair.

Class IIa

(a) MV repair is reasonable in experienced surgical centers for asymptomatic patients with chronic severe MR with preserved LV function (ejection fraction >0.60 and end-systolic dimension <40 mm) in whom the likelihood of successful repair without residual MR is >90%.

(b) MV surgery is reasonable for asymptomatic patients with chronic severe MR, preserved LV function, and new-onset atrial fibrillation.

(c) MV surgery is reasonable for asymptomatic patients with chronic severe MR, preserved LV function, and pulmonary hypertension (pulmonary artery, PA, systolic pressure >50 mm Hg at rest or >60 mm Hg with exercise).

(d) MV surgery is reasonable for patients with chronic severe MR due to a primary abnormality of the mitral apparatus and NYHA functional class III–IV symptoms and severe LV dysfunction (ejection fraction <0.30 and/or end-systolic dimension >55 mm) in whom MV repair is highly likely.

Class IIb

MV repair may be considered for patients with chronic severe secondary MR due to severe LV dysfunction (ejection fraction <0.30) who have persistent NYHA functional class III–IV symptoms despite optimal therapy for heart failure, including biventricular pacing.

Class III

(a) MV surgery is not indicated for asymptomatic patients with MR and preserved LV function (ejection fraction >0.60 and end-systolic dimension <40 mm) in whom significant doubt about the feasibility of repair exists.

(b) Isolated MV surgery is not indicated for patients with mild or moderate MR.

Adapted from 2006 Valve Disease ACC/AHA Valve Disease Guidelines.

to symptomatic improvement, but a survival benefit has not yet been demonstrated.

(4) Treatment of patients with **minimal or no symptoms but severe MR** is more complex. **The key is to identify patients before contractile dysfunction of the left ventricle becomes irreversible.** Watchful waiting until serious symptoms develop carries a risk for development of severe LV dysfunction and a poor prognosis. The feasibility of mitral valve repair with improved postoperative survival and ejection fraction (see later) has been another incentive in the push for earlier surgical intervention. If valve repair is not feasible, one may choose to wait longer before proceeding to surgical treatment. **The new valve guidelines have lowered the threshold to intervene in asymptomatic patients with repairable valves** when repair is performed in an experienced center where the likelihood of repair is >90% (Table 14.4).

b. Timing of surgery. A variety of clinical, echocardiographic, and invasively derived values appear to be predictive of the development of postoperative LV dysfunction, CHF, and death among patients with significant but asymptomatic MR. The timing of mitral valve surgery is a **decision that must be individualized** and depends on several variables including clinical signs and symptoms, echocardiographic findings, catheterization data, hemodynamic data, operative risk, and repairability of the mitral valve. Generally, the variables to be considered in patients whose MR is asymptomatic are (a) LV size and function; (b) exercise capacity and LV size and function at peak exercise; (c) repairability of the valve; (d) severity of MR, including presence of flail leaflet; (e) pulmonary artery pressures; (f) atrial fibrillation; and (g) age and other comorbidities.

(1) LV size and function. As noted previously, contractile impairment is often occult in severe MR using conventional indices of LV function. Elastance measured at the time of cardiac catheterization is the best load-independent measure of true contractile function in MR. However, as it requires the construction of a series of pressure–volume loops for its calculation, it is rarely performed outside research laboratories. Fortunately, conventional indices of LV size and function do provide useful information in MR. Therefore, **in severe primary MR, with normal contractile function, LV ejection fraction (LVEF) should be in the high-normal range. Studies have indicated that once the LVEF is <60%, the likelihood of impaired survival and permanent LV dysfunction postoperatively is high.** Therefore, consideration should be given to surgical intervention before the LVEF drops to below 60%. Increased LV size and volume in end-systole (more load independent than end-diastole) is also an indicator of increased likelihood of impaired survival and LV dysfunction postoperatively. When **LV end-systolic diameter is >4.0 cm, surgical intervention should be considered.**

(2) We have found that **exercise echocardiography** is very helpful in determining the likelihood of latent LV contractile dysfunction. **The ability of the left ventricle to cope with exercise is an indication of its contractile reserve.** In addition, **poor functional capacity** may indicate an adaptive response to MR (the patient was not truly asymptomatic) and may influence the decision to proceed with surgical treatment. We have found that a **failure to *increase* LVEF, or for end-systolic volume to *decrease* with stress, is predictive of postoperative LV dysfunction** and is a superior predictor of this eventuality than resting LVEF. In patients with severe asymptomatic MR, we perform stress echocardiography at 6 monthly intervals and recommend mitral valve surgery once end-systolic volume fails to decrease significantly at peak exercise or if LVEF fails to increase. This is particularly helpful in patients who wish to postpone surgical intervention as long as possible.

(3) The **feasibility of repair** depends on the cause of MR. This can be determined during the preoperative evaluation by echocardiography. **Repair in an experienced center is usually likely in MVP unless chordae to both leaflets are severed, severe damage from endocarditis has occurred, or there is extensive leaflet calcification.** Repair is usually feasible for a cleft valve and in less extreme forms of endocarditis such as leaflet perforation without chordal disruption, as well as in many cases of secondary MR (ischemic or dilated cardiomyopathy). Repair is more difficult to achieve in rheumatic involvement and when the valve leaflets or chordae are severely disrupted from any cause. Repair may be accomplished by a number of techniques, including resection or plication of a leaflet, patch to perforation, and chordal shortening or transposition, and usually involves insertion of an annuloplasty ring to decrease the size of the annulus and improve leaflet coaptation. **The threshold to intervene surgically is lower if repair appears feasible because of the lower surgical and long-term mortality and morbidity associated with it as compared with replacement.**

(4) The more severe the MR, the greater the volume load on the left ventricle usually, and the more likely that LV dysfunction will develop. One caveat here is that MR is not always holosystolic. Occasionally, apparently severe MR is seen without evidence of significant LV enlargement because the MR is occurring only in the latter part of systole.

The threshold to intervene surgically is lower as MR severity increases. In situations where MR severity is in doubt, a TEE should be performed and the quantitative assessment used as described previously. A flail leaflet usually (but not always) implies severe MR. A retrospective study suggested that earlier surgical intervention was associated with better long-term survival in patients with a flail leaflet, even if the condition was asymptomatic with flail being considered a surrogate for severe MR. More recent quantitative studies suggest that once ROA is >0.4 cm^2 that survival is better in those treated surgically, even in the absence of symptoms.

(5) Pulmonary pressures >50 mm Hg at rest or >60 mm Hg at peak exercise in the absence of another likely cause are an indication of severe MR and impaired survival, and **are considered ACC/AHA class IIa indications for surgical intervention.** These can be assessed noninvasively from the tricuspid regurgitant velocity at stress echocardiography.

(6) The occurrence of **atrial fibrillation** or flutter in the setting of severe MR is considered an indication (IIa) for surgical intervention. A concomitant maze procedure may be indicated, especially if atrial fibrillation has become persistent or frequent.

(7) Age and other comorbidities. Patients >75 years, those with concomitant coronary artery disease (CAD), or those with renal dysfunction have worse outcomes after surgical treatment. Patients with ischemic MR have a worse prognosis than those with regurgitation from other causes.

c. Medical therapy

(1) MR caused by LV dysfunction (with annular dilation) is managed with the agents used to manage heart failure.

(a) Afterload-reducing agents, particularly ACE inhibitors, minimize regurgitant volumes and maximize forward flow. These agents are also useful in managing MR from primary valvular disease in patients with symptoms who are awaiting surgical treatment.

(b) β-Blockers may also be beneficial in this group of patients and may be added once afterload reduction has been initiated.

(c) Diuretics and nitrates have a role in the management of pulmonary congestion.

(d) Ventricular rate-controlling agents and antiarrhythmics are used for atrial fibrillation. **Digitalis and β-blockers** are the mainstay of therapy for rate control.

(2) The role of medical therapy for **asymptomatic, chronic MR caused by primary valve disease** is not well established. There is no evidence that pharmacologic agents delay progression of the disease or prevent ventricular dysfunction. Patients with severe MR should be evaluated semiannually with echocardiography and stress echocardiography, if indicated. Patients with moderate MR should be evaluated annually.

(3) **In accordance with recent AHA guidelines,** endocarditis prophylaxis is not routinely indicated in patients with mitral regurgitation. These new guidelines recommend that prophylaxis be used only in patients with underlying cardiac conditions associated with the highest adverse outcome from infective endocarditis including prosthetic heart valves, previous infective endocarditis, certain classes of congenital heart disease, and in valvulopathy occurring post cardiac transplantation.

d. Surgical therapy

(1) Mitral valve replacement with transection of the subvalvular apparatus was once the only approach used in the surgical management of MR. Postoperative reduction of LV function and CHF were common sequelae.

Chordal preservation by leaving the subvalvular structures intact has been shown to reduce LV volumes and wall stress postoperatively, and is now the technique of choice.

(2) The increasing success of **mitral valve repair** has greatly reduced the morbidity and mortality associated with severe MR. Minimally invasive approaches further reduce morbidity.

(3) Although no randomized trials have compared repair with replacement, **comparative data suggest better postoperative LV function and survival with repair** (which in part reflects the selection of patients who are able to undergo repair). Long-term risk for thromboembolism and endocarditis are reduced with repair versus replacement, and need for reoperation is similar.

(4) **Minimally invasive** and **robotically assisted valve repair** can be considered in experienced centers and in selected patients. These approaches have the benefit of smaller incisions, resulting in more rapid postoperative recovery, but require considerable expertise. Complex surgeries, particularly if they require concomitant coronary artery bypass grafting (CABG) or multivalvular repair, are likely better handled with a standard operative approach at this point. These techniques may enjoy broader application in the future.

(5) Intraoperative echocardiography helps in **assessment of complications** of valve repair or replacement.

(a) Residual MR is the most common problem after a pump run. If further repair is feasible, a second pump run should be considered to correct residual MR (if 1+ or greater). If further repair is not possible, valve replacement may be needed. A second pump run does not appear to increase in-hospital mortality.

(b) Dynamic LV outflow obstruction is an important potential complication of MV repair. This is now uncommon in experienced centers. It is caused by anterior displacement of mitral leaflet coaptation point when the posterior leaflet is redundant (typically >1.5 cm in height). The result is systolic motion of the mitral leaflet into the outflow tract, with resultant pressure gradient across the outflow tract and the development of MR. This may be apparent immediately after surgery in the operating room with intraoperative echo or later in the course. It is exacerbated by increased inotropy and small LV size. Many instances resolve with cessation of the use of sympathomimetic agents and volume repletion. In the operating room, if these efforts fail to correct the condition, more surgery to reduce the height of the posterior mitral leaflet (sliding annuloplasty) or, rarely, mitral valve replacement may be necessary. In the postoperative patient, volume repletion and judicious use of β-blockade are often all that is necessary, although occasionally surgical revision of the repair is needed. The development of a new apical systolic murmur in the patient who has undergone postoperative mitral valve repair should prompt an echocardiogram to exclude this complication.

e. Postsurgical follow-up care

(1) Baseline echocardiography should be performed postoperatively. This is done ideally 4 to 6 weeks after the operation, but for the sake of convenience it is often done before hospital discharge (within 3 to 4 days).

(2) MR can recur because of failure of the repair or because of progression of the disease that caused MR. Patients should undergo clinical evaluations at least once a year. **Yearly echocardiography** after the operation to assess for MR and LV function is reasonable.

f. Percutaneous mitral valve repair. Percutaneous mitral valve repair is an emerging catheter-based treatment option in which coaptation of the mitral leaflets is achieved by devices deployed at the time of cardiac catheterization. The types of devices under investigation can be classed into two functional approaches.

(1) A **clip** can be used to approximate the center of the mitral valve leaflets, thus giving a double orifice valve in an approach that models the surgical Alfieri edge-to-edge repair.

(2) A **flexible ring** can be deployed and tightened in the coronary sinus in order to effectively reduce the mitral annulus area.

Clinical trials are underway using both approaches. The former is more suitable to repair of MVP, whereas the latter is felt to be more suited toward repair of functional regurgitation. Currently, these approaches are considered only in patients who are not ideal candidates for standard valve surgeries (i.e., high surgical risk, advanced age).

III. MITRAL VALVE PROLAPSE

A. Clinical presentation. MVP is also known as systolic click–murmur syndrome, myxomatous mitral valve, floppy valve syndrome, redundant cusp syndrome, and Barlow's syndrome. Prolapse exists when the mitral leaflets protrude into the left atrium during systole and the coaptation point of the leaflets lies superior to the plane of the annulus. A wide spectrum of pathologic changes and clinical symptoms occur, from mild degrees of prolapse diagnosed with echocardiography only, to clinically evident severe MR. MVP is the most common cause of MR in the United States. It affects approximately 2% of the population. Recent studies have suggested an equal prevalence among males and females, whereas earlier studies suggested a female preponderance. Males and older patients (age >45 years) are disproportionately likely to require surgical intervention and to develop other major complications such as endocarditis.

1. Signs and symptoms

a. Most patients with MVP have **no symptoms,** and the diagnosis is made by means of routine examination or echocardiography performed for other indications.

b. Although in the past many symptoms were attributed to MVP, including chest pain, panic attacks, and autonomic instability, more recent studies suggest that these occur no more frequently in patients with MVP than in control populations. Most symptoms associated with adverse prognostic implications occur when significant MR is present.

c. Arrhythmias are more common with MVP, even in the absence of MR. These include **supraventricular tachyarrhythmias, ventricular tachyarrhythmias, and bradyarrhythmias.** Sudden death occurs rarely in MVP, and its incidence in MVP is twice that of the normal population. It is more common in the setting of severe MR and/or flail valve leaflet.

d. Transient ischemic attack or stroke has been reported in MVP. The most recent studies in this area suggest no excess risk for cerebrovascular events among young patients with MVP.

e. When prolapse causes MR, symptoms referable to the valvular insufficiency may be present.

2. Physical findings

a. **Inspection.** There is a higher than expected incidence of **pectus excavatum** among patients with MV. Straight back and scoliosis also are found. Patients often have low body weight and relative hypotension.

b. The main **auscultatory** findings are summarized in Figure 14.4. The **midsystolic click** is the classic finding in prolapse. A systolic murmur is heard if MR is present.

c. Dynamic changes are elicited by **conditions that decrease LV size** (decreased venous return, increased contractility, or decreased systemic volume), which lead to earlier occurrence of prolapse, an earlier click, and increased duration of the murmur. These conditions include standing, the Valsalva maneuver, dehydration, and exposure to amyl nitrite.

d. Maneuvers that **increase LV size** by increasing venous return, decreasing contractility, or increasing systemic volume move the click and murmur later into systole. Examples include squatting and infusion of phenylephrine. The presence of a **click that responds to provocative maneuvers is sufficient**

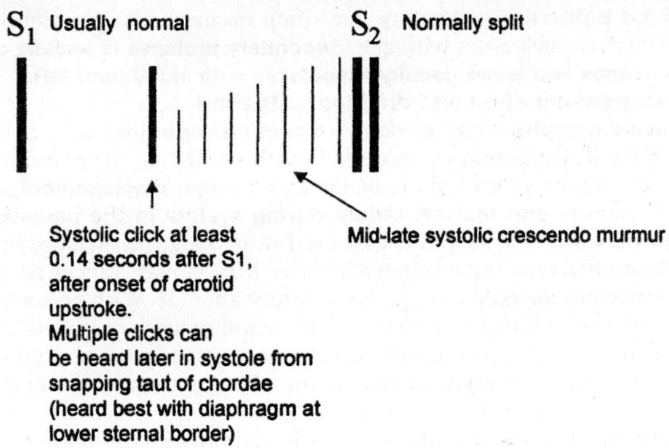

Figure 14.4. Auscultatory findings in mitral valve prolapse.

for the diagnosis of prolapse, even if an echocardiogram is not diagnostic (see **III.D.1**).

e. The **intensity of the murmur typically decreases with conditions that result in a later click and murmur.** An exception is exposure to amyl nitrite, which also reduces LV systolic pressure and the gradient that drives regurgitant flow. As such, the murmur is of lower intensity, although it occurs earlier in systole.

f. Aortic and pulmonic ejection sounds can produce systolic clicks. These occur earlier in systole than the click of mitral prolapse, and may be differentiated on the basis of timing in conjunction with the carotid upstroke. Other causes of midsystolic clicks include septal and free-wall aneurysms and mobile tumors such as myxoma. Clicks produced by these conditions do not change with maneuvers that alter LV volume.

B. Etiology and pathology. Prolapse may exist as a result of valvular abnormalities, deemed primary prolapse, or occur in the setting of normal leaflets (secondary prolapse).

1. Primary prolapse results from **myxomatous proliferation of the leaflets.** The middle layer of leaflet, the spongiosa, is unusually prominent. This produces redundant leaflets. The chordae usually are thickened and elongated. The annulus can be dilated. Recent studies suggest abnormalities in the proteoglycans in the valve tissue and reduced tensile strength and greater extensibility of the tissue. The chordae are more severely affected than the leaflets in terms of impaired tensile strength. Clinically, chordal elongation and leaflet prolapse are often followed by the development of chordal rupture with abrupt worsening of MR severity due to development of flail leaflet and complete loss of leaflet coaptation.

   a. Primary prolapse appears to have a genetic predisposition. There is a higher prevalence of MVP among family members of those affected, and an **autosomal dominant** mode of inheritance with variable penetrance has been postulated. Recent linkage studies suggest a site on chromosome 16 in some families with MVP. In addition, MVP is seen as part of disorders with more generalized abnormalities of the connective tissue, such as Marfan's syndrome, Ehlers-Danlos syndrome, pseudoxanthoma elasticum, and myotonic dystrophy.

   b. Most **complications** of prolapse, particularly severe MR, are associated with primary prolapse. Men in their sixth decade of life represent the most common demographic group with such a presentation.

2. In **secondary prolapse,** there is relatively **normal valvular structure.** A disproportion between leaflet size and LV cavity size produces mechanical forces that may lead to leaflet prolapse. This form of prolapse particularly affects **younger women.** It also may occur with atrial septal defect, hyperthyroidism, emphysema, and hypertrophic cardiomyopathy. Normalization of the relative disproportion

between leaflet size and cavity size often occurs with aging among women, so that incidence decreases with age. **Secondary prolapse is usually of little clinical significance and is not usually associated with significant MR.**

C. Laboratory examination and diagnostic testing

1. **Echocardiography.** M-mode demonstrates late or holosystolic bowing of the mitral valve leaflet 3 mm or more below the C-D line. In two-dimensional (2D) echocardiography prolapse is defined as >**2-mm displacement of one or both mitral leaflets into the left atrium during systole in the parasternal or apical long-axis views.** Caution must be used in making the diagnosis with the apical four-chamber view because normal valve leaflets may appear to prolapse in this view owing to the saddle shape of the mitral annulus. With primary causes of prolapse, increased leaflet thickness (>5 mm) and redundant leaflets and chordae are seen. Doppler echocardiography is used to assess the presence and severity of MR. Annual echocardiography is advised for those patients with moderate to severe MR.
2. **Electrocardiogram (ECG).** If there is severe MR, the findings described earlier are present. Otherwise, the ECG usually is normal or has nonspecific ST-T changes.
3. **Chest radiography.** Pectus excavatum or scoliosis can be present in some cases. If severe MR is present, the typical findings described earlier are seen. Otherwise, the **chest radiograph usually is normal.**

D. Therapy. For most patients, MVP carries a benign prognosis, and **periodic clinical follow-up examinations and reassurance** are all that is needed.

1. Endocarditis prophylaxis is not routinely indicated in patients with MVP.
2. Approximately 10% to 15% of patients, particularly those with redundant and thickened leaflets, eventually develop progressive MR. Chordal rupture is a contributing factor among these patients. **Management of MR** is outlined in **II.E.** Patients with evidence of primary MVP should avoid situations that might increase the stress on the chordae, such as sudden heavy lifting.
3. For patients with a history of **transient ischemic attacks, anticoagulant therapy with aspirin** (80 to 325 mg/day) is indicated. Warfarin is recommended for patients with poststroke MVP or for those who experience recurrent transient ischemic attacks while receiving aspirin therapy (international normalized ratio, INR; 2.0 to 3.0).
4. Patients who experience palpitations should be advised to abstain from caffeine, alcohol, and tobacco use. **β-Blockers** are useful in the management of premature atrial or ventricular contractions, and often alleviate symptoms. **Ambulatory electrocardiographic monitoring** is recommended for persistent palpitations. Ventricular tachycardia is an indication for **electrophysiologic testing** to assess risk for sudden death and possible need for **implantation of a defibrillator device.**

IV. MITRAL STENOSIS.

Although declining in incidence in the United States, rheumatic disease remains the predominant cause of MS. Other etiologic factors are listed in Table 14.5. In general, once symptoms begin, there follows a period of about 10 years before they become debilitating. Once significant limiting symptoms develop, the 10-year survival rate is <15%.

A. Clinical presentation

1. Signs and symptoms

a. There is often a **long asymptomatic course,** consisting of a couple of decades.
b. When symptoms do develop, **dyspnea** is common. Predominant symptoms are exertional dyspnea initially, then paroxysmal nocturnal dyspnea and orthopnea, which reflect elevated pulmonary venous pressure.
c. Precipitating factors, such as exercise, emotional stress, pregnancy, infection, or atrial fibrillation with a rapid ventricular response, can produce or dramatically worsen symptoms by generating increased transvalvular gradients and LA pressure. **Atrial fibrillation with rapid ventricular response is a classic exacerbating factor** and may produce pulmonary edema, even in those with mild MS. LA dilation is a predisposing factor to the development of atrial fibrillation.

TABLE 14.5	Causes of Mitral Stenosis
Rheumatic: most common cause	
Congenital	
Parachute mitral valve: single papillary muscle to which chordae to both leaflets attach; results in mitral stenosis or mitral regurgitation	
Supravalvular mitral ring	
Systemic diseases: can cause valvular fibrosis	
Carcinoid	
Systemic lupus erythematosus	
Rheumatoid arthritis	
Mucopolysaccharidosis	
Healed endocarditis	
Prior anorectic drug use	
Severe mitral annular calcification	

d. Hemoptysis can occur and likely represents rupture of small bronchial veins from elevated LA pressure.

e. Hoarseness occurs when the dilated left atrium impinges on the recurrent laryngeal nerve (Ortner's syndrome).

f. LA dilation and stasis, particularly in the context of atrial fibrillation (persistent or paroxysmal), may cause thrombus formation and embolic events. **Cerebrovascular events, coronary embolization, and renal emboli and infarction** are all possible sequelae. The malformed valve is predisposed to the development of **endocarditis.**

g. Fatigue is common because of reduced cardiac output.

h. With long-standing MS and elevated pulmonary pressure, symptoms of **RV failure** may develop.

i. Patients with elevated pulmonary pressures may have **angina-like chest pain,** as a reflection of increased RV oxygen demand.

2. Physical findings

a. Inspection and palpation. Patients may have a **malar facial flush.** The jugular venous pulse can demonstrate a **prominent *a* wave** if there is elevated pulmonary vascular resistance and the patient is still in sinus rhythm. **Jugular venous pressure is elevated with RV failure.** In advanced cases with low cardiac output, **peripheral cyanosis** occurs. The **carotid upstrokes usually are normal** but are of low amplitude if there is diminished cardiac output. The apex beat is not displaced and the impulse can have a tapping quality due to a palpable first heart sound. An apical diastolic **thrill** may be felt in the lateral decubitus position and has a quality that simulates a purring cat. If there is pulmonary hypertension, a **parasternal RV lift with a palpable P_2 is present.**

b. Auscultation. The main auscultatory findings are summarized in Figure 14.5

(1) The **opening snap** is the most characteristic auscultatory hallmark of MS. However, as the mitral valve becomes more calcified and immobile, the opening snap may be lost (just as S_1 becomes softer).

(2) The **murmur** of MS is typically a low-pitched rumbling mid-diastolic murmur, heard best with the bell of the stethscope with the patient in the left lateral decubitus position. Pre-systolic accentuation can be present whether or not the patient is in sinus rhythm (exact mechanism is unknown). Auscultation after a **brief period of exercise may accentuate the murmur** of MS as the increased output and heart rate increase the transvalvular gradient. The length of the murmur correlates better with the severity of MS than the loudness. **The longer the murmur and the shorter the time interval from S_2 to the opening snap, the more severe the MS.**

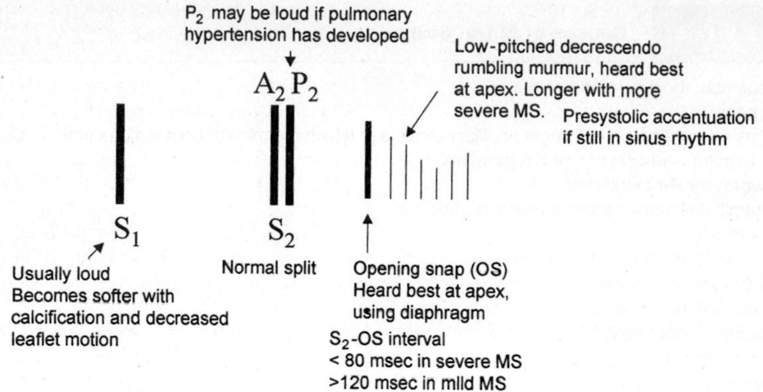

Figure 14.5. Auscultatory findings in mitral stenosis.

(3) Concomitant **conditions that result in decreased flow across the valve,** such as CHF, pulmonary hypertension, and aortic stenosis, may **reduce the diastolic murmur.** The presence of a loud S_1 may be the only clue to the presence of MS in these cases, particularly if pulmonary hypertension exists.

(4) Other **conditions that mimic** the clinical presentation of MS include LA myxoma and cor triatriatum. The tumor plop of myxoma may be mistaken for an opening snap, and tumor obstruction of the valve leads to a diastolic murmur. However, in this condition, the physical findings will vary with changes in position and from examination to examination. Other conditions in which a diastolic rumble may be present include atrial septal defect or VSD, the Austin-Flint murmur of aortic regurgitation (the murmur lessens with decreased afterload and is preceeded by an S_3, and the S_1 is normal), and tricuspid stenosis (the murmur is heard at the left sternal border and typically increases with inspiration; known as Carvallo's sign).

B. Etiology (Table 14.5)

1. In **rheumatic MS,** up to 50% of patients are not aware of a history of rheumatic fever.

a. In **acute** rheumatic fever, MR often predominates. Stenosis usually develops anywhere from 2 to 20 years later, and symptoms may not develop for many years thereafter. Although the incidence of rheumatic fever is roughly equal betweeen men and women, rheumatic mitral stenosis develops two to three times more frequently in women.

b. Thickening of leaflets with **fibrous obliteration** is a characteristic finding. Commissural and chordal fusion and chordal shortening contribute to the development of stenosis. Calcium deposition occurs on leaflets, chordae, and annulus, further restricting valvular function. These changes collectively produce a funnel-shaped mitral valve with a fish-mouth orifice.

C. Pathophysiology

1. The normal area of the mitral orifice is 4 to 6 cm^2. When the valve area is <2 cm^2, a **pressure gradient between the left atrium and the left ventricle in diastole occurs.** As orifice area declines, the transmitral pressure gradient and the LA pressure both increase, but these are also affected by the flow through the valve. **Although the transmitral pressure is a useful indicator of MS severity, it is critically affected by the cardiac output at any moment.** The **cross-sectional area of the mitral valve orifice is, for the most part, independent of flow considerations and thus is a more robust measure of the severity of MS.**

Typical findings indicative of the **severity of stenosis** as defined by the American Society of Echocardiography and endorsed by the recent ACC/AHA valve disease guidelines are as follows:

a. Severe stenosis is associated with a **mean** transvalvular gradient >**10** mm Hg, pulmonary artery (PA) pressures >50 mm Hg, and a valve **area** <**1.0 cm²**

b. Moderate stenosis is associated with a **mean** transvalvular gradient of **5 to 10** mm Hg, PA pressures of 30 to 50 mm Hg, and a valve area of **1.0 to 1.5 cm²**

c. Mild stenosis is associated with a **mean** transvalvular gradient of <**5** mm Hg, PA pressures <30 mm Hg, and a valve area >**1.5 cm²**.

The severity of the stenosis needs to be assessed not only in terms of the valve area but also of symptomatology and exercise capacity. Mixed MS and MR is often associated with greater symptomatic impairment than might be predicted from the severity of either lesion alone.

2. The **increased LA pressure is transmitted to the pulmonary vasculature,** resulting in symptoms of pulmonary congestion. The passive increase in pulmonary venous pressure may elevate pulmonary vascular resistance (reactive pulmonary hypertension). This condition usually is reversible if the stenosis is relieved. However, in long-standing, severe MS, obliterative changes in pulmonary vasculature may occur. Severe pulmonary hypertension can in turn lead to right-heart failure.

3. Up to 30% of patients have a **depressed LVEF.** This appears to result from decreased preload (decreased inflow into the left ventricle) or to a rheumatic myocarditis. The former will normalize after a corrective mitral valve procedure; the latter will not.

4. In severe MS there may be sufficiently low cardiac output to cause **symptoms of poor perfusion.** Chronically depressed cardiac output causes a reflex increase in systemic vascular resistance and increased afterload. This may further diminish LV performance.

D. Laboratory examination and diagnostic testing

1. Echocardiography has several critical roles in the evaluation of MS (all endorsed by ACC/AHA recommendations): initial diagnosis, determination of severity, evaluation of suitability for percutaneous balloon mitral valvuloplasty and identification of concomitant valve lesions.

a. M-mode findings include dense echoes on the mitral valve and decreased excursion of the mitral valve. **Poor leaflet separation in diastole, anterior motion of the posterior leaflet, and decreased E-F slope on the anterior leaflet** are M-mode hallmarks of MS.

b. 2D findings include restricted motion and diastolic doming of leaflets (hockey-stick sign) (Fig. 14.6). The leaflets and chordae are thickened and often are calcified in older patients.

c. Doppler echocardiography is **essential** in the assessment of stenosis severity.

(1) A **transmitral peak velocity** >1 m/s suggests MS. However, this is not specific because tachycardia, increased inotropy, MR, and VSD may cause increased flow in the absence of MS.

(2) The **transvalvular mean gradient** (assessed by means of tracing mitral inflow) provides an estimate of the severity of stenosis. A mean gradient <5 mm Hg is typical in mild stenosis. Moderate stenosis is associated with a mean gradient between 5 and 12 mm Hg. A gradient >12 mm Hg suggests severe MS.

d. Echocardiography is used to estimate **mitral valve area.**

(1) Direct planimetry of the orifice can be performed in the parasternal short-axis view.

(i) Optimal positioning is done by first obtaining a parasternal long-axis view and placing the mitral valve orifice in the center of the scan plane. The transducer is then rotated 90° to obtain the short-axis view. Measurements are obtained at the tips of the mitral leaflets.

(ii) Poor-quality 2D images and a thick, calcified subvalvular apparatus can make it difficult to obtain accurate measurements. Improper

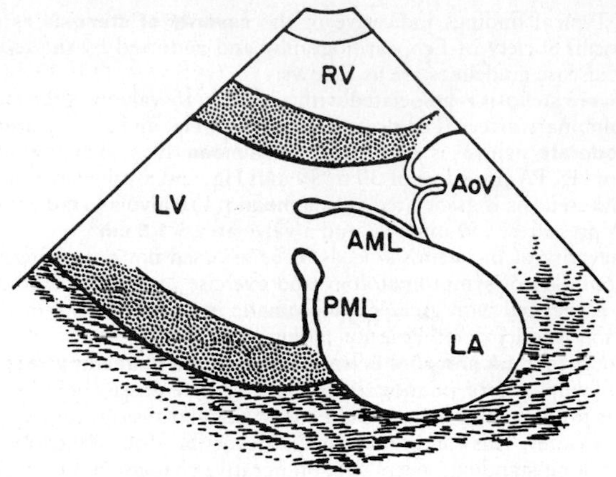

Figure 14.6. Two-dimensional echocardiographic scan in parallel long-axis view shows findings of mitral stenosis. Doming of leaflets is present. LV, Left ventricle; RV, right ventricle; AML, anterior mitral leaflet; PML, posterior mitral leaflet; LA, left atrium; *AoV,* aortic valve. (Reprinted from Wilkins GT, 1988, with permission.)

orientation of the scanning plane can produce oblique cuts across the valve and overestimation of valve area. Scanning up and down until the typical fish-mouth appearance is seen helps in this regard. Dense fibrosis or calcification at the margins of the valve orifice can lead to underestimation of valve area. Low-gain settings can cause dropout at the edges of the valve and overestimation of the valve area. High-gain settings can lead to underestimation. Planimetry is more difficult if commissurotomy has been performed. Despite the potential problems, planimetry is the preferred method to assess mitral valve area by means of echocardiography.

(2) Pressure half-time method. Impedance to LA emptying prolongs the decline in transvalvular pressure gradient. This prolongs pressure half-time (pressure to fall to one-half the starting value), which equates with the time for the velocity to decrease to 70% of peak velocity). The mitral inflow E wave is used in the calculation.

(i) Empiric pressure half-time has been shown to correlate with valve area:

$$\text{Mitral valve area (in cm}^2\text{)} = 220/\text{pressure half-time}$$

(ii) If a software package to perform the calculations is not available, pressure half-time can be found by means of measuring deceleration time and multiplying by 0.29. If atrial fibrillation is present, 5 to 10 consecutive beats are obtained and averaged.

(iii) It is important to have the **Doppler beam parallel to the direction of blood flow.**

(iv) The pressure half-time method **is inaccurate if there are rapid changes in LA hemodynamics,** such as immediately after balloon valvuloplasty.

(v) Obtaining a pressure half-time may be very difficult if sinus tachycardia is present (E-A fusion). **Severe aortic insufficiency also fills the left ventricle in diastole, decreases pressure half-time, and leads to overestimation of mitral valve area.**

e. Stress echocardiography is useful in the evaluation of patients with symptoms when the **resting study is discrepant with symptoms or clinical findings** (ACC/AHA class I). Gradients can be assessed during (supine bicycle) or immediately after (treadmill) exercise. Measurement of tricuspid regurgitation velocity is used to estimate pulmonary pressures with stress.

f. TEE is indicated to exclude LA thrombus and assess MR prior to valvuloplasty, or if the TTE data are suboptimal (ACC/AHA class I), but is not indicated routinely if TTE data are adequate (ACC/AHA class III).

g. Three-dimensional echocardiography (3DE) can obtain a 3D dataset to determine mitral valve area. This method can avoid error in measurement related to correct alignment of the cut-plane with the level of the mitral valve tips, and speeds up the time required for optimal planimetry. With the advent of real-time 3D transesophageal technology, visualization of the mitral valve en face from the left atrium or left ventricle is possible at the time of percutaneous balloon mitral valvuloplasty.

2. Cardiac catheterization. Hemodynamic measurements obtained in a cardiac catheterization laboratory are used to **assess severity of stenosis.** Simultaneous measurement of LV end-diastolic pressure, LA pressure [either directly or more commonly with pulmonary capillary wedge pressure (PCWP) as a surrogate], cardiac output (Fick method or thermodilution), heart rate, and diastolic filling period (seconds per beat) is required. LV pressure and pulmonary capillary wedge pressure (PCWP) (or LA pressure) tracings are made simultaneously (Fig. 14.7). A mean transmitral gradient is derived from the preceding (planimeter area between the left ventricle and PCWPs during diastole; this area is multiplied by the scale factor of the tracing in millimeters of mercury per centimeter to obtain the gradient). The PCWP tracing ideally should be realigned by 50 to 70 milliseconds to the left (with tracing paper) to account for the time delay in transmission of LA pressure to the pulmonary venous beds.

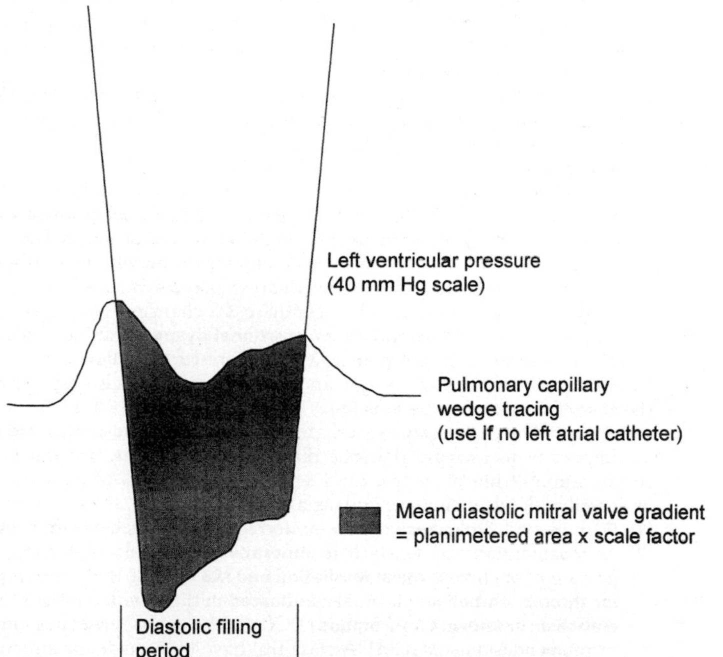

Figure 14.7. Simultaneous left ventricular and pulmonary capillary wedge pressure tracings used to measure mean gradient across mitral valve during diastole.

a. The **Gorlin formula**:

$$\text{Area} = \frac{\text{cardiac output/diastolic filling period} \times \text{heart rate}}{3.77 \times \sqrt{\text{(mean transmitral pressure gradient)}}}$$

Gorlin derived the empirical constant 37.7, which is the Gorlin constant (44.3) multiplied by 0.85 (the correction factor for the mitral valve).

b. A **simplified version of the Gorlin formula** proposed by Hakki et al. has been validated and provides a reasonable approximation of valve area.

$$\text{MVA} = \sqrt{\text{(mean mitral gradient)}}$$

c. Pitfalls. PCWP cannot be used if the patient has pulmonary venous occlusive disease or cor triatriatum. The catheter must be properly wedged. In addition, **thermodilution cardiac output is less accurate** if there is severe tricuspid regurgitation or low cardiac output. **Immediately after valvuloplasty** MR or atrial septal defect, flow may lead to inaccurate estimations of mitral flow.

d. Cardiac catheterization is indicated in evaluation of patients when echo-Doppler and clinical findings are discrepant (ACC/AHA class I), or when echo findings are internally discordant (class IIa) or if pulmonary hypertension is disproprtionate to severity of MS as assessed by echo (class IIa).

3. ECG. LA enlargement (P-mitrale) is usually present when sinus rhythm persists. Signs of RV hypertrophy are seen with pulmonary hypertension. Atrial fibrillation is common and the fibrillatory waves are usually coarse.

4. Chest radiography. LA enlargement is apparent with a **double density** along the right-heart border. A convexity can be apparent below the pulmonary artery, representing the LA appendage. Elevation of the left main bronchus and posterior displacement of the esophagus at barium swallow examination reflect LA enlargement. Kerley B lines may be present from increased pulmonary venous pressure. RV enlargement (decreased retrosternal air space on the lateral radiograph) may be present. Evidence of mitral valve calcification may be present. In rare instances, evidence of LA calcification can be seen.

E. Therapy. The overall management approach to the individual with mitral stenosis should integrate symptomatic status, degree of stenosis, and suitability of the valve for percutaneous balloon mitral valvuloplasty.

1. Medical therapy

a. Patients **without symptoms** who have mild MS (valve area >1.5 cm^2 and mean gradient <5 mm Hg) need no specific treatment and, **in accordance with recently revised AHA guidelines, do not require endocarditis prophylaxis.** In patients with rheumatic valve disease, guidelines for the **prevention of rheumatic fever** should be applied. Annual reevaluation is recommended, but a yearly echocardiogram is not indicated unless there is a change in clinical status.

b. Patients with only **mild symptoms of exertional dyspnea** can be treated with **diuretics** and salt restriction to lower LA pressure. **β-Blockers** blunt the chronotropic response to exercise and may improve exercise capacity. **Arterial vasodilators should be avoided.**

c. Atrial fibrillation can clearly exacerbate symptoms, and **rate control measures** are important to increase diastolic filling time. **Embolism** is a much-feared complication of mitral stenosis and occurs in up to 20% of patients; risk is increased with advancing age and atrial fibrillation.

(1) Digitalis and **β-blockers** are the preferred agents to achieve rate control.

(2) Anticoagulation with warfarin **is imperative** for patients with paroxysmal, persistent, or chronic **atrial fibrillation and MS** because they are at **high risk for thromboembolism** and is also**indicated** in those with a history of **prior embolism or known LA thrombus** (ACC/AHA class I). Newer less-emphatic recommendations (ACC/AHA class IIb) have been made for anticoagulation in MS patients with large atrial diameter ($\geq$55 mm) or those with severe MS and enlarged LA size and evidence of spontaneous contrast on echocardiogram. The targeted INR is typically between 2.0 and 3.0.

(3) Antiarrhythmic drug therapy may be used in an attempt to restore sinus rhythm, but long-term efficacy may depend on correction of the MS.

(4) The role of percutaneous balloon mitral valvuloplasty in patients with new-onset atrial fibrillation and moderate to severe MS who are otherwise asymptomatic is controversial.

2. **Percutaneous or surgical therapy** (Table 14.6). **If more than mild symptoms** (New York Heart Association [NYHA] class 2 or greater) are present due to mitral stenosis, the patient should be referred for surgical or percutaneous therapy. An asymptomatic patient, with moderate to severe MS and evidence of pulmonary hypertension at rest or with exercise, should also be referred for percutaneous therapy if the valve is suitable. Mortality increases substantially as symptoms progress. Results of natural history studies, conducted before valvotomy procedures were developed, indicate that young symptomatic patients have about 40% mortality at 10 years and almost 80% at 20 years. Elderly patients have 60% to 70% mortality at 10 years. Marked **pulmonary hypertension** (pulmonary arterial systolic pressure >60 mm Hg) is an indication for mechanical treatment, even in the absence of symptoms in moderate to severe MS. Rarely, for **patients with asymptomatic MS** who do not have pulmonary hypertension surgical or balloon intervention may be warranted. Instances where this is indicated include **women with severe MS contemplating becoming pregnant,** those with severe MS who will need a major surgical procedure with massive fluid shifts, or those with repeated embolism despite anticoagulation. In the last instance, surgical intervention is usually indicated, and LA appendage ligation is performed simultaneously.

TABLE 14.6 ACC/AHA Indications for Percutaneous Mitral Balloon Valvotomy

Class I

1. Percutaneous mitral valvotomy (PMV) is effective for symptomatic patients (New York Heart Association, NYHA, functional class II, III, or IV), with moderate or severe mitral stenosis (MS) and valve morphology favorable for PMV in the absence of left atrial thrombus or moderate to severe mitral regurgitation (MR).
2. PMV is effective for asymptomatic patients with moderate or severe MS and valve morphology that is favorable for PMV, who have pulmonary hypertension (pulmonary artery systolic pressure >50 mm Hg at rest or >60 mm Hg with exercise) in the absence of left atrial thrombus or moderate to severe MR.

Class IIa

PMV is reasonable for patients with moderate or severe MS who have a nonpliable calcified valve, are in NYHA functional class III–IV, and are either not candidates for surgery or at high risk for surgery.

Class IIb

1. PMV may be considered for asymptomatic patients with moderate or severe MS and valve morphology favorable for PMV who have new-onset atrial fibrillation in the absence of left atrial thrombus or moderate to severe MR.
2. PMV may be considered for symptomatic patients (NYHA functional class II, III, or IV) with mitral valve (MV) area >1.5 cm^2 if there is evidence of hemodynamically significant MS based on PA systolic pressure >60 mm Hg, pulmonary artery wedge pressure of 25 mm Hg or more, or mean MV gradient >15 mm Hg during exercise.
3. PMV may be considered as an alternative to surgery for patients with moderate or severe MS who have a nonpliable calcified valve and are in NYHA class III–IV.

Class III

1. PMV is not indicated for patients with mild MS.
2. PMV should not be performed in patients with moderate to severe MR or left atrial thrombus.

a. Percutaneous balloon mitral valvuloplasty is considered the treatment of choice for symptomatic patients with moderate to severe MS who have favorable valve morphology. The technique involves placement of a balloon-tipped catheter into the left atrium through a transseptal puncture and then across the mitral valve. The balloon is inflated and deflated to increasingly larger diameters until the desired result is obtained.

(1) Typically there is an increment in valve area of 1 cm^2, mainly as a result of splitting of the fused commissures. The mean valve area usually doubles with a 50% to 60% reduction in transmitral gradient.

(2) This procedure is **generally contraindicated in patients with >3+ MR** (the procedure normally increases MR by one grade) **or in whom there is an LA or appendage thrombus** (risk of procedural embolism). Severe tricuspid regurgitation (does not improve substantially) and severe pulmonary hypertension (if pulmonary artery pressures do not fall, then substantial risk of right-to-left shunt across procedural atrial septal defect) are relative contraindications to the procedure.

(3) An **echocardiographic score** has been developed to help select patients who may be candidates for percutaneous valvuloplasty. There are four parts to the assessment (mobility, leaflet thickening, subvalvular thickening, and calcification) (Table 14.7). In general, extensive subvalvular disease results in a poorer outcome with valvuloplasty. Patients with extensive fluoroscopically visible mitral valve calcification also have a worse outcome after percutaneous therapy.

(a) A total echocardiographic score (adding the four components) **higher than 11** is associated with a poorer outcome and a suboptimal increase in valve area, a higher incidence of heart failure and restenosis, and higher mortality. Patients with high scores **should not undergo valvuloplasty** unless surgical treatment is impossible.

(b) Echocardiographic scores of **9 to 11** represent a **gray zone** in which some patients have good results with valvuloplasty. Others have suboptimal results.

(c) Optimal results of balloon valvuloplasty are usually achieved when the echocardiographic score is **8 or less.**

TABLE 14.7 Echo Score Assessment for Percutaneous Valvuloplasty in the Management of Mitral Stenosis

MOBILITY (grade 0–4, 0 being normal)
1. Highly mobile with only leaflet tips restricted
2. Mild leaflet restriction; base portions have normal mobility
3. Valve moves forward in diastole, mainly from base
4. No or minimal diastolic movement of valve

SUBVALVULAR THICKENING (grade 0–4, 0 being normal)
1. Minimal thickening below leaflets
2. Chordal thickening up to one third of chordal length
3. Thickening extending to distal one-third of chords
4. Extensive thickening to papillary muscles

THICKENING OF LEAFLETS (grade 0–4, 0 being normal)
1. Near normal (4–5 mm)
2. Marginal thickening (5–8 mm) with normal thickness of midleaflets
3. Thickening of entire leaflet (5–8 mm)
4. Extensive thickening of all leaflet tissue (>8–10 mm)

CALCIFICATION (grade 0–4, 0 being normal)
1. Single area of echo brightness
2. Scattered areas of increased brightness along leaflet margins
3. Brightness extending to midportion of leaflets
4. Extensive brightness throughout leaflet tissue

From Wilkins GT, 1988, with permission. Br Heart J 1988;60:299–308.

TABLE 14.8	Complications of Balloon Valvuloplasty
Mitral regurgitation	
Cardiac perforation: incidence as high as 2% to 4%	
Embolization: incidence 2% in the National Heart, Lung, and Blood Institute registry	
Residual atrial septal defect: most close within 6 mo; can persist long term among as many as 10% of patients; generally small and well tolerated	

(4) TEE plays a critical role during valvuloplasty. The most immediate concern is to **rule out LA and appendage thrombi.** If thrombosis is present, anticoagulation for at least one month is undertaken with repeat TEE to confirm resolution before valvuloplasty. TEE can also help guide balloon positioning; after each inflation, the degree of MR and the gradient can be assessed. The degree of residual MS can be estimated with planimetry of the valve orifice before and after inflation. The pressure half-time method is unreliable until 24 to 48 hours after the procedure.

(5) Echocardiography is useful in the determination of immediate **postprocedural complications** (Table 14.8). Among these is MR with an incidence estimated at 3% to 8%, depending on series. The echocardiographic score is less predictive of the severity of postprocedural MR.

(6) The frequency of **restenosis of the valve** is variable, depending on the age of the patient and the immediate procedural increment in valve area. Data from the National Heart, Lung, and Blood Institute (NHLBI) registry of all functional classes of patients show an 84% survival rate 4 years after treatment. Advanced age, high NYHA functional class, presence of atrial fibrillation, smaller initial mitral valve area, higher pulmonary arterial pressure, and substantial tricuspid regurgitation are **associated with poorer long-term results.** These variables identify a population with more serious illness that frequently necessitates intervention and should not preclude valvuloplasty. More postprocedural MR and lower postprocedural mitral valve area are associated with poorer long-term results.

b. Surgical treatment. Closed **commissurotomy** was the earliest surgical approach used. This was performed through a thoracotomy (without a cardiopulmonary bypass) and atriotomy with a valve dilator. This procedure has been used rarely in the United States, since the development of the percutaneous approach and improvements in open-heart surgery. **Open mitral valvotomy** involves direct visualization of the mitral valve (with cardiopulmonary bypass), débridement of calcium, and splitting of fused commissures and chordae.

(1) Severe subvalvular disease or valvular calcification often leads to the choice of **surgical intervention over valvuloplasty.** Coexistent disease in other valves (e.g., aortic stenosis or aortic regurgitation) that necessitates treatment also favors surgical intervention.

(2) Mitral valve replacement

(a) Mitral valve replacement is often needed, particularly when there is **extensive fibrosis and calcification or concomitant MR.**

(b) The choice of **mechanical or bioprosthetic** valve replacement depends on weighing the risk of chronic anticoagulation associated with mechanical valves against the reduced longevity of the bioprosthetic valves.

(3) Mitral valve repair is more difficult but can be performed in selected cases with commissurotomy when there is mixed MS/MR.

(4) For patients with long-standing **atrial fibrillation,** a combined maze procedure has been used in conjunction with the valve operation.

c. Comparison of balloon valvuloplasty and open commissurotomy. Studies in ideal patients for balloon valvuloplasty and commissurotomy suggest equal improvement in valve area and symptoms immediately postprocedure, and in medium-term follow-up.

d. Postprocedural follow-up care. Patients who have undergone balloon valvuloplasty or operations for MS should undergo **baseline echocardiography,** preferably >72 hours after the procedure. In patients with a history of atrial fibrillation, warfarin should be restarted 2 to 3 days after the procedure. **Clinical follow-up examination** should be performed at least once a year, and more often if symptoms develop. It has become common practice at many centers for patients to undergo **follow-up echocardiography on a once-a-year basis,** although no firm guidelines have been developed for this.

Landmark Articles

Bargiggia GS, et al. A new method for quantification of mitral regurgitation based on color flow Doppler imaging of flow convergence proximal to regurgitant orifice. *Circulation* 1191;84:1481–1489.

Barlow JB, Bosman CK. Aneurysmal protrusion of the posterior leaflet of the mitral valve. An auscultatory-electrocardiographic syndrome. *Am Heart J* 1966;71:166–178.

Bonow RO, et al. ACC/AHA 2006 guidelines for the management of patients with valvular heart disease: a report of the American College of Cardiology/American Heart Association Task Force on Practice Guidelines (writing committee to revise the 1998 Guidelines for the Management of Patients With Valvular Heart Disease): developed in collaboration with the Society of Cardiovascular Anesthesiologists; endorsed by the Society for Cardiovascular Angiography and Interventions and the Society of Thoracic Surgeons. *Circulation* 2006;114:e84–e231.

Duran CG, Pomar JL, Revuelta JM. Conservative operation for mitral insufficiency: critical analysis supported by postoperative hemodynamic studies of 72 patients. *J Thorac Cardiovasc Surg* 1980;79:326–337.

Enriquez-Sarano M, Schaff HV, Orszulak TA, et al. Valve repair improves the outcome of surgery for mitral regurgitation: a multivariate analysis. *Circulation* 1995;91:1022–1028.

Enriquez-Sarano M, Tajik AJ, Schaff HV, et al. Echocardiographic prediction of survival after surgical correction of organic mitral regurgitation. *Circulation* 1994;90:830–837.

Enriquez-Sarano M, Tajik AJ, Schaff HV, et al. Echocardiographic prediction of left ventricular function after correction of mitral regurgitation: results and clinical implications. *J Am Coll Cardiol* 1994;24:1536–1543.

Farhat MB, Ayari M, Maatouk F, et al. Percutaneous balloon versus surgical closed and open mitral commissurotomy: seven year follow-up results of a randomized trial. *Circulation* 1998;97:245–250.

Freed LA, et al. Prevalence and clinical outcome of mitral-valve prolapse. *N Engl J Med* 1999;341:1–7.

Gillinov AM, et al. Durability of mitral valve repair for degenerative disease. *J Thorac Cardiovasc Surg* 1998;116:734–743.

Gorlin R, Gorlin G. Hydraulic formula for calculation of area of stenotic mitral valve, other cardiac values and central circulatory shunts. *Am Heart J* 1951;41:1.

Hatle L, Brubakk A, Tronsdal A, Angelsen B. Noninvasive assessment of pressure drop in mitral stenosis by Doppler ultrasound. *Br Heart J* 1978;40:131–140.

Leung DY, Griffin BP, Stewart WJ, et al. Left ventricular function after valve repair for chronic mitral regurgitation: predictive value of preoperative assessment of contractile reserve by exercise echocardiography. *J Am Coll Cardiol* 1996;28:1198–1205.

Levine RA, et al. Three-dimensional echocardiographic reconstruction of the mitral valve, with implications for the diagnosis of mitral valve prolapse. *Circulation* 1989;80:589–598.

Ling LH, Enriquez-Sarano M, Seward JB, et al. Clinical outcome of mitral regurgitation due to flail leaflet. *N Engl J Med* 1996;335:1417–1423.

Marks AR, et al. Identification of high-risk and low-risk subgroups of patients with mitral-valve prolapse. *N Engl J Med* 1989;320:1031–1036.

Reyes VP, Raju BS, Wynee J, et al. Percutaneous balloon valvuloplasty compared with open surgical commissurotomy for mitral stenosis. *N Engl J Med* 1994;331:961–967.

Wilkins GT, Weyman AE, Abascal VM, et al. Percutaneous balloon dilatation of the mitral valve: an analysis of echocardiographic variables related to outcome and the mechanism of dilatation. *Br Heart J* 1988;60:299–308.

Wilson W, et al. Prevention of infective endocarditis: guidelines from the American Heart Association: a guideline from the American Heart Association Rheumatic Fever, Endocarditis, and Kawasaki Disease Committee, Council on Cardiovascular Disease in the Young, and the Council on Clinical Cardiology, Council on Cardiovascular Surgery and Anesthesia, and the Quality of Care and Outcomes Research Interdisciplinary Working Group. *Circulation* 2007;116:1736–1754.

Key Reviews

Block PC. Percutaneous transcatheter repair for mitral regurgitation. *J Interv Cardiol* 2006;19:547–551.

Carabello BA. Mitral valve disease. *Curr Probl Cardiol* 1993;18:426–478.

Carabello BA, Crawford FA. Valvular heart disease. *N Engl J Med* 1997;337:32–41.

Hayek E, et al. Mitral Valve Prolapse. *Lancet* 2005;365:507–518.

Irvine T. Assessment of mitral regurgitation. *Heart* 2002;88:iv11–iv19.

Stewart WJ. Choosing the golden moment for mitral valve repair. *J Am Coll Cardiol* 1994;24:1544–1546.

Thomas JD. How leaky is that mitral valve? Simplified Doppler methods to measure regurgitant orifice area. *Circulation* 1997;95:548–550.

Thomas JD. Doppler echocardiographic assessment of valvular regurgitation. *Heart* 2002;88:651–657.

Relevant Book Chapters

Alpert JS, Sabik J, Cosgrove DM III. Mitral valve disease. In: Topol EJ, ed. *Textbook of cardiovascular medicine,* 2nd ed. Philadelphia: Lippincott–Raven Publishers, 2001:483–509.

Braunwald E. Valvular heart disease. In: Braunwald E, ed. *Heart disease: a textbook of cardiovascular medicine,* 5th ed. Philadelphia: WB Saunders, 1997:1007–1076.

Carabello B, Grossman W. Calculation of stenotic valve orifice area. In: Baim DS, Grossman W, eds. *Cardiac catheterization, angiography and intervention,* 5th ed. Baltimore: Williams & Wilkins, 1996:151–166.

Griffin BP, Stewart WJ. Echocardiography in patient selection, operative planning, and intraoperative evaluation of mitral valve repair. In: Otto CM, ed. *The practice of clinical echocardiography,* 2nd ed. Philadelphia: WB Saunders, 2002:417–434.

Grossman W. Profiles in valvular heart disease. In: Baim DS, Grossman W, eds. *Cardiac catheterization, angiography and intervention,* 5th ed. Baltimore: Williams & Wilkins, 1996:735–756.

Meier DJ, Landolfo CK, Starling MR. Role of echocardiography in the timing of surgical intervention for chronic mitral and aortic regurgitation. In: Otto CM, ed. *The practice of clinical echocardiography,* 2nd ed. Philadelphia: WB Saunders, 2002:389–416.

Reid CL. Echocardiography in the patient undergoing catheter balloon mitral commissurotomy. In: Otto CM, ed. *The practice of clinical echocardiography,* 2nd ed. Philadelphia: WB Saunders, 2002:435–450.

Stewart WJ. Intraoperative echocardiography. In: Topol EJ, ed. *Textbook of cardiovascular medicine.* Philadelphia: Lippincott–Raven Publishers, 1998:1492–1525.

Weyman AE. Left ventricular inflow tract. I. The mitral valve. In: Weyman AE, ed. *Principles and practice of echocardiography,* 2nd ed. Philadelphia: Lea & Febiger, 1994:391–470.

15 TRICUSPID VALVE DISEASE, PULMONARY VALVE DISEASE, AND DRUG-INDUCED VALVE DISEASE

Deepu Nair and Brian P. Griffin

TRICUSPID VALVE DISEASE

I. INTRODUCTION. The **tricuspid valve (TV) apparatus** consists of the three valve leaflets—septal, anterior, and posterior—along with the tricuspid annulus, the chordae tendineae, and the papillary muscles. Normally, the TV has an orifice area of 5 to 7 cm^2. Both tricuspid stenosis (TS) and tricuspid regurgitation (TR) can produce typical symptoms of right-sided congestive heart failure in their advanced stages. Tricuspid valve dysfunction can occur in both anatomically normal and abnormal valves.

II. TRICUSPID STENOSIS (TS). Tricuspid stenosis is rare as an isolated entity and is most commonly part of a multivalvular process, as described subsequently.

A. Etiology. Table 15.1 lists the causes of TS.

1. **Rheumatic heart disease (RHD)** is by far the most common cause of TS, accounting for >90% of cases. Isolated TS is uncommon in these patients, and most patients have a combination of TS and TR. Nearly all patients with rheumatic TS will have concurrent mitral valve (MV) involvement, and many will also have aortic valve involvement (i.e., trivalvular stenosis); however, clinically significant TS is present in only 5% of patients with RHD. Rheumatic TS is characterized by fibrosis, with contracture of the leaflets and commisural fusion.
2. **Carcinoid heart disease** is seen with metastatic carcinoid tumor to the liver and, while uncommon in general, is the second most common cause of TS. Once metastatic to the liver, this neuroendocrine malignancy secretes numerous vasoactive substances (e.g., serotonin, histamine, and bradykinins), which directly affect the right-sided heart valves. Carcinoid valvular disease is characterized by thickened, retracted, shortened, and even fixed tricuspid leaflets, causing a mixed picture of regurgitation and stenosis. The pulmonic valve may also be involved.

TABLE 15.1 Causes of Tricuspid Stenosis

Disease Entity
Congenital
Rheumatic
Infective endocarditis
Prosthetic valve failure
Carcinoid syndrome
Malignancy (e.g., myxoma, metastases)
Whipple's disease
Fabry's disease
Drug-induced (methysergide, ergot derivatives, anorexigenic agents)

The left-sided heart valves are usually spared, owing to clearance of the vasoactive substances by the lungs (in the absence of right-to-left shunt).

B. Pathophysiology

1. TS produced a **diastolic pressure gradient** between the right atrium and right ventricle, which is augmented when transvalvular flow increases. This typically occurs once the valve area falls below 1.5 cm^2. Therefore, the pressure gradient increases during inspiration or exercise and decreases during expiration.
2. A modest elevation of mean diastolic pressure gradient (i.e., $\geq$5 mm Hg) can raise right atrial pressure (i.e., >10 mm Hg) sufficiently to produce signs of **systemic venous congestion**, including ascites and edema.
3. The right atrial *a wave* may be very pronounced and may approach the level of the right ventricular systolic pressure.
4. Resting cardiac output may be markedly reduced and may fail to augment with exercise, due to limited right and left ventricular preload.
5. Development of atrial fibrillation results in higher right atrial pressures due to the absence of organized atrial contraction and emptying.

C. Clinical presentation

1. **Signs and symptoms.** The presentation of TS varies depending on the **severity of stenosis,** the presence of **concomitant cardiac lesions,** and the **etiology of the valvular disease.**
   - **a. Fatigue** is common and related to low and relatively fixed cardiac output.
   - **b. Right upper quadrant pain** can result from high systemic venous pressure and concomitant hepatomegaly, ascites, and abdominal distention.
   - **c.** Occasionally, patients will experience a **fluttering discomfort** in the neck, caused by the giant *a waves* transmitted to the jugular veins.
   - **d.** Severe TS may mask typical symptoms of other coexisting valvular lesions, such as mitral stenosis (MS). In the case of MS, the flow limitation across the TV can minimize the pulmonary congestion, orthopnea, and paroxysmal nocturnal dyspnea usually associated with MS.
2. **Physical findings.** The diagnosis of TS is often missed without a high index of suspicion. Clues that should raise suspicion of TS include the presence of **elevated jugular venous pressure** and **accentuation of a diastolic murmur along the left sternal border with inspiration** (not present in mitral stenosis).
   - **a.** Elevated central venous pressure may lead to marked hepatomegaly, ascites, and refractory edema. In sinus rhythm, a giant *a* wave in the jugular venous pulse at the first heart sound (S_1) results from impaired right atrial diastolic filling during atrial systole.
   - **b. Diastolic murmur.** The murmur of TS is **low pitched,** diastolic, and best heard along the left lower sternal border in the third to fourth intercostal space or over the xiphoid process. If the rhythm is sinus, the murmur is prominent at end-diastole (presystole). The murmur **intensity increases with inspiration**

(Rivero-Carvallo sign) or other preload augmenting maneuvers (e.g., leg raising, squatting), and may be accompanied by a thrill.

c. An **opening snap** (OS) may be heard at the left lower sternal border; however, this can be difficult to auscultate due to the commonly coexistent mitral OS.

d. Despite elevated neck veins and venous congestion, the patient may be comfortable laying flat due to the absence of pulmonary congestion. This apparent discrepancy between the severity of peripheral edema and the paucity of pulmonary congestion can help discriminate identify TS from other valvular lesions.

e. Respiratory variation in splitting of the second heart sound (S_2) may be absent in patients with TS due to the relatively fixed diastolic filling of the right ventricle despite respiration.

f. In patients with the carcinoid syndrome, symptoms related to neurohormonal release, such as flushing and diarrhea, are typically more common than symptoms attributable to TS.

D. Diagnostic testing. The hemodynamic expression of TS is a pressure gradient across the TV in diastole. A mean diastolic pressure gradient of 2 mm Hg across the TV establishes the diagnosis of TS during catheterization; however, in practice, TS is assessed by Doppler echocardiography;

1. **Electrocardiogram**—TS is suggested by the presence of right atrial enlargement on the electrocardiogram (ECG) (P wave amplitude >2.5 mV in lead II). Because of the common coexistence of MV disease, biatrial enlargement may be seen.
2. **Two-dimensional** (2D) **echocardiography**—The **echocardiogram is the most useful tool** in identifying TS. Typical findings **include reduction in the diameter of the TV orifice** and **thickening and diastolic doming of the tricuspid leaflets** (especially the anterior leaflet). Doppler interrogation of the TV will reveal increased transvalvular velocity; a mean pressure **gradient >5 mm Hg using continuous-wave (CW) Doppler i**s generally diagnostic of TS. Although it is possible to estimate the TV area by pressure half-time or planimetry, such measurements have limited utility in practice, as the severity of TS is more commonly described by the tricuspid diastolic pressure gradient. **Transesophageal echocardiogram (TEE)** is generally less useful than transthoracic echocardiogram (TTE) for assessing transvalvular gradients in TS, given that the TV is an anterior structure.
3. **Three-dimensional (3D) echocardiography**—Given the complex 3D structure of the TV, 3D echocardiography (transthoracic or transesophageal) may prove a useful adjunct to standard 2D echocardiography. Using this modality, all TV leaflets can be simultaneously imaged, potentially allowing for more accurate calculation of TV area.
4. Given the accuracy of modern echocardiographic techniques, cardiac catheterization can often be bypassed. **Right-heart catheterization can be used to confirm the diagnosis** already suggested by Doppler echocardiography, and can serve as a prelude to therapeutic balloon valvuloplasty. Cardiac output is typically low. The right atrial pressure is elevated and the *a wave* may be very tall, sometimes approaching the right ventricular systolic pressure in magnitude. Simultaneous measurement of the right atrial and right ventricular pressures with dual catheters (or a dual-lumen catheter) enables calculation of the diastolic pressure gradient (Fig. 15.1). The measured gradient is highly dependent on cardiac output and heart rate. Maneuvers such as lifting the legs or administration of atropine may accentuate the gradient.

E. Therapy

1. **Medical therapy** consists of intensive sodium restriction and diuretic therapy.
2. **Defining coexisting valvular lesions** is critical to properly managing TS. For instance, in patients with combined TS and MS, the former should not be corrected alone, as this may produce pulmonary congestion. If other valvular surgery is planned, concomitant treatment of TS should be considered if the gradient exceeds 5 mm Hg or the TV orifice area is <2.0 cm^2.
3. **Severe stenosis requires balloon valvuloplasty or TV replacement.** The indications for surgery or balloon valvuloplasty are usually determined by the

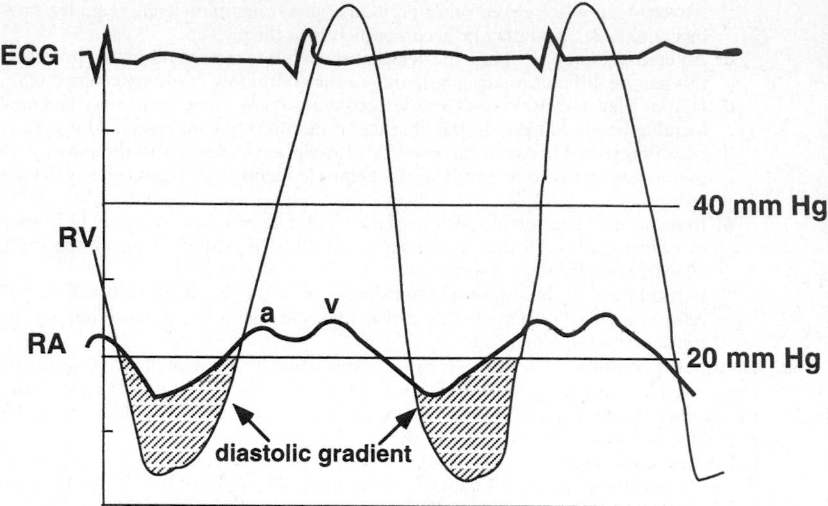

Figure 15.1. Tracings of simultaneous right atrial (RA) and right ventricular (RV) pressure waveforms in a patient with tricuspid stenosis.

severity of concomitant mitral or aortic valve disease. Limiting symptoms due to predominant TS are considered an indication for valvuloplasty or surgery. Balloon valvuloplasty appears to be successful both, from a symptomatic and hemodynamic standpoint, but can result in significant TR, potentially necessitating valve replacement.

4. **Bioprostheses are favored** when valve replacement is necessary at the tricuspid position, as **mechanical prostheses are more prone to thrombosis** at this location. Combined severe stenosis and regurgitation, as occurs with carcinoid disease, usually necessitates a surgical approach.

III. TRICUSPID REGURGITATION (TR)

A. Etiology and pathophysiology.

A. Etiology and pathophysiology. Any disease process that causes derangement of the TV apparatus (annulus, leaflets, chordae, and papillary muscles) can lead to TR. The most common cause of TR is not intrinsic valvular disease but rather dilation of the right ventricle, causing secondary (functional) TR. Table 15.2 lists the causes of TR.

1. TR with an **anatomically normal valve (i.e., secondary TR)** is more common and can occur in patients with pulmonary hypertension, cor pulmonale (e.g., chronic obstructive pulmonary disease, COPD), mitral stenosis, and left-heart failure. In each of these instances, TR reflects the presence of, and in turn aggravates, right ventricular failure.
2. TR with an **anatomically abnormal valve (i.e., primary TR)** can be a manifestation of congenital heart disease [e.g., Ebstein's anomaly, atrioventricular canal, ventricular septal defect (VSD)]. In addition, a variety of conditions such as rheumatic fever, myxomatous disease, carcinoid heart disease, radiation, endomyocardial fibrosis, and the hypereosinophilic syndrome can cause scarring/thickening of the TV apparatus, resulting in poor leaflet coaptation and TR.

B. Clinical presentation

1. **Signs and symptoms.** The spectrum of symptoms of TR is wide and depends on its etiology and chronicity. **Isolated TR is usually well tolerated.** When TR and pulmonary hypertension coexist, cardiac output declines and patients may manifest symptoms of right heart failure. Patients may present with painful **hepatic congestion and substantial peripheral edema. Fatigue** from reduced cardiac output is another common presentation. Patients may notice **pulsations in their**

TABLE 15.2 Causes of Tricuspid Regurgitation

Primary causes
Rheumatic
Ebstein's anomaly
Carcinoid
Connective tissue disease (e.g., Marfan's)
Tricuspid valve prolapse
Trauma
Tumor of tricuspid valve leaflet
Infective endocarditis
Papillary muscle dysfunction
Radiation injury
Myocardial infarction
Secondary causes
Right ventricular dilation (dilated annulus)
Pulmonary hypertension

MI, myocardial infarction; RV, right ventricular; TR, tricuspid regurgitation; TV, tricuspid valve.

neck due to the prominent *v wave* in the jugular venous pulse. TR often coexists with MV disease; in these patients, the symptoms associated with MV disease usually predominate.

2. **Physical findings**
   a. On general examination, patients with severe TR may have signs of weight loss, cachexia and jaundice, related to congestive hepatopathy and bowel edema.
   b. The neck veins will show loss of the usual *x* wave and a prominent systolic wave, usually referred to as a *c-v* wave, followed by a rapid *y* descent. The characteristics of the large *c-v* wave in the jugular venous pulse are dependent on TR severity. With significant TR, the prominent *c-v* wave has maximal height at S_2, and the rapid *y* descent is most prominent on inspiration. A venous systolic thrill and murmur in the neck may be present in severe TR. The RV impulse is often hyperdynamic.
   c. TR typically produces a **pansystolic murmur** at the third to fourth intercostal space along the left sternal border. The TR **murmur increases with inspiration (Carvallo sign).**
   d. A TR murmur that develops **in the presence of pulmonary hypertension is usually high pitched** and pansystolic, whereas a TR **murmur of primary etiology** (from endocarditis or trauma) is **short** (limited to first half of systole) **and low pitched.**
   e. TR causes an increase in diastolic flow across the TV. This may be heard as an **early diastolic rumble** (short and low pitched) along the left sternal border.
   f. With **severe, longstanding TR,** there is **ventricularization of the right atrium** (the pressure gradient across the TV is minimized), and the TR **may be barely audible or absent.**
   g. **Other findings.** A **right-sided third or fourth heart sound (S_3 or S_4) is often present along the left sternal border, which augments with inspiration. If pulmonary hypertension coexists, P_2** is accentuated. **Systolic pulsation** of the liver is often an associated physical finding, although this may be diminished once congestive cirrhosis develops.

C. **Laboratory examination**
   1. **Electrocardiography.** The findings are usually nonspecific. Incomplete right bundle-branch block may be seen. Atrial fibrillation is commonly found in association with severe TR.

2. **Echocardiography.** The most common views used for the detection of TR are the parasternal right ventricular inflow, basal short axis, and the apical four-chamber views.
   a. **Physiologic TR.** A small degree of TR is observed in about 70% of patients with structurally normal hearts, and the prevalence increases with age. Physiologic TR is usually represented by a small jet that does not extend >1 cm into the atrium.
   b. **Two-dimensional findings**
      (1) Leaflet thickening may be seen in TR due to rheumatic or carcinoid disease. In secondary TR, the leaflets may appear normal. Tricuspid prolapse often occurs in patients with MV prolapse and may cause significant TR. In Ebstein's anomaly, the septal leaflet of the TV is displaced apically. Vegetations are evident with endocarditis, and a flail valve leaflet may be seen with iatrogenic damage (e.g., after endomyocardial biopsy) or following papillary muscle rupture with right ventricular infarction.
      (2) With moderate to severe TR, a **right ventricular volume overload pattern** is seen, characterized by right ventricular enlargement, ventricular septal flattening or shift to the left in diastole, and paradoxical motion in systole. There is often associated dilation of the right atrium and inferior vena cava (IVC).
   c. **Doppler analysis.** Assessment of TR involves incorporation of all of the Doppler information obtainable: size of the color jet, presence or absence of a proximal convergence zone (on the right atrial side of the valve), velocity profile, and eccentricity of the TR jet. Eccentric, wall-hugging jets should are typically upgraded by one grade, as is done for mitral regurgitation, because they are generally not visualized fully by echocardiography.
      (1) TR direction and severity are assessed with color-flow Doppler. Severity of TR is estimated in several ways, including:
         (a) jet area—This measure is highly dependent on on echocardiographic settings, particularly the pulse repetition frequency (PRF), and the direction and eccentricity of the jet.
         (b) vena contracta—The narrowest portion of the jet just downstream from the valve orifice gives a rough estimate of the effective orifice area. A jet width of >0.7 cm suggests severe TR.
         (c) proximal flow convergence (see Chapter 14)
         (d) Continuous-wave Doppler—The signal intensity and contour of the TR jet by CW Doppler can help define TR severity. Severe TR produces a dense spectral recording along with a triangular, early peaking velocity.
         (e) hepatic vein flow—Systolic flow reversal in the IVC or hepatic veins is consistent with severe TR.
      (2) The RV systolic pressure (RVSP) is estimated by measuring the peak TR jet velocity by CW Doppler and applying the modified Bernoulli equation. In the absence of pulmonic stenosis, the pulmonary artery systolic pressure (PASP) can then be estimated as PASP = RVSP + RAP.
3. **Cardiac catheterization.** In the presence of moderate to severe TR, right-heart catheterization will show a dominant v wave in the right atrial pressure curve (Fig. 15.2), a right atrial pressure curve resembling that of the right ventricle, increased right ventricular end-diastolic pressure, and low cardiac output by thermodilution and Fick techniques. **Angiocardiography** involves injecting contrast into the right ventricle while viewing the right anterior oblique projection. This method allows for visualization and semiquantification of the TR jet but is rarely performed, as echocardiographic techniques are more reliable.

D. Therapy

1. In the absence of pulmonary hypertension, mild to moderate degrees of TR can be well tolerated for many years, and surgery is not recommended (ACC/AHA class III). If right ventricular failure develops, **medical therapy** should be targeted at diuretic therapy and afterload reduction, as in other heart failure states.

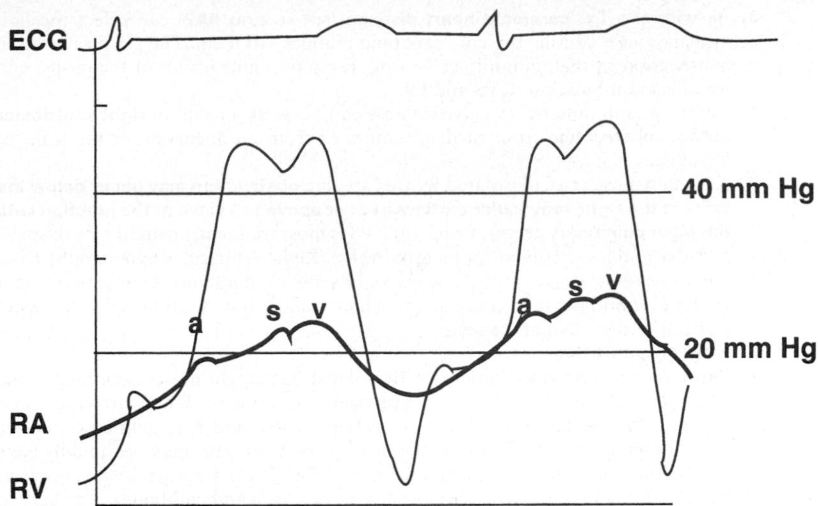

Figure 15.2. Tracings of simultaneous right atrial (RA) and right ventricular (RV) pressure waveforms in a patient with tricuspid regurgitation.

2. **Surgical therapy.** When there is an **organic (primary) cause** of moderate to severe TR, **surgical repair or replacement** may be necessary. Most commonly, surgery for TR is considered in combination with aortic or MV intervention. Tricuspid valve repair is recommended when there is severe TR in patients with MV disease requiring MV surgery (ACC/AHA class I). In patients with mitral stenosis and TR, a decision to repair the TV should be based on the severity of the TR, as well as the duration and severity of pulmonary hypertension (i.e., TR in the setting of longstanding pulmonary hypertension and MS is unlikely to improve with MV surgery alone). Usually tricuspid repair or annuloplasty is favored over prosthetic implantation where this is feasible. As severe TR may be well tolerated without symptoms for many years, indications for surgery in isolated severe TR are not well delineated. Generally, surgical intervention is recommended in severe TR for symptomatic deterioration (ACC/AHA class IIa), progressive enlargement of an already dilated right ventricle, or evidence of right ventricular contractile dysfunction.

PULMONARY VALVE DISEASE

I. INTRODUCTION. The pulmonary valve is a trileaflet valve that separates the right ventricle from the pulmonary vasculature. Dysfunction of the valve can have adverse effects on the right ventricle by producing pressure and/or volume overload. Like TR, a small degree of pulmonic regurgitation (PR) is a common finding in healthy adults. Acquired pulmonary valve disease is rare in comparison with other valvular disorders.

II. VALVULAR PULMONARY STENOSIS (PS)

A. Etiology

1. **Congenital** pulmonary stenosis is the most common pulmonary valve problem, occurring in approximately 10% to 12% of all adult patients with congenital heart disease. Valvular PS is typically an isolated abnormality, but it may occur in conjunction with VSD.
2. **Rheumatic** heart disease can affect the pulmonary valve, although this is uncommon and usually occurs in the setting of multivalvular involvement. This can result in thickening and fusion of the valve leaflets, resulting in pulmonary stenosis.

3. As with the TV, **carcinoid heart disease** (see section **IIA2**) can affect the pulmonary valve, causing typical "carcinoid plaques" to form. The plaques result in constriction of the pulmonic valve ring, retraction and fusion of the cusps, and usually a combination of PS and PR.
4. Rarely, pseudopulmonary valve stenosis can occur as a result of **right ventricular outflow obstruction** from cardiac tumors or from an aneurysm of the sinus of Valsalva.
5. Although most cases of isolated PS are valvular, **obstruction may occur below the valve in the right ventricular outflow tract or above the valve at the junction with the main pulmonary artery**. Congenital PS is most frequently caused by a dysplastic valve and less frequently a bicuspid valve. Right ventricular hypertrophy from the pressure overload of the PS on the right ventricle may cause concomitant right ventricular outflow tract obstruction, which usually reverses following successful dilation of the valvular stenosis.

B. Clinical presentation

1. **Signs and symptoms.** Patients with isolated PS present most commonly in the fourth or fifth decade of life with signs and symptoms of right heart failure and dyspnea on exertion. Of note, many patients with moderate pulmonic stenosis remain asymptomatic. When the stenosis is severe, patients may occsionally have retrosternal chest pain or syncope with exertion. If the foramen ovale is patent, right-to-left shunting may occur, producing cyanosis and clubbing.
2. **Physical findings**
   a. Pulmonary valve stenosis causes a systolic crescendo–decrescendo murmur, heard best in the third and fourth intercostal spaces, with delayed peaking of the murmur in severe PS. The murmur typically increases with inspiration. A thrill may be felt in the suprasternal notch and at the left upper sternal border. S_2 is often split widely, and the degree of the splitting increases with worsening stenosis due to delay of P_2. The intensity of P_2 may be increased in mild stenosis, but is usually diminished with severe stenosis. An ejection click can sometimes be heard along the left sternal border, and it may vary with respiration. As severity of PS increases, the click will move closer to S_1.
   b. The right ventricular impulse may be palpated at the left sternal border and be hyperdynamic.
   c. The jugular venous pressure can be normal. However, in patients with reduced right ventricular compliance, a prominent *a* wave may be seen in the venous pulse. A right-sided fourth heart sound (RV S_4) may be heard at the left lower sternal border.
   d. In advanced cases, evidence of right-sided heart failure may be present, including hepatic congestion and peripheral edema.

C. Diagnostic testing

1. **Electrocardiogram (ECG).** In patients with moderate to severe PS, the ECG may show right-axis deviation and right ventricular hypertrophy.
2. Chest radiography may reveal **poststenotic dilation** of the main pulmonary artery, and diminished pulmonary vascular markings.
3. **Echocardiography** is useful in diagnosing pulmonary valve stenosis and for quantifying the severity of the obstruction. The best images of the pulmonary valve are obtained from the short-axis view at the level of the base from the parasternal and subcostal windows. Transesophageal echocardiography is useful when the transthoracic echocardiogram images are suboptimal.
   a. **Leaflets.** In adults the leaflets can appear thickened and calcified with restricted motion. In children with congenital PS, the leaflets are noncalcified with doming of the valve.
   b. **Right ventricle.** The right ventricle can be normal, especially in children. Right ventricle dilation and hypertrophy can be seen in adults, depending on the severity and duration of the disease.
4. **Doppler echocardiography** is the preferred method for grading the severity of pulmonary stenosis. This method of quantifying pulmonary stenosis is well correlated with direct measurement by cardiac catheterization. The peak gradient

is measured across the pulmonary valve by using CW Doppler with the modified Bernoulli equation. The following levels of severity have been defined in the 2006 American College of Cardiology/American Heart Association (ACC/AHA) guidelines on the management of valvular heart disease:

(a) Severe stenosis: a peak jet velocity >4 meters per second (peak gradient >60 mm Hg)

(b) Moderate stenosis: peak jet velocity of 3 to 4 meters per second (peak gradient 36 to 60 mm Hg)

(c) Mild stenosis: peak jet velocity is <3 meters per second (peak gradient <36 mm Hg).

In determining need for intervention, no specific Doppler gradients have been proposed as guidelines.

D. Therapy

1. Mild to moderate pulmonary stenosis has a very good prognosis, and intervention is rarely necessary. Survival is excellent among patients with mild PS, with 94% still alive 20 years after diagnosis.
2. Patients with severe PS should have this stenosis relieved. In fact, only 40% of such patients do not require intervention by 10 years after diagnosis. The treatment of choice is **balloon valvuloplasty,** usually with a 75% decrement in the transvalvular gradient. The procedure is usually successful if the valve is mobile and pliant. Prognosis and morbidity subsequent to the procedure are largely based on right ventricular function at the time of the procedure. The hypertrophic subpulmonary stenosis that can accompany valvular stenosis usually regresses after successful valvuloplasty. Valve replacement may be necessary if the valve is severely calcified or if there is severe concomitant TR.
3. **ACC/AHA Guidelines for intervention** in congenital pulmonary stenosis are as follows:

   Class I: Balloon valvuloplasty is indicated in symptomatic patients with >30 mm Hg gradient (peak–peak) across the pulmonary valve at cardiac catheterization and in asymptomatic patients when this gradient is >40 mm Hg.

   Class II: Balloon valuloplasty may be reasonable if pulmonary valve gradient is 30 to 39 mm Hg by cardiac catheterization in an asymptomatic younger patient.

   Class III: Balloon valvuloplasty is not indicated in asymptomatic patients whose pulmonary valve gradient is <30 mm Hg at catheterization.
4. Pulmonary stenosis secondary to **carcinoid syndrome** has a very poor prognosis (with a median survival of 1.6 years), and the valve often does not respond to balloon valvuloplasty. **Valve replacement** is often necessary.

III. VALVULAR PULMONARY REGURGITATION (PR)

A. Etiology. PR is most commonly produced secondary to dilation of the valve ring due to pulmonary hypertension or dilation of the pulmonary artery.

1. Unlike pulmonary valve stenosis, **pulmonary regurgitation has rare congenital causes,** such as an absent, malformed, or fenestrated leaflet. In the setting of repaired tetralogy of Fallot, PR is a common and difficult problem, often contributing to progressive right ventricular dilation and dysfunction.
2. Acquired causes of pathologic pulmonary valve regurgitation are much more common. **The most common acquired cause is pulmonary artery hypertension,** followed by infective endocarditis. Carcinoid syndrome and rheumatic heart disease both can cause pulmonary regurgitation but are more likely to cause pulmonary stenosis. Marfan's syndrome can cause pulmonary valve regurgitation secondary to dilation of the pulmonary artery. Iatrogenic pulmonary regurgitation can be caused by placement of a pulmonary artery catheter.

B. Clinical presentation

1. **Signs and symptoms.** Like TR, PR causes volume overload of the right ventricle and may be tolerated well for many years, in the absence of pulmonary hypertension. Once symptomatic, patients with PR present with signs and symptoms of **right-heart failure and dyspnea on exertion.** In the setting of PR caused by infective endocarditis, patients may present with fevers and hypoxia due to septic pulmonary emboli.

2. **Physical findings**
   a. The murmur of pulmonary regurgitation is a relatively brief **low-pitched, diamond-shaped, diastolic murmur,** heard best in the third and fourth left intercostal spaces with a widening of S_2. The murmur increases with inspiration, and **P_2 is accentuated** in the presence of pulmonary artery hypertension.
   b. The **Graham Steell murmur** is a high-pitched, blowing decrescendo diastolic murmur starting immediately after P_2, which is accentuated by inspiration. This characteristic murmur occurs when pulmonary artery systolic pressure exceeds 70 mm Hg in the presence of pulmonary regurgitation.
   c. A right ventricular S_3 and S_4 may be audible in the fourth intercostal space and will be augmented by inspiration. Depending on the severity and duration of the regurgitant valve, signs and symptoms of right-heart failure may also be present on examination.

C. **Diagnostic testing.** The pulmonary valve is best evaluated with **echocardiography**, using the left ventricle short-axis view from the parasternal and subcostal windows. Minor degrees of pulmonary regurgitation are seen in 40% to 78% of normal individuals. Pathologic PR is relatively infrequent and should be diagnosed in the context of other structural abnormalities.
   1. **Anatomic assessment.** The right ventricular outflow tract and pulmonary valve should be interrogated for abnormalities such as leaflet hypoplasia, increased cusp number, and abnormal valve motion (i.e., doming).
   2. **Right ventricle.** Size and function of the RV can provide an indicator of the severity of PR (i.e., longstanding severe PR should be associated with RV dilation and/or hypertrophy).
   3. Color-flow Doppler will reveal a regurgitant jet toward the right ventricle during diastole. Jet length is determined largely by the pressure different between the pulmonary artery and right ventricular and, therefore, is an unreliable indicator of PR severity. The **vena contracta** is probably a better measure of PR severity.
   4. Continuous-wave Doppler will show a dense spectral signal and rapid equilibration of diastolic pressures in severe PR. Maintenance of the regurgitant velocity during diastole suggests that **pulmonary hypertension** is the cause of valve incompetence. Furthermore, increasing pulmonary artery pressures correlate with decreasing acceleration times of pulmonary artery flow. Pulmonary artery pressures can be obtained using Doppler flow measurements and the following equation. Pulmonary artery diastolic pressure (PADP) is only obtainable in the setting of pulmonary regurgitation:

$$\text{PADP} = 4(V_{\text{PR-E}})^2 + \text{RA}_{\text{PRESSURE}}$$

   where $V_{\text{PR-E}}$ is the end-diastolic pulmonary regurgitation velocity.

D. **Therapy**
   1. **Primary pulmonary valve regurgitation.** The prognosis is very good; rarely is correction of the defect necessary, except in cases of intractable right-heart failure.
   2. **Secondary pulmonary valve regurgitation.** The prognosis due to endocarditis, carcinoid, or pulmonary artery hypertension is tied to the prognosis and treatment of the primary disease. Treatment of the primary condition (e.g., repairing MV in the setting of pulmonary hypertension) often ameliorates the PR. Similarly, vasodilating therapies for pulmonary hypertension can reduce secondary PR. When treatment is necessary, **the preferred approach is valve replacement with a porcine bioprosthesis or a pulmonary allograft.** Percutaneous deployment of a prosthetic valve has been successfully accomplished in this setting and is under active investigation currently. Annulus repair is ideal in patients with coexisting left-sided valvular lesions.

DRUG-INDUCED VALVE DISEASE

I. **INTRODUCTION.** Most common forms of valve disease are inherited or acquired in response to a specific disease process. Over the last two decades, however, it has become clear that several prescribed drugs can produce a cardiac valvulopathy, which mimics other etiologies of valvular disease.

II. DRUGS KNOWN TO CAUSE VALVE DISEASE

A. Ergot alkaloid derivatives (ergotamine, methysergide) were reported to cause valve disease in the early 1990s.

B. In 1997, Connolly et al. reported that both **fenfluramine** and **dexfenfluramine,** the components of popular diet pills, were associated with valvular heart disease with a typical histologic appearance (described in subsequent text). This led to the withdrawal from the market of a number of common diet drugs. At their peak usage, about 14 million prescriptions had been written for these medications.

C. More recently, valvular heart disease was reported in 24% to 28% of patients undergoing treatment of Parkinson's disease with **ergot-derived dopamine agonists (pergolide, cabergoline).**

D. Thus far, there has not been convincing evidence of valvular heart disease with use of other serotonergic drugs (e.g., selective serotonin reuptake inhibitors [SSRIs]).

III. PATHOLOGY AND PATHOGENESIS

A. Surgically removed valves with these drugs are described as having a white, glistening appearance, with histologic evidence of a plaque-like process extending along the leaflet and encasing the chordae tendineae. These findings are **very similar to the findings seen in patients with valvular disease due to carcinoid tumors,** which also secrete vasoactive amines.

B. Subsequent research has indicated that valvulopathic drugs may act via their ability to stimulate the serotonergic receptors, particularly the 5-hydroxytryptamine $(5\text{-HT})_{2B}$ serotonin receptor. This receptor is plentiful in normal heart valves and appears to be essential for normal cardiac development. Stimulation of the 5-HT_{2B} receptor appears to cause mitogenic stimulation of normally quiescent valve cells, causing an "overgrowth" valvulopathy.

IV. PREVALENCE. Estimates of the prevalence of drug-induced valvular disease have varied widely. Initial studies based on case series suggested a prevalence of valve disease as high as 20% to 30% in the setting of fenfluramine exposure, but larger population-based studies suggest a much lower prevalence of around 10% to 12% (versus 5% to 6% in control group). **Factors that appear to be associated with a greater prevalence of valvular disease include duration of treatment, use of combination agents, and shorter time from cessation of drug treatment to evaluation.** The prevalence of disease is highest in those who have been on a valvulopathic medication for >6 months.

V. CLINICAL PRESENTATION. Most commonly, patients seek advice based on a history of taking ergot-derived medications or diet drugs, given the media attention associated with this condition and the legal action that has been mounted against the drug manufacturers. Patients may also present with symptoms of valve disease, such as dyspnea and fatigue. **The predominant findings on examination in patients with significant valve disease involve regurgitation of the aortic, mitral, or TVs.** Ergot derivatives and methysergide also affect mainly left-sided valves and cause regurgitation. Aortic regurgitation is reported with increased frequency in those with diet drug-induced disease than regurgitation at other valves.

VI. EVALUATION. Patients suspected of having valve lesions on examination or those in whom a cardiac examination is somewhat limited by obesity and who have been exposed to diet drugs should undergo echocardiography. The echocardiographic features simulate both rheumatic disease and carcinoid disease with **leaflet thickening and doming of the MV and thickening of the aortic or tricuspid valves leaflets.** Despite the apparent restriction of motion of the leaflets, **stenosis is rare.** Regurgitation, when present, may be of any grade of severity, although it is most commonly mild. However, severe regurgitation requiring surgery has been reported with diet drug–induced valve disease.

VII. TREATMENT. Once drug-induced valve disease is suspected, any drug associated with valve lesions should be discontinued immediately. In the case of diet drug–induced valve lesions, **some improvement in the severity of the valve regurgitation has been reported on echocardiography at follow-up intervals of 1 year in patients in whom the**

diet drugs were discontinued. Progression in the severity of valve disease following drug discontinuation is relatively uncommon. Indications for surgical intervention in drug-induced valve lesions are similar to those for other disease processes. However, watchful waiting is a prudent approach in these patients, given the potential for some reversibility of the valve lesions upon drug discontinuation. Endocarditis prophylaxis is not indicated in those with evidence of drug-induced valve disease, per the most recent American Heart Association guidelines.

VIII. FOLLOW-UP. Patients with valve disease should be evaluated both clinically and with echocardiography initially every 6 months. In those with mild stable lesions, yearly evaluation is appropriate.

ACKNOWLEDGMENTS

The authors thank Drs. Amy P. Scally and Marc Penn for their contributions to earlier editions of this chapter.

Suggested Readings

Antunes MJ, Barlow JB. Management of TV regurgitation. *Heart 2007*;93:271–276.

Brickner ME, Hillis LD, Lange RA. Congenital heart disease in adults—first of two parts. *N Engl J Med* 2000;342:256–263.

Connolly HM, Crary JL, McGoon MD, et al. Valvular heart disease associated with fenfluramine-phentermine. *N Engl J Med* 1997;337:581–588.

Gardin, JM, Weissman NJ, Leung C, et al. Clinical and echoicardiographi follow-up of patients previously treated with dexfenfluramine or phentermine/fenfluramine. *JAMA* 2001;286:2011–2015.

Jick H, Vasilakis C, Weinrauch LA, et al. A population-based study of appetite-suppressant drugs and the risk of cardiac-valve regurgitation. *N Engl J Med* 1998;339:719–724.

Redfield MM, Nicholson WJ, Edwards WD, et al. Valve disease associated with ergot alkaloid use: echocardiographic and pathologic correlations. *Ann Intern Med* 1992;117:50–52.

Roth BL. Drugs and valvular heart disease. *N Engl J Med* 2007;356:6–9.

Sadr-Ameli MA, Sheikholeslami F, Firoozi I, et al. Late results of balloon pulmonary valvuloplasty in adults. *Am J Cardiol* 1998;82:398–400.

Scully HE, Armstrong CS. Tricuspid valve replacement: fifteen years of experience with mechanical prosthesis and bio-prosthesis. *J Thorac Cardiovasc Surg* 1995;109:1035–1041.

Shively BK, Roldan CA, Gill EA, et al. Prevalence and determinants of valvulopathy in patients treated with dexfenflu-ramine. *Circulation* 1999;100:2161–2167.

Van Nooten GJ, Caes FL, Francois KJ, et al. The valve choice in tricuspid valve replacement: 25 years of experience. *Eur J Cardiothorac Surg* 1995;9:441–446.

Weissman NJ, Tighe JF Jr, Gottdiener JS, et al. Sustained-Release Dexfenfluramine Study Group. An assessment of heart-valve abnormalities in obese patients taking dexfenfluramine, sustained-release dexfenfluramine, or placebo. *N Engl J Med* 1998;339:725–732.

Zoghbi WA, Enriquez-Sarano M, Foster E, et al. Recommendations for the evaluation of native valvular regurgitation with two-dimensional and Doppler echocardiography. *J Am Soc Echocardiogr* 2003;16:777–802.

Relevant Book Chapters

Braunwald E. *Heart disease: a textbook of cardiovascular medicine,* 8th ed. Philadelphia: WB Saunders, 2007:1674–1681.

Cheitlin MD, Macgregor JS. Acquired tricuspid and pulmonary valve disease. In: Topol EJ, ed. *Textbook of cardiovascular medicine,* 2nd ed. Philadelphia: Lippincott–Raven Publishers, 2002:529–548.

Weyman AE. *Principles and practice of echocardiography,* 2nd ed. Philadelphia: Lea & Febiger, 1994:824–862.

PROSTHETIC HEART VALVES

Ron Jacob and Richard Troughton

16

I. INDICATIONS FOR IMPLANTATION

A. Types of prosthetic valves. Prosthetic valves are classified into two major categories: mechanical and bioprosthetic. Each model differs in its durability, thrombogenicity, and hemodynamic performance. Various mechanical and bioprosthetic valves are shown in Figure 16.1.

1. Bioprosthetic valves. These resemble native valves but have a slightly less optimal hemodynamic performance, owing to the reduction in flow profile by interposed stents and the sewing ring.

a. Heterografts

(1) Carpentier-Edwards valves are made of either bovine pericardium (aortic position), which have greater durability, or porcine leaflets mounted on a cloth-covered annular ring and supported by steel-alloy flexible stents at each of the commissures.

(2) The Hancock II porcine valve has stents manufactured from Delrin; the prosthetic sewing ring is supraannular to improve hemodynamic performance; and modern preservation techniques using low-pressure fixation and treatment with sodium dodecyl sulfate may increase longevity.

(3) For the **stentless porcine bioprostheses** (Medtronic Freestyle or St. Jude Medical), there are three different methods for implantation, with the subcoronary valve replacement being the most common. Although the stentless valves offer a better hemodynamic profile owing to the larger effective orifice area, convincing advantages in terms of mortality, left ventricular (LV) mass regression and durability (when compared with pericardial not porcine valves) have yet to be demonstrated.

b. Aortic homografts are cryopreserved cadaveric human aortic valves. These are typically implanted stentless, with a short segment of the donor's aortic root for support. The coronary arteries require reimplantation. The hemodynamic profile of the homograft is similar to that of the native valve. Availability of homografts is a limiting factor.

2. Mechanical valves

a. Single-leaflet tilting disk. These valves (e.g., Björk-Shiley, Medtronic Hall, and Omniscience) consist of a metallic sewing ring attached to a tilting disk made of pyrolytic carbon that rotates about an off-centered pivot axis with a range of about 60° to 85° from the occluded to the open position. When open, the prosthesis has two orifices separated by the occluder. The major orifice is formed as the disk swings downstream to the open position. The disk on the other side of the pivot axis swings proximally forming the minor orifice.

b. Bileaflet tilting disk. The St. Jude and Carbomedics valves have two semicircular pyrolytic carbon disks that rotate freely through 75° to 90°. Two large lateral orifices and a small central rectangular space are created in the open position. A built-in leakage volume is designed to reduce thrombus formation on disks.

c. Caged ball. The Starr-Edwards valve consists of a silicone ball within a cage attached to a metallic alloy ring. The ball is free to travel along the cage over a distance of 1 to 2 cm. Flow across the prosthesis is directed circumferentially around the ball. The hemodynamic profile is less favorable than that of the

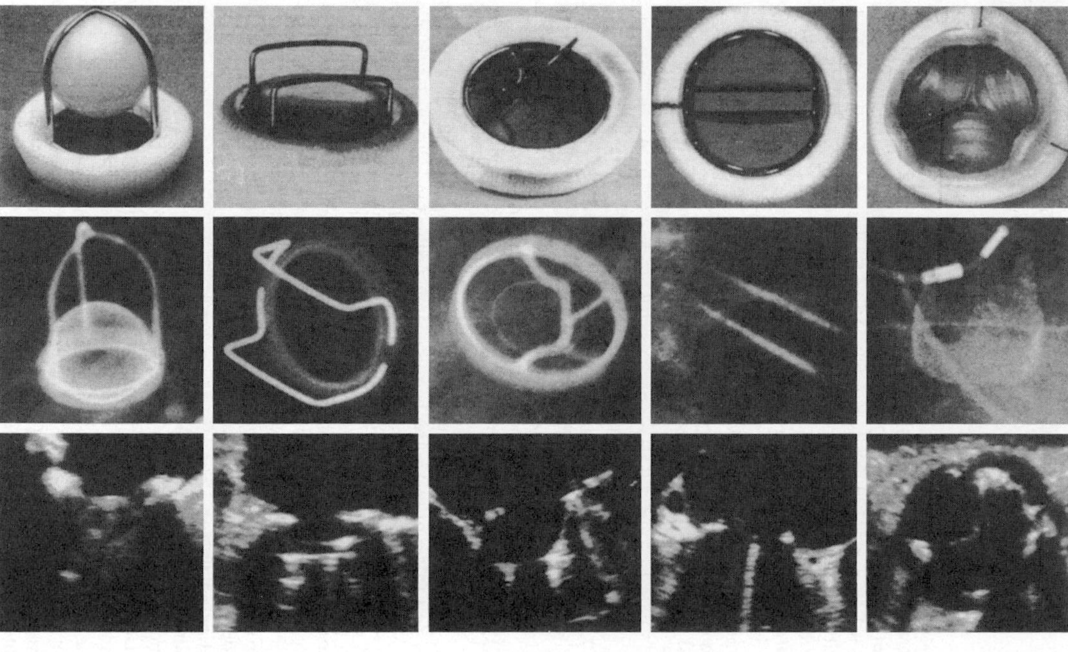

Figure 16.1. Photographic and radiographic appearance of different prosthetic heart valves. *From left to right*: Starr-Edwards caged ball, Kay-Suzuki caged disk, Björk-Shiley single tilting disk, St. Jude's bileaflet tilting disk mechanical valves, and Carpentier-Edwards xenograft. (From Garcia M. Principles of imaging. In: Topol EJ, ed. *Comprehensive cardiovascular medicine.* Philadelphia: Lippincott–Raven Publishers, 1998:610.)

TABLE 16.1 Clinical Factors Leading to Selection of a Bioprosthetic Versus a Mechanical Valve

Factors favoring bioprosthesis	Factors favoring homograft (aortic valve)	Factors favoring mechanical prosthesis
Age >70 y Bleeding diathesis High risk for trauma Poor compliance	Age <50 y Endocarditis Female considering pregnancy	Age <60 y Combined multivalvular placement Patients with other indications for chronic anticoagulation

tilting disk prosthesis.This is the valve with the greatest durability with a 30-year follow up in some studies.

B. Selection of valves. Table 16.1 summarizes the clinical factors that favor selection of a bioprosthetic versus a mechanical valve. The recommendation to use tissue valves in older patients and mechanical valves in younger patients are based on information obtained from older trials. There have been no randomized controlled trials after 1982 comparing mechanical with bioprosthetic valves, which makes the decision difficult, as newer bioprosthetic valves may be more durable than older ones.

1. **Valve repair.** The feasibility of native valve repair instead of replacement should always be considered prior to surgery (Table 16.2). Currently, the greatest experience is with mitral valve (MV) repair. If feasible, MV repair offers several potential advantages over replacement, including **preservation of LV function via conservation of the subvalvular apparatus, lower operative mortality, higher long-term survival rate, and freedom from anticoagulation.** Mitral valve repair may be considered for asymptomatic patients with severe mitral regurgitation if there is a high chance of repair at high volume centers. An aortic valve with predominant regurgitation due to prolapse, but without severe stenosis or calcification, can also be repaired, although the longterm durability of this approach is not as well established as it is for mitral repair.
2. **Bioprosthetic valves** are indicated in patients with **a contraindication to chronic anticoagulation** and preferred for **patients ≥ 65 years (70 years in the mitral position)** due to reasonable durability, favorable hemodynamic profile, and freedom from chronic anticoagulation. Approximately 30% of heterograft bioprostheses fail within 10 to 15 years of implantation, although the incidence of bioprosthesis failure is age dependent (Table 16.3). Overall complication rates for aortic bioprosthetic and mechanical valves are similar at 12 years, with a higher rate of reoperation for bioprosthetic valves and a higher rate of hemorrhage with mechanical valves. The advent of newer low-profile bioprostheses and the apparent improved durability of later models has led to an increase in their use, especially in patients who wish to avoid anticoagulation.

TABLE 16.2 Characteristics Favoring Valve Repair Versus Replacement

Favoring valve replacement	Favoring valve repair
Rheumatic valve disease	Mitral valve prolapse
Endocarditis	Excessive leaflet mobility
Inexperienced surgeon	Ischemic mitral valve regurgitation
Complex mitral valve morphology	Bicuspid aortic valve with prolapse
Calcified and fibrosed valve	Annular dilatation with normal leaflets
Extensive leaflet destruction	

TABLE 16.3 Heterograft Valve Failure Rate 10 Years after Valve Replacement Relative to the Patient's Age

Patient's age (year)	Failure rate at 10 years (%)
<40	40
40–49	30
50–59	20
60–69	15
≥70	10

Modified from Vongpatanasin W, Hillis LD, et al. Prosthetic heart valves. *N Engl J Med* 1996;335:412, by permission of the Massachusetts Medical Society.

3. **Homografts.** The homograft is the **valve of choice in aortic valve endocarditis** and has the lowest valvular gradient among the bioprosthetic valves. Durability was thought to be superior to that of heterografts, but recent studies throw some doubt on this. Only 10% are still functioning after 20 years. The primary operation is more difficult with homografts as the coronary arteries require implantation. Reoperation is also more complex, as the homograft frquently calcifies and is difficult to remove and replace. The main current indication for an aortic homograft is complex endocarditis involving a native valve, and especially in prosthetic valve endocarditis and abscess where the risk of reinfection of a new prosthesis is high. Another indication is in older patients with small aortic root and left ventricular outflow tract in order to maximize hemodynamics and minimize the transaortic gradient.
4. **Mechanical valves.** Mechanical valves are **more durable than bioprosthetic valves;** some last >20 years. Mechanical prostheses are generally recommended for **patients <60 years** because of greater durability, and for **patients already on permanent anticoagulation** for previous stroke or arrhythmia. The stroke risk of about 1% per annum for patients with a mechanical valve receiving appropriate anticoagulation management is similar to that for a bioprosthetic valve without anticoagulation. In **younger patients requiring combined aortic and mitral valve replacement,** mechanical valves are preferred, given the more rapid rate of prosthesis deterioration in the mitral position. **Pregnancy should be discouraged in patients with mechanical prostheses** because of the high risk to the mother and the fetus (see Chapter 38). Given their lower profile, mechanical prostheses may be preferred in **patients with small ventricles.** Issues of **compliance with anticoagulation and risks of trauma** should be integrated into the selection of a mechanical valve.
   a. St. Jude Medical and Medtronic-Hall valves are the most popular prosthetic valves because of their favorable hemodynamic performance, longevity, and low rates of complications. Loss of structural integrity has been reported in a small percentage of patients with St. Jude valves, whereas the primary concern with the Medtronic-Hall valve is the potential for occluder impingement during placement.
   b. Starr-Edwards valves are the most durable of all the prosthetic valves. However, they are less popular today because of their thrombogenicity and suboptimal hemodynamic performance in comparison with tilting disk valves.
   c. Manufacture of the Björk-Shiley valve was discontinued in 1986 following published reports of complications with **strut fracture**.

C. **Follow-up after valve surgery.** There is a **wide spectrum of clinical practices** in the follow-up of the asymptomatic patient after valve surgery. A **Doppler** study should be performed between 1 and 6 weeks following surgery as a baseline for future reference. For **mechanical valves, anticoagulation** should be monitored regularly for life. **Endocarditis prophylaxis** is imperative for prosthetic valves, and patients should

TABLE 16.4 Recommended Anticoagulation Therapy for Patients with Mechanical Prosthetic Valves

Level of risk	Prosthesis type	Recommended INR
Low	Single-tilting disk	3.0–4.0
	Double-tilting disk	2.5–3.0
High[a]	Caged disk	3.0–4.5
	Caged ball	3.0–4.5
	Multiple prostheses	3.0–4.5

INR, International normalized ratio.
[a]Patients with atrial fibrillation, left atrial thrombus, severe left ventricular dysfunction, or previous embolic events.

receive appropriate education. Annual or biannual echocardiography seems prudent **after the fifth postoperative year** for valve repair and replacement.

D. Anticoagulation. Table 16.4 summarizes the recommended targets for anticoagulation therapy in patients with prosthetic heart valves. The **embolic event rate is greater for mitral than for aortic** prostheses.

1. Immediate postoperative period

a. Mechanical valves. The approach to **postoperative anticoagulation** for mechanical prostheses varies widely. Early anticoagulation increases the risk of bleeding and tamponade. One approach is **warfarin, but not heparin, 3 to 4 days following surgery** when the epicardial wires are removed. Other centers recommend **low-dose intravenous heparin,** targeted for upper normal limits of activated partial thromboplastin time within 6 to 12 hours after valve replacement and **full-dose intravenous heparin once the chest tubes are removed. Warfarin** is initiated within 24 to 48 hours following valve replacement. **Chronic anticoagulation for mechanical valves is associated with rates** of minor hemorrhage of 2% to 4% per year, major hemorrhage of 1% to 2% per year, and death of 0.2% to 0.5% per year. The bleeding risk is 5% to 6% in patients aged ≥70 years. The target international normalized ratio (INR) is between 2.0 and 3.0 for mechanical valves (tilting disc and bileaflet) in the aortic position and 2.5 and 3.5 for mechanical valves in the mitral position. Patient-related risk factors for thromboembolism are older age, atrial fibrillation, and left ventricular dysfunction.

b. Bioprosthetic valves. The **need for anticoagulation** in bioprosthetic valves is **controversial.** The risk for embolism is greatest in the early postoperative period, declines after 3 months, and is greater for mitral (7%) than for aortic valves (3%). A reasonable approach is to anticoagulate patients with a **mitral** bioprosthesis for 3 months and then change to aspirin, 325 mg daily. Patients with **aortic prostheses** should receive aspirin, 325 mg daily, for 3 months unless there is another reason for anticoagulation. **Patients with prior embolic events, atrial fibrillation, or left ventricular dysfunction should be anticoagulated for the long term.**

2. Management of anticoagulation in patients with prosthetic valves undergoing noncardiac surgery. Although the risk of thromboembolism increases when anticoagulant therapy is briefly discontinued, the decision to suspend therapy should be individualized.

a. For **major procedures** in which substantial blood loss is expected, **warfarin should be discontinued at least 3 days prior to the procedure** to achieve an INR of 1.6 or less. Hospital admission for **intravenous heparin administration** is often recommended for patients with **caged-ball prosthetic valves, atrial fibrillation, left atrial thrombus, severe left ventricular dysfunction, or previous embolization. Postoperatively,** intravenous heparin therapy should be **resumed when it is considered safe and continued until therapeutic**

anticoagulation is achieved with warfarin. Low–molecular-weight heparin may be considered for patients with prosthetic valves as bridge therapy.

b. For **minor procedures** (e.g., dental extraction) where blood loss is minimal, anticoagulation can be continued.

3. Pregnancy (see Chapter 38). Pregnant women have an increased incidence of thromboembolic complications. The use of warfarin through the entire course of pregnancy is associated with warfarin embryopathy in as many as 6.4% of live births. Given its teratogenic effects, **warfarin should be discontinued (at least between 6 and 12 weeks of the pregnancy) when pregnancy is considered or detected during the first trimester. Subcutaneous heparin** 17500–20,000 U every 12 hours with a target-activated partial thromboplastin time of 1.5 to 2.0 times the control 6 hours after injection should be administered until at least between 6 and 12 weeks of pregnancy, at which time warfarin may be resumed and continued until the middle third trimester. Subcutaneous heparin 5000 U is then administered twice a day until delivery. Low-dose aspirin can be used in conjunction with anticoagulant therapy for women at higher risk for thromboembolism. Low–molecular-weight heparin (LMWH) or unfractionated heparin may be considered as an alternative for the entire course of the pregnancy. With LMWH the anti-Xa levels should be monitored to ensure therapeutic efficacy.

II. ASSESSMENT OF PROSTHETIC VALVES

A. Clinical presentation. The clinical presentations of prosthetic valve dysfunction vary substantially. Discussion of the various entities occurs in **III**.

1. History. This should include a thorough cardiovascular review in addition to questions pertinent to the function of the prosthesis.

a. The **indication** for placement of valve prosthesis, **position** of implantation, **type** of prosthesis, and the **year of implantation** should be elicited. The model and size of the prosthesis can be verified by the identification card provided by the manufacturer.

b. Other important questions involve **compliance with the anticoagulation** regimen, previous **endocarditis, thromboembolism, fever,** and perceived **change in the quality of the valvular click.**

2. Physical findings

a. The physical examination may be remarkable for a **new murmur, muffled prosthetic valve sounds, or evidence of embolic events.**

b. Prosthetic valves are associated with **distinct auscultatory events caused by prosthesis motion or altered flow patterns.** The prosthesis sounds may mask the normal heart sounds; significant valvular dysfunction may occur without audible changes. However, familiarity with the normal auscultatory findings in the prosthetic valve examination can provide valuable clues on prosthesis dysfunction prior to the more definitive imaging examination. Figure 16.2 summarizes the acoustic characteristics of each valve prosthesis.

B. Laboratory examination and diagnostic testing. The diagnosis of structural valve degeneration relies predominantly on echocardiographic findings, which can often identify degeneration prior to the onset of symptoms.

1. Two-dimensional echocardiography. The interrogation of the prosthetic valve requires a thorough evaluation of the native structures and a systematic approach to the following: prosthetic apparatus, peak and mean gradient, and regurgitant flow. Typically, **transesophageal echocardiography** (TEE) is performed to evaluate **patients whose disease is symptomatic or who are suspected of having endocarditis.** The two-dimensional assessment of prosthetic valves is similar to that of the native valve, but is **limited by reverberation artifacts and acoustic shadowing.** In general, echocardiographic evaluation should be done to assess the following:

a. Occluders and leaflets. Failure of the leaflet or occluder to open or coapt properly may result from pannus ingrowth (**IIIH**), **thrombus formation** (**IIIE**), **or calcification of bioprosthetic leaflets.** Imaging of leaflets and occluders may be suboptimal with transthoracic echocardiography (TTE). Multiplane TEE provides higher temporal and spatial resolution of the prosthesis than

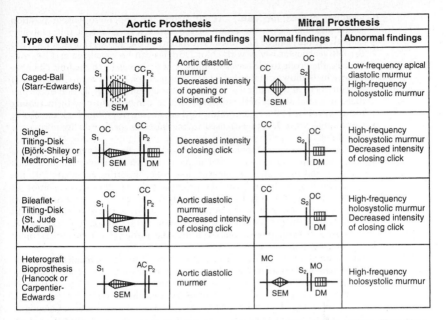

Type of Valve	Aortic Prosthesis		Mitral Prosthesis	
	Normal findings	Abnormal findings	Normal findings	Abnormal findings
Caged-Ball (Starr-Edwards)	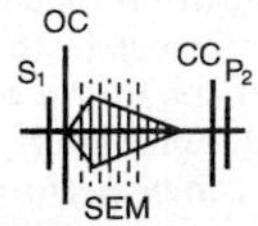 S_1 OC CC P_2 SEM	Aortic diastolic murmur Decreased intensity of opening or closing click	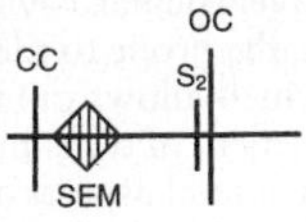 CC OC S_2 SEM	Low-frequency apical diastolic murmur High-frequency holosystolic murmur
Single-Tilting-Disk (Björk-Shiley or Medtronic-Hall)	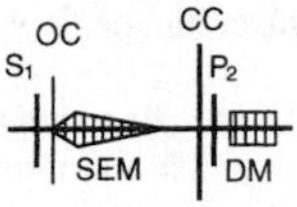 S_1 OC CC P_2 SEM DM	Decreased intensity of closing click	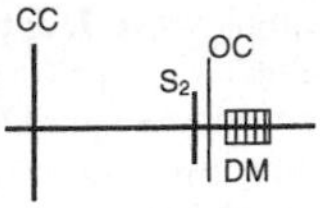 CC S_2 OC DM	High-frequency holosystolic murmur Decreased intensity of closing click
Bileaflet-Tilting-Disk (St. Jude Medical)	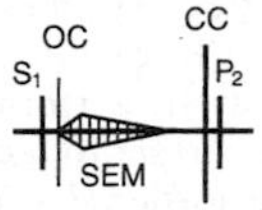 S_1 OC CC P_2 SEM	Aortic diastolic murmur Decreased intensity of closing click	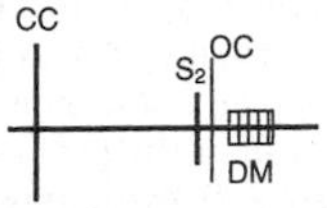 CC S_2 OC DM	High-frequency holosystolic murmur Decreased intensity of closing click
Heterograft Bioprosthesis (Hancock or Carpentier-Edwards)	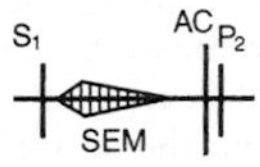 S_1 AC P_2 SEM	Aortic diastolic murmer	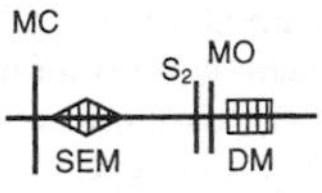 MC S_2 MO SEM DM	High-frequency holosystolic murmur

Figure 16.2. Acoustic characteristics of various mechanical and bioprosthetic valves. (From Vongpatanasin W, Hillis LD, et al. Prosthetic heart valves. *N Engl J Med* 1996;335:410.)

TTE and may allow measurement of valve area and mobility. Although the aortic prosthesis is less well visualized relative to the mitral prosthesis, TEE still provides a better visual inspection of the posterior aspect of the prosthesis and perivalvular structures than TTE. From 0° to 90° in the lower esophageal position, various aspects of the **mitral prosthesis** can be visualized. The mitral prosthesis can be imaged in cross-sectional view from the transgastric window. Mechanical valve leaflets in the aortic position can be challenging to assess especially when there are two mechanical valves.

b. Sewing ring. The orientation of the prosthetic valve in the annulus can be variable; however, **excessive motion** ("rocking") of the sewing ring is consistent with **dehiscence of the prosthesis. Adjacent echolucent structures** identified in the evaluation of endocarditis may represent abscess, fistula, or pseudoaneurysm. In general, **flow into an adjacent echolucent space is pathologic.** This may involve any portion of the annulus or the mitral–aortic intervalvular fibrosa.

2. Doppler evaluation. Doppler evaluation complements the two-dimensional examination and provides a **reliable indirect assessment of the prosthetic valve performance.** Color Doppler is useful in assessing regions of high velocity, proximal flow convergence, and regurgitant jets, whether they are valvular or perivalvular. Pulsed-wave and continuous-wave Doppler are used to assess transvalvular gradients, from which effective valve areas can be derived.

a. Imaging planes for TTE. Prosthetic mitral and aortic regurgitation can be visualized in the **parasternal long- and short-axis views.** Acoustic shadowing from the aortic and mitral prosthesis can interfere with the color Doppler display in the proximal portion of the aortic and mitral regurgitant jets. The apical views allow assessment of transvalvular pressure gradients but may underestimate the size of the mitral regurgitant jets due to acoustic shadowing. Pulmonary vein flows may not be available for the same reason. **Prosthetic aortic regurgitation** can be characterized from the **apical window.**

b. Imaging planes for TEE. At 40° from the upper esophageal position (cross-sectional view), the origin of the aortic regurgitant jet (intravalvular or perivalvular) can be identified. The extent of the aortic regurgitant jet into the left ventricular cavity with color Doppler can be visualized at 120°. Advancing the probe to the lower esophagus at 0° brings forth the four-chamber view, which allows unimpeded visualization of the mitral regurgitant jet and measurement of transmitral gradients. Color Doppler interrogation of the medial and lateral aspects of the mitral prosthesis can be performed by increasing the array toward 90° while rotating and advancing or pulling back the probe. Continuous-wave Doppler is used to measure the peak velocity across the prosthesis.

(1) Continuous-wave Doppler evaluation of the **aortic valve** may be performed at the lower esophageal level using the pinch maneuver (simultaneous ante- and right lateral flexion of the probe). Inserting the probe into the stomach at 5° to 10° with the probe anteflexed allows visualization of the origin of the mitral regurgitant jet. At 90° to 110°, continuous-wave Doppler evaluation of the aortic valve may be performed by left lateral flexion of the probe. Advancing the probe further to the deep transgastric view at 0° with anteflexion also brings the aortic valve in line for Doppler interrogation.

(2) Continuous-wave Doppler can also be used to assess **mechanical prosthesis regurgitation.** Advantages of continuous-wave Doppler include excellent temporal resolution to allow identification of specific periods in the cardiac cycle and the ability to indicate the severity of a regurgitant jet by its signal intensity. Using two-dimensional or color-flow imaging to guide, continuous-wave Doppler allows interrogation of different parts of the prosthesis and can help to detect eccentric jets. Color Doppler is useful if a view can be obtained where the ultrasound beam can enter the chamber receiving the regurgitant flow without traversing the prosthetic valve.

C. Normal Doppler findings

1. Prosthetic valve clicks. The opening and closure of mechanical valve leaflets creates a brief intense Doppler signal that appears as a narrow band on the spectral display.

2. Prosthetic valve velocities/pressure gradients. The systolic spectral Doppler contour is frequently triangular, with an earlier systolic peak velocity and a higher peak gradient than that of the mean gradient. The expected normal velocities and pressure gradients for commonly used prosthetic valves are shown in Table 16.5. However, there is a large variability in these numbers depending on flow and other factors. Therefore, a postoperative baseline study is indicated for patients with prosthetic valves.

3. Physiologic prosthetic valve regurgitation. Many prosthetic valves have regurgitant flow characterized by a uniform color without aliasing. For a mechanical prosthesis, the physiologic prosthetic regurgitant flow typically has a regurgitant jet area of <2 cm^2 and jet length of <2.5 cm in the mitral position, and a jet area of <1 cm^2 and jet length of <1.5 cm in the aortic position. **Most tissue valves exhibit minor regurgitant flow (closure volume) early after implantation.**

4. Assessment of prosthetic valve dysfunction. Loss of prosthetic valve clicks is a sensitive marker for prosthesis dysfunction.

a. Prosthetic valve stenosis

(1) Transvalvular gradients. Assessment of transvalvular gradients is the mainstay of the Doppler evaluation. **Each prosthetic valve is inherently stenotic and thus has a higher than normal peak velocity across it.** The continuous-wave Doppler gradient across the prosthesis obtained within weeks following implantation serves as a control for subsequent evaluations. High gradients may be also obtained in nonobstructive situations, such as high-output states, tachycardia, anemia, severe prosthetic leaks, or the pressure recovery phenomenon. Pressure recovery occurs secondary

TABLE 16.5 Normal Doppler Values of Prosthetic Valves

Prosthetic valve	Peak velocity (m/sec)	Mean gradient (mm Hg)
AORTIC POSITION		
Starr-Edwards	3.1 ± 0.5	24 ± 4
Björk-Shiley	2.5 ± 0.6	14 ± 5
St. Jude	3.0 ± 0.8	11 ± 6
Medtronic-Hall	2.6 ± 0.3	12 ± 3
Aortic homograft	0.8 ± 0.4	7 ± 3
Hancock	2.4 ± 0.4	11 ± 2
Carpentier-Edwards	2.4 ± 0.5	14 ± 6
MITRAL POSITION		
Starr-Edwards	1.8 ± 0.4	5 ± 2
Björk-Shiley	1.6 ± 0.3	5 ± 2
St. Jude	1.6 ± 0.3	5 ± 2
Medtronic-Hall	1.7 ± 0.3	3 ± 1
Hancock	1.5 ± 0.3	4 ± 2
Carpentier-Edwards	1.8 ± 0.2	7 ± 2

Modified from Nottestad SY, Zabalgoitia M. Echocardiographic recognition and quantitation of prosthetic valve dysfunction In: Otto CM, ed. *The practice of clinical echocardiography*. Philadelphia: WB Saunders, 1997:803

to flow acceleration through a narrowed orifice, especially with the mechanical bileaflet prosthesis in the aortic position. With this, the highest pressure measured through the prosthesis by Doppler overestimates the true pressure gradient by approximately one-third. With **prosthetic valve stenosis, pressure recovery becomes less evident.**

(2) Valve area calculations. Calculation of orifice area in prosthetic valves is difficult given the complexity of the orifice (struts/disks, and so forth), especially in mechanical prostheses. The following methods have been used to approximate orifice area:

(a) Continuity equation. The continuity equation can be used to estimate the functional orifice area of prosthetic aortic and mitral valves. For calculation of the prosthetic valve area in the aortic position:

$$\text{Area}_{\text{aortic prosthesis}} = (\text{diameter}_{\text{sewing ring}})^2 \times 0.785\ \text{TVI}_{\text{LVOT}}/\text{TVI}_{\text{aortic prosthesis}}$$

where TVI is time–velocity integral and LVOT is left ventricular outflow tract.

The LVOT diameter is replaced by the sewing ring inner diameter in the equation. The aortic prosthesis TVI is determined from continuous-wave Doppler velocity through the prosthesis. LVOT TVI is determined by pulsed-wave Doppler. Mitral valve prosthesis TVI is determined from continuous-wave Doppler. For the mitral position:

$$\text{Area} = (\text{LVOT diameter})^2 \times 0.785 \times \text{TVI}_{\text{LVOT}}/\text{TVI}_{\text{mitral prosthesis}}$$

(3) Pressure half-time (PHT). For a mitral valve prosthesis, the PHT method is useful for assessing prosthetic valvular stenosis. The empirical constant of 220 provides a reasonable approximation for mechanical prosthetic mitral valve area. The PHT method can also determine whether increased velocity is secondary to increased flow or to obstruction. If the peak velocity is increased but the PHT is not prolonged, then the increased velocity is most likely due to increased forward flow. However, PHT may overestimate the area of the mitral prosthesis.

(4) Dimensionless index. The LVOT and aortic valve prosthesis velocity ratio is possibly the most helpful index for the evaluation of prosthetic valve stenosis, particularly when the valve size is not known. The higher the index, the larger the effective orifice area, and vice versa. A value smaller than 0.23 suggests prosthesis stenosis.

$$\text{Dimensionless index} = \text{velocity}_{\text{LVOT}}/\text{velocity}_{\text{aortic prosthesis}}$$

b. Pathologic prosthetic valve regurgitation. The pathologic flow disturbance is **larger and wider than that seen with physiologic regurgitation.** Its **severity can be reliably quantified by TEE,** which can best identify periprosthetic regurgitation. Pathologic regurgitation may be related to a scarred/calcified annulus with disruption of the sutures securing the valve or a perivalvular abscess with adjacent tissue destruction. Single or multiple jets may be present.

(1) Severe mitral prosthetic regurgitation is suggested by increased peak early diastolic velocity ($\geq$2.5 m/s) and normal mitral inflow PHT ($\leq$150 m/s) (see Chapter 15).

(2) Severe aortic regurgitation is usually present when the PHT $\leq$250 meters per second or when flow reversal is detected in the descending aorta (see Chapter 14).

5. Cinefluoroscopy. Cinefluoroscopy is useful for assessing **mechanical prosthetic valves.** The image intensifier is moved to a position with x-rays parallel to the valve ring plane to determine the occluder's excursions in a caged valve. Despite the radiolucency of pyrolytic carbon disk valves, the opening angle can be measured from positioning the image intensifier parallel to the plane of the open leaflets. **The mitral prosthesis is best visualized from the right anterior oblique (RAO) cranial projections. The aortic prosthesis can be viewed from RAO caudal or left anterior oblique (LAO) cranial projection.**

a. Diminished motion of the disks suggests valve obstruction, whereas excessive rocking of the base ring (i.e., 7° for aortic prosthesis and 11° for mitral prosthesis) suggests partial dehiscence of the valve.

b. In the setting of **suspected strut fracture in a Björk-Shiley valve,** cinefluoroscopy evaluation of the prosthesis is best performed with the tunnel view profile. Increased incidence of strut fracture has been noted in patients with an opening angle of 70° or more.

6. Cardiac catheterization

a. Invasive assessment of the left ventricle can be performed safely in patients with bioprosthetic aortic valves. However, catheter-based evaluation of the mechanical aortic valve must be performed with a transseptal technique in patients with a mechanical prosthesis. It may be necessary for accurate measurement of the prosthetic mitral valve gradient, as catheter-based assessment overestimates the mitral valve gradient because of a dampening of the pressure contour and intrinsic delay in the pulmonary capillary wedge tracing.

b. Never cross the following prosthetic valves:

(1) Single or bileaflet tilting disk prosthesis

(2) Caged disk prosthesis

(3) Caged ball prosthesis

7. Magnetic resonance imaging (MRI) can be performed safely in patients with most prosthetic valves, as they are not ferromagnetic. It can identify **prosthetic regurgitation, periprosthetic fistulas, and abscess.** Prosthetic valves cause **imaging artifacts,** which preclude assessment of the leaflets of the prosthetic valve; however, dedicated sequences can provide information about **blood flow velocities,** and **regurgitant jets.**

8. Multislice cardiac CT may allow evaluation of leaflet motion in mechanical valves using four-dimensional reconstruction. Once the dataset is acquired, it can be reconstructed to view the motion of the valve in any selected plane. The utility of this method over conventional fluoroscopy remains to be evaluated.

III. VALVE DYSFUNCTION AND COMPLICATIONS RELATED TO PROSTHETIC VALVES

A. Atrial fibrillation. Up to 50% of patients undergoing valve surgery experience postoperative atrial fibrillation. Management of atrial fibrillation is discussed in Chapter 19.

1. In **patients without a previous history** of atrial fibrillation, the **arrhythmia is often self-limited.**
2. For patients with **persistent atrial fibrillation beyond 24 hours, anticoagulation, direct current cardioversion, and a short course of antiarrhythmic therapy** are warranted.
3. β-Blockade or amiodarone prophylaxis has been found to reduce the incidence of postsurgical atrial fibrillation.

B. Conduction disturbances. High-grade heart block requiring permanent pacemaker implantation has been described in 2% to 3% of patients after valve replacement and 8% following repeat valve surgery. It is caused by trauma to the bundle of His or from postoperative edema of the periannular tissue. Aortic or mitral annular calcification, preoperative conduction disturbance, advanced age, infectious endocarditis, and tricuspid valve surgery are associated with higher rates of postoperative conduction abnormalities leading to permanent pacemaker implantation.

C. Endocarditis. Approximately 3% to 6% of patients with prosthetic heart valves will experience prosthetic valve endocarditis. Prosthetic valve endocarditis is typically associated with large vegetations, since microorganisms are sheltered from the host defense mechanisms.

1. Early prosthetic valve endocarditis (<60 days following implantation) is typically caused by *Staphylococcus epidermidis*. The clinical course is often fulminant, with high mortality rates ranging from 20% to 70%.
2. Late prosthetic valve endocarditis occurs most commonly in patients with multiple prostheses and bioprosthetic valves, especially in the aortic position. Its clinical course resembles that of native valve endocarditis. Streptococci are the most common infectious agents, followed by gram-negative bacteria, enterococci, and *S. epidermidis*.
3. TEE is the imaging modality of choice, with sensitivity of 95% and specificity of 90% in diagnosis. It is useful also in detecting complications including abscess, tissue invasion, dehiscence, and fistula formation; and monitoring the efficacy of medical therapy.
4. **Therapy.** The mortality of patients managed with antibiotics alone is 61% versus 38% for those having valve replacement. (See Chapter 19 for more information on diagnosis, management, and antibiotic prophylaxis for endocarditis.)
   a. **Medical therapy.** Medical cure of prosthetic valve endocarditis caused by **staphylococci, gram-negative organisms, or fungi is rare. Streptococcal** prosthetic valve endocarditis responds to medical therapy alone in **50% of cases.** Patients with mechanical prosthetic valve endocarditis should **continue to receive anticoagulation.** In the absence of anticoagulation, prosthetic valve endocarditis is associated with an up to 50% incidence of stroke. Continuing anticoagulation for patients with prosthetic valve endocarditis is associated with a 10% incidence of cerebral embolization. There is no conclusive evidence for increased hemorrhage with warfarin in patients with prosthetic valve endocarditis. Careful surveillance of medically managed patients with prosthetic endocarditis is essential and should involve an infectious diseases consultant, multiple repeat cultures after the cessation of antibiotic treatment, and follow-up with TEE when needed. A high index of suspicion should be maintained for the presence of residual infection, and surgical reevaluation should be considered if medical treatment fails.
   b. **Surgical therapy.** Valve replacement surgery is indicated in the setting of:
      (1) Persistent bacteremia despite intravenous antibiotics
      (2) Tissue invasion or fistula formation
      (3) Recurrent embolization

(4) Fungal infection
(5) Prosthesis dehiscence or obstruction
(6) New or worsening heart block
(7) Congestive heart failure

D. Hemolysis. Subclinical hemolysis is present in many patients with mechanical valves but **rarely results in significant anemia.**

1. **Pathophysiology and etiology.** Clinical hemolysis occurs in 6% to 15% of patients with **caged ball valves** but is uncommon with normal bioprosthetic or tilting disk valves. Clinical hemolysis is also associated with **multiple prosthetic valves, small prostheses, periprosthetic leaks, and prosthetic valve endocarditis.** Mechanisms involved in the generation of hemolysis include high shear stress or turbulence across the prosthesis, interaction with foreign surfaces such as cloth, and rapid deceleration of erythrocytes following collision with adjoining structures (e.g., struts or cardiac walls).
2. **Laboratory examination and diagnostic testing**
   a. Diagnosis is made by **elevated lactate dehydrogenase, reticulocyte count, unconjugated bilirubin, urinary haptoglobin,** and presence of **schistocytes on blood smear.**
   b. Echocardiographic findings consistent with mechanical hemolysis include **abnormal rocking of the prosthesis or regurgitant jets of high shear stress** (e.g., eccentric or periprosthetic regurgitant jets or those impacting a solid surface such as the left atrial appendage).
3. **Therapy**
   a. **Medical therapy.** Mild hemolytic anemia can be managed with **iron, folic acid supplement, and blood transfusion. β-Blockade and blood pressure control** may reduce the severity of hemolysis.
   b. Surgical therapy. Repair of perivalvular leaks or valve replacement is indicated in **patients with severe hemolysis requiring repeated transfusions, or in those with congestive heart failure.**

E. Thrombosis. The annual incidence of mechanical prosthetic valve thrombosis is 0.2% to 1.8%. The incidence is highest in the tricuspid position, followed by the mitral then the aortic position. Thrombus is suspected in patients with **acute onset of symptoms, embolic event, or inadequate anticoagulation.** Thrombosis at bioprostheses is uncommon but may occur in low flow or prothrombotic states.

1. **Laboratory examination and diagnostic testing.** TEE is the most widely used diagnostic technique, although cinefluoroscopy can be used to document restriction in occluder mobility. No imaging modality, however, can clearly differentiate thrombus from pannus (see Section **III.H**). Frequently they coexist. Echocardiographic features suggestive of thrombus include soft, irregular, or mobile mass.
2. **Therapy.** The valve type or suspected duration of valve thrombosis does not influence the indications for treatment, although location of prosthetic valve does.
   a. **Priority of therapy**
      (1) Heparin is typically initiated early in the course of evaluation.
      (2) Warfarin is continued unless surgery is planned.
      (3) TTE, TEE, or cinefluoroscopy should be performed at 24 hours and, if the thrombus is still present, should be repeated serially.
   b. **Medical therapy**
      (1) Fibrinolytic therapy is considered the treatment of choice for **right-sided prosthetic valve thrombosis** because the consequences of distal embolization are less severe than in left-sided prosthesis. Streptokinase and urokinase are the most commonly used agents. Fibrinolytic therapy has an initial success rate of 82%, overall thromboembolism rate of 12%, and a 5% incidence of major bleeding episodes. For left-sided valves, there is a similarly high success rate (82%) with fibrinolytic therapy; however, the associated risks of death (10%) or systemic embolism (12.5%) are high. Thrombolysis should be considered for left-sided valves in patients with contraindications to sugery. Thrombolysis may be a reasonable alternative to surgery for

mitral or aortic prosthetic valve thrombosis in patients with a small thrombus burden, particularly if there is hemodynamic compromise.

(a) The classical regimen for **streptokinase** is a 500,000-IU bolus given over 20 minutes, followed by an infusion of 1.5 million IU infused over 10 hours.

(b) **rtPA (tissue plasminogen activator) 10 mg bolus followed by 90 mg an hour for 9 hours.**

(c) Thrombolysis should be stopped if there is no hemodynamic improvement after 24 to 72 hours. TEE is useful in assessment of progress.

(d) Following successful thrombolysis, close **follow-up of anticoagulation along with serial Doppler echocardiography** on an individual basis is recommended.

(2) Anticoagulation with heparin and warfarin is generally recommended for **small thrombus** ($\leq$5 mm). The regimen consists of intravenous heparin followed by subcutaneous heparin 17,000 U twice a day and warfarin (INR 2.5 to 3.5) for up to 3 months.

c. Surgical approach. The lowest surgical mortality reported has been approximately 5%. The risk profile of the individual patient must be balanced against the expertise and experience at each center.

(1) Valve replacement and débridement is generally performed for **left-sided prosthetic valve thrombosis,** unless the thrombus is small or the patient has a prohibitive surgical risk.

(2) Surgery is also indicated in the case of **unsuccessful thrombolysis** 24 hours following discontinuation of the infusion.

F. Dehiscence. Detachment of the sewing ring from the annulus may occur in the early postoperative period because of poor surgical techniques, excessive annular calcification, chronic steroid use, fragility of the annular tissue (particularly following prior valve operations), or infection. Late dehiscence occurs mainly from infectious endocarditis. **Abnormal rocking of the prosthesis** on echocardiography or cinefluoroscopy is an **indication for urgent surgery.** (Some rocking may occur with preservation of the mitral valve apparatus.)

G. Patient–prosthesis mismatch. All prosthetic valves, with the exception of stentless aortic homografts, have effective orifices that are smaller than that of native valves. There is an **inherent pressure gradient and relative stenosis with each prosthesis.** Occasionally, when an inappropriately small prosthesis is placed, the **ensuing low output may cause symptoms.** This mismatch occurs most frequently after valve placement for aortic stenosis.

1. In a patient with a **small annulus, a hemodynamically favorable prosthesis** like the aortic homograft or the tilting disk valve is preferred. Alternatively, the annulus may be enlarged surgically in order to accommodate a prosthesis of acceptable size.
2. Aortic prostheses <21 mm in diameter are not recommended for a large or physically active patient.
3. Surgery generally consists of replacement with a larger prosthesis and annular reconstruction or, in selected instances, homograft insertion.

H. Pannus formation. Valve obstruction occurs in up to 5% of mechanical valves per year. Valve thrombosis and pannus formation are responsible for the majority of mechanical prosthesis obstructions. Frequently, thrombus coexists with pannus. **Little is known about the causes** of fibroblastic proliferation in pannus formation. Foreign-body reactions to the prosthesis, inadequate anticoagulation, endocarditis, and blood flow turbulence in the mitral position have been implicated as potential causes. Pannus formation begins around the annulus of the valve and is more common in aortic than in mitral valve prostheses. A subacute presentation of fatigue or dyspnea in a patient who is well anticoagulated can suggest pannus formation. **TEE and/or cinefluoroscopy is generally required** to identify the cause of prosthetic valve obstruction.

I. Embolic stroke. Following an embolic stroke, the risk of recurrent stroke is approximately 1% per day for the first 2 weeks.

1. If no evidence of hemorrhage is detected on CT scan at 24 to 48 hours, **intravenous heparin** should be administered after a small to moderate embolic stroke. **Maintaining anticoagulation** reduces this risk of recurrent stroke to one-third but **carries an increased risk of hemorrhagic transformation** of 8% to 24%, particularly during the first 48 hours.
2. In patients with **larger infarcts, anticoagulation should be withheld for 5 to 7 days.**
3. Anticoagulation is withheld for 1 to 2 weeks in the setting of **hemorrhagic transformation.**
4. **Aspirin or clopidogrel** may be needed in the event of recurrent strokes, despite adequate anticoagulation.
5. Rarely, **reoperation with placement of a tissue valve** is needed for recurrent embolization.

J. Mechanical failure

1. Failure of **bioprostheses** is expected as the valves age. This may manifest as stenosis, regurgitation, or a combination, and is usually due to the deposition of calcium on the leaflets. The onset of mechanical failure is usually gradual. Leaflet tears may produce a sudden clinical deterioration with the onset of severe regurgitation. Bioprosthetic deterioration is managed expectantly with increasing frequency of evaluation as the valve ages and deterioration becomes more evident clinically, and on echo. Indications for reoperation are similar to those for native valve lesions, although the threshold to reoperate is somewhat higher given the greater mortality and morbidity associated with reoperation.
2. Failure of the current generation of **mechanical prostheses** is rare but may precipitate catastrophic hemodynamic compromise. Catastrophic failure occurs when a strut holding the occluder breaks, allowing the occluder to embolize, resulting in overwhelming regurgitation. Strut failure has been reported most commonly with the Björk-Shiley valve and results from fatigue of a metal weld in valves of specific sizes (larger) and year of manufacture (1981 to 1982 especially) in those younger than age 50 years at time of implantation. Explantation of those at highest risk has been recommended; in evaluating patients with Björk-Shiley valves, the risk/benefit of explanatation versus strut fracture should be determined, based on the excellent published literature on the topic.
3. In older ball-in-cage prostheses, ball **variance**, a structural deterioration of the occluder, can occur, giving rise to impaired occluder motion, sticking and thromboembolism. This is rarely seen nowadays with improved prosthetic materials.

ACKNOWLEDGMENTS

The authors thank Drs. Steve Lin and James Wong for their contributions to this chapter.

Landmark Articles

Acar J, Iung B, Boissel JP, et al. Multicenter randomized comparison of low-dose versus standard-dose anticoagulation in patients with mechanical prosthetic heart valves. *Circulation* 1996;94:2107–2112.

Akins CW. Results with mechanical cardiac valvular prosthesis. *Ann Thorac Surg* 1995;60:1836–1844.

Birkmeyer JD, Marrin CA, O'Connor GT. Should patients with Björk-Shiley valves undergo propyhlactic replacement? *Lancet* 1992;340:520–523.

Cannegieter SC, Rosendaal FR, Wintzen AR, et al. Optimal oral anticoagulant therapy in patients with mechanical heart valves. *N Engl J Med* 1995;333:11–17.

Davis EA, Greene PS, Cameron DE, et al. Bioprosthetic versus mechanical prosthesis for aortic valve replacement in the elderly. *Circulation* 1996;94:II-121–II-125.

Green CE, Glass-Royal M, Bream PR, et al. Cinefluoroscopic evaluation of periprosthetic cardiac valve regurgitation. *Am J Radiol* 1988;151:455–459.

Israel DH, Sharma SK, Fuster V. Antithrombotic therapy in prosthetic heart valve replacement. *Am Heart J* 1994;127:400–411.

Jaeger FJ, Trohman RG, Brener S, et al. Permanent pacing following repeat cardiac valve surgery. *Am J Cardiol* 1994;74:505–507.

Lengyel M, Fuster V, Keltai M, et al. Guidelines for management of left-sided prosthetic valve thrombosis: a role for thrombolytic therapy. *J Am Coll Cardiol* 1997;30:1521–1526.

Roudaut R, Lafitte S, Roudaut MF, Courtault C, et al. Fibrinolysis of mechanical prosthetic valve thrombosis: a single-center study of 127 cases. *J Am Coll Cardiol* 2003;41:653–658.

Van der Meulen JH, Steyerberg EW, Van der Graaf Y, et al. Age thresholds for prophylactic replacement of Björk Shiley convexo-concave heart valves. A clinical and economic evaluation. *Circulation* 1993;88:156–164.

Vogel W, Stoll HP, Bay W, et al. Cineradiography for determination of normal and abnormal function in mechanical heart valves. *Am J Cardiol* 1993;71:225–232.
Vongpatanasin W, Hillis LD, et al. Prosthetic heart valves. *N Engl J Med* 1996;335:407–416.

Key Reviews

Rahimtoola SH. Prosthetic heart valve performance: long-term follow-up. *Curr Probl Cardiol* 1992;6:334–406.
Zabalgoitia M. Echocardiographic assessment of prosthetic heart valves. *Curr Probl Cardiol* 1992;5:270–325.

Relevant Book Chapters

Garcia MJ. Prosthetic Valve Disease. In: Topol EJ, ed. *Textbook of cardiovascular medicine,* 3rd ed. Philadelphia: Lippincott–Raven Publishers, 2006:389–398.
Otto CM, Bonow RO. Valvular Heart Disease. In: *Braunwald's heart disease,* 8th ed. Philadelphia: Saunders, Elsevier, 2008:1625–1712.

INFECTIVE ENDOCARDITIS 17

Mateen Akhtar and Brian P. Griffin

I. INTRODUCTION

A. Infective endocarditis (IE) is **an infection of the cardiac endothelium,** macroscopically seen as vegetations. Despite modern medical and surgical therapy, IE is a serious and life-threatening condition. Mortality rates remain as high as 20% for both native and prosthetic valve endocarditis. The clinical diagnosis is based on multiple elements. Transesophageal echocardiography (TEE) has increased the diagnostic accuracy of IE. **Infective endocarditis is best managed via multidisciplinary collaboration among cardiologists, cardiothoracic surgeons, and infectious disease specialists.**

B. The incidence of IE has remained constant over the last 30 years, accounting for one case per 1000 hospital admissions. An estimated 10,000 to 15,000 new cases of IE are diagnosed each year in the United States. The incidence has increased in the elderly and in illicit injection drug users. There has also been an increase in the number of acute cases, prosthetic valve infections, and cases due to gram-negative, rickettsial, chlamydial, fungal, and fastidious infections.

C. Risk factors associated with infection include underlying cardiac structural abnormalities, immumunosuppressed status, underlying conditions that predispose patients to pacemaker-related infections, prolonged surgery, reoperation, catheter-related bacteremia, and sternal wound infection.

II. CLINICAL PRESENTATION

A. Signs and symptoms. The clinical manifestations of IE are highly variable, ranging from subtle symptoms to fulminant congestive heart failure with severe valvular regurgitation. **Acute IE** arises with marked toxicity and progresses over several days to weeks to valvular destruction and metastatic infection. **Subacute IE** evolves over several weeks to months with mild or modest toxicity and rarely causes metastatic infection. The rate of progression depends upon the virulence of the causative organism, the age and underlying health of the patient, and the nature and extent of the underlying valvular disease.

1. The **hallmarks of IE are fever and a new murmur** (more than 85%). However, fever may be absent in the elderly and the uremic or immunosuppressed population. Murmurs may be absent with right-sided or mural infections, or intracardiac device infection.

2. The patient often has nonspecific symptoms of fatigue, weight loss, malaise, chills, night sweats, and/or musculoskeletal aches.

B. **Physical findings.** A new murmur remains an important finding.

1. Congestive heart failure occurs in up to 55% of cases and tends to be more common in those with aortic valve disease (75%) than in those with mitral (50%) or tricuspid (20%) valve involvement.

2. Neurologic findings may include clinically apparent cerebral emboli (20%), encephalopathy (10%), mycotic aneurysm leak (less than 5%), meningitis, or brain abscess (less than 5%).

3. Additional physical findings reflecting **embolic or immune complex phenomena** include mucosal **petechiae** (20% to 40%), **splinter hemorrhages** (subungal dark linear streaks; 10% to 30%), **Osler's nodes** (painful, tender erythematous nodules on the pads of fingers or toes; 10% to 25%), **Janeway lesions** (erythematous, macular, nontender lesions on the fingers, palms, or soles; less than 5%), **clubbing** (10% to 20%), **arterial embolism** (peripherally or centrally), **splenomegaly** (30% to 50%), and **Roth's spots** (retinal hemorrhages; less than 5%). These classic physical findings are **neither sensitive nor specific** for the diagnosis of IE. Their frequency is continuing to diminish, due to a decrease in viridans *Streptococcus* IE and an increase in *Staphylococcus aureus* IE.

4. A formal **fundusscopic examination** should be routine in all patients with suspected or documented IE. It may reveal **chorioretinitis or endophthalmitis.**

5. **Systemic** embolization occurs in 25% to 50% of cases of IE and may mimic acute coronary syndrome (coronary artery emboli), peritonitis (embolization to spleen, kidney, or bowel), acute stroke (cerebral emboli), pulmonary embolism (from right-sided IE), or cause a cold extremity with reduced or absent pulse.

III. ETIOLOGY

Table 17.1 presents the various etiologic factors.

A. **Seventy percent to 75% of patients with IE have preexisting cardiac abnormalities. Mitral valve prolapse with regurgitation is the leading condition** underlying IE in adults. Rheumatic heart disease as a substrate for IE is decreasing, with congenital heart disease underlying 10% to 20% of IE cases.

B. The source of infection can only be identified occasionally (e.g., dental procedures, an infected vascular catheter, or an infected skin lesion). In many patients, there is no history of an antecedent localized infection.

C. **Native valve endocarditis**

1. The common microorganisms that cause native valve IE in adults (Table 17.2A) are viridans *Streptococcus* species, *S. aureus*, *Streptococcus bovis*, *Enterococcus*,

TABLE 17.1 Frequency of Organisms Causing Infective Endocarditis

Organism	NVE (%)	IDU (%)	Early PVE (%)	Late PVE (%)
Streptococci	60	15–25	5	35
Viridans *Streptococcus*	30–40	5–10	<5	25
S. bovis	10	<5	<5	<5
Enterococci	10	10	<5	<5
Staphylococci	25	50	50	30
Coagulase positive	23	50	20	10
Coagulase negative	<5	<5	30	20
Gram-negative (aerobes)	<5	5	20	10
Fungi	<5	<5	10	5
Culture negative	5–10	<5	<5	<5

IDU, intravenous drug use; NVE, native valve endocarditis; PVE, prosthetic valve endocarditis.
Adapted from Fuster V, Alexander RW, O'Rourke RA, eds. *Hurst's the heart,* 11th ed. McGraw Hill, New York: 2004.

TABLE 17.2A Duke Criteria: Definite Pathologic Diagnosis

A. Microorganisms, as demonstrated by culture or histology in Vegetation
   Vegetation that has embolized
   Intracardiac abscess
B. Pathologic lesions
   Vegetation or intracardiac abscess present, confirmed by histology showing active endocarditis

Adapted from Baddour LM, Wilson WR, Bayer AS, et al. Infective endocarditis: diagnosis, antimicrobial therapy, and management of complications. *Circulation* 2005;111:394–434.

as well as the HACEK group (*Haemophilus, Actinobacillus, Cardiobacterium, Eikenella*, and *Kingella*). The HACEK group, accounting for roughly 3% of cases, includes fastidious gram-negative organisms that are normal flora in the upper respiratory tract. *S. bovis* IE is often associated with colonic polyps and colonic cancer; as such, a colonoscopy is recommended for these patients.

2. Right-sided IE in injection drug users is usually due to *S. aureus* (60%), with a predilection for normal as well as abnormal cardiac valves. Despite the virulence of this organism, the disease tends to be **less severe** (mortality rates of 2% to 6%) than left-sided IE. The valve most commonly infected in injection drug users is the tricuspid (60% to 70% of cases), followed by the mitral (30% to 40%) and the aortic (5% to 10%). More than one valve is involved in 20% of these patients. Septic pulmonary emboli occur in up to 75% of injection drug users with tricuspid IE.
3. IE, from *Pseudomonas aeruginosa,* is both **destructive and poorly responsive to antibiotic therapy.** Therefore, many patients require surgery.
4. Enterococcal IE is increasing. The diagnosis must be considered in patients who have undergone recent genitourinary or obstetric procedures. These patients may not have underlying heart disease.
5. Other members of the Enterobacteriaceae *(Escherichia coli, Salmonella, Klebsiella, Enterobacter, Proteus, Serratia, Citrobacter, Shigella, and Yersinia)* are occasionally implicated in IE.
6. *Streptococcus pneumoniae* accounts for 1% to 3% of native valve IE, and it may present as part of the **"Austrian" triad**, which also includes pneumococcal pneumonia and meningitis. Alcoholics are typically affected, and mortality is high (30% to 50%).
7. The most common congenital heart anomalies predisposing to IE are bicuspid aortic valve, patent ductus arteriosus, ventricular septal defect, coarctation of the aorta, and tetralogy of Fallot. There is **no evidence** that secundum atrial septal defects increase the risk of IE.

D. Prosthetic valve endocarditis (PVE) has increased to account for about 10% to 20% of all cases of IE. The greatest risk is in the first 6 months after valve implantation. The risk appears to be **similar in mechanical or bioprosthetic valves.** Recent studies have suggested that infection occurs with similar frequency at mitral or aortic site.

1. Prosthetic valve endocarditis occurring within 2 months of surgery (early PVE) is commonly associated with intraoperative contamination and nosocomial infection, and usually implicates **coagulase-negative staphylococci** (30% of cases). The second most common pathogen in early PVE is *S. aureus* (20% of cases).
2. The microbiology of PVE with an onset more than 2 months after surgery (late PVE) reflects the pathogens of native valve IE, and is most commonly caused by streptococcal species, *S. aureus*, and *Enterococcus*. Coagulase-negative staphylococci cause less than 20% of infections in this period. Important to note fungi account for 10% to 15% of late PVE cases and are associated with a higher mortality. Among 270 cases of fungal endocarditis reported from 1965 to 1995, 135 (50%) occurred on prosthetic valves. These patients generally lacked an identifiable portal of entry for fungemia. Establishing the diagnosis of fungal PVE can be difficult due to the low yield from blood cultures. Despite aggressive

antifungal therapy, these patients remain at risk for the development of PVE months or years later. *Corynebacterium* species and other coryneform bacteria, often called diphtheroids, are also an important cause of PVE during the first year after surgery (5%). Although they are often blood culture contaminants, diphtheroids in multiple cultures should not be ignored.

E. Pacemaker/defibrillator endocarditis is increasing in clinical practice with the burgeoning number of devices implanted. The incidence of endocarditis following device therapy ranges from 0.2% to 7%. The infection may involve the generator or defibrillator pocket, the electrodes, and valvular or nonvalvular endocardium.

1. Pacemaker/defibrillator endocarditis occurring within 1 to 2 months of surgery is likely caused by direct microbial seeding intraoperatively. Late infection in the pocket produces a thinning of the overlying tissue and ultimately device erosion. The infection eventually may involve the electrodes and ultimately the endocardium. Hematogenous dissemination from distant sites of infection appears to be relatively rare, with exception of *S. aureus* bacteremia.

2. The majority of infections in PVE are caused by staphylococci: *S. aureus* and coagulase-negative staphylococci. More than 90% of early infections are caused by coagulase-negative staphylococci. Late infections are accounted for by *S. aureus* (50%) and coagulase negative staphylococci (50%). Infection by gram-negative bacilli, enterococci, or fungi is rare.

F. The incidence of **culture-negative endocarditis** may be as high as 10%. The most common cause is **previous antibiotic therapy**. Other causes include slow-growing or **fastidious organisms** (e.g., fungi, HACEK, anaerobes, *Legionella*, *Chlamydia psittaci*, *Coxiella*, *Brucella*, *Bartonella*, and nutritionally deficient streptococci), or **nonbacterial endocarditis** (Liebman-Sachs, marantic, antiphospholipid syndrome).

G. Fungal endocarditis (*Candida* and *Aspergillus*) usually occurs in association with **prosthetic valves, indwelling intravascular hardware, immunosuppression, or injection drug use.**

IV. PATHOPHYSIOLOGY.

The first step in the pathogenesis of vegetation is the formation of a **nonbacterial thrombotic endocarditis (NBTE)**, which usually results from endothelial injury followed by focal adherence of platelets and fibrin. Microorganisms circulating in the bloodstream in turn infect this sterile platelet-fibrin nidus.

A. The endothelium may be injured by regurgitant jets, leading to vegetation formation on the atrial surface of incompetent atrioventricular valves or the ventricular surface of incompetent semilunar valves. The foreign body, such as an intracardiac device, is not endothelialized initially and acts as a formation site for platelet-fibrin thrombi.

B. Bacteremia is the event that converts NBTE to IE when host defenses fail. The foreign material also impairs host defenses, rendering them more difficult to treat.

C. Vegetations often further impair valvular coaptation or cause perforation or chordal rupture, leading to worsening of regurgitation and congestive heart failure. Furthermore, the vegetations may dislodge, causing peripheral septic–nonseptic embolization.

D. The infection may extend to surrounding structures, such as the valve ring, the cardiac conduction system, the adjacent myocardium, or the mitral–aortic intravalvular fibrosa. Consequently, conduction defects, abscesses, diverticula, aneurysms, or fistula may develop. Infection involving prosthetic valves commonly invades paravalvular tissue, resulting in abscess formation or valve dehiscence.

V. LABORATORY EXAMINATION

A. Blood tests

1. Laboratory findings often reflect nonspecific acute inflammatory response, and manifest as a **modest leukocytosis,** a **normochromic normocytic anemia,** and a slightly increased or decreased **platelet count.** Other laboratory abnormalities may include an **elevated erythrocyte sedimentation rate (ESR),** C-reactive protein (CRP), rheumatoid factor, and/or a hypergammaglobulinemia.

2. Decreased complement and an elevated blood urea nitrogen (BUN) or creatinine may implicate renal dysfunction from an immune complex glomerulonephritis or drug toxicity.

3. Blood cultures are critical in the diagnosis and management of IE. However, if a patient is acutely ill **therapy should not be delayed for more than 2 to 3 hours,** as a fulminant infection may be rapidly fatal. In recent reports, cultures were negative in 2.5% to 31% of cases with established IE, despite the best modern methods.
   a. Three sets of cultures should be drawn at three different venipuncture sites before empiric antimicrobial therapy, if clinical condition allows. Each set should include two flasks, one containing an aerobic medium, and the other an anaerobic medium, into which at least **20 cm**^{3} (per tube) of blood should be placed. HACEK group bacteria are cultured routinely. Fungal cultures should be included when fungal infection is suspected.
   b. Intravascular infection leads to constant bacteremia originating from vegetations. Therefore, **it is unnecessary to await the arrival of a fever spike or chills to obtain blood cultures.**
   c. The laboratory should be alerted if a **culture-negative IE or a fastidious infectious agent** is suspected, as it may be necessary to enhance the culture medium or prolong the incubation period. For example, the HACEK group (see **III.C.1**) needs prolonged incubation of up to 21 days. The most common culture-negative IE organisms are *Coxiella burnetii*, *Bartonella* sp., *Tropheryma whipplei i*, HACEK group bacteria, *Brucella* sp., *Legionella* sp., *Mycoplasma* sp., *Mycobacterium*, or fungi. Serology for *Brucella*, *Legionella*, *Coxiella*, or *Psittacosis* may be revealing.

B. **Histologic evaluation.** Histopathology of resected valvular tissues remains the gold standard for the diagnosis of IE. It may demonstrate valvular inflammation, vegetations, and/or specific organisms. Detection of an etiologic agent in the vegetation by special stains or immunohistology can guide the choice of antimicrobial treatment. This is particularly useful in culture-negative IE, such as Q fever, *Bartonella* spp, or *T. whipplei* (Whipple's disease bacillus). **Good communication among cardiologists, surgeons, pathologists, and microbiologists helps ensure accurate diagnosis.**

C. **Urinalysis.** Microhematuria with or without proteinuria may be seen.

D. **Electrocardiography.** All patients with suspected IE should have baseline and follow-up electrocardiogram (ECGs).
   1. ECG may reveal **conduction disturbances** reflecting intramyocardial extension of infection, ranging from a prolonged PR interval to complete heart block (especially with PVE). A **new atrioventricular block** carries a 77% positive predictive value for abscess formation with 42% sensitivity.
   2. Myocardial infarction due to embolization of vegetations occurs rarely.

E. Chest x-ray may reveal **congestive heart failure or pleural effusions.** Right-sided IE may cause **nonspecific infiltrates** due to multiple septic pulmonary emboli.

VI. DIAGNOSTIC IMAGING TECHNIQUES

A. Echocardiography has a key role in both diagnosis and management of IE. The primary objective is to identify, localize, and characterize valvular vegetations and their effects on cardiac function. Vegetations may occur at intracardiac locations other than valves, such as the site of impact of a high-velocity jet or shunt. A limitation of echocardiography is that vegetations cannot always be distinguished from other noninfectious masses.
   1. All patients in whom IE is suspected should undergo baseline transthoracic echocardiography (TTE) to define underlying cardiac abnormalities, to determine the size and location of vegetations, and to explore the possibility of complications (e.g., aortic annular ring abscess). The sensitivity of TTE for detection of valvular vegetations is 65% to 70%. A repeat study is indicated for complications such as congestive heart failure or atrioventricular block, which herald progression of valvular and myocardial destruction.
   2. If IE is strongly suspected and the TTE is negative, then TEE should be performed because it is more sensitive in detecting vegetations, especially if TTE imaging is difficult. TEE is particularly useful for assessing posterior structures, abscesses, fistulae, perivalvular leaks, small vegetations, right-sided heart structures, masses on intracardiac devices, leaflet perforations, and prosthetic

valves. The ability to detect paravalvular abscesses, fistulae, and paraprosthetic leaks has a major impact on management strategy. Intraoperative TEE can be used to evaluate the success of surgical interventions and the need for potential modification of reparative cardiac surgical procedures. A postoperative TTE should also be done as a baseline measure of cardiac anatomy/function for long term follow-up.

a. A negative result on TEE indicates a low likelihood of IE (provided adequate images are available). However, it does not completely rule out the diagnosis. The negative predictive value is greater than 90%, but false negatives may occur early in endocarditis or if vegetations are small. Repeat TEE should be considered if clinical suspicion is high. Of importance to note, a negative TEE should never override strong clinical evidence of endocarditis in the diagnosis of PVE.

b. Myocardial abscesses are more reliably detected by TEE (87% sensitive) than by TTE (28% sensitive). A perivalvular abscesses is a serious complication and a strong indication for surgical intervention.

c. In the setting of PVE, TEE is superior (82% sensitive) to TTE (36% sensitive) in the detection of vegetations due to acoustic shadowing of prosthetic valves. **TEE should be performed if prosthetic valve endocarditis or pacemaker endocarditis is suspected but is not evident on TTE.**

3. Fungal endocarditis tends to cause larger vegetations than bacterial infections, whereas in Q fever vegetations are often absent. Care should be taken to differentiate bacterial vegetations from myxomas, papillary fibroelastomas, rheumatoid nodules, and inflammation involving degenerative valvular lesions, Lambl's excrescences, and nonbacterial endocarditis. **It is essential to interpret images in conjunction with clinical data.**

4. One meta-analysis showed that the risk of embolization in patients with large vegetations (greater than 10 mm) was nearly three times higher than in patients with no detectable vegetations or small vegetations. Prolapsing vegetations and involvement of extravalvular structures increase the overall risk of heart failure, embolization, and need for valve replacement. Vegetations that increase in size, despite appropriate therapy, are also more likely to be associated with adverse events needing surgery.

5. TEE is indicated in patients with suspected pacemaker or defibrillator endocarditis. The sensitivity of TTE for detecting valvular or lead vegetations is 30%, compared to 90% with TEE.

B. Cardiac catheterization. Left-heart catheterization with selective coronary angiography is indicated prior to surgical intervention if there is a suspicion of obstructive coronary disease. The abnormal rocking motion of a dehisced prosthetic valve may be noted on fluoroscopy. Care should be taken to avoid unnecessary coronary angiography or cardiac catheterization in aortic valve endocarditis because of the risk of embolization of vegetations.

C. Central nervous system (CNS) imaging. Computerized tomography (CT), magnetic resonance imaging (MRI), or cerebral angiography should be considered in any patient who has sustained a CNS complication, such as an embolic infarct, intracranial bleed, or mycotic aneurysm, or in the patient with persistent headaches.

D. Body imaging. CT or MRI may be useful in the detection of metastatic infection. The value of CT may increase in the future as spatial resolution improves. **MRI** does not currently have a significant role in assessing cardiac manifestations of IE, owing to intrinsic problems related to temporal resolution.

VII. DUKE CRITERIA. Given the complexity of IE, the diagnosis requires a high index of suspicion. The Duke schema is currently the most sensitive and specific diagnostic set of criteria available. It is particularly useful in diagnosing endocarditis in patients with *S. aureus* bacteremia, those with right-sided endocarditis, and those with negative blood culture results. However, these criteria have not been validated in PVE.

A. The criteria are broken into **definite** (pathologic or clinical), **possible,** and **rejected** diagnostic groups.

B. For a **definite pathologic diagnosis,** either (A or B) of the pathologic findings listed in Table 17.2a is sufficient.

C. For a **definite clinical diagnosis** (Table 17.2b), two major criteria, or one major and three minor, or five minor criteria are needed.

D. The **possible diagnostic** group has findings consistent with IE, including one major criteria and one minor criteria, or three minor criteria.

E. For a **rejected diagnosis,** there is a firm alternative diagnosis for clinical manifestations or resolution of clinical manifestations, with antibiotics for 4 days or less, or no pathologic evidence of IE at surgery or autopsy, after antibiotic therapy for 4 days or less.

VIII. THERAPY. A team approach (cardiologist, cardiothoracic surgeon, infectious diseases specialist, and pathologist) in the diagnosis and management of IE cannot be overemphasized due to the complexity of the disease. Effective therapy requires identification of the microbial cause, determination of a bactericidal regimen of proven efficacy, an understanding of the intracardiac pathology of IE and its implications for surgery, and effective management of extracardiac complications.

A. Medical therapy

1. Principles of therapy. Antibiotic regimens should be bactericidal and chosen in consultation with an infectious diseases specialist. **Measures of antibiotic effectiveness** include the minimum inhibitory concentration (MIC) of antibiotic required to inhibit growth, the minimum bactericidal concentration (MBC) of an antibiotic required to kill an organism, and the serum bactericidal titer (SBT), which is the highest dilution of a patient's serum that kills 99.9% of an inoculum. The SBT is especially helpful when treating unusual organisms, when using unusual antibiotic regimens, or when treatment is failing. The MIC and MBC are not routinely measured, but currently recommended antimicrobial regimens are based on these values for specific organisms.

a. Combination therapy using a β-lactam agent such as penicillin with an aminoglycoside has a synergistic bactericidal effect in streptococcal IE and is also somewhat effective in a subset of patients with staphylococcal IE. However, high-level aminoglycoside resistance represents the most common and grave obstacle to optimal therapy for enterococcal endocarditis.

b. A multidrug regimen is recommended for optimal management of staphylococcal PVE. Rifampin has a unique ability to kill staphylococci. However, staphylococci have a relatively high intrinsic mutation rate for the gene controlling the site of rifampin action. Therefore, when large populations of staphylococci are exposed to rifampin, selection of rifampin-resistant organisms is common. Often, antistaphylococcal agent(s) may be administered for 3 to 5 days to reduce the total number of staphylococci before the commencement of rifampin. A multidrug approach (two antibiotics that are known to be active against the staphylococcal isolate in addition to rifampin) may reduce the probability of developing rifampin-resistant subpopulations.

c. Renal function is an important consideration when using **aminoglycosides or vancomycin**. These antibiotics should be dosed according to estimated creatinine clearance. The following doses outlined are for normal renal function. A vancomycin dose should not exceed 2 g per 24 hours unless serum levels are monitored.

d. Anticoagulation does not prevent embolization related to IE. In fact, **simultaneous treatment with penicillin and heparin increases the risk** of fatal intracerebral hemorrhage. Warfarin may be given safely during the treatment of patients with PVE.

2. Empiric therapy for IE is often started and continued until the etiologic organism is identified and the antibiotic sensitivities are known. Occasionally, empiric therapy is administered as a therapeutic trial to help confirm a diagnosis. Empiric therapy for subacute IE consists of ampicillin and gentamicin per the standard regimen, for enterococcal endocarditis (Table 17.3B) with intravenous nafcillin, 12 g per 24 hours in six divided doses, added for acute IE. Vancomycin per standard dosing for enterococcal IE is added instead of nafcillin

TABLE 17.2B Duke Criteria: Definite Clinical Diagnosis

Major Clinical Criteria

1. Positive blood culture results for infective endocarditis
   A. Typical microorganisms (in two or more cultures)
      - Viridans *Streptococcus*
      - *S. bovis*
      - HACEK group
      - *S.* aureus
      - Community-acquired enterococci, in the absence of a primary focus

   B. Persistently positive blood culture
      - Recovery of a microorganism consistent with IE from two blood cultures drawn more than 12 h apart
        or
      - Recovery of a microorganism consistent with IE from all of three or a majority of four or more separate blood cultures, with the first and last draw at least 1 h apart
        or
      - Single positive blood culture for *Coxiella burnetii* or anti-phase 1 IgG antibody titer >1:800
2. Evidence of endocardial involvement
   A. Positive echocardiogram
      - Oscillating intracardiac mass, on valve or supporting structures, or in the path of regurgitant jets or on implanted material, in the absence of an alternative anatomic explanation
        or
      - Abscess
        or
      - New partial dehiscence of prosthetic valve
        or

   B. New valvular regurgitation (increase or change in preexisting murmur not sufficient)

Minor Clinical Criteria

1. Predisposition:
   - Predisposing heart condition
   - Injection drug use
2. Fever >38.0°C (100.4°F)
3. Vascular phenomena:
   - Major arterial emboli
   - Septic pulmonary infarcts
   - Mycotic aneurysm
   - Intracranial hemorrhage
   - Conjunctival hemorrhages
   - Janeway lesions
4. Immunologic phenomena:
   - Glomerulonephritis
   - Osler's nodes
   - Roth's spots
   - Rheumatoid factor
5. Microbiologic evidence
   - Positive blood culture but not meeting major criteria as noted above
   - Serologic evidence of active infection with organism consistent with infective endocarditis

HACEK, *Haemophilus, Actinobacillus, Cardiobacterium, Eikenella, Kingella;* IE, infective endocarditis.
Adapted from Baddour LM, Wilson WR, Bayer AS, et al. Infective endocarditis: diagnosis, antimicrobial therapy, and management of complications. *Circulation* 2005;111:394–434.

TABLE 17.3A Therapies for Native Valve Infective Endocarditis Due to Penicillin-susceptible Viridans *Streptococcus* or *S. Bovis*

Medication	Dosage	Duration of therapy (wk)
Penicillin G	12–18 million U per 24 h continuously IV or in 4–6 divided doses	4
or		
Ceftriaxone	2 g once daily IV or IM	4
or		
Penicillin G	12–18 million U per 24 h continuously IV or in 6 divided doses	2[a]
or		
Ceftriaxone *plus*	2 g once daily IV or IM	2
gentamicin*or,* if penicillin allergic:	3 mg/kg once daily IV or IM	2
Vancomycin	30 mg per 24 h in two divided doses	4

IM, Intramuscular; IV, intravenous.
[a]For relatively resistant viridans *Streptococcus* or *S. bovis,* or known cardiac or extracardiac abscess, or for those with creatinine clearance <20 mL/min, penicillin G dosing is extended to 4 weeks.
Adapted from Baddour LM, Wilson WR, Bayer AS, et al. Infective endocarditis: diagnosis, antimicrobial therapy, and management of complications. *Circulation* 2005;111:394–434.

if methicillin-resistant *S. aureus* is suspected, if the patient is penicillin allergic, or if a prosthetic valve is involved. Unless clinical or epidemiologic clues suggest an etiologic factor, treatment for culture-negative IE is the same.

3. It is important to point out that when initiating therapy for coagulase-negative staphylococcal PVE, the organism should be assumed to be methicillin-resistant until the laboratory definitively excludes this.
4. Antibiotic therapy **after surgery** is discussed in **VIII.B**.
5. Medical therapies for **specific organisms** are displayed in Tables 17.3A to 17.3F.

TABLE 17.3B Standard Therapies for Susceptible Enterococci, for Resistant and Nutritionally Variant Viridans *Streptococcus* Infective Endocarditis, and for Prosthetic Valve Endocarditis Due to Viridans *Streptococcus* or *S. Bovis*

Medication	Dosage	Duration of therapy (wk)
Penicillin G	24 million U per 24 h continuously IV or in 4–6 divided doses	6
or		
Ceftriaxone	2 g once daily IV or IM	6
with or without		
Gentamicin	3 mg/kg once daily IV or IM	2–6[a]
or, if penicillin allergic:		
Vancomycin	30 mg/kg IV per 24 h in 2 divided doses	6

IM, intramuscular; IV, intravenous.
[a]If penicillin-susceptible strain (minimum inhibitory concentration ≤0.12 μg/mL), duration of gentamicin in combination with ceftriaxone is 2 weeks; if penicillin relatively resistant or fully resistant strain (minimum inhibitory concentration >0.12 μg /mL), duration of gentamicin is extended to 6 weeks.
Adapted from Baddour LM, Wilson WR, Bayer AS, et al. Infective endocarditis: diagnosis, antimicrobial therapy, and management of complications. *Circulation* 2005;111:394–434.

TABLE 17.3C Therapies for Infective Endocarditis Due to Methicillin-sensitive *Staphylococcus* in the Absence of Prosthetic Material

Medication	Dosage	Duration of therapy
Nafcillin or oxacillin	2 g IV every 4 h	6 wk
plus		
optional gentamicin	1 mg/kg IV or IM every 8 h	3–5 d
or		
Cefazolin	2 g IV every 8 h	6 wk
plus		
optional gentamicin	1 mg/kg IV or IM every 8 h	3–5 d
or, if penicillin allergic		
Vancomycin[a]	30 mg/kg per 24 h in 2 divided doses	6 wk

IM, intramuscular; IV, intravenous.
[a]Recommended for methicillin-resistant *Staphylococcus.*
Adapted from Baddour LM, Wilson WR, Bayer AS, et al. Infective endocarditis: diagnosis, antimicrobial therapy, and management of complications. *Circulation* 2005;111:394–434.

TABLE 17.3D Therapy for Infective Endocarditis Due to Methicillin-sensitive *Staphylococcus* in the Presence of Prosthetic Material

Medication	Dosage	Duration of therapy (wk)
Nafcillin[a] or oxacillin	2 g IV every 4 h	>6
plus rifampin	300 mg orally every 8 h	>6
plus gentamicin	1 mg/kg IV or IM every 8 h	2

IM, intramuscular; IV, intravenous.
[a]For methicillin-resistant *Staphylococcus* or for the penicillin-allergic patient, vancomycin, 30 mg/kg per 24 h IV in two divided doses, is substituted for nafcillin.
Adapted from Baddour LM, Wilson WR, Bayer AS, et al. Infective endocarditis: diagnosis, antimicrobial therapy, and management of complications. *Circulation* 2005;111:394–434.

TABLE 17.3E Therapy for Infective Endocarditis Due to Hacek Microorganisms

Medication	Dosage	Duration of therapy
Ceftriaxone[a]	2 g once daily IV or IM	4
or		
Ampicillin-sulbactam[a]	3 g IV every 6 h	4
or		
Ciprofloxacin	1000 mg orally once daily *or* 400 mg IV every 12 h	4

HACEK, *Haemophilus, Actinobacillus, Cardiobacterium, Eikenella, Kingella;* IM, intramuscular; IV, intravenous.
[a]The third-generation cephalosporins or ampicillin-sulbactam therapy should be considered the drugs of choice. Length of therapy for prosthetic valve infective endocarditis should be 6 weeks. A fluoroquinolone should be considered as an alternative agent for patients unable to tolerate β-lactam therapy.
Adapted from Baddour LM, Wilson WR, Bayer AS, et al. Infective endocarditis: diagnosis, antimicrobial therapy, and management of complications. *Circulation* 2005;111:394–434.

TABLE 17.3F	Therapy for *Pseudomonas Aeruginosa* and Other Gram-negative Bacilli (Enterobacteriaceae)[a]
Extended-spectrum penicillin (ticarcillin or piperacillin) *or* third-generation cephalosporin *or* imipenem *plus* aminoglycoside	

[a]Combination therapy is recommended. The final choice of antibiotic therapy is to be made after sensitivity results are available.

6. **Fungal IE.** When fungal IE is diagnosed, the standard of care involves a **combined medical/surgical approach.**
   a. The mainstay of antifungal drug therapy is **amphotericin B** with or without **flucytosine** (a synergistic effect).
      (1) Amphotericin B is infused in 5% dextrose over 2 to 4 hours at a dose of 0.7 to 1.0 mg/kg daily. Larger doses (1 to 1.5 mg/kg daily) are recommended for management of PVE caused by *Aspergillus* spp.
      (2) The main toxicity of amphotericin B is **renal dysfunction.** Liposomal preparations may be less nephrotoxic.
      (3) The primary toxicity of flucytosine is **bone marrow suppression**; for this reason, flucytosine blood levels may be useful during therapy.
   b. After 1 to 2 weeks of full-dose amphotericin B therapy, surgery should probably be performed because effective penetration of the medicine into vegetations is unlikely. Valve replacement becomes necessary in almost all cases of fungal IE.
   c. Long-term oral suppressive therapy with antifungal agents such as fluconazole or itraconazole is commonly recommended to prevent relapse.

B. **Surgical therapy** (Table 17.4). Surgery is indicated in approximately 25% to 30% of cases during the acute phase of infection, and in another 20% to 40% in subsequent or secondary phases. Antibiotic therapy combined with valve replacement and cardiac reconstruction results in higher survival rates and fewer relapses or rehospitalizations, and lower late endocarditis–related mortality than does antibiotics alone in patients with complicated IE.
   1. The **fundamental principles** of operative procedures for IE involve débridement of infected tissue, removal of all nonviable tissue, reconstruction of the involved area, and restoration of valve competence. There is general consensus for surgical intervention in any of the following situations: refractory congestive heart failure due to significant valve dysfunction, uncontrolled infection, failed antimicrobial therapy with perivalvular extension of infection, most cases of prosthetic valve endocarditis, most cases of fungal IE, and established abscess. Debatable indications include the presence of more than one serious systemic embolic event or one embolus with a large residual vegetation. These indications are not absolute and must be implemented with a careful risk–benefit analysis.
   2. Congestive heart failure [New York Heart Association (NYHA) class III or IV] is the strongest indication for surgery in IE, as 90% of all deaths result from congestive heart failure. It should be remembered that the benefit of surgery persists even in the presence of comorbidities, such as acute renal failure.
   3. Prosthetic valve endocarditis usually requires a combined medical/surgical approach.
   4. **Patients with CNS infarcts or bleeds.** Special attention must be paid to the presurgical candidate who may have had a CNS infarct or bleed, since large doses of heparin are required for a cardiopulmonary bypass. Several studies report a significant risk for postoperative neurologic deterioration or even death in patients with recent CNS complication of IE. The best management in the scenario of hemodynamic instability and new-onset embolic stroke has not been addressed in randomized clinical studies. Where possible, cardiac surgery is

TABLE 17.4 Surgical Indications

CLEAR INDICATIONS
Uncontrolled congestive heart failure due to valve dysfunction
Unstable prosthesis
Uncontrolled/uncontrollable infection (e.g., by fungi, *Pseudomonas*, *Brucellae*)
S. aureus prosthetic valve endocarditis with an intracardiac complication
Relapse of prosthetic valve endocarditis after optimal therapy
Recurrent emboli
RELATIVE INDICATIONS
Perivalvular extension of infection (fistula/abscess)
Poorly responsive *S. aureus* native valve endocarditis
Relapse of native valve endocarditis after optimal antimicrobial therapy
Culture-negative endocarditis with persistent unexplained fever (≥10 d)
Large vegetations (>10 mm in diameter) with risk of embolization
Endocarditis caused by highly antibiotic-resistant enterococci

Adapted from Karchmer AW. Infectious endocarditis. In: Braunwald E, ed. *Heart disease: a textbook of cardiovascular medicine,* 7th ed. Philadelphia: WB Saunders, 2005:1633–1658.

delayed for at least 4 days, and ideally 10 days postinfarction in those with a CNS embolic infarct, and for 21 days following an intracranial hemorrhage. However, some patients may need early surgery despite a recent stroke if they are at high risk of recurrent emboli. **If a mycotic aneurysm is found, the timing of surgery should be reconsidered, and any prosthesis that requires postoperative anticoagulation should be avoided.** A ruptured mycotic aneurysm should be resected, clipped, or embolized **before** cardiac operation.

5. Metastatic infection, usually attributed to *S. aureus*, should be drained if accessible.
6. The optimal duration of **antibiotic therapy after surgery** for IE is not known.
   a. For **native valve IE** caused by an antibiotic-resistant organism with subsequent negative cultures, preoperative plus postoperative antibiotic therapy should consist of a full course of recommended treatment.
   b. For patients with **positive intraoperative cultures,** a full course of therapy should be given postoperatively.
   c. Patients with prosthetic valves who are undergoing surgery for IE should receive a full course of antibiotics postoperatively when organisms are discovered in resected material.

C. The optimal management of **pacer or defibrillator endocarditis** has been controversial in the literature, especially regarding the necessity of device removal.
   1. The success rate without removal of the entire device is low because typically the entire device is infected. Most studies suggest that the complete explantation of all hardware combined with antibiotic therapy is the optimal management.
   2. The optimal route or duration of antibiotics remains unclear in the literature. Experience suggests that a prolonged course of intravenous antibiotics is needed.
   3. The timing of device reimplantation is another dilemma. It is prudent to provide sufficient duration of antibiotic therapy to eradicate bacteremia and to suppress or eradicate endocardial infection prior to reimplantation in order to minimize the risk of reinfection of the new device. In the literature, reimplantation was successfully performed at a median of 7 days (5 to 25 days) after explantation.

IX. COMPLICATIONS

A. Table 17.5 lists the complications of IE.

B. Valve-ring abscess is a noteworthy complication of PVE, seen with mechanical and bioprosthetic valves and also occasionally seen in severe infection of native valves. Infection of the sutures used to secure the sewing ring to the periannular tissue may result in dehiscence of the valve. The clinical finding of a new perivalvular leak in a patient with PVE is worrisome. Risk factors for abscess formation include persistent

TABLE 17.5 Complications

CARDIAC COMPLICATIONS
Congestive heart failure (leading cause of death)
Abscess (pericardial, aortic annular, or myocardial)
Conduction abnormalities (due to invasive disease)
Coronary embolism
Mycotic aneurysm (often clinically silent)
Valvular regurgitaton (cusp/leaflet flail or perforation)
Valvular stenosis
Prosthetic dehiscence
Septal perforation (vertricular septal defect)
EXTRACARDIAC COMPLICATIONS
Systemic embolism (stroke, renal infarct, splenic infarct, or ischemic limb)
Mycotic aneurysm
Abscess
Immune complex deposition (glomerulonephritis)

fever, congestive heart failure, a history of intravenous drug use, infection with a virulent organism, and PVE.

X. RESPONSE TO THERAPY. Although a reduction in the size of vegetations during antimicrobial therapy suggests therapeutic success, vegetations may persist unchanged in the face of microbiologic cure. Significant enlargement of a vegetation during treatment indicates possible treatment failure and constitutes a relative indication for surgery.

A. Blood cultures should be obtained during therapy for IE to ensure eradication of the organism (see **V.A.3**).

B. Defervescence usually follows 3 to 7 days of successful antimicrobial therapy. **Persistent or recurrent fever may represent therapeutic failure, drug fever, a secondary nosocomial infection, or intracardiac or extracardiac abscess formation.** Generally, if fever persists for more than 7 days or if blood cultures are positive beyond the first week of antibiotic therapy, the treatment is considered a failure.

C. Relapses, should they occur, usually manifest clinically within 4 weeks and can be confirmed by blood cultures. With a combined medical and surgical approach, recurrent PVE occurs in 6% to 15% of patients.

D. The **frequency of emboli falls rapidly after 1 to 2 weeks of antibiotic therapy,** and the risk is considered to be greatest in the setting of large vegetations (larger than 10 mm in diameter) and specific infections (*S. aureus* and *Candida*).

E. Medical management is successful in many patients with IE; however, surgery is required in approximately 25% to 33% of cases.

XI. PROGNOSIS. The prognosis depends on **the virulence of the causative organism, the underlying health of the patient, the valvular structures, the duration of the infection, and the presence or absence of congestive heart failure.** The overall mortality of IE is around 20%. Notably, the mortality rates in early PVE (40% to 80%) are much higher than in late disease (20% to 40%). Five-year survival rates after surgery for PVE have ranged from 54% to 87%. In *S. aureus* IE, mortality has decreased from 50% to 60% to 15% to 30% in recent years. The presence of the factors in Table 17.6 should trigger an early and aggressive management plan.

XII. PROPHYLAXIS. Revised IE prophylaxis guidelines from the American Heart Association (AHA) concluded that **only those patients at highest risk for adverse outcome from IE require prophylaxis** prior to certain dental or surgical procedures (Tables 17.7A and 17.7B). This is based on studies suggesting that IE is more likely to occur from everyday activities such as flossing or brushing teeth than from dental procedures, and that an extremely small number of cases of IE might be prevented by antibiotic prophylaxis for dental, gastrointestinal, or genitourinary procedures. It is a standard practice (AHA guideline) that at-risk individuals be counseled and advised to carry a card with current prophylaxis recommendations. Failure to adhere to this practice

TABLE 17.6 Factors and Complications that Predispose to a Poor Outcome

Congestive heart failure (leading adverse prognostic factor)
Nonstreptococcal disease
Aortic valve involvement
Infection of a prosthetic valve
Older age
Abscess formation
HIV with CD4 count <200
Delayed diagnosis
CNS or coronary embolization
Recurrent infective endocarditis

CNS, central nervous system; HIV, human immunodeficiency virus.

may invite litigation. A recent study suggests that an echocardiographic report, stating the endocarditis risk and need for prophylaxis, improves compliance with AHA recommendations.

A. In deciding the need for antibiotic prophylaxis, two factors that must be considered are the risk associated with the specific valvular lesion (Table 17.7A) and the type of procedure to be performed (Table 17.7B). Patients for whom antibiotic prophylaxis for IE is recommended include those with **prosthetic heart valves, prior IE, post-cardiac transplantation valvulopathy, and certain patients with congenital heart disease** (Table 17.7A). Routine IE prophylaxis is no longer recommended in several cardiac conditions including mitral valve prolapse, rheumatic heart disease, bicuspid aortic valve, calcific aortic stenosis, atrial septal defect, ventricular septal defect, and hypertrophic cardiomyopathy.

B. Endocarditis prophylaxis following **dental or oral procedures** is directed primarily against viridans *Streptococcus;* following **genitourinary and gastrointestinal surgery** it is directed primarily against *Enterococcus* organisms.

C. **Routine antibiotic prophylaxis solely to prevent IE is no longer advised prior to gastrointestinal or genitourinary procedures.** This is based upon an increasing frequency of antimicrobial-resistant strains of enterococci and a lack of evidence conclusively linking these procedures to IE.

D. Available evidence supports a shift in emphasis away from a focus on dental procedures and antibiotic prophylaxis toward a greater **emphasis on maintaining good oral hygiene** and improved access to dental care in patients at risk for IE.

E. Prophylaxis against viridans *Streptococcus* is advised in patients at highest risk of IE who undergo **invasive procedures of the respiratory tract** that involve incision

TABLE 17.7A Cardiac Conditions Associated with the Highest Risk of Adverse Outcome from Infective Endocarditis

Prophylaxis for endocarditis recommended
Prosthetic heart valves
Previous infective endocarditis
Congenital heart disease (CHD)
Unrepaired cyanotic CHD (including palliative shunts or conduits)
Repaired CHD with residual defect at or adjacent to the site of repair
During the first 6 months after repair of congenital heart defects using prosthetic material or device
Cardiac transplantation recipients who develop cardiac valvulopathy

Adapted from Wilson W, Taubert KA, Gewitz M, et al. Prevention of infective endocarditis: guidelines from the American Heart Association. *Circulation* 2007;115:1–19.

TABLE 17.7B Recommendations for Prophylaxis in Dental or Surgical Procedures

Prophylaxis recommended only in patients at highest risk of adverse outcome from infective endocarditis (Table 17.7a)

OROPHARYNGEAL PROCEDURES

Dental procedures that involve manipulation of gingival tissue, the periapical region of teeth, or perforation of the oral mucosa

Tonsillectomy and/or adenoidectomy

RESPIRATORY PROCEDURES

Invasive procedures involving incision

MISCELLANEOUS

Procedures on infected skin or musculoskeletal tissue

Adapted from Wilson W, Taubert KA, Gewitz M, et al. Prevention of infective endocarditis: guidelines from the American Heart Association. *Circulation* 2007;115:1–19.

or biopsy (i.e., tonsillectomy or adenoidectomy). Routine endocarditis prophylaxis prior to **vaginal delivery** or hysterectomy is not recommended.

F. Incision and drainage or other procedures involving infected tissue may result in bacteremia. For nonoral soft-tissue infections, an antistaphylococcal penicillin or first-generation cephalosporin is an appropriate choice of prophylaxis.

G. Prophylaxis regimens are displayed in Table 17.7C. **Cardiac surgical patients** who undergo placement of prosthetic heart valves or other prosthetic material should receive antibiotic prophylaxis, primarily directed against *S. aureus*. A first-generation cephalosporin is commonly used, but the choice of antibiotic should be influenced by the antibiotic susceptibility pattern at each hospital. Prophylaxis should be started immediately before the procedure, repeated during prolonged procedures, and continued for no more than 48 hours. **A careful preoperative dental evaluation** is recommended so that, whenever possible, required dental treatment can be completed before cardiac valve surgery.

H. Patients after cardiac transplantation are at moderate risk for endocarditis because of continuous immunosuppression and the tendency for acquired valvular dysfunction (tricuspid regurgitation from endomyocardial biopsy or rejection).

I. Pneumococcal vaccination is recommended for all patients with prosthetic heart valves

TABLE 17.7C Prophylactic Regimens

Clinical situation	Antibiotic	Dose
Standard prophylaxis	Amoxicillin	2 g PO 1 h before procedure
Unable to take oral medications	Ampicillin	2 g IV or IM within 30 min before procedure
	or	
	Cefazolin or ceftriaxone	1 g IV or IM within 30 min before procedure
Penicillin allergy	Clindamycin	600 mg PO 1 h before procedure
	or	
	cephalexin	2 g PO 1 h before procedure
	or	
	Azithromycin *or* clarythromicin	500 mg 1 h before procedure

IM, intramuscular; IV, intravenous, PO, per oral.
Adapted from Wilson W, Taubert KA, Gewitz M, et al. Prevention of infective endocarditis: guidelines from the American Heart Association. *Circulation* 2007;115:1–19.

XIII. CONTROVERSIES

A. Therapy

1. Short courses of antibiotics (2 weeks) have shown some efficacy in the injection drug use population, as have oral antibiotics in the same population. However, intravenous antibiotics are indicated until conclusive data concerning attentive regimens are available. At least 5 to 7 days of inpatient therapy is advocated before considering outpatient treatment.
2. Correct timing of surgery is often the most difficult and critical decision in the management of IE. It is important to balance the need for medical stabilization with timely surgery.
3. Valve repair is a reasonable option for mitral, tricuspid, and, less often, aortic IE in which the infection has been controlled. The choice between mechanical, bioprosthetic, and biologic devices may be made according to the usual criteria. However, in the setting of aortic prosthetic endocarditis, a homograft or an autograft is less likely to become infected than either a xenograft or a mechanical valve, and is considered the optimal valve substitute.

ACKNOWLEDGMENTS

The authors thank Drs. Xiao-Fang Xu and Mark Murphy for their contributions to this chapter.

Landmark Articles

Chua JD, Wilkoff B, et al. Diagnosis and management of infections involving implantable electrophysiologic cardiac devices. *Ann Intern Med* 2000;133:604–608.
Durack DT. Prevention of infective endocarditis. *N Engl J Med* 1995;332:38–44.
Durack DT, Lukes AS, Bright DK. New criteria for diagnosis of infective endocarditis: utilization of specific echocardiographic findings. *Am J Med* 1994;96:200–209.
Knosalla C, et al. Surgical treatment of active infective aortic valve endocarditis with associated periannular abscesses with 11-year results. *Eur Heart J* 2000;21:490–497.
Sanders GP, Yeon SB, Grunes J, et al. Impact of a specific echocardiographic report comment regarding endocarditis prophylaxis on compliance with American Heart Association Recommendations. *Circulation* 2002;106:300–303.
Strom BL, Abrutyn E, Berlin JA, et al. Risk factors for infective endocarditis: oral hygiene and nondental exposures. *Circulation* 2000;102:2842–2848.
Wallace SM, et al. Mortality from infective endocarditis: clinical predictors of outcome. *Heart* 2002;88:53–60.
Wilson LE, et al. Prospective study of infective endocarditis among injection drug users. *J Infect Dis* 2002;185:1761–1766.
Wilson WR, Karchmer AW, Dajani AS, et al. Antibiotic treatment of adults with infective endocarditis due to streptococci, enterococci, staphylococci, and HACEK microorganisms. *JAMA* 1995;274:1706–1713.

Key Reviews

Adolf W, Longworth DL. Infection of intracardiac devices. *Infect Dis Clin North Am* 2002;16:477–505.
Baddour LM, Wilson WR, Bayer AS, et al. Infective endocarditis: diagnosis, antimicrobial therapy, and management of complications: A statement for healthcare professionals from the Committee on Rheumatic fever, Endocarditis, and Kawasaki Disease, Council on Cardiovascular Disease in the Young, and the Councils on Clinical Cardiology, Stroke, and Cardiovascular Surgery and Anesthesia, American Heart Association: Endorsed by the Infectious Diseases Society of America. *Circulation* 2005;111:394–434.
Bashore TM, Cabell C, Fowler V. Update on infective endocarditis. *Curr Probl Cardiol* 2006;31:274–352.
Krivokapich J, Child JS. Role of transthoracic and transesophageal echocardiography in diagnosis and management of infective endocarditis. *Cardiol Clin North Am* 1996;14:363–382.
Moreillon P, Que YA. Infective endocarditis. *Lancet* 2004;363:139–149.
Mylonakis E, Calderwood SB. Infective endocarditis in adults. *N Engl J Med* 2001;345:1318–1330.
Olaison L, Pettersson G. Current best practice and guidelines: indications for surgical intervention in infective endocarditis. *Infect Dis Clin North Am* 2002;16:453–475.
Sexton DJ, Spelman D. Current best practice and guidelines: assessment and management of complications in infective endocarditis. *Infect Dis Clin North Am* 2002;16:507–521.
Wilson W, Taubert KA, Gewitz M, et al. Prevention of infective endocarditis. Guidelines from the American Heart Association. *Circulation* 2007;115:1–19.

Relevant Book Chapters

Fuster V, Alexander RW, O'Rourke RA, eds. *Hurst's the heart,* 11th ed. New York: McGraw-Hill, 2004:2205–2242.
Mandell GL, Bennett JE, Dolin R, eds. *Principles and practice of infectious disease,* 6th ed. New York: Churchill Livingstone, 2005.
Karchmer AW. Infectious Endocarditis. In: Braunwald E, ed. *Heart disease: a textbook of cardiovascular medicine,* 7th ed. Philadelphia: WB Saunders, 2005:1633–1658.
Otto C. *The practice of clinical echocardiography,* 2nd ed. Philadelphia: WB Saunders, 2002:451–469.
Sexton DJ, et al. Infectious endocarditis. In: Topol EJ, ed. *Textbook of cardiovascular medicine.* Philadelphia: Lippincott–Raven Publishers, 2002:569–593.

RHEUMATIC FEVER

Stephen Gimple

18

I. INTRODUCTION. Rheumatic fever (RF) is a systemic autoimmune disorder related to prior streptococcal infection, which is a **leading cause of acquired heart disease in adults and children in many parts of the world**, although it has become markedly less common in industrialized nations over the last century.

A. The incidence of RF and prevalence of rheumatic heart disease **vary substantially among countries.** In many developing countries the incidence of acute RF approaches or exceeds 200 per 100,000, whereas in the Unites States it is estimated to be less than 1 per 100,000. In 2002, more than 3500 deaths were attributed to acute or chronic RF in the United States. Since the first half of this century, there has been a gradual decline in the incidence of RF in the United States, Japan, and most European countries. This is due to improved public health and living conditions, the development of modern antibiotics, as well as a shift in the endemic strains of group A *Streptococcus* (GAS). Localized outbreaks of RF have occurred in the United States as recently as the mid-1980s.

B. RF is more common among populations at high risk for streptococcal pharyngitis, such as military recruits, those in close contact with school-aged children, and persons of low socioeconomic status. It occurs commonly between the ages of 5 and 18 years and is rare before age 5, perhaps because a mature immune system is required. RF affects both sexes equally, except for Sydenham's chorea, which is more prevalent in females after puberty.

II. CLINICAL PRESENTATION. The clinical manifestations of RF **develop 3 weeks after a group A streptococcal (GAS) tonsillopharyngitis.** It is important to note that one-third of patients with RF do not remember having had a sore throat. Patients with RF present initially with a sudden onset of constitutional symptoms, including fever (101°C to 104°C), malaise, weight loss, and pallor. An exudative and proliferative inflammatory process involving collagen fibrils characterizes the acute phase of RF. **Multiple organ systems** such as the dermis, central nervous system, synovium, and heart, may be involved. In addition, manifestations may include serositis and involvement of the lungs, kidneys, and central nervous system.

A. Diagnostic criteria

1. The **Jones criteria,** last updated in 2002, are designed to aid in the diagnosis of the first episode of RF. It can be diagnosed when a **previous upper airway infection with GAS is detected in conjunction either with two major manifestations, or with one major and two minor manifestations.** Major manifestations include arthritis, carditis, chorea, erythema marginatum, and subcutaneous nodules. Minor manifestations include fever, arthralgias, high C-reactive protein (CRP) level or high erythrocyte sedimentation rate (ESR), and a prolonged PR interval on electrocardiogram (ECG) (Table 18.1).
2. In some circumstances, the **diagnosis of RF can be made without strict adherence to Jones criteria,** as in cases of indolent or recurrent carditis or isolated cases of chorea when other causes have been excluded.

B. Major manifestations (Table 18.1)

1. **Carditis.** This is the most serious and is often regarded as the most specific manifestation of RF, affecting 41% to 83% of patients. It may manifest as pancarditis affecting the endocardium, myocardium, and pericardium simultaneously.

TABLE 18.1 Diagnosis of Rheumatic Fever[a]

Gas infection	Major Jones criteria	Minor Jones criteria
Culture	Carditis	Fever
ASO titers	Arthritis	Arthralgia
anti-DNAse B	Sydenham's chorea	High ESR or CRP
Other antistreptococcal antibodies	Subcutaneous nodules	Prolonged PR
Streptococcal antigens	Erythema marginatum	

CRP, C-reactive protein; ESR, erythrocyte sedimentation rate; GAS, group A *Streptococcus.*
[a]The diagnosis of rheumatic fever requires confirmation of a previous ***GAS infection*** with at least one of the methods listed above together with either ***two major*** criteria or ***one major and two minor*** criteria.

a. Cardiac involvement **ranges from an asymptomatic presentation to progressive congestive heart failure and death.**

b. The most typical manifestations include **increased heart rate, rhythm disturbances, new murmurs or pericardial friction rub, cardiomegaly, and heart failure.**

c. Heart failure is rare in the acute phase; if present, it is usually the result of myocarditis.

d. The most characteristic component of rheumatic carditis is a valvulitis (endocarditis) involving the mitral and aortic valves.

(1) Mitral insufficiency is the hallmark of rheumatic carditis. Aortic insufficiency is less common and is almost always associated with mitral insufficiency.

(2) Acute mitral valve regurgitation produces an apical systolic murmur that may be accompanied by a mid-diastolic Carey-Coombs murmur of relative mitral stenosis (a high-pitched early diastolic murmur that varies from day to day). Right-sided valves are rarely involved.

(3) Those valvular lesions that are diagnosed by echocardiogram but are clinically silent, usually heal without scarring and have a good prognosis. Controversy exists whether echocardiographic findings of mitral regurgitation or aortic insufficiency constitute subclinical rheumatic carditis sufficient to meet the Jones criteria.

e. Pericarditis may cause chest pain, friction rubs, and distant heart sounds, but is often clinically silent.

2. **Arthritis.** This is the **most common manifestation of RF but it is the least specific.** It occurs in 80% of patients and is described as **painful, asymmetric, migratory, and transient. It involves large joints,** such as knees, ankles, elbows, wrists, and shoulders. It is **more common in older patients, and improves markedly with the use of salicylates** within 48 hours of treatment. Monoarthritis, oligoarthritis, and involvement of small joints of the extremities are less common. However, arthritis of the first metatarsophalangeal joint, enthesopathy, and axial involvement, especially of the cervical spine, have also been reported. The **arthritis of RF is benign and self-limiting** (lasting 2 to 3 weeks) and does not result in permanent sequelae. Inflammatory changes without signs of infection are seen in the joint fluid.

3. **Sydenham's chorea.** Also known as Saint Vitus' dance or chorea minor. This **extrapyramidal disorder is characterized by purposeless and involuntary movements** of face and limbs, muscular hypotonia, and emotional lability.

a. Initial manifestations include difficulty in writing, talking, or walking. Handwriting may deteriorate; speech may change to an explosive and halting tone; and the patient may become uncoordinated and easily frustrated.

b. Symptoms tend to be more evident when the patient is under stress or awake, and usually disappear during sleep.

c. Sydenham's chorea is a **delayed manifestation of RF,** usually appearing 3 months or more after an upper airway infection; it is often the sole manifestation of acute RF. Chorea has been reported in up to 30% of the patients. Most cases tend to follow a benign course with complete resolution of symptoms in 2 to 3 months, although cases in which symptoms persisted for more than 2 years have been reported.

d. It is important to **differentiate the symptoms of Sydenham's chorea from tics, athetosis, conversion reactions, hyperkinesia, and behavioral abnormalities.**

4. **Subcutaneous nodules.** These usually measure 0.5 to 2 cm, and are **firm, painless, and freely mobile nodules that can be isolated or found in clusters** over the **extensor surfaces** of joints (knees, elbows, and wrists), bony prominences, tendons, dorsum of foot, occipital region, and cervical processes. They are seen in up to 20% of patients with RF and last for a few days. The skin overlying the nodules is freely mobile and shows no signs of discoloration or inflammation.

5. **Erythema marginatum.** This is an **evanescent** erythematous **macular rash** with a pale center of irregular shape. It is **usually nonpruritic and tends to disappear after a few days.** It is highly specific, occurring in less than 5% of patients, and is obvious only in fair-skinned individuals. The lesions vary in size and affect mainly the trunk, abdomen, and inner aspect of arms and thighs, but not the face. The rash may be induced by application of heat. Its presence is **suggestive of coexisting carditis.**

C. **Minor manifestations.** Fever and arthralgias are common, but nonspecific findings of RF that can be used to support the diagnosis of RF when only a single major manifestation is present (Table 18.1).

1. Fever is encountered during the acute phase of the disease and does not follow a specific pattern.
2. Arthralgia is defined as pain in one or more large joints without objective findings of inflammation on physical examination.
3. Other clinical manifestations of RF include **abdominal pain, epistaxis, acute glomerulonephritis, rheumatic pneumonitis, hematuria, and encephalitis.** These are not included as diagnostic criteria for the diagnosis of RF.

III. ETIOLOGY AND PATHOPHYSIOLOGY

A. The association between tonsillopharyngitis–scarlet fever epidemics and acute RF in the 1930s, the findings of high levels of antistreptolysin O (ASO) in sera of patients with RF, and the confirmation of antibiotics as an efficient mode of prophylaxis of RF provide **strong evidence that GAS is the agent causing initial and recurrent attacks of RF.**

1. Acute RF might not be caused directly by the bacteria but rather through an immunologic mechanism. Specifically, it appears that patients who develop RF demonstrate a hyperimmune response to GAS, and the level of the immune response correlates with the severity of the RF manifestations. Supporting evidence includes onset approximately 3 weeks following an upper respiratory tract infection, rarity before age 5 when the immune system is still immature, and cross-reactivity between streptococcal cellular antigens and proteins present in human connective tissue.

   a. The most important antigenic structures (M, T, and R proteins) are localized in the external layer of the bacterial cell wall.

   b. The M protein is not only responsible for type-specific immunity; it has a powerful antiphagocytic action and is classically regarded as a marker of streptococcal rheumatogenic potential. Patients with acute RF possess high levels of antibodies targeted against this protein. Specific M serotypes of GAS have long been recognized as strong stimulators of a robust immune response and are associated with an increased risk for developing RF. Those M serotypes associated with impetigo or pyoderma may cause glomerulonephritis but are not associated with RF.

2. In epidemics of streptococcal pharyngitis, it is estimated that approximately **3% of untreated individuals will go on to develop RF.** However, recurrence of

RF is seen in about 50% of patients with a history of RF. For endemic GAS pharyngeal infections, the incidence of RF is much less common.

B. Numerous epidemiologic studies favor a **familial and even genetic predisposition.** A monoclonal antibody to B-cell alloantigen (D8/17) is almost universally detected in patients with RF, whereas this antibody is present in less than 14% of the general population. In addition, susceptibility to RF has also been linked with D-related human leukocyte antigen (HLA-DR) 1, 2, 3, and 4 haplotypes. These genetic markers may be useful in the future to identify individuals susceptible to acute RF.

IV. LABORATORY EXAMINATION AND DIAGNOSTIC TESTING. RF is a clinical diagnosis because there is no single laboratory study that is diagnostic of RF.

A. Supporting evidence of antecedent GAS infection can be obtained through cultures, antigen test, or serum antistreptococcal antibody test.

1. Although no consensus exists regarding which tests to order at what time, commonly ASO titers and cultures are initially obtained when RF is suspected. Other tests as detailed in subsequent text are useful only under certain conditions.
2. A negative throat culture is usually sufficient to withhold antibiotic treatment in most cases, especially if clinical suspicion of RF is low.
3. Elevated or rising ASO titers provide solid evidence for recent GAS infection. **A greater than twofold rise in ASO titers compared with convalescent titers is diagnostic.**
4. The probability of detecting a previous GAS infection can be increased by obtaining repeated ASO tests or by looking for antibodies to other streptococcal antigens, such as antideoxyribonuclease B **(anti-DNAase B).**
5. A slide agglutination test is commercially available, which measures antibodies to several streptococcal antigens. Although this test is simple to perform, it is **not well standardized and is not very reproducible.** Therefore, it is **not recommended** as a definitive test for prior GAS infection.

B. Biopsies

1. Aschoff's nodules, a form of granulomatous inflammation, can be seen in the proliferative stage and are considered pathognomonic for rheumatic carditis. They are encountered in 30% to 40% of biopsies from patients with primary or recurrent episodes of RF. Such nodules are most often found in the interventricular septum, the wall of the left ventricle, or the left atrial appendage.
2. The histologic findings of endocarditis include edema and cellular infiltration of valvular tissue. Hyaline degeneration of the affected valve results in the formation of verrucae at its edge, preventing the normal leaflet coaptation. If the inflammatory process persists, fibrosis and calcification develop, leading to valvular stenosis.
3. Endomyocardial biopsy does not help in diagnosing first attacks of rheumatic carditis. It is **useful in distinguishing chronic inactive rheumatic heart disease from acute rheumatic carditis.** As such, it is rarely indicated except in cases where recurrent carditis is suspected but cannot be confirmed otherwise.

C. Other blood tests

1. As in any inflammatory process, **leukocytosis, thrombocytosis, or hypochromic or normochromic anemia** may be noted.
2. The favored tests to measure acute phase response are ESR and CRP. Although these tests are nonspecific, they may be helpful in monitoring the inflammatory activity of the disease. These levels are **almost always elevated during the acute phase of RF in patients with arthritis and polyarthritis, and are usually normal in patients with chorea.**

D. Radiography. Chest radiography may identify increased cardiac size, increased pulmonary vasculature, or pulmonary edema.

E. Electrocardiography and echocardiography. In patients in whom **carditis is subtle and signs of valvular involvement may be mild or transient, a baseline echocardiogram and electrocardiogram** may help provide evidence of carditis.

1. The most common finding in the **electrocardiogram** is the presence of **PR prolongation and sinus tachycardia.** Myocarditis may prolong QT interval. In

cases of pericarditis, low-voltage QRS complexes and ST-segment changes in the precordial leads can be observed.

2. Echocardiography is likely to show mitral regurgitation or aortic insufficiency. Calcifications of the leaflets and subvalvular apparatus are present in the chronic, not acute, phase of rheumatic heart disease.

V. **THERAPY.** It is generally recommended that **patients with suspected RF be admitted for close observation and workup.**

A. **Arthritis.** Anti-inflammatory medications are usually needed for **3 weeks to achieve symptomatic relief.**

1. Pain resolves within 24 hours of starting therapy with salicylates.
2. If pain persists despite salicylate treatment, the **diagnosis of RF is questionable.**
3. The **recommended dose of salicylate** is 100 mg/kg per day, given in 4 or 5 divided doses. For optimal antiinflammatory effect, a serum salicylate level of 20 mg% is adequate.
4. Watch for toxic side effects, such as anorexia, nausea, vomiting, and tinnitus.
5. For patients who cannot tolerate salicylates, nonsteroidal anti-inflammatory drugs (NSAIDs) can be tried. However, there is no evidence that NSAIDs are more effective than salicylates. As with salicylates, improvement of symptoms is prompt.

B. **Carditis**

1. **Strenuous physical activity should be avoided.**
2. Congestive heart failure should be managed with standard therapy (Chapters 7 and 8).
3. In patients with significant cardiac involvement, corticosteroids are preferred over salicylates. The recommended dose of corticosteroid is 1 to 2 mg/kg per day (maximum of 60 mg/day). Salicylate or steroid therapy does not affect the course of the disease; therefore, the duration of anti-inflammatory therapy is somewhat arbitrary and is guided by the severity of disease and the response to therapy. Commonly, therapy is needed for 1 month in patients with relatively mild cardiac involvement. Therapy should be continued until there is sufficient clinical and laboratory evidence of disease inactivity.
4. After cessation of anti-inflammatory agents, relapse with mild symptoms may occur. **A gradual reduction in steroid dosing is necessary to avoid relapses.** If **symptoms are mild, they usually subside without specific treatment.** For **severe symptoms, treatment with salicylates** should be tried before restarting corticosteroids. Administering salicylate therapy (75 mg/kg per day) while tapering corticosteroids may reduce the likelihood of a relapse.
5. Corticosteroids, despite relieving symptoms or carditis, do not prevent valvular damage.

C. Sydenham's chorea. Although this was once thought to have a benign, self-limiting course, it is recognized today that some patients develop significant morbidity.

1. **Some investigators recommend haloperidol or valproate therapy.** Haloperidol is used in an initial dose of 0.5 to 1 mg/day, and 0.5 mg is added every 3 days for maximal effect or until a maximal dose of 5 mg/day is attained. Sodium valproate (15 to 20 mg/kg per day) is also effective.
2. In resistant cases, plasmapheresis, intravenous immunoglobulin, reserpine, and perphenazine have also been tried.
3. Steroid therapy is generally not effective in Sydenham's chorea.

VI. **PREVENTION.** See Table 18.2.

A. **Primary prevention.** The most important step in the management of RF is the eradication of GAS infection, which prevents chronic and repetitive exposure of antigenic streptococcal components to the host immune system. However, **no treatment can eradicate GAS completely in all patients because of high colonization rates.**

1. Early therapy is advisable because it reduces both morbidity and the period of infectivity. Studies have shown that antimicrobial therapy, even when started 9 days after the onset of acute streptococcal pharyngitis, is still effective in preventing primary attacks of RF.

TABLE 18.2 Prevention of Rheumatic Fever

Drug	Dosage	Route	Duration
Primary prevention			
Benzathine (penicillin G)	600,000 U (≤27 kg) 1.2 million U (≥27 kg) *or*	IM	Once
Penicillin V (children)	250 mg (2–3 times/d)	Oral	10 d
Penicillin V (adolescents and adults)	500 mg (2–3 times/d)	Oral	10 d
PENICILLIN-ALLERGIC PATIENTS			
Erythromycin ethyl succinate	40 mg/kg/d (2–4 times/day up to 1 g/d)	Oral	10 d
Erythromycin estolate	20–40 mg/kg/d (2–4 times/day up to 1 g/d)	Oral	10 d
Secondary prevention			
Benzathine (penicillin G)	1.2 million U	IM	q3–4 wk
or			
Penicillin V	250 mg	Oral	bid
or			
Sulfadiazine	0.5 g (≤27 kg) Oral 1.0 g (>27 kg)	qd	
PENICILLIN- AND SULFADIAZINE-ALLERGIC PATIENTS			
Erythromycin	250 mg	Oral	bid

bid, twice a day; IM, intramuscular; qd, every day.
Adapted from Dajani AS. Rheumatic fever. In: Braunwald E, ed. *Heart disease: a textbook of cardiovascular medicine,* 5th ed. Philadelphia: WB Saunders, 1997:1769–1775.

2. Penicillin is the agent of choice primarily for its narrow spectrum of activity, long-standing proven efficacy, and low cost.

a. Best results are achieved with a **single intramuscular dose of penicillin G benzathine.** An intramuscular regimen is preferred in patients unlikely to complete a 10-day course of oral therapy or for patients with personal or family history of RF or rheumatic heart disease. This preparation is painful; **preparations that contain procaine penicillin are less painful.**

b. In comparison with the intramuscular regimen, the oral regimen has several disadvantages, such as lower compliance due to its longer duration, more complicated dosing schedules, drug interactions, and, more importantly, socioeconomic factors. The oral antibiotic of choice is penicillin V (phenoxymethylpenicillin) (see Table 18.2 for dosage information). A broader-spectrum penicillin, such as amoxicillin, offers no microbiologic advantage over penicillin.

3. Patients allergic to penicillin:

a. Oral erythromycin can be used. The recommended dosage is erythromycin estolate or erythromycin ethyl succinate for 10 days. The maximum dose of erythromycin is 1 g/day.

b. Although uncommon in the United States, **strains resistant to erythromycin** have been found in some areas of the world and have caused treatment failures. The newer **macrolides, such as azithromycin,** have the advantage of a short treatment duration (5 days) and few gastrointestinal side effects. These can be used as second-line therapy for patients 16 years or older with GAS pharyngitis. The recommended dosage is 500 mg as a single dose on the first day followed by 250 mg once daily for 4 days.

c. Another alternative regimen for penicillin-allergic patients is a **10-day course with an oral cephalosporin.** A first-generation cephalosporin with a narrower spectrum of action (cefadroxil or cephalexin) is preferable to the broader-spectrum antibiotics such as cefaclor, cefuroxime, cefixime, and cefpodoxime. Several reports support the evidence that a 10-day course with oral cephalosporin is superior to 10 days of oral penicillin and a 5-day course with selected oral cephalosporins is comparable to a 10-day course of oral penicillin for eradication of GAS.

d. Sulfa-derived antibiotics **(sulfonamides, trimethoprim) do not eradicate GAS** in patients with pharyngitis, and **tetracycline should be avoided** because of the high prevalence of resistant strains.

B. Secondary prevention. Prophylaxis for preventing recurrences should **start as soon as RF or rheumatic heart disease is diagnosed,** as recurrences can sometimes be asymptomatic.

1. Penicillin in doses of 600,000 IU (patient's weight less than 27 kg) to 1.2 million IU (patient's weight more than 27 kg) every 4 weeks is the recommended regimen in most circumstances. The interval is reduced to 3 weeks for individuals at high risk for developing acute RF or living in endemic areas.
2. The duration of prophylaxis depends on the individual situation. Table 18.3 provides additional information.
   a. Prophylaxis for **recurrent RF in patients without cardiac manifestations** should be continued for 5 years after the last RF attack or up to age 21 years, whichever is longer.
   b. For **patients with RF and carditis but no residual valvular disease,** prophylaxis should extend for a period of 10 years or well into adulthood.
   c. Indefinite antibiotic prophylaxis is recommended in **patients with valvular heart disease.**
3. The success of **oral prophylaxis** depends on the patient's understanding and adherence to the prescribed regimen. Oral agents are **more appropriate for patients at lower risk for rheumatic recurrences.** Some favor switching patients to oral prophylaxis when they have reached late adolescence or young adulthood and have remained free of rheumatic attacks for at least 5 years.
   a. The preferred oral medication is penicillin V.
   b. For **patients with true or suspected allergy to penicillin, sulfadiazine** can be used (Table 18.2). **Erythromycin** is an alternative.
   c. It is important to keep in mind that even with optimal patient adherence, the **risk of recurrence is higher with an oral than with an intramuscular prophylactic regimen.**

C. Endocarditis prophylaxis. Updated guidelines from the American Heart Association (AHA) published in 2007 recommend against routine prophylaxis for endocarditis in patients with rheumatic valvular disease undergoing dental or other procedures. Antibiotic prophylaxis is recommended only for patients with prosthetic

TABLE 18.3 Duration of Therapy for Secondary Prevention of Rheumatic Fever

Disease state	Duration of therapy
RF + carditis + residual valvular disease	At least 10 y postepisode and at least until age 40. Lifelong prophylaxis may be required.
RF + carditis without valvular disease	10 y or beyond adulthood, whichever is longer.
RF without carditis	5 y or until age 21, whichever is longer.

RF, rheumatic fever.
Adapted from Dajani AS. Rheumatic fever. In: Braunwald E, ed. *Heart disease: a textbook of cardiovascular medicine,* 5th ed. Philadelphia: WB Saunders, 1997:1769–1775.

valves, previous endocarditis, certain forms of congenital heart disease and for heart transplant patients with vasculopathy (see Chapter 17).

D. Vaccines targeted against GAS. Several multivalent vaccines against GAS are currently in clinical trials. The M protein is the most promising target, but vaccine development has been complicated because there are multiple M-protein subtypes that are rheumatogenic. Use of a vaccine may prevent pharyngeal colonization, thereby removing population reservoirs, which allow for endemic disease.

ACKNOWLEDGMENTS

The author thanks Drs. Simone Nader and Mohammed Nasir Khan for their contributions to earlier editions of this chapter.

Landmark Articles

Bisno AL. Group A streptococcal infections and acute rheumatic fever. *N Engl J Med* 1991;325:783–793.

Dajani AS, Ayoub E, Bierman FZ, et al. Guidelines for the diagnosis of rheumatic fever: Jones criteria. Updated 1993. *Circulation* 1993;87:302–307.

Ferrieri P. Proceedings of the Jones Criteria Workshop. *Circulation* 2002;106:2521–2523.

Key Reviews

American Heart Association. Treatment of acute streptococcal pharyngitis and prevention of rheumatic fever. *Pediatrics* 1995;96:758–764.

Cilliers AM. Rheumatic fever and its management. *BMJ* 2006;333:1153–1156.

da Silva NA, de Faria Pereira BA. Acute rheumatic fever. *Pediatr Rheumatol* 1997;23:545–568.

Stollerman GH. Rheumatic fever. *Lancet* 1997;349:935–942.

Stollerman GH. Rheumatic fever in the 21st century. *Clin Infect Dis* 2001;33:806–814.

Relevant Book Chapter

Dajani AS. Rheumatic fever. In: Braunwald E, ed. *Heart disease: a textbook of cardiovascular medicine*, 7th ed. Philadelphia: WB Saunders, 2005:2093–2100.

19 CARDIAC TUMORS

Adam W. Grasso and Nitin Barman

I. INTRODUCTION. Cardiac neoplasms are **rare** in comparison with other forms of heart disease. Although secondary tumors of the heart are by definition malignant, primary tumors may be either benign or malignant. **Primary cardiac tumors occur 30 times less frequently than cardiac metastases.** In most autopsy studies, the reported prevalence of primary tumors of the heart ranges from 0.001% to 0.2%; about 75% are benign. Despite the relatively low prevalence, the advent of curative operative therapy has made antemortem diagnosis of these tumors more clinically relevant.

II. CLINICAL PRESENTATION. Cardiac tumors often present with very nonspecific signs and symptoms. Patient complaints may be attributable to constitutional manifestations, embolic phenomena, or direct cardiac invasion/mass effect.

A. Constitutional symptoms. Many tumors, especially myxomas, are associated with a wide variety of systemic manifestations. Fever, malaise, cachexia, and weight loss are not uncommon. Corresponding laboratory abnormalities, including thrombocytosis, hypergammaglobulinemia, and elevated erythrocyte sedimentation rate (ESR) and C-reactive protein (CRP) level, are frequently present as well. These findings are likely attributable to the constitutive production of **inflammatory cytokines** by the tumor. Myxoma cell production of **interleukin-6** and elevation of **antimyocardial antibodies** have been documented, with levels of these serum markers normalizing with tumor resection. Not surprisingly, patients with cardiac tumors often carry an incorrect antecedent diagnosis of collagen vascular disease, chronic infection, or noncardiac malignancy.

B. Embolic phenomena. Tumor embolization may account for the initial presenting symptom. The type of emboli is dependent on tumor **location** as well as the presence of intracardiac shunts. **Right-sided** tumors, and left-sided tumors with left-to-right shunts, result in pulmonary emboli, and if untreated may result in cor pulmonale. It may be difficult to clinically differentiate pulmonary tumor emboli from those due to venous thromboembolic disease. Chest radiography is usually not helpful. However, perfusion scanning often has two unique characteristics that help differentiate tumor emboli from venous thromboemboli. First, tumor emboli may result in completely unilateral defects. Second, defects caused by tumor emboli generally do not resolve with time. **Left-sided** tumor emboli may result in visceral infarction, limb ischemia, myocardial infarction, or transient ischemic attack/stroke. In addition, multiple vascular aneurysms may develop. Embolic findings in a young person, in sinus rhythm and without valvular disease or endocarditis, should raise suspicion for the presence of an intracardiac tumor.

C. Direct cardiac invasion/mass effect. Signs and symptoms are governed by tumor location. Intramyocardial tumors, which are most often found in the left ventricular free wall and intraventricular septum, can result in arrhythmias, conduction abnormalities, and sudden cardiac death. Impaired ventricular performance may mimic restrictive or hypertrophic cardiomyopathy. Rarely, ventricular rupture has been the initial presentation. Tumors of the left atrium, especially if mobile, may prolapse into the mitral valve, resulting in obstruction of atrioventricular (AV) blood flow. This results in signs and symptoms similar to mitral stenosis, such as dyspnea, orthopnea, paroxysmal nocturnal dyspnea (PND), edema, and fatigue. Importantly, **syncope and sudden death** may also occur.

III. PHYSICAL EXAMINATION. Physical examination may show signs of pulmonary venous congestion. A fourth heart sound (**S_4**) may be present, as may a widely split, **loud first heart sound** (S_1). The loud S_1 is caused by late closure of the mitral valve, when the left ventricular–left atrial pressure crossover occurs at a higher pressure. Although this finding is also seen with mitral stenosis and preexcitation, the absence of a diastolic rumble or a short PR on an electrocardiogram should raise the possibility of left atrial tumor. If the tumor obstructs the AV valve, a **presystolic crescendo murmur** may be present, which typically begins during ventricular systole as the tumor moves through the mitral orifice. This finding is present in approximately one-half of all patients with myxoma. The pathognomonic **tumor plop** manifests as an early diastolic sound, after an opening snap but before a third heart sound (S_3). Tumors of the **right atrium** often result in systemic venous congestion. Once significant pulmonary hypertension occurs, **systemic hypoxia, clubbing, and polycythemia** may develop as a result of right-to-left shunting. Right atrial tumors and intracavitary **right ventricular** tumors may present as right heart failure. A diastolic rumble that varies with inspiration may be noted and is due to tricuspid valve obstruction. The **P_2** is delayed and may have varying intensity. Jugular venous pressure waveform examination may demonstrate **prominent *a* waves** and **Kussmaul's sign**. Recurrent pulmonary emboli can potentiate pulmonary hypertension. **Left ventricular** tumors, when not intramural, typically result in signs and symptoms of pulmonary venous congestion or low-output states. Upon examination, findings may mimic aortic stenosis, subvalvular stenosis, or hypertrophic cardiomyopathy.

IV. DIAGNOSIS. Because no clinical sign or symptom is specific, more advanced diagnostic methodology is universally required.

A. Electrocardiography (ECG). In isolation, ECG provides little added clue to the diagnosis. However, changes in rhythm or voltage on serial tracings may be the first sign of either extension of a primary cardiac tumor or development of secondary cardiac involvement.

B. Radiography. Chest radiography may be helpful in identifying epicardial tumors. Cardiomegaly, mediastinal widening, or cardiac silhouette irregularities may suggest the diagnosis. Calcifications are seen occasionally. Pulmonary congestion or oligemia may be noted in patients with large left or right intracavitary tumors, respectively.

C. Echocardiography. M-mode and two-dimensional echocardiography help establish the diagnosis in most patients. If a tumor is strongly suspected or a mass is noted by transthoracic echocardiography (TTE), transesophageal echocardiography (TEE) should be performed. It provides improved sensitivity and specificity, particularly with atrial masses, and allows for superior visualization of anatomic details such as contour, cysts, calcification, and presence of a stalk.

D. Radionuclide imaging. Although gated blood-pool scanning has been used to identify cardiac tumors in the past, the inferior resolution and sensitivity has made this form of imaging uncommon in the workup.

E. Computerized tomography (CT). CT, especially multislice CT, is often used in the diagnosis and evaluation of cardiac masses. It can define tumor extension, although not as effectively as magnetic resonance imaging (MRI), and evaluates the adjacent extracardiac structures.

F. Magnetic resonance imaging (MRI). Like CT, MRI has an important role in the evaluation of cardiac tumors. Specifically, it characterizes size, shape, and surface features, as well as evaluates tissue composition. MRI has the highest soft tissue contrast of the imaging modalities, and it is particularly helpful in distinguishing thrombus from tumor. It is also the most sensitive imaging modality for the detection of tumor infiltration.

G. Angiography. Cardiac catheterization is **not necessary in most cases.** However, in the following scenarios, the risk and cost of angiography may be worthwhile: clarifying inadequate noninvasive imaging, defining blood supply for suspected malignant tumors, and evaluating coexistent valvular or coronary artery disease that could alter surgical approach. The major additional risk of angiography is embolization of tumor or thrombus. A transseptal approach is relatively contraindicated in cases of suspected left atrial myxoma given the high frequency of involvement of the fossa ovalis and the accompanying risk of embolization.

V. PRIMARY CARDIAC MALIGNANCIES

A. Benign neoplasms. A description of specific benign cardiac tumors is given in subsequent text. Relative proportions are given in Table 19.1.

1. **Myxomas.** Most benign cardiac tumors are myxomas, accounting for approximately 30% to 50% in most series. For **sporadic myxomas**, which account for nearly 90% of all myxomas, about 70% of patients are female, with a mean age of 56 years. Eighty-six percent of sporadic myxomas are found in the left atrium; 90% are solitary masses. When multiple tumors are present, they are not necessarily limited to one chamber. The typical site of attachment within the left atrium is on or near the **fossa ovalis**. Important to note is that tumors located on the posterior wall of the left atrium are usually not benign. Less frequently, myxomas may be found in the right atrium, either ventricle, or

TABLE 19.1 Relative Proportion of Benign and Malignant Tumors in Adults by Tumor Type

Benign tumor	% of group	Malignant tumor	% of group
Myxoma	46	Angiosarcoma	33
Lipoma	21	Rhabdomyosarcoma	21
Papillary fibroelastoma	16	Mesothelioma	16
Rhabdomyoma	2	Fibrosarcoma	11
Fibroma	3	Lymphosarcoma	6
Hemangioma	5	Osteosarcoma	4
Teratoma	1	Thymoma	3
AVN mesothelioma	3	Neurogenic sarcoma	3
Granular cell tumor	1	Leiomyosarcoma	1
Neurofibroma	1	Liposarcoma	1
Lymphangioma	1	Synovial sarcoma	1

AVN, atrioventricular nodal.

arising from the AV valves. **Familial myxomas**, although pathologically identical to sporadic myxomas, have a number of unique clinical features. They have a well-characterized **autosomal dominant** transmission, and they are often present within the construct of a larger syndrome. The **Carney complex**, or "syndrome myxoma," consists of both cardiac and noncardiac myxomas, spotty pigmentation (i.e., pigmented nevi), and endocrine overactivity (pituitary, adrenocortical, endocrine testicular tumors). Patients with the Carney complex typically present in the third decade, often have bilateral tumors, and have high recurrence rates following resection. If a myxoma syndrome is suspected, **screening echocardiography is recommended** for all first-degree relatives, particularly if the index patient is young, has multiple tumors, or has typical noncardiac features of the genetic syndrome.

Pathologically, cardiac myxomas are either smooth, round or gelatinous, or friable and irregular in appearance. They sometimes contain a hemorrhagic core, and may attach via a sessile or pedunculated base. The typical diameter at presentation is 4 to 8 cm. **Histologically**, myxomas have characteristic patterns of "lipidic" cells within glycosaminoglycan-rich myxoid stroma. **Ultrastructurally**, myxoma cells resemble embryonic mesenchymal cells. **Immunohistochemically**, they demonstrate variable activity for endothelial cell markers, with reliable positivity to vimentin, indicating a mesenchymal derivation.

2. **Lipomas.** These benign tumors occur at **all ages,** with men and women affected equally. Tumors range in size depending on their location. Seventy-five percent of tumors are found in the subendocardium or subepicardium, whereas the remainder are intramuscular. Many tumors are **clinically silent** and identified only at autopsy. Subendocardial tumors result in symptoms related to cavity obstruction, whereas subpericardial tumors can lead to compression of the heart and/or development of pericardial effusion. Intramyocardial tumors may result in arrhythmias or conduction disturbances. Lesions are generally **well encapsulated**. Without pathologic confirmation, lipomas can be confused with lipomatous hypertrophy of the interatrial septum.
3. **Papillary fibroelastomas.** The diagnosis of papillary fibroelastoma has increased with the more frequent use of TEE. Grossly, these benign tumors resemble sea anemones, with frond-like arms protruding off a central stalk. They are usually about 1 cm in length, single, and mobile in 40% of cases. The majority are located on the **ventricular surface of the aortic valve**, whereas the atrial side of the mitral valve is the second most common location. Rarely, they may present on the endocardial surfaces. Although these tumors are not associated with valvular dysfunction, in approximately 30% of cases thrombus, with subsequent emboli, develops. Surgical resection is generally recommended for patients with a symptomatic presentation with embolization or in an asymptomatic patient with large, mobile tumors (1 cm or greater in diameter). Anticoagulation may be considered if recurrent embolization occurs in a nonsurgical candidate. Fibroelastoma may be differentiated from Lambl's excrescences by their location on noncontact areas of the valve.
4. **Rhabdomyomas.** The most common benign tumor in **children** and **infants**, rhabdomyomas are frequently located within one of the ventricles. These tumors are nearly always **multiple**, and the majority of patients have at least one intracavitary, obstructing lesion. There is a clear association with **tuberous sclerosis**; 80% of rhabdomyoma patients have the disease, and 60% of tuberous sclerosis patients have rhabdomyomas.
5. **Fibromas.** Generally found in **pediatric** populations as well, these benign connective tissue tumors are almost universally **intramural.** They are usually firm, circumscribed but unencapsulated, and may grow to **several centimeters**. The **Gorlin's syndrome** includes cardiac fibromas, multiple basal cell carcinomas, jaw cysts, and skeletal abnormalities.
6. **Hemangiomas.** These tumors are **very rare** and consist of benign collections of endothelial cells. Usually they are located within the intraventricular septum or AV node, and as such may present as heart block, sudden cardiac death, or hemopericardium.

B. Malignant neoplasms. Histologically, **primary malignant tumors are virtually always sarcomas**. Suggestive **characteristics** include rapid growth, mediastinal invasion, hemorrhagic pericardial effusion, precordial pain, and pulmonary vein extension.

1. **Angiosarcomas.** Almost always found within the right atrium, angiosarcomas, which include Kaposi's sarcoma, have a **2:1 male-to-female predilection** and are almost exclusively seen in adults. Hemorrhagic pericardial effusions are not uncommon. These tumors have ill-defined vascular channels lined with atypical endothelial cells. The blood flow through the tumor may produce a continuous precordial murmur. Clinical deterioration is rapid.
2. **Rhabdomyosarcoma.** Like angiosarcomas, these tumors of striated muscle are **more common in men**. However, there is no specific chamber that is preferentially affected. Tumors are generally infiltrative, but on occasion they may develop polypoid extensions, which can cause them to be mistaken for myxomas. Prognosis is poor.
3. **Mesothelioma.** The typical location of primary cardiac mesothelioma is the **pericardium.** Generally very diffuse, these tumors lead to symptoms consistent with pericarditis or hemorrhagic effusion. They may occasionally infiltrate the **AV node**, leading to conduction disturbances, sudden cardiac death, or tamponade. Much like cardiac sarcomas, these tumors carry a very poor prognosis.
4. **Other.** Fibrosarcomas, lymphosarcomas, liposarcomas, and other undifferentiated sarcomas represent the remainder of primary cardiac malignancies. These tumors are very rare and are generally infiltrative, involving multiple cardiac chambers. A clinical syndrome mimicking hypertrophic cardiomyopathy has been observed.

VI. SECONDARY CARDIAC MALIGNANCIES.

As mentioned previously, most malignancies of the heart are secondary, and by definition, **metastatic**. The overwhelming majority of metastatic cardiac tumors occurs in the **pericardium** and are usually **carcinomas**, as opposed to sarcomas. Due to increased prevalence, **the most commonly found metastatic tumor to the heart is lung cancer**. The typical presentation is of pericardial effusion or tamponade, or pulmonary vein obstruction from direct extension. After metastatic lung cancer—breast cancer, lymphoma, and leukemia are the most common offenders. The tumor with **the greatest propensity to metastasize to the heart is melanoma,** followed by germ cell tumors and leukemia (Table 19.2). A new complaint referable to the heart in a patient with known extracardiac malignancy should prompt a thorough investigation to rule out cardiac malignancy. Unfortunately, prompt diagnosis usually does not favorably alter the prognosis.

VII. DIFFERENTIAL DIAGNOSIS.

Establishing the correct diagnosis is imperative. A thorough differential diagnosis of **nonmalignant conditions** must be considered and ruled out. Possibilities include pericardial cysts, teratomas, lipomatous hypertrophy of the

TABLE 19.2 Metastatic Tumors to the Heart by Absolute Number and Greatest Propensity

Primary tumor	By absolute no.	Primary tumor	No. per 100 tumors
Lung	180	Melanoma	46
Breast	70	Germ Cell	38
Lymphoma	67	Leukemia	33
Leukemia	66	Lymphoma	17
Esophagus	37	Lung	17
Uterus	36	Sarcoma	15
Melanoma	32	Esophagus	13
Gastric	28	Kidney	11
Sarcoma	24	Breast	10
Oral	22	Oral	9
Colon	22	Thyroid	9

interatrial septum, thrombus, and sarcoid. Unfortunately, the final diagnosis in many cases must still be made pathologically.

VIII. THERAPY AND PROGNOSIS. The primary therapy for benign tumors remains **operative resection**, given the associated risk of lethal obstruction, arrhythmia, or embolization. Most surgeons perform excision with extracorporeal circulatory support in order to directly visualize the tumor, as well as a careful search for metasynchronous tumors. In higher-risk patients, more extensive resection, including surrounding laser photocoagulation, is recommended. The femoral or azygous vein is usually cannulated, as opposed to the right atrium, to avoid potential tumor fragment embolization. Mitral valve repair or replacement is usually unnecessary in the absence of associated bacterial endocarditis. A recent analysis reviewing 106 operations for sporadic atrial myxomas noted only one perioperative death. Survival at 25 years is no different when compared to age- and sex-matched controls. There are limited data regarding the use of a minimally invasive approach to cardiac tumor resection. Small series suggest that parasternal or partial sternotomy access does not compromise safety or efficacy while allowing for shortened hospitalization and better cosmetic results. Long-term follow-up is not yet available for this approach.

Regardless of the type of surgical resection or whether the tumor is sporadic, annual **follow-up noninvasive imaging is recommended** in all patients after resection. Recurrence rates of 12% to 22% have been quoted in patients with family histories, syndromes, and multiple tumors at original presentation versus 1% for patients with sporadic, isolated myxomas. Primary malignant tumors generally portend dismal prognoses. They are rarely cured by surgery because of the large amount of cardiac tissue involved. Adjuvant therapy (i.e., chemotherapy, radiation) after resection does not affect the prognosis, although it may slow progression in individual cases. **Palliative resection** is advocated for obstructive symptoms. **Cardiac transplantation** has been performed for patients with both benign and malignant tumors, but thus far, series have been too small to reliably predict outcomes.

Landmark Articles

Burke A, Virmani R. Tumors of the heart and great vessels. In: *Atlas of tumor pathology*. Third Series. Fascicle 16. Washington, DC: Armed Forces Institute of Pathology, 1996:231.

Harvey WP. Clinical aspects of cardiac tumors. *Am J Cardiol* 1968;21:328.

Lam KY, Dickens P, Chan ACL. Tumors of the heart. A 20-year experience with review of 12485 consecutive autopsies. *Arch Pathol Med* 1993;117:1027–1031.

McAllister HA, Fenoglio JJ. Tumors of the cardiovascular system. In: *Atlas of tumor pathology*. Second Series. Fascicle 15. Washington, DC: Armed Forces Institute of Pathology, 1978.

Key Reviews

Abraham DP, Reddy V, Gattusa P. Neoplasms metastatic to the heart: review of 3314 consecutive autopsies. *Am J Cardiovasc Pathol* 1990;3:195–198.

ACC/AHA guidelines for the clinical application of echocardiography: cardiac masses and tumors. In collaboration with the ASE. March 1997.

Bear PA, Moodie DS. Malignant primary cardiac tumors. The Cleveland Clinic Experience, 1956–1986. *Chest* 1987;92:860–862.

Burke A, Jeudy J, Virmani R. Cardiac tumours: an update. *Heart* 2008;94:117–123.

Carney JA. Carney complex: the complex of myxomas, spotty pigmentation, endocrine overactivity and schwannomas. *Semin Dermatol* 1995;14:90.

Centofanti P, Di Rosa E, Deorsola L. Primary cardiac tumors: early and late results of surgical treatment in 91 patients. *Ann Thorac Surg* 1999;68:1236.

Ferrans VJ, Roberts WC. Structural features of cardiac myxomas. Histology, histochemistry, and electron microscopy. *Hum Pathol* 1973;4:111–146.

Monocada R, Baker M, Salinas M. Diagnostic role of CT in pericardial heart disease: congenital defects, thickening, neoplasms, and effusions. *Am Heart J* 1982;103:263–282.

Murphy MC, Sweeney MS, Putnam JB Jr. Surgical treatment of cardiac tumors: a 25-year experience. *Ann Thorac Surg* 1990;49:612–618.

Sun JP, Asher C, Yang XS. Clinical and echocardiographic characteristics of papillary fibroelastomas: a retrospective and prospective study in 162 patients. *Circulation* 2001;103:2687.

Williams DB, Danielson GK, McGoon DC. Cardiac fibroma: long-term survival after excision. *J Thorac Cardiovasc Surg* 1982;84:230–236.

Relevant Book Chapters

Colucci WS, Schoen FJ, Braunwald E. Primary tumors of the heart. In: Braunwald E, ed. *Heart disease: a textbook of cardiovascular medicine*, 5th ed. Philadelphia: WB Saunders, 1997:1464–1477.

Roberts WC. Cardiac Neoplasms. In: Topol EJ, ed. *Comprehensive cardiovascular medicine*. Philadelphia: Lippincott–Raven Publishers, 1998:917–933.

IV Arrythmias

20 TACHYARRHYTHMIAS

Ross A. Downey

I. INTRODUCTION. The mechanisms of tachyarrhythmias have been classically divided into those of disordered impulse formation, those of disordered conduction, and combinations of both.

A. Disorders of impulse formation. Disorders of impulse formation include deranged automaticity as well as triggered activity.

1. Automaticity refers to the ability of a fiber of cardiac tissue to generate pacemaker activity spontaneously. There are both normal and abnormal sources of automaticity.

a. An example of **normal** accelerated automaticity would be rapid firing rates of a normal pacemaker locus, such as the atrioventricular (AV) node or Purkinje system, due to ischemia, metabolic disturbance, or pharmacologic manipulation. A clinical example would be accelerated **sinus tachycardia** or **junctional rhythm.**

b. Abnormal automaticity refers to tissues that under normal circumstances do not demonstrate automaticity, but can become automatic in the setting of ischemia, metabolic disturbance, or pharmacologic manipulation. These latent or ectopic loci of cells generate automatic, spontaneous impulses that usurp control of the cardiac rhythm. A clinical example would be **accelerated idioventricular rhythm** (see **III.A.6**).

2. Triggered activity refers to pacemaker activity that is dependent on afterdepolarizations from a prior impulse or series of impulses. Afterdepolarizations are oscillations in the membrane potential. If these reach the threshold level for the surrounding cardiac tissue, they may trigger an action potential, thereby precipitating further afterdepolarizations and perpetuating the pacemaker activity.

a. Early afterdepolarizations (EADs) occur before repolarization of the cardiac tissue and may be the mechanism responsible for the ventricular arrhythmias of the **long QT syndromes,** as well as **torsade de pointes** ("twisting of the points") produced by class I and class III antiarrhythmics, sympathetic discharge, and hypoxia. Antibiotics such as macrolides, certain azole antifungal agents, some psychotropic medications such as haloperidol, and several nonsedating antihistamines have been shown to produce EADs. Rapid heart rates and the administration of magnesium have been shown to suppress EADs.

b. Delayed after depolarizations (DADs) occur after the repolarization of the surrounding tissue is complete, and are thought to be the mechanism of triggered atrial tachycardia and the arrhythmias of **digitalis toxicity.** These have been demonstrated in various cardiac tissues, including parts of the conducting system, myocardial cells, and valve tissues. Increases in intracellular calcium are associated with DADs, such as those caused by digitalis preparations or excessive sympathetic stimulation. Drugs that block the influx of calcium (such as calcium channel blockers and β-blockers) and drugs that decrease the sodium current (such as lidocaine and phenytoin) suppress the occurrence of DADs, whereas rapid heart rates augment DADs.

B. Disorders of impulse conduction. Disorders of impulse conduction include **reentry, which is the major cause of ventricular tachycardia** (VT) in the Western world. **Scar or ischemia** can produce regions anywhere in the heart that **conduct impulses inhomogeneously.** Therefore, the impulse can spread to an area that has already repolarized after being previously depolarized. This can set up a circular movement of the impulse resulting in sustained tachyarrhythmias such as VT. In order for reentry to occur, **three conditions** must be met:

1. Two functionally distinct conducting pathways
2. Unidirectional conduction block in one of the pathways
3. Slow conduction down the unblocked pathway, which allows the blocked pathway time to recover excitability and sustain the arrhythmia.

Elucidation of the mechanisms resulting in tachyarrhythmias has led to the development of catheter-based treatment strategies and more advanced medical therapy.

II. SUPRAVENTRICULAR TACHYARRHYTHMIAS

A. Sinus tachycardia

1. Clinical presentation. Sinus tachycardia manifests as sinus rhythm with a rate above 100 beats/min. Although the rate may be as high as 200 beats/min in younger individuals, it is generally **150 beats/min or less in older individuals.**

2. Pathophysiology

a. The sinus node is located along the lateral edge of the right atrium. Under normal circumstances the rate of sinus node discharge is governed by sympathetic and vagal stimulation.

b. Sinus tachycardia generally reflects **an underlying process, metabolic state, or medication effect,** such as fever, hypovolemia, shock, congestive heart failure (CHF), anxiety, pulmonary disease including pulmonary embolism, anemia, thyrotoxicosis, caffeine, nicotine, atropine, catecholamines, or withdrawal from alcohol or drugs (both therapeutic and illicit).

c. Sinus tachycardia can be appropriate, where it represents a physiologic response to maintain cardiac output, **or inappropriate,** as in defects in vagal or sympathetic tone or an intrinsic problem with the sinus node itself.

d. The **clinical consequences of sinus tachycardia vary** based on the presence or absence of underlying heart disease. Patients with significant coronary artery disease (CAD), left ventricular dysfunction, or valve disease may not tolerate sinus tachycardia. Patients with inappropriate sinus tachycardia may experience significant symptoms such as palpitations, dyspnea, and/or chest pain.

3. Diagnostic testing. Electrocardiography is the primary diagnostic test. The main differential is between sinus tachycardia, sinus node reentry tachycardia (see **II.B**), and inappropriate sinus tachycardia. Inappropriate sinus tachycardia is characterized by the following features: **(a) heart rate greater than 100 beats/min, (b) P-wave axis and morphology during tachycardia similar or identical to that during sinus rhythm, (c) exclusion of secondary causes of sinus tachycardia, (d) exclusion of atrial tachycardias, and (e) symptoms clearly documented to be related to resting or easily provoked sinus tachycardia.**

4. Therapy is directed generally at the elimination of the underlying cause whenever possible.

a. If withdrawal from a therapeutic medication is suspected, reinstitution or slow tapering of this medication can be attempted, if clinically appropriate.

b. In the case of **inappropriate sinus tachycardia, β-blockers and calcium channel blockers** may be necessary to control the heart rate.

c. In **medically refractory cases, catheter ablation for sinoatrial nodal modification** may have to be considered.

B. Sinus node reentry tachycardia (SNRT) accounts for 5% to 10% of all supraventricular tachyarrhythmias.

1. Clinical presentation. SNRT is most frequently seen in patients with structural heart disease or CAD, especially in inferior myocardial infarctions (MIs).

The rate varies from 80 to 200 beats/min. SNRT's abrupt onset and termination (paroxysmal nature) along with its ability to be induced and terminated by pacing distinguish it from sinus tachycardia and inappropriate sinus tachycardia.

2. **Pathophysiology.** Reentry occurs within or adjacent to the sinus node and then conducts via the normal conduction pathway to the rest of the heart. The morphology of the P wave is identical to the underlying sinus morphology. Block at the AV node may occur, but it does not slow the tachycardia. In fact, a Wenckebach-type block often occurs with this rhythm. The development of a bundle-branch block does not affect the cycle length or the PR interval.
3. **Therapy.** Vagal maneuvers or adenosine may successfully terminate this arrhythmia. **Rapid atrial pacing** can be used to induce and terminate this tachycardia. Various agents such as β-blockers, calcium channel blockers, and digoxin may help to prevent recurrences. Sinus node ablation or modification is rarely necessary.

C. Atrial fibrillation (AF) is the most common sustained arrhythmia, occurring in approximately 0.4% to 1.0% of the general population. The prevalence of AF increases with age, affecting up to 10% of the population older than age 80 (see Chapter 23).

D. Atrial flutter. Atrial flutter is the **second most common of the atrial tachyarrhythmias.** Its reported incidence varies from 0.4% to 1.2% in hospital reports of electrocardiogram (ECG) results. The **clinical significance of atrial flutter is generally due to its association with AF** (with all of the attendant risks of AF) and/or its association with rapid rates of ventricular response.

1. **Clinical presentation.** The clinical presentation may vary widely depending on the presence of underlying heart disease, the rate of ventricular response, and the overall condition of the patient. It is **occasionally reported to persist for days** and, less commonly, for weeks or longer. Careful examination of the jugular venous pulse may reveal **frequent, regular *a* waves** that correspond to the atrial flutter rate. Like AF, it is **commonly seen after open heart surgery, as well as with other conditions commonly associated with AF,** such as pulmonary disease, thyrotoxicosis, atrial enlargement due to any cause including mitral/tricuspid valve disease, and sinus node dysfunction.
2. **Pathophysiology.** "Typical" atrial flutter is the **result of a macroreentrant circuit in the right atrium.** Atypical atrial flutter generally involves other macroreentrant circuits around scar tissue or surgical incisions.
   a. **In typical flutter the reentrant circuit most commonly travels in a counter-clockwise rotation** down the right atrial anterolateral free wall across the cavotricuspid isthmus, and up the interatrial septum. Clockwise rotation of this circuit may also be seen.
   b. Atrial flutter has been classified into type I and type II based on the following characteristics:
      (1) Type I atrial flutter can be terminated with rapid atrial pacing and typically has an atrial rate in the range of 240 to 340 beats/min in the absence of drug therapy.
      (2) Type II atrial flutter cannot be terminated with rapid atrial pacing and typically has an atrial rate in the range of 340 to 440 beats/min in the absence of drug therapy.
      (3) Types I and II are not synonymous with typical and atypical. Type I atrial flutter can include typical and atypical atrial flutter. Type II atrial flutter is less well characterized than type I with respect to etiology and therapy; therefore, **we refer to type I atrial flutter throughout this discussion.**
3. **Laboratory examination**
   a. The **diagnosis can be difficult when the AV blockade is 2:1,** as the flutter waves may be superimposed on the QRS complex and/or the T waves. When the diagnosis is uncertain, one should **consider maneuvers or medications to slow the ventricular response,** thus revealing the atrial flutter complexes.
      (1) Vagal maneuvers include carotid sinus massage and Valsalva maneuver. **Caution must be exercised** in attempting carotid sinus massage **in patients with known or suspected carotid disease,** or vagal maneuvers in **patients with CAD who are at risk for ischemia.**

(2) Adenosine can be administered, 6 mg rapid IV push, followed by 12 mg if there is no response (a second 12-mg dose can be given if there is no response). The half-life of this medication is very short, approximately 9 seconds. This causes transient (lasting seconds), complete AV block. Alternative agents include the calcium channel–blocking agents **verapamil and diltiazem,** and the β-blockers **esmolol and metoprolol.**

(3) The clinician can place and record from a **transesophageal electrode** or record from a **temporary atrial epicardial pacing wire** (placed at open heart surgery). This results in an ECG with clearer atrial complexes, and simplifies diagnosis. This strategy also allows a method of delivering rapid atrial pacing in an attempt to terminate the atrial flutter.

b. On the surface ECG, typical counterclockwise atrial flutter shows the **classic negatively directed "sawtooth" waveform** in the inferior leads, II, III and aVF (Fig. 20.1). Conversely, the atrial depolarizations are positive in these leads in clockwise flutter (Fig. 20.2).

c. The **atrial rate** in the absence of drug therapy is **240 to 340 beats/min.**

d. The **QRS complex should be the same as that seen during sinus rhythm,** although aberrant conduction may occur, and the QRS may be slightly distorted by the atrial flutter waves.

e. The **ventricular response** can be irregularly irregular, due to varying degrees of block (2:1, 4:1, and so on), but is more **typically regular as a fixed ratio of the flutter rate.**

4. Therapy

a. Medical therapy differs very little from that for AF (see Chapter 23).

(1) Control of the ventricular response rate with a β-blocker, a calcium channel blocker, or digoxin, is critical prior to initiating therapy with agents such as the class IA or IC agents. These agents either enhance AV nodal conduction through their vagolytic effects, thereby enabling 1:1 (AV) conduction, or slow the atrial rate to a point where 1:1 conduction is facilitated.

(2) The conversion from atrial flutter to AF after cardioversion is substantially reduced by the administration of antiarrhythmic drugs prior to direct

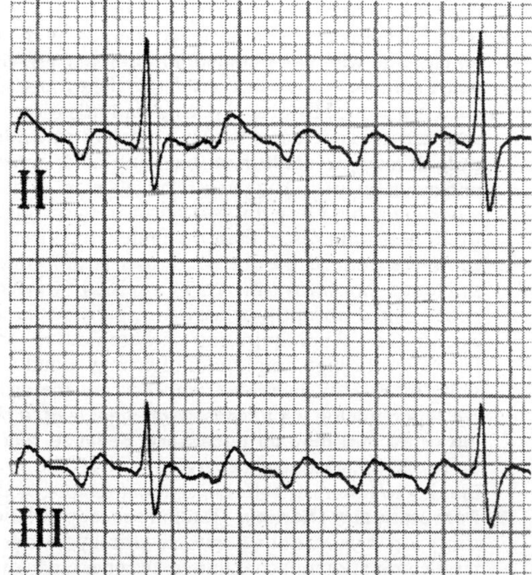

Figure 20.1. "Typical" atrial flutter, leads II and III.

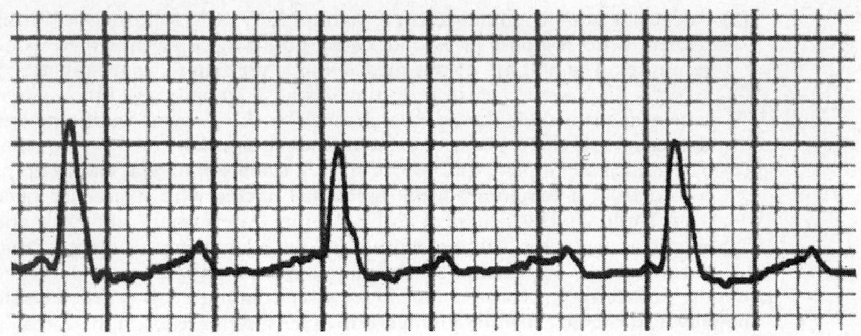

Figure 20.2. "Atypical" flutter, lead II.

current cardioversion (DCC), thereby increasing the chance of converting to sinus rhythm.

(3) Anticoagulation. There are no prospective data looking at the incidence of thromboembolic events with atrial flutter. However, retrospective data suggest an increased incidence of thromboembolic events. Recent ACCP (2004) and ACC/AHA/ESC (2006) guidelines recommend considering managing anticoagulation of atrial flutter in a manner similar to that for AF, including cardioversions. Optimal management is unclear and often needs to be individualized with the patients' profile for thromboembolic risk dictating the type and duration of therapy. We treat atrial flutter in a manner similar to that used for AF with regards to anticoagulation.

b. Direct current cardioversion

(1) DCC is the preferred and most effective therapy for most patients. The procedure is detailed in Chapter 55. A starting energy as low as 25 to 50 J is often effective. Because DCC may result in conversion from atrial flutter to AF, a second shock is sometimes necessary to convert AF to sinus rhythm.

(2) Rapid atrial pacing should be considered as the **first line of therapy for all patients who have epicardial atrial pacing wires in place after open heart surgery.** It may be considered via a transesophageal pacing lead or via a transvenously placed pacing lead in patients for whom DCC fails or who are not candidates for DCC. **Before attempting to rapidly pace the atria, it must be confirmed that ventricular capture is not inadvertently occurring** by first pacing at a relatively slow rate while observing for such a phenomenon. Once this is confirmed, the atrium is paced at a rate of 10 to 20 beats/min faster than the underlying atrial flutter rate. Once atrial capture is attained, the rate is increased steadily until the hallmark negative-sawtooth waveform converts to a positive waveform. The pacing is then either halted abruptly or slowed rapidly to an acceptable atrial pacing rate. In cases that require extremely rapid rates of pacing (more than 400 beats/min) or high amplitudes of pacing stimulus strength (more than 20 mA), there is an increased tendency for the atrial flutter to convert to AF. **When pacing via a transesophageal lead, a higher stimulus strength (up to 30 mA) may be necessary. Because this type of pacing can be quite painful,** a sufficient energy to convert the atrial flutter should be used initially to minimize the conversion attempts.

(3) Percutaneous therapy. Radiofrequency ablation of the cavotricuspid isthmus is often curative, with an efficacy greater than 90% for the long-term elimination of atrial flutter. Despite, the high success rate of catheter-based therapy a significant number of patients may subsequently develop AF.

E. Atrial tachycardias. This term encompasses a number of different types of tachycardia that originate in the atria. These tachycardias account for between 10% and 15% of the tachycardias seen in older patients, usually in the setting of structural or ischemic heart disease, chronic obstructive pulmonary disease, electrolyte imbalances, or drug toxicity (particularly digitalis).

1. Clinical presentation. These tachycardias are **infrequently seen in younger, healthy patients without underlying heart disease.** They are **typically paroxysmal,** but if incessant they can lead to a tachycardia-induced cardiomyopathy.

2. Diagnostic testing

a. ECG

(1) The **P-wave axis** or morphology is different from that of sinus rhythm.

(2) Atrial rhythm is regular, except with automatic atrial tachycardia, which displays a warm-up period (see **II.E.3.b**).

(3) A **QRS complex that is generally identical to sinus rhythm** (QRS can be wide if aberrant conduction occurs) follows each P wave.

(4) PR interval is within normal limits or prolonged.

(5) Nonspecific ST-T wave changes may be present.

(6) When an AV block is present, there is an **isoelectric baseline** between P waves in all leads.

b. Electrophysiologic study has become critical in determining the underlying mechanism of these tachycardias, as the clinical differences are subtle and overlapping.

3. Subclassifications. The current subclassifications are **based on mechanisms** and include intra-atrial reentry, automatic atrial tachycardia, and triggered atrial tachycardia.

a. Intra-atrial reentry is usually a disorder **seen in those with underlying heart disease or atrial arrhythmia history,** such as AF or atrial flutter. The mechanism is not well understood. The ventricular rate is typically 90 to 120 beats/min due to the frequent occurrence of 2:1 AV blocks, such that hemodynamic effects are generally minimal. This rhythm can be difficult to distinguish from other supraventricular tachyarrhythmias. One clue is that despite any AV conduction block, the rhythm continues. The ability to terminate with adenosine and β-blockers is variable. **Radiofrequency ablation may be effective,** with success rates greater than 75%. **Antiarrhythmics** (the same drugs as for AF and atrial flutter) **have been disappointing in the prevention of recurrence.**

b. Automatic atrial tachycardia appears to be generated by an ectopic atrial focus, which usually arises from regions around the crista terminalis in the right atrium and around the base of the pulmonary veins in the left atrium. The mechanism is not well understood. Automatic atrial tachycardia is **seen more often in younger patients,** displays a **warm-up phenomenon** (the supraventricular tachyarrhythmia accelerates after its initiation), **does not respond to vagal maneuvers, and is more likely to be incessant.** Automatic atrial tachycardia can be induced with treadmill testing or with administration of isoproterenol. Atrial stimulation during electrophysiologic study has no effect on either initiating or terminating this arrhythmia. **Propranolol** has been used successfully to suppress automatic atrial tachycardia. **Catheter ablation is the preferred therapy when the tachycardia is incessant.** Although adenosine may transiently slow automatic atrial tachycardia, it is unlikely to terminate it. Likewise, verapamil has been used without success.

c. Triggered atrial tachycardia is the least common of the atrial tachycardias and is virtually never incessant. It is more likely to appear in **older individuals.** It can be induced with rapid atrial pacing and is cycle-length dependent. The mechanism of triggered atrial tachycardia is thought to be due to delayed afterdepolarizations (see **I.A.2**) secondary to digitalis toxicity or sympathetic discharge. Catecholamines may play a role in the initiation of this arrhythmia, and thus exercise testing and isoproterenol may provoke it. Verapamil and adenosine have been shown to terminate triggered atrial tachycardia. β-Blockers have been less efficacious. Radiofrequency ablation (**RFA**) is preferred when the tachycardia is causing noticeable symptoms.

F. Multifocal atrial tachycardia

1. **Clinical presentation.** This atrial arrhythmia is uncommon and estimated to occur in 0.37% of hospitalized patients. The atrial rate is generally 100 to 130 beats/min. It occurs most often in elderly, critically ill patients and is frequently **associated with concurrent pulmonary disease, particularly chronic obstructive pulmonary disease.** It may also be seen in CHF and can degenerate into AF.
2. **Pathogenesis and diagnostic tests.** The mechanism appears to be abnormalautomaticity or triggered activity arising from distinct atrial sites. The diagnosis requires the following criteria: (1) atrial rate greater than 100 beats/min, (2) P waves with three or more different morphologies, (3) The P-P, P-R, and R-R intervals vary, and (4) the P waves are separated by isoelectric intervals. Loss of AV conduction of each P wave is uncommon, making it possible to distinguish multifocal atrial tachycardia from AF.
3. **Therapy is directed at the underlying illness, with little role for antiarrhythmics.** Calcium channel blockers in high doses may be useful, or amiodarone when antiarrhythmic therapy is deemed necessary. Maintenance of electrolyte balance, particularly potassium and magnesium, may suppress the occurrence of multifocal atrial tachycardia.

G. AV-node reentrant tachycardia (AVNRT)

1. **Clinical presentation.** AVNRT usually has a narrow QRS complex with a ventricular rate typically in the range of 150 to 250 beats/min, although faster rates are infrequently observed. AVNRT is generally seen in subjects without underlying heart disease. Palpitations and dyspnea are common presenting complaints. Angina, CHF, and rarely shock may be seen in those with a history of underlying heart disease. Syncope may occur due to rapid ventricular rates or due to the asystole or bradycardia occasionally seen when this tachycardia terminates.
2. **Pathophysiology.** The mechanism in AVNRT appears to be a reentrant circuit composed of separate fast and slow atrial pathways involving the AV node. In 50% to 90% of patients with "typical" AVNRT, the antegrade conduction to the ventricles travels over the slow pathway and the retrograde conduction to the atria occurs over the fast pathway. The initiating event may be either a premature atrial complex (PAC) or a premature ventricular complex (PVC). The PAC blocks the fast pathway antegradely and conducts down the slow pathway, then back up the now repolarized fast pathway. Less commonly, a PVC conducts retrogradely to the atria via the fast pathway and then returns to the ventricles via the slow pathway. In the remaining 5% to 10% of patients, with atypical AVNRT the antegrade conduction is down the fast pathway and retrograde via the slow pathway. The cycle length is thus dependent on the conduction velocity of the slow pathway as the fast pathway generally has rapid conduction. Termination of the tachycardia is often the result of a block in the slow pathway. However, AV dissociation may develop during the tachycardia because the ventricles are not involved in the reentry circuit. This does not affect the rate of tachycardia, nor does the development of bundle-branch block.
3. **Laboratory features and diagnosis.** P waves are generally hidden within the QRS complex or at the terminal portion of the QRS in typical AVNRT. This may be visible as a small pseudo-R′ in lead V_1, as depolarization of the atria occurs simultaneously with ventricular depolarization. The RP segment is generally less than 100 milliseconds. AVNRT is often induced abruptly by a PAC and its termination, which also tends to be abrupt, is often followed by a retrograde P wave. The termination may be followed by a brief period of asystole or bradycardia before the sinus node recovers from its tachycardia-induced suppression. The cycle length may vary, especially at the beginning and the end of the tachycardia.

This variation reflects the variable antegrade AV nodal conduction time. Vagal maneuvers may slow or terminate this tachycardia.

4. **Therapy.** Presently the success and safety of percutaneous catheter ablation has allowed this approach to be considered equally with medical therapy as first-line therapy for long-term management of AVNRT. The decision about treatment approach should be individualized according to the characteristics of each patient and his or her arrhythmia patterns.
   a. Radiofrequency ablation has the advantage of curing the arrhythmia in the majority of instances and eliminating the need for long-term suppressive therapy with medications. Cure rates with catheter ablation for AVNRT are in excess of 95%.
   b. **Medical therapy.** Medications that suppress AV node conduction such as β-blockers, calcium channel blockers, digoxin, and adenosine all slow or block conduction in the antegrade slow pathway, whereas class IA and IC antiarrhythmic drugs slow the conduction in the retrograde fast pathway. Adenosine may be considered as first-line drug therapy for acute termination of AVNRT. This medication is available in an intravenous form only and has a very short half-life of about 9 seconds. The use of intravenous or oral β-blockers or calcium channel blockers is an alternative if adenosine is unsuccessful. The onset of action of digoxin limits its usefulness in terminating these arrhythmias, although it may be useful to prevent recurrences. Recurrences may be prevented in patients with frequent sustained episodes with any of the above-named agents except adenosine. Antiarrhythmic drug therapy is not routinely necessary or desirable for AVNRT given the high success rates and low complication rates for catheter ablation.
   c. Direct current cardioversion should be considered for patients whose disease is unstable or highly symptomatic. Low energies of 10 to 50 J are usually sufficient to terminate AVNRT.

H. AV reentrant tachycardia (AVRT)

1. **Clinical presentation.** Similar to AVNRT, this is another example of an AV nodal–dependent supraventricular tachycardia. AVRT usually has a narrow QRS with ventricular rates similar to those of AVNRT, although it more often tends to have a ventricular rate greater than 200. The clinical features are very similar to those of AVNRT but are distinct on an electrophysiologic basis.
2. **Pathophysiology.** The mechanism in AVRT relies on the presence of an accessory pathway as one portion of the circuit and the AV node as the other portion. The atrium and the ventricle on the same side as the accessory pathway are necessary components of the circuit. AVRT may be orthodromic or antidromic. Orthodromic AVRT usually has a narrow-complex that uses the AV node as the antegrade limb and the accessory pathway as the retrograde limb of the circuit. Antidromic AVRT has a wide-complex that is the opposite of the orthodromic variety, such that the accessory pathway serves as the antegrade limb and the AV node as the retrograde limb of the circuit. AVRT is most often of the orthodromic type. Accessory pathways may be "concealed" (inapparent by ECG) due to having only retrograde (V to A) conduction properties or "manifest" (apparent on ECG as delta waves, i.e., Wolff-Parkinson-White pattern). **Unlike AVNRT, the AVRT circuit must involve one of the ventricles; therefore, the development of bundle-branch block on the side ipsilateral to the accessory pathway can prolong the cycle length of the tachycardia.** Bundle-branch block, particularly left bundle-branch block (LBBB), occurs more commonly in AVRT than in AVNRT. AVRT can be distinguished from AVNRT by electrophysiologic study. The presence of AV or ventricular–atrial block with continuation of the tachycardia should exclude the presence of an accessory AV pathway.
3. **Laboratory features and diagnosis.** The P waves of AVRT are frequently inscribed on the ST segment or T wave, as the atrial depolarization must occur after ventricular depolarization. The RP segment is generally greater than 100 milliseconds. Orthodromic AVRT is more common, accounting for about 95% of all AVRT, whereas antidromic AVRT accounts for only about 5%. Orthodromic

AVRT is usually characterized by a narrow QRS complex as opposed to antidromic AVRT, which is characterized by a wide-complex QRS.

4. **Therapy.** See discussion of therapy for Wolff-Parkinson-White syndrome (**I.5**).

I. Preexcitation syndromes. Preexcitation was originally used to describe premature activation of the ventricle in patients with WPW. The term has broadened to include all conditions in which antegrade ventricular or retrograde atrial activation occurs partially or totally via an anomalous pathway distinct from the normal cardiac conduction system. The incidence of preexcitation on ECG is approximately 1.5 per 1000, most of which occur in otherwise healthy subjects without organic heart disease. Seven percent to 10% of these patients have associated Ebstein's anomaly and are thus more likely to have multiple accessory pathways. There is a higher rate of preexcitation in males, with the **prevalence** decreasing with age, although the **frequency** of paroxysmal tachycardia increases with age.

1. **Clinical presentation.** Approximately 50% to 60% of patients with preexcitation report symptoms such as **palpitations, anxiety, dyspnea, chest pain or tightness, and syncope.** In approximately 25% of cases the disease will become asymptomatic over time. Those patients older than 40 whose disease has been asymptomatic are likely to remain symptom free. The absence of preexcitation on ECG despite the discovery of accessory pathways in patients with asymptomatic disease likely identifies a group of patients at low risk for developing symptoms.
2. **Pathophysiology.** Patients with preexcitation generally have an accessory pathway(s) that alters the conduction between the atria and ventricules. These accessory pathways are likely congenital, as relatives of subjects with preexcitation have an increased incidence of preexcitation. AVRT is the most common mechanism associated with preexcitation (80% to 85%) with permanent junctional reciprocating tachycardias (PJRT), Mahaim fiber tachycardias, and Lown-Ganong-Levine syndrome accounting for the remainder.
   a. **Wolff-Parkinson-White syndrome.** The basic abnormality lies in the existence of an accessory pathway of conducting tissue, outside of the normal conducting system, which connects the atria and ventricles. This accessory pathway permits the atrial impulse to bypass the normal pathway through the AV node to the ventricles. In the past these accessory pathways have been referred to as "bundles of Kent." An impulse from the atria can be conducted down both the accessory pathway and the AV node, arriving at the ventricle at nearly the same time. This results in preexcitation of the ventricle, which is really a fusion beat, as a portion of the ventricle is activated via the accessory pathway (giving rise to the delta wave; Fig. 20.3), and the remainder of the ventricle is activated by the normal activation pathway. If antegrade conduction occurs exclusively via the accessory pathway, the resultant QRS is maximally preexcited and is a wide complex. These accessory pathways may conduct rapidly, but frequently have longer refractory periods than the AV node. The inciting event for AVRT is frequently a PAC that is blocked in the accessory pathway and that conducts to the ventricles via the AV node, which has recovered more rapidly. The resultant QRS complex in this instance is normal in appearance. After the QRS complex, the accessory pathway has had sufficient time to recover excitability, and the impulse thus conducts retrogradely to the atria. A small but significant percentage (5% to 10%) of patients have multiple accessory pathways.

   b. The permanent form of junctional reentrant tachycardia is a variant of AVRT. It is often an incessant supraventricular tachyarrhythmia with an unusual accessory pathway. Here the accessory pathway behaves like the AV node in that it displays decremental retrograde conduction properties. Thus, the faster the stimulation of such an accessory pathway, the slower the conduction through the pathway. The accessory pathway is most often located in the posteroseptal region and acts as the retrograde limb of the reentrant circuit. The ventricular–atrial conduction is slowed by the decremental nature of the accessory pathway. Due to the incessant nature of this tachycardia, a tachycardia-induced cardiomyopathy may result.

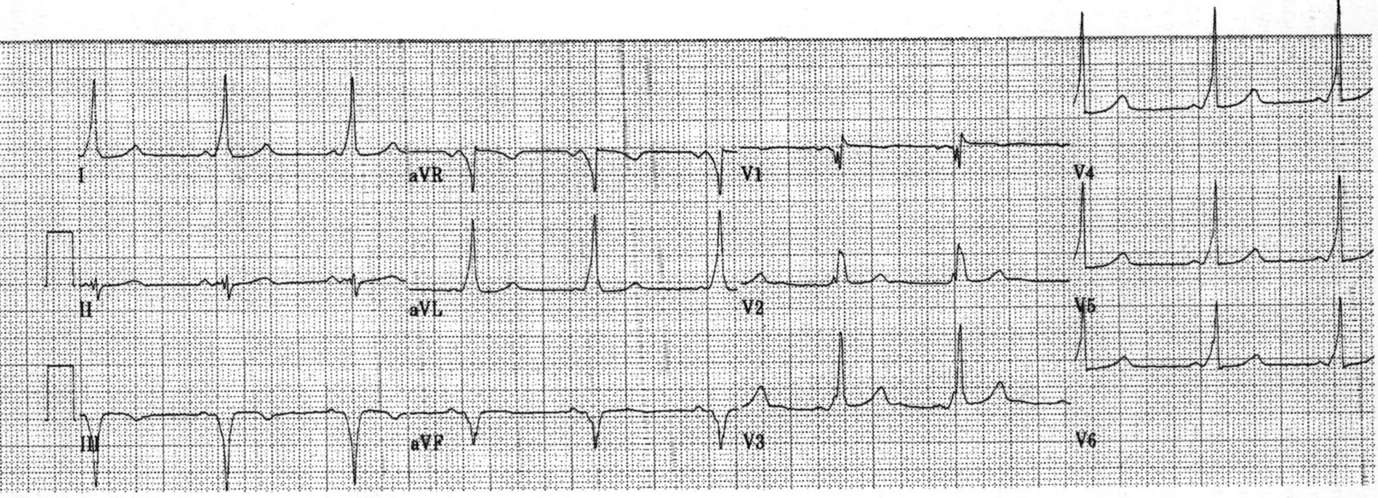

Figure 20.3. Wolff-Parkinson-White syndrome, with widespread delta waves seen at the upstroke of the QRS complexes.

c. **Mahaim tachycardias are another variant form of reentry.** The two most common varieties that are recognized are **atriofascicular** and **fasciculoventricular.** In the former, the accessory pathway is located within a few centimeters of the AV node and inserts into the right bundle branch. The reentrant tachycardia conducts antegrade via the accessory pathway, resulting in an LBBB morphology with left-axis deviation. The retrograde circuit is via the AV node. In the second form of Mahaim reentry, the accessory pathway arises in the His-Purkinje fibers and allows bypass of the distal conducting system.

d. Lown-Ganong-Levine syndrome is diagnosed by the presence of a short PR interval and a normal QRS complex on the surface ECG. LGL likely represents one end (enhanced) of the normal spectrum of AV nodal conduction properties, but in some cases it is impossible to exclude a distinct perinodal accessory pathway or an abnormality in conduction characteristics of the AV node. It is uncertain if this abnormality in AV conduction is itself associated with arrhythmias.

3. Diagnostic testing

a. The following electrocardiographic criteria are suggestive of an accessory pathway consistent with a Wolff-Parkinson-White pattern. The Wolff-Parkinson-White syndrome occurs in the setting of the Wolff-Parkinson-White pattern and supraventricular tachycardia.

(1) The PR interval is short, typically less than 120 ms.

(2) The QRS complex exceeds 120 milliseconds, with some leads showing the characteristic slurred upstroke known as a delta wave (Fig. 20.3), and a normal terminal QRS portion.

(3) The ST-T segment is directed opposite to the major delta and QRS vectors.

b. The most commonly seen tachycardia in Wolff-Parkinson-White syndrome is characterized by a normal QRS with a regular rate of 150 to 250 beats/min. Onset and termination are abrupt.

c. **Localization of accessory pathway.** The **surface electrocardiogram** may provide information that allows localization of the accessory pathway. The simplest classification is that of type A or B. **Type A** has a large R wave in lead V_1. It is due to a left-sided accessory pathway, which permits preexcitation to the posterobasilar segment of the left ventricle. **Type B** has an S or QS in V_1 and is due to a right-sided accessory pathway. When present, the morphology of a retrograde P wave can be helpful in predicting the location of the accessory pathway. More elaborate algorithms for localization are available. The **most precise localization method is electrophysiologic study** with ventricular pacing or during orthodromic AVRT (the latter condition is especially helpful as there is VA conduction purely through the accessory pathway and fusion with VA conduction through the AV node is, therefore, avoided). A positive P wave in V_1 during supraventricular tachyarrhythmia suggests a left free-wall pathway, whereas a negative P wave suggests a right-sided pathway.

d. Risk stratification should be considered for patients with Wolff-Parkinson-White pattern or ventricular preexcitation according to ECG. The appearance or disappearance of preexcitation on **serial ECGs is of no predictive value.** However, **the intermittent loss or appearance of preexcitation on a beat-to-beat basis is indicative of lower risk.** This may be assessed with ambulatory Holter monitoring during usual activities or with formal exercise stress testing. Such intermittent preexcitation suggests a pathway without the ability for rapid AV conduction and, therefore, low risk of sudden cardiac death (SCD). However, the reverse is not necessarily true in that most patients with persistent preexcitation may still be at low risk for SCD but these patients cannot be distinguished from those at risk. As the greatest danger to patients with preexcitation may be the development of AF; **the induction of AF may be most useful in risk stratification.** This can be done via transesophageal pacing; however, electrophysiologic study is the procedure of choice for risk stratification in patients with persistent ventricular preexcitation.

4. Therapy

a. Emergency management of acute tachycardic episodes. A patient demonstrating hemodynamic instability or extreme symptomatology should be cardioverted rapidly. Stable patients may be treated medically.

(1) Normal QRS width. Both types of AVRT (othrodromic and antidromic) are AV node–dependent and thus respond to AV nodal blocking therapies. Although it is reasonable to use vagal maneuvers and AV nodal blocking medications acutely in patients presenting with a narrow QRS (immediate synchronized DCC should be available should the rhythm degenerate), it is not safe in patients when they present with a wide QRS. Atrial pacing, either transvenous or transesophageal, is also quite efficacious for terminating these types of tachycardia. Adenosine, although effective in treating orthodromic and antidromic AVRT, may induce AF in up to 15% of cases and should, therefore, be used with caution. In patients with Wolff-Parkinson-White syndrome, AF is a potentially life-threatening arrhythmia, especially when the accessory pathway has a short anterograde refractory period capable of rapid ventricular conduction.

(2) Wide QRS width. Patients with accessory pathways can present with wide QRS complex resulting from (**1**) orthodromic AVRT with aberrant conduction, (**2**) antidromic AVRT or, **most importantly**, (**3**) atrial arrhythmias (AT/atrial flutter/AF) with anterograde conduction down an accessory pathway. Since it is often initially impossible to determine the mechanism of a wide QRS complex in patients with an accessory pathway, they should be treated with agents that slow conduction in the accessory pathways (procainamide, flecainide, sotalol, or amiodarone). Because atrial arrhythmias with anterograde accessory pathway conduction are **not** AV node–dependent, AV nodal blocking therapies are ineffective and potentially very dangerous. β-Blockers, calcium channel blockers, digoxin, and adenosine should be avoided in patients presenting with wide-complex tachycardias (WCTs), as they may encourage preferential conduction down accessory pathways and accelerate ventricular rates, precipitating ventricular fibrillation (VF). **If the tachycardia persists, synchronized DCC** is the treatment of choice. Energies of at least 200 J are likely to be required.

(3) If the patient develops AF, it has been observed that **definitive therapy for the AV reentrant circuit, such as ablation of the accessory pathway, often results in prevention of future episodes of AF.**

b. Long-term management

(1) Priority of therapy. Patients whose disease is asymptomatic at diagnosis are at low risk of sudden death. As such, it may not be justified to pursue medical or ablative therapy in these patients unless there is a family history of sudden death, or the patients are competitive athletes or are in a high-risk occupation. Patients whose disease is symptomatic or who have a history of AF or aborted sudden death may be at higher risk, and such patients warrant further study.

(2) Medical therapy. Medical therapy may be **appropriate for those with increased risk but no prior symptoms, those with accessory pathways located near the normal conduction pathway who might develop AV block with RFA,** or those at increased risk from invasive procedures. Single-drug therapy may be attempted with **amiodarone, sotalol, flecainide, or propafenone.** These drugs work to slow conduction in both the accessory pathway and the AV node. **Combination therapy** can be accomplished with drugs that work on the AV node (calcium channel blockers, β-blockers) with drugs that work exclusively on the accessory pathway (class IA antiarrhythmics).

(3) Percutaneous therapy. Radiofrequency ablation is effective 85% to 98% of the time, depending on the location of the accessory pathway. Recurrence rates are approximately 5% to 8%. Catheter ablation should be considered for any patient at high risk, patients with symptoms or tachycardias refractory to medical therapy, those who have intolerance to medical therapy, and those with high-risk occupations such as pilots.

III. VENTRICULAR TACHYARRHYTHMIAS. Sudden cardiac deaths are most frequently due to ventricular tachyarrhythmias. It is estimated that up to half of all cardiac deaths are sudden; therefore, ventricular tachyarrhythmias may be responsible for almost half of all cardiac deaths.

A. Ventricular tachycardia. Ventricular tachycardia is defined as three or more QRS complexes of ventricular origin at a rate exceeding 100 beats/min. The various types of VT and their course of disease are discussed in **III.A.5**.

1. **Clinical presentation.** The presentation can be varied and depends on the clinical setting, the heart rate, and the presence of underlying heart disease and other medical conditions. Some patients have no or minimal symptoms, whereas others may present with syncope or sudden death. The loss of normal AV synchrony may cause symptoms in a patient with decreased cardiac function at baseline. Heart rates less than 150 beats/min are surprisingly well tolerated in the short term, even in the most compromised individuals. Exposure to these rates for more than a few hours is likely to be associated with heart failure in patients with poor ventricular function, whereas those with normal ventricular function may tolerate prolonged periods at such rates. The range of 150 to 200 beats/min is tolerated variably, according to the factors noted previously. Once the rate reaches and exceeds 200 beats/min, there are symptoms in virtually all patients. **Nonsustained VT** (NSVT) is generally defined as VT of duration of less than 30 seconds. VT is **generally regular in rate and appearance,** although it can be polymorphic in appearance, slightly irregular with respect to rate, and may have capture and/or fusion beats within it.
2. **Differential diagnosis.** VT needs to be distinguished from **supraventricular tachyarrhythmia with aberrant intraventricular conduction, bundle-branch block, and morphologic changes of the QRS complex secondary to metabolic derangement or pacing.**
   a. **Brugada criteria.** Distinguishing VT from **supraventricular tachyarrhythmia with aberrancy** can be challenging. Various criteria have been proposed. A good rule of thumb is that any WCT in a patient with ischemic heart disease is VT until proven otherwise. Some have reported that more than 80% of WCTs in such patients are VTs. The **algorithm proposed by Brugada may be helpful in making this distinction, and the algorithm is both sensitive** (99%) **and specific** (96.5%) in patients without a preexisting bundle-branch block. As shown in Figure 20.4, a stepwise approach is applied. In the first step, the precordial leads are examined for the presence or absence of an RS complex. If an RS is uniformly absent, VT is established. If an RS is present in at least one precordial lead, one moves to the second step, which is measuring the interval from the onset of the QRS complex to the nadir of the S wave. If this distance is greater than 100 milliseconds in at least one precordial lead, then the diagnosis of VT is made. If there is no RS interval greater than 100 milliseconds, the third step is used. In the third step, one looks for evidence of AV dissociation. If there are more QRS complexes than P waves, then the diagnosis is VT. If not, then one moves to the fourth step, which involves examining the morphology of the QRS in the precordial leads V_1 and V_6. If the morphology criteria for VT (Fig. 20.5) are present in these leads, then the diagnosis of VT is established. If not, the diagnosis is supraventricular tachyarrhythmia with aberrant intraventricular conduction.
   b. The Brugada criteria have been further refined to distinguish between VT and supraventricular tachyarrhythmia with antegrade conduction over an accessory pathway. After applying the preceding criteria, a second stepwise algorithm is applied (Fig. 20.6). This **second algorithm has a sensitivity of 75% and a specificity of 100% to diagnose VT and exclude preexcited tachycardia.** In the first step, leads V_4 to V_6 are examined to see if the QRS is predominantly negative in these leads. If so, then VT is favored. If not, then the second step, examining leads V_2 to V_6 for the presence of a QR complex in one or more of these leads, is applied. If there is a QR complex in any of these leads,

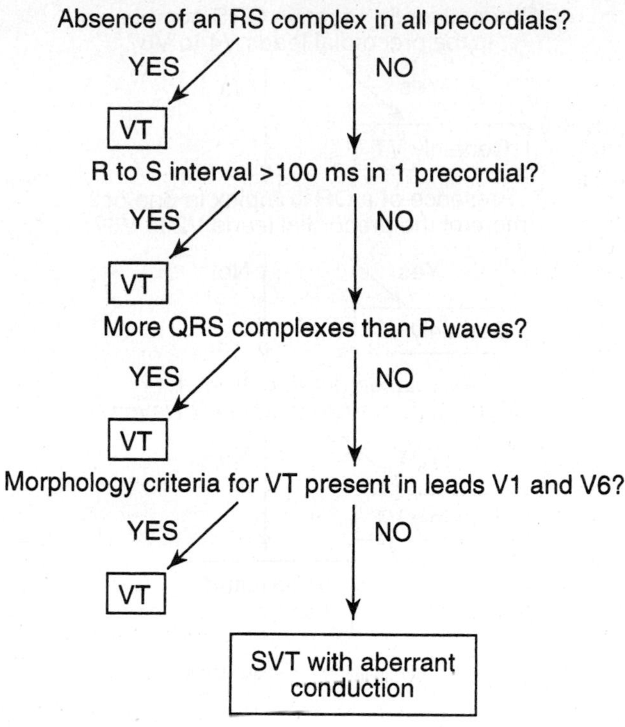

Figure 20.4. Brugada criteria for differentiating ventricular tachycardia from supraventricular tachycardia with aberrant intraventricular conduction.

1. QRS width > 0.14 s
2. Superior QRS axis
3. Morphology in precordial leads:

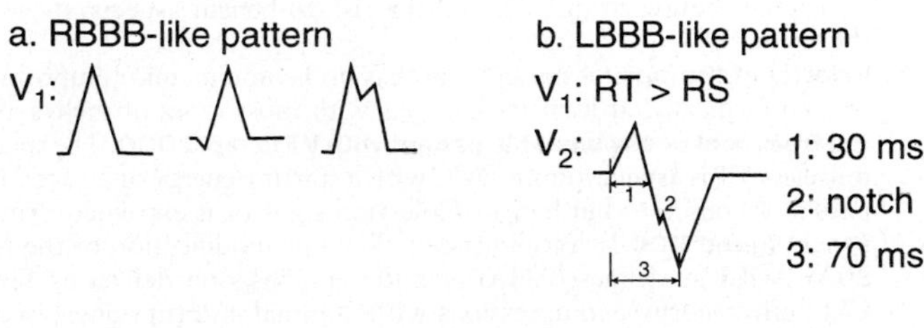

V_6: R/S ratio < 1 V_6: qR

4. AV dissociation, fusion, capture present

Figure 20.5. Classic morphology criteria for ventricular tachycardia.

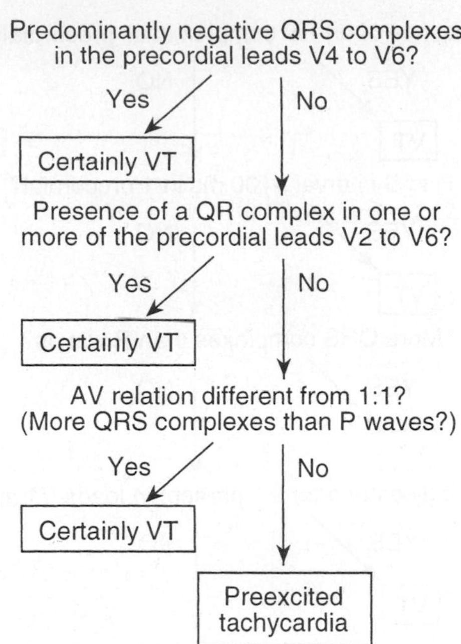

Figure 20.6. Brugada criteria for differentiating ventricular tachycardia from antidromic tachycardia over an accessory pathway.

then the diagnosis is VT. The third criterion, presence of AV dissociation, is 100% specific for VT. If there is no AV dissociation, then supraventricular tachyarrhythmia with antegrade accessory pathway conduction is favored.

3. Therapy

a. General management. The treatment of VT may involve DCC, discontinuation of offending proarrhythmic drugs, specific antiarrhythmic therapy with drugs, correction of electrolyte imbalances, implantable devices, ablation, revascularization, and surgery. The appropriate selection of the preceding therapies is aided by assessment of the patient, an understanding the etiology and mechanism of the VT, knowledge of any exacerbating medical conditions contributing to the VT, and the risk-to-benefit aspects of the available therapies.

b. Priority of therapy. A patient who has no hemodynamic compromise can be treated medically, at least initially. As with most types of tachyarrhythmias, **the treatment of any unstable patient with VT is rapid DCC**. The treatment for pulseless VT is asynchronous DCC with a starting energy of 200 to 360 J. If the patient is conscious but has unstable vital signs or is extremely symptomatic, **synchronized DCC** is recommended. The key modification of the November 2005 ACLS guidelines (AHA) was the emphasis on delivering high-quality CPR: effective chest compressions with minimal interruptions, rescue breaths given over 1 second with visible chest rise while avoiding hyperventilation (30:2 ratio before an advanced airway and 8–10 asynchronous breaths/min after airway is secured), and a **single** shock to attempt to defibrillate pulseless VT patients (as opposed to three stacked shocks) followed by immediate continuation of CPR. (See **III.B.3.** for treatment of pulseless VT/VF patients.)

c. Acute medical therapy. Intravenous amiodarone, lidocaine, procainamide, β-blockers, and other oral agents may be given initially depending on the clinical scenario. Amiodarone is the agent of choice for resistant VTs causing repeated episodes of VT, and also for pulseless VT/cardiac arrest. Amiodarone and lidocaine are the preferred agents in patients with LV dysfunction [left ventricular ejection fraction (LVEF) <40%]. Lidocaine is effective when VT is thought to be ischemic in nature. Procainamide is reasonable as the initial treatment in patients with stable monomorphic VT, as it more effectively provides early rate slowing and conversion than amiodarone. β-Blockers may be preferred for acute coronary syndrome (ACS), especially if not already being taken by the patient. Whenever possible, a **reversible cause for VT** should be sought. Elimination of **ischemia** and correction of **electrolyte abnormalities** is recommended. **Bradycardia** may cause frequent premature ventricular contractions or VT. Maneuvers and agents that increase heart rate should be employed for these bradycardias. **Hypotension** should be promptly corrected. Therapy for CHF should be optimized with the agents known to promote survival in this disorder. **Offending agents** should be stopped whenever possible, and **antidotes** should be administered in the case of overdosage and poisoning.

4. **Prevention and prophylactic treatment.** All antiarrhythmic agents to date, except β-blockers, have not been shown in randomized clincal trials to be effective as the primary management of patients with life-threatening ventricular arrhythmias or in the prevention of SCD. Since the CAST data have become available, there has been a shift away from the use of class I agents and toward the **use of class III agents and β-blockers for prophylactic maintenance therapy** of VT. The development of **curative catheter-based therapies and surgical procedures** has somewhat reduced the role of antiarrhythmics in the prevention of recurrence, especially for VT occurring in normal hearts, which has very high cure rates with catheter ablation. However, antiarrhythmic drug therapy remains the first-line treatment for VT, particularly for patients with cardiomyopathy. The greatest impact on survival in sudden death has been made by the implantable **cardioverter defibrillator.** Data from the Multicenter Unsustained Tachycardia Trial (MUSTT) investigations have shown that in **patients with coronary artery disease, an ejection fraction less than 40% and NSVT who have inducible sustained VT on testing are at substantially increased risk** over those who do not have inducible VT.

   a. **Medical therapy**

      (1) Although drug therapy continues to have a role in the prevention of VT and sudden death, this role has become more limited. The Electrophysiologic Studies Versus Electrocardiographic Monitoring (ESVEM) trial studied the efficacy of seven antiarrhythmics (imipramine, mexiletine, pirmenol, procainamide, propafenone, quinidine, and sotalol) in preventing the recurrence of sustained VT. Sotalol was seen to be the most effective, although even with sotalol the recurrence rate was disappointing. The European Myocardial Infarct Amiodarone Trial (EMIAT) and the Canadian Amiodarone Myocardial Infarction Arrhythmia Trial (CAMIAT) investigations were designed to study the effectiveness of empiric amiodarone for the prevention of VT after MI. Although both of these trials showed a decrease in arrhythmic deaths, no survival benefit was obtained. Therefore, the **role of antiarrhythmics remains uncertain,** and their use as the sole method of recurrence prevention should be questioned.

      (2) Combination therapy. Drug therapy is becoming **an adjunct to implantable cardioverter–defibrillator (ICD) therapy** in this high-risk population. At present, fully half of those with ICDs remain on antiarrhythmic therapy. The rationales for this combined therapy include preventing atrial tachyarrhythmias and reducing the frequency of VT, and thus the frequency of ICD discharge.

      (3) Calcium channel blockers are used primarily in the management of supraventricular tachyarrhythmia. However, some of the idiopathic monomorphic VTs described in **III.A.6** (the VTs originating in the right ventricular outflow tract (RVOT), with LBBB morphology, and VTs originating in the left ventricular apex, with right bundle-branch block, or RBBB, morphology) and the VTs of digitalis toxicity are responsive to calcium channel–blocking agents such as verapamil and diltiazem. Radiofrequency ablation is potentially curative for idiopathic VTs and should be considered despite effective termination with calcium channel blockers.

(4) β-Blockers may be effective, particularly for outflow tract VT. Idiopathic left ventricular VT may respond to calcium channel blockers.

b. Percutaneous therapy

(1) ICDs. Two large trials comparing ICDs with amiodarone in high-risk patients with prior infarction, the Multicenter Automatic Defibrillator Implantation Trial (MADIT) and the Antiarrhythmics Versus Implantable Defibrillator (AVID) trial, have recently been completed. High risk implies either an ejection fraction of 35% or less or the presence of inducible sustained VT at electrophysiologic study. Both trials showed a **decided advantage for ICDs,** with 30% to 50% reductions in mortality with ICDs. In fact, the AVID trial found no survival benefit from amiodarone, β-blockers, or any other antiarrhythmic agent. Newer ICDs often have antitachycardia pacing capabilities, can recognize monomorphic ventricular rhythms with rates of less than 200 beats/min, and can rapidly pace the ventricles to restore sinus rhythm, aborting the need for countershock (see Chapter 22). Data from MADIT II have shown that in patients with a prior MI and an ejection fraction less than 30%, the implantation of a defibrillator is associated with a significant improvement in survival.

(2) Catheter-based therapy. Radiofrequency ablation may be effective for eliminating VT. The success rate depends on the type of VT, with the highest success rates with normal heart VT that is in excess of 90%. VT associated with underlying cardiomyopathy has lower ablation success rates, particularly those with arrhythmogenic right ventricular dysplasia and ischemic cardiomyopathy. However, catheter ablation still remains an effective and feasible approach, even for these types of VT. Presently catheter ablation of VT does not obviate the need for an ICD in a patient with an indication for one.

5. Types of VT and their course of disease. The clinical presentation and course of VT can be divided into VT related to ischemia and nonischemic VT, including **torsade de pointes.**

a. Ischemic VT

(1) Etiology and pathophysiology. At the cellular level, ischemia may alter action potentials, prolong refractoriness of cells, and uncouple the cell-to-cell propagation of depolarization. The biochemical milieu in which the cells exist with respect to ion concentrations, acid–base balance, and so forth can be altered. Also, the damage of infarction is inhomogeneous. Therefore, scar tissue and functioning tissue are admixed in the region of the infarction. A reentrant circuit requires two functionally distinct pathways with unidirectional block in one pathway and slowed conduction down a second pathway. The changes associated with ischemia provide the anatomic substrate for reentry. The VT in the setting of ischemia tends to be **polymorphic.** Ischemia has been shown to prolong the QT interval in some subjects, often with associated T-wave inversion. The **QT interval in ischemic-mediated polymorphic VT is not as prolonged** as that in torsade de pointes, another polymorphic VT. Ischemia is by far the **most common cause of polymorphic VT with normal QT interval.**

(2) Predictors of VT. As might be expected, **larger infarcts with greater resultant impairment of left ventricular systolic function** are more likely to be associated with VT. In fact, left ventricular systolic function is the single most important predictor of sudden death due to arrhythmia. Similarly, the presence of an **open artery appears to reduce the occurrence of VT and other arrhythmias.** Other proposed predictors include syncope, abnormal signal averaged ECG (SAECG) result, NSVT, absence of heart rate variability, abnormal electrophysiologic study outcome, and T-wave alternans.

(3) **Laboratory examination and diagnostic testing.** The various tests for risk stratification (electrophysiologic study, SAECG, heart rate variability, T-wave alternans, and so forth) have shown poor specificity and positive predictive value for VT, **and thus should not be used alone to guide therapy but in combination with the rest of the clinical information.**

(4) Accelerated idioventricular rhythm (Fig. 20.7) is a form of VT seen almost exclusively in ischemic heart disease, particularly during an MI or after reperfusion of an occluded territory. It may also be seen with digitalis toxicity. The accelerated idioventricular rhythm often seen **after MI is rarely of clinical significance.**

(a) The electrocardiographic features include regular or slightly irregular ventricular rhythm, rate of 60 to 110 beats/min, a QRS morphology resembling that of premature ventricular complexes, and, often, AV dissociation as well as fusion beats and capture beats.

(b) **Pathophysiology.** The ectopic ventricular pacing focus competes with the sinus node and usurps control of the ventricular rate when the sinus rate slows or when sinoatrial or AV block occurs. Enhanced automaticity is the likely underlying mechanism.

(c) Accelerating the sinus rhythm with atropine or atrial pacing can be useful to suppress the accelerated idioventricular rhythm. **Therapy is rarely necessary unless** the loss of AV synchrony results in hemodynamic compromise, a more rapid VT intervenes, the accelerated idioventricular rhythm falls on the T wave of the preceding beat (R on T phenomenon), the ventricular rate is rapid enough to produce symptoms, or VF occurs.

b. **Nonischemic VT.** This category includes drug-induced VT, bundle-branch reentry, VT originating in the right or left ventricular outflow tracts, VT originating in the left ventricular apex, congenital long QT syndrome and other genetically associated VT, idiopathic polymorphic VT, arrhythmogenic right ventricular dysplasia, Wolff-Parkinson-White syndrome, and the VTs associated with various inflammatory and infectious conditions.

(1) **Drug-induced VT.** Drugs are a well-known cause of VT, both polymorphic and monomorphic. This is particularly true in ischemic or infarcted hearts. Phenothiazines, tricyclic antidepressants, digitalis, epinephrine, cocaine, nicotine, alcohol, and glue (inhaled) are some of the wide variety of drugs that have been implicated in the development of monomorphic VT. The CAST and other trials of the late 1980s showed an increase in mortality resulting from the use of class I antiarrhythmic agents employed to suppress asymptomatic ventricular ectopy after MI. NSVT and depressed left ventricular function remain risk factors for sudden death, and the agents studied in CAST did decrease the occurrence of ventricular ectopy; however, it is believed that these drugs (flecainide, encainide, and moricizine) generated VT, causing sudden death in recipients. These agents all have in common their sodium channel–blocking activities. Other drugs in this class, including procainamide, quinidine, disopyramide, lidocaine, tocainide, and mexiletine, have all been shown either experimentally or clinically to be associated with increased mortality compared with controls in the peri-infarction period. The results of CAST caused a major shift away from the sodium channel–blocking agents (class I antiarrhythmics) in the peri-infarction period.

(2) The generation of torsade de pointes due to effects on the QT interval is discussed in **III.A.5.c**.

(3) Digitalis toxicity can propagate delayed afterdepolarizations, which generate action potentials, leading to VT. The VT of digitalis toxicity is typically monomorphic and often responds to calcium channel blockers. Rarely, digitalis toxicity manifests as a bidirectional VT, meaning that it has a regular rhythm with an axis that alternates from –60 to –90° to +120 to +130°, with a ventricular rate from 140 to 200 beats/min. Because digitalis toxicity may have a narrow QRS complex and may respond

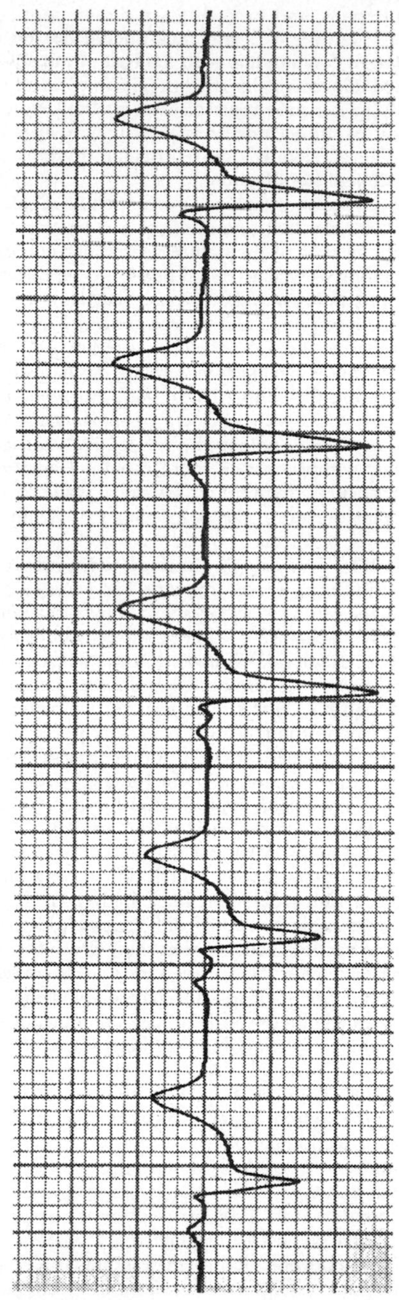

Figure 20.7. Accelerated idioventricular rhythm (beats 3 through 5), interspersed with normal sinus rhythm (beats 1 and 2), lead IV.

to calcium channel blockers, it may be confused with supraventricular tachyarrhythmia. This type of VT is best managed by removing the offending agent, digoxin, with its binding antibody. The treatment for digitalis toxicity is the same in the face of bidirectional VT.

(4) Bundle-branch reentry is commonly seen in patients with dilated cardiomyopathy. The presence of underlying His-Purkinje system disease and intraventricular conduction delay on surface ECG are universal findings in patients with bundle-branch reentry. This form of VT typically has an LBBB morphology, although the less common forms may have an RBBB morphology. The mechanism in the most common form involves antegrade conduction over the right bundle and retrograde conduction via the left bundle. The VT of bundle-branch reentry tends to be 200 beats/min or greater. The diagnosis needs to be confirmed by electrophysiologic study, although it may be suspected clinically.

(5) Idiopathic VT occurs in otherwise structurally normal hearts with no significant CAD, no family history of arrhythmia or sudden death, and normal surface electrocardiograms. It may be of LBBB morphology or RBBB morphology.

- **(a)** **VT** originating in the outflow tract is typically a monomorphic VT with an LBBB morphology and inferior rightward axis. This is likely a VT secondary to abnormal impulse formation, and may be triggered by delayed afterdepolarizations, perhaps during exercise or other periods of increased adrenergic stimulation. As such, it is often responsive to calcium channel blockers, which may lead to its being mistaken for supraventricular tachyarrhythmia. Other agents that may prove useful include β-blockers and class IA, IC, and III antiarrhythmics. **Adenosine** has often proven efficacious in terminating these VTs, which suggests that cyclic adenosine monophosphate may be a mediator in the sustainment of this type of VT. This fact may also lead to misinterpretation of the VT as a supraventricular tachyarrhythmia.
- **(b)** Repetitive monomorphic VT is a subtype of RVOT and has all of the properties of RVOT already discussed. It is generally not associated with any risk of sudden death; therefore, **therapy is undertaken only to alleviate symptoms. Catheter ablation** is often successful in curing these forms of VT.
- **(c)** VT of left ventricular apex origin is a second type of **monomorphic VT that occurs in otherwise normal hearts.** It has an RBBB morphology with a superior axis. It is also often **responsive to calcium channel blockers.** It most likely is a reentrant VT that originates in the left-sided His-Purkinje system, resulting in a fascicular tachycardia. When incessant, this type of VT **can lead to tachycardia-induced cardiomyopathy.** It is possible to cure this type of VT with catheter-based ablation, although this represents a complex ablation procedure.
- **(d)** Less commonly, the monomorphic VTs that occur in normal hearts are not typified by the characteristics of RBBB-shaped or LBBB-shaped VT. These too often respond to β-blockers and calcium channel blockers.

(6) Both dilated cardiomyopathy (DCM) and hypertrophic cardiomyopathy (HCM) have increased risk of VT and sudden death.

- **(a)** **Dilated cardiomyopathy.** Risk stratification is particularly difficult in patients with DCM as SAECG, microvolt T wave alternans (TWA), and an electrophysiologic study are not reliable predictors in this population, and asymptomatic ventricular arrhythmias are common. The DEFINITE and SCD-HeFT trials have influenced the current guidelines for implanting ICDs in patients with DCM. ICDs are recommended for patients who manifest life-threatening arrhythmias or syncope, and for primary prevention in patients who have a LVEF less than 35% and are New York Heart Association (NYHA) class I–III (less evidence exists for class I). All patients should be receiving chronic optimal medical therapy and have a life expectancy greater than 1 year. Bundle-branch reentrant tachycardia occurs most commonly in patients with DCM for which electrophysiologic testing is helpful in diagnosing and guiding ablative treatment. Although ablation may be curative if bundle-branch reentry is the mechanism, such patients should still be considered for ICD implantation.

(b) Hypertrophic cardiomyopathy. Supraventricular tachyarrhythmia and AF are particularly poorly tolerated by these patients, as is ischemia, and may lead to VT. No randomized trials have been done to date in this patient population regarding ICD therapy. Consequently, the precise risk stratifcation is debated. ICDs are recommended for patients who have sustained VT or VF, or both, and for primary prevention in patients who have either one of the preceding life-threatening arrythmias or one or more other major risk factors for SCD (nonsustained spontaneous VT, family history of premature SCD, unexplained syncope, LV thickness $\geq$30 mm, or abnormal exercise blood pressure). Again, all patients should be receiving chronic optimal medical therapy and have a life expectancy greater than 1 year. Electrophysiologic study may be helpful in stratifying risk for VT and sudden death. Patients at low risk with HCM include those with infrequent or brief episodes that are asymptomatic or mildly symptomatic. Although **amiodarone** may be beneficial in this population, an ICD is increasingly used in those considered to be at high risk.

(7) Muscular dystrophies, particularly Duchenne's muscular dystrophy and myotonic dystrophy, have been associated with frequent defects in the conduction system. Heart block and bundle-branch block as well as sudden death due to ventricular tachyarrhythmias are well-recognized complications of these muscular disorders.

(8) Structural abnormalities such as **repaired tetralogy of Fallot and mitral valve prolapse** have been associated with increased risk of VT and sudden death. In tetralogy of Fallot, the VT often originates in the RVOT, at the site of a previous repair. It can be cured by catheter ablation or surgical resection. Mitral valve prolapse has been uncommonly linked to sudden death, although ventricular arrhythmias are not uncommon. **The prognosis with respect to VT is quite good in mitral valve prolapse.**

(9) Arrhythmogenic right ventricular dysplasia is a cardiomyopathy that begins in the right ventricle and often progresses to involve the left ventricle. It results in right ventricular dilation with resultant poor contractile function. The right ventricular muscle becomes increasingly replaced by adipose and fibrous tissue as the disease progresses. VT arising in the right ventricle is often an early manifestation of this disorder. The **VT is a reentrant type and has an LBBB morphology;** although in sinus rhythm, there is often inversion of the T waves in the anterior leads and a slurring of the terminal portion of the QRS complex, known as an epsilon wave (Fig. 20.8). These patients frequently have a positive SAECG for late potentials. The combination of the scarring and the late potentials provides the anatomic substrate for reentry. During electrophysiologic study it may be possible to elicit VT of varying morphologies, due to the prolific scarring of the myocardium. The **risk of VT correlates with the extent of myocardial involvement.** Therapy with sotalol or high-dose amiodarone may be somewhat successful. Ablation via catheters is often successful, but only temporizing, as the generalized involvement tends to give rise to arrhythmias at a different locus later in the disease course. ICDs are often the only reliable therapy to prevent sudden death in this disorder.

(10) Wolff-Parkinson-White syndrome predisposes patients to very rapid rates of ventricular response during AF, which may result in VF. Curative therapy via catheter-based ablation is the best approach to this disorder, with success rates well in excess of 90% in most cases.

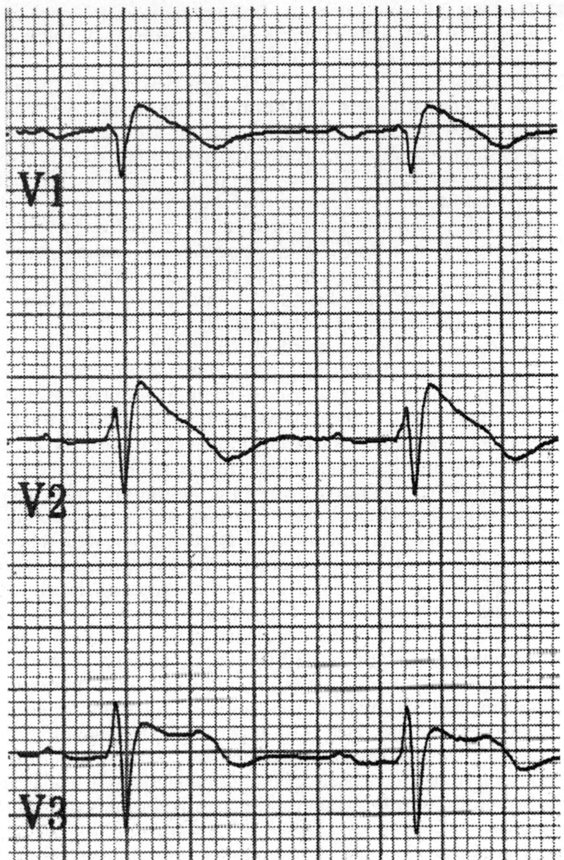

Figure 20.8. Leads V_1 through V_3, demonstrating large epsilon waves in the ST segment.

(11) Several inflammatory or infectious conditions have been associated with VT.

(a) Sarcoidosis is frequently cited as a cause of heart block, and may also cause VT and VF. **Amiodarone** and **sotalol** are the most efficacious agents in this disorder, although an ICD may be necessary in addition to the drug therapy.

(b) Acute myocarditis has been associated with both polymorphic and monomorphic VT. **Antiarrhythmic therapy and anti-Inflammatory therapy** are generally combined in the treatment of these patients.

(c) Chagas' disease, caused by the parasite *Trypanosoma cruzii,* is a well-known cause of cardiomyopathy, particularly in South and Central America. VT and other arrhythmias due to conduction system involvement are common complications. Therapy involves antiparasitic treatment, standard therapy for CHF, antiarrhythmics, and pacemaker or ICD implantation, as appropriate. Some patients require catheter ablation of refractory VT, which sometimes must be performed epicardially.

(12) The long QT syndrome is an uncommon disorder for which seven different genetic defects have thus far been identified. A full discussion of this syndrome can be found in Chapter 22.

(13) Idiopathic polymorphic VT has been described in patients with **structurally normal hearts and normal QT intervals.** Various characteristics have been described in these subjects. One group was noted to have persistent ST elevation (Brugada syndrome) despite any evidence for ischemia or CAD. Another group had reproducible arrhythmias with physical or emotional stress and were responsive to β-blocker therapy. A third group had polymorphic VT triggered by an early premature ventricular beat and a high incidence of sudden death that was not prevented by β-blocker therapy, although verapamil had some benefit.

(14) **Brugada syndrome.** Brugada syndrome is a condition associated with SCD in the setting of a structurally normal heart characterized by an electrocardiographic pattern of RBBB and ST-segment elevation in leads V_1 to V_3. It is inherited in an autosomal dominant pattern with a male predominance. It is a genetically heterogeneous disease with many mutations linked to the gene *SCN5A,* which encodes for a cardiac sodium channel. The diagnosis can be difficult because of the variable expression of the ECGs at baseline, changes in the ECG over time induced by a host of factors (temperature, heart rate, autonomic tone, medications), and widely ranging clinical manifestations of patients. The diagnosis should be considered in patients who have documented VF, self-terminating polymorphic VT, family members with ST-segment elevation, syncope, or family history of sudden death in the setting of the electrocardiographic findings noted previously. Currently, no medication has proved effective in preventing SCD in these patients. ICDs are currently the only available treatment, and are recommended in patients with previous cardiac arrest (class I), syncope with spontaneous ECG pattern (class IIa), and documented VT that has not resulted in cardiac arrest (class IIa). It is generally recommended to implant an ICD in **symptomatic** patients and clinically follow **asymptomatic** patients with an abnormal ECG only on pharmacologic provocation and no inducible ventricular arrhythmias.

(15) **Commotio cordis.** Commotio cordis is the sudden disturbance of heart rhythm occurring as a result of blunt, nonpenetrating impact to the precordial region, which is most commonly observed in young healthy persons during participation in sports. The blow likely falls within a small 10 to 30 millisecond window of ventricular vulnerabilty just prior to the peak of the T wave that results in polymorphic VT and sudden death. A 2002 case series of 128 individuals showed that only 16% of patients survived an episode of commotio cordis, with most returning to a baseline level of function. Prompt CPR/defibrillation was the only identifiable factor associated with a favorable outcome.

c. Torsade de pointes is a type of polymorphic VT associated with delayed myocardial repolarization, most often manifested as a prolonged QT interval. Alhough the duration of torsade de pointes is typically brief (less than 20 seconds), it can be sustained and can degenerate into VF. It generally has an irregular ventricular rate in excess of 200 beats/min and displays a polymorphic structure with an undulating appearance. The QRS complexes appear to twist around an isoelectric axis. Characteristics that distinguish torsade de pointes from other forms of VT include (1) prolonged QT interval, (2) initiation with a short-long-short sequence, and (3) typical "twisting of the points" appearance of the VT.

(1) **Etiology.** QT prolongation can be congenital or acquired.

(a) The **congenital** forms are seen in the long QT syndrome, discussed in Chapter 22.

(b) The **acquired forms are most often drug induced,** although polymorphic VT with a prolonged QT can be caused by electrolyte abnormalities, hypothyroidism, cerebrovascular events, MI or ischemia, starvation diets, organophosphate poisoning, myocarditis, severe CHF, and mitral valve prolapse.

The **most commonly implicated drugs have** been the **class IA drugs,** although less frequent occurrences have been reported with all subclasses of class I antiarrhythmics. The class III drugs, such as sotalol, dofetilide, and, less commonly, amiodarone, have been implicated. The incidence of torsade de pointes with sotalol is in the range of 2% to 5%. Ibutilide is a new antiarrhythmic agent for supraventricular tachyarrhythmias that is associated with an incidence of torsade de pointes at least as high as that of sotalol. Other drugs implicated include the phenothiazines, haloperidol, and the tricyclic antidepressants. Antibiotics, including erythromycin and other macrolides, as well as trimethoprim-sulfamethoxazole combinations, have been implicated. The macrolides are particularly prone to causing torsade de pointes when combined with certain antihistamines such as astemizole and terfenadine. These antihistamines have also been found to cause torsade de pointes when combined with certain azole antifungal agents such as ketoconazole. Ionic contrast and promotility agents such as cisapride have also been associated with torsade de pointes. Medications associated with increasing QT interval are listed on the following website: www.torsades.org. It is maintained by the University of Arizona Center for Education and Research on Therapeutics.

Bradycardia can promote torsade de pointes in patients with prolonged QT intervals, although it is not clear that bradycardia by itself predisposes to torsade de pointes. Specifically, pause-dependent VT occurs in the setting of bradycardia and a prolonged QT interval. Usually a long RR interval followed by a short RR interval followed by another long RR interval initiates the VT.

Electrolyte disorders. Hypokalemia is the electrolyte disorder most reliably linked to torsade de pointes. **Hypomagnesemia** has been proposed as a logical cause, as the administration of magnesium frequently terminates torsade de pointes. However, there is scant evidence to confirm this. Likewise, although **hypocalcemia** is associated with prolongation of the QT interval, there are only rare reports of torsade de pointes associated with hypocalcemia.

Short coupled VT. Polymorphic VT is initiated less than 400 milliseconds following the preceding QRS complex.

R-on-T phenomenon occurs when a defibrillation or pacing current or spike is delivered simultaneously with occurrence of the electrocardiographic T wave resulting in polymorphic VT.

A variety of **cerebrovascular events** have been associated with torsade de pointes, most notably subarachnoid hemorrhage. The prolongation of the QT interval sometimes seen with intracranial bleeding is usually transient, resolving within weeks.

(2) Therapy. Acute management is aimed at terminating the arrhythmia.

(a) If torsade de pointes is sustained or associated with hemodynamic compromise, prompt DCC should be carried out. Starting voltages are generally 50 to 100 J, and can be advanced to 360 J if necessary.

(b) Correction of hypokalemia, hypomagnesemia, and hypocalcemia should be undertaken promptly. Magnesium can be given in a bolus form at a dose of 1 to 2 g, with a total dose of 2 to 4 g given over 10 to 15 minutes. This successfully terminates torsade de pointes within 5 minutes in up to 75% of patients and within 15 minutes in virtually all patients.

(c) Bradycardia can be corrected with either isoproterenol infusion or temporary transvenous pacing. Pacing may be preferable when readily available, due to the potential complications of isoproterenol therapy (worsened ischemia, hypertension). Offending agents should be discontinued.

B. Ventricular fibrillation

1. Ventricular fibrillation is a **chaotic ventricular rhythm that reflects no organized electrical activity and hence no cardiac output** from the ventricle. It is devoid of the distinct elements that make up the usual electrical complex of ventricular activity. It is a **rapidly fatal rhythm, and if resuscitation is not begun within 5 to 7 minutes, death is virtually certain.** Ventricular fibrillation is often preceded by VT. Virtually all of the risk factors and conditions discussed for VT are applicable to VF. It may arise without any inciting cardiac rhythm or event.
2. **Course of disease.** Of patients who experience an out-of-hospital cardiac arrest, 75% have VF as their initial cardiac rhythm. Of those successfully resuscitated, 75% have significant CAD, and 20% to 30% have a transmural infarction. Patients without an ischemic etiology have an increased risk of further episodes of sudden death, whereas those who have an MI associated with sudden death have a 1-year recurrence rate of 2% for sudden death. Anterior MI complicated by VF represents a subgroup at high risk for recurrence of sudden death. Predictors of SCD include evidence of ischemia, decreased left ventricular systolic function, 10 or more premature ventricular complexes per hour on telemetry, inducible or spontaneous VT, hypertension and left ventricular hypertrophy, smoking, male sex, obesity, elevated cholesterol, advanced age, and excessive alcohol use.
3. **Therapy.** As noted previously, VF is a rapidly fatal rhythm, which virtually never terminates spontaneously. Cardiopulmonary resuscitation must be initiated promptly, and rapid, asynchronous DCC performed as soon as possible. A **single** shock of 200 to 360 J (biphasic, 200 J; monophasic devices, 360 J) should be given initially followed by immediate resumption of CPR for 2 minutes before checking for a pulse. If VF/pulseless VT persists, an immediate **second** shock (biphasic,-≥200 J; monophasic devices,-360 J) should be given followed by a vasopressor (1 mg of epinephrine every 3–5 minutes; single dose of 40 units of vasopressin may replace first or second dose of epinephrine). If VF/pulseless VT persists after 2 or 3 shocks, CPR, and a vasopressor, administration of an antiarrhythmic should be considered (amiodarone is preferred and lidocaine as an alternative). The emphasis should be on performing high quality CPR with interruptions in chest compressions **only** for ventilation (until an advanced airway is established), rhythm checks (pulse checks only if an organized rhythm is observed), and shocks.

   See Chapter 22 for a discussion about the long-term treatment of survivors of VF.

ACKNOWLEDGMENTS

The author thanks Drs. Keith Ellis and Thomas Dresing for their contributions to earlier editions of this chapter.

Key Reviews

Affirm Investigators. A comparison of rate control and rhythm control in patients with atrial fibrillation. *N Engl J Med* 2002;347:1825–1833.

American Heart Association. Medical/scientific statement. Management of patients with atrial fibrillation: a statement for healthcare professionals from the Subcommittee on Electrocardiography and Electrophysiology, American Heart Association, Eric N. Prystowsky MD, Chair. *Circulation* 1996;93:1262–1277.

Antiarrhythmics Versus Implantable Defibrillators (AVID) Investigators. A comparison of antiarrhythmic-drug therapy with implantable defibrillators in patients resuscitated from near-fatal ventricular arrhythmias. *N Engl J Med* 1997;337:1576–1583.

Antunes E, Brugada J, Steurer G, et al. The differential diagnosis of a regular tachycardia with a wide QRS complex on the 12-lead ECG: ventricular tachycardia, supraventricular tachycardia with aberrant intraventricular conduction, and supraventricular tachycardia with anterograde conduction over an accessory pathway. *PACE* 1994;17:1515–1524.

Buxton AE, Lee KL, DiCarlo L, et al. Electrophysiology testing to identify patients with coronary artery disease who are at risk for sudden death. *N Engl J Med* 2000;342:1937–1945.

Cairns JA, Connolly SJ, Roberts R, et al. Randomised trial of outcome after myocardial infarction in patients with frequent or repetitive ventricular premature depolarisations: CAMIAT. Canadian Amiodarone Myocardial Infarction Arrhythmia Trial Investigators. *Lancet* 1997;349:675–682. [Published erratum appears in *Lancet* 1997;349: 1776.]

Cardiac Arrhythmia Suppression Trial (CAST) Investigators. Preliminary report: effect of encainide and flecainide on mortality in a randomized trial of arrhythmia suppression after myocardial infarction. *N Engl J Med* 1989;321:406–412.

Cardiac Arrhythmia Suppression Trial II Investigators. Effect of the antiarrhythmic agent moricizine on survival after myocardial infarction. *N Engl J Med* 1992;327:207–233.

Chung MK, Martin DO, Sprecher D, et al. C-Reactive protein elevation in patients with atrial arrhythmias. Inflammatory mechanisms and persistence of atrial fibrillation. *Circulation* 2001;104:2886–2891.

Fontaine G, Fontaliran F, Lascault G, et al. In: Zipes DP, Jalife J, eds. *Cardiac electrophysiology: from cell to bedside,* 2nd ed. Philadelphia: WB Saunders, 1995:754–768.

Julian DG, Camm AJ, Frangin G, et al. Randomised trial of effect of amiodarone on mortality in patients with left-ventricular dysfunction after recent myocardial infarction: EMIAT. European Myocardial Infarct Amiodarone Trial Investigators. *Lancet* 1997;349:667–674. [Published errata appear in *Lancet* 1997;349:1180 and 1997;349: 1776.]

Klein AL, Grimm RA, Black IW, et al. Cardioversion guided by transesophageal echocardiography: the ACUTE pilot study. *Ann Intern Med* 1997;126:200–209.

Klein AL, Grimm RA, Murray DR, et al. Use of transesophageal echocardiography to guide cardioversion in patients with atrial fibrillation. *N Engl J Med* 2001;344:1411–1420.

Mason JW. A comparison of seven antiarrhythmic drugs in patients with ventricular tachyarrhythmias. Electrophysiologic Study versus Electrocardiographic Monitoring Investigators. *N Engl J Med* 1993;329:452–458.

Moss AJ, Hall WJ, Cannom DS, et al. Improved survival with an implanted defibrillator in patients with coronary disease at high risk for ventricular arrhythmia. Multicenter Automatic Defibrillator Implantation Trial Investigators. *N Engl J Med* 1996;335:1933–1940.

O'Keefe JH, Hammill SC, Freed M. *The complete guide to ECGs,* 2nd ed. Royal Oak, MI: Physicians Press, 2002.

Wellens HJ. Contemporary management of atrial flutter. *Circulation* 2002;106:649–652.

Wolf PA, Abbott RD, Kannel WB. Atrial fibrillation as an independent risk factor for stroke: the Framingham study. *Stroke* 1991;22:983–988.

Zipes DP, et al. In: Braunwald E, ed. *Braunwald's heart disease: a textbook of cardiovascular medicine,* 8th ed. Philadelphia: Saunders Elsevier, 2008.

BRADYARRHYTHMIAS, ATRIOVENTRICULAR BLOCK, ASYSTOLE, AND PULSELESS ELECTRICAL ACTIVITY 21

Gregory G. Bashian and Oussama Wazni

I. INTRODUCTION. Bradyarrhythmias and **conduction blocks** are common electrocardiographic findings. Many of these arrhythmias are asymptomatic and do not require specific therapy, whereas others can be life threatening, requiring rapid intervention. **Myocardial ischemia** is an important cause of acute and potentially dangerous bradyarrhythmia.

II. ANATOMY

A. Sinoatrial node. The sinus beat originates in the **sinoatrial node,** a focus of automatic cells near the junction of the superior vena cava and right atrium.

1. The blood supply to the sinoatrial node is from the **sinus node artery,** which arises from the proximal **right coronary artery** in 55% of the population (Fig. 21.1) and from the **circumflex artery** in 35%. The sinoatrial node receives a dual supply of blood from both the right coronary artery and the circumflex artery in 10% of the population.
2. The automaticity of the sinoatrial node is affected by both the parasympathetic and sympathetic nervous systems. If the sinoatrial node fails to generate an impulse, other foci in the atrium, atrioventricular node, or ventricle can act as "backup" pacemaker sites.

B. Atrioventricular node. The atrioventricular node is located in the anteromedial portion of the right atrium just anterior to the coronary sinus.

1. The impulse generated by the sinoatrial node progresses through the atrium to the atrioventricular node. The atrioventricular node is also innervated by both the parasympathetic and sympathetic nervous systems.

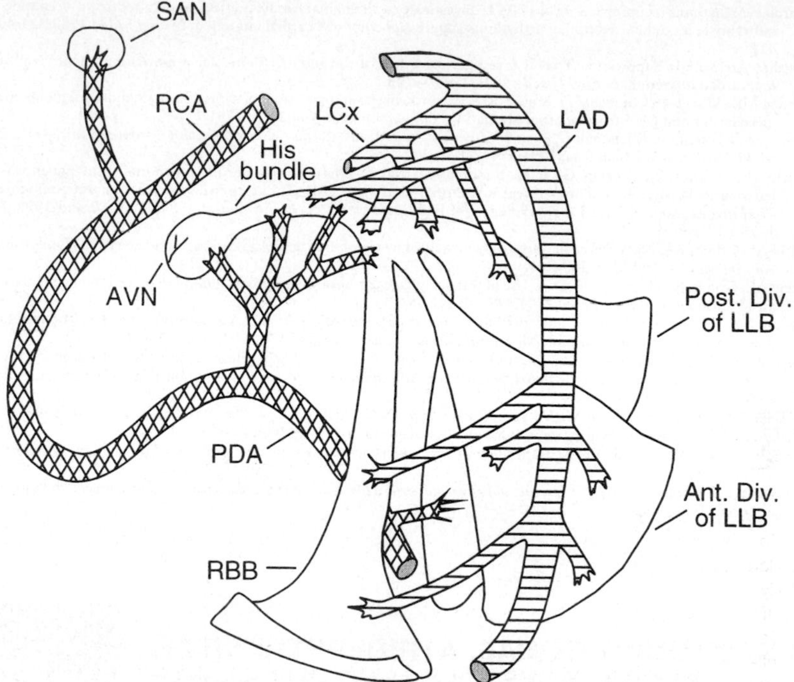

Figure 21.1. Diagrammatic representation of the conduction system and its blood supply.

2. The atrioventricular node receives its blood supply from the atrioventricular node artery, which arises from the posterior descending artery in 80% of the population (Fig. 21.1), from the circumflex artery in 10%, and from both arteries in 10%.
3. Collateral blood supply from the left anterior descending artery makes the atrioventricular node somewhat less prone to ischemic damage than the sinoatrial node.

C. His bundle and bundle branches

1. After a delay of less than 200 ms in the atrioventricular node, the electrical impulse is propagated down the His bundle to the right and left bundle branches. The **left bundle branch splits further into anterior and posterior fascicles.** The autonomic nervous system does not have a major effect on conduction below the atrioventricular node.
2. The **His bundle and right bundle branch** receive their blood supply from the atrioventricular node artery and from septal penetrating branches of the left anterior descending artery. The anterior fascicle of the **left bundle branch** receives blood from the septal perforating branches of the left anterior descending artery. The posterior fascicle has a dual blood supply from the septal perforating branches of the left anterior descending artery and branches of the posterior descending artery.

III. SINUS NODE DYSFUNCTION. Sinus node dysfunction encompasses any dysfunction of the sinus node and includes **inappropriate sinus bradycardia, sinoatrial exit block, sinoatrial arrest,** and **tachycardia–bradycardia syndrome.**

A. Clinical presentation. There is a wide range of presentations, and some patients' disease may be asymptomatic.

1. Syncope and **presyncope** are the most dramatic presenting symptoms. **Fatigue, angina,** and **shortness of breath** are more subtle consequences of sinus node dysfunction.
2. In the tachycardia–bradycardia syndrome, the primary complaint may be palpitation. Documentation of the arrhythmia may be difficult because of the sporadic and fleeting nature of the problem.

B. Etiology. The intrinsic and extrinsic causes of sinus node dysfunction are listed in Table 21.1. **Idiopathic degenerative disease** is the most common cause of intrinsic sinus node dysfunction, and the incidence increases with age. **Acute coronary syndromes** are a common cause of bradyarrhythmias, occurring in 25% to 30% of patients with myocardial infarction (MI) (Table 21.2).

C. Electrocardiographic findings

1. Inappropriate sinus bradycardia is defined as a sinus rate of less than 60 beats/min that does not increase appropriately with exercise. Inappropriate

TABLE 21.1 Etiologies of sinus node dysfunction

INTRINSIC CAUSES
Idiopathic degenerative disease
Coronary artery disease
Cardiomyopathy
Hypertension
Infiltrative disorders (amyloidosis, hemochromatosis, tumors)
Collagen vascular disease (scleroderma, systemic lupus erythematosus)
Inflammatory processes (myocarditis, pericarditis)
Surgical trauma (valve surgery, transplantation)
Musculoskeletal disorders (myotonic dystrophy, Friedreich's ataxia)
Congenital heart disease (postoperative or in the absence of surgical correction)

EXTRINSIC CAUSES
Drug effects
- β-Blocking agents
- Calcium channel blocking agents
- Digoxin
- Sympatholytic antihypertensives (clonidine, methyldopa, reserpine)
- Antiarrhythmic drugs
  - Type IA (quinidine, procainamide, disopyramide)
  - Type IC (flecainide, propafenone)
  - Type III (sotalol, amiodarone)
- Others (lithium, cimetidine, amitriptyline, phenytoin)

Autonomic influences
- Excessive vagal tone
- Carotid sinus syndrome
- Vasovagal syncope
- Well-trained athletes (normal variant, not dysfunction)

Electrolyte abnormalities
- Hyperkalemia
- Hypercarbia
- Endocrine disorders—hypothyroidism

Increased intracranial pressure
Hypothermia
Sepsis

From Topol EJ, ed. *Textbook of cardiovascular medicine.* Philadelphia: Lippincott–Raven, 1998, with permission.

TABLE 21.2 Incidence of Bradyarrhythmia in the Setting of Acute Myocardial Infarction

Rhythm	Incidence (%)
Sinus bradycardia	25
Junctional escape rhythm	20
Idioventricular escape rhythm	15
First-degree AV block	15
Second-degree, Mobitz type I AV block	12
Second-degree, Mobitz type II AV block	4
Third-degree AV block	15
Right bundle-branch block	7
Left bundle-branch block	5
Left anterior fascicular block	8
Left posterior fascicular block	0.5

AV, atrioventricular.

sinus bradycardia must be differentiated from a low resting heart rate, which may be normal in athletes and sleeping individuals.

2. Sinus arrest, or sinus pause, occurs when the sinus node fails to depolarize on time. Pauses of less than 3 seconds may be seen on Holter monitoring in up to 11% of normal adults (especially athletes) and are not a cause for concern. However, **pauses lasting longer than 3 seconds are generally considered abnormal and are suggestive of an underlying abnormality.**
3. Sinoatrial exit block, although similar to sinus arrest on the electrocardiographic tracing, may be distinguished by the fact that the **duration of the pause is a multiple of the sinus PP** interval. High-grade sinoatrial exit block cannot be differentiated from prolonged sinus arrest and is treated in the same manner.
4. Tachycardia–bradycardia syndrome, also referred to as "sick sinus syndrome," is characterized by episodes of sinus or junctional bradycardia interspersed with an atrial tachycardia, usually paroxysmal atrial fibrillation.

D. Diagnostic testing. Invasive testing is used when noninvasive methods have failed to yield a diagnosis and sinus node dysfunction is still strongly suspected.

1. Noninvasive testing

a. Electrocardiogram (ECG). In evaluating sinus node dysfunction, the initial workup should include a 12-lead ECG, followed by 24- to 48-hour ambulatory ECG monitoring, if necessary. Use of a diary during the recording period can help to correlate symptoms with the cardiac rhythm. For less frequent events, a loop recorder or event recorder may be used to assess symptoms over a 2- to 4-week period. Stress testing can help document the severity of chronotropic incompetence.

b. Autonomic testing includes physical maneuvers, such as carotid sinus massage and tilt-table testing, as well as pharmacologic interventions to test the autonomic reflexes.

(1) Carotid sinus massage distinguishes intrinsic sinus pause/sinus arrest from a pause due to **carotid sinus hypersensitivity,** which is a 3-second or longer pause and/or a $\geq$50 mm Hg or greater drop in blood pressure that occurs with massage of the carotid sinus (firm pressure applied to one carotid sinus at a time for 5 seconds). **Carotid sinus massage should not normally precipitate sinus pause/sinus arrest,** although it will decrease the rate of depolarization of the sinoatrial node and slow conduction in the atrioventricular node.

(2) Tilt-table testing may help to differentiate between syncope caused by sinus node dysfunction and that due to autonomic dysfunction.

Bradycardic episodes precipitated by tilt-table testing are usually caused by autonomic dysfunction and not sinus node dysfunction.

(3) Pharmacologic testing may be used to differentiate between sinus node dysfunction and autonomic dysfunction. Total autonomic blockade is achieved after administration of atropine 0.04 mg/kg and propranolol 0.2 mg/kg. The resulting intrinsic heart rate represents the sinus node rate, devoid of autonomic influences. Assuming that the normal intrinsic heart rate (in beats per minute) is defined by the formula:

$$\text{Intrinsic heart rate} = 118.1 - (0.57 \times \text{age})$$

then an intrinsic heart rate lower than predicted using this formula is consistent with sinus node dysfunction; an intrinsic heart rate close to the predicted rate in a patient with a clinical presentation of sinus node dysfunction is suggestive of an autonomic dysfunction as a cause of the bradyarrhythmia.

2. Invasive testing. The two most common tests use indirect measurements of sinoatrial node function. Direct measurement of sinoatrial node function is laborious and rarely performed.

a. Sinus node recovery time is the time it takes the sinoatrial node to recover following paced overdrive suppression of the node.

(1) **A delay of longer than 1400 ms is considered abnormal.** This measurement may be corrected by subtracting the intrinsic sinus cycle length (in milliseconds) from the recovery time. **A corrected sinus node recovery time of greater than 550 ms is suggestive of sinus node dysfunction.**

(2) The limitations of this test are:

(a) It is an indirect measurement of sinoatrial node function and reflects both sinoatrial node conduction time (SACT) and automaticity.

(b) It may be falsely shortened by sinoatrial node entrance block during atrial pacing (due to failure of the paced impulse to reset the sinus node) or falsely prolonged by a sinoatrial node exit block (the sinus node is normal but the impulse cannot leave the node).

(c) The sinus node recovery time is not prolonged in all patients with sinus node dysfunction.

b. SACT

(1) The steady-state atrial rate is determined (A_1–A_1 interval or the time between P waves). Then premature atrial **extra stimuli** (A_2) are introduced by pacing high in the right atrium, starting in late diastole at progressively shorter intervals until atrial refractoriness is found (i.e., A_2 does not result in a P wave). The duration before the next spontaneous atrial impulse (A_3) is measured and the baseline rate is subtracted.

$$\text{SACT} = (A_2 - A_3 \text{ interval}) - (A_1 - A_1 \text{ interval})$$

(2) The test assumes that sinoatrial node automaticity is not affected by pacing, that conduction time into the node is equal to conduction time out of the node, and that there is no shift in the principal pacemaker site.

E. Therapy. Treatment for symptomatic sinus node dysfunction may be pharmacologic, pacing, or a combination of both.

1. Indications for pacing in sinus node dysfunction are determined by symptoms (e.g., correlation with a documented arrhythmia; Table 21.3). Another common indication is when drug therapy that causes sinus node dysfunction cannot be stopped or changed.

2. Medications that suppress sinus node automaticity should be stopped if possible. If this is not possible, it may be necessary to place a temporary or permanent pacemaker (Table 21.3).

3. For patients with **tachycardia–bradycardia syndrome,** a pacemaker is often placed for management of the bradyarrhythmia, and antiarrhythmic drugs are added for treatment of the tachycardic episodes.

TABLE 21.3 Indications for permanent pacing

Indication	Class I	Class II	Class III
SND	1. SND documented in association with symptomatic bradycardia and due to factors that are irreversible, or due to essential drug therapy. 2. Symptomatic chronotropic incompetence.	IIa. No clear association between SND with heart rate <40 bpm and symptoms can be documented. IIb. In minimally symptomatic patients, chronic heart rate <30 bpm while awake.	1. SND with marked sinus bradycardia or pauses, but no associated symptoms including that due to long-term drug therapy. 2. SND in patients with symptoms suggestive of bradycardia that are clearly documented as not associated with a slow heart rate. 3. SND with symptomatic bradycardia due to nonessential drug therapy.
Acquired AV block	1. Third-degree AV block at any anatomic level, associated with any one of the following conditions: a. Bradycardia with symptoms presumed to be due to AV block b. Arrhythmias and other medical conditions that require drugs that result in symptomatic bradycardia. c. Documented periods of asystole ≥3.0 s or any escape rate <40 bpm in awake, symptom-free individuals. d. After catheter ablation of the AV junction. e. Postoperative AV block that is not expected to resolve. f. Neuromuscular diseases with AV block such as myotonic muscular dystrophy, Kearns-Sayre syndrome, Erb's dystrophy (limb girdle), and peroneal muscular dystrophy. 2. Second-degree AV block regardless of type or site of block, with associated symptomatic bradycardia.	IIa. 1. Asymptomatic third-degree AV block at any anatomic site with average awake ventricular rates ≥40 bpm. 2. Asymptomatic type II second-degree AV block. 3. Asymptomatic type I second-degree AV block at intra-His or infra-His levels found incidentally at EP study performed for other indications. 4. One-degree AV block with symptoms suggestive of pacemaker syndrome and documented alleviation of symptoms with temporary AV pacing. IIb. 1. Marked first-degree AV block (>0.30 s) in patients with LV dysfunction and symptoms of congestive heart failure in whom shorter AV interval results in hemodynamic improvement, presumably by decreasing left atrial filling pressure.	1. Asymptomatic one-degree AV block. 2. Asymptomatic type I second-degree AV block at the supra-His (AV node) level or not known to be intra- or infra-hisian. 3. AV block expected to resolve and unlikely to recur (e.g., drug toxicity, Lyme disease).

Postmyocardial infarction	1. Persistent second-degree AV block in the His-Purkinje system with bilateral bundle-branch block or third-degree AV block within or below the His-Purkinje system after acute myocardial infarction. 2. Transient advanced (second- or third-degree) infranodal AV block and associated bundle branch block. If the site of block is uncertain, an EP study may be necessary. 3. Persistent and symptomatic second- or third-degree AV block.	IIa. None IIb. 1. Persistent second- or third-degree AV block at the AV node level.	1. Transient AV block without intraventricular conduction defect. 2. Transient AV block in the presence of isolated left anterior fascicular block. 3. Acquired left anterior fascicular block in the absence of AV block. 4. Persistent first-degree AV block in the presence of bundle-branch block that is old or age indeterminate.
Chronic bifascicular and trifascicular block	1. Intermittent third-degree AV block. 2. Type II second-degree AV block.	IIa. 1. Syncope not proved to be due to AV block when other likely causes have been excluded, specifically ventricular tachycardia. 2. HV interval >100 ms. 3. Pacing induced block below the His that is not physiologic. IIb. None	1. Fascicular block without AV block or symptoms. 2. Fascicular block with first-degree AV block without symptoms.
Carotid sinus hypersensitivity (carotid sinus irritability) and neurally mediated syncope	1. Recurrent syncope caused by carotid sinus stimulation; minimal carotid sinus pressure induces ventricular asystole of >3 s duration in the absence of any medication that depresses the sinus node or AV conduction.	IIa. 1. Recurrent syncope without clear, provocative events and with a hypersensitive cardioinhibitory response. 2. Syncope of unexplained origin when major abnormalities of sinus node function or AV conduction are discovered or provoked in EP studies. IIb. 1. Neurally mediated syncope with significant bradycardia reproduced by a head-up tilt with or without isoproterenol and other provocative maneuvers.	1. A hyperactive cardioinhibitory response to carotid sinus stimulation in the absence of symptoms. 2. A hyperactive cardioinhibitory response to carotid sinus stimulation in the absence of symptoms. A hyperactive cardioinhibitory response to carotid sinus stimulation in the presence of vague symptoms such as dizziness, light-headedness, or both. 3. Recurrent syncope, light-headedness, or dizziness in the absence of a hyperactive cardioinhibitory response. 4. Situational vasovagal syncope in which avoidance behavior is effective.

Class I: Conditions for which there is evidence and/or general agreement that pacing is beneficial, useful, and effective.
Class II: Conditions for which there is conflicting evidence and/or a divergence of opinion about the usefulness/efficacy of pacing.
IIa: Weight of evidence/opinion is in favor of usefulness/efficacy.
IIb: Usefulness/efficacy is less well established by evidence/opinion.
Class III: Conditions for which there is evidence and or general agreement that pacing is not useful/effective and in some cases may be harmful.
SND, Sinus node dysfunction; AV, atrioventricular; LV, left ventricular; EP, electrophysiologic; HV, half-value.
Adapted from Gregoratos G, Chetlin MD, Conill A, et al. ACC/AHA guidelines for implantation of cardiac pacemakers and antiarrhythmia devices: a report of the American College of Cardiology/American Heart Association Task Force on Practice Guidelines (Committee on Pacemaker Implantation). *J Am Coll Cardiol* 1998;31:1175–1209.

4. Acute treatment for patients with **symptomatic sinus node dysfunction** includes:
   a. Atropine (0.04 mg/kg intravenous bolus).
   b. Temporary pacing for patients whose conditions fail to respond to drug therapy.
   c. Isoproterenol (starting at 1 μg/min intravenously), which may be used as a bridge to pacemaker placement. Isoproterenol is not indicated in most patients with cardiac arrest.

IV. **ATRIOVENTRICULAR CONDUCTION DISTURBANCES.** These disturbances are classified as first-, second-, or third-degree block, depending on the severity of the conduction abnormality.

A. **Classification**

1. First-degree atrioventricular block is characterized by prolongation of the PR interval beyond 200 ms. This finding may occur as a normal variant in 0.5% of asymptomatic young adults without overt heart disease. In older individuals, it is most often caused by idiopathic degenerative disease of the conducting system.
2. **Second-degree atrioventricular block**
   a. Second-degree atrioventricular block is characterized by **a failure of one or more, but not all, atrial impulses to conduct to the ventricles.** The block may be at any level of the atrioventricular conduction system.
   b. When more than one atrial impulse is present for each ventricular complex, the rhythm may be described as a ratio of the number of atrial impulses to the number of ventricular complexes (for three P waves preceding each QRS complex, 3:1 second-degree atrioventricular block is present).
      (1) Lesser degrees of atrioventricular block (i.e., 4:3 or 3:2) with a variable PR interval (typically prolonging) prior to a nonconducted atrial impulse are described as **Mobitz type I atrioventricular block** (also known as Wenckebach block).
         (a) The conducted impulse of a **Mobitz type I block** will generally be narrow, and the site of block is often in the atrioventricular node above the His bundle.
         (b) A Mobitz type I block with a bundle-branch block is still likely to be above the His bundle, but a His-bundle electrocardiogram is needed to confirm the level of block.
      (2) High-grade atrioventricular block (3:1, 4:1, or greater) is typically described as **Mobitz type II atrioventricular block.** The conducted impulses will generally be preceded by constant PR intervals and have a wide QRS morphology [right bundle-branch block (RBBB) or left bundle-branch block (LBBB) pattern]. The site of block often is below the atrioventricular node. A **Mobitz type II block** is usually intra- or infra-hisian and has a greater propensity for progressing to third-degree atrioventricular block.
      (3) Pure 2:1 conduction patterns cannot be reliably classified as Mobitz type I or type II.
3. Third-degree atrioventricular block, or **complete heart block,** may be acquired or congenital.
   a. Of patients with **congenital complete heart block,** 60% are female. Of children with congenital complete heart block, 30% to 50% of their mothers have connective tissue disease, usually systemic lupus erythematosus.
   b. Acquired atrioventricular block occurs most frequently in the seventh decade and more commonly affects males.

B. **Clinical presentation**

1. **Signs and symptoms**
   a. First-degree atrioventricular block is generally not a cause of symptoms.
   b. Second-degree atrioventricular block seldom results in symptoms, although high-grade second-degree atrioventricular block may progress to third-degree atrioventricular block, which can cause symptoms.
   c. Depending on the ventricular escape rate, patients with **third-degree atrioventricular block** may experience **fatigue** or **syncope.**

2. **Physical findings.** The amplitude of the arterial pulse and venous waveform varies, depending on the timing of atrial filling of the ventricles.
   a. Second-degree atrioventricular block is associated with a periodic change in amplitude. In patients with **third-degree atrioventricular block,** amplitude is constantly changing, for example, periodic appearance of cannon *a* waves (large-amplitude waves in the venous pulsations seen in the neck when the atria contracts against a closed tricuspid valve).
   b. Heart sounds are similarly affected by the change in filling duration of the ventricles.
      (1) **The first heart sound** (S_1) becomes softer as the PR interval is prolonged, resulting in a soft S_1 in first-degree atrioventricular block, a progressive softening of S_1 in type I second-degree atrioventricular block, and a constantly changing S_1 in third-degree atrioventricular block.
      (2) Third-degree atrioventricular block may also result in a functional systolic ejection murmur.

C. **Etiology.** The causes of atrioventricular block are listed in Table 21.4; the most common is **idiopathic fibrosis. Acute MI** results in atrioventricular block in 14% of patients with inferior infarction and 2% of those with anterior infarction, usually within the first 24 hours.

D. **Diagnostic testing**
   1. **First-degree atrioventricular block.** Measuring a PR interval longer than 200 ms in adults and 180 ms in children makes the diagnosis. A P wave precedes each QRS, and both the P and QRS are morphologically normal.
   2. **Second-degree atrioventricular block**
      a. The diagnosis of **Mobitz type I** is made when the following criteria are met on the ECG:
         (1) Sequential and gradual prolongation of the PR interval terminated by a nonconducted P wave
         (2) Prolongation of the PR interval occurring in progressively shorter increments in “typical” Wenckebach, which results in progressive shortening of the RR intervals prior to the nonconducted atrial impulse.
         (3) Duration of the pause following the nonconducted P wave is less than the sum of any two consecutively conducted beats
         (4) Decreased PR interval following the pause when compared to the prepause PR interval
         (5) “Grouped beating,” a pattern of repeated groups of QRS complexes characteristic of Wenckebach block
      b. Mobitz type II second-degree atrioventricular block is less common than type I.
         (1) The PR interval is constant with a sudden nonconducted P wave (Fig. 21.2), in contrast to nonconducted premature atrial contractions, which have a varying PR interval.
         (2) Each QRS complex may have multiple P waves, which are designated by the number of P waves before each conducted QRS (3:1, 4:1, etc.). The QRS complex typically is not narrow (a narrow QRS complex is suggestive of a Mobitz type I block).
   3. **Third-degree atrioventricular block** (Fig. 21.3)
      a. Third-degree atrioventricular block is characterized by identification of **complete dissociation of the atrial and ventricular electrical activity** (no temporal relationship exists between the P waves and the QRS complexes) with atrial activity more rapid than ventricular activity. Using calipers, it is possible to march out the progression of the P waves to determine the atrial rate.
      b. Third-degree atrioventricular block is only one cause of atrioventricular dissociation; **not all atrioventricular dissociation is third-degree atrioventricular block.**

E. **Therapy.** Patients with first-degree and Mobitz type I atrioventricular block usually do not require therapy. Permanent pacing is indicated for Mobitz type II

TABLE 21.4 Causes of atrioventricular block

- Drug effects
  - Digoxin
  - β-Blockers
  - Certain calcium channel blockers (non-dihydropyridines)
  - Membrane-active antiarrhythmic drugs
- Ischemic heart disease
  - Acute myocardial infarction
  - Chronic coronary artery disease
- Idiopathic fibrosis of the conduction system
  - Lenegre's disease
  - Lev's disease
- Congenital heart disease
  - Congenital complete heart block
  - Ostium primum atrial septal defect
  - Transposition of the great vessels
  - Maternal systemic lupus erythematosus
- Calcific valvular disease
- Cardiomyopathy
- Infiltrative disease
  - Amyloidosis
  - Sarcoidosis
  - Hemochromatosis
- Infectious/inflammatory diseases
  - Endocarditis
  - Myocarditis (Chagas' disease, Lyme disease, rheumatic fever, tuberculosis, measles, mumps)
- Collagen vascular diseases (scleroderma, rheumatoid arthritis, Reiter's syndrome, systemic lupus erythematosis, ankylosing spondylitis, polymyositis)
- Metabolic
  - Hyperkalemia
  - Hypermagnesemia
- Endocrine—Addison's disease
- Trauma
  - Cardiac surgery
  - Radiation
  - Catheter trauma
  - Catheter ablation
- Tumors
  - Mesothelioma
  - Hodgkin's disease
  - Malignant melanoma
  - Rhabdomyosarcoma
- Neurally mediated
  - Carotid sinus syndrome
  - Vasovagal syncope
- Neuromyopathic disorders
  - Myotonic muscular dystrophy
  - Slowly progressive X-linked muscular dystrophy

From Topol EJ, ed. *Textbook of cardiovascular medicine*. Philadelphia: Lippincott–Raven, 1998, with permission.

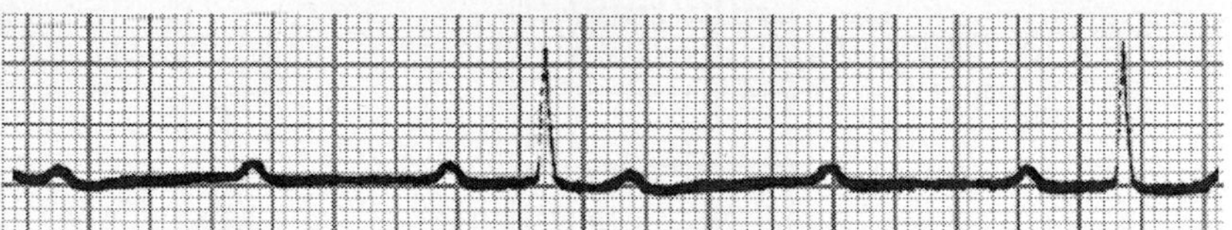

Figure 21.2. Mobitz type II second-degree atrioventricular block with 3:1 conduction.

atrioventricular block and third-degree atrioventricular block. See Table 21.3 for complete indications for pacing.)

1. Medical therapy may be used as a bridge to pacing but has no role in long-term treatment.
   a. The principal drug used as a bridge to pacing is **atropine,** which:
      (1) Reduces heart block due to hypervagotonia but not due to atrioventricular node ischemia
      (2) Is more useful for atrioventricular block in inferior MI than anterior MI
      (3) Does not increase infranodal conduction (will not improve third-degree atrioventricular block or second-degree atrioventricular block that is below the atrioventricular node)
      (4) Is ineffective in the denervated hearts of transplantation patients
      (5) Is used with caution (if at all) in Mobitz type II atrioventricular block due to a possible paradoxical decrease in heart rate (as atrial rate increases, atrioventricular conduction decreases, and a 2:1 block with an atrial rate of 80 and a ventricular rate of 40 may be converted to a 3:1 block with an atrial rate of 90 and a ventricular rate of 30)
   b. Digoxin-specific Fab fragments may be used to treat patients with symptomatic atrioventricular blocks related to use of digitalis. The number of vials = weight (kg) × digoxin serum concentration (ng/mL) ÷ 100.
2. **Pacing**
   a. Third-degree atrioventricular block as a complication of inferior MI is usually temporary, and thus usually only requires **temporary pacing.**
   b. However, complete heart block as a result of anterior MI often requires **permanent pacing** (Table 21.3).
   c. Acquired third-degree atrioventricular block usually requires pacing, but patients with congenital third-degree atrioventricular block often have a sufficiently rapid escape rhythm to prevent symptoms and avoid permanent pacemaker implantation.

V. JUNCTIONAL RHYTHMS. Junctional rhythms arise from the area surrounding the atrioventricular node, including the approaches to the node, the node itself, and the bundle of His. This area has an intrinsic rate of 30 to 60 beats/min and serves as an escape mechanism to prevent ventricular asystole in case of complete atrioventricular block. Junctional rhythm that is faster than the sinus rhythm is referred to as **accelerated junctional rhythm.**

A. Clinical presentation. Patients usually do not develop symptoms directly attributable to accelerated junctional rhythm. The **physical findings of atrioventricular dissociation may be noted** and are the same as those seen in third-degree atrioventricular block.

B. Etiology

1. Accelerated junctional rhythm is seen in approximately **10% of patients with acute MI.** More than one-half of these patients have inferior MI and about one-third have anterior infarctions.
2. Digitalis toxicity by itself does not seem to cause accelerated junctional rhythm, as evidenced in persons with normal hearts who take accidental overdoses of digoxin. **Concomitant heart disease** is required to develop accelerated junctional rhythm.

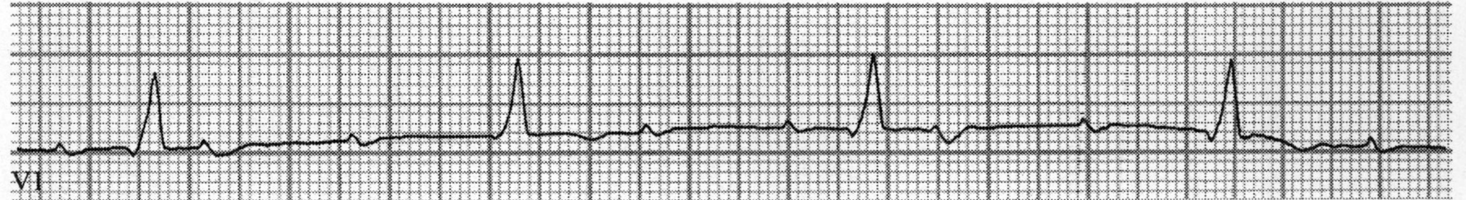

Figure 21.3. Third-degree atrioventricular block with sinus tachycardia and right bundle-branch block.

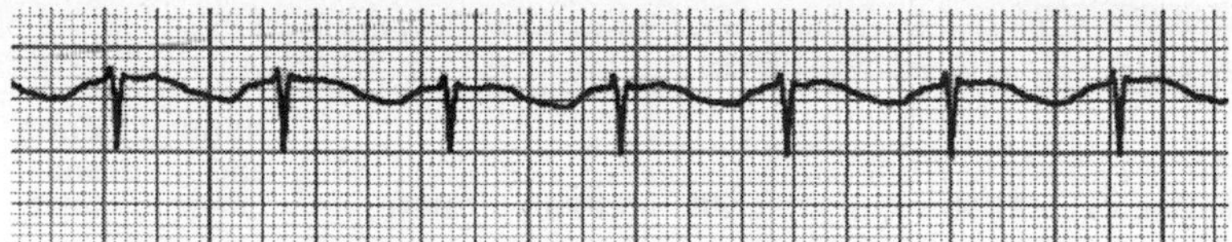

Figure 21.4. Accelerated junctional rhythm.

3. Other causes of accelerated junctional rhythm are valve surgery, acute rheumatic fever, direct current cardioversion, cardiac catheterization, serious infection, chronic obstructive pulmonary disease, systemic amyloidosis, and uremia with hyperkalemia.

C. ECG findings

1. **Accelerated junctional rhythm**
   a. **Unless the junctional rhythm causes retrograde activation of the atria,** the P wave is normal in morphologic characteristics. The QRS complex has a normal duration, unless there is concomitant bundle-branch block. The distinguishing characteristic of accelerated junctional rhythm is the atrioventricular dissociation and changing PR interval (Fig. 21.4).
   b. **The difference between accelerated junctional rhythm and third-degree atrioventricular block is the fact that the ventricular rate is faster than the atrial rate in accelerated junctional rhythm and slower than the atrial rate in third-degree atrioventricular block.**
2. **Junctional rhythm.** In the absence of a sinus beat, the atrioventricular node can act as a back-up pacemaker. The ECG findings are an absence of P waves (or retrograde P waves immediately before or after the QRS complex), a narrow QRS complex, and a rate of 30 to 60 beats/min.

D. Therapy

1. Therapy for junctional rhythm secondary to sinoatrial node failure or atrioventricular block is as previously outlined for atrioventricular conduction disturbances.
2. Patients with accelerated junctional rhythm do not usually require therapy for the arrhythmia, although management of the underlying cause is indicated.
3. Suppression of accelerated junctional rhythm may be achieved by **increasing the atrial rate with drugs** (e.g., atropine, adrenergics, and so forth) or **pacing.**
4. Digoxin-induced accelerated junctional rhythm is an indication to stop digoxin but does not usually require administration of digoxin-specific Fab fragments.

VI. INTRAVENTRICULAR CONDUCTION DISTURBANCES. Conduction disturbances due to block below the atrioventricular node are classified on the basis of the intraventricular conduction system. An intraventricular conduction disturbance does not itself cause bradyarrhythmia, but it may be associated with any of the other rhythms that cause bradycardia. When associated with an acute MI, an intraventricular conduction disturbance predicts a worse outcome.

A. Etiology

1. The causes of intraventricular conduction disturbances are similar to those that cause atrioventricular block (Table 21.4); **idiopathic degenerative conduction disease** and **acute ischemic syndromes** are the most common causes.
2. Intraventricular conduction disturbances increase with age and affect up to 2% of individuals older than age 60 years.
3. The incidence of intraventricular conduction disturbances is increased in persons with structural heart disease, especially those with coronary artery disease.

B. ECG findings

1. The ECG findings of intraventricular conduction disturbances are summarized in Table 21.5, and examples are presented in Figs. 21.5 to 21.8 As shown,

TABLE 21.5 **Electrocardiographic features for the fascicular and bifascicular blocks**

ECG Finding	LBBB	LAFB	LPFB	RBBB	RBBB and LAFB	RBBB and LPFB
QRS axis		≥–45°	+90° to +120°		–60° to –120°	≥ +120°
QRS duration	≥120 ms	Normal	Normal	≥120 ms	≥120 ms	≥120 ms
Leads I/aVL	Broad monophasic R	qR	rS	qRS with wide terminal S	qR	rS
Leads II, III, aVF		rS	qR		rS	qR
Leads VI and V2	rS or QS			rsR′ or rSR′	rsR′ or rSR′	rsR′ or rSR′
Leads V5 and V6		S	no Q's	qRS		

ECG, electrocardiography; LAFB, left anterior fascicular block; LBBB, left bundle-branch block; LPFB, left posterior fascicular block; RBBB, right bundle-branch block.

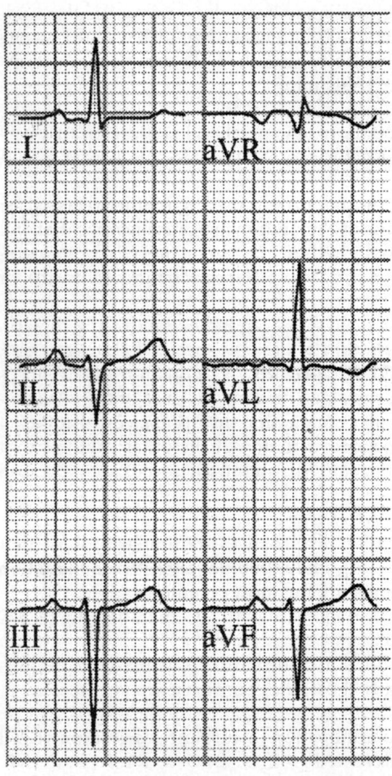

Figure 21.5. Left anterior hemiblock.

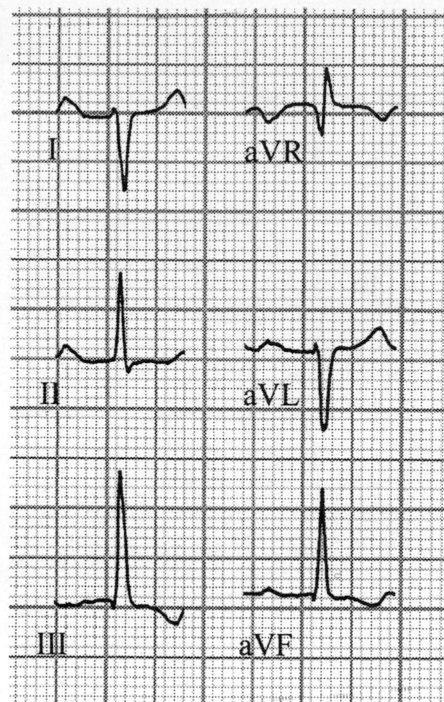

Figure 21.6. Left posterior hemiblock.

intraventricular conduction disturbances may be further classified by the number of fascicles they affect.

2. **Fascicular blocks**
   a. Unifascicular blocks affect only one of the three fascicles. Examples are RBBB, left anterior fascicular block, and left posterior fascicular block.
   b. Bifascicular block is present when conduction disturbances affect two of the fascicles, most commonly the right bundle branch and the left anterior fascicle. Approximately 6% of these patients progress to complete heart block. RBBB with left posterior fascicular block is less common, but the progression to complete heart block is more common.
   c. Trifascicular block is said to be present when there is a combination of bifascicular block and first-degree atrioventricular block (Fig. 21.8).

C. **Therapy.** Pacing is indicated in patients with bifascicular block who have intermittent symptomatic complete heart block and in patients with bifascicular or trifascicular block with asymptomatic intermittent Mobitz type II atrioventricular block (Table 21.3).

VII. POSTSURGICAL BRADYARRHYTHMIAS

A. **Etiology.** Bradyarrhythmias following cardiac surgery are common.
   1. Valvular surgery and septal myectomy can cause mechanical damage to the conduction system, leading to atrioventricular blocks and intraventricular conduction disturbances.
   2. Prolonged ischemic time during cardiac transplantation can lead to sinus node damage.

B. **Therapy.** Because postsurgical bradyarrhythmias may be only temporary, the decision to proceed to **permanent pacing** should be made after 5 to 7 days. The same criteria listed in Table 21.3 are used to determine the need for a pacemaker.

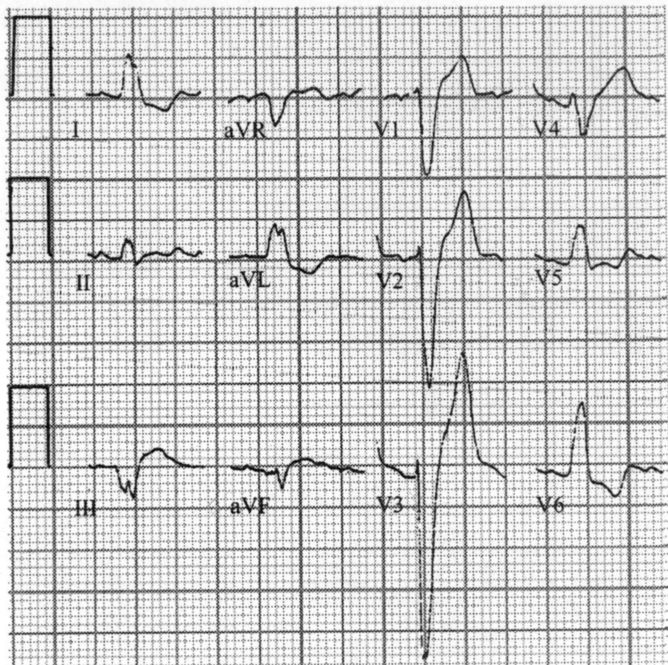

Figure 21.7. Left bundle-branch block.

Permanent pacing is required in 2% to 3% of patients following valve surgery and in upward of 10% of transplantation patients.

VIII. PULSELESS ELECTRICAL ACTIVITY. Pulseless electrical activity is defined as the absence of a pulse or blood pressure measured by usual methods, with the continued presence of electrical activity of the heart.

A. Etiology

1. Pulseless electrical activity may result from a variety of **rhythm disturbances,** such as electrical mechanical dissociation, idioventricular rhythms, and

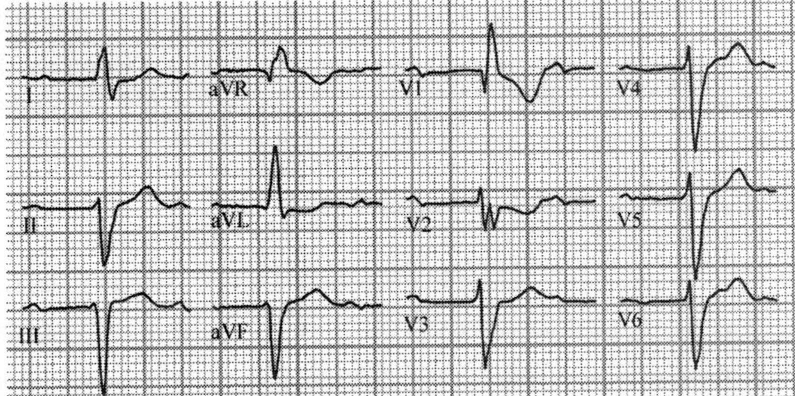

Figure 21.8. First-degree atrioventricular block with right bundle-branch block and left anterior hemiblock.

ventricular tachycardias. When the electrical activity is organized and within the physiologic range, the term **electrical mechanical dissociation** is used.

2. A variety of clinical situations are also associated with pulseless electrical activity, a potentially manageable condition if certain actions are undertaken rapidly (Table 21.6).

B. Therapy

1. Specific management of the underlying cause is most likely to result in a successful outcome (Table 21.6).

2. Emergency intervention should be initiated at once, including:

a. Cardiopulmonary resuscitation and airway management with intubation to treat any possible hypoxia

b. Epinephrine, 1 mg intravenous push every 3 to 5 minutes

c. Atropine, 1 mg intravenously, if the rate is less than 60 beats/min; may be repeated every 3 to 5 minutes to a total dose of 0.03 to 0.04 mg/kg

d. Empiric intravenous volume infusion

TABLE 21.6 Conditions that cause pulseless electrical activity

Condition	Clues	Management
Hypovolemia	History, flat neck veins	Volume infusion
Hypoxia	Cyanosis, blood gases, airway problems	Ventilation
Cardiac tamponade	History (trauma, renal failure, malignancy), no pulse with CPR, vein distention; impending tamponade—tachycardia, hypotension, low pulse pressure	Pericardiocentesis
Tension pneumothorax	History (asthma, ventilator, chronic obstructive pulmonary disease, trauma), no pulse with CPR, neck-vein distention, tracheal deviation	Needle decompression
Hypothermia	History of exposure to cold, central body temperature, ECG	Gradual warming
Massive pulmonary embolism	History, no pulse felt with CPR	Pulmonary arteriogram, surgical embolectomy, thrombolytics
Drug overdose (tricyclics, digoxin, β-blockers, calcium channel blockers)	Bradycardia, history of ingestion, empty bottles at the scene, pupils, neurologic examination	Drug screens, intubation, lavage, activated charcoal, lactulose per local protocols
Hyperkalemia	History of renal failure, diabetes, recent dialysis, medications, ECG	Calcium chloride (immediate); then combination of insulin, glucose, sodium bicarbonate; then sodium polystyrene sulfonate/sorbitol; dialysis (long term)
Preexisting acidosis	Renal failure	Sodium bicarbonate, hyperventilation
Acute massive MI	History, ECG, enzymes	Treat for cardiogenic shock

CPR, cardiopulmonary resuscitation; ECG, electrocardiogram; MI, myocardial infarction.

IX. ASYSTOLE

A. Clinical presentation. Asystole is defined as the absence of myocardial electrical activity. It should be confirmed by switching between several leads or changing the position of the defibrillation paddles.

1. Most patients with asystole present in a code situation. Persons outside of the hospital who are found to have asystole by the initial responding team usually have it as a result of **profound myocardial ischemia.** The possibility of a successful outcome in this situation is extremely small.
2. Hospital inpatients monitored by telemetry, on the other hand, may have a favorable outcome.

B. Etiology. Asystole may be due to profound parasympathetic suppression of both atrial and ventricular activity, stunning of the myocardium due to electrical defibrillation, complete heart block, or prolonged myocardial ischemia.

C. Therapy. Management consists of **cardiopulmonary resuscitation, intubation,** and **atropine** to unmask the possibility of profound parasympathetic suppression of both atrial and ventricular activity.

1. Routine shocking is strongly discouraged. Electrical shocks have not been demonstrated to have any benefit in the management of asystole and may in fact produce a stunned myocardium, leading to a delay in the return of a rhythm.
2. Pacing for asystole is controversial. If pacing is to have any effect, it must be initiated early. Patients with asystole due to myocardial ischemia are unlikely to respond to pacing, but those with asystole due to other causes might respond.

X. CAROTID SINUS HYPERSENSITIVITY.

Carotid sinus hypersensitivity, defined as a sinus pause of 3 seconds or more and/or a drop in blood pressure of 50 mm Hg or more with carotid sinus massage, is common, affecting up to one-third of older men with coronary artery disease. Carotid sinus hypersensitivity may be purely cardioinhibitory, purely vasodepressive, or a combination of both. **Carotid sinus syndrome** is present when carotid sinus hypersensitivity is accompanied by syncope or near-syncope.

A. Etiology and pathophysiology

1. The **cause of carotid sinus hypersensitivity and carotid sinus syndrome is unknown.** It is more common in older individuals, particularly those with atherosclerotic disease. Carotid sinus syndrome may be precipitated by the patient stretching his or her neck (such as with shaving or turning the head) or wearing a tight collar, but often a precipitating event cannot be found.
2. Sites of potential lesions causing carotid sinus hypersensitivity are the sternocleidomastoid muscle, the central nervous system, and the feedback loops between the cardiovascular and central nervous systems.
3. It has been demonstrated that the **carotid sinus function is intact** and the sinus is not hypersensitive in the true sense. Some investigators have suggested that carotid sinus syndrome be renamed carotid sinus irritability to better reflect its pathophysiology.

B. Diagnostic testing. A patient with suspected carotid sinus hypersensitivity/carotid sinus syndrome should be tested lying down with ECG and blood pressure monitoring.

1. Carotid sinus massage is performed by placing firm manual pressure over the carotid sinus located at the bifurcation of the carotid artery for no more than 5 seconds. Only one sinus at a time is compressed, and the temporal artery should be lightly palpated to ensure that complete occlusion of the artery does not occur.
2. Potential risks of carotid sinus massage are transient ischemic attack and stroke. This test should not be performed if a carotid bruit is present. Tilting the patient to an upright position will increase the diagnostic yield of the test but may also result in false-positive outcomes.

C. Therapy

1. Carotid sinus hypersensitivity by itself generally does not require treatment. However, therapy is warranted if carotid sinus hypersensitivity is demonstrated to be the cause of syncope or near-syncope.

2. For purely cardioinhibitory or the mixed type of carotid sinus syndrome, the therapy of choice is pacing (Table 21.3).
3. Management of vasodepressive carotid sinus syndrome is more difficult, and pacing is generally ineffective.

ACKNOWLEDGMENT

The authors thank Dr. Christopher Cole for his contributions to earlier editions of this chapter.

Landmark Articles

American College of Cardiology/American Heart Association. Guidelines for pacemaker implantation after acute myocardial infarction. What is persistent advanced block at the atrioventricular node? *Am J Cardiol* 1997;80:770–774.

Gregoratos G, Abrams J, Epstein AE, et al. ACC/AHA/NASPE guideline update for implantation of cardiac pacemakers and antiarrhythmia devices: summary article. A report of the American College of Cardiology/American Heart Association Task Force on Practice Guidelines (ACC/AHA/NASPE Committee to Update the 1998 Pacemaker Implantation). *Circulation* 2002;106:2145.

Kusumoto FM, Goldschlager N. Cardiac pacing. *N Engl J Med* 1996;334:89–97.

Maloney JD, Jaeger FJ, Rizo-Patron C, et al. The role of pacing for the management of neurally mediated syncope: carotid sinus syndrome and vasovagal syncope. *Am Heart J* 1994;127:1030–1037.

Rotman M, Wagner GS, Wallace AG. Bradfarrhythmeas in acute myocardial infarction. *Circulation* 1972;45:703–722.

22 SUDDEN CARDIAC DEATH

Bryan Baranowskl, Mandeep Bhargava, and Robert A. Schweikert

I. DEFINITION AND EPIDEMIOLOGY. Sudden cardiac death (SCD) accounts for an unanticipated natural death from a cardiac cause occurring shortly after the onset of symptoms. The incidence of SCD in the United States is estimated to be approximately 300,000 to 400,000 cases annually, possibly accounting for more than one-half of all cardiovascular deaths in this country. It is estimated that about 80% of patients who present with SCD have coronary artery disease (CAD). High-risk subgroups of patients include those with reduced left ventricular ejection fraction (LVEF), patients with a history of congestive heart failure (CHF), and survivors of out-of-hospital cardiac arrests. SCD is the primary presentation of cardiovascular disease in approximately 25% of patients. The malignant rhythm most commonly associated with SCD is ventricular tachycardia (VT), ventricular fibrillation (VF), or VT degenerating to VF (85% of cases). Bradyarrhythmias account for about 7% of SCD cases.

Survival in SCD is poor. Approximately 80% of victims of SCD do not survive to hospital discharge. This statistic underscores the importance of primary prevention of SCD.

II. ETIOLOGY: SUBSTRATE AND TRIGGERS

A. Coronary artery disease. The majority of episodes of SCD occur in individuals with CAD. However, the extent to which acute ischemia plays a role in initiating a trigger for SCD has been unclear due to conflicting data. Autopsy data have demonstrated a recent occlusive thrombus in only about 15% to 20% of patients while evidence of a remote infarct is identified in 40% to 70% of cases. The majority (80%) of SCD episodes in patients with CAD are considered to be primary (i.e., no precipitating factor can be identified). Secondary causes like myocardial ischemia/infarction, drug toxicity or proarrhythmia, decompensated heart failure, or electrolyte imbalance can be identified in the minority.

In most situations, SCD is triggered by VF. If rhythm identification occurs within 4 minutes of SCD, the culprit arrhythmia is found to be VF in 95% of cases and asystole in only 5% of the cases. As the time elapsed increases, the proportion of cases triggered by VF decreases, suggesting that asystole and electromechanical dissociation are the result of prolonged VF and hypoxia. At about 7 minutes the incidence of VF decreases to about 70%. There is not much evidence to suggest that VF in such situations is preceded by monomorphic VT. The incidence of bradyarrhythmia-related deaths is slightly higher in patients with advanced heart failure, although tachycardia still predominates.

B. Cardiomyopathies

1. **Idiopathic dilated cardiomyopathy (DCM).** DCM represents the second largest group of patients who experience SCD, accounting for approximately 10% of cases. The overall mortality from DCM is very high (about 25% at 2.5 years), with SCD accounting for about 30% of all deaths in this population. The presence of nonsustained VT, history of syncope, and advanced heart failure are markers of a high risk of SCD in these patients. There is also a higher incidence of sudden deaths related to bradyarrhythmias and electromechanical dissociation in patients with advanced disease. Primary prevention with the implantation of a cardiac defibrillator was recently evaluated in the Sudden Cardiac Death in Heart Failure Trial (SCD-HeFT), which demonstrated a clear mortality benefit.
2. **Hypertrophic cardiomyopathy (HCM).** The incidence of SCD in patients with *hypertrophic cardiomyopathy* is 2% to 4% per year in adults and 4% to 6% per year in children and adolescents. The factors identifying the high-risk population in patients with HCM are a previous history of SCD, a family history of SCD, a diverse genotype (α-tropomyosin and β-myosin heavy chain mutations), sustained or nonsustained VT, recurrent syncope, marked septal hypertrophy ($\geq$30 mm), and a younger age at diagnosis. SCD is usually triggered by ventricular arrhythmias, but may also be precipitated by atrial fibrillation, atrioventricular block, rapid conduction over accessory pathways, or myocardial ischemia.
3. **Arrhythmogenic right ventricular cardiomyopathy (ARVD).** *ARVD* is also an important cause of SCD. A familial disorder with autosomal dominant inheritance, it is characterized by fibrous and fatty infiltration of the ventricles. The incidence of SCD is approximately 2% per year and is mainly related to the risks of ventricular tachyarrhythmia. Patients are identifiable by epsilon waves on the electrocardiogram (ECG) and characteristic fatty myocardial infiltration on magnetic resonance imaging (MRI).

C. Primary electrophysiologic (EP) disorders

1. ***The congenital long QT syndrome (LQTS).*** *LQTS* is a familial disease characterized by an abnormally long QT interval, leading to the development of early afterdepolarization. Several genetic disorders have been identified. Most involve either the sodium (Na) or potassium (K) ion channels and result in either increased Na influx or decreased K efflux. These mutations prolong depolarization and predispose the patient to torsade de pointes. Most episodes are stress mediated. The two variants of the syndrome include the more common autosomal dominant form (Romano-Ward syndrome) and the less common recessive form (Jervell and Lange-Nielsen syndrome) associated with congenital deafness. To date, mutations at nine different LGTS susceptibility genes have been identified. The most common, accounting for 30% to 35% of cases, is a mutation in the gene encoding the delayed rectifier potassium channel. This mutation produces LQT1 syndrome, which is characterized clinically by broad-based T waves and exercise-induced arrhythmic events (especially swimming). LQT2 syndrome (25% to 30% of cases) presents with low-amplitude T waves and auditory arrhythmogenic triggers, whereas LQT3 syndrome usually manifests a long ST isoelectric segment and SCD events during sleep.

The mortality rate for LQT syndrome is estimated to be about 1% per year. High-risk patients include those with a corrected QT interval greater than 500 ms, a history of syncope or SCD, female sex, and the LQT2 or LQT3 genotype. In general patients are treated with β-blocker therapy. Symptomatic patients who are either refractory to or intolerant of medical therapy, or who have other high-risk markers for SCD, should be considered for implantation of a cardiac defibrillator.

2. **Brugada syndrome.** The Brugada syndrome is an autosomal-dominant arrhythmogenic disorder caused by a mutation (SCNA5) in the cardiac sodium channels, which predisposes patients to develop polymorphic VT or VF. The arrhythmias commonly occur at rest or during sleep, and the risk of SCD is up to 30% at 3 years in untreated patients. Symptomatic patients and asymptomatic patients with a family history with SCD should be considered for implantation of a cardiac defibrillator.
3. **Wolff-Parkinson-White (WPW) syndrome.** The risk of SCD is also higher in patients with *WPW,* especially if they have rapidly conducting accessory pathways, which can conduct as rapidly as 250 milliseconds or less in atrial fibrillation. The incidence of SCD is lower than 1 per 1000 patient-years, and is more common in males in their second and third decades, but the phenomenon is easily identifiable and manageable.

D. Others. Less frequent causes, whereby a low but definitive risk of SCD has been identified as higher than in the normal population, include subgroups of patients with severe aortic stenosis, mitral valve prolapse, left ventricular hypertrophy, anomalous origin of the coronary arteries, myocardial bridging, myocarditis, and trained athletes.

III. DIAGNOSTIC AND PROGNOSTIC TESTING. Survivors of SCD should have a detailed cardiovascular evaluation. Reversible precipitating factors must be identified and corrected. Underlying diseases must be identified and managed, and the risk of recurrent SCD must be determined. Diagnostic and prognostic testing appropriate for the survivor of SCD includes the following:

A. Electrocardiogram for evidence of myocardial infarction (MI) or ischemia, intraventricular conduction delay, accessory pathway (WPW syndrome), prolonged QT interval, epsilon waves, and left ventricular hypertrophy.

B. Laboratory data to rule out reversible causes, such as cardiac enzymes [creatine kinase–myocardial band (CK-MB), troponin T, troponin I], abnormal electrolytes, antiarrhythmic drug levels for toxicity, and urine screening for illicit drugs such as cocaine.

C. ECG monitoring to assess frequency, duration, and symptomatology of arrhythmias.

D. Twenty-four-hour ambulatory electrocardiography can be useful in predicting the risk of SCD, especially for primary prophylaxis in high-risk patients. The absence of ventricular ectopy correlates better with a low risk of SCD.

E. Echocardiography for assessment of left ventricular function, valvular disease, cardiomyopathy, and hypertrophy. Nuclear or angiographic determinations of left ventricular function may be used but do not provide as much information as echocardiography. The LVEF continues to be the most potent predictor of SCD. An LVEF of less than 40% is predictive of a risk of SCD, with a sensitivity of 68% and a specificity of 69%. In the Multicenter Post Infarction Program study, an LVEF of less than 30% was associated with a higher risk of SCD.

F. Coronary angiography for assessment of CAD or coronary anomalies.

G. Exercise or pharmacologic stress testing with radionuclide imaging or echocardiography if CAD is present and myocardial ischemia and/or viability is in question.

H. EP testing. For the survivor of SCD, the need for EP testing is somewhat controversial, especially in light of the superiority of the ICD over antiarrhythmic drugs in this population. There are some electrophysiologists who advocate EP testing for the survivor of SCD prior to implantation of an implantable cardioverter–defibrillator (ICD) to identify and characterize an inducible tachyarrhythmia, particularly one that may be cured with catheter ablation techniques, or to rule out a supraventricular arrhythmia that might complicate management of an ICD. In addition, EP testing may guide the clinician in selecting a particular ICD, in programming the tachyarrhythmia therapy, and in identifying the need for concomitant cardiac pacing. For primary prophylaxis, the role of programmed electrical stimulation (PES) remains debatable. Wilber et al. had shown that inducibility of sustained monomorphic VT by programmed electrical stimulation reliably identifies patients with left ventricular dysfunction and CAD for guiding subsequent therapy. Their study revealed that patients with inducible sustained monomorphic VT despite antiarrhythmic drugs had a risk of SCD of up to 50% in the succeeding 2 years. In patients who had suppression of the tachycardia with drugs, the risk was around 11%, and in those with no inducible tachycardia, the risk was 2% to 6%. There has been no prospective randomized trial to show that inducibility with PES predicts mortality over LVEF or that suppression of inducibility confers benefit. It is also recognized that among patients with SCD, inducible sustained monomorphic VT on PES is present in only about 30% of the patients. The role of an EP study in nonischemic dilated cardiomyopathy is even less established than in patients with CAD.

I. Cardiac MRI. Particularly for the patient with normal left ventricular function, cardiac MRI may be useful to evaluate for arrhythmogenic right ventricular cardiomyopathy.

IV. THERAPY

A. Acute therapy for SCD

1. **Cardiopulmonary resuscitation (CPR).** Early response is crucial. The two most critical components of out-of-hospital cardiac resuscitation are the availability of a rapid response system and citizen bystander CPR. Survivors of SCD are more likely to be discharged from the hospital if they are witnessed and have received early CPR from bystanders. There is an increasing drive to train police personnel, students, and even the common person in resuscitation and defibrillation techniques. There have also been strong efforts in providing easy accessibility to automated external defibrillators.
2. **Advanced cardiac life support (ACLS).** Early defibrillation is crucial to improved survival. Approximately 40% of SCD victims are found to have VF upon arrival of paramedical personnel, and this figure is almost doubled if the rhythm can be detected in the first 7 minutes after collapse. The key to survival in any resuscitative effort is early defibrillation. If this is achieved within 3 minutes, up to 74% of patients may survive, versus less than 40% if delayed beyond that point. The trials have also shown that amiodarone is more effective than lidocaine in shock-resistant VF.
3. **Automated external defibrillation and public access defibrillation.** An automated external defibrillator is designed to be used by emergency personnel and perhaps even minimally trained lay rescuers, particularly for victims of out-of-hospital SCD. The device monitors the patient's electrocardiogram via self-adhesive defibrillation electrode pads applied to the chest wall and is programmed with a VF detection algorithm. When the device detects VF, an alarm is emitted, followed by delivery of a defibrillation shock or an indicator for the rescuer to press a button to deliver the shock. There is evidence that the use of these devices results in more rapid delivery of a defibrillation shock than that achieved with manual defibrillation, particularly in those areas served by personnel with less training. Efforts to provide automated external debrillators at specific locations for public access defibrillation, including airplanes, airports, and shopping malls, have made a significant impact on improving the success rates of out-of-hospital cardiac resuscitation.
4. **Survival to hospital.** Some centers in the United States with rapid emergency medical response and early bystander CPR have reported that of the 40% of SCD victims found in VF, up to 60% to 70% survive to be admitted to the hospital, and approximately 25% are subsequently discharged from the hospital (therefore, only approximately 10% of SCD victims survive overall). As most cities in the United States do not achieve quite as rapid a response, it is clear that

primary prevention of SCD would be a more effective focus. The improvement in community resuscitation is likely to be contingent on the widespread availability of the automated external defibrillator and on placing its use not only in the hands of paramedics and the police but also in those of the first responders. However, even the best survival rates continue to be low, and this determines the importance of primary prevention of SCD.

B. Primary prevention of SCD

1. Identifying individuals at risk for SCD. No single factor has been identified that accurately predicts the occurrence of SCD, although combinations of factors have been more useful. In general, the specificity and positive predictive value of these tests are poor, whereas the negative predictive value is much better (particularly for combinations of tests). Overall the most potent predictor of survival continues to be LVEF, but other tools may add to further prognosticating the patients and guide subsequent therapy. Other tools for predicting the risk of SCD, especially EP testing, ambulatory electrocardiography, signal-averaged electrocardiography, assessment of baroreceptor sensitivity, measurement of heart rate variability, and measurement of the circadian variation of heart rate variability, have been used to identify the high-risk groups, but none have been shown to be of convincing value. Although a combination of different tests improves their predictive value, the positive predictive accuracy rarely reaches more than 40%. A two-step strategy of using LVEF ($\leq$40% and ventricular arrhythmias on Holter monitoring ($\geq$20 premature ventricular contractions per hour, $\geq$10 ventricular couplets per day, or VT with a cycle length $\leq$600 ms) and then EP testing, can improve the positive predictive accuracy to moderate levels. T wave alternans is also a potential investigative tool that may prove useful.
2. Pharmacologic agents and surgical/percutaneous techniques. Because the majority of episodes of SCD occur in patients with CAD, agents that reduce myocardial ischemia, prevent or limit the extent of MI, or alter ventricular remodeling after MI should reduce the incidence of SCD. The use of statins, too, in reducing the incidence of CAD and its complications cannot be overemphasized. Early studies of surgical myocardial revascularization have shown a reduction in SCD for patients with triple-vessel CAD and left ventricular dysfunction compared with those patients treated medically. Combined surgical revascularization and aneurysmectomy to remove the arrhythmogenic myocardial substrate had variable results. Catheter-based VT mapping and ablation methods continue to be investigated and may have a role in select patient populations, particularly in patients with incessant arrhythmias, despite optimal antiarrhythmic drug and/or implantable device therapy. More recently, myocardial reperfusion and revascularization with thrombolytic agents and/or percutaneous interventions have decreased the mortality from SCD, especially in acute coronary syndromes.

   Several studies have demonstrated the efficacy of β-blockers for the prevention of all-cause mortality, as well as a trend toward reduction in SCD in survivors of MI. An analysis of 31 β-blocker trials showed that in 13 of them SCD was reduced by 43% to 51%. Angiotensin-converting enzyme inhibitors also decrease progression to heart failure and SCD in MI survivors by 30% to 54%. Aldosterone receptor blockers are also of benefit in reducing the incidence of heart failure and SCD.

   More than a decade ago, ventricular ectopy in survivors of MI was recognized as a risk factor for SCD. Suppression of ventricular ectopy with antiarrhythmic drugs in such patients was, therefore, thought to be beneficial. However, the Cardiac Arrhythmia Suppression Trial (CAST) investigation demonstrated that the proarrhythmic and/or adverse effects of the class IC antiarrhythmic drugs is greater than the benefit achieved through arrhythmia suppression and that the use of these drugs in the post-MI population caused an increased mortality. Other studies have demonstrated that survivors of MI with poor left ventricular function are particularly at risk for proarrhythmia or excess mortality from certain antiarrhythmic drugs, including the class IC agent encainide and the class III agent *d*-sotalol in the Survival With Oral *d*-Sotalol

(SWORD) study. To date, only amiodarone of all the antiarrhythmic drugs has been shown to reduce SCD, and the evidence for amiodarone has been mixed. Initial small trials of amiodarone therapy for survivors of MI (including a meta-analysis of these trials) suggested a reduced mortality with amiodarone use but this has not been corroborated by larger prospective controlled trials. The European Myocardial Infarct Amiodarone Trial (EMIAT) was designed to study the efficacy of amiodarone in reducing mortality for survivors of MI with left ventricular dysfunction (EF, 40%). There was no difference in all-cause or cardiac mortality, although there was a significant reduction in arrhythmic deaths. The Canadian Amiodarone Myocardial Infarction Arrhythmia Trial (CAMIAT) was designed to study the efficacy of amiodarone in reducing mortality for survivors of MI with frequent ventricular ectopy. There was no difference in all-cause mortality, but again there was a significant reduction in a composite endpoint of resuscitated VF or arrhythmic deaths.

Amiodarone treatment for the prevention of SCD in patients with CHF has also been studied, with conflicting results. The Grupo de Estudio de la Sobrevida en la Insuficiencia Cardiaca en Argentina (GESICA) trial studied the efficacy of amiodarone for the prevention of SCD in patients with severe CHF. There was a significant reduction in all-cause mortality and SCD for the patients treated with amiodarone. However, this trial has been criticized for its nonblinded design and the lack of uniform follow-up strategies among the study groups. The Survival Trial of Amiodarone in Patients with Congestive Heart Failure (CHF-STAT) did not demonstrate a difference in SCD or all-cause mortality with prophylactic amiodarone therapy for patients with CHF, left ventricular dysfunction (EF, 40%), and asymptomatic ventricular ectopy. However, in a subgroup analysis, patients with nonischemic cardiomyopathy showed a trend towards reduction in SCD.

3. **Implantable devices.** In light of the evidence for the inefficacy and hazards of antiarrhythmic drugs for the prevention of SCD, attention shifted to the ICD. Several randomized trials comparing ICD and medical therapy for the primary prevention of SCD have shown benefit of ICD. In the Multicenter Automatic Defibrillator Implantation Trial (MADIT), the ICD was more effective than conventional antiarrhythmic drug therapy in the primary prevention of SCD for patients with nonsustained VT, poor left ventricular function after MI, and inducible ventricular arrhythmia at the time of EP testing that was not suppressed with procainamide. The Multicenter Unsustained Tachycardia Trial (MUSTT) randomized patients with coronary artery disease and an EF 40% or less to receive electrophysiologically guided therapy in three arms: ICD therapy, drug therapy, or no therapy. This trial not only showed a 50% reduction of mortality in patients with ICDs, but it also showed that drug therapy was worse than no therapy at all.

   The Coronary Artery Bypass Graft (CABG) patch trial demonstrated that prophylactic ICD implantation at the time of CABG for patients with left ventricular dysfunction and an abnormal signal-averaged ECG did not improve survival. This trial suggested that coronary revascularization may have decreased the triggers for arrhythmias, and that signal-averaged electrocardiography could not replace invasive EP testing.

   The MADIT II trial assessed the importance of risk stratification of patients for SCD on the basis of LVEF alone. In this trial, patients with an old MI and an LVEF of less than 30% were randomized to receive either an ICD or conventional therapy. During an average follow-up of 20 months, the ICD group had a mortality of 14.2%, versus 19.8% in the conventional therapy group. The reduction in the all-cause mortality in the ICD group was 21% at the end of 1 year and 28% at the end of 2 and 3 years, respectively.

   MADIT, MUSTT, and MADIT II studied patients with remote (>3 weeks) ischemic events. The Defibrillator in Acute Myocardial Infarction Trial (DINAMIT) assessed whether the benefits of ICD therapy would also be seen in those with more recent ischemic events. The trial enrolled patients with both impaired LV function (EF <35%), and impaired autonomic dysfunction, 6 to 40 days post-MI who were randomized to receive optimal medical therapy or ICD. There was no significant mortality difference between the two groups at 30 months. The reason for this result remains unclear; however, the results are reflected in the Centers for Medicare & Medicaid Services ICD guidelines, which exclude the implantation of an ICD within 40 days of an MI or within 3 months of a cardiac revascularization procedure.

Although MADIT, MUSTT, and MADIT II helped to establish the role for ICD therapy for the primary prevention of SCD in patients with CAD, they did not address patients with nonischemic cardiomyopathy (CM). This was addressed in The Defibrillators in Nonischemic Cardiomyopathy Treatment Evaluation (DEFINITE) trial and the SCD-HeFT. The DEFINITE study enrolled patients with nonischemic CM with and EF less than 36%; New York Heart Association (NYHA) class I, II, or III CHF; and a history of nonsustained VT or frequent premature ventricular contractions (PVCs). The patients were randomized to receive either standard medical therapy or an ICD. At the end of a 29-month mean follow-up period, there was a 34% relative risk reduction in all-cause mortality for those patients who received an ICD. The greatest benefit occurred in those patients with NYHA class III CHF. In part based on this study, the Centers for Medicare & Medicaid Services expanded reimbursment for ICDs to include patients with nonischemic CM, an EF 35% or less, and NYHA class III or IV CHF.

The SCD-HeFT randomized patients with either ischemic or nonischemic CM, an EF of 35% or less, and NYHA class II or III CHF to receive either therapy with placebo, amiodarone, or an ICD. ICD therapy significantly reduced all-cause mortality (23%) compared to placebo, whereas amiodarone did not change survival compared to placebo. Subgroup analysis of the study suprisingly demonstrated that the mortality benefit of ICD therapy occurred exclusively in the NYHA class II patients. This finding was in contrast with the results of DEFINITE, which demonstrated the most benefit in NYHA class III patients. As a result of SCD-HeFT, Medicare and Medicaid coverage for ICD was expanded to include patients with nonischemic CM, an EF of 35% or less, and NYHA class II CHF.

4. **Cardiac resynchronization therapy.** Approximately 30% of patients with advanced heart failure (EF ≤35%) have an associated ventricular conduction delay resulting in a QRS 120 milliseconds or greater. Delayed ventricular conduction can result in dyssynchronous contraction of both the left and right ventricle, which in turn reduces stroke volume and cardiac output. Delayed ventricular conduction in patients with advanced heart failure is associated with increased mortality. Biventricular pacemaker (BiV) technology attempts to restore cardiac synchronization by pacing both the right and left ventricles via a lead placed in the coronary sinus. Biventricular pacing has been shown to improve quality of life, exercise capacity, and ejection fraction in patients with advanced CHF. The Comparison of Medical Therapy, Pacing, and Defibrillation in Heart Failure (COMPANION) trial was the first to assess the mortality effect of biventricular pacing (BiV) and ICD therapy in patients with advanced ischemic or nonischemic CM. The study randomized patients with NYHA class III or IV CHF, and EF of 35% or less and a QRS greater than 120 ms to receive either optimal medical therapy, a BiV pacemaker, or a BiV pacemaker with ICD. At the end of a 12-month follow-up, the risk of the combined endpoint of death or hospitalization for CHF was reduced by 34% with BiV pacing alone and 40% with combined BiV pacing and ICD therapy. The Cardiac Resynchronization in Heart Failure (CARE-CHF) trial assessed the risk of all-cause mortality and hospitalization for a cardiovascular event in patients with NYHA class III or IV CHF, and EF of 35% or less and a QRS duration of greater than or equal to 120 milliseconds. Patients were randomized to receive either standard medical therapy or BiV pacing (no ICD). The relative risk of all-cause mortality and hospitalization for a cardiovascular event was reduced by 37% in the BiV

group. The study's secondary endpoint looked at all-cause mortality alone and demonstrated a relative risk reduction of 36% with BiV therapy. These results, which were similar to COMPANION, caused some to question the need for ICD therapy in addition to BiV pacing in select patients with severe CHF. Subgroup analysis of the CARE-CHF trial, however, suggested that SCD accounted for 35% of the deaths in the BiV pacing group. Presumably a significant portion of these were caused by malignant arrhythmias, which could have been prevented with ICD therapy.

C. Secondary prevention

1. Pharmacologic agents. As with primary prevention of SCD, the disappointment regarding the efficacy and safety of class I antiarrhythmic drugs also shifted attention to non–class I antiarrhythmic drugs for the secondary prevention of SCD. In the Cardiac Arrest in Seattle Conventional Versus Amiodarone Drug Evaluation (CASCADE) study, amiodarone was demonstrated to be superior to conventional class I antiarrhythmic drugs in the secondary prevention of SCD. In addition, the Electrophysiologic Study Versus Electrocardiographic Monitoring (ESVEM) trial demonstrated that the class III antiarrhythmic drug sotalol was more efficacious than several class I agents in the reduction of total mortality, cardiac mortality, arrhythmic mortality, and VT recurrence for patients with a history of VT, VF or syncope, ventricular ectopy by Holter monitoring of more than 10 premature ventricular contractions per hour, and reproducibly inducible ventricular arrhythmias by EP testing. These studies supplied further evidence supporting the abandonment of class I antiarrhythmic drugs as first-line therapy for malignant ventricular arrhythmias. However, emergence of the ICD led to randomized trials comparing the efficacy of best medical therapy and ICDs for the secondary prevention of SCD.

2. Implantable devices. The Antiarrhythmics Versus Implantable Defibrillators (AVID) trial was designed to study the efficacy of ICD therapy versus the antiarrhythmic drugs amiodarone or sotalol for the secondary prevention of SCD for patients with a history of VF or sustained VT and left ventricular dysfunction or hemodynamically compromising VT. Less than 10% of patients randomized to antiarrhythmic drug therapy received sotalol. The trial was prematurely terminated due to a 29% mortality benefit in patients with an ICD when compared with drug therapy.

Two other large trials of secondary prevention of SCD have shown similar results for the role of ICDs in the secondary prophylaxis of SCD. The Cardiac Arrest Study Hamburg (CASH) study was designed to assess the efficacy of the ICD versus propafenone, amiodarone, or metoprolol in the secondary prevention of SCD. The propafenone arm of the study was terminated in 1992 due to excess mortality in this group compared with the ICD group. There was a 37% relative reduction is all-cause 2-year mortality in those patients who received an ICD compared to those who were treated medically with metoprolol or amiodarone. Interestingly, there was no significant difference in mortality between the amiodarone and metoprolol groups. The Canadian Implantable Defibrillator Study (CIDS) was similar to the AVID trial in its investigation of the efficacy of ICD versus amiodarone for the secondary prevention of SCD. The results from this trial showed a modest improvement in survival in the ICD group (approximately 20% reduction in total mortality). Of note, a potentially important difference between the AVID and CIDS investigations is that the latter included patients with undocumented syncope and either inducible sustained VT at EP study or 10 seconds of VT by monitor.

V. SUMMARY: ANTIARRHYTHMIC DRUGS VERSUS ICDs. Indications for ICD therapy are summarized in Table 22.1. From the available data there is good evidence that many antiarrhythmic drugs are not efficacious and may be harmful in the primary prevention of SCD. The ICD has been proven to be highly effective in the termination of malignant ventricular arrhythmias and is more effective than antiarrhythmic medications for the prevention of SCD in patients with CAD and a reduced LVEF. The value of EP testing is debatable, but it may be moderately efficacious in stratifying patients for

TABLE 22.1 Iindications for ICD Therapy

Class I

1. Cardiac arrest due to ventricular fibrillation (VF) or VT not due to a transient or reversible cause.
2. Spontaneous sustained VT in association with structural heart disease.
3. Syncope of undetermined origin with clinically relevant, hemodynamically significant sustained VT or VF induced at EP study when drug therapy is ineffective, not tolerated, or not preferred.
4. NSVT in patients with CAD, prior MI, LV dysfunction, and inducible VF or sustained VT at EP study that is not suppressible by a Class I antiarrhythmic drug.
5. Spontaneous sustained VT in patients who do not have structural heart disease that is amenable to other treatments.

Class IIa

1. Patients with LVEF $\leq$30%, at least one month post MI and 3 months post CABG.

Class IIb

1. Cardiac arrest presumed to be due to VF when EP testing is precluded by other medical conditions.
2. Severe symptoms (e.g., syncope) attributable to ventricular tachyarrhythmias in patients awaiting cardiac transplantation.
3. Familial/inherited conditions with a high risk for life-threatening ventricular tachyarrhythmias such as long-QT syndrome or HCM.
4. NSVT with CAD, prior MI, LV dysfunction, and inducible sustained VT or VF at EP study.
5. Recurrent syncope of undetermined etiology in the presence of ventricular dysfunction and inducible ventricular arrhythmias at EP study when other causes of syncope have been excluded.
6. Syncope of unexplained etiology or family history of SCD in association with typical or atypical RBBB and ST-segment elevations (Brugada syndrome).
7. Syncope in patients with advanced structural heart disease in which thorough invasive and noninvasive investigation has failed to define a cause.

Class III

1. Syncope of undetermined cuase in a patient without inducible ventricular tachyarrhythmias and without structural heart disease.
2. Incessant VT or VF.
3. VF or VT resulting from arrhythmias amenable to surgical/catheter ablation (e.g., WPW syndrome, RVOT VT, fascicular VT).
4. Ventricular tachyarrhythmias due to a transient or reversible disdorder (e.g., AMI, electrolytes, drugs, or trauma) when correction of the disorder is considered feasible and likely to substantially reduce the risk of recurrent arrhythmia.
5. Significant psychiatric illnesses that may be aggravated by device implantation or may preclude symptomatic follow-up.
6. Terminal illnesses with projected life expectancy <6 months.
7. Patients with CAD with LV dysfunction and prolonged QRS duration in absence of spontaneous or inducible VT who are undergoing CABG.
8. NYHA Class IV drug-refractory CHF in patients who are not candidates for cardiac transplantation.

Adapted from 2002 ACC/AHA/NASPE Pacemaker/ICD Guideline Update.

the risk of SCD. However, the results of the MADIT II trial and the SCD-HeFT would suggest that LVEF alone may be sufficient to guide ICD therapy for primary prevention. The high-risk group of patients with other diseases predisposing to SCD, such hypertrophic cardiomyopathy, arrhythmogenic right ventricular dysplasia, Brugada syndrome, and congenital long QT syndrome, may also benefit from long-term ICD therapy. The bradyarrhythmias respond well to pacemaker therapy. Radiofrequency catheter ablation is the therapy of first choice in patients with Wolff-Parkinson-White syndrome and is an effective synergistic therapy in patients with VT who have recurrent

ICD shocks, especially in bundle-branch reentry tachycardias. There has been growing enthusiasm for the use of biventricular pacemaker–defibrillators in patients with refractory heart failure, and this significantly reduces SCD and heart failure morbidity.

The treatment of survivors of SCD is much less controversial. The evidence from several recent randomized trials demonstrates the superiority of the ICD over antiarrhythmic drugs for the population requiring secondary prophylaxis. Perhaps more controversial for this group of patients is the type of ICD to implant, given the fact that the majority of these patients require only protection from sudden death. The choice of device and its associated technologic features should be considered on an individual basis.

VI. KEY SUGGESTIONS

A. Thorough evaluation of the SCD survivor for reversible triggers of the episode, particularly myocardial ischemia, is crucial.

B. Risk stratification for recurrent SCD is also important, especially determination of left ventricular function and the extent and severity of CAD.

C. If CAD is present, stress testing with radionuclide or echo imaging to detect myocardial ischemia and/or viability may be indicated.

VII. FUTURE. Several areas of research will have an impact on the occurrence of SCD. The majority of episodes of SCD are secondary to underlying CAD. Therefore, efforts to prevent CAD and improve treatment modalities for myocardial ischemia and MI may have the greatest impact on the incidence of SCD. Advances in the understanding of the mechanisms and triggers of SCD may lead to more specific and efficacious treatments aimed at prevention, such as new medications, gene therapies, or advanced catheter ablation techniques. Technologic advances will continue to improve the efficacy and safety of the ICD, and improved telemetry storage within these devices for arrhythmic events may provide valuable insight into the mechanisms of SCD. Large-scale, controlled randomized trials designed to investigate the therapeutic strategies for populations at risk for SCD will continue to be important.

Landmark Articles

Bigger JT Jr. Prophylactic use of implanted cardiac defibrillators in patients at high risk for ventricular arrhythmias after coronary artery bypass graft surgery. Coronary Artery Bypass Graft (CABG) Patch Trial Investigators. *N Engl J Med* 1997;337:1569–1575.

Bristow MR, Saxon LA, Boehmer J, et al. Cardiac-resynchronization therapy with or without an implantable defibrillator in advanced chronic heart failure. *N Engl J Med* 2004;350:2140–2150.

Buxton AE, Fisher JD, Josephson ME, et al. Prevention of sudden death in patients with coronary artery disease: the Multicenter Unsustained Tachycardia Trial (MUSTT). *Prog Cardiovasc Dis* 1993;36:215–226.

Cairns JA, Connolly SJ, Roberts R, et al. Randomized trial of outcome after myocardial infarction in patients with frequent or repetitive ventricular premature depolarizations: CAMIAT. Canadian Amiodarone Myocardial Infarction Arrhythmia Trial Investigators. *Lancet* 1997;349:675–682.

Cardiac Arrhythmia Suppression Trial (CAST) Investigators. Preliminary report: effect of encainide and flecainide on mortality in a randomized trial of arrhythmia suppression after myocardial infarction. *N Engl J Med* 1989;321:406–412.

Cardiac Arrhythmia Suppression Trial II Investigators. Effect of the antiarrhythmic agent moricizine on survival after myocardial infarction. *N Engl J Med* 1992;327:227–233.

Connolly SJ, Gent M, Roberts RS, et al., for the CIDS Investigators. Canadian Implantable Defibrillator Study: a randomized trial of the implantable cardioverter defibrillator against amiodarone. *Circulation* 2000;101:1297–1302.

Doval HC, Nul DR, Grancelli HO, et al. Randomised trial of low-dose amiodarone in severe congestive heart failure. Grupo de Estudio de la Sobrevida en la Insuficiencia Cardiaca en Argentina (GESICA). *Lancet* 1994;344:493–498.

Freemantle N, Cleland JG, Young P, et al. Beta-blockade after myocardial infarction: systematic review and meta regression analysis. *BMJ* 2001;318:1730–1737.

Gregoratos G, Abrams J, Epstein AE, et al. ACC/AHA/NASPE 2002 guideline update for implantation of cardiac pacemakers and antiarrhythmia devices: summary article: a report of the American College of Cardiology/American Heart Association Task Force on Practice Guidelines (ACC/AHA/NASPE Committee to Update the 1998 Pacemaker Guidelines). *Circulation* 2002;106:2145–2161.

Hinkle LE Jr, Thaler HT. Clinical classification of cardiac deaths. *Circulation* 1982;65:457–464.

Julian DG, Camm AJ, Frangin G, et al. Randomised trial of effect of amiodarone on mortality in patients with left ventricular dysfunction after recent myocardial infarction: EMIAT. European Myocardial Infarct Amiodarone Trial Investigators. *Lancet* 1997;349:667–674.

Kadish A, Dyer A, Daubert JP, et al. Prophylactic defibrillator implantation in patients with nonischemic dilated cardiomyopathy. *N Engl J Med* 2004;350:2151–2158.

Kim SG, Fogoros RN, Furman S, et al. Standardized reporting of ICD patient outcome: the report of a North American Society of Pacing and Electrophysiology Policy Conference, February 9–10, 1993. *PACE* 1993;16:1358–1362.

Kober L, Torp-Pedersen C, Carlsen JE, et al. A clinical trial of the angiotensin-converting-enzyme inhibitor trandolapril in patients with left ventricular dysfunction after myocardial infarction. Trandolapril Cardiac Evaluation (TRACE) Study Group. *N Engl J Med* 1995;333:1670–1676.

Kuller LH, Lilienfeld A, Fisher R. Epidemiological study of sudden and unexpected deaths due to arteriosclerotic heart disease. *Circulation* 1966;34:1056–1068.

Mason JW. A comparison of seven antiarrhythmic drugs in patients with ventricular tachyarrhythmias. Electrophysiologic Study versus Electrocardiographic Monitoring Investigators. *N Engl J Med* 1993;329:452–458.

Mason JW. A comparison of electrophysiologic testing with Holter monitoring to predict antiarrhythmic-drug efficacy for ventricular tachyarrhythmias. Electrophysiologic Study versus Electrocardiographic Monitoring Investigators. *N Engl J Med* 1993;329:445–451.

Moss AJ, Hall WJ, Cannom DS, et al. Improved survival with an implanted defibrillator in patients with coronary disease at high risk for ventricular arrhythmia. Multicenter Automatic Defibrillator Implantation Trial Investigators. *N Engl J Med* 1996;335:1933–1940.

Moss AJ, Zareba W, Hall WJ, et al. Prophylactic implantation of a defibrillator in patients with myocardial infarction and reduced ejection fraction. *N Engl J Med* 2002;346:877–883.

Siebels J, Kuck KH. Implantable cardioverter defibrillator compared with antiarrhythmic drug treatment in cardiac arrest survivors (the Cardiac Arrest Study Hamburg). *Am Heart J* 1994;127:1139–1144.

Singh SN, Fletcher RD, Fisher SG, et al. Amiodarone in patients with congestive heart failure and asymptomatic ventricular arrhythmia. Survival Trial of Antiarrhythmic Therapy in Congestive Heart Failure. *N Engl J Med* 1995;333:77–82.

The Antiarrhythmics versus Implantable Defibrillators (AVID) Investigators. A comparison of antiarrhythmic-drug therapy with implantable defibrillators in patients resuscitated from near-fatal ventricular arrhythmias. *N Engl J Med* 1997;337:1576–1583.

The CASCADE Investigators. Randomized antiarrhythmic drug therapy in survivors of cardiac arrest (the CASCADE study). *Am J Cardiol* 1993;72:280–287.

The Encainide–Ventricular Tachycardia Study Group. Treatment of life-threatening ventricular tachycardia with encainide hydrochloride in patients with left ventricular dysfunction. *Am J Cardiol* 1988;62:571.

Waldo AL, Camm AJ, deRuyter H, et al. Effect of *d*-sotalol on mortality in patients with left ventricular dysfunction after recent and remote myocardial infarction. The SWORD Investigators. Survival With Oral *d*-Sotalol. *Lancet* 1996;348:7–12. [Published erratum appears in *Lancet* 1996;348:416.]

Wilkoff BL, Cook JR, Epstein AE, et al. Dual-chamber pacing or ventricular backup pacing in patients with an implantable defibrillator: the Dual Chamber and VVI Implantable Defibrillator (DAVID) Trial. *JAMA* 2002;288:3115–3123.

Key Reviews

Domanski MJ, Zipes DP, Schron E. Treatment of sudden cardiac death. Current understandings from randomized trials and future research directions. *Circulation* 1997;95:2694–2699.

Furberg CD. Effect of antiarrhythmic drugs on mortality after myocardial infarction. *Am J Cardiol* 1983;52:32C–36C.

Myerburg RJ, Interian A Jr, Mitrani RM, et al. Frequency of sudden cardiac death and profiles of risk. *Am J Cardiol* 1997;80:10F–19F.

Priori SG, Aliot E, Blomstrom-Lundqvist L, et al. Task force on sudden cardiac death of the European Society of Cardiology. *Eur Heart J* 2001;22:1374–1450.

Yusuf S, Peto R, Lewis J, et al. Beta blockade during and after myocardial infarction: an overview of the randomized trials. *Prog Cardiovasc Dis* 1985;27:335–371.

Zipes DP, Wellens HJ. Sudden cardiac death. *Circulation* 1998;98:2334–2351.

23 ATRIAL FIBRILLATION

Carlos Alves

I. INTRODUCTION. Atrial fibrillation (AF) is the most common sustained tachyarrhythmia, and is associated with increased cardiovascular morbidity, mortality, and preventable stroke, accounting for approximately one-third of cardiac hospitalizations for cardiac rhythm disturbances. The incidence and prevalence of atrial fibrillation increase with age, with a prevalence of 0.4% to 1% in the general population and as high as 8% in patients older than 80 years of age. In addition the age-adjusted incidence in the Framingham study increased significantly from the 1960s to the present. It is estimated that 2.2 million people in America and 4.5 million people in Europe have either paroxysmal or persistent AF. AF is associated with increased risk of stroke, heart failure exacerbation, and all-cause mortality, especially in women. The mortality rate in patients with AF is about twice that of patients in normal sinus rhythm.

A. Classification: AF may be classified as lone, idiopathic, first detected, recurrent, paroxysmal, persistent, and permanent. **Lone AF** is used to describe patients experiencing AF without clinical or echocardiographic evidence of cardiopulmonary disease. **Idiopathic AF** refers to the uncertainty of AF origin without considering age or underlying cardiovascular pathology. During a patient's first detected episode of AF, it should be noted whether it is self-limited, or the patient symptomatic with the arrhythmia. When a person has experienced two or more episodes of AF it is considered **recurrent,** and once recurrent AF is terminated it is referred to as **paroxysmal.** Paroxysmal episodes are usually self-terminating, and at least initially, do not usually require direct current cardioversion (DCC). **Persistent AF** usually lasts longer than 7 days and requires cardioversion for its termination. AF becomes **permanent** once cardioversion, either electrical or chemical, is unsuccessful.

B. Clinical presentation. As with all arrhythmias, the clinical presentation of AF can vary widely and p**atients may be asymptomatic,** despite rapid rates of ventricular response. Common symptoms include **palpitations, fatigue, dyspnea and/or shortness of breath, dizziness, and diaphoresis.** Less commonly, patients may present with extreme manifestations of hemodynamic compromise, such as **chest pain, pulmonary edema, and syncope.** AF is often noted in patients presenting with a new thromboembolic stroke, with reported rates of 10% to 40%.

C. Differential diagnosis. AF needs to be **distinguished from multifocal atrial tachycardia**, **frequent premature atrial contractions,** and **automatic atrial tachycardias**.

D. Etiology. AF is **most commonly associated with advanced age, hypertension, valvular heart disease, congestive heart failure (CHF), and coronary artery disease (CAD).** Pathophysiologically these entities result in left atrial fibrosis, pulmonary vein dilation, and reduced atrial contractility, which in turn result at a cellular level in abnormal intracellular calcium handling, atrial myolysis, connexin downregulation, and altered sympathetic innervation. These cellular changes cause atrial conduction abnormalities, and increase ectopic atrial activity and favor the development and establishment of micro-reentrant circuits, which lead to the establishment of AF.

AF has been associated with physiologic stress, drugs, pulmonary embolism, chronic lung disease, hyperthyroidism, caffeine, infectious processes, and various metabolic disturbances. AF has also been linked with obesity, and this phenomenon seems to be mediated by left atrial dilation. Other less-common cardiac associations include Wolff-Parkinson-White (WPW) syndrome, pericarditis, and cardiomyopathy. Surgery, particularly **cardiac surgery, is associated with a high risk of postoperative AF** that depends on the type of cardiac surgery and is highest for mitral valve surgery, and which may reach 35% to 50%. Persistence of AF has been correlated with elevated C-reactive protein levels, which raises the question of a role for inflammation in this condition, and atrial natriuretic peptide has been found to be elevated in people with acute AF. This hormone, which is released by myocardial tissue in response to increased wall stress, promotes diuresis and vasodilation. However, with long-standing AF, atrial natriuretic peptide levels remain within the normal range and patients do not experience its useful hemodynamic effects.

E. Pathophysiology

1. The role of the pulmonary veins as a source of triggers and/or drivers in AF is increasingly appreciated. A previous model proposed by Moe et al. in 1962, had described multiple reentrant wavelets within the atrial tissue (substrate) that contributed to the maintenance of AF. Recent data support a focal mechanism involving both increased automaticity and multiple reentrant wavelets, occurring predominantly in the left atrium around the pulmonary veins. A new model incorporates these mechanisms of initiators/drivers of AF and atrial substrate conditions for AF maintenance. This in turn may be affected by various modulating factors, such as autonomic tone, medications, atrial pressure, and catecholamine levels.

AF is a very complex arrhythmia, and this mechanistic model simply serves to provide a conceptual framework from which to gain insight into the arrhythmia.

2. Paroxysmal, persistent, or chronic AF presents a **considerable risk for thromboembolism;** lone AF is presently thought to also increase the risk, but to a lesser extent. **The risk of stroke becomes more pronounced with increased age.** An increased risk for stroke has been shown to be associated with AF in the presence of any of the following: **age greater than 65 years, history of diabetes, history of hypertension, history of CHF, history of prior stroke, or transient ischemic attacks.** Left ventricular systolic dysfunction predicts ischemic stroke in patients with AF who do not receive antithrombotic therapy.

F. Laboratory examination and diagnostic testing. The initial evaluation of a patient with new-onset AF includes at a minimum a detailed history and physical examination to define the clinical type of AF; frequency, duration, and precipitating factors; and to delineate the presence and nature of symptoms associated with AF. In addition, evaluation should include:

1. **12-Lead electrocardiogram** (ECG) to identify the rhythm (that is to verify AF), underlying left ventricular (LV) hypertrophy, presence of preexcitation, and diagnose the existence of coronary artery disease and any other atrial arrhythmias. A 12-lead EKG may also be used to measure and follow PR, QRS, and QT intervals during treatment with antiarrhythmic therapy. In AF the P waves are absent. Atrial activity is chaotic and fibrillatory **(F) waves are present.** The baseline of the ECG is often undulating and may occasionally have coarse, irregular activity that can resemble atrial flutter, but it is not as stereotypical from wave to wave as atrial flutter. AF is distinguished from multifocal atrial tachycardia (MAT) by the presence in MAT of at least three different morphologic types of P waves. **Ventricular rhythm is usually irregularly irregular, and if AF is suspected with a regular ventricular response, then either some form of heart block is present or a junctional or ventricular tachycardia is present.** The **atrial rate** is generally in the **range of 400 to 700 beats/min,** with a ventricular response generally in the range of 120 to 180 beats/min in the absence of drug therapy. Ventricular response in excess of 180 beats/min, especially if the regular suggests the presence of an accessory pathway.
2. **Transthoracic echocardiogram** is uaually performed to identify the presence of valvular heart disease, and atrial and ventricular size and function, and to document coexistent pulmonary hypertension. Echocardiography can also be used as a prognostic tool to predict the development of systemic complications from AF and to help in the decision to initiate antithrombotic therapy. Echocardiographic predictors of increased thromboembolic risk include mitral stenosis, left atrial enlargement, reduced LV systolic function, decreased left atrial appendage emptying velocities, and evidence of spontaneous contrast ("smoke") or thrombus in the left atrium or left atrial appendage.
3. **Tests of thyroid, renal, and hepatic function.** Hyperthyroidism should always be considered and especially when the ventricular rate is difficult to control.
4. Additional investigation in selected patients with AF may include ambulatory electrocardiogram monitoring (e.g., Holter), or a 6-minute treadmill walk test to document the appropriateness of rate control.

G. Therapy. The therapy of choice in any unstable patient is immediate DCC. The term "unstable" should include the patient who is highly symptomatic (e.g., chest pain, pulmonary edema), as well as the patient who is hemodynamically unstable. **General management of AF centers on three areas: control of the ventricular response, minimization of the thromboembolic risk, and restoration and maintenance of sinus rhythm.**

1. **Control of the ventricular response.** The ventricular response is generally **controlled through drugs** that slow conduction through the atrioventricular (AV) node. AF that presents in the setting of WPW syndrome usually has evidence of preexcitation on ECG and is treated differently from AF conducting down the AV node alone. As noted previously, **intravenous calcium channel blockers, β-blockers, adenosine, and lidocaine are contraindicated in patients with AF and WPW**

syndrome associated with preexcitation because they facilitate conduction down the accessory pathway, causing acceleration of the ventricular rate, hypotension, and ventricular fibrillation. In the hemodynamically stable patient, class I antiarrhythmic medications such as procainamide may be administered intravenously, which diminishes antegrade conduction down the accessory pathway and decreases the degree of preexcitation, and may convert the AF entirely. For patients without evidence of preexcitation, the following agents are available to control the ventricular rate.

a. β-Blockers have a **rapid onset of action,** as well as **short half-lives in both the oral and intravenous forms.** These medications should be used cautiously in patients who have known decreased systolic function or evidence of heart failure. Intravenous preparations of metoprolol, esmolol, and propranolol have their onset of action in approximately 5 minutes. Orally available β-blockers of varying durations of action can be used for rate control. These include metoprolol and propranolol, as well as atenolol, nadolol, and a number of less commonly used agents (see Appendix: Drug Index for details). Amiodarone is an antiarrhythmic medication with β-blocking properties and can be used both for rate and rhythm control in the acute setting. Sotalol is another class III antiarrhythmic with β-blocking properties, which can be used for both rate and rhythm control; however, this medication is available in oral form only, and is more proarrhythmic then amiodarone.

b. Calcium channel blockers such as diltiazem and verapamil are available in both intravenous and oral forms. The intravenous forms are rapidly effective and have a short duration of effect. **In appropriate patients, they provide rapid control of the ventricular response.** Both oral diltiazem and verapamil are available in short-acting and sustained-release preparations.

c. Digitalis has long been used for rate control. Given its relatively long onset of action, **digoxin is ideally used in patients with decreased LV function, or where a contraindication exists to the use of β-blockers or calcium channel blockers** (e.g., brochospastic airway disease, asthma, or hemodynamic instability). Digoxin is usually **effective at controlling the resting heart rate;** however, it is **less effective at lowering the ventricular response to activity.** Because of this it is recommended that if digoxin alone is used in rate control, the patient should undergo monitored exercise and the exertional heart rate be verified to be under 110 beats/min.

Digoxin can be administered intravenously or orally. The **onset of action of digoxin is slow** (1 to 4 hours). Initially dosing of digoxin is 0.25 mg intravenously every 6 hours for a total of 1 mg every 24 hours. Then a maintenance dose is given that is based on the patient's renal function. Digoxin is **generally well tolerated, although it is associated with adverse effects,** such as gastrointestinal toxicity and neurotoxicity, and because of its long half-life (38 to 48 hours) is more likely to be associated with symptomatic bradycardia requiring intervention such as temporary pacing.

d. Angiotensin-converting enzyme (ACE) inhibitors and angiotensin receptor antagonists may decrease the incidence of AF by decreasing left atrial pressure and reducing the frequency of atrial premature beats. These medications may also reduce atrial fibrosis and decrease the recurrence of AF. Withdrawal from ACE inhibitors is associated with postoperative AF in patients undergoing coronary artery bypass grafting (CABG) surgery, and concurrent therapy with ACE inhibitors and antiarrhythmic agents enhances the maintenance of sinus rhythm.

e. HMG Co-A reductase inhibitors: "Statins" decrease the risk of AF recurrence following cardioversion. The mechanisms underlying this are poorly understood but probably include an inhibitory effect on the progression of coronary disease as well as their pleotropic anti-inflammatory and antioxidant properties.

f. Antiarrhythmics such as dofetilide and ibutilide are effective for conversion of atrial flutter and AF but are not effective for the control of ventricular rate alone. Propafenone, which is a class Ic antiarrhythmic drug, exerts addition mild beta-blocking effects, and may slow conduction across the AV node, although this is seldom sufficient to control the rate in patients with AF and may paradoxically cause an increase in AV nodal conduction and accelerate the ventricular rate response. Flecainide is another class IC agent, which is very effective in converting AF in structurally normal hearts but like propafenone requires concomitant AV nodal blockage.

2. Thromboembolic risk management

a. Current recommendations regarding the use of antithrombotic therapy to prevent the development of thromboembolism in patients with AF are to use antithrombotic therapy in all patients with AF except those with lone AF or with contraindications to antithrombotic agents. Lone AF is defined as that occurring in a structurally normal heart, in a patient younger than 65 years of age. The **American Heart Association** (AHA) recommends the individualized selection of appropriate antithrombotic agents depending on the patient's risks for stroke and bleeding. Factors associated with the highest risk of stroke in patients with AF include a history of prior thromboembolism [stroke, transient ischemic attack (TIA), systemic embolism] and rheumatic mitral stenosis. Moderate risk factors for stroke include age older than 65 years of age, CAD, CHF, female gender, hypertension, diabetes mellitus, and renal insuficiency. Presence of more than one moderate risk factor suggests the use of a vitamin K antagonist with a goal international normalized ratio (INR) of 2.0 to 3.0. Aspirin in doses of 81 to 325 mg daily is recommended as an alternative to vitamin K antagonism in low-risk patients or in those with contraindications to oral anticoagulation. The most recent guidelines also suggest similar use of antithrombotic therapy in patients with atrial flutter. Table 23.1 outlines one method of selecting the appropriate antithrombotic therapy for any given patient.

Based on the multivariate analysis from randomized controlled trials (RCTs), there have been several clinical scores developed to stratify the risk of systemic complications. The most well known of these is called the CHADS (Cardiac Failure, Hypertension, Age, Diabetes, and Stroke) risk index, which is a point system and assigns 2 points for history of TIA or stroke, 1 point

TABLE 23.1 Adapted from ACC/AHA Practice Guidelines

Risk category	Recommended therapy
No risk factors	Aspirin, 81 to 325 mg daily
One moderate-risk factor	Aspirin, 81 to 325 mg daily, or warfarin (INR 2.0 to 3.0, target 2.5)
Any high risk factor or more than 1 moderate-risk factor	Warfarin (INR 2.0 to 3.0, target 2.5)[a]

Less validated or weaker risk factors	Moderate-risk factors	High-risk factors
Female gender	Age greater than or equal to 75 y	Previous stroke, TIA or embolism
Age 65 to 74 y	Hypertension	Mitral stenosis
Coronary artery disease	Heart failure	Prosthetic heart valve*
Thyrotoxicosis	LV ejection fraction 35% or less	
	Diabetes mellitus	

[a]If mechanical valve, target international normalized ratio (INR) greater than 2.5.
INR, indicates international normalized ratio; LV, left ventricular; and TIA, translent ischemic attack.

TABLE 23.2 Anticoagulation Strategies in Patients Who Require Cardioversion

Length of time in atrial fibrillation	Elective cardioversion?	Timing and anticoagulation strategy
Less than 48 hours	Yes	Depends on the presence of risk factors for thromboembolism
Less than 48 hours	No	Immediate DCC may be performed without delay or need to start anticoagulation.
More than 48 hours, or unknown	Yes	A goal INR 2.0 to 3.0 for at least 3 weeks prior to and 4 weeks following DCC
More than 48 hours, or unknown	Yes	A TEE can be performed while the patient is on IV heparin with a goal appt ratio of 1.5 to 2.0, and if no identifiable thrombus is present, DCC can safely be performed, followed by 4 weeks of oral coumadin with goal INR 2.0 to 3.0.
More than 48 hours, or unknown	Yes	If the TEE demonstrates a thrombus, then anticoagulation with Coumadin with a goal INR 2.0 to 3.0 for a period of 3 weeks prior to a repeat TEE to assess for thrombus resolution. If no identifiable thrombus is visible on repeat TEE, then DCC should be followed by at least 4 weeks of anticoagulation with INR 2.0 to 3.0 post DCC.

for each of the following risk factors: age older than 75 years, hypertension, diabetes, or recent heart failure. This risk factor index was evaluated retrospectively in patients with ages older 65 years, and with nonvalvular AF, and the stroke risk varied between 1.8% per year in the lowest risk group with a CHADS score of 0, to 18.2% per year for those with an index score of 6.

Warfarin should be continued until sinus rhythm has been maintained for at least 4 weeks to allow for recovery of the atrial transport mechanism and for the recurrence of AF. **If cardioversion cannot be postponed for 3 weeks, patients should be anticoagulated (Table 23.2) with intravenous heparin and should undergo transesophageal echocardiography (TEE)** to rule out atrial thrombus; **then warfarin** is used for 4 weeks after cardioversion.

b. A number of major trials have attempted to compare the benefits of aspirin and warfarin in minimizing the stroke risk in patients with AF. Overall, warfarin has shown an annual average 68% reduction in relative risk for stroke, with aspirin showing a reduction anywhere from 0% to 44% (mean, ~30%). A recent trial has shown that clopidogrel reduces the risk for embolic stroke similar to that of aspirin.

The decision to anticoagulate patients with AF depends both on the risk of thromboembolic complications as well as the risk of bleeding. In younger patients at low risk for stroke (younger than 65 years, without other risk factors), and who generally lead active lifestyles that place them at increased risk for bleeding, **aspirin** may be an acceptable alternative to warfarin. **Older patients at greater risk for stroke (age 65 and older, with or without other risk factors)** should be anticoagulated with **warfarin to maintain an INR of 2 to 3. The risk of thromboembolism increases rapidly at INR levels even slightly less than 2, and the risk of bleeding increases at INR levels greater than 3.** Studies of fixed low-dose warfarin and aspirin have shown ineffective protection from thromboembolic risk as compared to anticoagulation with warfarin to maintain an INR of 2 to 3, and are not recommended. **Patients who have contraindications to warfarin** therapy should be treated with **aspirin. Risk for thromboembolism increases with longer duration of AF. Current guidelines recommend that patients who have been in AF for longer than 48 hours**

should be systemically anticoagulated whenever possible. This can be accomplished quickly with intravenous heparin. Cardioversion should be delayed in patients with AF of more than 48 hours duration who have not been anticoagulated as described in the AHA guidelines discussed previously unless a patient is sufficiently unstable that more rapid cardioversion is necessary, in which case screening of the atria for presence of thrombus with TEE is appropriate.

c. TEE is highly effective in the detection of thrombus in the atria and the left atrial appendage, and is more sensitive in this regard than transthoracic echocardiography (TTE). The ACUTE (Assessment of Cardioversion using Transesophageal Echocardiogram) study compared the use of TEE screening of patients with AF prior to cardioversion with a conventional approach based on 3 weeks of anticoagulation therapy. In the TEE group, those patients without thrombus on TEE underwent immediate cardioversion after therapeutic anticoagulation had been initiated and without waiting for 3 weeks. Patients were continued on warfarin for 4 weeks after the cardioversion as in the conventional group. No significant difference was noted in the embolic event rate or in the likelihood of maintenance of normal rhythm. TEE cardioversion is now considered an acceptable alternative when the conventional approach is not possible.

d. Cardiac output may be decreased after cardioversion in up to one-third of patients, and this can persist for as long as a week. Rarely, this leads to pulmonary edema as soon as 3 hours after cardioversion. Atrial function also declines immediately after cardioversion, even after that occurring spontaneously or pharmacologically. Cardiac output should return to baseline within 4 weeks. The risk of thromboembolism is thus still increased during this time period, and that is why warfarin therapy is recommended for a minimum of 4 weeks after cardioversion.

e. After 4 weeks of therapy, the decision to continue anticoagulation is based on each patient's individual risk for recurrence of AF. **Patients who cannot be successfully cardioverted should be anticoagulated for the long term,** as should patients with frequent recurrences/paroxysms.

3. Rate control during AF. Patients with AF may have controlled heart rates at rest but which accelerate even with mild exercise. Hence it is useful in patients with chronic AF to evaluate the heart rate response to submaximal or maximal exercise or to monitor the heart rate over an extended period (such as a 24-hour Holter monitor). The criteria defining adequate rate control vary with age but usually involve achieving a ventricular rate between 60 and 80 beats/min at rest and between 90 and 110 beats/min during moderate exercise.

4. Restoration and maintenance of sinus rhythm. There is debate as to whether restoration to sinus rhythm is beneficial for patients whose disease is asymptomatic as compared with a combined strategy of simply controlling the ventricular response and minimizing the thromboembolic risk. Data from nonrandomized trials show an increase in mortality in patients on long-term antiarrhythmic therapy for AF. The Atrial Fibrillation Follow-up Investigation of Rhythm Management (AFFIRM) trial is a recently reported study comparing two treatment strategies in patients with asymptomatic or tolerable AF. It compared outcomes in two groups of patients. One group was treated with antiarrhythmic drugs and cardioversion as necessary to maintain sinus rhythm. The other group was allowed to remain in AF with control of the ventricular rate alone. Both groups received anticoagulation therapy. There was no difference in survival or embolic event rate between the two groups. However, those treated with rhythm control alone had a lower incidence of adverse side effects.

a. Direct current cardioversion (DCC). When restoration of sinus rhythm is deemed necessary, this is most effectively carried out with DCC. **DCC is successful at least 80% of the time,** whereas pharmacologic rates of successful cardioversion are lower and depend on the antiarrhythmic drug used and the clinical scenario. Whenever possible, **DCC should be carried out under sedation, with appropriate cardiac and hemodynamic monitoring, and in the**

TABLE 23.3 Intravenous Medications used for the Cardioversion of AF

Drug name	Vaughn Williams class	Dose	Adverse side effects
Amiodarone	III	5 to 7 mg/kg over 30–60 min, followed by 1.2 to 1.8 g/d until 10 g, then 200–400 mg daily for maintenance.	Hypotension, bradycardia, hyperthyroidism, hepatits, skin discoloration, phlebitis
Ibutilide	III	1 mg over 10 min, repeat as needed.	Torsades de pointes, increased QTc
Propafenone	Ic	1.5 to 2.0 mg/kg over 20 min	Hypotension, atrial flutter with RVR
Flecanide	Ic	1.5 to 3.0 mg/kg over 10 to 20 min	Hypotension, atrial flutter with RVR

presence of personnel skilled in airway control/management. See Chapter 55 for the details of DCC, including sedation and methods.

b. Pharmacologic cardioversion

(1) The "drugs first" approach may promote more successful DCC and/or maintenance of sinus rhythm after DCC, if the attempt at pharmacologic cardioversion is unsuccessful. Similarly, it is reasonable to **attempt chemical cardioversion on any patient who fails DCC,** especially before repeated attempts at DCC.

(2) Table 23.3 shows the currently available intravenous agents available in the United States for the pharmacologic cardioversion of AF to sinus rhythm.

(i) Procainamide is a class IA antiarrhythmic that is often considered **the first line of therapy** for the pharmacologic conversion of AF occurring in the postoperative period after cardiac surgery.

(ii) Amiodarone is considered a class III antiarrhythmic drug, although it has properties of all of the four Vaughn Williams classes. Like procainamide, amiodarone is commonly used intravenously in the postoperative period for AF after cardiac surgery, particularly for those patients with renal insufficiency or failure who are not candidates for procainamide.

(iii) Ibutilide is an agent recently approved for the pharmacologic conversion of AF. The incidence of torsade de pointes [see **III.A.6.c(1)(b)**] is at least 1% to 2% with ibutilide, which is higher than that seen with procainamide or amiodarone. Ibutilide is available in only the intravenous form and is, therefore, not an option for long-term maintenance of sinus rhythm.

(3) A number of **oral agents** are available for the pharmacologic cardioversion of AF. **In appropriate patients the class IC agents, such as flecainide and propafenone, may be particularly effective for pharmacologic cardioversion**. In the text to follow are some other agents that may be used in the long term for maintenance of sinus rhythm in patients with AF. It should be kept in mind that initiation or upward dose titration of antiarrhythmic drugs should be done with caution, and in many instances should be performed in a hospital setting on a cardiac monitor. This is particularly true for the class III agents sotalol and dofetilide. On the other hand, in patients without structural heart disease, the class IC agents flecainide and propafenone may be considered for initiation on an outpatient basis. Table 23.4 outlines the presently available orally acting medications to treat AF.

TABLE 23.4 Oral Agents Available for Rhythm Control in Atrial Fibrillation

Drug name	Vaughn Williams class	Cardioversion dose		Daily maintenence dose
Amiodarone	III	600 to 800 mg in bid or tid dosing daily until 10 g, then		200 to 400 mg
Dofetelide	III	Based on CrCl (mL/min):	Dose: (μg bid)	Same. Dosing also adjusted for adjusted QTc
		>60 mL/min	500	
		40 to 60	250	
		20 to 40	125	
		<20	contraindicated	
Propafenone	Ic	600 mg		450 mg to 900 mg
Flecanide	Ic	200 to 300 mg		Same
Sotalol	III	160 to 320 mg		Same

(i) **Class IA agents.** These agents have seen a decline in their use, primarily due to a high incidence of intolerance because of side effects but also due to evidence of possible increased mortality for those patients with structural heart disease.

- **Procainamide.** This medication has not been used as frequently now for long-term treatment of AF, especially due to the potential for gastrointestinal, hematologic, and immunologic (e.g., lupus-like syndrome) side effects. An active metabolite of this drug, *n*-acetylprocainamide (NAPA), is cleared renally and has class III antiarrhythmic properties. Blood levels of both procainamide and NAPA need to be followed to prevent toxicity, especially in the setting of renal and/or hepatic insufficiency.
- **Quinidine.** Another class IA drug that has not been used as frequently in recent years, again primarily due to a relatively high incidence of side effects, such as gastrointestinal, hematologic, and neurologic effects. In addition, quinidine interacts with several cardiac and noncardiac medications.
- **Disopyramide.** This antiarrhythmic medication may have a "niche" for the treatment of vagally mediated AF, or AF that occurs in the setting of hypertrophic cardiomyopathy. However, its **negative inotropic effects** are greater than those of other class IA drugs, and it is associated with **greater anticholinergic effects** such as constipation and urinary retention.

(ii) **Class IC agents.** This group has become the preferred antiarrhythmic drugs for the management of AF in patients without structural heart disease, especially those patients with "lone" AF. These medications should not be used in patients with structural heart disease, especially patients with known or suspected ischemic heart disease. **Flecainide** was shown in the Cardiac Arrhythmia Suppression Trial (CAST) to be associated with increased mortality when used for suppression of ventricular arrhythmias in patients with LV dysfunction following myocardial infarction (MI). This has led to much concern over the use of the class IC agents in any patient with CAD and even in other types of structural heart disease.

- **Flecainide.** This is a well-tolerated medication that has a low incidence of neurologic side effects. This medication is approved both in oral form and intravenous form for the acute cardioversion of AF. Randomized trials with this drug show that it converts 60% to70% of patients with new onset AF at 4 hours and close to 90% at 8 hours. Oral and intravenous administration were equally efficacious, but the average response to the intravenous loading is seen within 1 hour, whereas it is 3 hours with the oral loading dose.

- **Propafenone.** This is also a well-tolerated medication. Its β-blocking properties limit its use in patients intolerant of such medications. Like sotalol, this property allows for its use as a single agent for AF suppression and ventricular rate control.

(iii) Class III agents. This group has become the preferred treatment for AF in patients with structural heart disease.

- Sotalol also has β-blocking properties, which makes it useful as a **single-agent therapy** for AF suppression and ventricular rate control. However, these properties also are responsible for the intolerance seen with this drug and may contribute to exacerbation of heart failure in some patients. **The dose must be reduced with renal insufficiency**.
- **Dofetilide.** This is the latest antiarrhythmic drug to be approved by the Food and Drug Administration (FDA) for management of AF. This drug is generally well tolerated and has been shown to be safe for patients with structural heart disease, in particular those patients who have had an MI and those with CHF. **This drug has been associated with proarrhythmia, especially in the setting of renal dysfunction. The prescription of the drug is tightly controlled, and only those certified in its use may prescribe it**.
- **Amiodarone.** This is a unique medication in that it has properties of all four Vaughn Williams classes. It is also unique with regard to its very long elimination half-life (up to 120 days). Amiodarone is effective for management of AF but is generally reserved for patients in whom other antiarrhythmic drugs have been ineffective or poorly tolerated, due to the important potential organ toxicities that may occur, predominantly to the liver, lungs, thyroid, and eyes. It is recommended that patients treated with amiodarone have baseline and then regular screening tests such as ophthalmologic examination, pulmonary function study, chest x-ray, and blood tests for liver and thyroid function.
- **Azimilide.** New class III antiarrhythmic drug not yet FDA approved for the management of AF.

(4) Figure 23.1, adapted from American Heart Association/American College of Cardiology/European Society of Cardiology (AHA/ACC/ESC) guidelines, outlines strategies used in the maintenance of sinus rhythm.

c. Atrio-Ventricular Nodal Ablation (AVN Ablation) in conjunction with permanent pacemaker.

(1) Symptomatic refractory AF, especially when the ventricular rate is uncontrollable or such control is limited by underlying bradycardia, may be amenable to ablation of the AV node and implantation of a **rate-responsive single-chamber permanent pacemaker.** These patients still require systemic anticoagulation. A recent meta-analysis of 21 studies that included 1100 patients who underwent AV nodal ablation for highly symptomatic AF, concluded that AV nodal ablation and subsequent pacemaker implantation significantly improved quality of life, exercise capacity, and LV function, and decreased symptoms of AF. In a small subset of 56 patients who had impaired LV function (an ejection fraction <40%) and AV nodal ablation, permanent pacemaker implantation caused an average improvement in ejection fraction of 8%, and complete normalization of the ejection fraction in one-third of the patients. The remaining patients with persistent LV dysfunction after AV nodal ablation had a 5-year survival rate of

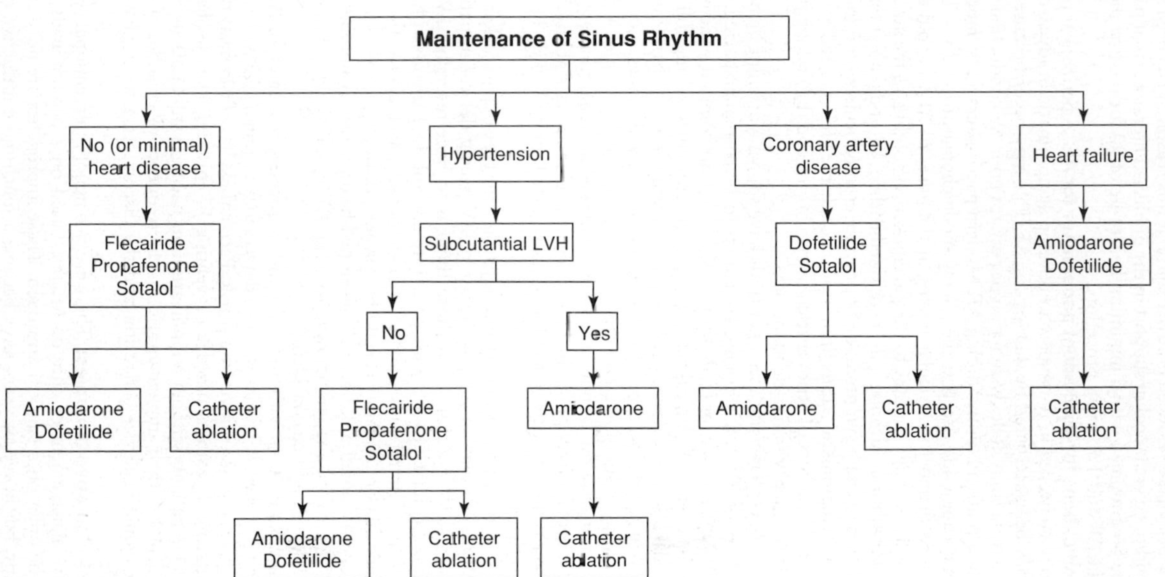

Figure 23.1. Therapeutic approach to the maintenance of sinus rhythm. Adapted from American College of Cardiology/American Heart Association (ACC/AHA) practice guidelines.

less than 40%. The 1-year mortality rate after AV nodal ablation and permanent pacemaker implantation is approximately 6.3%, which includes a high 2% risk of sudden cardiac death (SCD), which is thought to be related to early post pacemaker implantation R-on-T phenomenon caused by pacemaker-induced bradycardia. For this reason, it has been suggested, without a great deal of support in the published literature, that pacemakers be programmed with a minimum heart rate of 90 for the first month after the AV nodal ablation procedure.

(2) Indications for permanent pacemaker for AF. A permanent pacemaker may be needed in patients who develop symptomatic bradycardia, which may be exacerbated by therapy for AF. This may occur because of an underlying sinus node dysfunction or perhaps poor AV conduction leading to slow ventricular rates during AF. Modern pacemakers have **"mode switching"** capabilities, so that the pacing mode changes from dual-chamber to single-chamber ventricular pacing at the onset of AF to avoid rapid ventricular pacing rates due to the pacemaker responding to the atrial activity.

(3) Limitations. Although, as mentioned earlier, AV nodal ablation has been shown to cause symptomatic improvement in patients with refractory and very symptomatic AF, its limitations include the lifelong need for anticoagulation, the loss of atrioventricular synchrony, and the lifelong pacemaker dependence with its attendant risks.

Several recent pacemaker trials have shown worsening hemodynamic effects of RV apical pacing compared to biventricular pacing. The Post AV Nodal Ablation Evaluation (PAVE) trial randomized patients to right ventricular (RV) apical pacing versus biventricular pacing following AV nodal ablation for permanent AF. At an average follow-up of 6 months, the biventricular-paced group had longer 6 minute walk times, increased peak oxygen consumption, and reported improved quality of life. Although LV ejection fraction did not differ between the groups at baseline, at follow-up, the ejection fraction in the biventricular pacing group stabilized, whereas the ejection fraction in the RV apically paced group had declined significantly.

Current recommendations regarding the type of pacemaker following AV nodal ablation suggest the use of RV pacing devices in patients with normal LV function or in those thought to have reversible LV dysfunction secondary to AF with poor rate control. In patients with impaired LV function not caused by AF, a biventricular pacemaker with or without defibrillator capability should be considered. In patients who have undergone AV nodal ablation and developed heart failure symptoms following RV apical pacing, an upgrade from an RV apical system to biventricular system should be considered.

d. Implantable devices with treatment and suppressive strategies for AF are now available for selected patients. Some devices may terminate AF with rapid atrial burst pacing or a cardioversion shock. Pacemakers have become available that have pacing algorithms aimed at preventing AF episodes. The use of such pacemakers in patients without an indication for pacing is still under investigation. A difficulty in their implementation is the frequency of episodes of AF in patients requiring device activation and the discomfort associated with shock delivery.

e. Invasive curative therapies: There are two major interventional approaches for the management or cure of AF, one based on a percutaneous approach and the other on a surgical approach. These approaches are not yet first-line therapy, but in recent years have become a much more attractive option for patients with troublesome AF in whom antiarrhythmic treatment has been ineffective or poorly tolerated.

(1) Catheter ablation of AF with pulmonary vein isolation (PVI). In 1998, Haissaguerre and colleagues described the presence of isolated foci in the left atrium and pulmonary veins and their role in the initiation of AF. They also were able to demonstrate that ablation of these foci could successfully terminate AF. Based upon this early work, the field of AF ablation was born. Initial experiences with AF ablation attempted to mimic the surgical Maze procedure. Since that time, ablation has undergone various changes in both philosophy and technique.

Currently, approaches to AF ablation can be separated into two broad categories: anatomical and substrate/electrogram based. Anatomic ablation techniques use recently developed three-dimensional (3D) mapping systems to demonstrate the anatomy of the left atrium and the pulmonary veins. Various anatomic techniques including the isolation of each of the four veins, individually or via isolation of two veins at a time, have been developed. In addition, anatomic lines extended to the mitral isthmus or involving the room of the left atrium have been utilized. Purely anatomic procedures do not check for complete isolation of the pulmonary veins from the left atrium, and in most cases there are demonstrable gaps present post procedure.

Electrogram-based techniques require the use of a second (ring) mapping catheter. After circumferential isolation, the mapping catheter is used to evaluate for the presence of gaps in the ablation line and these gaps are then ablated. There have also been experiences using electrogram-based approaches to perform additional ablation points in other areas of the heart including the coronary sinus, the superior vena cava, and the right atrium after performing pulmonary vein isolation.

Advances in techniques have improved the efficacy and safety of the procedure. One major advance has been the development of protocols that ablate outside the ostia of the pulmonary veins to help reduce the incidence of postprocedure pulmonary vein stenosis.

Patient Preparation and Procedural Considerations

Prior to ablation considerations including access, conscious sedation, and choice of anticoagulation regimen should be made on an individual patient basis. The presence of multiple catheters in the left atrium requires patients to be given full anticoagulation. Prior to the procedure, some centers require patients to be therapeutic on warfarin for 4 to 6 weeks. Patients not anticoagulated prior to the procedure should undergo transesophageal echocardiogram to exclude the presence of left atrial thrombus. Regardless of preprocedural anticoagulation status, patients are fully anticoagulated with unfractionated heparin during the procedure to achieve a prespecified targeted active clotting time.

Catheters are placed in the right atrium and coronary sinus, typically via sheaths in the right and left femoral veins, and an additional sheath is often needed if intracardiac echo is used. The left atrium is accessed via transeptal puncture. Great care is needed, using fluoroscopic guidance to assure successful transeptal puncture, and many centers use intracardiac echo to assist in safely achieving transeptal puncture. After placement in the left atrium, circular "lasso" mapping and ablation catheters are used to approach the pulmonary veins. If used, intracardiac echo can assist 3D mapping techniques in identifying the pulmonary vein ostia.

End point for ablation differs depending on technique used. At completion of electrogram-based ablation, success is demonstrated by the development of entry block in the antrum of the pulmonary veins. However, anatomic-based procedures do not require the demonstration of block.

Centers performing ablation should have backup available of physicians experienced in pericardiocentesis and cardiothoracic surgery, secondary to the development of hemorrhagic pericardial effusion or atrial appendage rupture.

The identification of the pulmonary veins as the predominant source of ectopic foci that trigger AF has led to catheter-based ablation strategies to electrically isolate the pulmonary veins by delivering radiofrequency energy at their ostium. In the initial series, foci of increased automaticity within the pulmonary veins were targeted and ablated; in this initial series of 45 patients with proximal AF, 62% became free of symptomatic AF over a mean follow-up of 8 months. However 70% of the patients required multiple procedures. In a subsequent study using the same approach, the success rate (defined as the return of symptomatic AF) was 86% over a 6-month follow-up.

Continued research into the substrate for AF has demonstrated that there are many potentials that can contribute to the initiation and maintenance of AF, and that these may arise in multiple areas of the right and left atrium. Thus, procedures have been developed to incorporate linear lesions in the roof of the left atrium and mitral valve isthmus ablation to account for these. Using this approach in a series of 70 patients with symptomatic AF, 70% of the patients were found to be free from AF following pulmonary vein isolation without antiarrhythmic medications at 4 months of follow-up. The procedure continued to advance with the development of the circular mapping catheter, which allowed for more accurate mapping and isolation of the pulmonary veins.

At the time of this writing, the accumulated published experience in pulmonary vein isolation involves nearly 4000 patients, with an approximately 90% success rate in patients with paroxysmal AF and 80% success rate in patients with persistent AF. It must be noted that the success rates in patients with depressed ejection fraction is much lower than that in patients with normal systolic function.

A newer approach to radiofrequency catheter ablation of AF involves the ablation of complex fractionated electrograms, which has a 91% efficacy reported at one year. This study also showed that restoration of sinus rhythm following catheter-based ablation of AF caused a significant improvement in exercise capacity, quality of life, and LV systolic function.

Presently, the long-term efficacy of catheter-based ablation is not known and requires further study. Long-term follow-up from randomized controlled trials are presently either lacking in patient numbers, or marred by high crossover rates or by antiarrhythmic use. The current ACC/AHA/ESC guidelines allow for the use of PVI in the treatment of symptomatic AF following intolerance to, depending on the susbstrate, at least one drug and as many as three antiarrhythmic drugs.

Complications

Major complications from catheter-based ablation have been reported in about 6% of patients and include pulmonary vein stenosis, systemic thromboembolism, atrial esophageal fistula, and the development of atypical left atrial flutter.

The incidence of **pulmonary vein stenosis** has diminished by the judicious use of radiofrequency ablation energy to target areas just outside the pulmonary veins so as to isolate the ostia of the pulmonary veins from the remainder of the left atrium. The use of intracardiac echocardiography to detect microbubble formation as a means to measure the magnitude of radiofrequency energy delivered has been reported to reduce the instance of pulmonary vein stenosis. This complication often presents as dyspnea and breathlessness in the weeks to months following catheter-based ablation, with radiographic evidence of asymmetric pulmonary edema or pulmonary emboli, as it results in obstructive venous outflow from a single pulmonary lobe. This diagnosis is best made by the use of CT venography, but it can also be made through the use of transesophageal echocardiography with the finding of high-velocity flow in the affected pulmonary vein.

Systemic embolic events including embolic stroke are among the most serious complications of catheter-based ablation of AF, and the reported incidence varies from 0 to 5%. A trial comparing heparin-dosing regimens found that increasing the intensity of anticoagulation reduces the probability of forming left atrial thrombi from 11% to 3%, when the activated clotting time (ACT) was increased from 250 to more than 300 seconds.

Atrial esophageal fistula is a relatively rare complication of pulmonary vein isolation, and is more likely to occur when extensive ablation occurs over the posterior left atrial wall where it abuts the esophagus. Typical symptoms include nausea, vomiting, fever and sudden neurologic deterioration (from systemic embolization), and which occur in the days to weeks following ablation. Successful treatment of this condition requires prompt recognition of its clinical signs, as delay in the treatment often leads to death.

The development of **atypical left atrial flutter** is thought to be related to the development of scar in the left atrium, which creates the substrate for reentry required for this arrhythmia. The most important predictor of the development of left atrial flutter is the presence of an incomplete line of ablation, and it has been found that extending the ablation line to the mitral valve annulus may reduce the frequency of this complication. This arrhythmia, as is the case with right atrial flutter, is amenable to further catheter-based ablation.

(2) Cox Maze procedure is a surgical approach that has been developed over the last 25 years, and that tested the original hypothesis that reentry is the predominant mechanism for the development and maintenance of AF. It has undergone multiple revisions through the years, and now it has evolved to include techniques that surgically isolate the pulmonary veins, and connect these dividing lines to the mitral valve annulus. The surgical procedure uses atrial incisions in critical locations to create barriers to the propagating wavelets that are responsible for the initiation and maintenance of AF, and that consequently eliminate the macro-reentrant circuits in the atrium necessary to maintain AF.

The Maze procedure has changed over the last two decades, and present techniques use transmural lesions to isolate the pulmonary veins, and to connect these dividing lines to the mitral valve annulus, as well as lesions to create barriers in the right atrium. The reported success of the combined three developmental stages of the Cox-Maze procedure is 93% in patients with symptomatic AF who were intolerant of antiarrhythmic drugs. This long term report included 178 patients, and there was a 2.2% risk of peri-procedure death, and a 6% risk of pacemaker requirement in the patients undergoing a Cox-Maze I procedure. Other, more current studies have reported lower success rate of around 70%. This procedure maintains the atrial transport function, and especially when allied with left atrial appendage ligation reduces substantially the risk of postoperative thromboembolic events.

Procedure risks include a **death** risk, which is dependent on the patient's comorbidities but it is usually estimated to be less than 1% as an isolated procedure, the need for a **pacemaker**, **impaired atrial transport function**, and delayed **atrial arrhythmias** including atrial flutter.

The Maze procedure has not had widespread acceptance as a means for treatment of AF, except in patients undergoing open heart surgery. Even in these patients, the additional intraoperative time and complexity of the procedure has limited its widespread surgical application. Currently under development are less invasive approaches, including thoracoscopic and catheter-based epicardial techniques.

The Maze procedure is often associated with significant edema formation, probably due to atrial natriuretic peptide derangements. This is effectively mitigated by the use of aldosterone antagonists such as spironolactone for the first 4 to 6 weeks postoperatively. All procedures used to restore normal sinus rhythm in patients with AF have had a variable effect on the restoration of atrial transport function, depending on the duration of fibrillation before the procedure and the rhythm maintained following the procedure. The need for long-term anticoagulation following these procedures is generally assessed on an individual basis.

II. SPECIAL CONSIDERATIONS

A. Postoperative AF. AF is common postoperatively. The incidence of AF postoperatively varies with the type of surgery and is highest following open-heart surgery during, which time it ranges between 20% and 50%. It usually occurs in the first 5 days. Risk factors for perioperative AF include age, a history of AF, COPD, valvular heart disease (especially mitral valve disease), atrial enlargement, perioperative heart failure, and withdrawal from a β-blocker or ACE inhibitor. Postoperative AF is a major determinant of length of stay and thus of cost. It is associated with all the risks associated with AF in the nonpostoperative setting including hemodynamic compromise and thromboembolism.

1. Therapy. Postoperative AF is usually self-limited, and direct current cardioversion is usually not needed. There are a variety of antiarrhythmic agents available for cardioversion in postoperative patients. In a small trial, ibutilide was more effective than placebo for the treatment of postoperative AF. Sotalol is particularly effective acutely in patients with preserved LV systolic function, because the risk of proarrhythmic toxicity is small, and also because its β-blocker action contributes to slowing the ventricular rate.

AF carries an increased risk of stroke in post-CABG patients, and so anticoagulation with heparin followed by oral anticoagulants is recommended if AF persists for longer than 48 hours. The choice of antiarrhythmic therapy, AV node blocking agents and the use of either heparin and/or oral anticoagulants depends on the individual patient, the time from surgery, and the specific type of surgery.

2. Prevention. There is evidence supporting the prophylactic administration of β-blocker medications in patients undergoing cardiac surgery to prevent the development of AF. Sotalol has also been studied, but there is at present conflicting evidence regarding its effectiveness. Amiodarone when given either prophylactically before cardiac surgery or following open-heart surgery has been found to significantly reduce the incidence of postoperative AF. In the Prophylactic Oral Amiodarone for the Prevention of Arrhythmias that began Early after Revascularization (PAPABEAR) trial, oral amiodarone, dosed at 10 mg/kg beginning 6 days before and continuing for 6 days after surgery, decreased the incidence of postoperative AF by 50%. This efficacy was present in patients irrespective of whether CABG, valve surgery, or a combination was performed. Preoperative treatment with procainamide has yielded inconsistent results, as has treatment with either digoxin or verapamil.

At present there are limited data supporting the use of atrial overdrive pacing as opposed to single-chamber pacing in the prevention of postoperative AF. In a randomized trial involving 132 patients undergoing CABG, postoperative biatrial pacing significantly reduced incidence of AF by 12.5% compared to left atrial pacing, right atrial pacing, or no pacing. A meta-analysis of ten randomized trials also concluded that biatrial atrial and right atrial pacing reduced the incidence of AF after CABG surgery.

B. AF in acute MI. The incidence of AF following acute myocardial infarction varies depending on the population sampled as well as the type of myocardial infarction, but ranges between 10% and 20% at 30 days. AF is more commonly associated with acute MI in older patients as well as those with a higher Killip class and more severe LV dysfunction. Patients with AF in the setting of an acute MI have a worse outcome at 30 days than those in sinus rhythm [29.3% with AF versus 19% in normal sinus rhythm (NSR)]. Stroke rates are also increased in patients with post-MI AF.

The guidelines presently recommend urgent direct current cardioversion in patients with acute myocardial infarction who present with AF, especially if in rapid ventricular response with intractable ischemia or evidence of hemodynamic instability including congestive heart failure. Intravenous β-blockade is indicated for rate control to reduce myocardial oxygen consumption and demand, and digoxin is an alternative in patients with severe left surgical dysfunction and heart failure. Anticoagulation is recommended in patients with large anterior myocardial infarctions and those in which the AF becomes persistent. Post-MI ACE inhibitors seem to reduce the incidence of AF in patients with significant LV dysfunction. Post-MI use of carvedilol also seems to diminish the incidence of AF and atrial flutter.

C. AF and Wolff-Parkinson-White (WPW) syndrome. The most feared complication of the WPW syndrome is the development of ventricular fibrillation and sudden cardiac death secondary to antegrade conduction of the AF into the ventricles. The incidence of sudden cardiac death in patients with a WPW syndrome is around 0.6% per year, and risk factors for sudden cardiac death include having a short antegrade bypass tract refractory period (less than 250 ms), short RR intervals during preexcited AF, and the presence of multiple accessory pathways.

It is important to avoid AV node blocking agents in a patient who presents with a preexcited tachycardia, as this has the potential to increase the refractory period of the AV node and facilitate conduction down the accessory pathway. Administration of AV node blocking agents such as verapamil, diltiazem, and digoxin are contraindicated in this setting. Intravenous β-blockers are ineffective in this setting and may have adverse hemodynamic consequences.

Flecainide, a class IC antiarrhythmic, can be used to slow the ventricular rate in patients who have AF with rapid ventricular rates associated with preexcitation by shortening the shortest preexcited cycle length during AF.

Patients with WPW syndrome and syncope or with a short antegrade bypass tract refractory period, require immediate direct current cardioversion followed by catheter-based ablation of the accessory pathway as the preferred therapy. Ablation of the bypass tract does not necessarily prevent recurrence of the AF, it should be noted, but following this ablation the management of AF is similar to that of patients without preexcitation.

D. Atrial fibrillation in pregnancy. AF occurs infrequently during pregnancy and when it does usually has an identifiable cause, such as mitral valve disease, thyroid disease, or pulmonary processes. The ventricular rate can be controlled with digoxin, β-blockers, or a nondihydropyridine calcium channel blocker. Currently available antiarrhythmic medications cross the placenta and are excreted in breast milk and should be avoided if possible in the pregnant and lactating individual, but amiodarone, sotalol, and flecainide have all been used successfully during pregnancy in selected instances. Quinidine has the longest safety record of any antiarrhythmic in pregnancy and remains the agent of choice for pharmacologic conversion of AF. In the hemodynamically unstable patient, direct current cardioversion can be performed without any concerns of fetal damage.

Anticoagulation should also be given high priority during pregnancy, given the risk of thromboembolic disease during pregnancy, and only those patients with lone AF at low risk for thromboembolic complications should not receive anticoagulants.

The oral anticoagulant warfarin is generally avoided during the first trimester of pregnancy because of teratogenic effects, and also during the last month of pregnancy because of bleeding concerns during delivery. Administration of unfractionated heparin either by continuous intravenous infusion in a dose sufficient to increase the activated partial thromboplastin time (aPTT) to 1.5 to 2 times control, or by intermittent subcutaneous injection of 10,000 to 20,000 units every 12 hours adjusted to prolong the mid-interval APTT to 1.5 times control is appropriate. Low–molecular-weight heparin may also be considered during the first trimester and last month of pregnancy, although there are limited data on clinical outcomes with its use.

E. Atrial fibrillation and hypertrophic obstructive cardiomyopathy (HOCM). Patients with atrial fibrillation and hypertrophic obstructive cardiomyopathy have a high risk of systemic embolic events. For this reason it is recommended to maintain oral anticoagulation therapy in the range of an INR of 2.0 to 3.0 in patients with HOCM and AF. Antiarrhythmic medications can be used to prevent recurrent episodes of AF, and although there are insufficient data comparing the various antiarrhythmics, anecdotal evidence seems to support the use of disopyramide in combination with a β-blocker or a nondihydropyridine calcium channel blocker.

F. Atrial fibrillation and pulmonary disease. AF commonly develops in patients with COPD exacerbations. General recommendations include the treatment of the underlying lung process, correction of hypoxia, and of the acid–base imbalances. Medications commonly used to treat bronchospastic airway disease such as theophylline and

β-adrenergic agonists can precipitate AF and decrease the ability of medications to control the ventricular rate. Antiarrhythmic medications with β-blocking properties such as sotalol, propafenone, and adenosine can worsen bronchospasm, and are contraindicated in patients with severe bronchospastic airway disease. Ventricular rate control is usually achieved with a nondihydropyridine calcium channel blockers such as verapamil and diltiazem.

Guidelines

Valentin Fuster, et al. ACC/AHA/ESC 2006 guidelines for the management of patients with atrial fibrillation. *Circulation* 2006;114;257–354.

Landmark Articles

The Atrial Fibrillation Follow-up Investigation of Rhythm Management (AFFIRM) investigators. A comparison of rate control and rhythm control in patients with atrial fibrillation. *N Engl J Med* 2002;347:1825–1833.

Cox JL, Boineau JP, Schuessler RB, et al. Electrophysiologic basis, surgical development, and clinical results of the Maze procedure for atrial flutter and atrial fibrillation. *Adv Card Surg* 1995;6:1–67.

Cox JL, Schuessler RB, D'Agostino HJ Jr, et al. The surgical treatment of atrial fibrillation, III: development of a definitive surgical procedure. *J Thorac Cardiovasc Surg* 1991;101:569–583.

Doshi RN, Daoud EG, Pires L, et al. for the PAVE Study Group (2005). Left Ventricular-Based Cardiac Stimulation Post AV Nodal Ablation Evaluation (The PAVE Study). *J Cardiovasc Electrophysiol* 2005;16:1160–1165.

Haissaguerre M, Jais P, Shah DC, et al. Right and left atrial radiofrequency catheter therapy of paroxysmal atrial fibrillation. *J Cardiovasc Electrophysiol* 1996;7:1132–1144.

Haissaguerre M, Jais P, Shah DC, et al. Spontaneous initiation of atrial fibrillation by ectopic beats originating in the pulmonary veins. *N Engl J Med* 1998:339:659–666.

Mitchell LB, Exner DV, Wyse D, et al. Prophylactic Oral Amiodarone for the Prevention of Arrhythmias That Begin Early After Revascularization, Valve replacement, or Repair: PAPABEAR: A Randomized controlled trial. *JAMA* 2005;294:3093–3100.

Oral H, Knight BP, Tada H, et al. Pulmonary vein isolation for paroxysmal and persistent atrial fibrillation. *Circulation* 2002;105:1077–1081.

Pappone C, Oreto G, Rosanio S, et al. Atrial electroanatomic remodeling after circumferential radiofrequency pulmonary vein ablation. Efficacy of an anatomic approach in a large cohort of patients with atrial fibrillation. *Circulation* 2001;104:2539–2544.

Pappone C, Rosanio S, Augello G, et al. Mortality, morbidity, and quality of life after circumferential pulmonary vein ablation for atrial fibrillation: outcomes from a controlled nonrandomized long-term study. *J Am Coll Cardiol* 2003;42:185–197.

V VASCULAR AND PERICARDIAL DISEASES

24 VENOUS THROMBOEMBOLISM AND HYPERCOAGULABLE STATES

Esther S. H. Kim and John R. Bartholomew

I. VENOUS THROMBOEMBOLISM AND HYPERCOAGULABLE STATES

A. Venous thromboembolism. Deep vein thrombosis (DVT) and pulmonary embolism (PE) represent different manifestations of the same clinical entity referred to as venous thromboembolism (VTE). It is a common, lethal disease that affects hospitalized and nonhospitalized patients, which recurs frequently, is often overlooked, and can result in long-term complications including chronic thromboembolic pulmonary hypertension (CTPH) and the postthrombotic syndrome (PTS). Although PE is the third most common cause of hospital-related death in the United States, only one-third of all hospitalized patients at risk for VTE receive adequate prophylactic treatment. Most hospitalized patients have at least one or more risk factors for VTE, and without prophylaxis, the incidence of hospital-acquired DVT is 10% to 20% among medical patients and even higher among surgical patients (15% to 40%).

1. **DVT.** The lower extremities are the most common sites for DVT, but other affected sites include the upper extremities and the mesenteric and pelvic veins. The main goal in the management of DVT is the prevention of PE and the PTS. **Proximal lower-extremity DVTs (popliteal vein and above) have an estimated risk for PE of 50% if not treated. Approximately 25% of calf vein thrombi propagate (in the absence of treatment)** to involve the popliteal vein or above.
2. **Pathogenesis and risk factors.** **Virchow's triad** still forms the best framework for understanding the pathogenesis of VTE. The triad includes **stasis, hypercoagulability, and injury to the vessel wall.** They are both inherited and acquired risk factors for hypercoagulability. The most common inherited risk factors include **factor V Leiden and prothrombin gene mutation (G20210A); deficiency of the natural anticoagulants proteins C, S, and antithrombin; hyperhomocystinemia; and elevated factor VIII levels.** Acquired risk factors include immobilization, surgery, trauma, pregnancy, use of oral contraceptives or hormone replacement therapy, malignancy, antiphospholipid syndrome (lupus anticoagulant and/or anticardiolipin antibodies), heparin-induced thrombocytopenia (HIT), myeloproliferative disorders, obesity [body mass index (BMI) >30], inflammatory bowel disease, central venous catheters or pacemakers and the nephrotic syndrome.
3. **Clinical manifestations.** Typical symptoms of DVT in the upper and lower extremities include pain and swelling. Signs of DVT on physical examination may include increased warmth, tenderness, edema, the presence of dilated veins (collaterals), erythema, and, in extreme situations, cyanosis or gangrene. Various signs such as Homans' sign (dorsiflexion of the ankle with the knee at 30° flexion causing calf pain), Louvel's sign (worsening of pain with coughing or sneezing), and Lowenberg's sign (more pain on the affected leg after inflation of a sphygmomanometer around each calf) have been described, but these are neither sensitive nor specific for the diagnosis. A limb-threatening manifestation of DVT, **phlegmasia cerulea dolens,** occurs most often in the setting of malignancy, HIT, or other hypercoagulable conditions in which the thrombus completely occludes venous outflow causing massive limb swelling, hypertension in the capillary bed, and eventually ischemia and necrosis. Phlegmasia cerulea dolens is a vascular emergency requiring leg elevation, anticoagulation, and in select cases, thrombolysis or surgical or catheter-based thrombectomy. Fasciotomy may also be required to relieve associated compartmental syndromes.
4. **Diagnosis**
   a. **Clinical examination** is unreliable in the diagnosis of DVT, as symptoms and signs are often insensitive and nonspecific. Pretest probability scores improve the utility of further testing. For example, using the **Wells score** (Table 24.1), patients in the low pretest probability category have a 96% negative predictive value for DVT (99% if the D-dimer is negative as well), but the positive predictive value in patients with a high pretest probability is less than 75%, supporting the need for further diagnostic testing to identify patients with thrombosis.
   b. **Venography** has been the gold standard test for the diagnosis of DVT in the past. The presence of an intraluminal filling defect is diagnostic, although abrupt cutoffs, nonfilling of the deep venous system, and/or demonstration of collateral flow may also serve as evidence for the presence of DVT. However, because venography is invasive and requires the use of potentially harmful contrast agents, it has largely been replaced by noninvasive tests such as duplex ultrasonography.
   c. **Duplex ultrasonography** has a sensitivity and specificity of about 95% and 98%, respectively, for the detection of DVT in symptomatic patients; however,

TABLE 24.1 Pretest Probability of Deep Vein Thrombosis (DVT) (Wells Score)

Clinical feature[a]	Score
Active cancer (treatment ongoing or within previous 6 months of palliative	1
treatment)	1
Paralysis, paresis, or recent plaster immobilization of the lower extremities	1
Recently bedridden for more than 3 days or major surgery, within 4 weeks	1
Localized tenderness along the distribution of the deep venous system	1
Entire leg swollen	1
Calf swelling by more than 3 cm when compared with the asymtpomatic leg	1
(measured 10 cm below tibial tuberosity)	1
Pitting edema (greater in the symptomatic leg)	–2
Collateral superficial veins (nonvaricose)	
Alternative diagnosis as likely or greater than that of deep vein thrombosis	
Score	
High	3 or greater
Moderate	1 or 2
Low	0 or less
Modified score (adds one point if there is a previously documented DVT	
Likely	2 or more
Unlikely	1 or less

[a]In patients with symptoms in both legs, the more symptomatic leg is used.
Reproduced from Wells et al. *Lancet* 1997;350:1795 *(Copyright © 1997 Elsevier. All rights reserved.)* and Wells et al. *N Engl J Med* 2003;349:1227 *(Copyright © 2003 Massachusetts Medical Society. All rights reserved.)*

it is operator dependent and is less sensitive in asymptomatic individuals and for thrombi located in the calf veins. An inability to compress the vein with the ultrasound transducer is diagnostic for DVT. Other findings suggestive, but not diagnostic, of an acute DVT include venous distention or absent or decreased spontaneous flow. Diagnosis of recurrent DVT is more challenging, given the high incidence of persistently noncompressible veins after an initial event. Other limitations of compression ultrasonography include the difficulty in detecting isolated thrombi in the iliac veins or superficial femoral veins within the abductor canal. False positives may occur when pelvic abscesses or neoplasms result in isolated noncompressiblility of the common femoral veins.

d. D-Dimer. The sensitivity and negative predictive value of this test are high. **The combination of a low pretest probability and a negative D-dimer has an extremely high negative predictive value for VTE (approximately 99%).** A positive D-dimer, however, does not confirm the diagnosis of DVT.

e. Other diagnostic tests less frequently used to detect DVT include magnetic resonance venous imaging (MRVI) and computed tomography (CT).

5. Treatment

a. The main goals of treatment for DVT include prevention of PE, CTPH, the PTS, and recurrent VTE. Once DVT is suspected, anticoagulation should be started immediately, unless there is a contraindication, and continued once the diagnosis is confirmed. Initial therapy should include heparin, low–molecular-weight heparin (LMWH), or fondaparinux followed by an oral anticoagulant (vitamin K antagonist or VKA). LMWH and fondaparinux are renally cleared, and although the LMWHs can be given in patients with renal insufficiency after dose adjustment, both are contraindicated in patients requiring dialysis.

Weight-based dosing of unfractionated heparin (UFH) [80 U/kg bolus followed by 18 U/kg per hour intravenous (IV) infusion] has been shown to achieve a therapeutic activated partial thromboplastin time (aPTT) more rapidly than fixed-dose regimens. The target aPTT has traditionally been 1.5 to 2.5 times the control aPTT; however, the actual aPTT in seconds varies among laboratories because of their use of different aPTT reagents. The American Coollege of Chest Physicians (ACCP) and the College of American Pathologists (CAP) now advocate the use of an anti-factor Xa assay to establish a heparin dose-response curve for the aPTT ratio (of each laboratory), using concentrations that correlate to therapeutic heparin levels of 0.3 to 0.7 IU/mL determined by factor Xa inhibition. The aPTT should not be followed in patients with an abnormal baseline aPTT (e.g., in patients with lupus anticoagulant), in patients who require unusually high doses of heparin such as antithrombin deficiency, or in individuals with an underlying malignancy or during pregnancy. In these situations, also referred to as heparin resistance, the anti-factor Xa assay should be used. UFH can also be administed subcutaneously as an alternative to IV administration, and several dosing nomograms have been recommended. One approach is to give an initial IV bolus of 5000 U followed by a subcutaneous dose of 17,500 U twice daily on the first day. Blood for an aPTT is drawn 6 hours after the initiation dose, and subsequent doses are adjusted accordingly to achieve an aPTT 1.5 to 2.5 times the control. Another recently derived nomgram recommends a subcutaneous loading dose of 333 U/kg followed by fixed doses of 250 U/kg subcutaneously every 12 hours without the need for aPTT monitoring.

LMWH is administered as a weight-based subcutaneous injection. Enoxaparin, the most commonly used agent in the United States, is given either as a once daily injection (1.5 mg/kg per day) or twice per day (1 mg/kg every 12 hours). No monitoring is required except in obese, pediatric, or pregnant patients or patients with renal insufficiency. The anti-Xa level using LMWH as a reference standard should be measured 4 hours after an injection, and the therapeutic range is 0.5 to 1.0 IU/mL for the 12-hour regimen and ≥1.0 IU/mL for the daily dose.

Once anticoagulation with UFH or LMWH is begun, a VKA may be initiated. The overlap should be continued for a minimum of 4 to 5 days and until the international normalized ratio (INR) is within the target range of 2.0 to 3.0 for two consecutive days to permit adequate depletion of vitamin K–dependent coagulation factors.

Fondaparinux, an indirect factor Xa inhibitor, is approved by the U.S. Food and Drug Administration (FDA) for use as DVT prophylaxis in patients undergoing orthopedic procedures (total hip and knee arthroplasty) and abdominal surgery. It is also approved as treatment of acute DVT and PE when used in combination with a VKA. Its efficacy and safety in comparison to LMWH for the treatment of acute DVT and in comparison with IV UFH for the treatment of PE has been shown in large randomized controlled trials. Fondaparinux is administered as a once-daily subcutaneous injection of 2.5 mg for DVT prophylaxis, and 5 mg, 7.5 mg, or 10 mg based on body weight (<50 kg, 50 to 100 kg, and >100 kg, respectively) for the treatment of DVT or PE. Fondaparinux is contraindicated in patients with severe renal impairment (creatinine clearance <30 mL/min) and bacterial endocarditis. When used as DVT prophylaxis, fondaparinux is also contraindicated in patients with body weight <50 kg who are undergoing hip fracture, hip replacement or knee replacement surgery, and abdominal surgery.

Thrombolytic therapy for DVT may be beneficial in select individuals and can be administered systemically or locally under catheter guidance. Both routes carry an increased risk of systemic hemorrhage compared to standard anticoagulation alone. Although it has been suggested that use of thrombolytics promote early recanalization and minimizes the incidence of the PTS, their role in DVT without a threatened limb is still unclear. The current ACCP guidelines recommend against their routine use in patients with DVT, except for those patients (without contraindication) with a massive ileofemoral DVT or individuals at risk of limb gangrene secondary to venous occlusion.

Damage to the venous valves from DVT and venous hypertension can lead to the development of the PTS, which is characterized by edema, skin changes including increased pigmentation and lipodermatosclerosis, pain, and, in severe cases, stasis ulceration. The incidence of this complication is drastically reduced with the use of **compression stockings**, and current guidelines recommend the use of stockings at a pressure of 30 to 40 mmHg at the ankle for 2 years after an episode of DVT. In addition, early ambulation as tolerated after diagnosis is encouraged, as mobile patients with DVT do not require bed rest.

b. **Vena caval interruption.** Current guidelines recommend against the routine insertion of inferior vena cava (IVC) filters for the treatment of DVT. **Indications for placement of IVC filters are: contraindication to anticoagulation, complication from anticoagulation, or recurrent thromboembolization despite adequate anticoagulant therapy.** Relative indications for IVC filters are massive PE, iliocaval DVT, free floating proximal DVT, cardiac or pulmonary insufficiency, high risk of complications from anticoagulation (frequent falls, ataxia), or poor compliance. Retrievable filters can be considered for situations for which anticoagulation is temporarily contraindicated or there is a short duration of PE risk. IVC filter alone is not effective therapy for DVT, and resumption of anticoagulation as soon as possible after placement is recommended.

c. **Duration of treatment.** The duration of treatment following the diagnosis of DVT is dependent on the risk of recurrence. Risk factors for recurrence include an idiopathic DVT, underlying hypercoagulable states (listed in subsequent text), and malignancy. In addition, placement of a permanent IVC filter, elevated D-dimer levels, advanced age, male sex, and increased BMI also place individuals at a higher risk for recurrence. The risk of recurrence decreases with longer durations of anticoagulation; however, clinicians must weigh the risk of bleeding against the risk of new thrombosis.

Current guidelines recommend 3 months of anticoagulation with a VKA targeting an INR of 2 to 3 for patients with a first episode of DVT secondary to a transient cause. Anticoagulation with a VKA for at least 6 to 12 months with a target INR of 2 to 3 is recommended for patients with a first episode of idiopathic DVT, although consideration should also given for indefinite anticoagulation in this situation. Patients with the antiphospholipid syndrome, homozygous for factor V Leiden, or doubly heterozygous for factor V Leiden and prothrombin gene mutation should be considered for indefinite anticoagulation. Long-term (indefinite) anticoagulation is also recommended in patients with malignancy, as long as the cancer remains active, and in patients who have unexplained recurrent DVTs.

6. **Calf vein thrombosis.** Anticoagulation is generally indicated for symptomatic calf DVT or when there is propagation into the popliteal vein or proximally. Current guidelines recommend 3 months of treatment with a VKA targeting an INR of 2 to 3 for patients with a first episode of symptomatic DVT confined to the calf veins secondary to a transient cause. Monitoring calf vein thrombosis for propagation into the proximal veins with serial ultrasonography (once or twice weekly for 2 to 3 weeks) without anticoagulation represents an alternative approach to treatment for individuals with a contraindication to anticoagulation.
7. **Superficial venous thrombosis** frequently occurs as a complication of an intravenous line, but may occur spontaneously. Anticoagulation is generally not required due to the lower risk of PE, unless the thrombosis propagates into the deep venous system or if the event is spontaneous. Guidelines recommend intermediate doses of heparin or LMWH for at least 4 weeks for spontaneous superficial thrombophlebitis.
8. **Upper extremity DVT.** Upper extremity DVT is most often related to central venous catheter placement and/or pacemaker devices. Other less common causes include thoracic outlet syndrome, Paget-von Schröetter (also referred to

as effort thrombosis), and hypercoagulable conditions including malignancy. Patients may be asymptomatic but more frequently complain of arm swelling and pain. Anticoagulation is indicated if there are no contraindications. Thrombolysis should be considered in younger patients with a low risk of bleeding and symptoms of acute onset. Determination of the length of anticoagulation with a VKA should be decided using the same processes described for acute lower extremity DVTs.

B. PE. It is difficult to approximate the true incidence of PE, but there are estimates that as many as 300,000 Americans have a fatal PE each year and as many as 34% of affected individuals present with sudden death. The majority of patients die because of a failure in diagnosis rather than inadequate therapy. In fact, the mortality rate for PE without treatment is approximately 30%, whereas it is only 2% to 8% with adequate treatment. Pulmonary embolism remains the most common preventable cause of hospital death in the United States.

1. **Pathophysiology and symptoms.** Hemodynamic collapse related to pulmonary embolism results from a combination of vascular obstruction from thrombus and vasoconstriction caused by inflammatory mediators and hypoxia. Elevated pulmonary vascular resistance results in decreased right ventricular outflow, leading to a decrease in preload and cardiac output resulting in hypotension. To overcome an obstruction of 75% and maintain pulmonary perfusion, the right ventricle must generate a systolic pressure in excess of 50 mmHg and a mean pulmonary artery pressure greater than 40 mmHg. The normal right ventricle is unable to generate these pressures, and right heart failure and cardiac collapse ensues. In addition, elevated right ventricular wall tension can lead to decreased right coronary artery flow and ischemia. Cardiopulmonary collapse from pulmonary embolism is more common in patients with coexisting coronary artery disease or underlying cardiopulmonary disease.

   Pulmonary embolism may present as one of the following three syndromes: (a) acute cor pulmonale, (b) pulmonary infarction, or (c) dyspnea. Patients presenting with acute cor pulmonale, as manifested by the sudden development of dyspnea, cyanosis, shock, or syncope, usually have a massive PE leading to cardiovascular collapse. Patients with pulmonary infarction usually present with pleuritic chest pain, dyspnea, and hemoptysis, and an audible friction rub may be heard. The majority of patients present with generalized symptoms of chest pain, dyspnea, and malaise.

2. **Diagnosis**
   - **a.** Several pretest probability scores have also been developed for the diagnosis of PE similar to those for DVT. In a validation study of the Wells clinical decision rule, only 0.5% of patients who were unlikely to have PE and had a negative D-dimer went on to have subsequent nonfatal VTE.
   - **b. Troponin.** Cardiac troponins have been evaluated in the setting of acute PE, and elevated levels correlate with electrocardiographic and echocardiographic findings of right ventricular pressure overload. Elevations in this marker can be seen in patients with and without CAD, but overall mortality and in-hospital complications are higher in patients with acute PE and elevated cardiac troponin than in patients without.
   - **c. Brain natrluretic peptide (BNP)** elevation in the absence of renal dysfunction is also a marker of right ventricular dysfunction in patients with PE. Like elevated troponin levels, elevated levels have also been shown to be predictors of adverse outcome in patients with acute PE.
   - **d. Arterial blood gas.** Pulmonary embolism can result in signficant hypoxia, but in the Prospective Investigation of Pulmonary Embolism Diagnosis (PIOPED) study, 26% of patients with angiographically proven PE had PaO_2 >80 mm Hg. Similarly, a normal alveolar–arterial gradient does not preclude the diagnosis of PE. Therefore, a normal PaO_2 cannot rule out PE; however, hypoxia in the absence of cardiopulmonary disease should raise the suspicion for this diagnosis. In patients with cardiopulmonary collapse, a normal PaO_2 suggests that PE is an unlikely cause.

e. **Chest radiography** may be more helpful in establishing other diagnoses. When present, findings are nonspecific and include pleural effusion, atelectasis, and consolidation. The classic signs including the Westermark sign (regional oligemia), Hampton's hump (pleural based, wedge-shaped shadow), and Palla's sign (enlarged right inferior pulmonary artery) are uncommon.

f. **Electrocardiography.** Like chest radiography, the major utility of the electrocardiogram (ECG) in the diagnosis of PE is to rule out other major diagnoses, such as acute myocardial infarction (MI). The most specific finding on an electrocardiogram is the classic $S_1Q_3T_3$ pattern, but the most common findings are nonspecific ST-segment and T-wave changes. Other commonly reported findings include sinus tachycardia, atrial fibrillation, and right bundle-branch block. In a study of electrocardiograms in patients with acute PE and increased right ventricular end-diastolic dimension and tricuspid regurgitation, three or more of the following abnormalities were seen in more than three-fourths of the patients: (a) incomplete or complete right bundle-branch block, (b) S waves >1.5 mm in lead I and aVL, (c) shift in transition zone to V_5, (d) Q waves in leads III and aVF but not II, (e) right axis deviation greater than 90 or indeterminate axis, (f) low-voltage QRS in limb leads, and (g) T-wave inversion in leads III and aVF or leads V_1 through V_4.

g. **Echocardiography.** More than 50% of hemodynamically stable patients with PE will not have evidence of right ventricular dysfunction on transthoracic echocardiography (TTE). Patients with hemodynamic collapse, however, will generally have severe right ventricle dysfunction, and TTE can provide rapid bedside assessment in these critically ill patients. TTE findings include right ventricular dilation, right ventricular hypokinesis, tricuspid regurgitation, septal flattening, paradoxical septal motion, diastolic left ventricular impairment secondary to septal displacement, pulmonary artery hypertension, lack of inspiratory collapse of the inferior vena cava, and occasionally direct visualization of the thrombus. **In patients with large PE, it has been observed that despite moderate or severe right ventricular free-wall hypokinesis there is relative sparing of the apex. This finding is referred to as McConnell's sign and has a specificity of 94% and a positive predictive value of 71% for PE.** McConnell's sign may be useful in discriminating right ventricular dysfunction due to PE versus other causes.

h. **Ventilation–perfusion ($\dot{V}/\dot{Q}$) scanning.** $\dot{V}/\dot{Q}$ scanning is now a second-line imaging method for the diagnosis of PE. $\dot{V}/\dot{Q}$ scans are helpful in patients who have normal chest radiography or who are unable to have CT scanning, such as those with renal insufficiency, contrast allergy, or pregnancy. The results of PIOPED suggest that $\dot{V}/\dot{Q}$ scanning is helpful if the scan is normal or at high probability for PE (87% of patients with high-probability scans had PE, but only 4% of patients with normal scans had PE). Intermediate-probability or low-probability scans are the most common finding, however, occurring in approximately 70% of patients in the PIOPED study. In addition, **patients who had a high or intermediate clinical suspicion for PE but a low-probability scan still had a 40% and 16% rate, respectively, of PE diagnosed by pulmonary angiography.** Hence, it is currently advised that patients with a high or intermediate clinical suspicion for PE but a low-probability $\dot{V}/\dot{Q}$ scan have additional tests to confirm or refute the diagnosis.

i. **CT scanning.** Because of its wide availablility and the ability to directly visualize thrombus, CT imaging has become the standard imaging technique for the diagnosis of acute PE. It is especially useful in evaluating central PE (thrombus is seen as an intraluminal filling defect), and although the diagnostic yield for peripheral or subsegmental PE was low initially, newer multiple-slice CT scans have improved this diagnostic ability as well. CT scanning also allows direct imaging of the inferior vena cava, pelvic and leg veins, as well as identifying other pathologies that may be mimicking symptoms of acute PE. The major disadvantages of CT are radiation exposure, higher cost, and the possibility of contrast-induced nephrotoxicity. A meta-analysis of 23 studies, including 4657 patients with a suspicion of PE who had normal CT scans, found that only 1.4% went on to develop VTE and 0.51% developed fatal PE by 3 months. These rates are similar to those in other studies involving patients who had suspected PE but were found to have normal pulmonary angiograms.

j. **Pulmonary angiography** remains the gold standard diagnostic test for PE, but it is used infrequently due to the advent of CT scanning. Four injections with four views (right and left anteroposterior, and right and left oblique) are performed. In some situations where a lung scan shows perfusion abnormalities and is nondiagnostic for PE, selective angiography of the abnormal area may be considered so as to limit the amount of contrast needed. In experienced centers, associated morbidity and mortality are low.

k. **Magnetic resonance angiography** (MRA) may be an alternative to CT for the diagnosis of PE in patients who have contrast allergy or for whom avoidance of radiation exposure is desired. Reports of sensitivity and specificity are varied, but compared to CT, MRA has been reported to be both less sensitive and specific and limited by interoberserver variability.

3. **Treatment.** Anticoagulation with heparin, LMWH, and, more recently, fondaparinux followed by the addition of a VKA and supportive care has remained the standard of care in the management of acute PE. Current guidelines recommend initial treatment with anticoagulants for patients with a high clinical suspicion for PE while awaiting the results of diagnostic testing. For patients with nonmassive PE, subcutaneous LMWH, IV UFH, or fondaparinux are recommended as initial treatment. In patients with acute nonmassive PE, LMWH is recommended over UFH. A VKA may be initiated together with IV UFH, LMWH, or fondaparinux, and should be continued for a minimum of 4 to 5 days and until the INR is stable and $\geq$2.0. The outpatient use of LMWH in the management of PE has not yet received approval from the FDA.

a. **Thrombolysis** for the treatment of acute PE is highly individualized, as there have been no clearly established short-term mortality effects. Because of favorable outcomes with prompt recognition and anticoagulation for PE, thrombolysis should be reserved for hemodynamically unstable patients with acute massive PE and a low risk of bleeding. It is unclear whether there is any benefit for thrombolytic therapy in patients who are hemodynamically stable but who have echocardiographic evidence of right ventricle dysfunction. Streptokinase, urokinase (no longer available in the United States), and tissue plasminogen activator are the current agents approved by the FDA. Current guidelines recommend the use of systemic thrombolytic therapy in patients who are hemodynamically unstable. Local administration of thombolytic therapy via a catheter is not suggested, owing to the risk of hemorrhage at the insertion site.

b. **Pulmonary embolectomy** was the first definitive therapy to be performed for PE. There have been no randomized trials evaluating embolectomy, and the primary use of this procedure is in patients with shock and a contraindication to thrombolysis. Other investigational therapies include catheter-based embolectomy procedures that utilize aspiration, fragmentation, or rheolytic therapy. As of yet, there are currently no guidelines for the use of these therapies.

II. **HYPERCOAGULABLE CONDITIONS.** Conditions that predispose persons to an increased risk for thrombosis are referred to as hypercoagulable states or thrombophilia. These conditions are being identified more frequently and may be classified as inherited or acquired. Patients who should have hypercoagulable profiles peformed are those individuals with an idiopathic VTE, women with thrombosis while on oral contraceptives, receiving hormone replacement therapy or during pregnancy, family history of clotting, a first thrombotic event before the age of 50, thombosis at unusual locations, resistance to anticoagulation, and those with recurrent thromboses.

A. **Factor V Leiden and prothrombin gene mutation.** Activated protein C inactivates factors Va and VIIIa and is one of the mechanisms by which the balance between clotting and bleeding are maintained. The autosomal dominant acquisition of a single-point mutation (factor V Leiden) in the factor V gene renders the protein factor V resistant to inactivation by activated protein C. Both homozygous and heterozygous states are at an increased risk for venous thrombosis, with a 50- to 100-fold increase in the homozygous state and a 3- to 7-fold increase in the heterozygous state. The factor V Leiden mutation (FVL) is more prevalent in persons of European and Scandinavian ancestry. The prothrombin gene mutation G20210A (PT G20210A) is also inherited as an autosomal-dominant mutation and may lead to a higher plasma level of prothrombin. It is also more common in those of Caucasian ancestry and confers a 2.8-fold increased risk for VTE. The role of FVL and PT G20210A mutations in arterial thrombosis is unclear. There is only a modest association between inherited thrombophilias and major arterial thromboses such as MI, stroke, or peripheral arterial disease (PAD). Therefore, routine screening for these mutations is not warranted in most patients with arterial thrombosis. In young persons who develop arterial events, however, abnormalities in hemostasis may play a role particularly in the presence of other risk factors such as smoking and oral contraceptive (OCP) use, and additional testing may be warranted. Factor V Leiden and PT G20210A are associated with VTE during pregnancy, oral contraceptive use, and hormone replacement therapy (HRT). For example, the annual risk for DVT is 3 per 10,000 in women without FVL who use OCPs, 5.7 per 10,000 in women with FVL who do not use OCPs, and 28.5 per 10,000 in women with FVL who use OCPs. FVL can be identified by evaluating for activated protein-C resistance in plasma or by gene analysis using polychromase chain reaction. The prothrombin gene mutation is also identified by genetic analysis. There are no clear evidence-based guidelines for managing patients with thrombosis in the setting of these thrombophilias. In general, acute thrombosis should be managed in a standard fashion, but the duration of therapy is less clear, and the benefits of long-term anticoagulation must be weighed against the risks of bleeding. Current guidelines recommend long-term therapy for patients who are homozygous for FVL or who are doubly heterozygous for FVL and PT G20210A, as well as individuals with the antiphospholipid syndrome. Patients with asymptomatic disease should receive prophylaxis in high-risk situations.

B. Defects in the natural anticoagulants [protein C (PC), protein S (PS), and antithrombin (AT)]. Deficiency of any of the three natural anticoagulants is associated with an increased risk for venous thrombosis. All are inherited as autosomal dominant defects and are further subclassified based on reduction in their levels or defective quality of the protein. PS acts as a cofactor in the inactivation of factors Va and VIIIa by activated PC. It is bound to C4-binding protein (an acute-phase reactant) in the plasma. Levels of PS and PC are lower in conditions such as disseminated intravascular coagulation (DIC), inflammatory states, nephrotic syndrome, acute thrombosis, and liver disease. Pregnancy and oral contraceptive use can also decrease levels of PS. Both PC and PS levels are lowered by warfarin therapy and, therefore, these tests should not be assayed in patients who are receiving VKAs. Similarly, initiation of warfarin therapy without concomitant anticoagulation in the setting of acute VTE may lead to warfarin-induced skin necrosis (manifested as painful necrosis of the skin, primarily in fatty areas including the breast, buttocks, and thighs). Treatment includes stopping warfarin, administering vitamin K and fresh frozen plasma to replete levels, and using an alternative anticoagulant. AT is produced by the liver and endothelial cells and functions by inactivating thrombin, factor Xa, and factors IXa, XIa, and XIIa. Homozygous states are incompatible with life. Levels are also low in those with DIC, sepsis, liver disease, nephrotic syndrome, with the use of oral contraceptives, and during pregnancy. As previously discussed, patients with AT deficiency may have resistance to heparin because it exerts its anticoagulant effect through AT. AT concentrates are available and can be used temporarily to correct this deficiency.

C. Homocysteine. Hyperhomocysteinemia is a risk factor for venous and arterial thrombosis. It may be inherited, and genetic defects causing a deficiency of cystathionine β-synthase or a mutation in methylenetetrahydrofolate reductase (MTHFR) have been reported. Acquired causes include deficiencies in vitamin B_{12}, B_6, or folate; smoking; and liver or renal failure. Treatment with folate in doses between 0.5 and 5 mg is usually effective in reducing the levels of homocysteine, but whether this reduces the risk of thrombosis is unknown.

D. Heparin-induced thrombocytopenia. Heparin-induced thrombocytopenia (HIT) is a common, underrecognized but potentially devastating condition in patients who receive heparin or LMWH. The reported incidence is between 3% and 5% in patients exposed to UFH and lower (<1%) in patients exposed to LMWH. The pathogenesis of HIT involves the formation of antibodies (usually IgG) against a heparin–platelet factor 4 (PF4) complex. The HIT antibodies then trigger procoagulant effects through platelet and endothelial cell activation, as well as thrombin generation leading to both micro- and macrovascular thrombosis. The clinical spectrum of HIT ranges from isolated thrombocytopenia without thrombosis (referred to as isolated HIT) to HIT(T), which is associated with both arterial and venous thromboses. Other manifestations of HIT may include hypotension from adrenal hemorrhage secondary to adrenal vein thrombosis and ensuing infarction, skin necrosis at injection sites, or venous limb gangrene. HIT should be suspected in any patient who develops thrombycytopenia while receiving heparin or LMWH; any patient who develops a greater than 50% decline in platelet count after the initiation of either anticoagulant; or any patient who develops new thrombosis or extension of an existing thrombosis while receiving either of these agents. In patients with HIT and de novo exposure to heparin, thrombocytopenia (platelet count <150,000 per μL) usually occurs between day 5 and 14 (with day of heparin exposure being day 0). In patients with a recent exposure to either agent (generally within the last 100 days), HIT may develop sooner and is referred to as rapid-onset HIT. This complication may also develop 9 to 40 days after heparin or LMWH has been discontinued and is known as delayed-onset HIT. Laboratory tests to aid in the diagnosis of HIT include functional assays (detection of heparin-dependent platelet activation in the presence of the UFH or LMWH), such as heparin-induced platelet aggregation and serotonin-release assays (SRA), and antigen assays (immunoassays), which detect immunoglobulin G (IgG), IgM, or IgA antibodies that bind UFH to PF4. The SRA has the highest sensitivity and specificity for the diagnosis of HIT. The first step in the treatment of HIT is the prompt discontinuation of all sources of heparin or LMWH including heparin flushes, heparin-coated catheters, any intermittent use of heparin during dialysis, and patients receiving total parenteral nutrition or angiography. However, approximately 20% to 53% of patients with HIT will develop thrombosis (many within the first month) when treated only with discontinuation of heparin or LWMH alone. Therefore, the initation of an alternative anticoagulant, unless contraindicated, is recommended. **Direct thrombin inhibitors (DTI)** including lepirudin and argatroban (both approved by the FDA), may be used initially. Lepirudin has a longer half-life and is metabolized primarily by the kidney. The aPTT can be used to monitor therapy with a target range of 1.5 to 2.5 times the baseline level measured 4 to 6 hours after dose adjustments. Argatroban has a shorter half-life than lepirudin and is primary metabolized in the liver. The goal for the aPTT is 1.5 to 3.0 times the baseline level. There are no agents available that reverse the effects of either drug; therefore, if bleeding develops, prompt discontinuation should be considered. Once platelet counts are more than 100,000 to 150,000 mm^3, warfarin may be started at a low dose (2.5 to 5 mg preferred). Early introduction or higher doses of warfarin may lead to venous limb gangrene or warfarin-induced skin necrosis. Overlapping the DTI with the VKA should be continued for at least 5 days and not discontinued until the INR is therapeutic for two consecutive days. **Argatroban falsely elevates the INR**; therefore, it should not be discontinued until the INR is greater than 4, as recommended by the manufacturer. After cessation of argatroban, the INR should be rechecked within a few hours to confirm that it is between 2 and 3. The duration of anticoagulation for patients with HIT is generally determined by the location and type of thrombosis. In patients without thrombosis (isolated HIT), the duration of anticoagulation is less clear, but given the high incidence of thrombosis within the first month, it is reasonable to continue anticoagulation for at least a month in the absence of contraindications.

E. Antiphospholipid antibodies are a heterogeneous group of autoantibodies, that, if present in a patient with thrombosis, lead to the antiphospholipid syndrome. Antiphospholipid antibodies can be divided into two large groups: (a) anticardiolipin antibodies and (b) lupus anticoagulants. They are often associated with other autoimmune conditions and can cause recurrent pregnancy loss, as well as arterial or venous thrombosis. Thrombocytopenia is also an occasional feature of this syndrome. Anticardiolipin antibodies are detected and quantified using an enzyme-linked immunosorbent assay (ELISA) and may be IgG, IgM, or IgA. IgG titers have been correlated more often with thrombosis. Lupus anticoagulants prolong phospholipid-dependent blood clotting times, and it has been reported that there is about a fivefold increase risk for thrombosis in patients with this finding. Once a thrombotic event occurs, long-term therapy with warfarin must be considered. A higher target INR had been considered necessary in the past (approximately $\geq$3.0), but is no longer considered necessary as more recent data have suggested that most patients can be maintained with a target INR of 2.0 to 3.0. In those individuals that are suspected of failing adequate therapy, one strategy is to correlate the INR to factor II and factor X levels (of $\leq$20% to 30%) to ensure adequate anticoagulation. Patients with recurrent miscarriages should receive aspirin and LMWH during pregnancy.

F. **Malignancy.** Many malignancies induce a hypercoagulable state, and in patients with idiopathic VTE a search for age- and gender-specific malignancies may be necessary.

G. **Other conditions.** Elevated factor VIII levels and the dysfibrinogenemias have also been associated with thrombosis; however, the role for deficiencies of plasminogen, tissue plasminogen activator (of the fibrinolytic system), and factor XIII polymorphisms as emerging risk factors for hypercoagulability are less clear.

ACKNOWLEDGMENT

The authors thank Dr. Vijay Nambi for his contribution to earlier editions of this chapter.

Landmark Articles

Benotti JR, Dalen JE. The natural history of pulmonary embolism. *Clin Chest Med* 1984;5:403–410.

Bratzler DW, Raskob GE, Murray CK, et al. Underuse of venous thromboembolism prophylaxis for general surgery patients: physician practices in the community hospital setting. *Arch Intern Med* 1998;158:1909–1912.

Carson JL, Kelley MA, Duff A, et al. The clinical course of pulmonary embolism. *N Engl J Med* 1992;326:1240–1245.

Lensing AW, Prandoni P, Brandjes D, et al. Detection of deep-vein thrombosis by real-time B-mode ultrasonography. *N Engl J Med* 1989;320:342–345.

Mattos MA, Londrey GL, Leutz DW, et al. Color-flow duplex scanning for the surveillance and diagnosis of acute deep venous thrombosis. *J Vasc Surg* 1992;15:366–375; discussion 375–376.

Moser KM, LeMoine JR. Is embolic risk conditioned by location of deep venous thrombosis? *Ann Intern Med* 1981;94:439–444.

Ribeiro A, Lindmarker P, Juhlin-Dannfelt A. Echocardiography Doppler in pulmonary embolism: right ventricular dysfunction as a predictor of mortality rate. *Am Heart J* 1997;134:479–487.

Sandler DA, Martin JF, Duncan JS, et al. Diagnosis of deep-vein thrombosis: comparison of clinical evaluation, ultrasound, plethysmography, and venoscan with X-ray venogram. *Lancet* 1984;2:716–719.

Sreeram N, Cheriex EC, Smeets JL. Value of the 12-lead electrocardiogram at hospital admission in the diagnosis of pulmonary embolism. *Am J Cardiol* 1994;73:298–303.

Stein PD, Goldhaber SZ, Henry JW. Alveolar-arterial oxygen gradient in the assessment of acute pulmonary embolism. *Chest* 1995;107:139–143.

Stein PD, Terrin ML, Hales CA, et al. Clinical, laboratory, roentgenographic, and electrocardiographic findings in patients with acute pulmonary embolism and no pre-existing cardiac or pulmonary disease. *Chest* 1991;100:598–603.

Value of the ventilation/perfusion scan in acute pulmonary embolism. Results of the Prospective Investigation of Pulmonary Embolism Diagnosis (PIOPED). The PIOPED Investigators. *JAMA* 1990;263:2753–2759.

Vandenbroucke JP, Koster T, Briet E, et al. Increased risk of venous thrombosis in oral-contraceptive users who are carriers of factor V Leiden mutation. *Lancet* 1994;344:1453–1457.

Wells PS, Anderson DR, Bormanis J, et al. Value of assessment of pretest probability of deep-vein thrombosis in clinical management. *Lancet* 1997;350:1795–1798.

Suggested Readings

Birdwell BG, Raskob GE, Whitsett TL, et al. Predictive value of compression ultrasonography for deep vein thrombosis in symptomatic outpatients: clinical implications of the site of vein noncompressibility. *Arch Intern Med* 2000;160:309–313.

Blum A, Bellou A, Guillemin F, et al. Performance of magnetic resonance angiography in suspected acute pulmonary embolism. *Thromb Haemost* 2005;93:503–511.

Buller HR, Agnelli G, Hull RD, et al. Antithrombotic therapy for venous thromboembolic disease: the Seventh ACCP Conference on Antithrombotic and Thrombolytic Therapy. *Chest* 2004;126[Suppl 3]:401S–428S.

Buller HR, Davidson BL, Decousus H, et al. Fondaparinux or enoxaparin for the initial treatment of symptomatic deep venous thrombosis: a randomized trial. *Ann Intern Med* 2004;140:867–873.

Buller HR, Davidson BL, Decousus H, et al. Subcutaneous fondaparinux versus intravenous unfractionated heparin in the initial treatment of pulmonary embolism. *N Engl J Med* 2003;349:1695–702.

Crowther MA, Ginsberg JS, Julian J, et al. A comparison of two intensities of warfarin for the prevention of recurrent thrombosis in patients with the antiphospholipid antibody syndrome. *N Engl J Med* 2003;349:1133–1138.
de Moerloose P, Boehlen F. Inherited thrombophilia in arterial disease: a selective review. *Semin Hematol* 2007;44:106–613.
Geerts WH, Pineo GF, Heit JA, et al. Prevention of venous thromboembolism: the Seventh ACCP Conference on Antithrombotic and Thrombolytic Therapy. *Chest* 2004;1263[Suppl]:338S–400S.
Goldhaber SZ. Echocardiography in the management of pulmonary embolism. *Ann Intern Med* 2002;136:691–700.
Heit JA. Venous thromboembolism: disease burden, outcomes and risk factors. *J Thromb Haemost* 2005;3:1611–1617.
Kaufman JA, Kinney TB, Streiff MB, et al. Guidelines for the use of retrievable and convertible vena cava filters: report from the Society of Interventional Radiology multidisciplinary consensus conference. *J Vasc Interv Radiol* 2006;17:449–459.
Kearon C, Ginsberg JS, Julian JA, et al. Comparison of fixed-dose weight-adjusted unfractionated heparin and low-molecular-weight heparin for acute treatment of venous thromboembolism. *JAMA* 2006;296:935–942.
Konstantinides S, Geibel A, Olschewski M, et al. Importance of cardiac troponins I and T in risk stratification of patients with acute pulmonary embolism. *Circulation* 2002;106:1263–1268.
Moores LK, Jackson WL, Jr., Shorr AF, et al. Meta-analysis: outcomes in patients with suspected pulmonary embolism managed with computed tomographic pulmonary angiography. *Ann Intern Med* 2004;141:866–874.
Tamariz LJ, Eng J, Segal JB, et al. Usefulness of clinical prediction rules for the diagnosis of venous thromboembolism: a systematic review. *Am J Med* 2004;117:676–684.
U.S. Food and Drug Administration. Prescribing Information, Arixtra (fondaparinux sodium) Injection 2005; GlaxoSmithKline, Research Triangle Park, NC 27709.
van Beek EJ, Brouwerst EM, Song B, et al. Clinical validity of a normal pulmonary angiogram in patients with suspected pulmonary embolism—a critical review. *Clin Radiol* 2001;56:838–842.
van Belle A, Buller HR, Huisman MV, et al. Effectiveness of managing suspected pulmonary embolism using an algorithm combining clinical probability, D-dimer testing, and computed tomography. *JAMA* 2006;295:172–179.
Wells PS, Anderson DR, Rodger M, et al. Derivation of a simple clinical model to categorize patients probability of pulmonary embolism: increasing the models utility with the SimpliRED D-dimer. *Thromb Haemost* 2000;83:416–420.
Wells PS, Anderson DR, Rodger M, et al. Evaluation of D-dimer in the diagnosis of suspected deep-vein thrombosis. *N Engl J Med* 2003;349:1227–1235.
Wells PS, Owen C, Doucette S, et al. Does this patient have deep vein thrombosis? *JAMA* 2006;295:199–207.
Wolde M, Tulevski, II, Mulder JW, et al. Brain natriuretic peptide as a predictor of adverse outcome in patients with pulmonary embolism. *Circulation* 2003;107:2082–2084.

AORTIC ANEURYSM AND AORTIC DISSECTION

25

Kamran I. Muhammad and Maran Thamilarasan

I. INTRODUCTION

A. Aorta. The aorta is the **principal conductance vessel** in the body, and is divided into the ascending, arch, descending thoracic, and abdominal components.

1. The **ascending aorta** includes the aortic root, which contains the sinuses of Valsalva. The left and right coronary arteries arise from the left and right coronary sinuses, respectively.
2. The **aortic arch** gives rise to the great vessels of the head and arms. These include the brachiocephalic (innominate), the left common carotid, and the left subclavian arteries.
3. The **descending thoracic aorta** provides the intercostal vessels as it courses through the posterior mediastinum. The vascular supply to the anterior spinal artery is included among these vessels.
4. The **abdominal aorta** begins just after the aorta crosses the diaphragm. It provides the splanchnic and renal arteries before bifurcating to become the common iliac arteries.

B. Histology. The aorta comprises **three layers:** the intima, the media, and the adventitia.

1. The **intima** is the internal lining layer of the aorta and is easily damaged.

2. The **media** is the main structural layer of the aorta. It consists primarily of laminar layers of elastic tissue and smooth muscle in varying amounts. This structure allows for the high tensile strength and elasticity required to withstand the pressure changes of each heartbeat throughout the life of the individual.
3. The **adventitia** is the thin outer layer that anchors the aorta within the body, in addition to providing nourishment to the outer half of the wall through the vasa vasorum.

C. Physiology

1. The **elasticity of the aortic wall allows it to distend** under the pressure created during ventricular systole. In this way the kinetic energy that was developed during ventricular systole is stored as potential energy in the distended aortic wall. Then, during ventricular diastole, the potential energy is converted back to kinetic energy by elastic recoil of the wall. Therefore, forward blood flow is maintained throughout the cardiac cycle.
2. The aorta aids in the control of **systemic vascular resistance (SVR).** Pressure receptors in the ascending aorta and aortic arch signal the vasomotor centers of the brain via the vagus nerve. When blood pressure is elevated, the reflex response is to lower heart rate and decrease SVR. The converse is true when blood pressure is decreased.

D. Acute aortic syndromes including aortic dissection, aortic intramural hematoma, and penetrating atherosclerotic ulcer are life-threatening disorders that require prompt diagnosis and treatment.

II. AORTIC DISSECTION

A. Etiology and pathology

1. **Aortic dissection occurs when a tear in the intima results in separation of the intima from the aortic wall resulting in the formation of a false lumen. Acute aortic dissection usually results from a pathologic weakening of the aortic wall due to cystic medial necrosis, atherosclerosis, or inflammation.** There are many risk factors for aortic dissection, the most common of which is systemic hypertension (found in up to 72% of patients). Younger patients are more likely to have Marfan's syndrome, bicuspid aortic valve, and/or prior aortic surgery.
   a. Increased age and uncontrolled hypertension (found in up to 80%) are two of the most commonly associated factors.
   b. Tobacco use, dyslipidemia, and use of cocaine are important risk factors.
   c. Hereditary connective tissue disorders associated with an increased risk of aortic dissection include Marfan's syndrome and Ehlers-Danlos syndrome.
   d. Hereditary conditions such as bicuspid aortic valve and coarctation of the aorta are also established risk factors, as they have been found to be associated with a diffuse aortopathy.
   e. Disorders that result in vascular inflammation (i.e., aortitis), including giant cell arteritis, Takayasu arteritis, syphilis, and Behçet's disease, may also result in medial degeneration, thereby increasing the risk of aortic dissection.
2. There is an **association between pregnancy and dissection**. Up to 50% of dissections that occur in women <40 years of age occur in the third trimester or postpartum period [12% in International Registry of Aortic Dissection (IRAD)]. This is especially true of women with Marfan's syndrome and preexisting aortic root dilation.
3. Direct trauma is also associated with dissection. Blunt trauma causes transection or mural hematoma more commonly; however, it also rarely causes dissection. Instrumentation with arterial catheterization or intraaortic balloon pump can cause intimal damage and dissection, as may cardiac surgery (at the site of cannulation, cross clamping, or graft insertion).

B. Epidemiology. The incidence of aortic dissection is approximately 2000 cases per year in the United States. The male-to-female ratio is 2:1, with the peak incidence in the sixth and seventh decades of life. The mortality for untreated acute aortic dissection is largely determined by the location of the dissection, but overall mortality for untreated acute aortic dissection is approximately 1% per hour within

TABLE 25.1 Aortic Dissection Classification Systems

Classification	Pathologic description
STANFORD	
Type A	Any dissection involving the ascending aorta
Type B	Any dissections *not* involving the ascending aorta
DEBAKEY	
Type I	Entry point in the ascending aorta, extends to the aortic arch and often beyond
Type II	Confined entirely to the ascending aorta
Type III	Entry in the descending aorta (distal to left subclavian); extends distally (usually) or proximally (rarely)

the first 48 hours. Approximately 65% of dissections originate in the ascending aorta (just above the right or noncoronary sinus), 20% in the descending thoracic aorta, 10% in the aortic arch, and the remainder in the abdominal aorta.

C. Classification schemes

1. Currently in use are **three classification schemes** based on anatomy. These are the DeBakey, Stanford, and anatomic classifications. (See Table 25.1 and Fig. 25.1 for a description of the DeBakey and Stanford classifications; anatomic classification refers to the portion(s) of aorta involved.)

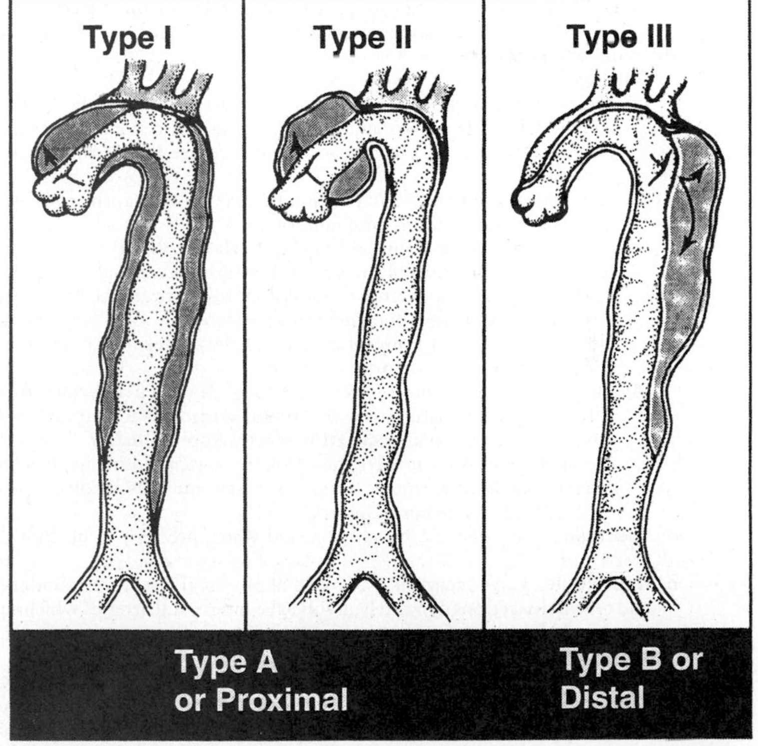

Figure 25.1. Anatomic appearance of three different aortic dissection classifications.

2. Dissections are further classified according to chronicity: acute (less than 2 weeks from onset) or chronic (greater than 2 weeks). The mortality curve for untreated type A aortic dissection rises during the first 2 weeks and levels off at 75% to 80%, thereby providing a natural breakpoint.
3. Anatomic involvment and chronicity of dissection affect the optimal treatment approach.

D. Clinical presentation

1. Signs and symptoms

a. Aortic dissection may present with a wide range of clinical manifestations. As noted by IRAD, severe sharp pain of sudden onset is the single most common presenting symptom. This is in contrast to the pain of myocardial infarction (MI), which is more gradual in onset. Localization of pain may help in classifying the dissection: chest pain is typically more common in type A dissection, whereas back and abdominal pain are more common in type B dissection. The classic description of tearing, ripping, or stabbing pain is well-known but, according to large registry studies of aortic dissection, does not represent the typical pain on presentation.

b. Less common presentations include congestive heart failure (CHF), usually due to severe aortic insufficiency (AI) in proximal dissection, syncope (up to 13% of cases—due to rupture into pericardial space with resultant tamponade, cerebral hypoperfusion, or activation of cerebral baroreceptors), myocardial infarction (MI), cardiovascular accident (CVA), paraplegia, or cardiac arrest.

c. **In contrast to younger patients (younger than 40 years of age), elderly patients** (older than 70 years of age) are less likely to present with typical symptoms. Women are more likely to present later and more likely to present with neurologic symptoms (altered mental status or coma).

2. Physical examination

a. Cardiac

(1) Hypertension is often seen with aortic dissection, frequently as the cause and occasionally as a complication. In distal dissections, which involve the renal artery, the increase in blood pressure is a response to renal ischemia.

(2) Hypotension can be seen in proximal dissection with aortic root involvement, hemopericardium, and tamponade.

(3) Pseudohypotension occurs when the subclavian artery is involved with resultant compression of the vessel. Pressure differential in the left and right arms may also occur if blood flow is compromised to one of the arms. Because of this phenomenon, measurement of bilateral brachial blood pressures is an important part of the physical examination of a patient with suspected aortic dissection.

(4) The diastolic murmur of **AI** (16% to 67%) often indicates root involvement, with disturbance of normal aortic valve coaptation. CHF symptoms can occur if acute AI is severe. Approximately 1% to 2% of proximal dissections involve the coronary ostia, resulting in an acute MI picture. The right coronary ostium is most commonly involved, producing a picture of inferior ST-elevation MI.

b. **Vascular.** Pulse deficits, which wax and wane, are seen in up to 30% of cases.

c. **Neurologic.** CVA occurs in 3% to 6% of proximal dissections. Both type A and type B dissections can rarely involve the intercostal arteries which supply the spinal blood supply, resulting in transient or permanent paraplegia.

E. Diagnostic testing

1. **Evaluation.** Figure 25.2 provides an algorithm to aid in diagnosis. The following characteristics are important in defining the extent of aortic dissection: ascending versus descending aortic involvement; site of the intimal tear; presence or absence of AI; presence/absence of pericardial effusion/tamponade; coronary involvement; involvement of blood vessels to visceral organs. The relative

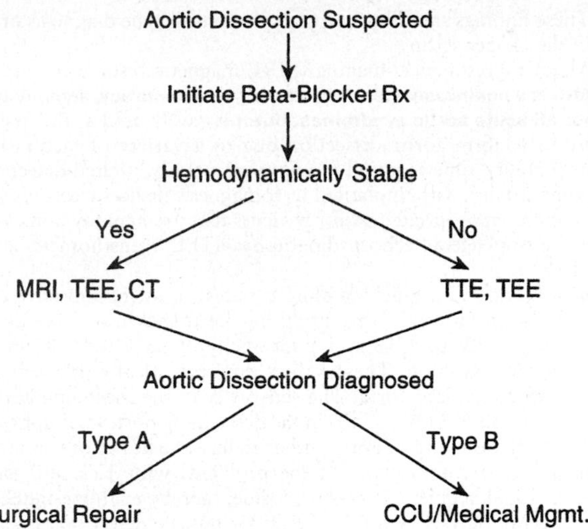

MRI–magnetic resonance imaging; TEE–transesophageal echocardiography; CT–computed tomography; TTE–transthoracic echocardiography. (See text for details)

Figure 25.2. Aortic dissection diagnostic/therapeutic algorithm.

advantages and disadvantages of the four modalities are outlined in Table 25.2. **The technique chosen should be based on local expertise and clinical availability to facilitate rapid diagnosis.**

2. A 12-lead ECG should be performed in all patients with suspected aortic dissection to facilitate differentiation from acute MI, although these conditions may coexist and require further testing to fully define. Up to one-third of patients with coronary involvement will have a normal ECG.
3. Chest radiograph findings are suggestive of dissection in more than 80% of cases. Findings include a widened aortic silhouette (80% to 90% of cases), widened mediastinum, or the calcium sign (displacement of intimal calcium greater than 1 cm from outer aortic soft tissue), pleural effusion, and CHF.

TABLE 25.2 Comparison of Imaging Modalities in Aortic Dissection

Factor	Angiography	CT	MRI	TEE
Intimal tear definition	++	+++	+++	++
False lumen thrombus +/–	+++	+++	+++	+
Involvement of branch vessels	+++	++	++	+
Pericardial effusion	–	+++	+++	+++
Coronary involvement	+++	–	–	++
AI presence	+++	–	+	+++
Overall sensitivity (%)	88	100	98	98
Overall specificity (%)	95	98	98	95

AI, aortic insufficiency; CT, computed tomography; MRI, magnetic resonance imaging; TEE, transesophageal echocardiography.

Modified from Isselbacher EM, Eagle RA, DeSanctis RW. Diseases of the aorta. In: Braunwald E, ed. *Heart disease: a textbook of cardiovascular medicine*, 5th ed. Philadelphia: WB Saunders, 1997:1546–1581.

These findings should prompt one to consider the diagnosis of aortic dissection in the proper setting.

4. Magnetic resonance imaging (MRI)/magnetic resonance angiography (MRA). **MRI is a noninvasive test with the highest accuracy, sensitivity, and specificity for all acute aortic syndromes, but it is** rarely used as the first imaging modality to confirm aortic dissection due to a variety of factors including limited availability, time required to complete a study, limited detection of AI, and incompatibility with implanted ferromagnetic devices (see subsequent text). MRI is not an appropriate test for patients that are hemodynamically unstable.
5. Transesophageal echocardiography (TEE)/transthoracic echocardiography (TTE)
   a. TTE allows a quick (within minutes), easy, noninvasive evaluation at the bedside. However, this study has been shown to have an overall sensitivity of 59% to 85% and a specificity of 63% to 96% for the detection of aortic dissection. These values are dramatically different in the ascending and descending aorta. The sensitivity in the ascending aorta is 78%, but it drops off to 31% to 55% in the descending portion. Emphysema, mechanical ventilation, and obesity further reduce the utility of this technique.
   b. TEE overcomes many of the problems with TTE and has the advantage of rapid acquisition at the bedside, thereby enabling immediate triage. The overall sensitivity for TEE is 98%, but the detection of an intimal tear and intramural thrombus have been reported to be between 68% and 73%. Detection of AI and/or pericardial effusion is 100%. The reported specificity of TEE for detection of dissection has varied in the literature, and is dependent on the experience of the operator and the number of criteria used to define the diagnosis. A recent systematic review and meta-analysis by Shiga et al. suggests a specificity of 95%; however, significant heterogeneity was found.
6. **Computed tomography (CT).** Contrast-enhanced cardiac-gated multidetector CT is now the most commonly used imaging modality for the detection of aortic dissection, with excellent sensitivity and specificity, both nearly 100%. This modality has many advantages, including rapid scan and interpretation times, but does involve contrast and radiation exposure.
7. Aortography was the first means available to evaluate patients with suspected dissection. Visualization of the false lumen or intimal flap are considered diagnostic; and studies comparing aortography to newer modalities—including CT, MRI, and TEE—show the overall sensitivity and specificity to be 88% and 95%, respectively. False negatives can occur with thrombosis of the false lumen, intramural hematoma, or equal filling of the false lumen.
   a. Advantages of aortography include definition of coronary anatomy, branch vessel involvement, and extent of the dissection, as well as wide availability.
   b. Disadvantages, beyond its low sensitivity, are risks of an invasive procedure, contrast administration, and prolonged time to diagnosis and treatment.
8. **Comparison**
   a. CT and TEE offer the most rapid answer in most emergency situations. Multidetector CT has become the preferred modality given its high sensitivity and specificity, noninvasive nature, rapid scanning times, nondependence on operator skill/experience, and ability to characterize the full extent of a dissection. CT will not provide information regarding AI but this can be easily obtained with TTE.
   b. MRI allows the most detail and has the highest sensitivity and specificity. In the unstable setting of acute dissection, however, limited availability and length of the procedure make this a less desirable alternative. **MRI is best suited for serial evaluation of chronic dissection, whether treated medically or surgically.**
   c. Aortography is the most difficult to obtain rapidly in an emergent situation and may simply delay a life-saving surgical procedure. Therefore, **aortography should be reserved for when a definitive diagnosis is not obtained with other studies or definition of coronary anatomy is imperative** to surgical planning.

F. Predictors of death. Data from IRAD:

1. Type A dissection. Predictors of death are age 70 years or older, abnormal electrocardiogram (ECG), pulse deficit, acute renal failure and the composite of hypotension, shock, or tamponade.
2. Type B dissection. Predictors of death are branch vessel involvement, absence of chest or back pain, and hypotension/shock. Recent data suggest that continued patency of the false lumen predicts a worse outcome in type B aortic dissection with highest survival when there is complete thrombosis of the false lumen, intermediate survival with fully patent false lumens, and poorest survival with partial false lumen thrombosis.

G. Therapy. Death in aortic dissection results from vascular compromise, tamponade, or aortic rupture. **Proximal (type A) aortic dissection is universally believed to mandate immediate surgical treatment.** This greatly reduces the risk of poor outcomes (acute AI, CHF, tamponade, and neurologic sequelae) from progression of the dissection and halts the 1% per hour mortality rate. There is no proven superiority of surgical management over medical management for **patients with stable distal (type B) aortic dissections**. Surgical interventions are reserved for complications of dissection or treatment failure. Endovascular stent-grafting for unstable type B aortic dissection has been proposed and found to be technically feasible and effective. Further studies are needed directly comparing this approach to the traditional surgical approach. In addition, studies are underway comparing aortic stent-grafting to best medical therapy for stable type B aortic dissection. Table 25.3 recommends course of treatment for various types of dissections. The 5-year survival rate for patients leaving the hospital with appropriate treatment (medical or surgical) for type B dissection ranges from 75% to 82%.

1. **Priority of therapy.** The initial management of patients with suspected aortic dissection is directed to **reducing dP/dt** and lowering blood pressure. Close hemodynamic monitoring with an arterial line and sufficient venous access for volume replacement should be established simultaneously. This initial aggressive dP/dt and blood pressure management applies to all patients regardless of the type of dissection or the long-term management (medical or surgical).
2. **Medical therapy** (see Table 25.4)
   a. β-Blockers should be initiated immediately if aortic dissection is being considered in the differential diagnosis. They should be titrated to effect (heart rate <60, mean arterial pressure 60 to 70 mm Hg). In patients who are

TABLE 25.3 Surgical Versus Medical Therapy for Aortic Dissection

Medical therapy	Surgical therapy	Endovascular therapy
Uncomplicated type B dissection	Acute, type A dissection	Malperfusion syndrome associated with type B dissection
Stable, lone arch dissection	Acute, complicated type B dissection	Possibly as an alternative to surgical therapy for complicated type B dissection
Stable, chronic type B dissection (more than 2 wk after onset of symptoms)	End-organ dysfunction	Possibly as an alternative to medical treatment uncomplicated type B dissection
	Rupture/impending rupture Aortic insufficiency Associated with Marfan's syndrome Retrograde extension into the ascending aorta	

TABLE 25.4 Intravenous Dosing for Acute Medical Management of Acute Aortic Syndromes

Drugs	Loading dose	Maintenance dose
FIRST-LINE AGENTS		
Propranolol	1 mg IV q 3–5 min (max. 6.15 mg/kg)	2 to 6 mg IV q 4–6 h
Labetalol	10 mg IV over 2 min, then 20–80 mg q 10–15 min (max 300 mg)	2 mg/min IV drip titrate to 5–20 mg/min
Esmolol	30 mg IV bolus	3 to 12 mg/min drip
Metoprolol	5 mg IV q 5 min to effect	5 to 10 mg IV q 4–6 h to effect
SECOND-LINE AGENTS IN PATIENTS WITH CONTRAINDICATIONS FOR β-BLOCKERS		
Enalaprilat	0.625 mg IV	0.625 mg IV q 4–6 h
Diltiazem	0.25 mg/kg IV over 2 min. 0.35 mg/kg IV after 15 min if no effect	5 mg/hr titrate by 2.5- to 5-mg/h increments; max 15 mg/h
Verapamil	0.075–0.1 mg/kg to 2.5–5 mg/kg over 2 min	5 to 15 mg/h IV drip

IV, intravenous.

intolerant of β-blockers, calcium channel blockers are acceptable alternatives (see Table 25.4).

b. Once the target heart rate has been achieved, sodium nitroprusside can be initiated for further blood pressure control. It is an effective, rapid-onset, intravenous medication that can be easily titrated. Initial infusion is at 20 μg/min, with titration to maintain a mean arterial pressure of 60 to 70 mm Hg.

3. Surgical therapy

a. Patients with type A dissection should be taken to surgery emergently upon diagnosis.

b. Patients with type B who have evidence of rupture or end-organ involvement, should receive surgical repair. Traditionally it has been held that patients with type B dissections with recurrent pain and/or hypertension that cannot be controlled medically should undergo surgical therapy. However, a study by Januzzi et al. suggests that a significant number of patients with type B dissection (64%) have recurrent pain and refractory hypertension without imaging evidence of dissection extension, impending or active rupture or branch vessel compromise. Furthermore, mortality, need for surgery, and length of hospital stay were not increased in these patients, and conservative management should be continued unless there is objective evidence of complications resulting from aortic dissection.

c. Perioperative risk. Data from IRAD suggests that pre-operative stability—defined as the absence of cardiac tamponade, shock, congestive heart failure, cerebrovascular accident, coma myocardial ischemia, myocardial infarction, acute renal failure, and mesenteric ischemia—predicts a significantly lower surgical mortality for type A dissection (17%) as compared to those who are unstable (31%).

d. Surgical repair. Details are beyond the scope of this book. The general approach is to remove the intimal flap, oversew the entry and exit sites of the false lumen, and usually reinforce the aorta with a Dacron graft. In the event that the aortic valve cannot be repaired or resuspended, a Bentall procedure is performed with a prosthetic valve sewn onto a Dacron graft and used to replace the native valve. The coronary arteries are reimplanted into the graft. In similar fashion, the visceral arteries and T_8 to L_2 intercostal/lumbar arteries are reimplanted if needed.

e. Complications from this procedure include bleeding, infection, ischemic acute tubular necrosis, paraplegia, and mesenteric ischemia.

(1) Paraplegia is one of the most feared complications in repair of descending thoracic dissections. Paraplegia results from the disruption of blood flow to the anterior spinal artery via the intercostal arteries.

(2) Late complications include progressive AI (if the valve was not replaced at surgery), anastomotic aneurysm formation, and recurrent dissection at the previous or a secondary site.

4. **Percutaneous therapy.** Percutaneous therapies have been used for the treatment of acute vascular complications/malperfusion syndromes caused by dissection, as well for nonsurgical treatment of unstable type B dissection via aortic stent-grafting. Studies comparing aortic stent-grafting for stable type B aortic dissection with traditional medical therapy are currently underway.

   a. In the setting of aortic dissection, end-organ ischemia may occur because of progressive enlargement of the false lumen (where there is no distal re-entry) with resultant compression of the true lumen and impairment of blood flow to branch vessels. Percutaneous balloon fenestration and/or stent-grafts may be used in such cases to decompress the false lumen, thereby improving flow in the true lumen.

   b. Percutaneous aortic stent-grafting has been employed as an alternative to surgical therapy for the treatment of unstable type B aortic dissection. The purpose of this procedure is to close the site of blood flow entry into the false lumen—the intimal tear—thereby decompressing the false lumen and causing its thrombosis. In this way, blood flow into the true lumen and branch vessels is reestablished. This technique has been shown to be technically feasible and effective. Studies are needed to directly compare this approach with traditional surgical therapy.

   c. Percutaneous aortic stent-grafting for stable type B aortic dissection is an area of active study. The Investigation of STEnt grafts in patients with type B Aortic Dissection (INSTEAD) trial and the Acute Dissection Stent-grafting OR Best Medical Treatment (ADSORB) trial are two studies that are underway and compare this approach to best medical therapy. Preliminary results from INSTEAD suggest improved survival in those receiving stent-grafts.

5. **Complications**

   a. **Hypotension.** The most likely causes are aortic wall rupture or tamponade. In either event, **aggressive volume replacement should be initiated and the patient taken to the operating room promptly.** In a small nonrandomized series of seven patients who developed pericardial tamponade as a result of aortic dissection, three of the four who underwent pericardiocentesis died suddenly 5 to 40 minutes after the procedure. All three of the patients who went to the operating room without the procedure survived. It is possible that the hemodynamic improvement that was seen after pericardiocentesis, with its accompanying increase in dP/dt, caused rapid and fatal progression of the dissection. If pericardiocentesis becomes an absolute requirement to get the patient to the operating room, enough fluid to raise the blood pressure to an acceptable level, but no more, should be removed. **If vasopressors are required for hemodynamic stabilization, norepinephrine and phenylephrine are the drugs of choice, as neither has a demonstrable effect on dP/dt. Epinephrine and dopamine should be avoided.**

   b. Acute MI can be seen in association with a type A dissection. In this setting, **thrombolysis is absolutely contraindicated.** Lack of flow in the proximal coronary artery or a flap obstructing the coronary artery may be visible on TEE. In the acute setting, coronary angiography is a higher-risk procedure with low yield. Downstream thromboembolism and mechanical progression of the dissection are possible complications. **A time delay to surgical repair with the resultant increase in preoperative mortality is a complication of angiography in the acute setting.**

6. Long-term management of type B dissection is the same for all patients, regardless of whether they had surgical repair, and is an extension of the acute management.

a. Aggressive blood pressure control is obtained with oral agents such as atenolol, metoprolol, labetalol, or diltiazem.

(1) Vasodilators, such as hydralazine or minoxidil, which increase dP/dt, **should be used only in conjunction with a negative inotrope** (β-blocker).

(2) In the event of treatment failure, these patients should always be considered for surgical treatment. Failure is defined as evidence of aortic leak, progression with visceral organ involvement, possibly recurrent pain, or AI.

b. Monitoring should be performed for the early detection of secondary aneurysms. In about 30% of cases, late deaths are caused by rupture of a secondary aneurysm or recurrence of the dissection. A majority of these secondary aneurysms will develop within 2 years of the initial treatment. Serial imaging of the aorta is critical, and either CT or MRI are acceptable. MRI may be the test of choice for serial imaging as it does not require contrast or radiation. Imaging should be performed at 1, 3, 6, and 12 months after discharge and at least annually thereafter.

H. Atypical variants of dissection

1. Intramural hematoma may be caused by rupture of the vasa vasorum leading to hemorrhage within the aortic wall. This can result in secondary dissection in a minority of cases, but pure intramural hematomas lack an identifiable dissection flap or false lumen. Intramural hematomas have a natural history similar to that of classic aortic dissection. Therefore, management for this entity mirrors therapy for true dissection. Specifically, intramural hematomas in the ascending aorta should be treated surgically, whereas those in the descending aorta should be treated with aggressive medical management.

2. Penetrating atherosclerotic ulcer is an atherosclerotic plaque that ulcerates into the media, potentially leading to an intramural hematoma, aortic dissection, or perforation. Risk factors for this process include older age, extensive atherosclerosis, and uncontrolled hypertension. The descending aorta is the most common site. The presentation may be similar to other types of dissection, with sudden-onset back and/or chest pain, but penetrating atherosclerotic ulcer may also be an incidental finding on imaging done for other reasons in an asymptomatic patient. Complications include development of intramural hematoma, local dissection, pseudoaneurysm formation, true aneurysm formation, and transmural erosion with rupture. The diagnostic study of choice for this process is aortography, which defines the presence of contrast protruding into an atherosclerotic plaque. CT, MRI and TEE can help to characterize the penetrating ulcer. The natural history and outcomes of this entity are not well elucidated, and treatment is tailored to the patient. In the event that a patient presents with this process with hemodynamic instability, urgent surgical repair is necessary. Otherwise, medical management with β-blockers and frequent radiologic follow-up for signs of progression should be undertaken. Follow-up studies should be performed every 6 to 12 months, or more frequently if clinically indicated. Endovascular therapies for treatment for penetrating atherosclerotic ulcer have been advocated.

III. AORTIC ANEURYSM. An aortic aneurysm is defined as a pathologic dilation to more than 1.5 times the normal diameter of the aorta. The aneurysm can be either fusiform (symmetric dilation) or saccular (asymmetric outpouching). Pseudoaneurysms, which are well-defined pockets of blood and connective tissue resulting from contained aortic rupture, must be distinguished from true aneurysms. Overall, 13% of patients with a single aneurysm have one or more additional aneurysms, and 25% of patients with a thoracic aneurysm have abdominal aneurysms as well. There are no well-defined guidelines for screening other vascular beds in patients upon diagnosis of aortic aneurysm. However, given the high incidence of multiple aneurysms, a chest and abdominal CT scan on diagnosis to rule out other sites would be reasonable.

A. Abdominal aortic aneurysms (AAAs) are much more common than thoracic aortic aneurysms (TAAs), and **up to 75% of aortic aneurysms involve the abdominal aorta.** The prevalence of the disease in men 65 years of age or older is about 5%

compared to the prevalence of AAA in women, which has been cited to about 1.0% to 2.2% in some epidemiologic studies. Risk factors for the development of AAA include current or past history of tobacco use, male gender, age, first-degree relative with AAA, hypertension, hyperlipidemia, and atherosclerosis in other vascular beds. Diabetes seems to have a protective effect against the formation of AAA, possibly due to vascular calcification and negative remodeling associated with diabetes. The incidence of AAA increases after age 55 in men and age 70 in women. There is a **male-to-female ratio of 9:1,** and most cases (95%) involve the infrarenal aorta.

1. **Clinical presentation.** The majority of AAAs are discovered incidentally on physical examination or during radiologic or ultrasound evaluation of the abdomen.
   a. **Signs and symptoms.** Most patients are asymptomatic; therefore, the diagnosis of AAA should be considered in patients with an appropriate risk profile.
      (1) The predominant symptom associated with rapid enlargement or rupture/impending rupture is severe back or flank pain. This is often described as sudden in onset, constant, and not affected by movement or position. Occasionally, there is radiation to the legs, buttocks, or groin.
      (2) Findings consistent with shock (hypotension, pallor, diaphoresis, oliguria, and obtundation) can develop rapidly with a ruptured aneurysm.
   b. **Physical examination**
      (1) A palpable, pulsatile mass may be felt on examination, variably extending from the xiphoid process to below the umbilicus. This is more difficult to palpate in obese individuals. Accurate sizing is nearly impossible on physical examination. Palpation should be gentle, especially if the aneurysm is tender, as tenderness can be an indication of impending rupture.
      (2) Often evidence of **associated vascular disease** can be found (abdominal or femoral bruits) or decreased pulses.
      (3) Physical evidence of **thromboembolism** is sometimes found. Either atheromatous material or mural thrombus can embolize and livedo reticularis, painful blue toes, hypertension, and renal insufficiency can ensue.
2. **Etiology**
   a. Atherosclerosis has long been considered the underlying etiologic factor for abdominal aneurysms, but evidence of active inflammation found within the wall of aortic aneurysms on pathologic specimens has supported the theory that immunologic factors, in conjunction with genetic, environmental, and hemodynamic factors, play an important role in the pathophysiology of AAA. Matrix metalloproteinases and other proteinases that are locally produced by smooth muscle may degrade elastin and collagen and lead to aneurysm formation. Specifically, elevated levels of matrix metalloproteinases (MMP)-2, MMP-9 and MMP-14 have been found in walls of human aortic aneurysms. A large proportion of patients with AAA have elevated circulating levels of MMP-9, and levels have been shown to decrease after repair.
   b. Genetic factors may also play a role, with family studies showing up to 28% of patients having a first-degree relative with an abdominal aneurysm. First-degree male relatives of patients with AAA have a 12 times greater risk of having an aneurysm.
   c. Less common causes include infection *(Salmonella, Staphylococcus aureus), vasculitis,* and trauma.
3. **Clinical course**
   a. The risk of rupture is proportional to aneurysm size.
      (1) Available data suggest that aneurysms larger than 6.0 cm have greater than 20% per year risk of rupture, whereas those between 5 and 6 cm have approximately 6% risk of rupture per year.
      (2) Enlargement rate is dependent on the diameter of the AAA and can range from 0.2 cm/year to more than 3 cm/year. The majority of aneurysms

enlarge at a rate of 2.6 mm/year. The larger the aneurysm grows, the faster it will continue to expand.

b. Laplace's law defines the parameters for growth of aneurysms.

$$\text{Wall tension (WT)} = \text{transmural pressure (TP)} \times \text{radius } (r)$$

Therefore, with luminal dilation (increased r), the wall tension will increase at a given blood pressure (TP). This leads to a further increase in radius and to a self-perpetuating cycle of growth of the aneurysm.

c. Rupture usually occurs into the left retroperitoneal space (80%). This may initially be contained; ultimately it will extend, causing shock and death if untreated.

d. AAA can also rupture into the inferior vena cava (causing aortovenous fistula formation) and the gastrointestinal tract (causing aortoenteric fistula formation). Hence, **the patient with gastrointestinal bleed and history of AAA or AAA repair should always be suspected of potentially having an aortoenteric fistula.**

e. Ruptured AAA is associated with high mortality. 25% of patients die before reaching the hospital, 50% die without undergoing surgery, and of those who survive to undergo surgery, the **operative mortality approaches 50%.**

4. Diagnostic testing

a. Abdominal ultrasound is the most commonly used screening tool for AAA. It has the capacity to obtain both longitudinal and transverse images of the aneurysm.

(1) Advantages. Ultrasound has been verified to accurately measure size to within ±0.3 cm. It is widely available, relatively low in cost, and does not involve radiation exposure. It is a reasonable choice to follow aneurysm growth serially.

(2) Disadvantages. Abdominal ultrasound cannot adequately define involvement of branch vessels and, therefore, is insufficient for preoperative evaluation.

b. CT

(1) Advantages. CT allows for a **more accurate evaluation of the aneurysm shape** and its spatial relations to the branch vessels. The technique allows for evaluation of extravasated blood in acute or subacute rupture, as well as for measurements that have been validated to within ±0.2 cm. It also allows for evaluation of branch vessel involvement, diagnosis of complications such as penetrating ulcer, and relationship of the aneurysm to other structures. The ability to create multiple oblique sections of the aorta as well as three-dimensional reconstructions from the acquired CT data set can be helpful in designing an appropriate management strategy.

(2) Disadvantages. CT uses ionizing radiation and requires intravenous contrast. The significant radiation dose associated with CT scans of the aorta limit its utility in follow-up of chronic aortic dissection (see Chapter 47).

c. Aortography

(1) Advantages include its ability to define suprarenal and iliofemoral involvement, as well as branch vessel impingement. Although aortography previously was used commonly for evaluation of aortic pathology, it has largely been replaced by multidector CT scanning. Aortography is now generally reserved for planning endografting in some centers and is less useful as an initial diagnostic modality.

(2) Disadvantages. Aortography tends to underestimate size, especially when mural thrombus is present. In addition, it is invasive, expensive, and involves the use of intravenous contrast and ionizing radiation.

d. MRI/MRA

(1) Advantages. MRI allows for **excellent definition of aneurysm size** as well as suprarenal and iliofemoral extension. MRA allows for improved visualization of compromised flow to branch vessels. The techniques have an advantage over aortography in that they are noninvasive and require no intravenous contrast.

(2) Disadvantages. MRA lacks sensitivity to absolutely define obstruction in the renal vessels. It is expensive, and there is a limited availability of scanners and qualified physicians to interpret the results.

5. Therapy

a. Medical therapy

(1) β-Blockers have been shown to decrease the rate of enlargement and risk of rupture in at least one clinical trial (Gadowski, et al., *J Vasc Surg* 1994), although other studies have not confirmed this effect.

(2) Aggressive risk factor modification with control of hypertension and hypercholesterolemia is **imperative to prevent adverse events from atherosclerotic disease in other vascular beds. Smoking cessation should be strongly advocated.**

(3) Serial ultrasound or CT scanning is indicated in patients with aortic diameters of 2.5 cm and greater and without symptoms. Studies should be obtained yearly when the aortic diameter reaches 3.0 cm, every 6 months for dimensions between 4 and 5 cm and every 3 to 6 months for aneurysms 5.0 to 5.5 cm. Ultrasound is generally preferred for surveillance of small AAAs, owing to lack of radiation exposure.

b. Endovascular therapy is a less-invasive option for the repair of AAA. Under fluoroscopic guidance, the proximal and distal ends of the stent-graft are affixed to normal segments of the aorta above and below the aneurysmal portion, thereby sealing off the aneurysm. Suitable anatomy is necessary for stent-grafting, and some favorable characteristics include normal diameter of aorta distal to the renal arteries and proximal to the aneurysmal segment, minimal angulation, freedom from severe obstructive lesions, and patency of side branches and distal iliac vessels. Only 30% to 60% of patients will have anatomy suitable for endovascular repair.

Several randomized trials, including the Dutch Randomized Endovascular Aneurysm Management (DREAM) trial, the Endovascular Aneurysm Repair 1 (EVAR-1) trial, Eindhoven Stent Prosthesis for Aneurysm Study (ESPAS), and a study by Soulez, have compared endovascular repair to open repair and found lower operative mortality of endovascular repair over open repair. Mid-term follow-up (2 to 4 years) from DREAM, EVAR-1 and Soulez's study revealed that this early mortality difference had disappeared and no difference in mid-term all-cause mortality between endovascular and open repair was seen. Data regarding long-term survival with endovascular repair as compared to open repair are not yet available.

Endovascular Aneurysm Repair 2 (EVAR-2) trial compared endovascular repair to observation in patients for whom open repair was recommended but deemed too high risk because of medical comorbidities. This study failed to show any survival benefit with endovascular repair—a disappointing finding as the clearest indication for endovascular repair was traditionally thought to be for those at high risk for open repair. However, EVAR-2 has received significant criticism, owing to high crossover and procedural mortality rates, and further studies will likely be needed to definitively address this important issue.

One of the common complications of endovascular repair is endoleak, which occurs as a result of failure of the stent-graft to completely exclude the aneurysm, and results in persistent flow into the aneurysm, thereby increasing the risk for aneurysm expansion and rupture. Endoleaks occur in 10% to 20% of cases and are associated with more frequent reinterventions than open repair and the requirement of life-long periodic follow-up imaging. For these reasons and unavailability of long-term outcome data, endovascular repair has generally been limited to older and high risk patients.

c. **Surgical therapy.** The technical details of repair are beyond the scope of this book. The basic premise is for a Dacron tube graft to be inserted in place of the diseased aorta. The major branches are then reimplanted to the graft.

(1) **Preoperative evaluation.** Given the strong association of coronary artery disease and AAA, and the high operative mortality with untreated severe coronary artery disease, **all patients being considered for surgical repair of AAA need preoperative risk assessment.**

(2) **Timing**

(a) Perioperative mortality in elective procedures is 4% to 6% (less than 2% in low-risk patients).

(b) Two randomized trials, the United Kingdom Small Aneurysm Trial (UKSAT) and the Aneurysm Detection and Management (ADAM) Veterans Affairs Cooperative Study, have shown that there is no long-term survival benefit associated with repair of AAAs that are less than 5.5 cm in diameter. Therefore, surgery is indicated for an aneurysm that is rapidly expanding (>1 cm/year) or 5.5 cm or greater in diameter. Women have a higher risk of rupture and rupture at smaller aortic diameters. Therefore, it is the recommendation of some vascular societies that women should undergo elective repair at aortic diameters 4.5 to 5.0 cm. Symptomatic patients should also be referred for repair.

B. TAAs are much less common than AAAs (incidence 5.9 per 100,000 person-years). Thoracic aneurysms include those aneurysms that involve the aorta from the level of the aortic root to the diaphragmatic crura. Extension of a descending thoracic aneurysm below the diaphragm creates a thoracoabdominal aneurysm.

1. **Clinical presentation.** Most patients with the thoracic aneurysm are asymptomatic at the time of diagnosis, and the condition is often discovered as an incidental finding on imaging done for other reasons.

a. **Signs and symptoms**

(1) **Vascular complications of the aneurysm** include AI with left ventricular dilation and CHF, myocardial ischemia due to coronary artery compression, sinus of Valsalva rupture into the right atrium/ventricle with left-to-right shunt and CHF, or thromboembolic phenomena.

(2) **Compression of external structures by the aneurysm** causes superior vena cava syndrome, dysphagia from esophageal compression, or hoarseness from recurrent laryngeal nerve compression. In addition, compression of the trachea or mainstem bronchus can lead to wheezing, dyspnea, tracheal shift, cough, or hemoptysis. Chest or back pain from compression and bony involvement is described as constant, boring, and deep.

(3) **Rupture** presents with sudden, severe, sharp chest or back pain. In order of decreasing frequency, TAAs rupture into the left pleural space, the pericardium (presenting as tamponade), and the esophagus (presenting as hematemesis).

(4) **Aortic dissection.** (See preceding section.)

b. Physical examination. Specific physical findings directly referable to the TAA **are usually absent.**

(1) **Cardiac.** The diastolic murmur of AI (classically right lower sternal border) and a laterally displaced point of maximum impulse are sometimes noted with chronic ascending aortic dilation. Signs of CHF can be seen in these circumstances. Unilateral jugular venous distention can be seen in patients with venous compression.

(2) **Vascular.** Rarely, a pulsatile mass can be palpated in the suprasternal notch. Differential pulses in the extremities can sometimes be found. Evidence of thromboembolic events can be seen upon examination of the digits. If the aneurysm compresses the venous return, evidence of superior vena cava syndrome or lower extremity edema may be found.

(3) **Pulmonary.** If the aneurysm compresses part of the bronchial tree, decreased air movement or stridor is auscultated.

TABLE 25.5 Causes of Thoracic Aortic Aneurysm

Etiology	Aortic segment involved	Pathophysiology
Cystic medial degeneration	Ascending aorta, aortic arch	*De novo* cystic medial degeneration
Marfan's syndrome	Ascending aorta and root, aortic arch	Defective fibrillin; secondary cystic medial degeneration
Ehlers-Danlos syndrome, type IV	Ascending aorta, predominantly aortic arch	Defective collagen; secondary cystic medial degeneration
Bicuspid aortic valve	Ascending aorta and root	Inadequate production of fibrillin; cystic medial degeneration
Familial thoracic aortic aneurysm syndrome	Ascending aorta	Autosomal dominant, 3p24.2-25, 5q13-15, 11q23.2-q24
Turner's syndrome	Ascending aorta and root	Cystic medial degeneration
Advanced age		Cystic medial degeneration
Atherosclerotic	Descending aorta	Atherosclerotic plaques, weakening vessel walls
Traumatic	Aortic isthmus, proximal descending aorta	Damaged vessel wall, intramural hematoma
Inflammatory	Variable	Takayasu's arteritis, giant cell arteritis, HLA-B27-associated spondyloarthropathies, others
Infectious	Aortic root (syphilis), variable (mycotic)	CMD (syphilis), inflammatory changes (mycotic)
Poststenotic	Ascending (aortic stenosis), descending (coarctation)	Hemodynamic insult
Postsurgical	Aortic valve replacement, status post aortic anastomosis	Weakening of the anastomotic walls
Chronic aortic dissection	Variable	Weakening of false lumen over time

2. Etiology

a. Table 25.5 gives the various classifications of TAAs as well as the segment involved and pathophysiology. The most common cause of TAA formation is cystic medial necrosis, which is characterized by loss of elastic fibers and smooth muscle within the aortic media, with replacement of tissue with interstitial cysts of basophilic ground substance leading to a cystic appearance.

b. Approximately 5% to 10% of patients undergoing surgery for AI are secondary to **annuloaortic ectasia,** which is a variant of cystic medial necrosis. Annuloaortic ectasia is a clinicopathologic diagnosis in which the aortic root, ascending aorta, and aortic annulus dilate, resulting in AI. This is more common in men and is typically seen in the fourth, fifth, and sixth decades of life.

3. Pathophysiology and clinical course. The natural history and progression of TAA is not as well defined as that of AAA.

a. The rate of dilation, as well as the TAA's propensity to rupture, may be related to its underlying cause. Onset of symptoms usually heralds a more rapid course, as do larger dimensions at baseline.

b. There appears to be a dichotomy in the rate of growth according to data from Dapunt et al. In looking at all TAAs, aneurysms smaller than 5.0 cm at baseline have a mean growth rate of 0.17 cm/year, whereas those larger than 5.0 cm grew at a mean rate of 0.79 cm/year.

c. Rupture is the most common cause of death in these patients. Data from the Yale group found median size at rupture for an ascending aortic aneurysm was 6.0 cm, and 7.2 cm for a descending aortic aneurysm.

4. Diagnostic testing

a. The **chest radiograph** frequently shows widening of the mediastinum, unusual aortic contours, or displacement of the trachea or bronchi in the presence of a large TAA.

b. CTA and MRA both allow for good definition of the size and extent of aneurysmal involvement. CTA is the preferred modality for serial follow-up after surgical or endovascular repair, whereas MRA is the preferred modality when visualization of the aortic root is necessary, as it is more accurate than CTA for this purpose.

c. TTE and TEE. TTE is of limited use in evaluating the thoracic aorta, except for the aortic root and proximal ascending portion. TEE can be used to visualize the entire thoracic aorta, but given the availability of noninvasive imaging to diagnose TAA, TEE is not routinely used for this purpose.

d. MRI and MRA are also useful for detecting and defining the extent of aneurysmal involvement. They allow for evaluation of the entire aorta, branch vessels, aortic valve, and pericardium. Disadvantages and other advantages are similar to those noted for in **II.E.3**.

e. Aortography allows for evaluation of the segment involved by the aneurysm as well as the branch vessels off the aorta. This procedure is currently reserved for preoperative evaluation to establish branch vessel patency.

5. Therapy

a. Medical therapy. Long-term data on medical management for TAA are lacking. Based on one small prospective trial of patients with Marfan's syndrome, which showed a slower rate of dilation in patients treated with propranolol, β-blockers are generally recommended for all patients with TAA, with or without Marfan's syndrome. Recent trials are investigating the efficacy of angiotensin-converting enzyme inhibitors to slow aneurysm growth in patients with Marfan's syndrome.

b. Endovascular therapy. Use of percutaneous aortic stent-grafts has been reported for descending thoracic aneurysms. Larger studies and longer follow-up must be evaluated before widespread use of this technology can be encouraged. It is currently reserved for patients who are at high risk for open repair and those with ideal aortic anatomy.

c. Surgical therapy. The **timing of surgical repair is less clear than in AAA.**

(1) Several factors contribute to this lack of clarity. First, **availability of data is limited** on natural history, progression of dilation, and short- and long-term surgical outcomes. Second, **significant risks and complications are associated with repair,** especially if the aneurysm involves the arch or descending aorta.

(2) Currently, there are no specific American Heart Association/American College of Cardiology (AHA/ACC) guidelines for surgery for such aneurysms. Current practice has been to consider surgery for ascending aneurysm in the 5.0 to 5.5 cm range, and certainly for those larger than 5.5 cm. Practice patterns are more variable for intervention in the descending thoracic aorta, with some groups adovocating intervention when greater than 6.0 cm. Body size must be taken into account as well, with lower cutoffs suggested for those of shorter stature. Special considerations are for those with Marfan's syndrome and bicuspid aortic valves. These patients are prone to complications at relatively smaller sizes. Our institutional practice has been to recommend surgery for the ascending aorta in patients with Marfan's syndrome when the ratio of the cross-sectional area of the aorta at its greatest dimension to the patient's height in meters exceeds 10 cm^2/meter. Smaller aneurysms can be followed with serial CT scanning. The frequency of evaluation is controversial and depends on the aneurysm size. Usually every 6 to 12 months is sufficient if the patient is not having symptoms.

(3) The technical details of repair are beyond the scope of this text. However, the basic premise is for a Dacron tube graft to be inserted in place of the diseased aorta. The main branches are reimplanted to the graft (coronary arteries, great vessels, mesenteric, and T_8 to L_2 intercostals/lumbricals). When the aortic valve is involved with aortic root dilation, a modified **Bentall procedure** (composite prosthetic aortic valve with Dacron graft) or **aortic valve homograft** is performed. The aortic valve homograft is a cryopreserved cadaveric aortic valve with a portion of the original ascending aorta intact. Aneurysms involving both the ascending and descending aorta can be treated by a two-staged approach, with an **elephant trunk** procedure.

(4) Overall perioperative survival is reported to be 90% to 95% for elective repair (ascending aorta) in most institutions.

(5) The **major complications** associated with TAA repair include MI (7.2%), CVA (4.8%), acute renal failure (2.4%), perioperative hemorrhage (7.2%), and paraplegia (6.0%) due to perioperative ischemia of the anterior spinal cord. Even with proper reimplantation of the T_8 to L_2 arteries, the reported rate of paraplegia is 5% to 6% during repair of descending TAA.

(6) Factors associated with increased surgical risk include emergent surgery, greater age, prolonged cross-clamp time, diabetes, previous aortic surgery, and intraoperative hypotension.

IV. CONTROVERSIES

A. There has been considerable interest in screening for AAA given the possibility of reduction in mortality from aneurysm rupture. Several large randomized trials have explored the potential benefits of screening for AAA with ultrasound. A recent systematic review of four large randomized trials of screening for AAA with ultrasound suggests that there is a benefit to be derived from screening in men ages 65 to 79 years, with reduced mortality from AAA. This benefit did not extend to women. The cost-effectiveness of this screening strategy was deemed to be acceptable. The rate of surgery was significantly higher in those undergoing screening, and these studies provided few data on quality of life or complications from surgery.

The U.S. Preventative Services Task Force (USPSTF) currently recommends one-time screening for AAA by ultrasound in men aged 65 to 70 years who have ever smoked and makes no recommendation for screening for men aged 65 to 70 years who have never smoked. The USPSTF recommends against routine screening for AAA in women.

Further investigation is needed to refine the concept of screening for AAA, particularly in women.

B. As discussed previously, there is some emerging debate regarding the optimal management strategy for stable type B aortic dissection. Although medical therapy is the currently accepted standard of care for the management of stable type B dissection, two studies are underway (INSTEAD and ADSORB) comparing best medical therapy with endovascular repair plus medical therapy in this population. Preliminary data from INSTEAD suggest more favorable survival in those treated with endovascular repair.

Suggested Readings

Blankensteijn J, de Jong SECA, et al. Two-year outcomes after conventional or endovascular repair of abdominal aortic aneurysms. *N Engl J Med* 2005;352:2398–2405.

Cigarroa JE, Isselbacher EM, et al. Diagnostic imaging in the evaluation of suspected aortic dissection. *N Engl J Med* 1994;328:35–43.

Coady MA, Rizzo JA, et al. What is the appropriate size criterion for resection of thoracic aortic aneurysms? *J Thorac Cardiovasc Surg* 1997;113:476–491.

Coselli JS, de Figueiredo LFP. Natural history of descending and thoracoabdominal aortic aneurysms. *J Cardiovasc Surg* 1997;12[Suppl]:285–291.

Cosford PA, Leng GC. Screening for abdominal aortic aneurysm. *Cochrane Database Syst Rev* 2007, Issue 2. Art. No.: CD002945.

Cuypers PW, Gardien M, et al. Randomized study comparing cardiac response in endovascular and open abdominal aortic aneurysm repair. *Br J Surg* 2001;88:1059–1065.

Dapunt OE, et al. The natural history of thoracic aortic aneurysms. *J Thorac Cardiovasc Surg* 1994;107:1323–1332.

Eggebrecht H, Nienaber CA, et al. Endovascular stent-graft placement in aortic dissection: a meta-analysis. *Eur Heart J* 2006;27:489–498.

Elefteriades JA. Natural history of thoracic aortic aneurysms: indications for surgery, and surgical versus nonsurgical risks. *Ann Thorac Surg* 2002;74:S1877–1880; discussion S1892–S1878.

Erbel R, Alfonso F, Boileau C, et al. Diagnosis and management of aortic dissection. *Eur Heart J* 2001;22:1642–1681.

Erbel R, et al. Echocardiography in the diagnosis of aortic dissection. *Lancet* 1998;1:457–461.

Estrera AL, Miller CC, et al. Outcomes of medical management of acute type B aortic dissection. *Circulation* 2006;114[Suppl I]:I384–I389.

EVAR Trial Participants. Comparison of endovascular aneurysm repair with open repair in patients with abdominal aortic aneurysm (EVAR 1 trial), 30-day operative mortality results: randomised controlled trial. *Lancet* 2004;364:843–848.

EVAR Trial Participants. Endovascular aneurysm repair and outcome in patients unfit for open repair of abdominal aortic aneurysm (EVAR trial 2): randomised controlled trial. *Lancet* 2005;365:2187–2192.

Fleming C, Whitlock EP, et al. Screening for abdominal aortic aneurysm: a best-evidence systematic review for the U.S. Preventative Services Task Force. *Ann Intern Med* 2005;142:203–211.

Furthmayr H, Francke U. Ascending aortic aneurysm with or without features of Marfan syndrome and other fibrillinopathies: new insights. *Semin Thorac Cardiovasc Surg* 1997;9:191–205.

Fuster V, Halperin JL. Aortic dissection: a medical perspective. *J Cardiovasc Surg* 1994;9:713–728.

Gadowski GR, Pilcher DB, Ricci MA. Abdominal aortic aneurysm expansion rate: effect of size and blockade. *J Vasc Surg* 1994;19:727–731.

Greenberg R, Resch T, et al. Endovascular repair of descending thoracic aortic aneurysm: an early experience with intermediate-term follow-up. *J Vasc Surg* 2000;31:147–156.

Hagan PG, Nienaber CA, et al. The International Registry of Acute Aortic Dissection: new insights into an old disease. *JAMA* 2000;283:897–903.

Januzzi JL, Isselbacher EM, et al. Characterizing the young patient with aortic dissection: results from the International Registry of Aortic Dissection. *J Am Coll Cardiol* 2004;43:665–669.

Kiell CS, Ernst CB. Advances in management of abdominal aortal aneurysm. *Adv Surg* 1993;26:73–98.

Kouchoukos NT, Dougenis D. Surgery of the thoracic aorta. *N Engl J Med* 1997;336:1876–1888.

Lawrence-Brown MM, Norman PE, et al. Initial results of ultrasound screening for aneurysm of the abdominal aorta in Western Australia: relevance for endoluminal treatment of aneurysm disease. *Cardiovasc Surg* 2001;9:234–240.

Lederle FA, Kane RL, et al. Systematic review: repair of unruptured abdominal aortic aneurysm. *Ann Intern Med* 2007;146:735–741.

Lederle FA, Wilson SE, et al. Immediate repair compared with surveillance of small abdominal aortic aneurysms. *N Engl J Med* 2002;346:1437–1444.

Lindholt JS, Juul S, et al. Hospital costs and benefits of screening for abdominal aortic aneurysms. Results from a randomised population screening trial. *Eur J Vasc Endovasc Surg* 2002;23:55–60.

Lindholt JS, Juul S, et al. Screening for abdominal aortic aneurysms: single centre randomised controlled trial. *BMJ* 2005;330:750–753.

Lindsay J Jr. Diagnosis and treatment of diseases of the aorta. *Curr Probl Cardiol* 1997;22:485–548.

Lottman PE, Laheij RL, et al. Health-related quality of life outcomes following elective open or endovascular AAA repair: a randomized controlled trial. *J Endovasc Ther* 2004;11:323–329.

Miller DC. The continuing dilemma concerning medical versus surgical management of patients with acute type B dissections. *Semin Thorac Cardiovasc Surg* 1993;5:33–46.

Mitchell RS, Dake MD, et al. Endovascular stent-graft repair of thoracic aortic aneurysms. *J Thorac Cardiovasc Surg* 1996;111:1054–1062.

Multicentre Aneurysm Screening Study Group. The Multicentre Aneurysm Screening Study (MASS) into the effect of abdominal aortic aneurysm screening on mortality in men: a randomised controlled trial. *Lancet* 2002;360:1531–1539.

Multicentre Aneurysm Screening Study Group. Multicentre aneurysm screening study (MASS): cost effectiveness analysis of screening for abdominal aortic aneurysms based on four year results from randomised controlled trial [comment]. *BMJ* 2002;325:1135.

Nienaber CA, et al. The diagnosis of thoracic aortic dissection by noninvasive imaging procedures. *N Engl J Med* 1993;328:1–9.

Nienaber CA, von Kodolitsch Y, Nicholas V, et al. The diagnosis of thoracic aortic dissection by noninvasive imaging procedures. *N Engl J Med* 1993;328:1–9.

Nienaber CA, Zannetti S, et al. Investigation of stent grafts in patients with type B aortic dissection: design of the INSTEAD trial—a prospective, multicenter, European randomized trial. *Am Heart J* 2005;149:592–599.

Norman PE, Jamrozik K, et al. Population based randomised controlled trial on impact of screening on mortality from abdominal aortic aneurysm. *BMJ* 2004;329:1259–1264.

Parodi J. Endovascular repair of abdominal aortic aneurysms and other arterial lesions. *J Vasc Surg* 1995;21:549–555.

Parodi JC. Endovascular repair of abdominal aortic aneurysms and other arterial lesions. *J Vasc Surg* 1995;21:549–557.

Penn MS, Smedira N, et al. Does coronary angiography before emergency aortic surgery affect in-hospital mortality? *J Am Coll Cardiol* 2000;35:889–894.

Pitt MPI, Bonser RS. The natural history of thoracic aortic aneurysm disease: an overview. *J Cardiovasc Surg* 1997;12[Suppl]: 270–278.

Pretre R, Von Segesser LK. Aortic dissection. *Lancet* 1997;349:1461–1464.

Prinssen M, Verhoeven ELG, et al. A randomized trial comparing conventional and endovascular repair of abdominal aortic aneurysms. *N Engl J Med* 2004;351:1607–1618.

Scott RA, Wilson NM, et al. Influence of screening on the incidence of ruptured abdominal aortic aneurysm: 5-yr results of a randomized controlled study. *Br J Surg* 1995;82:1066–1070.

Shiga T, Wajima Z, et al. Diagnostic accuracy of transesophageal echocardiography, helical computed tomography, and magnetic resonance imaging for suspected thoracic aortic dissection: systematic review and meta-analysis. *Arch Intern Med* 2006;166:1360–1356.

Slonim SM, Nyman U, et al. Aortic dissection: percutaneous management of ischemic complications with endovascular stents and balloon fenestration. *J Vasc Surg* 1996;23:241–253.

Svensson LG. Natural history of aneurysms of the descending and thoracoabdominal aorta. *J Cardiovasc Surg* 1997;12[Suppl]:279–284.

Svennson LG, Khitin L. Aortic cross-sectional area/height ratio timing of aortic surgery in asymptomatic patients with Marfan syndrome. *J Thorac Cardiovasc Surg.* 2002;123:360–361.

Tsai TT, Evangelista A, Nienaber CA, et al; International Registry of Acute Aortic Dissection. Partial Thrombosis of the false lumen in patients with acute type B aortic dissection. *N Engl J Med* 2007;357:349–359.

Tsai TT, Fattori R, et al. Long-Term survival in patients presenting with type B acute aortic dissection: insights from the International Registry of Acute Aortic Dissection. *Circulation* 2006;114:2226–2231.

Tsai TT, Nienaber CA, Eagle KA. Acute Aortic Syndromes. *Circulation* 2005;112:3802–3812.

The United Kingdom Small Aneurysm Trial Participants. Mortality results for randomised controlled trial of early elective surgery or ultrasonographic surveillance for small abdominal aortic aneurysms. *Lancet* 1998;352:1649–1655.

The United Kingdom Small Aneurysm Trial Participants. Health service costs and quality of life for early elective surgery or ultrasonographic surveillance for small abdominal aortic aneurysms. *Lancet* 1998;352:1656–1660.

The United Kingdom Small Aneurysm Trial Participants. Long-term outcomes of immediate repair compared with surveillance of small abdominal aortic aneurysms. *N Engl J Med* 2002;346:1445–1452.

Williams DM, Lee DY, et al. The dissected aorta. Percutaneous treatment of ischemic complications: principles and results. *J Vasc Intervent Radiol* 1997;8:605–625.

Relevant Book Chapters

Gornik HL, Creager MA. Diseases of the aorta. In: Topol EJ, ed. *Textbook of cardiovascular medicine,* 3rd ed. Philadelphia: Lippincott Williams and Wilkins, 2006:1473–1491.

Isselbacher, EM. Diseases of the aorta. In: Braunwald E, ed. *Braunwald's heart disease: a textbook of cardiovascular medicine,* 8th ed. Philadelphia: Saunders Elsevier, 2005:1457–1490.

26 PERICARDIAL DISEASE

Deborah H. Kwon

I. INTRODUCTION. The pericardium is a fibrous sac composed of two layers. The inner monocellular visceral layer is composed of mesothelial cells and is adherent to the myocardium. The outer parietal layer is a fibrous layer less than 2-mm thick that consists mostly of collagen and elastin. It is joined to adjacent intrathoracic structures by means of ligaments. Interspersed between the two layers is a small amount of serous pericardial fluid, generally about 15 to 35 mL. **The normal pericardium is distensible and permits unimpeded expansion of the ventricles during diastole. Normally, changes in intrathoracic pressure are easily transmitted to the heart**, resulting in increased venous return to the right side of the heart with inspiration and increased pulmonary venous return to the left side of the heart with expiration.

The pericardium helps to maintain the position of the heart within the chest cavity, acts to reduce friction during the cardiac cycle, and also acts as a barrier to infection and inflammation. The pericardium secretes prostaglandins that can modulate cardiac reflexes and coronary tone.

A. Acute pericarditis is a clinical syndrome caused by **inflammation of the pericardium** and is associated with **chest pain, a friction rub, and characteristic electrocardiographic changes.** The incidence of acute pericarditis is 2% to 6% in autopsy series, although it is diagnosed clinically in only 1 in 1000 admissions. It is more **common in adults (20 to 50 years of age) and in men.**

B. Constrictive pericarditis is caused by **fibrous thickening of the pericardium** secondary to **chronic inflammation** from a variety of causes.

C. Pericardial effusion is a **fluid collection in the pericardial space.** The clinical presentation may range from being **asymptomatic to life-threatening** hemodynamic compromise, depending on the **underlying cause of the effusion** and the **rate of accumulation**, as discussed later in detail.

D. Cardiac tamponade is a clinical emergency that arises when a pericardial fluid collection impairs diastolic filling sufficiently to produce a low cardiac output state.

II. ACUTE PERICARDITIS.

There are a large number of potential etiologies of acute pericarditis. In practice, these are classified into the following groups: idiopathic, infectious, inflammatory, uremic, post-myocardial infarction (MI), neoplastic, and traumatic (Table 26.1).

A. Etiology

1. **Idiopathic.** Most cases of acute pericarditis are **idiopathic**, although many of these may be **viral in orlgin.**
2. **Viral pericarditis.** The most common viruses involved are coxsackievirus B and echovirus. A **prodrome of upper respiratory tract symptoms** preceding the onset of chest pain, along **with a fourfold or higher rise in viral convalescent antibody titers,** supports the diagnosis. Most cases are self-limited; infrequent complications include myocarditis (i.e., myopericarditis), recurrent pericarditis, pericardial effusion, tamponade, and constrictive pericarditis.
3. **Purulent pericarditis.** Purulent pericarditis usually occurs as a **complication of pneumonia or empyema** caused by staphylococci, pneumococci, or other streptococci. Early diagnosis of purulent pericarditis is paramount, as **cardiac tamponade often develops and is associated with high mortality. Purulent pericarditis** is characterized by **acute onset of fever, shaking chills, night sweats, and dyspnea** of a few days duration. **Chest pain or pericardial friction rub is not necessarily present.**
4. **Tuberculous pericarditis.** Although uncommon in the United States, this entity should be considered in patients with fever and pericardial effusion, particularly

TABLE 26.1 Causes of Pericarditis

IDIOPATHIC (nonspecific)
Viral infections: coxsackievirus A, coxsackievirus B, echovirus, adenovirus, mumps virus, infectious mononucleosis, varicella, hepatitis B virus, acquired immunodeficiency syndrome
Bacterial infections: *Pneumococcus, Staphylococcus, Streptococcus,* gram-negative septicemia, *Neisseria meningitidis, Neisseria gonorrhoeae,* tularemia, *Legionella pneumophila, Mycobacterium tuberculosis*
Fungal infections: histoplasmosis, coccidioidomycosis, *Candida,* blastomycosis
UREMIA
Neoplasm: lung cancer, breast cancer, leukemia, Hodgkin's disease, lymphoma
RADIATION
Autoimmune diseases: acute rheumatic fever, systemic lupus erythematosus, rheumatoid arthritis, scleroderma, mixed connective tissue disease, Wegener's granulomatosis, polyarteritis nodosa
Inflammatory disease: sarcoidosis, amyloidosis, inflammatory bowel disease, Whipple's disease, temporal arteritis
DRUGS
Hydralazine, procainamide, phenytoin, isoniazid, phenylbutazone, doxorubicin, penicillin
TRAUMA
Postmyocardial–pericardial injury syndromes: postmyocardial infarction (Dressler's syndrome), postpericardiotomy syndrome
Dissecting aortic aneurysm

Adapted from Lorell BH. Pericardial disease. In: Braunwald E, ed. *Heart disease: a textbook of cardiovascular medicine,* 5th ed. Philadelphia: WB Saunders, 1997:1482.

if there is an underlying immunocompromised state. Pericardial involvement occurs in 1% to 2% of cases of pulmonary tuberculosis. **If the clinical suspicion is high, the patient should be hospitalized and started on triple-drug therapy,** while definitive diagnostic testing is undertaken [acid-fast bacilli (AFB) testing, pericardial/pleural biopsy].

5. Post-MI pericarditis occurs most often after a large anterior-wall MI. Because post-MI pericarditis is a marker for extensive myocardial necrosis, these **patients are at increased risk for congestive heart failure and mortality at 1 year after MI.** It is notable that the rate of post-MI pericarditis has declined since the introduction of successful reperfusion therapies.
6. **Dressler's syndrome** usually **occurs weeks to several months after MI,** with an incidence of about 1%. It presents as **malaise, fatigue, and chest pain** that can be concerning for recurrent MI. The cause of Dressler's syndrome is unclear, although it has been proposed to be autoimmune in nature.
7. **Postpericardiotomy syndrome.** Although similar to Dressler's syndrome in presentation, it **usually occurs within the first 6 to 8 weeks following cardiac surgery.** The incidence varies from 10% to 40%, and the syndrome is believed to be caused by an autoimmune reaction.
8. Uremic pericarditis typically develops in patients who are just beginning renal replacement therapy with hemodialysis. The majority present with a **rub**, and the associated **pericardial effusions tend to be large.** The cause is unknown but does not seem to be related to the level of circulating uremic catabolites or toxins.
9. **Neoplastic pericarditis.** Tumors involving the pericardium are typically metastatic in nature (lung, breast, Hodgkin's and non-Hodgkin's lymphoma, and leukemia). It is important to **suspect cardiac tamponade in patients with a known malignancy who present with symptoms of relatively acute onset fatigue, dyspnea, or edema.**
10. **Auto-immune and inflammatory.** Lupus, rheumatoid arthritis, vasculitis, and other rheumatologic disorders are also associated with pericarditis.

B. Clinical presentation

1. Signs and symptoms

- **a.** Chest pain from pericarditis is described as a severe, sharp retrosternal pain that may radiate to the neck, shoulders, and back with worsening when lying supine, coughing, or during inspiration. The pain may be alleviated when the patient leans forward.
- **b.** There may be a **prodrome of fever and myalgias.**
- **c.** Dyspnea may result from shallow breathing due to inspiratory chest pain.
- **d.** Patients with **purulent pericarditis** may appear toxic with **high fevers, shaking chills, and night sweats.**
- **e.** Tuberculous pericarditis is characterized by gradual onset of symptoms with chronic, nonspecific, constitutional symptoms such as **fever, chills, and night sweats.**

2. Physical findings

- **a.** The **pericardial friction rub is the major clinical finding in pericarditis** but is not present in all cases. It is described as a **scratchy, grating, and high-pitched sound.** The rub is often evanescent, changes in quality and intensity on serial examinations, and may be accentuated with deep respiration. Classically, it has **three components**, corresponding to atrial systole, ventricular systole, and early ventricular diastole. Most often, however, it is a **biphasic** rub consisting of the atrial and ventricular systolic components.
- **b. Auscultation of the rub is ideally performed** using the diaphragm of the stethoscope **at the left lower sternal border** during inspiration, with the patient leaning forward.

C. Laboratory examination and diagnostic testing. Pericarditis is a **clinical diagnosis based on history, physical examination, chest radiograph, and serial electrocardiographic changes.** Based on the clinical scenario, some patients may require further testing, such as tuberculin skin testing, fungal tests, viral serologies, cold agglutinins,

TABLE 26.2 Typical Electrocardiographic Evolution of Acute Pericarditis

Stage	J-ST	T waves	PR segment
"EPICARDIAL" LEADS (I, II, AVL, AVF, V_3–V_6)			
I	Elevated	Upright	Depressed or isoelectric
II early	Isoelectric	Upright	Isoelectric or depressed
II late	Isoelectric	Low to flat to inverted	Isoelectric or depressed
III	Isoelectric	Inverted	Isoelectric
IV	Isoelectric	Upright	Isoelectric
"ENDOCARDIAL" LEADS (AVR, Often V_1, Sometimes V_2)			
I	Depressed	Inverted	Elevated or isoelectric
II early	Isoelectric	Inverted	Isoelectric or elevated
II late	Isoelectric	Shallow to flat to upright	Isoelectric to elevated
III	Isoelectric	Upright	Isoelectric
IV	Isoelectric	Inverted	Isoelectric

Modified from Spodick DH. Electrocardiographic changes in acute pericarditis. *Am J Cardiol* 1974;33:470.

thyroid function tests, heterophile antibodies, antinuclear antibodies (ANAs), rheumatoid factor, bacterial culture, and cytology.

1. **Electrocardiography.** The associated electrocardiographic changes evolve through **four stages** (Table 26.2). Although these changes occur in most patients, their **absence does not exclude acute pericarditis,** particularly in patients with neoplastic or tuberculous pericarditis.
   a. The first stage usually occurs within hours of the onset of chest pain and is diagnostic of acute pericarditis (Fig. 26.1). The presence of **stage 1 electrocardiographic changes is most useful in confirming the diagnosis of acute pericarditis,** yet such changes are often **difficult to distinguish from changes associated with early repolarization and acute infarction.** There is **diffuse ST-segment elevation with upright T waves** in all leads except aVR and V_1. **PR-segment depression** is seen in all leads except aVR and V_1. There is often PR-segment elevation in lead aVR (the "knuckle" sign).
   b. Stage 2, which occurs several days later, is characterized by resolution of PR/ST segments to baseline and T-wave flattening.
   c. The T-wave inversions mark **stage 3.**
   d. Stage 4 occurs when T waves become upright again, which may take days to weeks.
   e. With a large **effusion,** the electrocardiogram (ECG) may show **electrical alternans or low voltage.**
2. A chest radiograph may reveal **cardiomegaly** and may yield important information in support of tuberculous or neoplastic processes.
3. Blood cultures along with sputum and gastric aspirate for tuberculosis should be done where such a diagnosis of purulent or tuberculous pericarditis is suspected (including in immunosuppressed, immigrants). Pericardial or pleural biopsy may be necessary to diagnose tuberculosis.
4. Blood tests may reveal leukocytosis or an elevated erythrocyte sedimentation rate (ESR), which are nonspecific markers of inflammation. Mild **elevations in the** creatinine kinase-myocardial band (**CK-MB) fraction or cardiac troponin levels can be seen** and suggest a more extensive acute inflammatory process involving the epicardium; significant elevations in these markers should raise suspicion for more extensive myocardial involvement, referred to as **myopericarditis.**

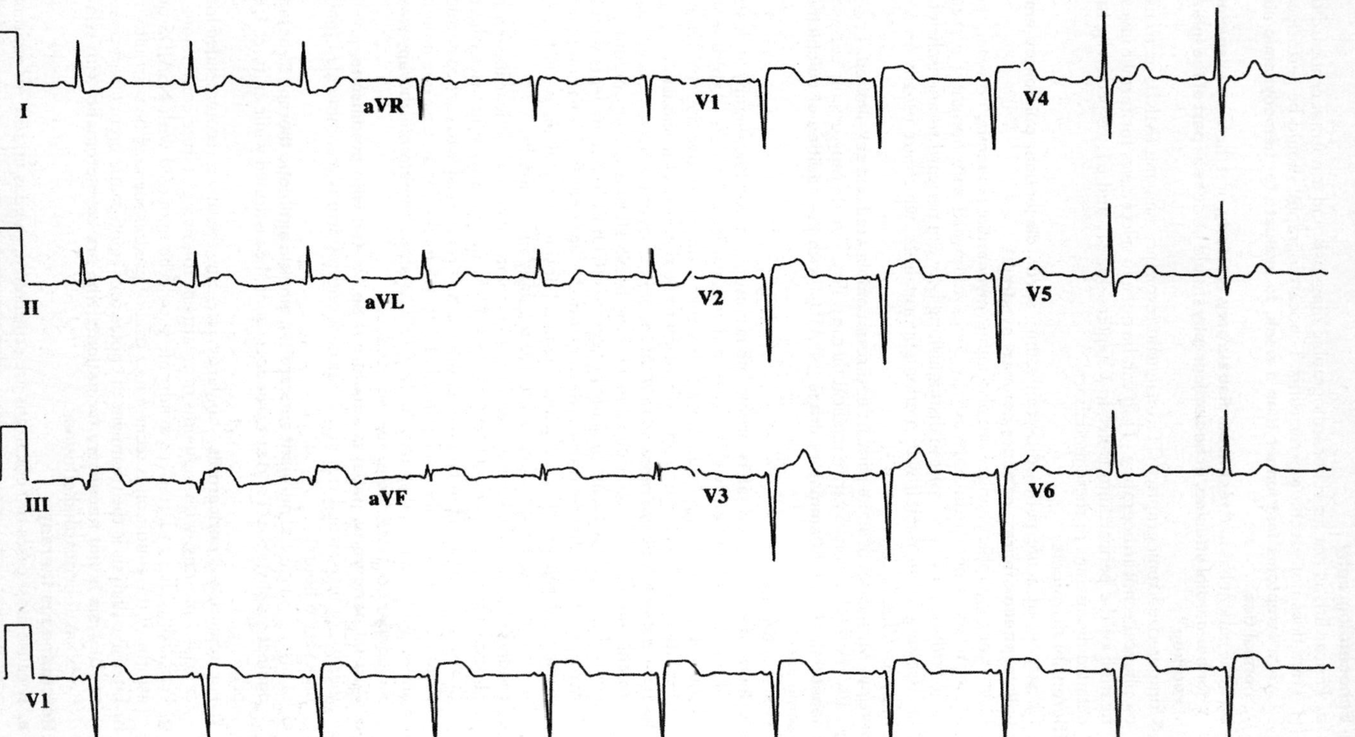

Figure 26.1. Stage 1 electrocardiographic changes in acute pericarditis. Note PR segment elevation in lead aVR, and diffuse ST elevation and the upsloping nature of ST segments as compared to acute myocardial infarction.

5. **Echocardiography**
   a. Pericarditis is not an echocardiographic diagnosis and a normal echocardiogram does not preclude pericarditis. Echocardiography should be performed when **symptoms last longer than a week, to evaluate for hemodynamic abnormalities.**
   b. If the patient has had **recent cardiac surgery,** is **elderly,** or if there is a **suspicion for pericardial effusion, echocardiography** should be done as **part of the initial workup.**
6. Computerized tomography (CT), magnetic resonance imaging (MRI), or transesophageal echocardiography (TEE) can be done in select cases for further investigation of the pericardium (refer to Chapters 46, 47, and 61, respectively, for detailed discussions of these modalities).

D. **Differential diagnosis**
   1. Chest pain of acute pericarditis can mimic **aortic dissection, pulmonary embolism, pneumothorax, or acute coronary syndrome.**
   2. Electrocardiographic changes can also mimic **myocardial ischemia;** however, the ST segments of pericarditis are usually concave upward with upright T waves. Echocardiography may assist in distinguishing between pericarditis and ischemia by assessing for segmental wall-motion abnormalities, which are usually absent in pericarditis.

E. **Therapy.** Most cases of acute pericarditis are **uncomplicated and self-limited.** These typically respond to conservative medical therapy. First-line therapy usually consists of **nonsteroidal anti-inflammatory drugs** (NSAIDs) **with the addition of colchicine in some cases.**
   1. **Medical therapy**
      a. **Ibuprofen** has a good safety profile and is reasonable first-line therapy at doses of 600 to 800 mg orally three times a day for at least 2 weeks. A**spirin** 650 mg orally every 6 to 8 hours for 2 to 4 weeks is an alternative therapy. Other NSAID agents, including naproxen, seem to be similarly efficacious.
      b. If the **patient does not respond to NSAIDs**, or in cases of recurrent pericarditis, **colchicine** should be considered in addition to NSAIDs. A recent randomized controlled trial colchicine in acute pericarditis (COPE) of 120 patients with a first episode of acute pericarditis demonstrated superior efficacy of a combined regimen of aspirin with colchicine. The usual dosing of colchicine is 1.0 to 2.0 mg for the first day and then 0.5 to 1.0 mg daily for 3 months.
      c. **Prednisone** should only be used in patients with recurrent pericarditis with persistent symptoms despite NSAIDs and colchicine therapy, or in cases where there is an underlying inflammatory disease that is responsive to corticosteroid therapy. Prednisone should be dosed at 1 to 1.5 mg/kg for at least one month and should be tapered slowly. In the COPE trial, **corticosteroid therapy was an independent risk factor for recurrence.**
      d. **Post-MI pericarditis patients should *not* be treated with prednisone**, given the risk of myocardial rupture. Treatment with aspirin is recommended (650 mg every 6 hours).
      e. In cases of suspected **purulent pericarditis, empiric antibiotic therapy directed against staphylococci and streptococci** should be instituted while cultures are pending.
      f. For **tuberculous pericarditis,** standard triple-drug therapy is recommended for at least 9 months, with 6 months of treatment following culture conversion.
      g. Pericarditis due to Dressler's syndrome should be managed with NSAIDS or aspirin. If the condition is recurrent, a trial of prednisone may be warranted.
      h. Intensive dialysis is the treatment of choice for symptomatic uremic pericarditis. **Dialysis is not necessary for patients who are asymptomatic** with relatively small pericardial effusions.
   2. **Percutaneous therapy**
      a. Because most cases of pericarditis are self-limited, there is no role for routine pericardiocentesis, intrapericardial administration of steroids, or pericardial biopsy.

b. In cases complicated by tamponade or suspected purulent effusion or neoplasm, pericardiocentesis should be performed. Pericardiocentesis should be reserved for large, hemodynamically compromising pericardial effusions or when fluid is needed for diagnostic purposes.

c. If the etiology is uncertain, **pericardial fluid should be sent for a hematocrit and a white blood cell count with differential, glucose, protein, cytology, and microbiology (e.g., culture for various organisms and AFB staining).** If there is a clinical suspicion of purulent pericarditis, pericardiocentesis should be performed promptly and the fluid sent for culture. If the pericardial fluid is **serosanguineous or grossly bloody,** the clinician should send it for cytologic examination, culture, and AFB.

3. **Surgical therapy**

a. Subxiphoid pericardiostomy is usually performed for neoplastic pericarditis with rapidly recurrent pericardial effusions. Sclerotherapy with tetracycline has been performed in severe cases of neoplastic pericarditis; however, the procedure is painful and is associated with arrhythmias and risk for constrictive pericarditis.

b. Pericardiectomy is reserved for severe recurrent pericarditis. More commonly it is employed in the management of constrictive pericarditis, as will be discussed later in this chapter.

F. **Follow-up**

1. Most patients with idiopathic or viral pericarditis **should receive 1-month follow-up** to ensure that their symptoms have resolved and that no evidence of constrictive pericarditis exists.

2. Patients with pericardial effusions should have serial echocardiograms to assess for recurrence or an increase in the size of the effusion.

G. **Complications**

1. **Recurrent pericarditis** can occur after an episode of acute idiopathic pericarditis, open heart surgery, cardiac trauma, or Dressler's syndrome. Natural history studies suggest that recurrent pericarditis occurs in 20% to 30% of patients. Recurrent pericarditis may be very bothersome. However, with appropriate management of exacerbations and prophylaxis, it frequently responds favorably and eventually peters out.

a. Clinical presentation is similar to that of acute pericarditis, with **variable onset** from months to years after the initial episode.

b. **Therapy.** NSAIDS and colchicine should be administered. **Only if patients fail to respond should prednisone be administered** (1–1.5 mg/kg) for at least one month and tapered slowly. Intravenous methylprednisolone can be given depending on the severity of symptoms. Most patients respond within a few days but may have recurrence with cessation of steroids. **Surgical pericardiectomy is reserved for patients with persistent recurrent pericarditis accompanied by severe chest pain despite aggressive medical therapy. It too may fail as it is difficult to remove all of the pericardium surgically.**

c. **Prevention.** The COPE trial has shown that **colchicine is safe and effective in the prevention of recurrent pericarditis.**

2. Cardiac tamponade will occur in about 15% of patients, most commonly after a cardiac surgical intervention or with neoplasm.

3. **Constrictive pericarditis.** Approximately 9% of patients develop mild constrictive physiology. However, this usually resolves after 3 months. Some patients develop a subacute picture of **effusive–constrictive disease,** with both an effusion and pericardial thickening. This may progress to symptomatic pericardial constriction. When it does so, the interval of onset of severe constrictive findings is much more rapid than in constriction without effusive changes.

III. **CONSTRICTIVE PERICARDITIS** results from **a fibrous thickening of the pericardium** secondary to chronic inflammation from a variety of injuries. Essentially, the **heart is encased by the rigid pericardium**, leading to a decrease in diastolic filling, an increase in intracardiac pressures, and a **dissociation of intracardiac pressure from intrathoracic pressure. The hallmark of pericardial constriction is the equalization of end-diastolic**

TABLE 26.3 Common Causes of Constrictive Pericarditis

Idiopathic
Infectious diseases
Tuberculosis
Bacterial
Viral (e.g., coxsackievirus B, echovirus)
Fungal
Parasitic
Trauma (including cardiac surgery)
Radiation
Inflammatory/immunologic disorder
Rheumatoid arthritis
Systemic lupus erythematosus
Scleroderma
Sarcoidosis
Neoplastic disease
Breast cancer
Lung cancer
Lymphoma
Mesothelioma
Melanoma
End-stage renal disease

pressures in all four cardiac chambers. The elevated cardiac pressures and diminished diastolic filling lead to increased venous pressure, both pulmonary and systemic, and thus to progressive **signs and symptoms of right and left heart failure.** Although constrictive pericarditis is a relatively uncommon cause of heart failure, recognition of this entity is important, as its **prevalence appears to be increasing and the diagnosis is often missed.**

A. Causes of constrictive pericarditis. The **factors involved in the development of constrictive pericarditis are varied,** and are similar to those of acute pericarditis (Table 26.3). However, there is **a common pathophysiologic pathway** leading to **chronic inflammation and pericardial fibrosis.** Neoplastic disease is an exception because tumor infiltration of the pericardium is often responsible for constriction. The causes of constrictive pericarditis in decreasing order of frequency are idiopathic factors, radiation therapy, postsurgical therapy, and infectious disease. This represents a significant change from a century ago when infectious disease, specifically tuberculosis, predominated.

1. Since the advent of effective antitubercular medications, the **number of cases attributable to tuberculosis has dropped precipitously in the United States.** However, tuberculosis remains the primary cause of constrictive pericarditis in most developing regions of the world.
2. Similarly, **bacterial infections of the chest** continue to represent a large number of cases on a global scale but **have largely disappeared in the United States** following the introduction of antibiotics and improved drainage procedures.
3. Most **"idiopathic"** cases are **likely infectious in nature,** due to viral infections such as **coxsackievirus and echovirus**; however, a clear etiologic link is rarely established. Less common infectious causes include fungal and parasitic organisms.
4. Constrictive pericarditis is a **late complication of radiation therapy,** generally occurring **many years after the administration of radiation.** Risk factors for developing constrictive pericarditis include duration of therapy, total amount of radiation administered, and volume of the heart in the radiation field. In contrast to other causes of constrictive pericarditis, where the myocardium is typically normal in structure and function, there may be **associated radiation damage to the myocardium.**

5. Constrictive pericarditis is a well-documented **late complication of cardiac surgery, including** coronary artery bypass grafting and valvular surgery. **Risk factors** for development of postoperative constrictive pericarditis include **intraoperative hemorrhage into the pericardium, postoperative pericarditis,** and the occurrence of **postpericardiotomy syndrome.**
6. End-stage renal disease, neoplastic disease (primarily breast, lung, and lymphoma), and connective tissue disease are less common causes that must be considered in the initial differential.

B. Pathophysiology. In constrictive pericarditis there is **thickening and fibrosis of the pericardium,** often with superimposed calcification, resulting in **decreased ventricular compliance** (Ventricular compliance = end-diastolic volume/end-diastolic pressure). However, in a small percentage of patients with constrictive pericarditis, the pericardium may not appear thickened on noninvasive imaging.

As the pericardium thickens and limits ventricular compliance, there is an **increased end-diastolic pressure for any given end-diastolic volume.** This increase in pressure **affects both ventricles equally**, and effectively decreases diastolic filling and thus end-diastolic volume of both ventricles. The increased pressure is transmitted backward and results in elevated pulmonary venous and systemic venous pressures. **Equalization of end-diastolic pressures in all four cardiac chambers then ensues and is the hallmark of contrictive pericarditis.**

1. The myocardium is generally normal in structure and function; therefore, **systole is unimpaired.**
2. Diastolic function, on the other hand, **is markedly altered** by the constrictive process. In early diastole, the ventricles expand normally, and there is rapid filling secondary to the elevated pulmonary and systemic pressures. Once the **ventricles reach the confines of the rigid pericardium,** there is an **immediate increase in ventricular pressure** and **diastolic filling comes to an abrupt halt.**
3. The result is that **nearly all ventricular filling occurs in the second phase of diastole (early filling)** with little contribution from the third phase (diastasis) and the fourth phase (atrial systole).

C. Physical signs and symptoms

1. The **early symptoms** of constrictive pericarditis are often insidious, and the patient may have nonspecific complaints such as **malaise, fatigue, and decreased exercise tolerance.**
2. As the disease progresses, **symptoms consistent with systemic congestion and low cardiac output,** such as **marked jugular venous distention, ascites, peripheral edema, and worsening exercise tolerance,** may predominate. Symptoms due to right-sided failure usually predominate over left-sided failure due to equalization of pressures.
3. **Examination of jugular veins.** Nearly all patients have **jugular venous distention,** which simply reflects the elevated right-sided pressures. Many patients demonstrate an inspiratory increase in venous distention known as **Kussmaul's sign.** This finding is sensitive but lacks specificity as other conditions such as right ventricular hypertrophy and right ventricular infarction also produce this sign. Observation of the jugular venous pulsations reveals a **prominent *y* descent that is produced by the rapid ventricular filling in early diastole.** The jugular venous pressure is sometimes so high in constrictive physiology that the level is not evident in the neck on examination with the patient at a 45-degree angle and the diagnosis is, therefore, missed. Appreciation of the height of the pressure may only be evident on examining the patient upright.
4. **Cardiac examination.** Cardiac auscultation may reveal **muffled heart sounds** due to decreased transmission through the thickened pericardium. Because the mitral and tricuspid valves are nearly closed by the end of diastole, there may be a **soft first heart sound (S_1). Occasionally, one may hear a pericardial knock** in early diastole [60 to 120 msec after the second heart sound (S_2)]. This represents the abrupt cessation of diastolic filling that occurs when further ventricular relaxation is impeded by the rigid pericardium. The pericardial knock **must be differentiated from other early diastolic sounds** such as an opening snap, third

heart sound (S_3), and tumor plop. In general, the **pericardial knock is of a higher frequency, is heard best with the stethescope diaghragm, and occurs slightly earlier than an S_3.** An opening snap may be similar in frequency and timing, but is nearly always followed by a diastolic rumble.

5. **Pulmonary examination.** Auscultation of the lung fields may reveal **decreased breath sounds at the bases,** attributed to pleural effusions.
6. **Abdominal examination.** The abdominal exam may reveal evidence of right-sided heart failure, with **hepatomegaly and splenomegaly** frequently noted. In **severe cases, there may be** liver dysfunction and **ascites.**
7. **Examination of the extremities.** Elevated central venous pressures due to right ventricular impairment and sodium retention due to left ventricular (LV) impairment contribute to the development of **peripheral edema.**

D. Diagnostic testing. Confirming the diagnosis of constrictive pericarditis often presents a challenge, since no gold-standard test exists. **The clinician must rely on a collection of findings from multiple diagnostic modalities to detect both anatomic and pathophysiologic abnormalities.** Perhaps the greatest challenge lies in differentiating constrictive pericarditis from restrictive cardiomyopathy.

1. **Electrocardiography.** Low voltage is frequently seen with **generalized flattening of the T waves.** There may be **left atrial enlargement. Atrial fibrillation** is a common finding.
2. **Chest radiograph.** Pericardial calcification is relatively common in advanced disease. The calcification is usually best appreciated with a lateral film and frequently involves the right ventricle and atrioventricular groove. **Pleural effusions** occur frequently, and there may be evidence of both **left and right atrial enlargement.**
3. **Two-dimensional echocardiography**
   a. **Septal bounce.** This is the sudden cessation of septal motion as the heart abruptly stops filling upon meeting the rigid pericardium.
   b. **Ventricular interdependence.** This is due to the fixed space in cardiac filling occurs. Preferential filling of the right ventricle on inspiration causes the septum to move to the left, whereas on expiration the augmentation of LV filling causes the septum to move to the right.
   c. **Inferior vena cava (IVC) plethora.** The IVC is typically dilated and does not collapse, due to elevated right-sided pressures.
4. **Doppler echocardiography.** Although imaging findings may suggest pericardial constriction, most of the findings described previously are relatively low in sensitivity and specificity. Doppler assessment of diastolic flow patterns and the respiratory changes in these patterns may provide **significant evidence for the presence of constrictive physiology** and assists in helping **exclude competing diagnoses,** such as restrictive cardiomyopathy.
   a. **Respiratory variation in mitral and tricuspid flow.** In constrictive pericarditis, the thickened pericardium isolates the cardiac chambers from respiratory changes in intrathoracic pressures.
      (1) During **inspiration,** the drop in intrathoracic pressure is transmitted to the pulmonary veins, but not to the left ventricle. This reduces the pressure gradient required for diastolic filling of the left ventricle; therefore, a **decrease in mitral flow is observed during inspiration.** Conversely, there is an **increased tricuspid flow during inspiration. Findings suggestive of constrictive physiology include:**
         (a) Mitral valve inflow. Peak E velocity decreased by 33% (Fig. 26.2).
         (b) Tricuspid valve inflow. Peak E velocity increased by 44% and peak A velocity increased by 38% (Fig. 26.3).
      (2) Opposite changes are seen with expiration. Increased intrathoracic pressure is transmitted to the pulmonary veins and thus increases the driving pressure for LV filling. There is a **decreased tricuspid flow. The wide respiratory variation in peak E velocities helps to differentiate constrictive pericarditis from restrictive cardiomyopathy, in which *minimal* respiratory variation occurs** (Figs. 26.2 and 26.3).

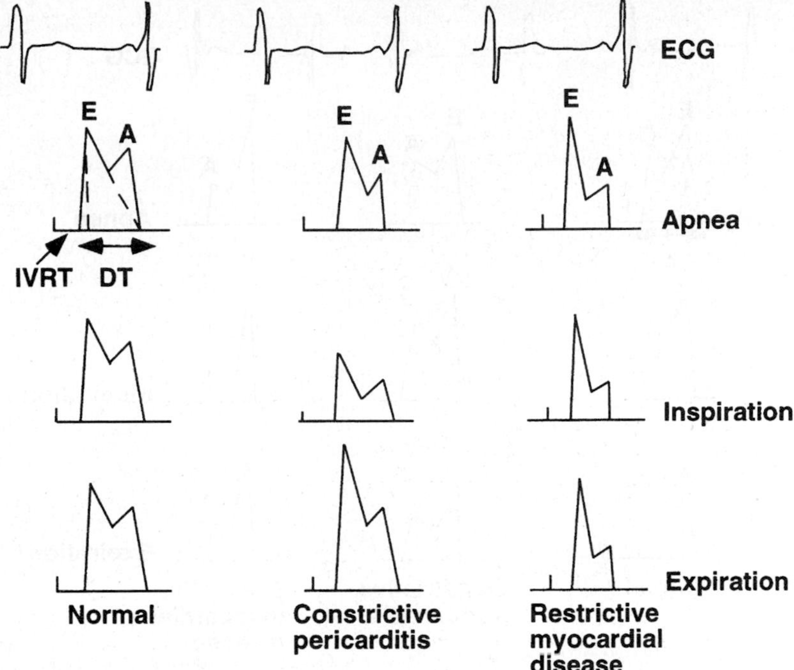

Figure 26.2. Respiratory variation in flow across the mitral valve in normals, constrictive pericarditis, and restrictive cardiomyopathy. The peak early diastolic filling velocity is denoted as E and the peak late diastolic filling velocity (from atrial contraction) is denoted as A. The isovolumetric time (IVRT) is the period between aortic valve closure and mitral valve opening. The deceleration time (DT) is the time it takes to go from peak E velocity to cessation of flow. In constrictive pericarditis, expiration results in a decreased IVRT and a marked increase in peak E and peak A velocities across the mitral valve. Similar changes are not observed in normals and those with restrictive disease. Patients with restriction have an increased E/A and shortened DT; however, there is no significant respiratory variation. (Adapted from Klein AL, et al. Differentiation of constrictive pericarditis from restrictive cardiomyopathy by Doppler transesophageal echocardiographic measurements of respiratory variations in pulmonary venous flows. *J Am Coll Cardiol* 1993;22:1935–1943.)

b. **Pulmonary venous flow.** In a healthy individual, pulmonary venous flow consists of a peak velocity during ventricular systole (S wave) and a smaller peak velocity during ventricular diastole (D wave). There is normally little respiratory variation in these velocities. In constrictive pericarditis, there is an increase in early diastolic flow manifested as a larger D wave; therefore, the **pulmonary systolic/diastolic (S/D) flow ratio is decreased.** In addition, **both systolic and diastolic pulmonary venous flow are markedly increased during** ***expiration.*** This increase in expiratory pulmonary venous flow assists in distinguishing constrictive pericarditis from restrictive cardiomyopathy (Fig. 26.4).

c. **Respiratory variation in hepatic vein flow.** Hepatic venous flow reflects right-sided filling in much the same manner that pulmonary venous flow reflects left-sided filling. It is represented similarly by an S wave and a D wave, as well as a reversal in flow in atrial systole (AR wave) and a reversal in flow due to late ventricular systole (VR wave). Individuals with constrictive pericarditis and those without have a more prominent systolic flow than a diastolic flow; however, individuals without constrictive pericarditis have little respiratory variation in these flow velocities. **In constrictive pericarditis there is a**

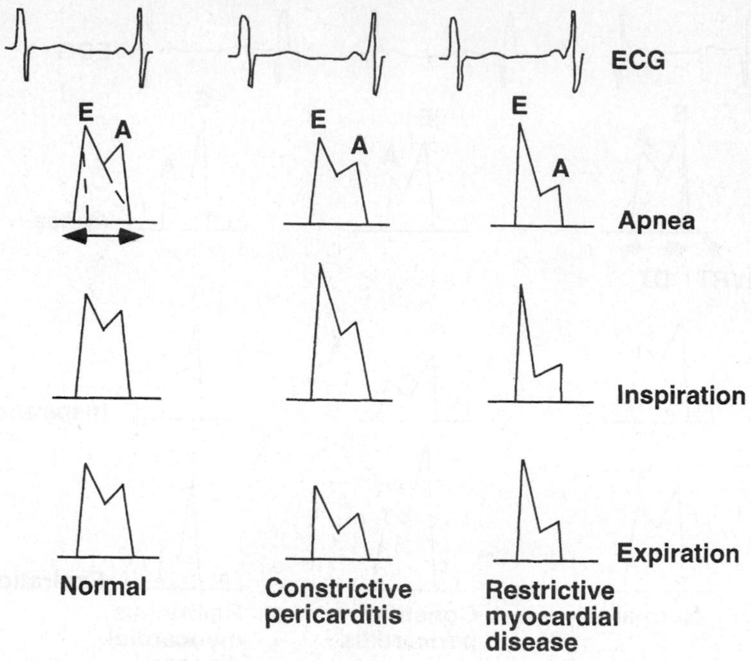

Figure 26.3. Respiratory variation in flow across the tricuspid valve in normals, constrictive pericarditis, and restrictive cardiomyopathy. Constrictive pericarditis results in changes in flow across the tricuspid valve that are opposite to those described for the mitral valve in Figure 26.2. In constrictive pericarditis, inspiration results in increased peak E and peak A velocities across the tricuspid valve. Similar changes are not observed in normals and those with restrictive cardiomyopathy. Patients with restriction have an increased E/A and shortened DT; however, there is no significant respiratory variation. (Adapted from Klein AL, et al. Differentiation of constrictive pericarditis from restrictive cardiomyopathy by Doppler transesophageal echocardiographic measurements of respiratory variations in pulmonary venous flows. *J Am Coll Cardiol* 1993;22:1935–1943.)

marked increase in the D wave during inspiration and a significant blunting during expiration. Expiration also results in prominent diastolic flow reversal demonstrated by increase in AR and VR. In restrictive disease there is a reversal in systolic-to-diastolic flow ratios, and no respiratory variation exists in these flow velocities (Fig. 26.5).

d. Doppler tissue imaging

a. Myocardial relaxation is relatively preserved in constriction unless the myocardium is also involved. Therefore, the Doppler velocities of the mitral valve annulus in early diastole are **normal or slightly increased** in constrictive pericarditis.

b. In restrictive cardiomyopathies, the early diastolic annular velocity is characteristically **low** (<8 cm/sec).

5. Cardiac catheterization. The hemodynamics obtained in the catheterization laboratory assist in both diagnosing constrictive pericarditis and differentiating it from restrictive cardiomyopathy. In general, both right and left heart catheterization are performed to obtain simultaneous ventricular pressure readings.

a. Atrial pressures. The right atrial pressure waveform has been described as having a **W-shaped configuration.** This morphology is produced by a prominent *a* wave as the atria contract against an elevated ventricular pressure, an exaggerated *x* descent, and a steep *y* descent, due to rapid ventricular filling in early diastole (Fig. 26.6).

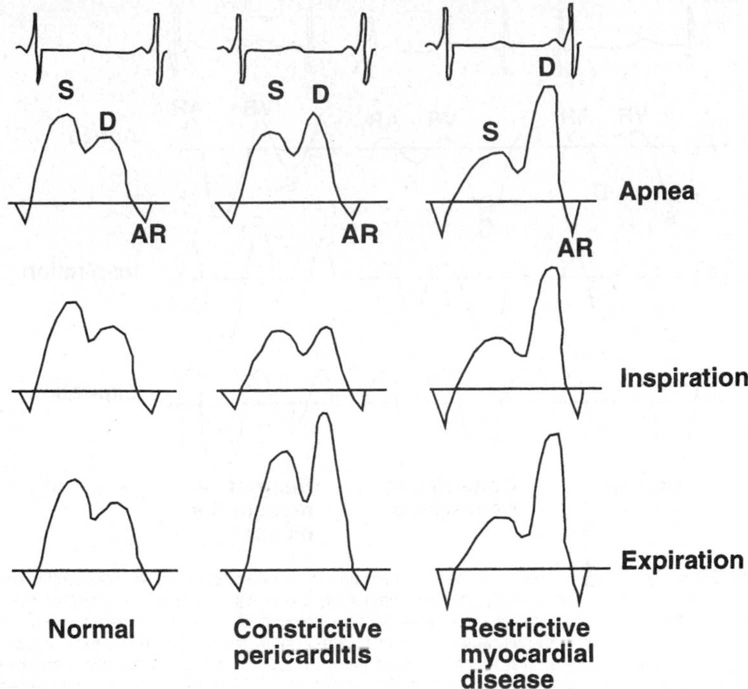

Figure 26.4. Respiratory variation in pulmonary venous flow in normal circumstance, constrictive pericarditis, and restrictive cardiomyopathy. The peak pulmonary venous velocities during systole are denoted as the S wave and peak diastolic velocities are denoted as the D wave. The AR wave represents the small reversal in flow noted with atrial contraction. In constrictive pericarditis, there is a slight decrease in the S/D ratio and a marked increase in both velocities during expiration as compared to inspiration. This respiratory variation in pulmonary venous flows is not observed in normal individuals or those with restrictive disease. (Adapted from Klein AL, et al. Differentiation of constrictive pericarditis from restrictive cardiomyopathy by Doppler transesophageal echocardiographic measurements of respiratory variations in pulmonary venous flows. *J Am Coll Cardiol* 1993;22:1935–1943.)

b. Ventricular pressures

(1) Ventricular pressure waveforms demonstrate the classic **dip-and-plateau** physiology, commonly referred to as the **square root sign** (Fig. 26.7). The initial downward deflection reflects the drop in pressure during the isovolumetric relaxation period. The subsequent upward deflection reflects early diastolic filling. The terminal plateau represents the cessation of flow that occurs once the limit of the rigid pericardium has been reached.

(2) The end-diastolic pressures of both ventricles are not only elevated but also equal, with a less than 5 mm Hg difference between the two. The right ventricular systolic pressure is generally less than 55 mm Hg, with a right ventricular end-diastolic pressure that is one-third greater than the right ventricular systolic pressure. **These findings assist in differentiating constrictive pericarditis from restrictive cardiomyopathy, where RV systolic pressure is often elevated to greater than 55 mm Hg.**

E. Therapy. Pericardiectomy is preferred in most cases, although there are certain patient populations in which medical therapy is appropriate.

1. Medical therapy

a. Patients who have NYHA class I symptoms may initially be treated with diuretics and a low-sodium diet. One case series of 36 patients demonstrated

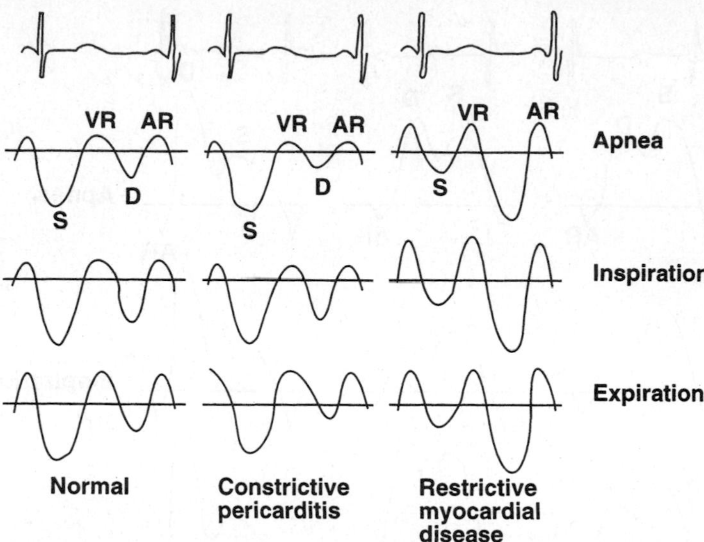

Figure 26.5. Respiratory variation in hepatic vein flow in normals, constrictive pericarditis, and restrictive cardiomyopathy. Similar to pulmonary vein flow, the S wave represents peak systolic flow velocity and the D wave represents peak diastolic flow velocity. VR denotes reversal in flow noted in late systole, and AR is the reversal in flow due to atrial contraction. In both normal subjects and those with constrictive pericarditis, there is an increase in both S and D waves with inspiration. In expiration, there is little change in normal subjects; however, those with constrictive pericarditis will have a marked drop in both S and D waves and an increase in both VR and AR. (Adapted from Klein AL, et al. Differentiation of constrictive pericarditis from restrictive cardiomyopathy by Doppler transesophageal echocardiographic measurements of respiratory variations in pulmonary venous flows. *J Am Coll Cardiol* 1993;22:1935–1943.)

resolution of pericardial contriction with the use of NSAIDs, colchicine, and/or steroids. However, most of these patients ultimately require pericardiectomy.

b. Medical therapy is also appropriate in **patients with severe comorbid illnesses** that limit life expectancy and/or place them at an unacceptably high risk for operative mortality.

2. **Surgical therapy**

a. The treatment of choice is pericardiectomy. More than 90% of patients will report symptomatic improvement following the procedure.

b. However, pericardiectomy carries an **operative mortality** reported to range from **5% to 20%.** The etiology of constrictive pericarditis can predict perioperative mortality. Patients who have constriction due to viral or idiopathic pericarditis have better outcomes than those who have radiation-induced constriction. Those patients with a poor preoperative functional class are at highest risk for perioperative death; therefore, most physicians advocate **early surgical intervention.**

IV. **PERICARDIAL EFFUSION** is a common clinical entity that is routinely diagnosed by echocardiography. It may be asymptomatic or present as life-threatening tamponade. **The presenting syndrome depends on the volume, rate of accumulation, and characteristics of the fluid.** Large effusions may be found unexpectedly and be asymptomatic, whereas rapidly accumulating small effusions may result in tamponade. An unstretched pericardium accommodates only 80 to 200 mL of rapidly accumulating fluid, without a significant change in hemodynamics. In contrast, the pericardial space may accumulate up to 2 L of fluid without any hemodynamic or clinical sequelae if this occurs slowly.

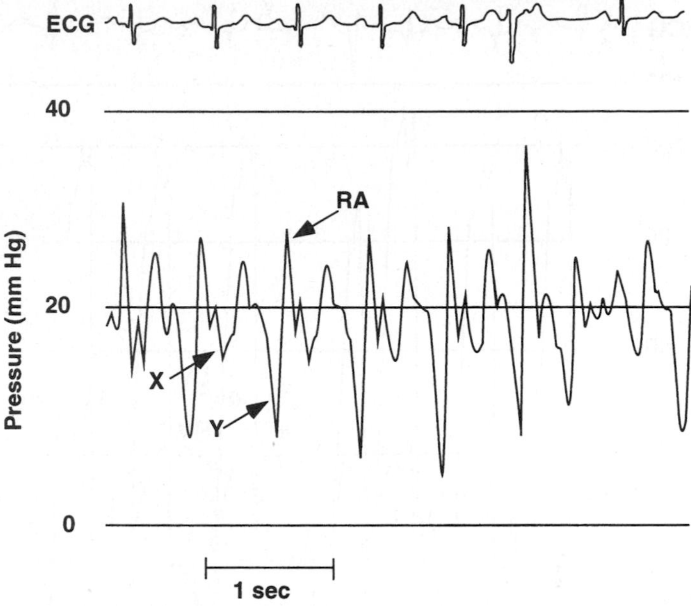

Figure 26.6. Right atrial pressure waveform in constrictive pericarditis. The preserved *x* descent and the prominent *y* descent contribute to the classic W-shaped atrial waveform. (Adapted from Lorell BH, Grossman W. Profiles in constrictive pericarditis, restrictive cardiomyopathy and cardiac tamponade in cardiac catheterization. In: Baim DS, Grossman W, eds. *Angiography and intervention,* 5th ed. Baltimore: Williams & Wilkins, 1996:801–822.)

Compressive physiology may occur with rapid accumulation of smaller amounts of fluid if the pericardium is stiff from fibrosis or infiltration by a tumor.

A. Clinical presentation

1. Slowly developing pericardial effusions, with no elevation of intrapericardial pressures, are **usually asymptomatic.**
2. Patients may complain of a **constant dull ache or pressure in the chest.**
3. There may also be a variety of symptoms from the space-occupying effects of the pericardial fluid on other organs in the chest. These include **dysphagia** from esophageal compression, **dyspnea** from lung compression and atelectasis, **hiccups** from compression of the phrenic nerve, and **nausea and abdominal fullness** from pressure on adjacent abdominal organs.
4. Large-volume effusions may be associated with muffled heart sounds, Ewart's sign (dullness to percussion, bronchial breath sounds, and egophony below the angle of the left scapula), and rales in the lung field secondary to compression.
5. **Sinus tachycardia and hypotension are signs of hemodynamic compromise.**
6. **Patients with tamponade will have a pulsus paradoxus greater than 10 mm Hg.** The total intrapericardial volume is fixed; therefore, during inspiration, filling of the right ventricle pushes the septum into the left ventricle. This impairs left-sided filling, and there is a drop in systolic pressure during inspiration. Pulsus paradoxus is **not specific for cardiac tamponade** and may be seen in severe obstructive pulmonary disease, right ventricular infarction, pulmonary embolism, or asthma.
7. Patients with tamponade will have jugular venous distention, and the *x* descent is typically the predominant wave form. **Beck's triad** includes jugular venous distention, distant heart sounds, and hypotension.

B. Etiology. Any cause of acute or chronic pericarditis (Table 26.4) may lead to the development of a pericardial effusion. Common causes of large chronic effusions

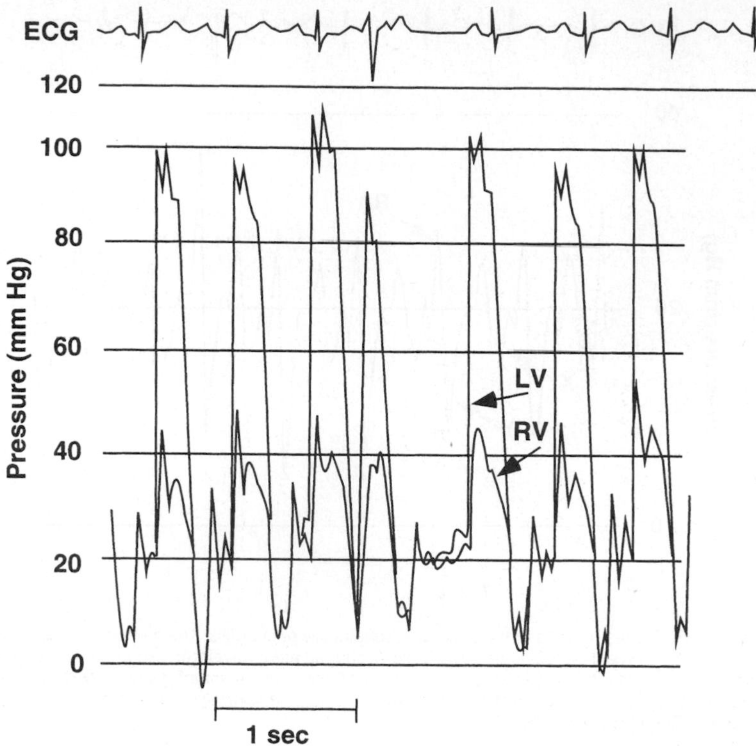

Figure 26.7. Right and left ventricular waveforms in constrictive pericarditis. Note the equalization of left ventricular and right ventricular end-diastolic pressures, generally within 5 mm Hg of one another. The rapid early diastolic filling and subsequent abrupt cessation of flow due to the rigid pericardium produces a dip-and-plateau waveform (square root sign) appreciated best in this waveform following the premature ventricular contraction (PVC). (Adapted from Lorell BH, Grossman W. Profiles in constrictive pericarditis, restrictive cardiomyopathy and cardiac tamponade in cardiac catheterization. In: Baim DS, Grossman W, eds. *Angiography and intervention,* 5th ed. Baltimore: Williams & Wilkins, 1996:801–822.)

include idiopathic pericarditis, uremia, pericarditis from malignancy or myxedema, congestive heart failure, nephrotic syndrome, cirrhosis, hypothyroidism, postcardiac surgery, and certain medications.

C. Laboratory examination and diagnostic testing

1. ECG. The classic electrocardiographic finding consists of a **low-voltage tracing. Electrical alternans** is a marker of a massive pericardial effusion.

2. Chest radiography. **Cardiomegaly may occur if more than 250 mL of fluid has accumulated.** Cardiomegaly with a large prominent superior vena cava, azygous vein, and decreased pulmonary vascularity should suggest the diagnosis of pericardial effusion.

3. Transthoracic echocardiogram (TTE) is the **modality of choice** for diagnosing and following pericardial effusions. It allows for accurate diagnosis, ensures the adequacy of drainage procedures, and enables a qualitative assessment in following pericardial effusions. Echocardiography is **not** useful in differentiating among the different etiologic factors.

a. Two-dimensional echocardiographic findings are as follows:

(1) An **echo-free space** is found between the visceral and parietal pericardium in both systole and diastole.

TABLE 26.4 CAUSES OF PERICARDIAL EFFUSION

- Idiopathic
- Acute myocardial infarction
- Delayed postmyocardial–pericardial injury syndromes:
  - Postmyocardial infarction (Dressler's) syndrome
  - Postpericardiotomy syndrome
- Metabolic
  - Uremia
  - Myxedema
  - Hypoalbuminemia
- Radiation
- Dissecting thoracic aneurysm
- Trauma
  - Pericardiotomy
  - Indirect trauma to the chest
  - Percutaneous cardiac interventions
  - Perforation of the heart by indwelling catheters
- Viral infections
  - Coxsackieviruses A, B5, B6
  - Echovirus
  - Adenovirus
  - Mumps virus
  - Hepatitis B virus
  - Infectious mononucleosis
  - Influenza
  - Lymphogranuloma venereum
  - Varicella
  - Human immunodeficiency virus
- Bacterial infections
  - *Staphylococcus*
  - *Streptococcus*
  - *Pneumococcus*
  - *Haemophilus influenzae*
  - *Neisseria gonorrhoeae*
  - *Neisseria meningitidis*
  - *Legionella hemophilia*
  - Tuberculosis
  - *Salmonella*
  - Psittacosis
  - Tularemia
  - Bacterial endocarditis
- Fungal infections
  - Histoplasmosis
  - Aspergillosis
  - Blastomycosis
  - Coccidioidomycosis
  - Fungal endocarditis
- Other *Infections*
  - Amebiasis
  - *Echinococcus*
  - Lyme disease
  - Mycoplasma pneumonia
  - Rickettsia
- Tumors
  - Primary
    - Mesothelioma
    - Teratoma
    - Fibroma
    - Leiomyofibroma and sarcoma
    - Lipoma angioma
  - Metastatic
    - Breast carcinoma
    - Bronchogenic carcinoma
    - Lymphoma
    - Leukemia melanoma
    - Others
- Immunologic/inflammatory disorders
  - Rheumatic fever
  - Systemic lupus erythematosus
  - Ankylosing spondylitis
  - Rheumatoid arthritis
  - Vasculitis
  - Wegener's granulomatosis
  - Polyarteritis nodosa
  - Scleroderma
  - Dermatomyositis
  - Sarcoidosis
  - Inflammatory bowel disease
  - Whipple's disease
  - Behçet's syndrome
  - Reiter's syndrome
  - Temporal arteritis
  - Amyloidosis
  - Familial Mediterranean fever
- Drugs
  - Procainamide
  - Hydralazine
  - Heparin
  - Warfarin
  - Phenytoin
  - Phenylbutazone
  - Cromolyn sodium
  - Dantrolene
  - Methysergide
  - Doxorubicin
  - Penicillin
  - Minoxidil
  - Colony-stimulating factor
  - Interleukin-2

(2) The **motion of the parietal pericardium is decreased.**

(3) When the effusion is large, the **entire heart swings in the pericardium.** This swinging or rocking may occur along both the anteroposterior and the mediolateral axes of the heart, and is thought to be the mechanism for electrical alternans seen on the electrocardiogram.

b. The Doppler echo findings in cardiac tamponade are described subsequently.

(1) Small effusions (less than 100 mL) tend to localize at the posterior wall distal to the atrioventricular ring. These tend to be less than 1 cm in width.

(2) Moderate effusions (100 to 500 mL). A moderate effusion could also be classified as one that surrounds the heart **but is 1 cm or less at its greatest width.**

(3) Large effusions (more than 500 mL). Here, although the posterior accumulation continues, the heart seems to settle posteriorly with a greater expansion of the pericardial space laterally, apically, and anteriorly. The **effusion is greater than 1 cm at its widest.**

c. The following may mimic a pericardial effusion on two-dimensional echocardiography.

(1) Pericardial fat tends to be **localized anteriorly.** Unless loculated, a pericardial effusion localized to the anterior wall is very rare.

(2) Seventy percent of **pericardial cysts** are found adjacent to the right cardiophrenic junction and adjacent to but separate from the right atrium in the apical four-chamber view.

(3) A pleural effusion can be differentiated from a pericardial effusion by virtue of the **position of the descending thoracic aorta in the parasternal long-axis view.** If the fluid is based in the pericardium, the aorta is displaced posteriorly to the effusion, away from the posterior wall of the left atrium. If the fluid is pleural based, the aorta retains its position immediately below the left atrium. Lung parenchyma may be seen in the pleural fluid.

(4) Other mimics of pericardial effusions are pericardial fibrous bands and pericardial calcification, anterior mediastinal tumors, peritoneal fluid, and a giant left atrium.

4. **MRI.** Although not usually required, MRI offers high sensitivity in the detection of pericardial effusions. It outlines the distribution and provides an estimate of the pericardial fluid volume that correlates well with echocardiography. It is very effective in facilitating detection of loculated pericardial effusions and pericardial thickening. Because of its high tissue contrast, MRI allows the visualization of the pericardium in multiple planes. It can also differentiate simple from complex effusions and pericardial fat from pathologic thickening.

5. **CT.** Using high-resolution axial images, CT provides excellent visualization of the pericardium. The size and distribution of the pericardial effusion is easily obtained using this technique. Moreover, differentiation among blood, exudate, chyle, and serous fluid may be achieved owing to the different attenuation coefficients for these substances.

6. Diagnostic pericardiocentesis and pericardial fluid examination should be considered in patients with large effusions without clear etiology. Aspirated pericardial fluid should be carefully inspected and immediately placed in sterile tubes for biochemical, microbiologic, and cytologic examination.

D. **Therapy.** The management of pericardial effusions depends on the underlying etiologic factor, volume, and hemodynamic significance.

1. **Pericardiocentesis.** Although the cause of the effusion is important, it can often be determined without pericardiocentesis by virtue of the clinical, systemic, and laboratory features of the presenting condition.

a. Pericardiocentesis is **indicated if malignancy, bacterial, mycobacterial, or fungal pericardial effusion is suspected.**

b. **Pericardiocentesis is indication in the setting of large pericardial effusion with associated pericardial tamponade (see subsequent text).**

c. With large effusions of recent onset, close clinical and echocardiographic follow-up is warranted. Pericardiocentesis **may be warranted in large asymptomatic pericardial effusions** when there is echocardiographic concern for early signs of tamponade.

2. Anticoagulation is best avoided until the effusion has resolved.

V. Cardiac tamponade occurs when an increase in pericardial fluid raises intrapericardial pressure and impairs diastolic filling. Cardiac tamponade is characterized by **elevated intracardiac pressures, a progressive limitation of ventricular diastolic filling, and a reduction in cardiac output.**

A. **Pathophysiology**

1. There appears to be an **inverse relationship between the volume of the pericardial effusion and cardiac output once a critical volume is reached.** Beyond this, small increments in pericardial volume result in large increases in intrapericardial pressure. This critical volume depends on the compliance of the pericardium, the rate of fluid accumulation, and the status of the pericardial lining (infiltrations, calcification, or fibrosis).
2. The raised intrapericardial pressure results in a **decreased transmural distending pressure that results in decreased diastolic filling.**
3. The **cardiac output is initially maintained** by a heightened adrenergic tone resulting in a resting tachycardia and peripheral vasoconstriction.
4. In severe tamponade, the compensatory mechanisms fail, resulting in a decreased cardiac output. Reduced coronary perfusion may cause subendocardial hypoperfusion, further compromising the stroke volume and cardiac output. The finite space around the heart chambers also results in the equalization of filling pressures with that in the pericardium.
5. Following cardiac surgery, localized **pericardial hematoma** rather than fluid may impair filling of the heart. This most commonly occurs around the right atrium, is easily overlooked, and is difficult to diagnose by TTE. TEE should be considered in cases where **pericardial hematoma** is suspected but TTE images are nondiagnostic.

B. **Clinical presentation.** The signs and symptoms of cardiac tamponade all reflect a low cardiac output: **restlessness, agitation, drowsiness or stupor; decreased urine output; dyspnea; chest discomfort, syncope or near syncope;** and **weakness, anorexia, and weight loss with a chronic effusion.**

1. **Physical findings**

a. Raised central venous pressure. Characterized by a prominent *x* descent and an attenuated, or absent, *y* descent.
b. Tachypnea. Reflects elevated pulmonary venous pressure.
c. Tachycardia. Compensatory due to the low-output state.
d. Diminished heart sounds. Decreased transmission through the fluid-filled pericardium. A pericardial friction rub may present in some cases.
e. Pulsus paradoxus as described previously.
f. **Hypotension (in severe cases).**

C. **Laboratory examination and diagnostic testing**

1. TTE should always be performed when the diagnosis of cardiac tamponade is suspected. An ECG may suggest findings consistent with cardiac tamponade, but the clinical diagnosis requires **synthesis of both bedside and echocardiographic findings.**

a. Echocardiographic signs of cardiac tamponade include the following:

(1) **Pericardial effusion.**
(2) Right atrial diastolic collapse typically begins in late diastole and continues into ventricular systole. It is best seen in the parasternal short-axis view, the subcostal view, and the apical four-chamber view. It is a **very sensitive sign, but its specificity is 82%,** with a positive predictive value of 50%. **The longer the duration of diastolic collapse, the more specific it is for tamponade.**
(3) Right ventricular early diastolic collapse (or right ventricular diastolic inversion). **Although very sensitive in medical patients, it is less so in**

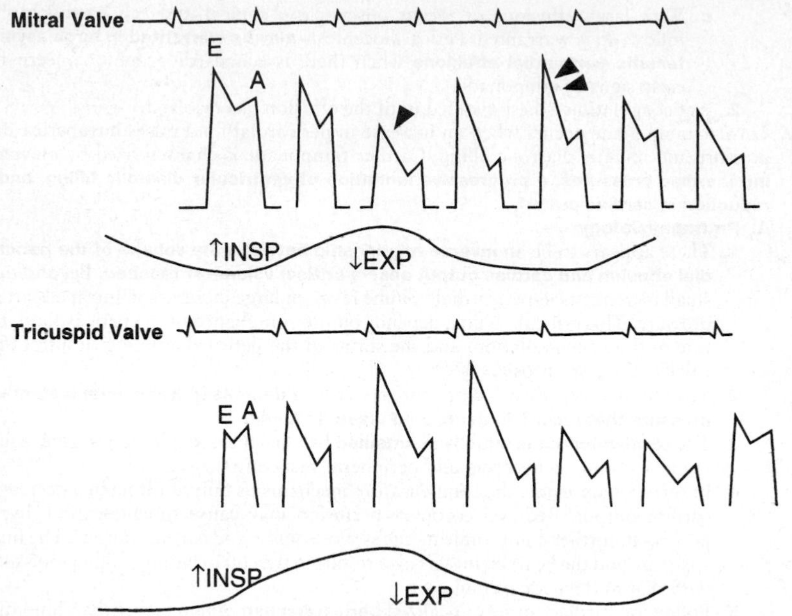

Figure 26.8. Pulsed-wave Doppler for the mitral and tricuspid valves in a patient with cardiac tamponade. Note the marked respiratory variation of the inflow pattern, which in tamponade is a typical physiologic finding.

surgical patients due to the loculated nature of these effusions and the presence of adhesions. When present, the collapse is described as a persistent posterior or inward movement of the right ventricular free wall in diastole. It is seen most commonly in the anterior right ventricular free wall and infundibulum with patients in the supine position. The parasternal long- and short-axis views of the heart are the best for evaluating this sign; M-mode recording through the right ventricle helps to outline the timing and duration of the event. **Isolated right ventricular diastolic collapse appears to occur before the onset of clinical tamponade.** Conditions that raise right ventricular intracavity volume and right ventricular pressure (pulmonary hypertension, right ventricular hypertrophy, and right ventricular infarction) delay the occurrence of right ventricular diastolic collapse until higher intrapericardial pressures are reached.

(4) Left atrial diastolic collapse—a rare but specific sign of tamponade

(5) Abnormal inspiratory increase of **right ventricular dimensions** with abnormal inspiratory decrease of LV dimensions.

(6) Respiratory variation in atrioventricular valve flow pattern, with an abnormal inspiratory increase in tricuspid valve flow and abnormal inspiratory decrease of mitral valve flow (Fig. 26.8). Normally inspiration causes a decrease in mitral valve flow of up to 10% and an increase in tricuspid valve flow of up to 7%. **A decrease on inspiration of the transmitral E wave of more than 25% is highly suggestive of significant tamponade.** A reduction of the tricuspid E wave of more than 40%, together with prominent hepatic venous flow reversal in expiration, also suggests tamponade.

(7) Inferior vena cava plethora. Failure to decrease the proximal diameter by at least 50% on sniff or deep inspiration has 97% sensitivity but only 40% specificity for tamponade physiology.

2. TEE is indicated in the postoperative patient with clinical signs of tamponade and inadequate surface images or in whom fluid is not present in the pericardium. TEE is highly sensitive for detecting hematoma in this setting.

3. Right-heart catheterization (RHC) is not necessary in patients for whom clinical and echocardiographic findings are consistent with tamponade and, in fact, may produce a delay in definitive treatment for these patients. However, RHC may be helpful in certain "borderline" cases for confirmation of the diagnosis of tamponade, quantitation of the hemodynamic compromise, and continuous assessment following pericardiocentesis. This is especially the case if pericardiocentesis is technically challenging.

a. The **hemodynamic findings** include **equalization (within 4 mm Hg) of the right arterial pressure, pulmonary capillary wedge pressure (PCWP), pulmonary artery diastolic pressure, and right ventricle mid-diastolic pressure,** which are raised usually between 10 and 30 mm Hg; the right arterial pressure reveals a **preserved *x* descent with an absent or attenuated *y* descent;** during expiration, the PCWP is slightly greater than the intrapericardial pressure that promotes filling of the left heart. With inspiration, the PCWP decreases (transiently), rendering a low or negative pressure gradient between the pulmonary venous circulation and the left heart.

b. Following pericardiocentesis, there is an initial decrease in all pressures (right atrium, right ventricular diastolic, intrapericardial, PCWP, and LV end-diastolic). As the intrapericardial pressures continue to fall below the right atrial pressure, the *y* descent recovers to baseline. This may take as little as 50 mL of fluid aspiration, due to the steep nature of the pressure-volume curve of the pericardium. These changes are accompanied by an increase in blood pressure and abolition of the pulsus paradoxus. Only with adequate hemodynamic monitoring, including arterial line and right heart catheterization, can these changes be followed.

D. Therapy

1. Priority of therapy. Once the diagnosis of tamponade is made, one needs to consider immediate **drainage.** The timing and method of drainage ultimately depend on the etiology of the effusion, the patient's level of acuity, and the availability of trained physicians. The options include needle pericardiocentesis and surgical drainage (subxiphoid pericardiectomy, pericardial window, and subtotal pericardiectomy).

2. Medical therapy. Optimal medical management is important and includes volume expansion, inotropic support if the patient is hypotensive, and avoidance of diuretics or vasodilators.

3. Percutaneous therapy

a. Pericardiocentesis allows the rapid drainage of pericardial fluid. Advantages are that it **can be performed quickly, is less invasive than other drainage methods, and requires minimal preparation.** Complications include laceration of the heart, coronary arteries, or lung. There is also the possibility of recurrent effusions or incomplete drainage. Pericardiocentesis is not recommended for small (<1 cm) effusions, or for those characterized by loculation, adhesions, or fibrinous stranding (see Chapter 54).

b. Percutaneous balloon pericardiotomy is a technique involving balloon dilation of the pericardium after securing access to the pericardial space with a transcutaneous approach. It has been used for large pericardial effusions, particularly when caused by malignancy.

4. Surgical therapy. Surgical drainage allows for more complete drainage and is preferred if there is a high likelihood of recurrence. In addition, a surgical approach permits direct examination of the pericardium, access to the pericardial tissue for histopathologic and microbiologic diagnosis, and the capability to drain loculated effusions. Surgical drainage is associated with more pain, a longer recovery time, and more periprocedural morbidity.

ACKNOWLEDGMENTS

The author thanks Drs. Jenny Wu, Stanley Chetcutti, and Joel Reginelli for their contributions to earlier editions of this chapter.

ACUTE PERICARDITIS

Landmark Articles

Imazio M, M Bobbio, et al. Colchicine in addition to conventional therapy for acute pericarditis: results of the COlchicine for acute PEricarditis (COPE) trial. *Circulation* 2005;112:2012–2016.

Lange RA, Hillis D. Acute pericarditis. *N Engl J Med* 2004;351:2195–2202.

Troughton RW, Asher CR, Klein AL. Pericarditis. *Lancet* 2004;363:717–727.

Key Reviews

Lange RA, Hillis D. Acute Pericarditis. *N Engl J Med* 2004;351:2195–2202.

Troughton RW, Asher CR, Klein AL. Pericarditis. *Lancet* 2004;363:717–727

Shabetai R, ed. Diseases of the pericardium. *Cardiol Clin* 1990;8:579–716.

Spodick DH. Pericarditis, pericardial effusion, cardiac tamponade, and constriction. *Crit Care Clin* 1989;5:455–475.

CONSTRICTIVE PERICARDITIS

Landmark Articles

Hansen AT, et al. Pressure curves from the right auricle and the right ventricle in chronic constrictive pericarditis. *Circulation* 1961;3:881–888.

Hatle LK, et al. Differentiation of constrictive pericarditis and restrictive cardiomyopathy by Doppler echocardiography. *Circulation* 1989;79:357–370.

Key Reviews

Brockington GM, Zebede J, Pandian NG. Constrictive pericarditis. In: Shabetai R, ed. Diseases of the pericardium. *Cardiol Clin* 1990;8:645–661.

Fowler N. Constrictive pericarditis: its history and current status. *Clin Cardiol* 1995;18:341–350.

Klein AL, et al. Differentiation of constrictive pericarditis from restrictive cardiomyopathy by Doppler transesophageal echocardiographic measurements of respiratory variations in pulmonary venous flows. *J Am Coll Cardiol* 1993;22:1935–1943.

Relevant Book Chapters

Braunwald E, Lorell BH. Pericardial diseases. In: Braunwald E, ed. *Heart disease: a textbook of cardiovascular medicine,* 7th ed. Philadelphia: WB Saunders, 2005:1757–1780.

Topol EJ, Klein AL, Asher, CR. Diseases of the pericardium, restrictive cardiomyopathy, and diastolic dysfunction. In: Topol EJ, ed. *Textbook of cardiovascular medicine,* 3rd ed. Philadelphia: Lippincott–Raven Publishers, 2007:420–459.

PERICARDIAL EFFUSION/TAMPONADE

Landmark Articles

Appleton PA, Hatle LK, Popp RL. Cardiac tamponade and pericardial effusion: respiratory variation and transvalvular flow velocities studied by Doppler echocardiography. *J Am Coll Cardiol* 1988;11:1020.

Burstow DJ, Oh JK, Bailey KR, et al. Cardiac tamponade: characteristic Doppler observations. *Mayo Clin Proc* 1989;64:312.

Singh S, Wenn LS, Schuchard GH, et al. Right ventricular and right atrial collapse in patients with cardiac tamponade: a combined echocardiographic and hemodynamic study. *Circulation* 1984;70:960.

Key Reviews

Little WC, Freeman GL. Pericardial disease. *Circulation* 2006;113:1622–1632.

Roy CL, Minor MA, Brookhart MA, et al. Does this patient with a pericardial effusion have cardiac tamponade? *JAMA* 2007;297:1810–1818.

Relevant Book Chapters

Feigenbaum H. Pericardial disease. In: Feigenbaum H, ed. *Echocardiography,* 5th ed. Baltimore: Williams & Wilkins, 1994:511–555.

Lorell BH, Grossman W. Profiles in constrictive pericarditis, restrictive cardiomyopathy and cardiac tamponade in cardiac catheterization. In: Baim DS, Grossman W, eds. *Angiography and intervention,* 5th ed. Baltimore: Williams & Wilkins, 1996:801–822.

PERIPHERAL ARTERY DISEASE

Thomas J. Helton

27

I. INTRODUCTION. Peripheral artery disease (PAD) describes the pathologic states that lead to stenoses and aneurysms in the noncoronary arterial circulation. This chapter will focus on the diseases of the **arterial supply to the extremities** and the **renal vasculature** (disease states involving the aorta and cerebral vasculature are discussed elsewhere in this volume). PAD can be classified as occlusive or aneurysmal. **Atherosclerosis is the most common cause of PAD.** In **aneurysmal** states, weakening of the arterial media results in focal dilation of the artery to at least 1.5 times the normal diameter. These aneurysmal segments can subsequently dissect, rupture, or thrombose, with catastrophic consequences. In addition to atherosclerosis, there are several less common pathologies that can cause PAD, including vasculitis, arterial injury, entrapment syndromes, and cystic adventitial disease. These disorders are beyond the scope of this chapter.

II. LOWER EXTREMITY PERIPHERAL ARTERY DISEASE

A. Etiology and natural history. Atherosclerosis is the most common cause of lower extremity PAD. Traditional risk factors include age, smoking history, diabetes mellitus, hyperlipidemia, and hypertension. Emerging risk factors include elevated markers of inflammation such as C-reactive protein, fibrinogen, and interleukin (IL)-6, chronic kidney disease, hypercoagulable states such as hyperhomocysteinemia, and possibly a genetic predisposition to PAD. African Americans have a twofold increase in risk of developing PAD. The prevalence of PAD increases significantly with age such that the prevalence is 2% to 3% in persons aged ≤50 years and up to 20% in persons age >70 years. **Fibromuscular dysplasia**, a noninflammatory and nonatherosclerotic process, can also affect the lower extremities by causing hyperplastic cell growth and luminal narrowing, although it predominantly affects the renal and carotid arteries. Patients with lower extremity PAD may present with leg symptoms or may be entirely asymptomatic. Approximately 50% of patients >55 years old with PAD, with or without claudication symptoms, when followed for 5 years, will remain stable or improve with exercise and lifestyle modifications. The remaining 50% will have progressive worsening of symptoms, and approximately 4% will require major amputation if they do not undergo revascularization. The highest risk of amputation occurs in those patients who are diabetic and continue to smoke. **Cardiac disease accounts for the majority of deaths in patients with PAD, in whom the relative risk of death from cardiac causes is increased more than sixfold. Approximately one-third to one-half of all patients with PAD will have concomitant coronary disease depending on the diagnostic criteria utilized, and thus PAD is considered a coronary artery disease risk equlvalent.**

B. Clinical manifestations

1. Signs and symptoms. Rest perfusion of the lower extremities may be adequate; however, if the arterial stenosis is severe, then exercise may precipitate ischemia and **claudication.** Symptoms may include pain, discomfort, or fatigue of the buttock, thigh, or calf musculature, and are usually gradual in onset. The amount of exercise required to precipitate pain is roughly related to the severity of the stenosis. Pain is usually manifested one segment below the area of severe stenosis (Table 27.1), and the most frequently involved artery in intermittment claudication is the superficial femoral artery. The symptoms are usually promptly relieved with rest or standing. More severe stenosis or more distal atherosclerotic lesions may

TABLE 27.1 Localization of Peripheral Arterial Disease

Location of pain	Likely involved segment
Buttock and thigh	Aortoiliac
Thigh	Aortoiliac, common and/or profunda femoral artery
Calf	Superficial femoral or popliteal artery[a]
Foot	Tibial or peroneal arteries

[a]Most commonly involved artery.

result in **limb-threatening ischemia with foot pain at rest, tissue ulceration, or gangrene.** There are two terms frequently used to describe this condition that should be differentiated: critical limb ischemia and acute limb ischemia. **Critical limb ischemia** is resting limb pain that results from severe atherosclerotic disease that compromises distal blood flow of the involved limb. This term typically is used to describe chronic lesions such ischemic rest pain, ischemic ulcers, or gangrene, and is caused by a slow progression of atheroslcerotic disease. **Acute limb ischemia** occurs abruptly and threatens the viability of the involved tissue. Acute limb ischemia is usually the result of an embolic event or arterial thrombosis.

2. **Physical examination.** Characterization of **femoral, popliteal, dorsalis pedis, and posterior tibial pulses**; **auscultation for bruits** in the abdomen and bilateral groins; and palpation for **aneurysm** in the abdomen and over the popliteal arteries are all a part of a comprehensive lower extremity vascular examination. A complete cardiac examination and auscultation of carotid arteries should also be perfromed to assess for concurrent abnormalities, given the common atherosclerotic pathogenesis of cerebral, myocardial, and peripheral arterial disease. Signs of lower extremity arterial insufficiency can include coolness, dry skin and scaling, pallor that is worsened with leg elevation, and ulcerations. Rarely muscular atrophy can be seen. The evaluation of a patient with possible acute limb ischemia should include the "5 P's": pain, pallor, pulselessness, parasthesias, and paralysis. These clinical features have prognostic value in acute limb ischemia. (Table 27.2)

C. **Diagnostic evaulation** (Fig. 27.1)

1. **Ankle–brachial index (ABI).** The ABI is a measurement of lower extremity perfusion, which compares the blood pressure in a pedal artery to the higher of two brachial artery blood pressures. The ABI cannot localize stenosis, but it is a simple and accurate measure of disease severity (Table 27.3). In general, ABI value correlates poorly with symptoms, and two patients with the same ABI may have remarkably different complaints. **Symptoms at rest rarely occurs unless the ABI is less than 0.4 (i.e., critical limb ischemia).** The ABI has limited use in noncompressible, calcified vessels. In patients with noncompressible ankle vessels (ABI >1.3) the toe–brachial index can be used in conjunction with pulse-volume recordings (PVRs) to document PAD. Measuring the ABIs before and after exercise can help diagnose PAD when the resting ABI is normal but there is a high clinical suspicion for PAD. It can also help differentiate between true claudication and nonarterial leg pain (pseudoclaudication).

2. **Pulse-volume recordings (PVRs).** PVRs detect changes in the volume (arterial flow) of the limb during the cardiac cycle. Blood pressure cuffs are placed at the thigh (one or two cuffs), calf, ankle, midfoot, and toe. The change in volume of the respective cuff during the cardiac cycle identifies the presence of arterial stenosis by reduction in the pulsatile flow as detected by changes in pulse contour and amplitude at that cuff, as documented by the PVR waveform (Fig. 27.2). Segmental blood pressure measurements may be taken along

TABLE 27.2 Categorizing Acute Limb Ischemia

Category	Prognosis	Sensory loss	Muscle weakness	Arterial doppler signal	Venous doppler signal
Viable	Not immediately threatened	None	None	Audible	Audible
Threatened marginally	Salavgeable if promptly treated	Minimal (toes) or none	None	Often inaudible	Audible
Threatened immediately	Salavgeable with immediate revascularization	More than toes, rest pain	Mild, moderate	Usually inaudible	Audible
Irreversible	Major tissue loss or permanent nerve damage	Profound anesthesia	Profound paralysis	Inaudible	Inaudible

Adapted from Katzen BT. Clinical diagnosis and prognosis of acute limb ischemia. *Rev Cardiovas Med* 2002;3[Suppl 2]:S2–S6.

the leg with the segmental PVR tracings for localization of disease. Unlike ABIs, arterial calcification does not effect PVR tracings, and PVR can often be helpful in the diabetic patient with a foot ulcer and suspected arterial calcification. The benefit of PVR over ABI is its ability to qualitatively identify the level of stenosis.

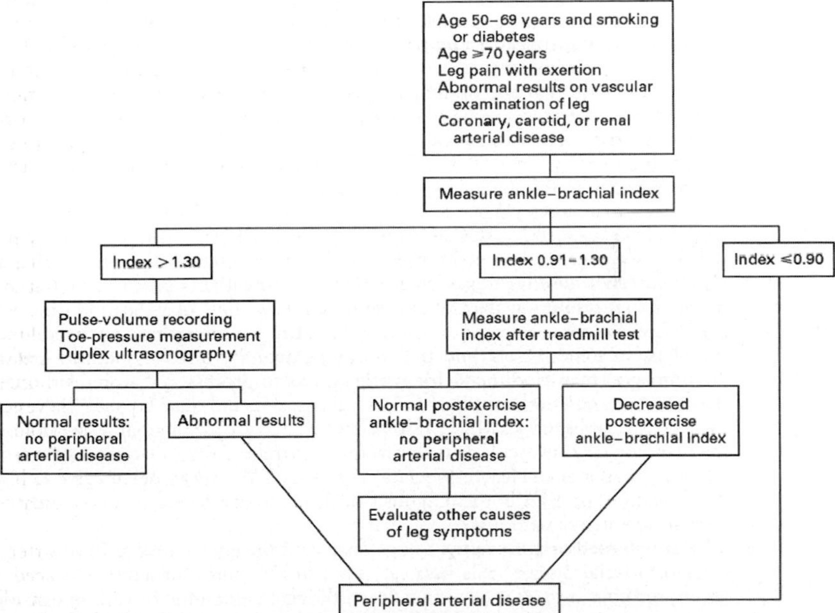

Figure 27.1. ***Evaluation of patients in whom peripheral arterial disease is suspected*** (Reproduced from Hiaat WR. Medical treatment of peripheral arterial disease and claudication. *N Engl J Med* 2001;344:1608, with permission.)

TABLE 27.3 Evaluating Disease Severity with the Ankle–Brachial Index (ABI)

ABI	Interpretation
1.3	Noncompressible vessel
1.0–1.29	Normal
0.91–0.99	Equivocal
0.4–0.90	Mild to moderate PAD
<0.4	Severe PAD

3. **Duplex ultrasound.** The arterial duplex renders an anatomic assessment of the arterial system using a combination of B-mode ultrasound imaging and Doppler frequency spectral analysis. Doppler complements the standard qualitative ultrasound imaging by allowing waveform analysis and assessment of Doppler velocities. Using the concept that velocity of blood flow inceases as it flows through a stenotic lesion, peak systolic and end-diastolic velocities are measured and used to estimate the severity of a stenosis.
4. **Magnetic resonance angiography (MRA).** The MRA signal is a reflection of the velocity and flow patterns of protons within the artery. The noninvasive nature of MRA and its ability to generate three-dimensional (3D) reconstructions are the main advantages of MRA over conventional angiography. Its limitations include a tendency to overestimate lesion severity secondary to flow turbulence, imaging artifact with metal clips or stents, and its association with nephrogenic systemic fibrosis (2.5% to 5.0%) in patient's with a glomeralular filtration rate <30 mL/min. Despite these limitations MRA still has a class I indication to diagnose the anatomic location and severity of stenosis in patients with PAD.
5. **Computed tomographic angiography (CTA).** CTA is a rapidly progressing technology that uses an intravenous contrast agent and a multidetector scanner to obtain images that are of similar quality to those of coventional angiography. New 64 detector scanners allow the simultaneous aquistion of 64 cross-sectional image slices; this has dramatically reduced radiation and contrast doses required to obtain adequate images. CTA has the advantage of being capable of reconstructing 3D images in virtually any oblique projection to help evaluate eccentric stenoses. Other advantages of CTA included better visualization of collaterals to distal vessels, identification of aneurysms, and cystic adventitial disease, which may not be picked up by conventional angiography. CTA also has several disadvantages when compared to catheter-based angiography: lower spatial resolution than digital subtraction, venous opacification can preclude visualization of arterial filling, asymmetric leg filling may miss the arterial phase in some vessels, and the enormous quantity of data obtained (up to 2000 images) may be difficult for workstations to process and store. Although the accuracy and effectiveness of CTA in diagnosing and quantifying PAD is not as well as established as MRA, it appears to have great potential, especially in the planning of a revascularization strategy. Currently, the American College of Cardiology/American Heart Association (ACC/AHA) PAD guidelines give a class IIb indication for CTA in the diagnosis of the anatomic location and severity of stenosis in patients with PAD.
6. **Catheter-based angiography.** Long considered the gold standard for the diagnosis of arterial disease, this invasive procedure requires intraarterial vascular access and contrast (often nonionic dye, although gadolinium or carbon dioxide can be used). It is recommended for the evaluation of patients for whom revascularization procedures are planned (those with lifestyle-limiting claudication, rest pain, ischemic ulceration, or gangrene), or for when noninvasive techniques are inconclusive. Because contrast angiography demonstrates only the arterial

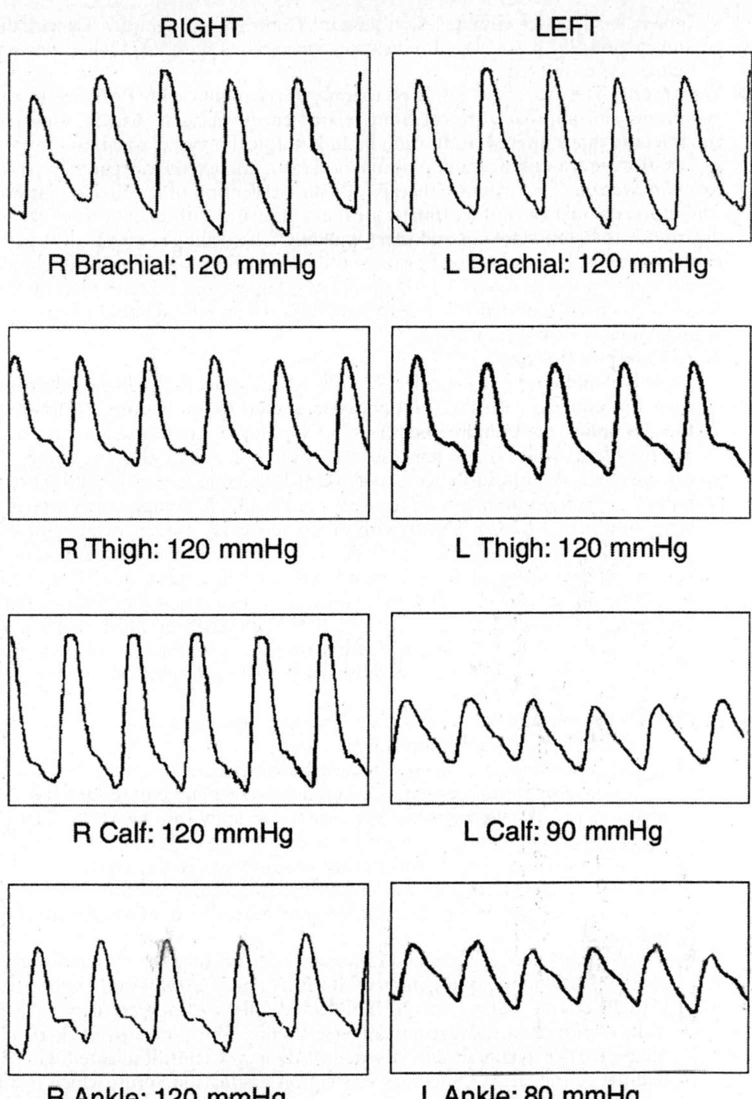

Figure 27.2. ***Pulse-volume recording (PVR) of the lower extremities***. This PVR was obtained from a 42-year-old man with a history of diabetes mellitus and tobacco use who developed new left calf cramping with exertion. It demonstrates moderate disease (ankle–brachial index = 0.66) of left femoropopliteal segment and a normal recording on the right lower extremity. He was advised to begin both a tobacco cessation program and a walking regimen.

lumen, it can underestimate lesion severity. Contrast angiography (Ia) with digital subtraction (Ib) has a class I indication for patients with PAD when revascularization is considered.

D. Treatment. The two main goals of therapy for patients with PAD are to relieve symptoms and improve survival from related cardiovascular disease. Options for treatment of intermittent claudication include surgical revascularization ("bypass"), percutaneous revascularization, pharmacotherapy, and exercise. Aggressive risk factor modification is the primary therapy for the prevention of cardiovascular events. Therefore, the mainstay of treatment for many patients with mild to moderate claudication is to **"stop smoking and start walking."** Accordingly, a trial of supervised exercise therapy is given a class I recommendation as the initial therapy of choice for claudication in the ACC/AHA PAD guidelines. Supervised exercise therapy ("PAD rehab") has been reported to increase walking distance by up to 130% to 180% among patients with claudication.

1. **Antiplatelet therapy**

   Aspirin/clopidogrel. Antiplatelet therapy reduces mortality and cardiovascular events in patients with PAD. **All patients should be on aspirin (75 to 325 mg) therapy unless contraindicated** (class I). Clopidogrel can be used in the setting of aspirin allergy (class I) and has also been shown in subset analysis of the Clopidogrel versus Aspirin in Patients at Risk of Ischaemic Events (CAPRIE) trial to reduce the composite major adverse events by 23.8% compared to aspirin in a large cohort of 19,185 patients with atherosclerotic vascular disease, of whom 6,452 had symptomatic PAD. More direct comparative trial data are needed before clopidogrel alone can be considered as the first-line agent for PAD. In terms of dual antiplatelet therapy, the Clopidogrel and Aspirin versus Aspirin Alone for the Prevention of Atherothrombotic Events (CHARISMA) trial failed to show a significant additive reduction in cardiovascular events with dual antiplatelet therapy in patients with asymptomatic cardiovascular disease or multiple cardiovascular disease risk factors.

2. **Risk factor modification.** PAD is a coronary risk equivalent and as such, aggressive risk factor modification is warranted.

   a. Cigarette **smoking** has been associated with progression of atherosclerosis. Physician counseling is essential, as **tobacco cessation can reduce the 5-year amputation risk and decrease the 5-year mortality rate by 50%**. The importance of this intervention cannot be underestimated. Whenever possible, extensive counseling and referral to formal smoking cessation programs should be offered (class I). In addition, several pharmacologic therapies are available (buproprion, nicotine replacement, varenicline) and should be prescribed when indicated.

   b. Current guidelines recommend treatment of **hypertension** to goal blood pressure <140/90 mm Hg in patients with PAD and <130/80 mm Hg in patients with PAD and diabetes or chronic kidney disease to prevent the development of future cardiovascular adverse events. The use of β-blockers as antihypertensive agents in patients with PAD is *not* contraindicated. Given the findings of the Heart Outcomes Prevention Evaluation Study, which included patients with PAD, it is reasonable to treat patients with symptomatic PAD, irrespective of diabetes, with an angiotensin-converting enzyme (ACE) inhibitor to reduce cardiovascular events (class IIa).

   c. Aggressive treatment of **hyperlipidemia** should include therapy with 3-hydroxy-3-methylglutaryl coenzyme A reductase inhibitors (statins) whenever possible to achieve a low-density lipoprotein (LDL) goal of <100 mg/dL in patients with PAD (class I). For patients at especially high risk for ischemic events, a LDL goal of <70 mg/dL may be desirable (class IIa). Patients with normal LDL cholesterol, low high-density lipoprotein (HDL) cholesterol and elevated triglycerides may derive benefit from a fibric acid derative (class IIa).

   d. The management of **diabetes** in patients with PAD is important given their increased risk of amputation (overall 20%) and increased mortality (estimated to be 50% at 5 years). Current recommendations advocate daily assessment of the feet to aid in the early identification of complications of ischemia, such as foot ulcers (class I). The recommended target HbA1c is <7.0% (class IIa). Aggressive risk-factor modification is a critical component of management for diabetic patients with PAD, and these patients should be treated with antiplatelet therapy, lipid lowering agents, and ACE inhibitors in the absence of contraindication.

3. **Treatment of claudication**
   a. **Exercise is an inexpensive, low-risk option in comparison with invasive therapies and pharmacotherapies for intermittent claudication.** Potential mechanisms by which exercise improves symptoms include augmentation of collateral flow, improved rheologic characteristics of blood, decreased reliance on anaerobic metabolism, and greater extraction of oxygen. Supervised exercise programs have been shown to improve pain-free walking distance up to 180% from resting values. For patients with symptomatic claudication, current guidelines recommend a supervised exercise program for 30 to 45 minutes three times a week for at least 12 weeks (class I). For patients who do not have a supervised exercise program available to them, a self-directed structured walking program should be encouraged.
   b. **Cilostazol** is a type 3 phosphodiesterase inhibitor that suppresses platelet aggregation and acts as a direct arterial vasodilator. Cilostazol also beneficially increases HDL, decreases triglycerides, and inhibits vascular cell adhesion molecule-1 expression, thereby decreasing vascular smooth cell proliferation. Randomized controlled trials of patients with moderate to severe claudication have demonstrated 40% to 60% increases in maximal walking distances with 12 to 24 weeks of therapy with cilostazol 100 mg twice daily. A trial of cilostazol, 100 mg twice daily, is recommended in all patients with PAD and intermittent claudication to relieve symptoms and improve walking distance (class I). Cilostazol is contraindicated in patients with congestive heart failure, owing to an increased risk of sudden death associated with related phosphodiesterase inhibitors. Common side effects associated with cilostazol include diarrhea, palpitations, and headaches.
   c. **Pentoxifylline.** Oral pentoxifylline, 400 mg three times daily, can be considered as a second-line alternative to cilostazol in patients with symptomatic claudication (class IIb). Pentoxifylline is a methylxanthine derivative that functions as a vasodilator, an antiplatelet agent, and reduces blood viscosity and improves deformability of erythocytes and leukocytes to exert it effects. Trials have been divergent on the efficacy of pentoxifylline, and it is felt to result in only marginal improvements in maximal walking distance and symptoms.
4. **Revascularization.** Revascularization is indicated for "lifestyle-limiting" claudication (after failed medical therapy), rest pain, ischemic ulceration, or gangrene. It may be **performed surgically or percutaneously.**
   a. **Percutaneous therapy.** In carefully selected patients, catheter-based revascularization is an attractive alternative to conventional surgical management. Percutaneous revascularization has a class I indication for individuals with lifestyle-limiting claudication when there is a reasonable likelihood of procedural success and there has been an inadequate response to conservative therapy. Percutaneous revascularization is recommended according to the TransAtlantic inter-Society Consensus II (TASC II) guidelines, which divide lesion anatomy according to location, distribution, length and likelihood of procedural success. TASC type A lesions are those in which endovascular therapy is recommended, and type B lesions are those in which endovascular therapy is preferred in most cases. For instance, TASC type A disease in the aortoiliac system is defined as unilateral or bilateral disease in the common iliac or external iliac arteries of short length (<3 cm). In the femoral popliteal region, a type A lesion is defined as a single stenosis ≤10 cm in length or a single occlusion ≤5 cm in length. Translesional pressure gradients (criteria:

threshold peak systolic difference 5 to 10 mm Hg prevasodilation and 10 to 15 mm Hg postvasodilation) should be obtained for angiographic lesions that appear moderately stenotic (e.g., 50% to 75%) prior to intervention (class I). The treatment of choice for focal aortoiliac disease is angioplasty with or without stenting. This approach has a technical success rate of 90%, 2-year patency rate of 73% to 84%, a complication rate of less than 10% (usually related to the arterial access site), and periprocedural mortality rate of less than 1%. For femoropopliteal disease, patency rates with percutaneous therapies are lower than in iliac disease; therefore, angioplasty is utilized to manage focal disease after failure of medical therapy. Direct stenting as a primary therapy is not recommended for femoral, popliteal or tibial arteries; however, stenting may be effective as salvage therapy after suboptimal or failed baloon angioplasty (class I).

b. Surgical. Similarly, surgical revascularization also has a class I indication for individuals with lifestyle-limiting claudication when there is a reasonable likelihood of procedural success and there has been an inadequate response to conservative therapy. Surgery is used to bypass long segments of diffuse disease (particularly involving the femoropopliteal segment) or when endovascular therapy fails. Various conduits, such as reversed or in situ saphenous vein, Dacron, and polytetrafluoroethylene, are used. For severe disease below the popliteal artery, both percutaneous and surgical revascularization approaches have marginal outcomes with regard to limb salvage. In patients younger than 50 years of age, the efficacy of surgical intervention for symptomatic claudication is not well established due to the aggressive nature of their atherosclerosis and limited graft durabiltiy (class IIb). Given the coincidence of coronary artery disease in these patients, a thorough preoperative assessment of cardiac risk should be performed prior to vascular surgery.

III. LOWER EXTREMITY ANEURYSMS. Aneurysms of the peripheral arteries, as in the aorta, are most commonly due to atherosclerotic disruption of the arterial media. Up to 70% of lower extremity aneurysms involve the popliteal arteries. The incidence of bilateral involvement in lower extremity aneurysm is high (45% to 68%). The majority of patients (62%) with popliteal aneurysms have been reported to have concomitant abdominal aortic aneurysms (AAAs), and this co-prevalence increases to 85% in patients with femoral artery aneurysms. Accordingly, patients diagnosed with peripheral arterial aneurysms, especially femoral or popliteal, should be screened with ultrasound for AAA and for the presence of contralateral lower extremity disease (class I). The greatest concern with lower extremity aneurysms is thrombosis and thromboembolism. Lower extremity aneurysms infrequently rupture (7% to 12%), but up to 60% will have an ischemic complication; therefore, acute limb ischemia is the most common presenting symptom. As an aneurysm increases in size it can compress adjacent venous and lymphatic structures causing lower extremity edema. Given the risk of thrombosis, it is recommended that popliteal aneurysms greater than 2.0 cm (class I) and femoral artery aneurysms greater than 3.0 cm be repaired. Unless symptomatic, aneurysms of smaller caliber should be followed by annual arterial duplex ultrasound examinations (class IIa).

IV. UPPER EXTREMITY ARTERIAL DISEASE. In addition to atherosclerosis, the most common cause of upper extremity PAD, other pathologic states can result in stenosis of the upper extremity arteries. These disorders include vasculitis (particularly Takayasu and giant cell arteritis), fibromuscular dysplasia, thoracic outlet syndrome, ionizing radiation, and repetitive injury. Associated clinical symptoms include arm and hand claudication, digital ulceration, and neurologic symptoms caused by vertebral–subclavian steal. The diagnostic modalities are similar to those in lower extremity arterial disease. The simple clinical maneuver of checking blood pressure measurements in both arms is an excellent screening test for significant upper extremity PAD. Risk-factor modification and revascularization (for symptomatic patients) are the mainstays of therapy. Finally, a high index of suspicion for concurrent cardiovascular and cerebrovascular disease should be maintained.

V. RENAL ARTERY DISEASE

A. Clinical manifestations. Renal artery stenosis (RAS) is commonly associated with two clinical syndromes: hypertension and ischemic nephropathy. Clues to the presence of RAS include the following: **abrupt onset of hypertension** (before age 30, often due to fibromuscular dysplasia; or after 55, often due to atherosclerotic disease); **previously well-controlled essential hypertension that becomes resistant to medical therapy** (three-drug regimen including a diuretic); **azotemia**, which is unexplained or induced by angiotensin-converting enzyme inhibitor administration; **recurrent flash pulmonary edema**, often with normal left ventricular function (due to renin–angiotensin-mediated volume overload and peripheral vasoconstriction). Physical examination in RAS may reveal hypertension, epigastric bruits, and evidence of atherosclerosis in other vascular beds (e.g., carotid or femoral bruits, diminished pedal pulses). Renal imaging can reveal an atrophic kidney or a size discrepancy between the two kidneys.

B. Etiology and natural history. The most common causes of RAS are atherosclerosis and fibromuscular dysplasia. Atherosclerosis accounts for 90% of RAS and usually involves the ostium and proximal third of the main renal artery. The prevalence of atherosclerotic RAS increases with age, particularly in patients with diabetes, aortoiliac disease, coronary artery disease, or hypertension. Studies have suggested the prevalence of RAS in patients with PAD may be as high as 59%. It is the most common cause of secondary hypertension, may account for 1% to 5% of all cases of hypertension, and may be the cause of end-stage renal failure in up to 20% of new dialysis patients. RAS is an independent risk factor for mortality in patients with other vascular disease. Moreover, end-stage renal disease due to RAS is associated with the highest mortality (median survival of 2.7 years) among all dialysis dependent patients. Fibromuscular dysplasia (FMD), which usually results from muscular dysplasia of the arterial media, accounts for less than 10% of cases of RAS, but should be suspected in younger patients without atherosclerotic risk factors who present with RAS. It more frequently affects women ages 15 to 50 years, involves the distal two-thirds of the main renal artery and its branches, and has a characteristic "string of beads" appearance on angiography. The cause of fibromuscular dysplasia is unknown. Rarer causes of RAS include vasculitis, neurofibromatosis, congenital bands, extrinsic compression, and ionizing radiation.

C. Diagnostic evaluation

1. **Laboratory studies.** Blood urea nitrogen (BUN) and serum creatinine are readily available and are often used in practice as screening tools. Although azotemia and increased serum creatinine are neither sensitive nor specific for RAS, they may be the first clue to the disease. Urinalysis in RAS usually reveals proteinuria and a bland sediment. Because of the advent of sensitive and specific noninvasive imaging modalities, plasma renin activity and selective renal vein renin measurements are not recommended as screening test to diagnose RAS (class III).
2. **Duplex ultrasonography (DUS).** Arterial duplex uses a combination of B-mode ultrasound imaging and Doppler frequency spectral analysis. As blood flows through a stenotic lesion its velocity increases, and thus the measured velocity is used to estimate the severity of RAS. The ratio of the peak systolic velocity to the aortic velocity, the renal-to-aortic ratio (RAR), can be used to estimate the degree of stenosis. In addition, DUS allows for calculation of the renal resistive index (renal parenchymal peak systolic velocity minus end-diastolic velocity divided by the peak systolic velocity), which is a potential marker of renal parenchymal disease. Some data suggest that patients with an elevated resistive index may not improve after revascularization. DUS is inexpensive, widely available, and highly sensitive and specific for RAS when compared to angiography (reported sensitivities between 84% to 98% and reported specificities between 62% to 99%). It is also highly useful for surveillance of renal arteries after stenting, as flow through a stent can be easily detected, in contrast to MRA, which is limited by metal artifact. Duplex ultrasonography for RAS must be performed in

experienced centers. The test may be limited by difficulty in obtaining measurements due to excess bowel gas or obesity. It also has lower sensitivity (64%) for identifying accessory renal arteries, narrowing of which which could also lead to the signs of RAS.

3. **Renal scintigraphy.** Radionuclide renal imaging is used to assess differential renal blood flow and has been used in conjunction with captopril renography to attempt to diagnose RAS. Captopril renography precipitates an angiotensin-converting enzyme (ACE) inhibitor–mediated fall in glomerular filtration to amplify differences in renal perfusion consistent with RAS. Due to a relative lack of sensitivity (74%) and specificity (59%) compared to catheter-based angiography, captopril renography is no longer recommended for the screening of RAS (class III).
4. **Magnetic resosance angiography (MRA).** MRA now has a class I indication as a test for the diagnosis of RAS with reported sensitivity and specificity from 90% to 100% and 76% to 94%, respectively, when compared to angiography. MRA is noninvasive and has the ability to generate 3D reconstructions. Its limitations include expense, limited availability, lack of resolution in the setting of high-grade stenosis (often appearing as an occlusion or loss of signal), a tendency to overestimate lesion severity, and difficulty with post-stent imaging due to artifact. It is also less sensitive for the detection of FMD given that the typical arterial beading may be subtle and resolution of MRA is still limited, particularly of the distal renal vasculature. In addition, in patients with advanced renal insufficiency or renal failure, gadolinium-containing contrast agents have been linked to nephrogenic systemic fibrosis (NSF) in 2% to 3% of patients (see Chapter 46). This has complicated the use of contrast-enhanced MRI in patients with RAS and renal insufficiency.
5. **Computed tomographic angiograpy (CTA).** Like MRA, CTA has the capability of producing excellent 3D images of the renal arteries as well as the aorta and other visceral vessels. CTA has a sensitivity and specificity for detecting significant RAS ranging from 59% to 96% and 82% to 99%, respectively. Contrast administration (100 to 150 mL) and radiation dose remain limitations of CTA. Unlike MRA, CTA does not have significant imaging artifact with metal clips or stents, and, therefore, can be used to detect in-stent restenosis.
6. **Renal arteriography.** This is the gold standard for the diagnosis of RAS. It allows for excellent visualization of the main renal and acessory renal arteries and their branches, Arteriography allows for assessment of the degree of stenosis visually and adds the ability to obtain hemodynamic measurements (gradients) across the stenotic lesions. Disadvantages include the requirement for intraarterial access and nephrotoxic radiocontrast.

D. Treatment. Despite antihypertensive therapy, RAS tends to progress and may be associated with renal ischemia and loss of renal function (i.e., renal insufficiency). Atherosclerotic nephropathy is complex and not simply related to stenosis of the renal artery. Examination of renal histology in patients with atherosclerotic nephropathy reveals other potential mechanisms for loss of function, including small-vessel occlusion from atheroemboli, intrarenal arterial stenoses, and preexisting hypertensive nephrosclerosis. Importantly, as with other peripheral vascular disease processes, a high index of suspicion for concurrent cardiovascular and cerebrovascular disease should be maintained.

1. **Medical therapy.** Aggressive antihypertensive therapy using multiple agents remains the mainstay of RAS therapy and is often the control arm of randomized trials of interventional approaches to RAS. ACE inhibitors, angiotensin receptor blockers, diuretics, β-blockers, calcium-channel blockers, and various other antihypertensives have been shown to be effective in treating hypertension associated with RAS. ACE inhibitors and angiotensin-receptor blockers should not be used in patients with bilateral RAS or a solitary kidney with RAS. However, these agents can be highly effective in the management of hypertension in patients with unilateral RAS (class I). Patients with RAS should be treated to blood

pressure targets consistent with the Seventh Report of the Joint National Committee on Prevention, Detection, Evaluation and Treatment of Hypertension. Aggressive atherosclerotic disease risk factor modification should be part of a comprehensive treatment plan.

2. **Percutaneous revascularization.** The principle behind revascularization is that early restoration of renal artery patency in patients with atherosclerotic RAS may improve hypertension management and minimize progressive renal dysfunction; however, there is a paucity of data from controlled clinical trials to show that revasucularization for RAS improves hypertension or delays renal dysfunction. Two small randomized trials demonstrated that patients treated with percutaneous renal artery angioplasty had improved systolic blood pressure and/or blood pressure control (as measured by a reduction in the number or dose of antihypertensive agents used) compared to patients treated with antihypertensive therapy alone. The response is better among patients with fibromuscular dysplasia than those with atherosclerotic RAS, a finding that may be expected given the pathology that is seen at multiple levels in renal vasculature with atherosclerotic RAS. Congestive heart failure (CHF) and chronic obstructive pulmonary disease (COPD) have been shown to be independent predictors of increased mortality in patients undergoing renal artery stenting; however, baseline azotemia remains the strongest predictor of long term mortality (70% 5-year mortality rate with serum creatinine >2.5 mg/dL).

   Revascularization for RAS has been shown to stabilize or improve renal function in patients with symptomatic RAS up to 1 year after intervention. In the ACC/AHA PAD Guidelines, the only class I indication for percutaneous renal artery revascularization is hemodynamically significant RAS in patients with recurrent unexplained pulmonary edema or congestive heart failure. Other clinical scenarios in which percutaneous renal artery revascularization for hemodynamically significant RAS can be considered (class IIa) are uncontrolled/malignant hypertension, progressive chronic kidney disease with bilateral RAS, RAS in a solitary functioning kidney, or unstable angina with RAS. A hemodynamically significant lesion in RAS is defined as any lesion with greater than 70% stenosis or a lesion that has 50% to 70% stenosis with a translesional pressure gradient of more 20 mmHg or mean gradient greater than 10 mm Hg. In terms of revascularization technique, renal artery stent placement has a class I indication for ostial atherosclerotic RAS. Stenting is also recommended as bail-out therapy following failed angioplasty in renal FMD, although angioplasty alone is generally successful in this disorder. Predictors of poor outcomes with RAS interventions include significant proteinuria (>1 g/day), renal atrophy, parenchymal renal disease and diffuse renal arterial disease.

3. **Surgical revascularization.** Vascular surgery approaches to RAS include surgical bypass (aortorenal, celiac-renal, or mesenteric-renal) and endarterectomy. Perioperative mortality rates range from 1% to 5%. The comparable procedural success with percutaneous approaches and fewer major complications have led to a decline in the number of vascular surgeries for RAS. In the setting of RAS and aortic disease (either aneurysmal or occlusive), surgical revascularization with renal artery bypass grafting is the preferred approach (class I). Surgical revascularization is also recommended for patients with significant atherosclerotic RAS and clinical indications for intervention with multiple renal arteries or early branching main renal artery (class I). In patients with FMD, surgical revascularization is recommended for RAS associated with macroaneurysms or complex disease involving segmental renal arteries (calss I).

4. **Controversies.** Among existing revascularization procedures for peripheral vascular disorders, renal artery stenting is possibly the most widely applied and poorly tested. To date, there are no published randomized, controlled trials demonstrating the superiority of renal artery stenting over optimal medical therapy (risk factor modification, aggressive antihypertensive therapy, lipid reduction therapy, and aspirin) for RAS. In addition, the ability of renal artery stenting to decrease mortality or progression to dialysis, or to provide prolonged benefits

in blood pressure control remains uncertain. The National Institutes of Health (NIH)–sponsored Cardiovascular Outcomes with Renal Atherosclerotic Lesions (CORAL) trial is the first large randomized controlled trial comparing medical therapy versus medical therapy plus renal artery stenting for the treatment of patients with systolic hypertension and RAS. CORAL is currently enrolling patients (1080 patients anticipated) with expected completion in 2010, and it is hoped that this trial will provide much needed data to determine the optimal management of RAS.

ACKNOWLEDGMENT

The author thanks Dr. Frank J. Zidar for his contributions to earlier editions of this chapter.

Landmark Articles

Antiplatelet Trialists' Collaboration. Collaborative overview of randomised trials of antiplatelet therapy—I: Prevention of death, myocardial infarction, and stroke by prolonged antiplatelet therapy in various categories of patients. *BMJ* 1994;308:81–106.

Bhatt DL, Fox KA, Hacke W, et al. Clopidogrel for and aspirin versus aspirin alone for the prevention of atherothrombotic events (CHARISMA) trial. *N Engl J Med* 2006;354:1706.

CAPRIE Steering Committee. A randomised, blinded, trial of clopidogrel versus aspirin in patients at risk of ischaemic events (CAPRIE). *Lancet* 1996;348:1329–1339.

Criqui MH, Langer RD, Fronek A, et al. Mortality over a period of 10 years in patients with peripheral arterial disease. *N Engl J Med* 1992;326:381–386.

Dotter CT, Judkins MP. Transluminal treatment of arteriosclerotic obstruction. Description of a new technique and a preliminary report of its application. 1964. *Radiology* 1989;172:904–920.

Hirsch AT, Criqui MH, Treat-Jacobson D, et al. Peripheral arterial disease detection, awareness, and treatment in primary care. *JAMA* 2001;286:1317–1324.

Hirsch AT, Haskal ZJ, Hertzer NR, et al. ACC/AHA 2005 Practice Guidelines for the management of patients with peripheral arterial disease (lower extremity, renal, mesenteric, and abdominal aortic): a collaborative report from the American Association for Vascular Surgery/Society for Vascular Surgery, Society for Cardiovascular Angiography and Interventions, Society for Vascular Medicine and Biology, Society of Interventional Radiology, and the ACC/AHA Task Force on Practice Guidelines (Writing Committee to Develop Guidelines for the Management of Patients With Peripheral Arterial Disease): endorsed by the American Association of Cardiovascular and Pulmonary Rehabilitation; National Heart, Lung, and Blood Institute; Society for Vascular Nursing; TransAtlantic Inter-Society Consensus; and Vascular Disease Foundation. *Circulation* 2006;113:e463–e654.

Holm J, Arfvidsson B, Jivegard L, et al. Chronic lower limb ischaemia. A prospective randomised controlled study comparing the 1-year results of vascular surgery and percutaneous transluminal angioplasty (PTA). *Eur J Vasc Surg* 1991;5:517–522.

Lundgren F, Dahllof AG, Lundholm K, et al. Intermittent claudication—surgical reconstruction or physical training? A prospective randomized trial of treatment efficiency. *Ann Surg* 1989;209:346–355.

Norgren L, Hiatt WR, Dormandy JA, et al. TASC II Working Group. Inter-Society Consensus for the Management of Peripheral Arterial Disease (TASC II). *Eur J Vasc Surg* 2007;33[Suppl 1]:S1–S75.

Perkins JM, Collin J, Creasy TS, et al. Exercise training versus angioplasty for stable claudication. Long and medium term results of a prospective, randomised trial. *Eur J Vasc Endovasc Surg* 1996;11:409–413.

Plouin PF, Chatellier G, Darne B, et al. Blood pressure outcome of angioplasty in atherosclerotic renal artery stenosis: a randomized trial. Essai Multicentrique Medicaments vs Angioplastie (EMMA) Study Group. *Hypertension* 1998;31:823–829.

Rundback JH, Sacks D, Kent KC, et al. Guidelines for the reporting of renal artery revascularization in clinical trials. American Heart Association. *Circulation* 2002;106:1572–1585.

Van Jaarsveld BC, Krijnen P, Pieterman H, et al. The effect of balloon angioplasty on hypertension in atherosclerotic renal artery stenosis. Dutch Renal Artery Stenosis Intervention Cooperative Study Group. *N Engl J Med* 2000;342:1007–1014.

Webster J, Marshall F, Abdalla M, et al. Randomised comparison of percutaneous angioplasty vs continued medical therapy for hypertensive patients with atheromatous renal artery stenosis. Scottish and Newcastle Renal Artery Stenosis Collaborative Group. *J Hum Hypertens* 1998;12:329–335.

Weibull H, Bergqvist D, Bergentz SE, et al. Percutaneous transluminal renal angioplasty versus surgical reconstruction of atherosclerotic renal artery stenosis: a prospective randomized study. *J Vasc Surg* 1993;18:841–850; discussion 850–852.

Whyman MR, Fowkes FG, Kerracher EM, et al. Is intermittent claudication improved by percutaneous transluminal angioplasty? A randomized controlled trial. *J Vasc Surg* 1997;26:551–557.

Wilson SE, Wolf GL, Cross AP. Percutaneous transluminal angioplasty versus operation for peripheral arteriosclerosis. Report of a prospective randomized trial in a selected group of patients. *J Vasc Surg* 1989;9:1–9.

Wolf GL, Wilson SE, Cross AP, et al. Surgery or balloon angioplasty for peripheral vascular disease: a randomized clinical trial. Principal investigators and their Associates of Veterans Administration Cooperative Study Number 199. *J Vasc Interv Radiol* 1993;4:639–648.

Key Reviews

Almahameed A. Peripheral arterial disease: recognition and management. *Cleve Clin J Med* 2006;73:621–626, 628, 632–634.

Almahameed A, Bartholomew JR. Peripheral arterial disease: recognition and contemporary management. *Cleve Clin J Med* 2006;73[Suppl 4]:S1–S51.

Balk E, Raman G, Chung M, et al. Effectiveness of management strategies for renal artery stenosis: asystematic review. *Ann Intern Med* 2006;145:901–912.

Hiatt WR. Medical treatment of peripheral arterial disease and claudication. *N Engl J Med* 2001;344:1608–1621.

Mahmud E, Cavendish JJ, Salami A. Current treatment of peripheral arterial disease. *J Am Coll Cardiol* 2007;50:473–490.

Mukherjee D, Yadav JS. Update on peripheral vascular diseases: from smoking cessation to stenting. *Cleve Clin J Med* 2001;68:723–733.

Safian RD, Textor SC. Renal-artery stenosis. *N Engl J Med* 2001;344:431–442.

Helpful Websites

http://www.acc.org/clinical/**guidelines**/pad/index.pdf
www.tasc-2-pad.org/
http://www.padcoalition.org/wp
http://www.aboutpad.org
http://www.coralclinicaltrial.org
http://www.vdf.org

CAROTID ARTERY DISEASE 28

Adnan K. Chhatriwalla and Christopher T. Bajzer

I. EPIDEMIOLOGY AND ETIOLOGY OF STROKE

A. There are more than 700,000 strokes in the United States annually, and 15 million strokes wordwide annually, making it the **third leading cause of death** in Western societies.

B. The cause of ischemic stroke can be classified into two broad categories.

1. **Embolic:** may be arterial (e.g., aortic atheroma or large-vessel atherosclerosis in the carotid, vertebral, or basilar arteries) or cardiac in origin [e.g., left ventricular thrombus postmyocardial infarction (MI), atrial fibrillation, valvular disorders, and cardiac tumors].
2. **Thrombotic:** may be caused by stenosis of smaller intracerebral arteries, a hypercoagulable state, or a systemic inflammatory condition causing vasculitis.

II. NORMAL CAROTID ANATOMY

A. The aortic arch normally gives rise to the innominate artery (a.k.a., brachiocephalic artery), the left common carotid artery (CCA), and the left subclavian artery (Fig. 28.1). The innominate artery bifurcates into the right common carotid artery and the right subclavian artery. The **left common carotid arises from the aortic arch in 70% of people and from the innominate artery in 20% (bovine arch variant).**

B. The aortic arch can be classified into three types based on the distance of the origin of the great vessels from the top of the arch (Fig. 28.2). The widest diameter of the left common carotid is used as a reference unit. If all the great vessels originate **within an arc of the aortic arch subtended by a line parallel to a horizontal reference line at the top of the arch and separated from the top reference line by the reference unit**, it is classified as a **type 1 arch**. In a **type II arch**, all the great vessels originate within an arc **within two reference units** from the top of the arch, and in a **type III** arch the great vessels **originate within an arc beyond two reference units** from the

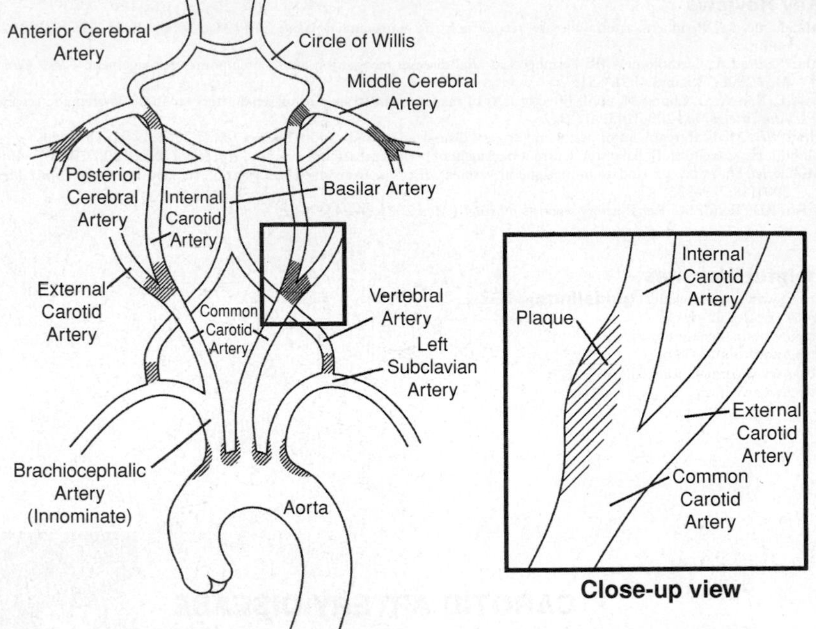

Figure 28.1. Normal anatomy of the aortic arch, great vessels, and circle of Willis. The *shaded areas* depict the areas most prone for the development of atherosclerosis.

top of the arch. Type III arches are harder to access during percutaneous intervention than type I arches.

C. The CCAs divide into the internal and external carotids at the C4-5 level in 50% of patients. In approximately 40% of patients, the bifurcation is higher, and it is lower in the remaining 10%.

D. The external carotid artery (ECA) provides flow to the facial muscles, scalp, and thyroid. It has a complex system of collaterals, and symptoms from stenosis are rare.

E. The circle of Willis provides collateral flow between the left and right hemispheres of the brain and connects the anterior and posterior circulation.

III. RISK FACTORS FOR CAROTID ATHEROSCLEROSIS

A. **Smoking and age** are the two most important risk factors for developing carotid atherosclerosis. The others, in order of importance, are **hypertension, diabetes, gender (men more than women if younger than 75 years; women more than men if older than 75 years), and hyperlipidemia**. As with coronary artery disease (CAD), inflammation likely plays a major role in carotid disease. African American men and Hispanic Americans appear to have a higher incidence of carotid atherosclerosis. Some data suggest a role for chronic infection in the development of carotid disease.

B. Between 30% and 60% of patients with peripheral arterial disease have carotid disease, and approximately 50% to 60% of patients with carotid disease have severe CAD. However, only 10% of patients with CAD have severe carotid disease.

C. Increased carotid intimal-media thickness (IMT) is strongly associated with the presence of CAD and the risk of MI.

IV. PATHOPHYSIOLOGY

A. As with coronary disease, atherosclerotic carotid disease usually develops at branch points and bends, especially at the bifurcation of the CCA and origin of the internal carotid artery (ICA) (Fig. 28.1).

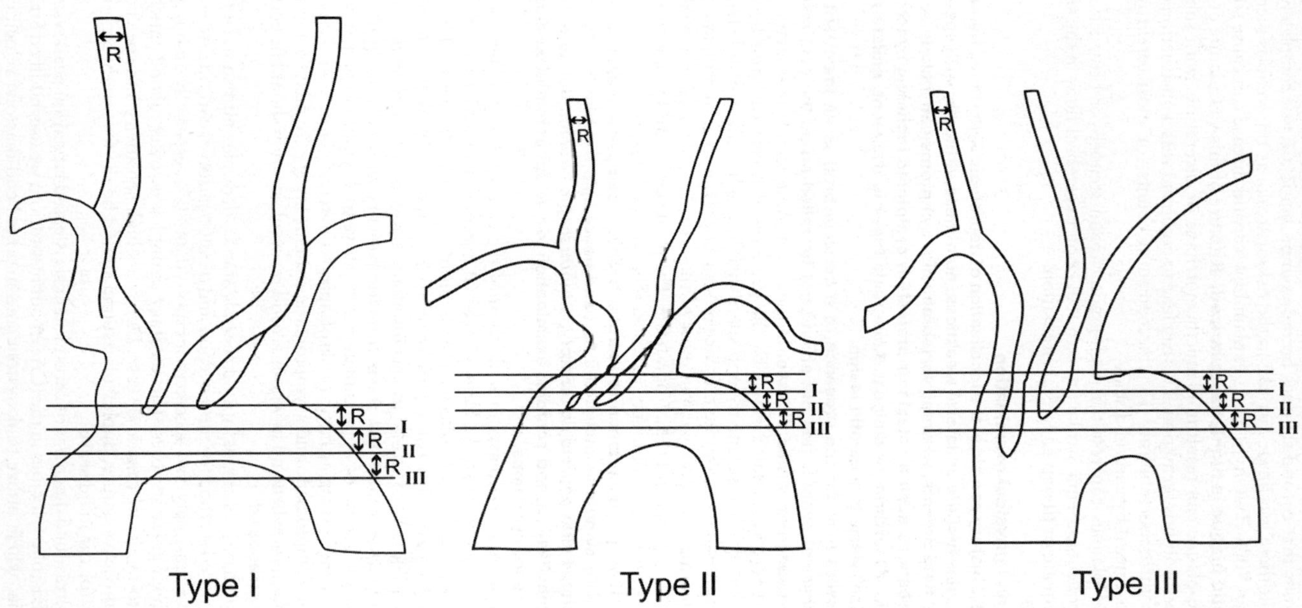

Figure 28.2. Aortic arch classification. The classification system is based on the distance of the origin of the great vessels from the top of the arch.

B. Plaque is most often localized at the carotid bifurcation and tends to extend from the outer wall of the carotid bulb into the ICA origin (Fig. 28.1).

C. The reasons that carotid stenoses become symptomatic are not completely understood, but there is a linear increase in the risk of stroke as the stenosis increases to more than 70%. Two hypotheses explain how carotid disease can cause stroke.

1. **Carotid plaque is highly vascularized.** Rupture of this vasculature or rupture of the plaque can result in plaque hemorrhage or ulceration, with subsequent *in situ* thrombus formation. This can lead to complete vessel obstruction or distal atherothromboembolism. This mechanism accounts for most cerebrovascular events caused by carotid disease.
2. Larger plaques can result in high-grade carotid stenosis or obstruction, with subsequent ischemic stroke due to a reduction in cerebral flow, in the setting of inadequate or absent collateral circulation.

V. DIAGNOSIS

A. History and physical examination

1. **Careful history can aid in the localization of neurologic symptoms. Hemispheric symptoms include unilateral weakness, numbness, difficulty with speech, and visual field defects, whereas vertebrobasilar symptoms can include cerebellar disturbances such as ataxia or brainstem symptoms including syncope, dysphagia, dysarthria, or diplopia. Amaurosis fugax is transient, unilateral vision loss ipsilateral to a carotid lesion.**
2. **An assessment for the presence of a cervical bruit is an important part of the physical examination but should not be relied on as the sole marker for the presence of carotid disease.** In the North American Symptomatic Carotid Endarterectomy Trial (NASCET), the presence of a cervical bruit had an approximately 60% sensitivity and specificity for high-grade carotid stenosis. In the Framingham study, the presence of a carotid bruit in asymptomatic patients doubled the risk of stroke, but most of these strokes occurred in vascular beds different from that of the carotid bruit. The presence of a bruit may be a general marker for patients at higher risk of cerebrovascular events.
3. **In addition to auscultation for carotid bruits, a complete evaluation in a patient with symptoms includes a focused neurologic examination to correlate symptoms with neurologic territory, a funduscopic examination to detect retinal embolization, and a cardiac examination to rule out potential cardioembolic sources for symptoms.**
4. All patients should have an evaluation of the carotid arteries after a stroke or transient ischemic attack (TIA). The risk of a second stroke is elevated for several years after the first stroke or TIA. Symptomatic patients with 70% or more stenosis have an 8% risk of stroke at 30 days and a 13% annual incidence of stroke. The risk of stroke in asymptomatic patients increases as the degree of carotid stenosis increases. Asymptomatic patients with 60% or more stenosis have a stroke risk of approximately 2% per year. Asymptomatic patients with 80% or more stenosis have a risk of approximately 5% per year. These stroke rates in symptomatic and asymptomatic patients lay the foundation for a logical paradigm for when and in whom carotid revascularization should be performed.

B. Duplex ultrasound

1. Although carotid angiography is the gold standard, duplex ultrasound is the most widely used method for the detection and quantification of carotid artery disease. It has a sensitivity and specificity of more than 80%, especially among patients with high-grade stenoses. The accuracy of duplex is lower among patients with mild-to-moderate carotid disease. Due to its high sensitivity and specificity and it noninvasive nature, duplex ultrasound should be the first study performed to assess for carotid disease.
2. The ultrasound diagnosis of carotid stenosis is based largely on peak systolic and end-diastolic velocities in the ICA. At our institution, we use modified Strandness criteria, which utilize peak systolic and maximal end-diastolic velocities in the ICA, along with the ratio of ICA/CCA peak systolic velocities to discern higher levels of stenosis (Table 28.1). Duplex ultrasound criteria for carotid stenosis vary by institution, and each vascular laboratory must assess the accuracy of its

TABLE 28.1 Duplex Criteria for Classification of Carotid Stenosis

% Diameter stenosis	PSV	EDV	Plaque?
0–19%	<105 cm/sec	—	No
20–39%	<105 cm/sec	—	Yes
40–59%	105–150 cm/sec	—	Yes
60–79%	151–240 cm/sec	—	Yes
80–99%	>240 cm/sec	>135 cms/sec	Yes
Occluded	No flow -"thump" prior to occlusion	No flow	Yes

PSV = peak-systolic velocity; EDV = end-diastolic velocity.
ICA/CCA <2.0, not significant stenosis; PSV ICA/CCA >4.0 suggests stenosis.

criteria for stenosis in a quality assurance program. Compared with angiography, duplex ultrasound is noninvasive, less expensive, and can be done at the bedside. Limitations include the inability to image intracranial disease, limited ability to assess collateral flow, occasional inaccuracy in distinguishing high-grade stenoses ("string sign") from complete obstructions, and the need for an experienced sonographer. Conditions that may elevate intravascular flow velocities, such as common carotid disease, contralateral carotid disease, or presence of a carotid stent, may result in an artificially high estimate of ICA stenosis. The ability of ultrasound to assess the posterior carotid circulation is limited.

C. Computed tomography angiography

1. Computed tomography angiography (CTA) offers high sensitivity and specificity for the identification of carotid artery disease (77% and 95%, respectively in a recent meta-analysis). CTA allows for visualization of the carotid artery lumen as well as adjacent bony and soft-tissue structures. Advantages include high sensitivity (particularly for carotid artery occlusion), reproducibility, and the ability to visualize the entire carotid artery including the extracranial and intracranial portions. Disadvantages include cost and the need for contrast injection, which may be unsuitable for patients with chronic kidney disease or volume overload.

D. Magnetic resonance angiography

1. Contrast-enhanced magnetic resonance angiography (CEMRA) is rapidly gaining acceptance as a sensitive (80% to 90%) and specific (60% to 90%) test for carotid disease. Advantages include high sensitivity, reproducibility, and the ability to visualize the entire carotid artery including the extracranial and intracranial portions. Disadvantages include the potential for misdiagnosis of severe stenoses as occlusions, overestimation of stenosis severity due to artifact, high cost, and inability to study critically ill patients, claustrophobic patients, or patients with metallic implants such as pacemakers.

2. The combination of CEMRA and Doppler ultrasound results in a lower number of misclassifications and higher sensitivity and specificity for the diagnosis of severe ICA stenosis. When there is concern regarding the accuracy of one study, it is justifiable to perform both.

E. Contrast angiography

1. Contrast angiography with digital subtraction angiography (DSA) is the gold standard for assessment of carotid atherosclerosis. It allows the simultaneous assessment of the aortic arch, subclavian arteries, vertebral arteries, and intracranial circulation. Angiography enables the accurate assessment of collateral circulation. This is important because the presence of collateral circulation in medically treated patients with high-grade stenosis reduces the risk of ipsilateral stroke.

2. The risk of neurologic events during carotid angiography has historically been cited as low as 0.5% for major events to as high as 4% for all events. In the hands of an experienced interventional cardiologist, the risk of stroke in one study was found to be approximately 0.5%. In our institution, one stroke was

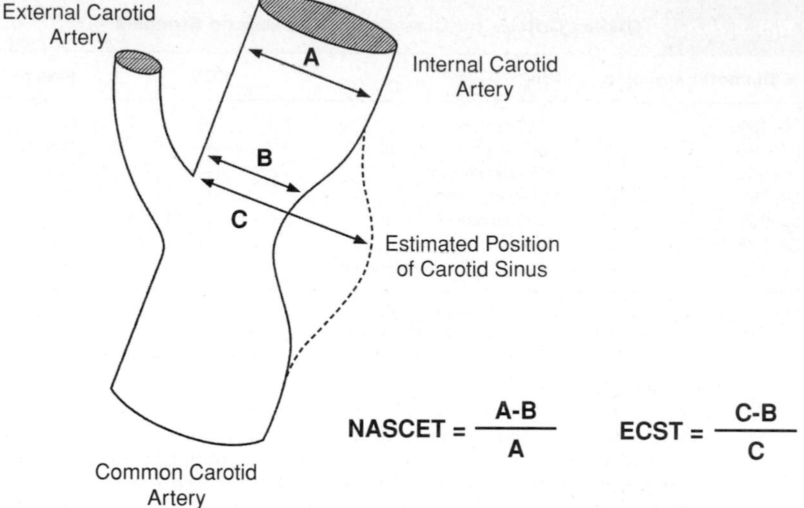

Figure 28.3. The North American Symptomatic Carotid Endarterectomy Trial (NASCET) and European Carotid Surgery Trialists' Collaborative Group (ECST) criteria for determining the degree of carotid stenosis.

observed in 580 consecutive diagnostic carotid catheterizations. Nonetheless, the risk–benefit ratio of performing carotid angiography must be carefully evaluated for each patient.

3. Two criteria are used to quantify carotid stenosis angiographically: the North American Symptomatic Carotid Endarterectomy Trial (NASCET) criteria and the European Carotid Surgery Trialists' Collaborative Group (ECST) criteria (Fig. 28.3). According to the NASCET criteria, the normal reference internal carotid diameter is the maximum diameter of the ICA distal to the lesion and distal to the carotid bulb. According to the ECST criteria, however, the normal reference diameter is defined by the estimated position of the external wall of the carotid bulb. The same lesion has a higher percentage of stenosis using the NASCET criteria compared with the ECST criteria. The NASCET criteria, however, are difficult to apply in subtotal occlusions with collapse of the distal ICA due to underfilling. The NASCET criteria inherently have less variability and are now recommended as the standard for reporting of angiographic carotid stenosis in Medicare physician quality initiatives.

4. Technique

a. Complete cerebral angiography involves angiography of the aortic arch and carotid arteries, intracerebral angiography, and angiography of the vertebral arteries and posterior circulation. A three-vessel study including angiography of both carotid arteries and the dominant vertebral artery is often sufficient.

b. A low-osmolar or iso-osmolar, nonionic, heparinized contrast agent should be used. In the absence of contraindications, the patient should be anticoagulated with 50 U/kg of intravenous heparin. The patient's head is often put in a holder or immobilizer to prevent inadvertent movement, and the patient is advised to look at the ceiling or keep his or her eyes closed. DSA should be used, if available, to improve resolution and minimize the amount of contrast needed. Before obtaining each cine angiogram, the patient should be instructed not to move, breathe, or swallow during image acquisition.

c. Aortic arch angiography is performed using an angled pigtail catheter. Using a 0.035-inch guidewire, the pigtail catheter is positioned in the midportion of the ascending aorta, and a cine angiogram of the aortic arch is obtained in a left anterior oblique projection (approximately 45 degrees).

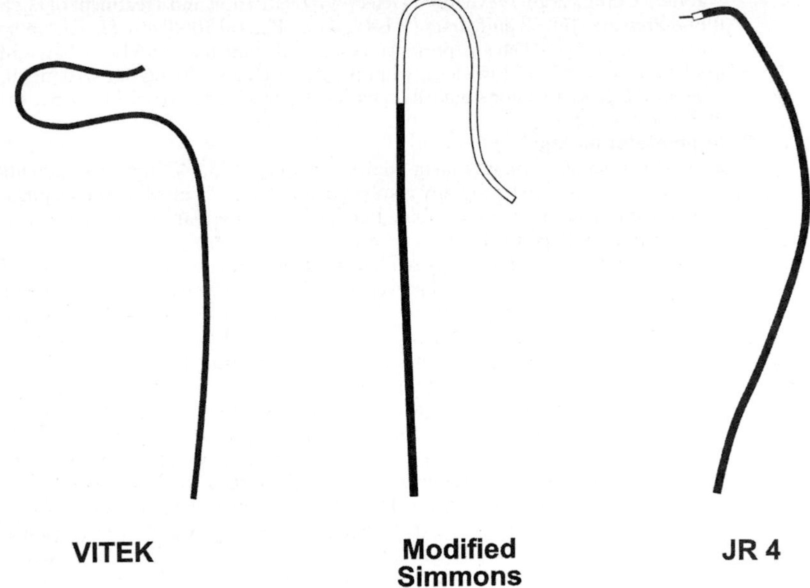

Figure 28.4. The three most common types of catheters used for carotid angiography.

d. Carotid angiography can be safely performed using a Judkins Right (JR4) or a Headhunter catheter. Alternatively, a Vitek catheter can be used with bovine anatomy or type II or III arch. The Simmons catheter is useful in cases of severe tortuosity but requires reshaping in the aortic arch, which can lead to higher complication rates (Fig. 28.4). In the left anterior oblique projection, the JR4 catheter is positioned in the superior portion of the ascending aorta and rotated counterclockwise until it is positioned in the innominate artery. Non-selective cine angiography of the innominate, right subclavian, right carotid, and right vertebral arteries can then be performed with the image train in the right anterior oblique projection. In the right anterior oblique projection, a 0.035-inch wire (e.g., Stiff-Angled Glide, Magic Torque, Wholey) is used to advance the JR4 catheter to selectively engage the right common carotid. Two basic views should be obtained for each carotid: an ipsilateral oblique view (30 to 45 degrees) and a cross-table lateral view. The table should be positioned so that the carotid bifurcation is in the middle of the screen, and shutters and filters should be used to optimize image quality.

e. For cerebral angiography, the patient's head is positioned in the center of the screen. Cine angiography is performed in the posteroanterior and lateral projections. It is important to continue the cine until the venous runoff has been captured to assess for intracranial arterial venous malformations (AVMs) and anomalous venous drainage. To selectively engage the left carotid, the catheter is positioned in the innominate artery so that the tip is pointing superiorly. The catheter is slowly pulled back, ensuring that the tip remains pointed superiorly, until the catheter tip exits the innominate and engages the left common carotid. The same views can then be obtained for the left carotid.

VI. MANAGEMENT OF CAROTID DISEASE

A. Medical management

1. Risk factor modification. Aggressive cardiovascular risk-factor modification is recommended to reduce the risk of stroke and prevent the progression of existing disease, regardless of whether revascularization is indicated. Smoking cessation, blood pressure control to levels recommended by Seventh Report of the Joint

National Committe on Prevention, Detection, Evaluation and Treatment of High Blood Pressure (JNC7) guidelines [<140/90 mm Hg, <130/80 mm Hg if chronic kidney disease or diabetes is present), control of diabetes (HbA1c <7%), and lipid management [goal low-density lipoprotein (LDL) <100 mg/dL, <70 mg/dL if high CAD risk] are important treatment goals for which to strive in any patient with carotid disease.

2. **Antiplatelet therapy**
   a. The Antiplatelet Trialist's meta-analysis including 73,247 high-risk patients found that antiplatelet therapy resulted in a 27% (25% attributed to aspirin) relative reduction in the combined endpoint of vascular death, myocardial infarction (MI), or stroke.
   b. **Aspirin** is the most extensively studied antiplatelet drug for the prevention of stroke and other cardiovascular events, and should be initiated in all patients with evidence of carotid atherosclerosis. Men whose 10-year risk for the development of stroke or MI is ≥10% or greater should be started on low-dose (75 to 160 mg/day) aspirin for primary prevention. Women ≥65 years of age or older should be started on aspirin therapy (75 to 325 mg/day) for the primary prevention of MI and stroke. Aspirin therapy is also recommended in women younger than 65 years for the prevention of stroke when the benefits of ischemic stroke prevention outweigh the adverse effects of aspirin therapy.
   c. The **Clopidogrel** versus Aspirin in Patients at Risk of Ischaemic Events (CAPRIE) trial demonstrated a decrease in the combined endpoint of vascular death, stroke, or MI with clopidogrel therapy compared with aspirin (5.32% vs. 5.83%) among patients with a history of stroke, MI, or symptomatic peripheral vascular disease. These data represented an 8.7% relative risk reduction ($p= 0.043$). Currently there is no consensus on the use of clopidogrel for the primary prevention of stroke. Clopidogrel may be an option for the primary prevention of stroke in patients with moderate carotid stenosis who cannot tolerate aspirin.
   d. The MATCH study, which evaluated dual antiplatelet therapy with aspirin and clopidogrel in stroke patients with concomitant cardiovascular disease, patients who suffered a stroke while on a single antiplatelet agent, and those with severe aortic arch disease, demonstrated an insignificant trend toward improved efficacy with dual antiplatelet therapy; however, there was a highly significant increase in life-threatening bleeding events.
   e. Low-dose aspirin (25 mg twice daily) plus dipyridamole (200 mg twice daily) has been found to be more beneficial than aspirin alone or dipyridamole alone for the secondary prevention of stroke in the European Stroke Prevention Study 2 (ESPS 2) study. Similarly, in the European/Australian Stroke Prevention in Reversible Ischemia Trial (ESPRIT), extended-release dipyridamole administered with aspirin was superior to aspirin alone in the prevention of MI, stroke, or vascular death.
   f. The Ticlopidine Aspirin Stroke Study (TASS) found a significant reduction (19% vs. 17%, $p = 0.048$) in the incidence or nonfatal stroke or death in stroke patients treated with ticlopidine versus aspirin. Ticlopidine is now seldom used due to the availability of clopidogrel, which has a superior safety profile.
   g. According to the AHA/ASA Guidelines for the Prevention of Stroke in Patients with Ischemic Stroke or TIA, the accepted treatment strategies for the secondary prevention of noncardioembolic stroke include the following:
      (1) Aspirin (50 to 325 mg daily)
      (2) Aspirin (25 mg) and extended-release dipyridamole (200 mg twice daily)
      (3) Clopidogrel (75 mg daily), especially for patients with aspirin allergy or resistance
3. **Antihyperlipidemic agents**
   a. Epidemiologic data have shown higher stroke rates among patients with high LDL and low high-density lipoprotein (HDL) cholesterol levels. Several studies have consistently shown carotid plaque regression in patients treated

with statins, and clinical trials have shown a reduction in stroke among patients treated with statins. In the Scandinavian Simvastatin Survival Study (4S), nonembolic strokes were significantly reduced in statin arm. The Stroke Prevention by Aggressive Reduction in Cholesterol (SPARCL) study demonstrated a 16% relative risk reduction in stroke with statin therapy in 4731 patients with prior stroke or TIA randomized to atorvastatin versus placebo. In a meta-analysis of 20,438 patients in 13 trials, a 31% relative risk reduction in stroke was observed among patients treated with statins.

b. The beneficial effects of statins in reducing strokes are highest among patients at the highest risk for stroke. For primary prevention, all high-risk patients (e.g., diabetes, peripheral vascular disease, CAD) should be treated with statins. For secondary prevention, all patients with a history of MI, TIA, and stroke should be on statin therapy. Statin therapy should be considered for all asymptomatic patients with documented carotid stenosis of more than 50% or an estimated risk of stroke of 2% or higher per year.

c. The benefits of lipid lowering with nonstatin agents is less robust; however, some data have demonstrated a reduction in stroke with nicotinic acid (niacin) and fibrate therapy.

4. Antihypertensive agents

a. Hypertension is the single most modifiable risk factor in the prevention of stroke, and epidemiologic data suggest that approximately 60% of all strokes are attributable to hypertension. It is unclear which antihypertensive agents have the greatest impact on stroke rates. In the Losantan Intervention for Endpoint Reduction (LIFE) study, the angiotensin receptor blocker losartan was associated with a 15% reduction in stroke, whereas in the Antihypertension and Lipid-lowering Treatment to Prevent Heart Attack Trial (ALL-HAT) study, ACE-inhibitor therapy was associated with a 15% greater stroke risk than thiazide diuretic or dihydropyridine calcium channel blocker therapy. However, in the PROGRESS study, the ACE-inhibitor perindopril was associated with a 43% reduction in stroke.

b. The JNC-7 guidelines recommend that all patients with prehypertension (systolic blood pressure 120 to 139 mm Hg or diastolic blood pressure 80 to 89 mm Hg) undergo lifestyle modifications to lower blood pressure. Furthermore, all patients with blood pressure greater than 140/90 mm Hg (or >130/80 with diabetes or chronic kidney disease) should receive antihypertensive drug therapy to achieve their blood pressure goal. ACE inhibitors and diuretic agents remain first-line therapy in patients with cerebrovascular disaese.

5. Anticoagulation

a. There are no data specifically addressing the use of warfarin for primary stroke prevention in patients with documented carotid stenosis. However, one study has suggested that **low-dose warfarin may attenuate carotid plaque progression** in men. The use of warfarin for the secondary prevention of noncardioembolic strokes (including patients with carotid stenosis) is controversial. There was no clear benefit for low- and medium-dose oral warfarin therapy (INR, 2.0–3.0) for the secondary prevention of noncardioembolic stroke in the Warfarin-Aspirin Symptomatic Intracranial Disease (WASID) trial, and a significant increase in adverse effects, including death, major hemorrhage, and MI with warfarin use. High-dose warfarin (INR, 3.0 to 4.5) for the secondary prevention of noncardioembolic stroke results in a high rate of bleeding complications, including hemorrhagic stroke, and should not be used.

B. Surgical management: carotid endarterectomy

Carotid endarterectomy (CEA) is the standard of care for the reduction of stroke or TIA in patients with high-grade symptomatic or asymptomatic carotid stenosis. Several trials have firmly established the utility of CEA in preventing stroke in the presence of severe carotid stenosis as compared with medical therapy. It is important to keep in mind that high-risk patients were not enrolled in these trials. Because the risk of surgery among such patients probably would be higher than reported in these trials, extrapolation of these data to high-risk patients must be done with caution.

1. Major trials

a. Asymptomatic, low-risk patients

(1) Asymptomatic Carotid Atherosclerosis Study (ACAS)

(a) A total of 1659 patients with asymptomatic carotid stenosis of 60% or more were randomized to CEA or medical therapy. All patients were treated with aspirin (325 mg daily).

(b) At a median of 2.7 years of follow-up, the incidence of stroke or death was 5.1% in the surgical arm and 11% in the medically treated arm ($p = 0.004$). The annual risk of stroke among patients in the medical arm was 2.2%. The perioperative stroke or death rate was 2.3%.

(2) Veterans Affairs Asymptomatic Carotid Stenosis Study

(a) In this study, 444 patients with 50% or more carotid stenosis were randomized to CEA or to medical therapy with aspirin. There was a nonsignificant trend toward better outcomes (stroke or death) with surgery compared with medical therapy (4.7% vs. 9.7%).

b. Symptomatic, low-risk patients

(1) North American Symptomatic Carotid Endarterectomy Trial (NASCET)

(a) In this trial, 659 patients with severe carotid stenosis (70% to 99%), ipsilateral hemispheric or retinal TIA, amaurosis fugax, or nondisabling stroke within 120 days were randomized to CEA or medical therapy.

(b) The 30-day risk of stroke or death was 3.3% in the medical group and 5.8% in the surgical group. Two-year risk of any stroke was 26% in the medical group and 9% in the surgical group ($p < 0.001$), and the risk of major stroke or death was 18.1% in the medical group and 8% in the surgical group ($p < 0.001$). Patients with the most severe stenoses had the most benefit.

(c) In a separate arm of the study, 2267 patients with 30% to 69% stenosis, ipsilateral hemispheric or retinal TIA, or nondisabling stroke within 120 days were randomized to CEA or medical therapy. Patients with 50% to 69% stenosis had a 5-year stroke rate of 22.2% in the medical group and 15.7% in the surgical group ($p = 0.045$). Patients with 30% to 49% stenosis had a 5-year stroke rate of 18.7% in the medical group and 14.9% in the surgical group ($p = 0.16$).

(2) Veterans Affairs Cooperative Study

(a) In the Veterans Affairs Cooperative Study, 189 men with greater than 50% internal carotid stenosis with ipsilateral symptoms were randomized within 120 days of a neurologic event to CEA or medical therapy.

(b) At a mean of 11.9 months' follow-up, the incidence of stroke or TIA was 19.4% in medical arm and 7.7% in the surgical arm ($p = 0.011$). The 30-day stroke or death rate was 6.6% in the surgical group and 2.2% in the medical group.

(3) European Carotid Surgery Trialists' (ECST) Collaborative Group

(a) A total of 2518 patients with symptomatic carotid stenosis were randomized to CEA or medical therapy. Patients ($n = 374$) with mild stenosis (0–29%) had low rates of ipsilateral stroke overall, and 3-year benefits of surgery were small and outweighed by operative risk. The ipsilateral stroke rate at 3 years of follow-up for patients with stenoses between 705 and 99% ($n = 778$) was 16.8% in the medical arm and 10.3% in the surgical arm.

2. Complications and management of patients after CEA

a. Major complications of CEA include MI, stroke, and death. Other complications include bleeding and wound hematoma, cranial nerve injury, wound infection, bradycardia, hyper- or hypotension, and, rarely, seizures and intracerebral hemorrhage.

b. After CEA and in the absence of contraindications, all patients should be treated with antiplatelet therapy.

3. American Heart Association (AHA) recommendations for Carotid Endarterectomy

a. CEA is recommended in symptomatic patients with ipsilateral carotid stenosis of greater than 70% by a surgeon with a perioperative morbidity and mortality of less than 6%. CEA is recommended in symptomatic patients with ipsilateral carotid stenosis 50% to 69% depending on age, gender, comorbidities, and severity of initial symptoms. CEA is inappropriate in patients with stroke or TIA and ipsilateral carotid stenosis of less than 50%.

b. Among asymptomatic patients, the presence of carotid stenosis of more than 60% is a proven indication for CEA if the surgical risk is less than 3% and the patient's life expectancy is more than 5 years. If the surgical risk is between 3% and 5%, it is acceptable to recommend CEA in patients with *bilateral* carotid stenosis greater than 75%. If the surgical risk exceeds 5%, asymptomatic patients should not be referred for CEA.

4. Combined CEA and coronary artery bypass grafting (CABG)

a. Patients with severe coronary disease may have severe carotid disease, and surgery in this population is a high-risk procedure. The optimal treatment strategy remains unclear.

b. Options include simultaneous CEA and CABG, staged CEA followed by CABG, or staged CABG followed by CEA. In staged procedures, CEA first increases risk of perioperative MI, and CABG first increases risk of perioperative stroke.

c. Some investigators have reported better results with simultaneous procedures, but patient selection is likely an important factor in achieving satisfactory outcomes. Recent studies have suggested adverse outcomes with this approach. A meta-analysis of 16 studies with a total of 844 combined-procedure and 920 staged-procedure patients reported a higher risk of death, stroke, or MI among patients undergoing combined compared with staged procedures. Percutaneous intervention may be a better choice for this patient population, and this is an area that requires further investigation.

C. Percutaneous carotid intervention

1. Since carotid angioplasty was first described in 1980, a number of registry studies and trials have been published reporting high rates of procedural success. However, percutaneous carotid angioplasty is rarely performed as a standalone procedure because of unacceptably high rates of recoil, restenosis, and adverse procedural outcomes due to distal embolization. Carotid stenting has become the standard of care for patients undergoing percutaneous carotid intervention.

2. Compared with angioplasty alone, carotid stenting improves procedural success rates, decreases periprocedural complications (including carotid artery dissection), and decreases restenosis. Embolic protection devices reduce the incidence of distal embolization and should be used in all cases.

3. Several manufacturers have stents approved for use in the carotid artery. Balloon-expandable stents are generally not used for carotid stenting because of the potential for structural deformation that can occur as a result of external forces such as those caused by neck movement. Self-expanding stents, such as the Wallstent (Boston Scientific Corp, Quincy, MA), Acculink carotid stent (Abbott Vascular Devices, Redwood City, CA, formerly Guidant Corp), Xact carotid stent (Abbott Vascular Devices, Redwood City, CA) and the carotid SMART stent (Cordis Endovascular, Warren, NJ) are preferred, as they continue to exert outward radial force after deployment and resist crushing.

4. Trials

a. The CAVATAS study compared carotid angioplasty (without stenting) with CEA among patients with more than 50% carotid stenosis and found similar rates of procedural bleeding, major stroke, or death between the two treatment strategies at 30 days and 1 year. However, the CEA cohort did have a

TABLE 28.2 Registry Studies of Carotid Artery Stenting

Study	Number of patients	Technical success (%)	30-day minor stroke (%)	30-day major stroke (%)	30-day death (%)	Late strokes (%)	Restenosis rate (%)
Diethrich et al.[a]	110	99	4.2	1.7	0.9	0	1.7
Yadav et al.[b]	107	100	7	2	1	0	4.9
Shawl et al.[c]	170	99	2	0.5	0	0	2
Gupta et al.[d]	100	100	5	1	0	0	1
Roubin et al.[e]	528	98	4.8	1	1.6	3.2	—
Wholey et al.[f]	4749	98.4	2.48	1.36	0.79	1.39	2.27
White et al.[g]	747	98	2.5	1.0	1.5	—	—
Safian et al.[h]	419	97.4	1.0	3.5	1.9	—	—
Gray et al.[i]	3500	—	2.9	2.0	1.8	—	—

[a]Diethrich EB, Ndiaye M, Reid DB. Stenting in the carotid artery: initial experience in 110 patients. *J Endovasc Surg* 1996;3:42–62.
[b]Yadav JS, Roubin GS, Iyer S, et al. Elective stenting of the extracranial carotid arteries. *Circulation* 1997;95:376–381.
[c]Shawl F, Kadro W, Domanski MJ, et al. Safety and efficacy of elective carotid artery stenting in high-risk patients. *J Am Coll Cardiol* 2000;35:1721–1728.
[d]Gupta A, Bhatia A, Ahuja A, et al. Carotid stenting in patients older than 65 years with inoperable carotid artery disease: a single-center experience. *Catheter Cardiovasc Interv* 2000;50:1–8, discussion 9.
[e]Roubin GS, New G, Iyer SS, et al. Immediate and late clinical outcomes of carotid artery stenting in patients with symptomatic and asymptomatic carotid artery stenosis: a 5-year prospective analysis. *Circulation* 2001;103:532–537.
[f]Wholey MH, Wholey M, Mathias K, et al. Global experience in cervical carotid artery stent placement. *Catheter Cardiovasc Interv* 2000;50:160–167.
[g]White CJ, Iyer SS, Hopkins LN, et al. Carotid stenting with distal protection in high surgical risk patients: The BEACH trial 30 day results. *Catheter Cardiovasc Interv* 2006;67:503–512.
[h]Safian RD, Bresnahan JF, Jaff MR, et al. Protected carotid stenting in high-risk patients with severe carotid artery stenosis. *J Am Coll Cardiol* 2006;47:2384–2389.
[i]Gray WA, Yadav JS, Verta P, et al. The CAPTURE registry: Results of carotid stenting with embolic protection in the post approval setting. *Catheter Cardiovasc Interv* 2007;69:341–348.

higher number of patients whose surgery was complicated by cranial nerve injury.

b. Several registry studies have been published on the outcomes of carotid stenting (Table 28.2). Most patients enrolled in these studies were high-risk patients, and most would not have been eligible for CEA trials such as NASCET because of comorbidities. Their surgical complication rates would likely have been higher than those reported in the large CEA trials. Despite the high-risk nature of these patients, the results of these studies show very high procedural success rates with stenting, excellent angiographic results, low periprocedural complication rates, low rates of restenosis, and low rates of long-term adverse events.

c. The SAPPHIRE trial was the first multicenter, randomized, controlled trial comparing carotid stenting to CEA in high-risk patients. Using the PRECISE nitinol stent (Cordis, Warren, NJ) and the AngioGuard (Cordis, Warren, NJ) distal protection device, 307 patients were randomized, 156 to carotid stenting and 151 to CEA. An additional 409 patients were enrolled in a stent registry. The combined endpoint of death, stroke, or MI at 1 year was reached in 12.2% of patients in the stenting arm and in 20.1% of patients in the CEA arm ($p = 0.004$ for noninferiority and $p = 0.053$ for superiority). This is the first randomized trial to show noninferiority of carotid stenting compared to CEA.

d. The CARESS trial was a phase I multicenter, prospective randomized trial comparing carotid stenting to CEA in a broad-risk group of symptomatic (with >50% stenosis) and asymptomatic patients (with >75% stenosis). The combined primary endpoint of stroke and death was 3.6% for CEA and 2.1% for carotid stenting at 30 days, and 13.6% for CEA and 10.0% for carotid stenting at 1 year. The authors concluded that carotid stenting was equivalent to CEA in both symptomatic and asymptomatic patients at 1 year.

e. The SPACE trial was a multinational, multicenter randomized trial evaluating carotid stenting with optional distal embolic protection versus CEA in 1200 patients with symptomatic carotid artery stenosis. Unlike the SAPPHIRE trial, the SPACE trial was not limited to high-risk surgical patients. The SPACE trial was unable to demonstrate noninferiority of carotid stenting compared to CEA, as the rate of death or ipsilateral ischemic stroke at 30 days from procedure was 6.84% with carotid stenting versus 6.34% with CEA ($p = 0.09$). A criticism of the SPACE trial was that embolic protection devices were not required, and were only utilized in 27% of cases. However, no significant difference in the primary endpoint was observed with or without the use of embolic protection devices.

f. The EVA-3S trial was a multicenter, randomized, noninferiority trial comparing carotid stenting to CEA in symptomatic patients with 605 to 99% carotid stenosis. The EVA-3S trial enrolled moderate-risk surgical patients. EVA-3S was stopped prematurely after enrollment of 527 patients, due to higher rates of stroke and death at 1 month (9.6% vs. 3.9%, $p = 0.01$) and 6 months (11.7% vs. 6.1%, $p = 0.02$) with carotid stenting versus CEA. A criticism of the EVA-3S trial was the lack of experience of the operators taking part in the study, as the interventionalists were required to have completed only two procedures with any device prior to its use in the trial. Furthermore, the use of embolic protection devices was optional at the onset of the trial, and a significant difference in the 30-day outcome of stroke and death was present between patients treated with and without embolic protection devices (7.9% vs. 25% respectively).

D. Complications and management

1. The major periprocedural complications during carotid stenting are stroke, MI, and death. Other complications include TIAs, access site bleeding, bradycardia, hypotension, seizures, and intracranial hemorrhage. **Advanced age and long or multiple stenoses have been found to be independent predictors of periprocedural stroke**. In one study, stenting in the presence of a contralateral occlusion, stenting after a previous CEA, or combined carotid and coronary interventions **did not** increase the risk of adverse outcomes.

2. Periprocedural cerebrovascular events occur largely because of embolization of plaque debris and thrombus into the cerebral circulation during manipulation of the carotid plaque. Such emboli have been documented by the use of transcranial Doppler, and the amount of embolization has been correlated with the size of infarct during CEA. Emboli protection devices decrease the volume of distal embolization.

3. Several emboli protection devices are being studied (Figs. 28.5 and 28.6), and they fall into three general categories: distal occlusion balloon protection, distal filter, and proximal occlusion balloon. The PercuSurge GuardWire (Medtronic, Minneapolis, MN) system provides occlusion of distal flow during carotid stenting, enabling the removal of embolized debris (Fig. 28.5). The AngioGuard (Cordis, Warren NJ) is one example of a filtration umbrella mounted on a 0.014-inch guidewire, which is positioned distal to the plaque during stenting (Fig. 28.6). At the end of the procedure, the filter is removed using a retrieval catheter. Proximal occlusion balloon systems create reversal of flow in the ICA, preventing embolization of debris into the cerebral vasculature.

4. Bradycardia and hypotension occur often during carotid stenting because of instrumentation and stretching of the carotid sinus baroreceptors. These hemodynamic effects are usually transient but can persist for up to 24 hours after

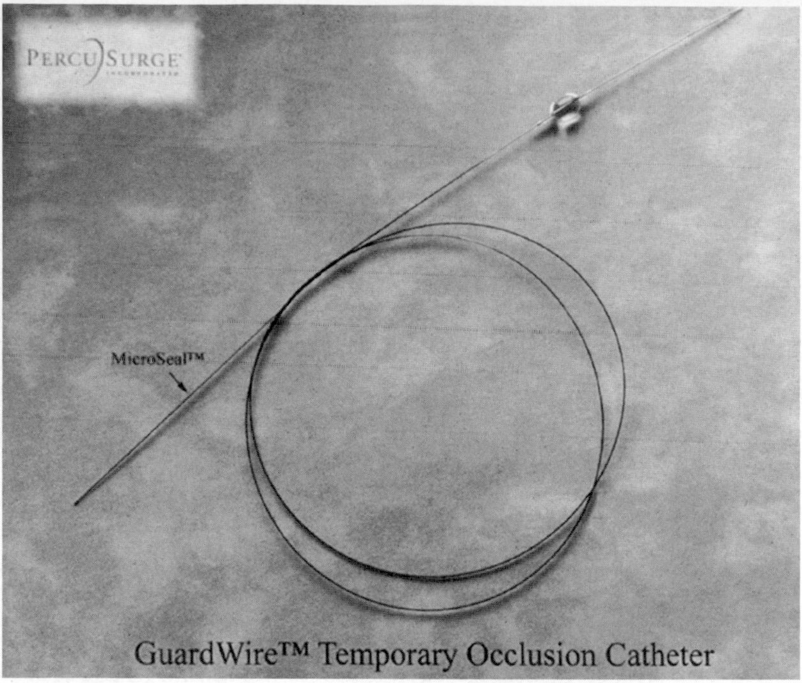

Figure 28.5. The PercuSurge GuardWire (Medtronic, Minneapolis, MN) system.

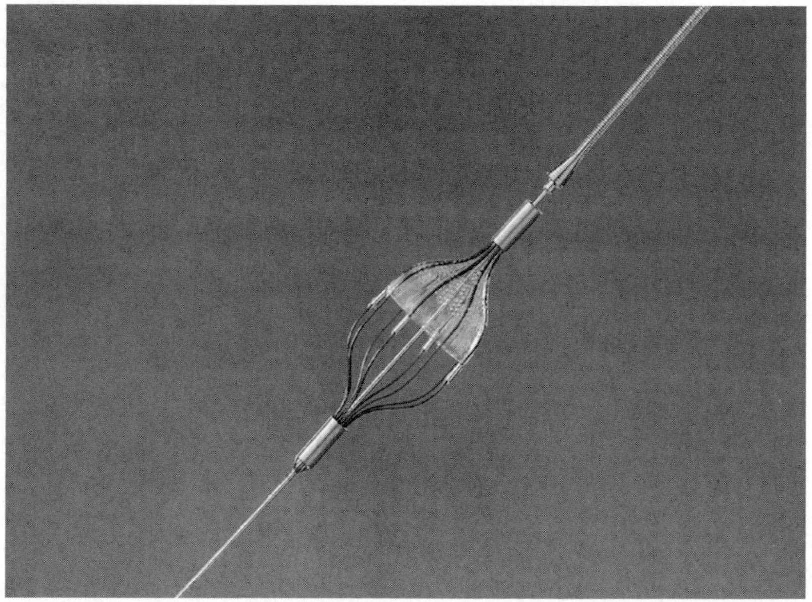

Figure 28.6. The AngioGuard (Cordis, Warren, NJ) emboli protection device.

intervention. **Symptomatic patients** should be managed with **IV crystalloid infusion and potentially a low-dose infusion of an inotropic agent (e.g., dopamine) or temporary pacing as required**. Unless the patient is hypertensive, antihypertensive and negative-inotropic medications are usually withheld immediately preprocedure and postprocedure, as patients generally have a normal to low blood pressure and pulse. Telemetry monitoring should be continued for 24 hours, and the nursing staff should perform frequent neurologic checks post-procedure. All patients should undergo a thorough and well-documented neurologic examination before and after the procedure. Standardized stroke scales are often utilized (e.g., NIHSS, Barthel, modified Rankin).

5. **Hyperperfusion syndrome**, manifested by stroke-like symptoms and signs, can occur because of the rapid return of flow to a chronically underperfused cerebral vascular bed with resultant disordered autoregulation. Risk factors include **severe hypertension, critical carotid stenosis, and contralateral carotid occlusion**. Cerebral hemorrhage is a dreaded complication of the hyperperfusion syndrome.
6. Patients undergoing carotid stenting should be pretreated with aspirin (325 mg daily) and clopidogrel (75 mg daily) for 3 days before the procedure if possible. After the procedure, **lifelong aspirin therapy should be instituted**, and **clopidogrel (75 mg daily) should be continued for at least 4 to 6 weeks**. For patients with recurrent symptoms, clopidogrel should be continued indefinitely. The incidence of restenosis after carotid stenting is lower than after coronary stenting and ranges between 1% and 6% per year.
7. The routine use of adjunctive glycoprotein (GP) IIb/IIIa inhibitors has not been well studied in the setting of carotid stenting. Initial observational data suggest that their use may be safe. However, because of the potential for intracranial hemorrhage, especially among patients with hypertension or hyperperfusion syndrome after carotid stenting, and without clear evidence of benefit, GP IIb/IIIa inhibitors are not routinely used. Further studies are needed to better define the use of these agents in this arena; however, incremental benefit above and beyond the use of mechanical embolic protection devices may be difficult to demonstrate.
8. Patients with carotid stenosis frequently have concomitant CAD. Successful combined carotid stenting and percutaneous coronary intervention has been reported as a simultaneous procedure, and the two are frequently performed as staged procedures with satisfactory outcomes.

VII. FUTURE DIRECTIONS

A. Despite a growing body of literature supporting percutaneous carotid intervention, the clinical equivalence of carotid stent outcomes compared to CEA remains a subject of debate. Furthermore, clinical trials to date have been relatively small, and have not allowed complete evaluation of carotid stenting in prespecified subgroups. The SAPPHIRE trial showed a lower 30-day adverse event rate, with carotid stenting utilizing embolic protection compared with CEA in high-risk patients while the CARESS trial demonstrated equivalence of carotid stenting to CEA in a broad-risk group. In contrast, the SPACE trial and the EVA-3S trial failed to demonstrate the noninferiority of carotid stenting, largely without embolic protection, in moderate-risk surgical patients.

B. The Carotid Revascularization Endarterectomy versus Stent Trial (CREST) and the International Carotid Stent Study (CAVATAS-2) are multicenter trials randomizing low-risk patients to carotid stenting with distal emboli protection or to CEA. The results of these trials may potentially expand the indications for carotid stenting. Until the results of these and other trials are reported, caution is advocated for the use of carotid stenting for the treatment of severe carotid stenosis in low- and medium-risk patients.

Key Reviews

Bates ER, Babb JD, Casey DE, et al. ACCF/SCAI/SVMB/ASITN 2007 Clinical Expert Consensus Document on Carotid Stenting. *J am Coll Cardiol* 2007;49:126–170.

Biller J, Feinberg WM, Castaldo JE, et al. Guidelines for Carotid Endarterectomy: A Statement for Healthcare Professionals from a Special Writing Group of the Stroke Council, American Heart Association. *Stroke* 1998;29:554–562.

Blauw GJ, Lagaay AM, Smelt AH, et al. Stroke, statins, and cholesterol. A meta-analysis of randomized, placebo-controlled, double-blind trials with HMG-CoA reductase inhibitors. *Stroke* 1997;28:946–950.

Cho L, Yadav JS. Embolization in atherosclerosis. *Neuroimaging Clin N Am* 2002;12:365–372.

Daniel, GK. Update of carotid stent trials. *Catheter Cardiovasc Interv* 2006;68:803–811.

Fayed AM, White CJ, Ramee SR, et al. Carotid and cerebral angiography performed by cardiologists: cerebrovascular complications. *Catheter Cardiovasc Interv* 2002;55:277–280.

Mathur A, Roubin GS, Iyer SS, et al. Predictors of stroke complicating carotid artery stenting. *Circulation* 1998;97:1239–1245.

Mohr JP, Albers GW, Amarenco P, et al. American Heart Association Prevention Conference. IV. Prevention and Rehabilitation of Stroke. Etiology of stroke. *Stroke* 1997;28:1501–1506.

Moore WS, Barnett HJ, Beebe HG, et al. Guidelines for carotid endarterectomy. A multidisciplinary consensus statement from the Ad Hoc Committee, American Heart Association. *Circulation* 1995;91:566–579.

Rothwell PM, Eliasziw M, Gutnikov SA, et al. Analysis of pooled data from the randomised controlled trials of endarterectomy for symptomatic carotid stenosis. *Lancet* 2003;361:107–116.

Sacco RL, Adams R, Albers G, et al. Guidelines for Prevention of Stroke in Patients with Ischemic Stroke of Transient Ischemic Attack: A Statement for Healthcare Professionals From the American Heart Association Council on Stroke: Co-Sponsored by the Council on Cardiovascular Radiology and Intervention: The American Academy of Neurology affirms the value of this guideline. *Stroke* 2006;37:577–617.

Wolf PA, Kannel WB, Sorlie P, et al. Asymptomatic carotid bruit and risk of stroke. The Framingham study. *JAMA* 1981;245:1442–1445.

Landmark Articles

A randomised, blinded, trial of clopidogrel versus aspirin in patients at risk of ischaemic events (CAPRIE). CAPRIE Steering Committee. *Lancet* 1996;348:1329–1339.

Barnett HJ, Taylor DW, Eliasziw M, et al. Benefit of carotid endarterectomy in patients with symptomatic moderate or severe stenosis. North American Symptomatic Carotid Endarterectomy Trial Collaborators. *N Engl J Med* 1998;339:1415–1425.

Beneficial effect of carotid endarterectomy in symptomatic patients with high-grade carotid stenosis. North American Symptomatic Carotid Endarterectomy Trial Collaborators. *N Engl J Med* 1991;325:445–453.

Char D, Cuadra S, Ricotta J, et al. Combined coronary artery bypass and carotid endarterectomy: long-term results. *Cardiovasc Surg* 2002;10:111–115.

Chimowitz MI, Lynn MJ, Howlett-Smith H, et al. Comparison of warfarin and aspirin for symptomatic intracranial arterial stenosis. *N Engl J Med* 2005;352:1305–1316.

Collaborative overview of randomised trials of antiplatelet therapy. I. Prevention of death, myocardial infarction, and stroke by prolonged antiplatelet therapy in various categories of patients. Antiplatelet Trialists' Collaboration. *BMJ* 1994;308:81–106.

Corti R, Fuster V, Fayad ZA, et al. Lipid lowering by simvastatin induces regression of human atherosclerotic lesions: two years' follow-up by high-resolution noninvasive magnetic resonance imaging. *Circulation* 2002;106:2884–2887.

Diener HC, Cunha L, Forbes C, et al. European Stroke Prevention Study 2. Dipyridamole and acetylsalicylic acid in the secondary prevention of stroke. *J Neurol Sci* 1996;143:1–13.

Diethrich EB, Ndiaye M, Reid DB. Stenting in the carotid artery: initial experience in 110 patients. *J Endovasc Surg* 1996;3:42–62.

Endovascular versus surgical treatment in patients with carotid stenosis in the Carotid and Vertebral Artery Transluminal Angioplasty Study (CAVATAS): a randomised trial. *Lancet* 2001;357:1729–1737.

Executive Committee for the Asymptomatic Carotid Atherosclerosis Study. Endarterectomy for asymptomatic carotid artery stenosis. *JAMA* 1995;273:1421–1428.

Hass WK, Easton JD, Adams HP Jr, et al. A randomized trial comparing ticlopidine hydrochloride with aspirin for the prevention of stroke in high-risk patients. Ticlopidine Aspirin Stroke Study Group. *N Engl J Med* 1989;321:501–507.

Henderson RD, Eliasziw M, Fox AJ, et al. Angiographically defined collateral circulation and risk of stroke in patients with severe carotid artery stenosis. North American Symptomatic Carotid Endarterectomy Trial (NASCET) Group. *Stroke* 2000;31:128–132.

Hobson RW 2nd, Weiss DG, Fields WS, et al. Efficacy of carotid endarterectomy for asymptomatic carotid stenosis. The Veterans Affairs Cooperative Study Group. *N Engl J Med* 1993;328:221–227.

Kapadia SR, Bajzer CT, Ziada KM, et al. Initial experience of platelet glycoprotein IIb/IIIa inhibition with abciximab during carotid stenting: a safe and effective adjunctive therapy. *Stroke* 2001;32:2328–2332.

Mas JL, Chatellier G, Beyssen B, et al. Endarterectomy versus stenting in patients with symptomatic severe carotid stenosis. *N Engl J Med* 2006;355:1660–1671.

Mayberg MR, Wilson SE, Yatsu F, et al. Carotid endarterectomy and prevention of cerebral ischemia in symptomatic carotid stenosis. Veterans Affairs Cooperative Studies Program 309 Trialist Group. *JAMA* 1991;266:3289–3294.

Mohr JP, Thompson JL, Lazar RM, et al. A comparison of warfarin and aspirin for the prevention of recurrent ischemic stroke. *N Engl J Med* 2001;345:1444–1451.

Nederkoorn PJ, Mali WP, Eikelboom BC, et al. Preoperative diagnosis of carotid artery stenosis: accuracy of noninvasive testing. *Stroke* 2002;33:2003–2008.

O'Holleran LW, Kennelly MM, McClurken M, et al. Natural history of asymptomatic carotid plaque. Five year follow-up study. *Am J Surg* 1987;154:659–662.

Randomised trial of cholesterol lowering in 4444 patients with coronary heart disease: the Scandinavian Simvastatin Survival Study (4S). *Lancet* 1994;344:1383–1389.

The SPACE Collaborative Group. 30 day results from the SPACE trial of stent-protected angioplasty versus carotid endarterectomy in symptomatic patients: a randomized non-inferiority trial. *Lancet* 2006;368:1239–1247.

Yadav JS, Wholey MH, Kuntz RE, et al. Protected carotid-artery stenting versus carotid endarterectomy in high-risk patients. *N Engl J Med* 2004;351:1493–1501.

ADULT CONGENITAL HEART DISEASE

VI

ATRIAL SEPTAL DEFECT AND PATENT FORAMEN OVALE

29

Kellan E. Ashley

I. INTRODUCTION

A. Atrial septal defects (ASDs) constitute approximately 5% to 10% of congenital heart disease. Excluding bicuspid aortic valve and mitral valve prolapse, ASD is the most common form of congenital heart defect found among adults and is the most common acyanotic shunt lesion in adults as well.

B. Often, an atrial communication may go unrecognized into adulthood because the clinical symptoms and physical manifestations can be subtle.

C. Although survival into adulthood is the rule, the overall life expectancy is decreased in patients with an unrepaired ASD. Long-term exposure to chronic right-heart volume overload can have deleterious effects, such as atrial arrhythmias, pulmonary vascular disease, and right-heart failure. These clinical findings are directly related to patient age, with almost all patients becoming symptomatic by the fifth or sixth decade. The presence of an atrial communication is also a potential source of paradoxical embolus.

D. A patent foramen ovale (PFO) is a form of interatrial communication that does not represent a congenital ASD.

E. Atrial septal aneurysms are congenital outpouchings of the atrial septum, near the fossa ovalis. These can perforate, resulting in an ASD with left-to-right shunting of blood. Atrial septal aneurysms can be detected in up to 10% of patients undergoing echocardiography and in up to 30% of patients with cryptogenic stroke.

II. ANATOMY AND EMBRYOLOGY.

The primitive atrium is first partitioned into right and left atria by growth of the septum primum, a thin, crescent-shaped membrane, from the roof of the primitive atrium toward the endocardial cushions. An atrial communication initially persists as the foramen primum, composed of the free edge of the septum primum and the endocardial cushions. Before closure of the foramen primum, fenestrations develop in the septum primum that coalesce to form the ostium secundum. As the foramen primum then fuses with the endocardial cushions, the ostium secundum maintains right-to-left atrial flow important in the fetal circulation. Failure of this fusion results in the development of a primum ASD. A second septum, the septum secundum, then forms to the right of the septum primum, growing toward the endocardial cushions and usually closing the ostium secundum. **Failure to close the ostium secundum results in the formation of a secundum ASD.**

The septum secundum forms an incomplete partition of the atria, leaving a foramen ovale (i.e., fossa ovalis). The remaining septum primum tissue on the left atrial side becomes a flap valve, or valve of the foramen ovale, and allows for the continued right-to-left shunting in the fetal circulation. At birth, when left atrial pressure increases, the septum primum flap closes and eventually fuses to anatomically seal the atrial septum. A "true ASD" results from a deficiency in septal development or from resorption of atrial tissue, whereas a **PFO results from failure of this septum primum flap to adequately seal the fossa ovalis.** At autopsy, a "probe" PFO can remain in 25% to 30% of patients.

During development, if there is overabundant or weakened septal tissue, the septum becomes very mobile. This can be visualized at echocardiography, and the degree of excursion can be measured. If the maximal excursion of the interatrial septum is **15 mm or more**, this abnormality is called an **atrial septal aneurysm**. If the amount of septal excursion is less than 15 mm, it is referred to as a redundant atrial septum.

ATRIAL SEPTAL DEFECTS

I. ASD TYPES (Fig. 29.1)

A. Ostium secundum defects constitute the most common type of ASD, accounting for 60% to 70%. This defect, a true defect of the atrial septum, is located in the midportion of the atrial septum, within or including the fossa ovalis. Defects result from deficient septum primum or an abnormally large foramen secundum. This type of ASD is two times more common in female patients. Isolated secundum ASD has been associated with mitral valve prolapse and other forms of congenital heart disease. It may also be associated with rheumatic mitral stenosis (i.e., Lutembacher syndrome).

B. Ostium primum defects account for 15% to 20% of ASDs and are part of the spectrum of atrioventricular (AV) septal defects (also known as AV canal defects or endocardial cushion defects). These defects occur in the inferior–anterior portion of the atrial septum and are frequently associated with a cleft in the anterior leaflet of the mitral valve, leading to varying degrees of mitral regurgitation. In their

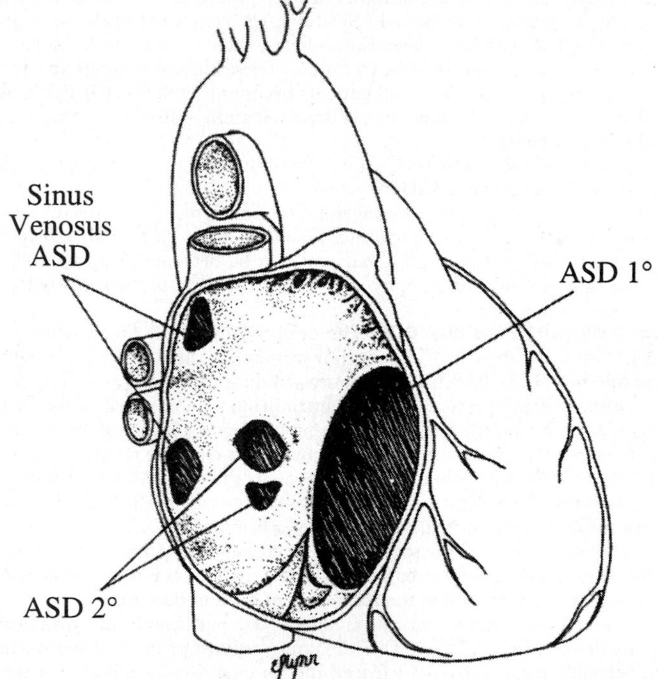

Figure 29.1. Diagrammatic representation of common atrial septal defects. ASD, atrial septal defect; 1°, primum; 2°, secundum. (Reproduced from Fyler DC, ed. *Nadas pediatric cardiology.* Philadelphia: Hanley & Belfus, 1992, with permission.)

complete form, they include a large ventricular septal defect and a common AV valve. Depending on the severity of dysfunction of the mitral valve, these patients may become symptomatic at a younger age. This defect in the inlet septum is the most common ASD associated with Down's syndrome.

C. Sinoseptal defects constitute the remaining 5% to 10% of septal defects. Distinct from the true ASDs described previously, these lesions involve the portion of the atrial wall derived from the sinus venosus (i.e., there is no direct communication between the right and left atria). **Sinus venosus defects** are typically at the orifice of the superior vena cava (SVC) at the junction of the right atrium or, less frequently, in the region of the inferior vena cava (IVC). These sinus venosus defects are frequently associated with partial anomalous pulmonary venous drainage of the right pulmonary veins and require a high index of suspicion for diagnosis because they are typically difficult to visualize by standard transthoracic echocardiography. Transesophageal echocardiography is needed in adults, and magnetic resonance imaging (MRI) or computed tomography (CT) may be required for their diagnosis. These defects should be considered in any patient with unexplained right atrial (RA) or right ventricular (RV) dilation. An uncommon sinoseptal defect is the partially or completely **unroofed coronary sinus**, which is located inferior and slightly anterior to the fossa ovalis. These defects are commonly associated with other forms of congenital heart disease, such as complete atrioventricular septal defect, or can be associated with an absent coronary sinus and a left SVC that drains into the left atrium.

II. PATHOPHYSIOLOGY. The magnitude and direction of the shunt through the ASD depends on the size of the defect as well as the diastolic filling properties of the ventricles. Any condition that causes reduced left ventricular (LV) compliance, such as LV hypertrophy or LV scar, or increased left atrial (LA) pressure, such as mitral stenosis, will increase the degree of left-to-right shunting. Conversely, conditions that cause reduced RV compliance, such as pulmonary hypertension or pulmonary stenosis, or increased RA pressure, such as tricuspid stenosis, will reduce the degree of left-to-right shunting and, in some instances, lead to shunt reversal. In general, the ASD must be at least 10 mm in greatest dimension to cause a significant shunt, although this can be hard to measure because most ASDs are not circular. A left-to-right shunt is considered significant when the ratio of pulmonary-to-systemic blood flow, or shunt fraction (Q_p/Q_s), is greater than 1.5/1.0, or when right heart chamber dilation is present.

III. CLINICAL MANIFESTATIONS. The clinical presentation of a patient with an ASD results from the effects of long-term left-to-right shunting and subsequent volume loading of the right heart. The age at which symptoms occur is variable and does not necessarily depend on the size of the defect.

A. Exercise intolerance with **fatigue** and **dyspnea** may occur, but it is frequently not appreciated by the patient until after the defect has been closed. Late findings include **supraventricular arrhythmias**, such as atrial fibrillation or flutter, severe irreversible **pulmonary vascular disease**, and, eventually, **right heart failure**. Occasionally, a **paradoxical embolus** causing a stroke or transient ischemic attack is the first clue to an ASD.

B. The physical findings may include a hyperdynamic cardiac impulse, the characteristic **widely or fixed split second heart sound**, and a **soft systolic murmur at the second left intercostal space** due to increased flow across the pulmonary valve. If the shunt is more than a shunt fraction (Q_p/Q_s) of 2.5 to 1, there may be a diastolic murmur secondary to increased flow across the tricuspid valve. A loud P_2 component of the second heart sound indicates pulmonary hypertension, which can affect up to 20% of patients; if cyanosis is present, this generally indicates advanced pulmonary hypertension with reversal of shunt flow (**Eisenmenger syndrome**). An important clue to the presence of Eisenmenger syndrome is an oxygen saturation that generally does not improve with supplemental oxygen administration. Another physical examination finding that may be encountered is a holosystolic murmur characteristic of mitral regurgitation, which is often heard in a patient with a primum ASD.

IV. LABORATORY EXAMINATION

A. Electrocardiogram (ECG). The ECG can provide clues to the possibility of an ASD. The rhythm may be sinus, but may also be atrial fibrillation or atrial flutter. Inverted P waves in the inferior leads suggest an absent or nonfunctional sinus node, as may be seen in a sinus venosus defect.

1. Secundum ASD

- **a.** RSR^1 pattern in lead V_1
- **b.** QRS duration less than 0.11 second (incomplete right bundle-branch block)
- **c.** Right axis deviation
- **d.** RV hypertrophy
- **e.** First-degree atrioventricular block (20%)
- **f.** RA enlargement (about 50%) with a prominent P wave in lead II

2. Primum ASD

- **a.** RSR^1 pattern in lead V_1
- **b.** Left axis deviation
- **c.** First-degree atrioventricular block

B. Chest radiograph may reveal cardiomegaly due to right heart enlargement. With large left-to-right shunts, the central pulmonary arteries and vascular markings may appear prominent. In the setting of advanced pulmonary vascular disease, however, the pulmonary arteries may appear large but have oligemic peripheral lung fields, so called "vascular pruning."

V. DIAGNOSTIC STUDIES

A. Echocardiography is the primary means by which an ASD is diagnosed. Transthoracic echocardiography (TTE) can document the size of the defect as well as the direction of the shunt flow, and occasionally the location of the pulmonary veins in the younger patient. In the adult, transesophageal studies are generally required. An ASD should be suspected when right-sided chamber enlargement is noted on echocardiography and no other cause is identified.

1. Typical transthoracic views for imaging an ASD include the parasternal short-axis view, apical four-chamber view, and the subcostal coronal and sagittal views. Findings include RA and RV enlargement, which indicate the functional importance of the defect. An estimate of RV pressure should be measured via the jet of tricuspid insufficiency, and evidence for RV pressure and volume overload noted via observation of septal motion in systole and diastole, respectively. Evidence of left-to-right (or right-to-left) shunting across the defect should be demonstrated using color Doppler techniques. Evidence of RA and RV enlargement in the absence of an obvious cause on echocardiography, such as tricuspid regurgitation or an ASD, should prompt a search for a sinus venosus defect and/or anomalous pulmonary venous drainage. Intravenous contrast (i.e., agitated saline) and transthoracic echocardiography can identify a shunt, but transesophageal echocardiography (TEE) is usually required to demonstrate a sinus venosus defect.

2. TEE is usually required in the adult patient for further anatomic definition and to determine whether the defect is amenable to percutaneous closure. Contrast studies with agitated saline are helpful in confirming the presence and location of atrial shunting. The mid-esophageal four-chamber and bicaval views are preferred, with injection of agitated saline through an upper extremity vein. Injection into the left arm may be particularly helpful to establish the presence of a persistent left SVC that drains to the coronary sinus or directly to the left atrium. In the diagnosis of a sinus venosis defect, care must be taken to evaluate the location of the pulmonary veins for evidence of anomalous drainage.

B. Cardiac catheterization is typically not required for diagnostic purposes except to assess pulmonary pressures and resistance, to assess for coronary artery disease before planned surgical closure in the adult patient, or as part of transcatheter device closure. Catheterization can be performed in most cases using a standard end-hole catheter. The lateral camera is helpful in directing the catheter posterior before advancing across the ASD. Our standard is to perform a complete right heart catheterization, including oximetry measurements and hemodynamic assessment.

1. Oximetry samples obtained during catheterization demonstrate a step-up within the right atrium due to shunting across the defect. Careful interrogation of innominate vein saturation and SVC saturation is important to exclude a step-up in the SVC that would support the existence of associated partial anomalous pulmonary venous drainage. Desaturation in the left atrium systemically confirms right-to-left shunting and should prompt further investigation of RV and pulmonary artery pressures. Other diagnoses producing a similar picture include large ventricular septal defects with tricuspid regurgitation, partial or complete atrioventricular canal defects, or systemic arteriovenous fistulas.

   The significance of the defect can be assessed by calculating the **shunt fraction (Q_p/Q_s)**, which is the ratio of pulmonary blood flow (Q_p) to systemic blood flow (Q_s). Oximetry values, obtained at right heart catheterization and used previously to determine if a step-up is present, can be helpful for shunt calculation as follows:

$$Q_p/Q_s = \frac{(\text{aortic saturation} - \text{mixed venous saturation})}{(\text{pulmonary vein saturation} - \text{pulmonary artery saturation})}$$

   The mixed venous saturation is obtained in the setting of an ASD, by multiplying the SVC saturation by 3, adding the IVC saturation, and then dividing the sum by 4. If the pulmonary vein saturation is not directly measured, it can be assumed to be 95%.

2. Hemodynamic assessment may reveal modest elevations in RV and pulmonary artery pressures. An important assessment is comparison of RV pressure to systemic pressure and measurement of pulmonary vascular resistance. If pulmonary pressures are elevated, the response to oxygen or other vasodilators should be assessed. Examples of the usual catheterization findings with and without pulmonary vascular disease are illustrated in Figure 29.2.

   Using a derivative of Ohm's law, P = Q × R, an ASD will increase the flow (Q) to the lungs, and, therefore, increase the pulmonary pressure (P) without a significant change in resistance (R). Findings that may preclude eventual ASD

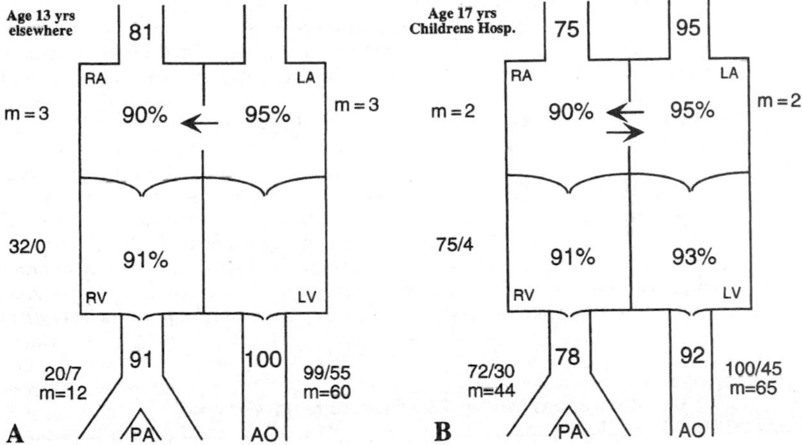

Figure 29.2. Catheterization data derived from two studies of the same female patient. The data obtained at age 13 **(A)** were interpreted as compatible with a small atrial septal defect of insufficient size to require closure. Some years later, she had developed pulmonary vascular obstructive disease **(B)** and was no longer shunting enough to recommend surgery. Death occurred 5 years later. AO, aorta; LA, left atrium; LV, left ventricle; PA, pulmonary artery; RA, right atrium; RV, right ventricle; numeric values within the schematic, oxygen saturation (%); numeric values outside the schematic, pressure (mm Hg). (Adapted from Fyler DC, ed. *Nadas pediatric cardiology.* Philadelphia: Hanley & Belfus, 1992.)

closure include one or more of the following: a peak pulmonary pressure of more than 60 mm Hg, pulmonary vascular resistance more than one-half of the systemic vascular resistance, or an indexed pulmonary vascular resistance of more than 7 Wood units/m^2.

3. Angiography is typically not necessary for diagnostic purposes. Some transcatheter closure-device protocols include angiography, typically performed in the right pulmonary vein or levophase from a main pulmonary artery injection in the left anterior oblique and cranial projections. This may be an important way to confirm the absence of additional defects, such as partial anomalous pulmonary venous drainage, before proceeding with transcatheter device closure.

C. Cardiac MRI can be helpful, as it can provide additional information beyond echocardiography. MRI provides an excellent assessment of RV size and function, especially if views obtained with echocardiography are not diagnostic. MRI is also excellent at determining the location of the pulmonary veins as well as calculating ventricular volumes and shunt fraction.

VI. MEDICAL THERAPY. Medical intervention is typically not required preoperatively, because many patients are asymptomatic. Congestive symptoms may be improved with standard diuretic therapy. Rhythm disturbances such as atrial fibrillation require attention with respect to rate control and anticoagulation. Endocarditis antibiotic prophylaxis is not required in the setting of an isolated ASD before surgery, but is warranted for 6 months after surgical or device closure.

A. Surgical or transcatheter therapy. The mainstay of therapy is closure of the defect by surgical or transcatheter techniques. Because of the reduced life expectancy associated with an ASD, closure is recommended on diagnosis if there is evidence of a hemodynamically significant shunt ($Q_p/Q_s \geq 1.5{:}1$), evidence of right heart dilation, or associated symptoms. In the setting of pulmonary hypertension, pulmonary reactivity to vasodilators should be documented and a net left-to-right shunt shown at catheterization before consideration for closure. Alternatively, the defect can be temporarily balloon-occluded at the time of catheterization, and the hemodynamic effects directly measured. It has also been argued that an ASD in the setting of a cryptogenic stroke or likely embolic stroke is another indication for closure, even if it does not meet additional indications for correction. Situations in which ASD closure should not be pursued are listed in Table 29.1 and include advanced pulmonary hypertension (Eisenmenger syndrome) and severe LV dysfunction.

B. Primary surgical closure has been the standard approach for many years. Generally, surgical closure is the treatment of choice for ostium primum and sinus venosus defects. Patients with secundum ASDs and anatomy that is not amenable to percutaneous closure (stretched ASD >36 mm; inadequate septal rims to permit device deployment; or close proximity to AV valves, coronary sinus, or vena cavae) are also candidates for open surgical closure. Depending on the defect size and location, the secundum ASD can be closed by primary suture or, if needed, by use of an autologous pericardial or synthetic patch. Ostium primum defects require patch closure as well as repair of the likely cleft mitral valve. Repair of sinus venosus defects is more

TABLE 29.1 Conditions Where ASD Closure is not Favored

Defect is too small to be hemodynamically significant
Pulmonary hypertension is too advanced
Severe LV dysfunction, where ASD is acting as "pop-off" valve for the left ventricle
In most cases where ASD is diagnosed in pregnancy, closure can be postponed until 6 months after delivery

ASD, atrial septal defect; LV, left ventricular.

technically challenging, as the pulmonary veins often have anomalous drainage and require re-routing.

1. Important preoperative risk factors include older age at operation, presence of atrial fibrillation, and elevated pulmonary pressures and resistance.
2. Postoperatively, patients are at risk for heart block, which is a significant complication in these cases. They are also at risk for postpericardiotomy syndrome, more so than after other surgery for congenital defects. Atrial arrhythmias may persist in short- and long-term follow-up because the right atrial and ventricular sizes may take time to return to normal. In some centers, prophylactic β-adrenergic blockade is advocated empirically for 3 to 6 months after surgery.

C. Transcatheter closure of a secundum ASD has become an attractive alternative to surgical closure and is considered the treatment of choice. Any patient with an isolated secundum ASD may be suitable for transcatheter closure, which is generally assisted with TEE or intracardiac echocardiography in addition to fluoroscopy. Catheter closure decreases hospital length of stay, avoids surgical wounds and their possible complications, and speeds postprocedure recovery. With the devices available today, defects with a resting diameter less than 30 mm may be considered. In general, the stretched diameter of the defect is approximately 6 to 8 mm greater than the resting diameter. The defect must be located centrally with adequate room for the device to be positioned, without interference of other intracardiac structures such as the atrioventricular valves, coronary sinus, or right pulmonary veins. The U.S. Food and Drug Administration (FDA) has approved two devices for the closure of secundum ASDs: the Amplatzer Septal Occluder (AGA Medical Corporation, Golden Valley, MN) and the Helex septal occluder (WL Gore & Associates, Flagstaff, AZ). Studies have proven the safety and efficacy of catheter-based closure of a secundum ASD compared with surgical closure. The Amplatzer device consists of two disks made of Nitinol wire separated by a narrow, 3- to 4-mm waist. It is inserted percutaneously through a 6F to 12F sheath, depending on the device size required. Major complications, such as cardiac perforation or device embolization, happen very rarely (generally fewer than 1% of cases), and successful closure of the defect is achieved in up to 95% of all patients. After closure, antiplatelet therapy, frequently aspirin and clopidogrel, are prescribed for a minimum of 6 months, after which time the device is generally endothelialized.

VII. PROGNOSIS. Hemodynamically significant ASDs are associated with increased morbidity and mortality. Long-term outcomes can be improved by closing these defects, especially if done early in life. Atrial arrhythmias are common, especially in older patients, and are the result of long-standing right atrial stretch. These arrhythmias, particularly atrial flutter and fibrillation, contribute to a significant portion of the morbidity and mortality of older patients, especially with the risk of systemic embolization and resultant stroke. It has been demonstrated that age at the time of surgical repair is inversely related to risk of atrial fibrillation or flutter after repair and argues for earlier closure. Some have advocated for consideration of a concomitant ablation procedure in high-risk patients.

The functional capacity of patients improves dramatically after closure of the ASD. Often a patient will not realize how severely their functional capacity has been affected until after the defect is closed. In addition, improvements in LV filling and systemic cardiac output are seen rapidly after defect closure. Reduced RA and RV volumes can be seen within 24 hours and continue to improve over the course of the first year following closure.

PATENT FORAMEN OVALE (PFO) AND ATRIAL SEPTAL ANEURYSM

I. PATHOPHYSIOLOGY. Prevalence of PFOs in the adult population tends to decrease as patients age, implying that these defects may close spontaneously if given time. Generally, PFOs result in right-to-left shunting of blood flow, usually when RA pressure exceeds LA pressure. These defects generally do not cause significant hemodynamic derangements. The clinical importance of an atrial septal aneurysm or a PFO is its impact on the risk of stroke. PFO features that increase the risk of a paradoxical embolus include large tunnel lengths (≥4 mm), high mobility of the valve of the foramen ovale, a well-formed eustachian valve, and a resting right-to-left shunt.

II. CLINICAL MANIFESTATIONS. Generally these defects are **asymptomatic**, most often coming to attention in patients with cryptogenic (unexplained) stroke. PFO is about three times more common in patients with cryptogenic stroke than in the general population. PFO should be suspected in young patients who sustain a stroke, as more than one-half of stroke patients younger than 45 years have a PFO. Once a patient with a PFO has an embolic event, there is a higher risk for recurrence, especially if a concomitant atrial septal aneurysm is present. The presence of both abnormalities is also more common in patients with cryptogenic stroke, seen up to six times more frequently in these patients than in the general population.

Other less-common clinical associations with PFO include migraine headaches, platypnea–orthodeoxia syndrome, and decompression illness in divers and those who work in high altitudes.

III. DIAGNOSTIC STUDIES. Echocardiography can easily differentiate between an ASD and a PFO if the interatrial septum can be visualized. If this is not possible via a transthoracic approach, a TEE may be necessary. A simple way to determine if a shunt is present is the "**bubble study**," which is the injection of agitated saline via an upper extremity vein. The patient then performs the Valsalva maneuver. If bubbles can be seen in the LA or LV within three cardiac cycles on transthoracic echocardiography, the diagnosis of an interatrial right-to-left shunt is established.

TEE will likely be required in most adults for better visualization of the interatrial septum. TEE helps to differentiate between a PFO and a secundum ASD, both of which can have positive bubble studies. TEE also allows assessment of other potential sources of emboli, such as atheroma in the aortic arch, thrombus in the LA appendage, or cardiac tumors.

IV. THERAPY. Unfortunately, there is no clear consensus on primary or secondary prevention measures for patients found to have a PFO or atrial septal aneurysm. Most patients with neurologic events are treated with antiplatelet agents (either aspirin or a thienopyridine, or both), anticoagulants (warfarin), and percutaneous or surgical closure, although no clear consensus exists. Primary surgical closure is generally not pursued, unless the patient needs concomitant surgery for other conditions. Patients with cryptogenic stroke in the presence of atrial septal aneurysm and a PFO represent a high-risk subgroup, and may be candidates for aggressive treatment strategies, including percutaneous closure. There are currently two devices available for percutaneous closure: the CardioSeal (NMT Medical, Boston, MA) and the Amplatzer PFO occluder. Neither is FDA-approved and both are currently used in an "off-label" fashion or investigationally in this patient population. Generally, percutaneous closure is considered in patients with recurrent cryptogenic stroke who have failed medical therapy. Contraindications to percutaneous closure are noted in Table 29.2. Additional data from ongoing randomized, controlled studies are needed before making a more definitive recommendation.

TABLE 29.2 Contraindications to Percutaneous PFO Closure
Presence of an alternative source of emboli
Severe pulmonary hypertension
Recent gastrointestinal bleeding
Presence of congenital heart defect that needs surgical repair
Venous thrombus or vena cava filter precluding passage of catheter
Hypersensitivity or contraindication to anti-platelet or anticoagulant therapy
Unexplained fever or infection

There are few data to support PFO closure in patients with migraine headaches. The MIST (Migraine Intervention with STARFlex Technology) trial randomized 147 participants with severe migraine headaches and right-to-left shunt consistent with PFO to either percutaneous closure or a sham procedure, and then followed the patients for 6 months. There was no significant difference in the primary endpoint of complete cessation of migraine headache or in the host of secondary endpoints such as change in severity, quality, and frequency of headache as well as quality of life.

Patients with platypnea–orthodeoxia syndrome (acute arterial desaturation with change in position from supine to upright), however, should be considered for closure, as oxygen saturation improves with elimination of the right-to-left shunt.

ACKNOWLEDGMENTS

The author would like to gratefully acknowledge the contributions of Niranjan Seshadri and J. Donald Moore to previous editions of this manuscript.

Key Reviews/Trials

Brickner ME, Hillis LD, Lange RA. Medical progress: congenital heart disease in adults: first of two parts. *N Engl J Med* 2000;342:256–263.

Connelly MS, Webb GD, Sommerville J, et al. Canadian Consensus Conference on Adult Congenital Heart Disease 1996. *Can J Cardiol* 1998;14:395–452.

Dowson A, Mullen MJ, Peatfield R, et al. Migraine Intervention With STARFlex Technology (MIST) trial: a prospective, multicenter, double-blind, sham-controlled trial to evaluate the effectiveness of patent foramen ovale closure with STARFlex septal repair implant to resolve refractory migraine headache. *Circulation* 2008;117:1397–1404.

Du ZD, Hijazi ZM, Kleinmann CS, et al. Comparison between transcatheter and surgical closure of secundum atrial septal defect in children and adults: results of a multicenter nonrandomized trial. *J Am Coll Cardiol* 2002;39:1836–1844.

Ebeid MR. Percutaneous catheter closure of secundum atrial septal defects: a review. *J Invasive Cardiol* 2002;14:25–31.

Gatzoulis MA, Freeman MA, Siu SC, et al. Atrial arrhythmia after surgical closure of atrial septal defects in adults. *N Engl J Med* 1999;340:839–846.

Krasuski RA. When and how to fix a 'hole in the heart': Approach to ASD and PFO. *Cleve Clin J Med* 2007;74:137–147.

Latson LA. Per-Catheter ASD Closure. *Pediatr Cardiol* 1998;19:86–93.

Mandelik J, Moodie DS, Sterba R, et al. Long-term follow-up of children after repair of atrial septal defects. *Cleve Clin J Med* 1994;61:29–33.

Mas JL, Arquizan C, Lamy C, et al. Recurrent cerebrovascular events associated with patent foramen ovale, atrial septal aneurysm, or both. *N Engl J Med* 2001;345:1740–1746.

Webb G, Gatzoulis MA. Atrial septal defects in the adult: recent progress and overview. *Circulation* 2006;114:1645–1653.

Relevant Book Chapters

Brecker SJD. Atrial septal defect. In: Redington A, Shore D, Oldershaw P, eds. *Congenital heart disease in adults: a practical guide*. London: WB Saunders, 1994;103–110.

Perloff JK. Survival patterns without cardiac surgery or interventional catheterization: a narrowing base. In: Perloff JK, Child JS, eds. *Congenital heart disease in adults*, 2nd ed. Philadelphia: WB Saunders, 1998:15–53.

Webb GD, Smallhorn JF, Therrien J, et al. Congenital heart disease. In: Zipes DP, Libby P, Bonow RO, Braunwald E, eds. *Braunwald's heart disease: a textbook of cardiovascular medicine*, 7th ed. Philadelphia: Elsevier Saunders, 2005:1505–1509.

30 VENTRICULAR SEPTAL DEFECT

Samuel Unzek

I. INTRODUCTION

A. Ventricular septal defect (VSD) is one of the most common congenital heart defects in both children and adults, although the true incidence is difficult to determine due to the tendency for spontaneous closure in some cases. VSDs are frequently associated with other congenital defects, and 15% to 20% spontaneously close by 6 months of age. The incidence of VSD is about 2 per 1000 live births, and isolated VSDs account for about 25% of all congenital heart defects in childhood. Males and females appear to be affected equally.

B. Isolated VSDs are found in approximately 10% of adult patients with congenital heart disease. This reflects the natural tendency for spontaneous closure and an improved diagnosis in childhood with subsequent surgical closure.

C. Natural history

1. **Spontaneous closure** occurs most commonly with smaller VSDs and usually happens before the age of 2 years. In general, nearly 35% of perimembranous defects close spontaneously, and 75% to 80% of all small VSDs close spontaneously by 10 years of age. These high rates in some series are a reflection of the ability to diagnose smaller defects with newer and more sensitive echocardiographic modalities. For large and nonrestrictive defects, spontaneous closure rates are much lower, roughly 10% to 15%; for malalignment defects, spontaneous closure is rare. The defects close by two mechanisms: (1) by muscular septum growth, or (2) by "aneurysmal tissue" from a septal leaflet of the tricuspid valve in the case of perimembranous defects. Of VSDs that persist, a restrictive nature can protect the patient from pulmonary vascular injury.
2. **Endocarditis** remains a risk because of the presence of a high-velocity, turbulent jet into the right ventricle, and most frequently involves the tricuspid valve apparatus. The risk of endocarditis is roughly 4% to 10% for the first 30 years of life.
3. A large VSD during childhood is associated with significant **left-to-right shunt** and eventual development of congestive heart failure. Children with very large defects usually present during infancy or early childhood with heart failure and pulmonary hypertension. Patients with moderate-sized VSDs can survive to adulthood before detection. In these patients, the excess right-sided flow may lead to pulmonary vascular disease and Eisenmenger's physiology if left untreated. As pulmonary vascular resistance increases, the left-to-right shunt changes to a right-to-left flow. The murmur often disappears during this transition. After this physiology has developed, patients rarely survive beyond the fourth decade. Complications in patients with Eisenmenger's syndrome or irreversible pulmonary hypertension include pulmonary hemorrhage, endocarditis, cerebral abscess (from hypoxemia), ventricular arrhythmias, and the complications associated with erythrocytosis. Poor prognostic factors in this population include syncope, congestive failure, and hemoptysis.
4. Risk factors for decreased survival include cardiomegaly seen on the chest radiograph; elevated pulmonary artery systolic pressure (more than 60 mm Hg and/or more than one-half of the systemic pressure); cardiovascular symptoms such as shortness of breath, fatigue, or dyspnea on exertion; and progressive aortic insufficiency. Good prognosticators include normal left ventricular (LV) size and function, small left-to-right shunt, normal pulmonary pressures or resistance,

an intact vasodilator response in the pulmonary vasculature, and a lack of symptoms.

5. Genetic factors play a significant role in this disease, as in other forms of congenital heart disease. Having an affected father increases the risk of VSD in the offspring to 2%, but having an affected mother appears to confer a higher risk of recurrence in offspring—as high as 6%.

6. Overall, the 25-year survival for all patients with a VSD is 87%. Mortality increases with the size of the VSD.

II. ANATOMY

A. Embryology. Partitioning of the ventricular mass begins as a muscular ridge in the floor of the ventricle near the apex. This ridge later undergoes active growth, which forms the muscular ventricular septum. Concomitantly, the endocardial cushions fuse, and the two regions meet, completing closure of the interventricular foramen. See Figure 30.1 for anatomic localization of VSDs.

B. Defect size. The consequences of a VSD depend on the size of the defect and the pulmonary vascular resistance. Smaller defects provide higher resistance to flow and may have little impact on right-sided flow. The VSD is described as small when the defect is less than one-third of the size of the aortic root, moderate when the defect is less than one-half of the size of the aortic root, and large when the defect is equal to or larger than the size of the aortic root. However, other indirect measures, including clinical signs and symptoms and echocardiographic features, must be taken into consideration when determining the size and clinical significance of a VSD. VSD size is often classified on the basis of its hemodynamic consequences:

1. Restrictive VSDs produce a significant pressure gradient between the left and right ventricles (e.g., pulmonary/aortic systolic pressure ratio <0.3) and are associated with a small shunt ($Q_p/Q_s < 1.4/1$)

2. Moderately restrictive VSDs produced an intermediate interventricular gradient and produce a moderate shunt ($Q_p/Q_s = 1.4/2.2$).

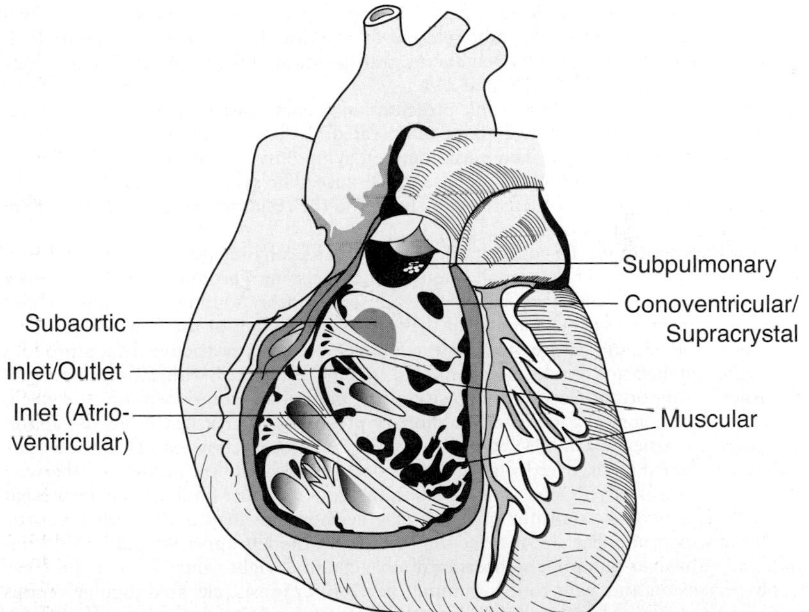

Figure 30.1. Anatomic localization of VSDs.

3. **Nonrestrictive** VSDs are usually larger than 1.0 cm^2 and are associated with a very large shunt (Q_p/Q_s >2.2). The pressures in the left ventricle and right ventricle will approach equalization, and the amount of flow across the defect will be determined by the ratio of pulmonary to systemic vascular resistance.

C. VSD types

1. **Membranous** defects are the most common type, accounting for approximately 70% to 80%. The membranous septum is the area under the aortic valve on the left side and next to the septal leaflet of the tricuspid valve on the right side. Most of these defects extend into the infundibular region and are then referred to as perimembranous. Membranous defects are less likely to be associated with additional intracardiac defects and have a high rate of spontaneous closure. However, when there is malalignment of the defect, spontaneous closure is unlikely.
2. **Muscular** defects account for approximately 5% to 20% of VSDs and can be single or multiple (i.e., Swiss cheese septum). These defects, when single, also have a high spontaneous closure rate.
3. **Inlet or atrioventricular (AV) canal–type** defects account for approximately 5% to 8% of cases. These defects rarely close spontaneously, are usually large, and are associated with abnormalities of the AV valves. These abnormalities range from cleft mitral and tricuspid valves to the common AV valve, as seen in complete AV canal defect. This type of defect in the inlet ventricular septum is commonly associated with Down's syndrome (trisomy 21).
4. **Supracristal or subaortic** defects account for approximately 5% to 7% of cases and are located immediately beneath the pulmonary and aortic valves. These defects vary in size but are often small. Of patients who present with a VSD, 5% to 10% will develop aortic regurgitation because of poor support of the right coronary cusp and the Venturi effect caused by the VSD jet, resulting in prolapse of one of the aortic valve leaflets.

D. Associated lesions. Among adults who present with a small VSD, a **bicuspid aortic valve** and **coarctation of the aorta** are the most commonly associated lesions. Discrete fibrous subaortic stenosis and right ventricular (RV) outflow tract obstruction are less common associations. Less than 10% develop subvalvular pulmonary stenosis or an obstructive muscle bundle referred to as a double-chamber right ventricle. It can also be associated with open ductus, transposition of the great arteries, tetralogy of Fallot, or trisomia 13, 18, and 21.

III. CLINICAL PRESENTATION. Adult presentation occurs most frequently in small, restrictive VSDs or, occasionally, in large unoperated VSDs with Eisenmenger's complex.

A. Signs and symptoms. The most common symptoms in adult patients with VSD are dyspnea on exertion and exercise intolerance. The symptoms are related to the degree and chronicity of left-to-right shunt and the resultant increase in pulmonary pressure and resistance.

B. Physical findings. The auscultatory findings classically include a holosystolic murmur of varying intensity. Smaller muscular defects may produce a high-frequency early systolic murmur that ends before the second heart sound (S_2) because of closure from muscular contraction of the septum. The pitch of the murmur can be a clue to the size and nature of the defect. Smaller and more restrictive defects produce higher-pitched and louder murmurs and may be associated with a palpable thrill. Another important feature is intensity of the pulmonary component of, S_2, which, if increased, suggests increased pulmonary pressures. An RV heave may be appreciated in patients with RV volume overload. A diastolic flow rumble at the apex may be heard in large left-to-right shunts due to increased flow across an otherwise normal mitral valve. Depending on associated lesions, other findings may be present such as a diastolic murmur of aortic insufficiency that may occur with subaortic defects. A prominent systolic ejection murmur at the left upper sternal border suggests subvalvar pulmonic stenosis or double-chamber right ventricle. As pulmonary hypertension and right-to-left shunting develop, cyanosis, elevated jugular venous pressure, enlarged and pulsatile liver, clubbing, and a decrease in murmur intensity may occur. A systolic murmur in this setting often reflects concomitant tricuspid insufficiency. Of importance to note, the murmur of a large VSD is often less harsh and more blowing in nature than that of a small VSD, because of the absence of a significant pressure gradient across the larger defect.

C. The **differential diagnosis** on examination includes tricuspid regurgitation, acyanotic tetralogy of Fallot with a pulmonary outflow murmur, isolated subvalvar pulmonic stenosis, and hypertrophic cardiomyopathy.

IV. LABORATORY TESTS

A. The **electrocardiogram (ECG)** may be unremarkable with small defects, or reveal left atrial and LV enlargement in the larger defect. An inlet or AV canal defect can be diagnosed from the ECG based on the presence of marked left-axis deviation. Right-axis deviation suggests elevated RV and pulmonary artery pressure. After surgical repair, right bundle-branch block may occur.

B. A **chest radiograph** is often helpful in determining the degree of left-to-right shunt. A small or normal-sized heart with normal pulmonary vascular markings on the chest radiograph suggests a hemodynamically insignificant lesion, whereas cardiomegaly and left atrial and LV enlargement are seen with large left-to-right shunts. A large defect associated with a small heart and oligemic lung fields should raise the suspicion of pulmonary vascular disease.

V. DIAGNOSTIC TESTING

A. **Echocardiography** is the diagnostic modality of choice for VSDs and associated lesions. Transthoracic echocardiographic imaging is almost always sufficient in the child and young adult, but transesophageal echocardiographic imaging may be required the some adult patients. Defect size and location should be defined using two-dimensional and color Doppler techniques. Complete scans of the ventricular septum should be made to rule out additional defects. Optimal images are usually obtained from the parasternal long- and short-axis views and the apical four-chamber view; other views may fail to visualize the VSD jet, owing to perpendicular alignment of the echocardiographic probe and the jet. In the younger patient, subcostal coronal and sagittal views may also be helpful. Measurements of left atrial and LV size are key in determining the amount of volume load and magnitude of the left-to-right shunt. Echocardiographic features of pulmonary hypertension are helpful in confirming the reversal of the shunt. Quantification of shunt velocity provides an estimate of the restrictive nature of the defect. The higher the velocity, the more restrictive the defect and the less likely the patient has experienced pulmonary vascular insult. Systemic blood pressure should be noted when the velocity across the VSD is measured. Assuming no LV outflow obstruction, RV pressure can then be estimated based on the gradient across the VSD. This pressure can also be estimated if tricuspid insufficiency exists. A perimembranous VSD is often associated with a ventricular septal aneurysm formed by the septal leaflet of the tricuspid valve bowing into the defect. Similarly, supracristal VSDs are associated with aortic insufficiency caused by prolapse of the right or left coronary cusps into the VSD. A complete evaluation is always indicated to exclude other associated findings such as aortic coarctation, atrial septal defect, patent ductus arteriosus, and RV or left-heart outflow tract obstruction.

B. **Catheterization** is seldom needed in the management of isolated VSD in the infant or child. Surgical correction, when indicated, proceeds in most cases based on echocardiographic evaluation. In the adult, catheterization should be considered if anatomic questions remain despite transthoracic and transesophageal echocardiography, or if pulmonary hypertension is suspected based on these studies. Hemodynamic assessment should include quantification of cardiac index and careful oximetric definition of the shunt level and quantity. An elevated pulmonary artery saturation confirms persistent left-to-right shunt across the defect and should correlate with acceptable pulmonary artery pressures and resistance. Evidence of low pulmonary artery saturations is expected with elevations of pulmonary resistance. Simultaneous comparison of RV pressure to systemic pressure is mandatory in these cases, along with documentation of changes in response to oxygen or nitric oxide administration. Left ventriculography performed with **left anterior-oblique and cranial angulation** demonstrates the defect in most cases. If an inlet-type defect is present, the hepatoclavicular view (about 40 degrees left anterior-oblique and 40 degrees cranial) is usually adequate. Right ventriculography does not adequately opacify the left ventricle unless there is suprasystemic RV pressure. Coronary angiography should be performed during the case in patients felt to be at risk for coronary artery disease. Aortography can be helpful in eliminating the possibility of an associated ductus arteriosus or coarctation of the aorta.

C. Cardiac **computed tomography** (CT) can be used to assess VSD anatomy in patients with suboptimal echocardiographic images but, unlike magnetic resonance imaging (MRI), does not provide added information about shunt fraction (see Chapter 47) and carries additional risk associated with radiation and contrast material.

D. **Magnetic resonance imaging,** using spin-echo and velocity-encoded cine sequences, can be used to delineate VSD location and shunt fraction in patients with complex associated lesions (see Chapter 46).

VI. THERAPY. Factors supporting intervention include cardiomegaly on the chest radiograph, significant left-to-right shunt (pulmonary-to-systemic flow ratios greater than 1.5:1), elevated but responsive pulmonary vascular resistance, symptoms of congestive failure or associated lesions such as aortic insufficiency, RV or LV outflow tract obstruction, and recurrent endocarditis. Management of VSD after myocardial infarction is discussed separately in Chapter 3.

A. **Medical management** in symptomatic cases without Eisenmenger's physiology involves anticongestive measures such as the use of diuretics and digoxin. Efforts should then be focused on addressing suitability for surgical closure. Endocarditis is a recognized complication of VSD. In the patient with culture-proven endocarditis, 4 to 6 weeks of antibiotics should be administered parenterally before consideration of intervention. This must be tailored to the individual patient's clinical status and the infective organism's identification and sensitivity. Recent data suggest that selective pulmonary vasodilators, including nitric oxide, prostacyclin analogs, and endothelin-receptor antagonists, may be beneficial in these patients. Phosphodiesterase-5 inhibitors may have benefit as well (see Chapter 32).

B. **Transcatheter device closure** of VSDs is being performed on an investigational or compassionate-use basis in selected medical centers. Perimembranous defects pose particular problems for transcatheter closure. However, newer device technology and design has made this a viable treatment option. It is technically difficult to approach these defects because of the proximity of the conduction system and the AV and semilunar valves. The devices can technically close many muscular defects, although the long-term outcome of this approach has yet to be determined. Initial studies using the Amplatzer VSD Occluder (Fig. 30.2) or the CardioSEAL devices for closure of muscular VSDs have shown promise. The rate of complete closure for the Amplatzer membranous device at 6 months is 96% and is 100% for the muscular occluder at 3 to 96 months follow-up according to a phase I clinical trial. Complications with these devices include arrhythmia, tricuspid valve damage resulting in stenosis or regurgitation, and mechanical device failure during deployment. Active investigation and device development for this purpose continues. Transcatheter closure of VSDs after ventricular septal rupture in the setting of myocardial infarction has been performed in selected individuals who are considered high-risk surgical candidates, or when the defect is not close to vital structures.

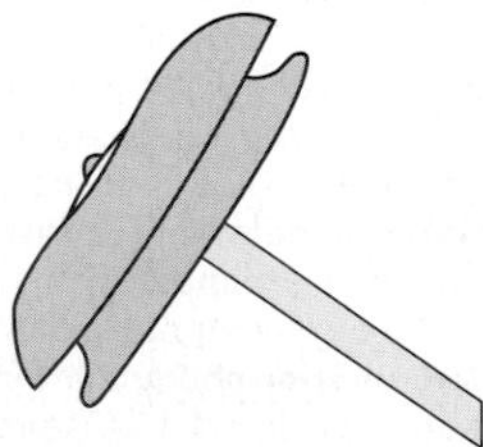

Figure 30.2. Amplatzer VSD Occluder.

C. Surgical closure is the primary means of repair. Outcome after VSD closure is good in children, with low mortality rates of 2% to 3%. Repair of VSDs in patients with evidence of increased pulmonary artery pressure is generally performed before the age of 2 years and, in many centers, in the first year of life.. Surgical closure in the symptomatic adult appears to be well tolerated, with acceptable mortality and improved functional status. Irreversible pulmonary vascular disease with Eisenmenger's physiology, however, is a general contraindication for surgical closure because right heart failure will often develop thereafter. Pulmonary artery banding (performed to limit pulmonary blood flow) was more frequently done in the past and is now reserved for the few patients who are very small, have lung disease, or who have complex, multiple VSDs. Postoperative sequelae include residual patch leaks, as well as supraventricular and ventricular arrhythmias. More recent studies have shown the presence of a residual shunt following surgical closure in 5% to 31% of patients depending on the type of VSD that is being repaired.. Recent reports suggest that postsurgical residual VSDs less than 2 mm close spontaneously within 1 year in the majority (83%) of patients.

D. According to new American Heart Association (AHA) guidelines, **antibiotic prophylaxis** is recommended in three situations in relation to congenital heart disease: (1) unrepaired cyanotic defect (.i.e, VSD with right-to-left shunt), (2) repaired defect (i.e., VSD) with prosthetic material/device for the first 6 months, and (3) repaired defect (i.e., VSD) with residual defect at the site of a prosthetic patch/device.

E. Eisenmenger's syndrome is usually referred to in the context of irreversible pulmonary hypertension from long-standing exposure of the pulmonary vasculature to left-to-right shunting across a VSD. However, this physiology can occur as a result of any left-to-right shunt, including patent ductus arteriosus and, less commonly, isolated atrial septal defect. As a result of the elevated pulmonary pressures, the direction of shunting is reversed across the defect, producing systemic cyanosis and its associated complications. **Pregnancy is poorly tolerated and is contraindicated in the presence of Eisenmenger's syndrome** (see Chapter 38).

F. Follow-up is indicated in patients whose VSDs were repaired late in life, since the majority of patients already have some degree of pulmonary hypertension or LV dysfunction., or both. Patients with residual shunt after repair, arrhythmias or conduction blocks, also require continued follow-up.

ACKNOWLEDGMENT

The author thanks Dr. J. Donald Moore and Dr. Matthew Hook for contributions to earlier editions of this chapter.

Landmark Articles

Birnbaum Y, Fishbein MC, Blanche C, et al. Ventricular septal rupture after acute myocardial infarction. *N Engl J Med* 2002;347:1426–1432.

Brickner ME, Hillis LD, Lange RA. Medical progress: congenital heart disease in adults: first of two parts. *N Engl J Med* 2000;342:256–263.

Bridges ND, Perry SB, Keane JF, et al. Preoperative transcatheter closure of congenital muscular ventricular septal defects. *N Engl J Med* 1991;324:1312–1317.

Chessa M, Carminati M, Cao QL, et al. Transcatheter closure of congenital and acquired muscular ventricular septal defects using the Amplatzer device. *J Invasive Cardiol* 2002;14:322–327.

Connelly MS, Webb GD, Sommerville J, et al. Canadian Consensus Conference on Adult Congenital Heart Disease 1996. *Can J Cardiol* 1998;14:395–452.

Dodge-Khatami A, Knirsch W, Tomaske M, et al. Spontaneous closure of small residual ventricular septal defects after surgical repair. *Ann Thorac Surg* 2007;83:902–906.

Ellis JH, Moodie DS, Sterba R, et al. Ventricular septal defect in the adult: natural and unnatural history. *Am Heart J* 1987;114:115–120.

Folkert M, Szatmari A, Utens E, et al. Long-term follow-up after surgical closure of ventricular septal defect in infancy and childhood. *J Am Coll Cardiol* 1994;24:1358–1364.

Hein R, Buscheck F, Fischer E, et al. Atrial and ventricular septal defects can safely be closed by percutaneous intervention. *J Interv Cardiol* 2005;18:515–522.

Landzberg MJ, Lock JE. Transcatheter management of ventricular septal rupture after myocardial infarction. *Semin Thorac Cardiovasc Surg* 1998;10:128–132.

Lock JE, Block PC, McKay RG, et al. Transcatheter closure of ventricular septal defects. *Circulation* 1988;78:361–368.

Mahoney LT. Acyanotic congenital heart disease: atrial and ventricular septal defects, atrioventricular canal, patent ductus arteriosus, pulmonic stenosis. *Cardiol Clin* 1993;11:603–616.

Milo S, Ho SY, Wilkinson JL, et al. Surgical anatomy and atrioventricular conduction tissues of hearts with isolated VSDs. *J Thorac Cardiovasc Surg* 1980;79:244.

Minette MS, Sahn DJ. Ventricular Septal Defects. *Circulation* 2006;114:2190–2197.
Neumayer U, Stone S, Somerville J. Small ventricular septal defects in adults. *Eur Heart J* 1998;19:1573.
O'Fallon MW, Weidman WH, eds. Long-term follow-up of congenital aortic stenosis, pulmonary stenosis, and ventricular septal defect. Report from the Second Joint Study on the Natural History of Congenital Heart Defects (NHS-2). *Circulation* 1993;87[Suppl II]:II-1–II-126.
O'Laughlin MP, Mullins CE. Transcatheter closure of ventricular septal defect. *Catheter Cardiovasc Diagn* 1989;17:175–179.
Pesonen E, Thilen U, Sandstrom S, et al. Transcatheter closure of post-infarction ventricular septal defect with the Amplatzer Septal Occluder device. *Scand Cardiovasc J* 2000;34:446–448.
Somerville J. How to manage the Eisenmenger syndrome. *Int J Cardiol* 1998;63:1–8.
Szkutnik M, Quareshi SA, Kusa J, et al. Use of the Amplatzer muscular ventricular septal defect occluder for closure of perimembranous ventricular septal defects. *Heart* 2007;93:355–358.
Walsh MA, Coleman DM, Oslizlok P, et al. Percutaneous closure of postoperative ventricular septal defects with the Amplatzer device. *Catheter Cardiovasc Interv* 2006;67:445–451.

Relevant Book Chapters

Brecker SJD. Ventricular septal defect. In: Redington A, Shore D, Oldershaw P, eds. *Congenital heart disease in adults: a practical guide.* London: WB Saunders, 1994:111–117.
Driscoll DJ, eds. *Moss and Adams' heart disease in infants, children, and adolescents, including the fetus and young adult,* 6th ed. Philadelphia: Lippincott Williams & Wilkins, 2001:636–651.
Gumbiner CH, Takao A. Ventricular septal defect. In: Garson A, Bricker JT, Fisher DJ, Neish SR, eds. *The science and practice of pediatric cardiology,* 2nd ed. Baltimore: Williams & Wilkins, 1998:1119–1140.
McDaniel NL, Gutgesell HP. Ventricular septal defects. In: Allen HD, Gutgesell HP, Clark EB, et al., eds. Survival patterns without cardiac surgery or interventional catheterization: a narrowing base. In: Perloff JK, Child JS, eds. *Congenital heart disease in adults,* 2nd ed. Philadelphia: WB Saunders, 1998:15–53.
Ritter SB, eds. *Echocardiography in pediatric heart disease,* 2nd ed. St. Louis: Mosby, 1997:246–265.
Snider AR, Serwer GA, Ritter SB. Defects in cardiac septation. In: Snider AR, Serwer GA, Ritter SB, eds. *Echocardiography in pediatric heart disease*, 2nd ed. St. Louis: Mosby, 1997:246–265.

31 PATENT DUCTUS ARTERIOSUS AND COARCTATION OF THE AORTA

Matthew A. Kaminiski and Arman T. Askari

I. PATENT DUCTUS ARTERIOSUS–INTRODUCTION

A. The ductus arteriosus is a fetal communication between the descending aorta just distal to the left subclavian artery and the main pulmonary artery near its bifurcation. A patent ductus arteriosus (PDA) occurs when the ductus arteriosus fails to close after birth. PDA occurs in approximately 1 of 2000 live births but is relatively uncommon among the adult population. In infants, it accounts for 10% to 12% of all congenital heart disease.

B. Natural history. The natural history depends on the size of the PDA, the direction of the shunt, and the development of any associated complications. At birth, 95% of patients with isolated PDA have left-to-right shunts and normal, or near-normal, pulmonary pressures. Patients with normal pulmonary artery pressures and no evidence of chronic left ventricular volume overload have a better prognosis. If untreated, life expectancy of patients with PDA is shortened; one-third of patients with PDA die by age 40 years, and almost two-thirds die by age 60 years. With a PDA, **congestive heart failure (CHF) can occur** because of chronic left heart volume overload. In patients with death related to PDA, CHF is the most common cause. Development of right-to-left shunting is also an ominous sign because it reflects the development of advanced pulmonary vascular disease and associated elevation in right-sided cardiac pressures (see Chapter 32 for discussion of Eisenmenger's syndrome).

C. Risk factors for PDA include maternal rubella infection, birth at high altitude, premature birth, female sex, and genetic factors. In infants born at less than 28 weeks of gestation, there is a 60% incidence of PDA. PDAs are two to three times more common in female infants than in male infants, and have a hereditary component. In a family in which one child has a PDA, there is approximately a 3% risk of having a PDA in subsequent offsping.

II. ANATOMY AND PATHOPHYSIOLOGY

A. Embryology. The ductus arteriosus is a **normal and essential component** of cardiovascular development that originates from the distal sixth left aortic arch. Variations in the side on which the arch is situated or branch vessels originate can cause abnormally positioned or bilateral ductus arteriosus. A PDA is most commonly funnel-shaped with the larger aortic end (ampulla) narrowing down to the pulmonary end.

B. Fetal circulation. The presence of the ductus arteriosus in the fetal circulation is essential to allow **preferential shunting of nutrient-rich, oxygenated blood from the placenta to the fetal systemic circulation, thereby bypassing the fetal pulmonary circuit.** In the normal fetal circulation, oxygenated blood travels from the mother through the placenta to the fetus. The oxygen-rich blood traverses the fetal inferior vena cava, right atrium, right ventricle, and main pulmonary artery. The fetal pulmonary arteries are constricted and have high pulmonary vascular resistance. Oxygenated blood bypasses the fetal pulmonary circulation and enters through the ductus arteriosus to the lower-resistance systemic circulation. Oxygenated blood then enters the fetal aorta distal to the left subclavian artery, perfuses the fetal systemic circulation, becomes deoxygenated, and returns to the maternal circulation. **In the fetus, the ductus arteriosus is maintained open by low arterial oxygen content and placental prostaglandins.**

C. Birth. Several **changes occur at birth** to initiate normal functional **closure of the ductus arteriosus within the first 15 to 18 hours of life.** Spontaneous respirations result in increased blood oxygen content. Prostaglandin levels decrease because of placental ligation and increased metabolism of prostaglandins within the pulmonary circulation. The combination of increased oxygen content and lowered circulating prostaglandin levels usually results in closure of the ductus arteriosus. Generally, the ductus arteriosus is hemodynamically insignificant within 15 hours and completely closed by 2 to 3 weeks. The **fibrotic remnant** of this structure persists in the adult as the **ligamentum arteriosum. Spontaneous closure of a PDA is unlikely in term infants after 3 months and in preterm infants after 12 months.**

III. CLINICAL PRESENTATION

A. Symptoms. Severity of symptoms depends on the size of the PDA, ductal resistance, cardiac output, as well as the systemic and pulmonary vascular resistances. Between 25% and 40% of patients with PDA are asymptomatic, especially those with a small PDA. With larger PDAs, symptoms may develop. The most common symptom is exercise intolerance followed by dyspnea, peripheral edema, and palpitations. As is often the case in adult congenital heart disease, a previously well-tolerated PDA may become manifest in the setting of acquired heart disease such as ischemia, essential hypertension, and valvular disease.

B. Physical examination. Patients with PDAs may present with a wide range of physical findings. Pulse pressure may be wide because of diastolic runoff into the PDA, and peripheral pulses may be bounding. The jugular venous pressure is often normal with a small PDA, whereas with a large PDA, prominent *a* and *v* waves may be present. Precordial palpation often reveals a normal precordial impulse with a small PDA and a prominent left ventricular impulse with a large PDA. A **harsh, continuous murmur may be heard at the left first or second intercostal space.** The murmur envelops the second heart sound (S_2) and decreases in intensity during diastole. A small PDA has a soft, high-frequency, continuous murmur, whereas a large PDA classically has a machinery-like, loud murmur. With a large PDA, a mid-diastolic apical murmur may occur because of increased diastolic flow across the mitral valve. If **pulmonary hypertension** is present, a right ventricular lift may be present, and the pulmonic component of S_2 has increased intensity. The duration of the diastolic murmur reflects pulmonary artery pressures. Elevated pulmonary artery pressures lead to a decreased gradient for left-to-right flow through the PDA during diastole, which results in a shorter diastolic murmur. As pulmonary pressures further increase, the systolic component of the murmur then shortens. Right-to-left flow may not generate a systolic murmur. For patients with a right-to-left shunt, a pathognomonic physical finding is **differential cyanosis of the lower extremities and left hand.**

C. Complications of PDA include **CHF, infective endocarditis**, and **pulmonary hypertension.** CHF occurs through volume overload of the left side of the heart and may be accompanied by **atrial fibrillation**. Vegetations generally develop on the pulmonary side of the PDA, and septic lung emboli may occur. Untreated PDAs with audible murmurs have a risk of infective endocarditis of 0.45% per year after the second decade. Spontaneously occurring **aneurysms of the ductus arteriosus** have been reported, although typically in association with endarteritis or among very young or very old patients. Pulmonary hypertension develops as a result of increased pulmonary vascular flow from a large PDA with significant left-to-right flow. Elevation in right-sided pressures may eventually result in Eisenmenger's physiology, right-to-left flow, and isolated cyanosis and clubbing of lower extremities (occuring in 5% of unrepaired PDA patients) with signs of pulmonary hypertension.

D. Differential diagnosis of PDA includes ventricular septal defect associated with aortic insufficiency, aortopulmonary window, pulmonary atresia with systemic collateral vessels, innocent venous hum, and arteriovenous malformations such as pulmonary arteriovenous fistula, coronary artery fistula, systemic arteriovenous fistula, and ruptured sinus of Valsalva.

IV. LABORATORY TESTING

A. Blood work results are generally unremarkable, although compensatory erythrocytosis may be present in the setting of long-standing cyanosis resulting from a right-to-left shunt.

B. Electrocardiogram (ECG) is neither sensitive nor specific for PDA. The ECG for a patient with a small PDA often is normal. Depending on the duration and hemodynamic significance of the PDA, electrocardiographic criteria for left atrial enlargement or left ventricular hypertrophy may be present. If pulmonary hypertension exists, the ECG may demonstrate right ventricular hypertrophy or right atrial enlargement.

C. Chest radiography is neither sensitive nor specific for PDA. A normal chest radiograph implies a small, hemodynamically insignificant PDA. With a large PDA, left atrial and left ventricular enlargement may be present, as well as increased pulmonary vascularity. With right-to-left shunting from pulmonary hypertension, the main pulmonary artery is frequently enlarged. The PDA occasionally appears as a separate convexity between the aortic knob and pulmonary trunk. Calcification of the PDA may be visualized in older individuals.

V. DIAGNOSTIC TESTING.

Standard transthoracic echocardiography (TTE) is the preferred initial diagnostic modality because of its low cost and noninvasive nature. Transesophageal echocardiography (TEE) may be required in subjects with suboptimal echocardiographic windows. Cardiac catheterization is typically reserved for therapeutic intervention.

A. TTE has a 42% sensitivity and 100% specificity for the diagnosis of PDA. The suprasternal notch views are usually the best views for demonstrating the PDA, especially its aortic origin. The complete course of a PDA may be difficult to follow in some patients because of its tortuosity. Color Doppler imaging often can reveal flow between the descending aorta distal to the left subclavian artery and the pulmonary trunk. It is imperative to demonstrate color Doppler flow within the pulmonary artery, typically on a high parasternal short-axis view. Color Doppler and continuous-wave Doppler help determine direction of flow in the PDA. The timing of flow (systolic or diastolic) depends on pressure gradients between the systemic and pulmonary circulation. Quantitative assessment of shunt velocity is valuable to estimate degree of restriction across the PDA. This measurement becomes important in planning transcatheter intervention. Diastolic flow reversal is seen in the descending aorta if the shunt is significant. Associated left atrial and left ventricular enlargement also suggests a hemodynamically significant lesion.

B. TEE may be required if TTE windows are suboptimal or nondiagnostic. TTE and TEE have nearly 100% specificity for diagnosis of PDA, but TEE has much higher sensitivity (97%) than TTE (42%).

C. Cardiac catheterization is usually not needed for diagnostic purposes. Rarely, PDAs undiagnosed by physical examination or noninvasive testing may be diagnosed during left heart or right heart cardiac catheterization by recognizing the unexpected course of the catheter as it crosses the PDA, or by measuring a step-up in the oxygen saturation at the level of the left pulmonary artery.

1. A PDA is best demonstrated by a **descending aortogram** performed in the **lateral projection** with a standard angiographic catheter positioned just below the ductal ampulla. If biplanar imaging is used, the right anterior-oblique cranial projection is sometimes helpful.
2. A PDA can be crossed antegrade from the main pulmonary artery or can be crossed retrograde from the descending aorta, best guided by the lateral projection. Oximetric sampling typically demonstrates an increase in saturation in the main pulmonary artery compared with the right ventricle. Pulmonary artery and right ventricular pressures may be slightly elevated but typically remain below systemic levels. The presence of systemic pulmonary pressures indicates the possibility of pulmonary arterial vascular disease, pulmonary venous stenosis, mitral stenosis, or left ventricular failure.

D. Magnetic resonance imaging and computed tomography may be useful in defining the anatomy in patients with unusual PDA geometry and in patients with associated abnormalities of the aortic arch.

VI. THERAPY. Because of the natural history of persistent PDA, **closure of all PDAs is recommended at the time of diagnosis in adults.** The exception is a small PDA without an audible murmur (i.e., silent PDA) without left heart enlargement in an asymptomatic patient that is discovered incidentally on TTE. Whether such PDAs should be closed is controversial, but given the safety and efficacy of percutaneous closure methods, it is reasonable to pursue this treatment strategy to prevent the development of left ventricular volume overload or endarteritis. Successful closure of PDA results in a good prognosis and may prevent adverse left ventricular remodeling as a result of volume overload.

The shape and size of a PDA determine the mode of therapy. Small- or moderate-caliber PDAs are generally closed percutaneously with coils. Large PDAs may require the Amplatzer duct occluder (ADO) or surgery. Heavily calcified PDAs represent a relative contraindication to surgical closure because of an increased risk for bleeding and incomplete closure with surgery. Cardiopulmonary bypass may be required for heavily calcified PDAs. PDAs with significant right-to-left shunts and Eisenmenger's physiology are generally not closed unless the patient has had a prior episode of infective endarteritis. In patients with pulmonary vascular resistance greater than 8 U/m^2, lung biopsy has been recommended to determine candidacy for closure. However, even histologically severe pulmonary vascular disease may resolve after closure of the PDA. Reactivity of the pulmonary vascular bed to pulmonary vasodilating agents or significant reduction in pulmonary artery pressure during test occlusion may signal reversibility of pulmonary hypertension, but the absence of these findings does not rule out the possibility of reversibility in the long term.

A. Since the early 1990s, **transcatheter techniques** have become the **first-line therapy for most PDAs**. Many centers use single or multiple stainless steel coils to achieve complete closure. Numerous devices have been adapted or are under clinical investigation to allow transcatheter closure of larger defects. These procedures can often be performed on an outpatient basis, and complete closure rates at follow-up generally exceed 90% to 95% in most studies. The mortality rate is typically less than 1% at experienced centers. Success has been reported even when ductal calcification has been apparent, but large clinical series are lacking. Brief descriptions of percutaneous therapies follow.

1. **Percutaneous coil occlusion.** Percutaneous coils were developed in 1992 and are the **preferred treatment for older children and adults with small or medium-sized PDAs** (<3.5 mm). Embolization coils have thrombogenic strands spanning

the coils and are placed across the PDA to occlude flow. Advantages include low cost, small-caliber venous access, and easy implantation. Advances include detachable coils and development of a snare-assisted technique, both of which allow assessment and fine-tuning of correct coil position before actual release of the coil. The coils are loaded at the tip of a catheter, the catheter is placed in the PDA under fluoroscopic guidance, and the coils then deployed. Coil sizes are 2 to 2.5 times the narrowest diameter of the PDA. With moderate- or large-sized PDAs, multiple coils may be used. However, as PDA size becomes larger (>3.5 to 4.0 mm), percutaneous, 0.038-inch coils become a less desired closure option, and alternative therapies become preferred. Although with children complete closure is usually accomplished with a single coil, multiple coils are frequently needed for complete closure in the adult. Although coil embolization may occur, the snare-assisted technique is almost always successful at percutaneous removal of the coil.

2. The **Amplatzer Ductal Occluder (ADO)**, a cone-shaped plug occluder made of thrombogenic wire mesh delivered with a 5F to 7F venous system, is the **preferred device for percutaneous closure of moderate to large PDAs.** The ADO stents the PDA, and blood is forced to flow through the center of the device, which is lined with thrombogenic wire mesh. The PDA then essentially clots off. Advantages include simple implantation, ability to retract the ADO into the sheath and redeploy if needed, and high success rates. There is an 89% occlusion rate day 1 postprocedure and 97% to 100% complete occlusion after 1 month.
3. **Complications** of transcatheter closure are rare. The most common complication is embolization of the coil or device. Embolized coils are usually able to be retrieved, but even when this is impossible, adverse consequences are rare. Other potential complications include flow disturbance in the pulmonary artery or aorta from device protrusion, hemolysis from high-velocity residual shunting, vascular access complications, and infection.

B. **Surgical closure.** In 1938, the first successful closure of a PDA was performed (the first repair of a congenital heart defect). Surgical closure is the most effective method for complete closure and is usually performed without cardiopulmonary bypass by double ligation and division of the PDA. Ligation may be performed without division, but there is then a risk of recanalization of the PDA of up to 20%. In neonates and premature infants, ligation without division is performed because of the small size of the structures. With continued advances in percutaneous closure devices, **surgery has become second-line therapy for most adults with PDAs**. If surgery is necessary, the procedure is more than 95% successful and has a low complication rate. The operative mortality rate is less than 1%. However, the thoracotomy approach can be painful for adults and necessitates inpatient recovery. Newer surgical techniques such as transaxillary thoracotomy and video-assisted thorascopic ligation have improved surgical morbidity.

C. **Medical therapy.** In adults, medical therapy is ineffective to close a PDA. Medical therapy is indicated to prevent and treat complications of PDA, including heart failure, atrial arrhythmias, and pulmonary hypertension**. The most recent guidelines from the American Heart Association (AHA)** recommend antibiotic prophylaxis for endarteritis **ONLY** in the setting of transcutaneous closure of the PDA for 6 months after the procedure.

D. **Follow-up.** If immediate duct closure is demonstrated after the procedure, a 6-month follow-up with transthoracic echocardiography should suffice to assess for residual flow through the PDA. If residual shunt exists after the procedure, transthoracic echocardiography should be performed every 2 to 3 months, and early repeat attempt of complete closure considered, depending on the size of the residual shunt. For long-term follow-up, annual transthoracic echocardiograms are adequate.

VII. **COARCTATION OF THE AORTA–INTRODUCTION.** Coarctation of the aorta (CoA) has been found at necropsy in approximately 1 of every 1550 individuals. It accounts for 5% to 10% of congenital heart disease and occurs more frequently in whites (7:1) and males (2:1). The disorder is typically diagnosed in childhood but may go undetected well into adulthood. Most patients develop persistent systemic hypertension, often as children, and are at risk for premature coronary artery disease. Cases usually occur sporadically, but an autosomal-dominant inheritance pattern has been observed. It is frequently associated with bicuspid aortic valve, and coarctation should be excluded in patients with bicuspid aortic valve and hypertension. Coarctation also commonly occurs in patients with Turner's syndrome (15% to 35%). Potential catastrophic complications include aortic rupture or dissection and cerebral berry aneurysm rupture. The mean survival for untreated patients is 35 years, with a 25% survival rate beyond 50 years.

VIII. ANATOMY.

CoA usually consists of a **narrowing in the region of the ligamentum arteriosum**, the remnant of the ductus arteriosus, just distal to the origin of the left subclavian artery. Most coarctations, therefore, are juxtaductal. The exact anatomy, however, varies, and the coarctation may include a long segment, the transverse arch, or the abdominal aorta. Rarely, tortuosity of the arch is identified. The main anatomic substrate is a prominent posterior shelf of the aorta, composed predominantly of thickened media.

A. Embryology. The exact embryonic origin remains uncertain, but two main theories exist. The first suggests that the narrowing is caused by aberrant ductal tissue that constricts the aorta at time of ductal closure. The second proposes that aortic hypoplasia develops as a consequence of reduced blood flow in utero.

B. Associated cardiac defects include **bicuspid aortic valve** in 50% to 85% of cases, valvular and subvalvular aortic stenosis, ventricular septal defects, patent ductus arteriosus, and congenital malformations of the mitral valve (i.e., smaller orifice, supravalvular ring, and parachute mitral valve resulting from a single papillary muscle). Multiple left-sided heart lesions may be associated with CoA and are often referred to as the Shone complex.

C. Associated extracardiac defects include intracranial aneurysms, especially within the circle of Willis (3% to 5% of cases), hemangiomas, hypospadias, and ocular defects.

IX. CLINICAL PRESENTATION

A. Symptoms. For patients with CoA who survive to adulthood, symptoms are usually negligible and nonspecific. Patients may complain of headaches, nosebleeds, cool extremities, leg weakness, or claudication with exertion. More serious manifestations include angina and heart failure.

B. Physical examination

1. A thorough cardiovascular examination may identify a systolic ejection murmur at the left upper sternal border that radiates to the intrascapular area, located immediately anterior or posterior to the CoA. The murmur may be longer in systole and even continue into diastole, depending on the degree of obstruction. Increased flow through the collateral intercostal arteries can produce a continuous murmur appreciated diffusely over the precordium. In the setting of a bicuspid aortic valve, a systolic click may be appreciated, or systolic and diastolic murmurs of aortic stenosis/regurgitation.
2. Upper extremity hypertension is often present, usually in conjunction with **diminished and delayed femoral pulsations.** CoA should always be considered in the differential diagnosis of refractory hypertension, especially in younger patients.
3. Funduscopic examination may demonstrate a "corkscrew" tortuosity of the retinal arterioles.

X. DIAGNOSTIC TESTING

A. The **electrocardiogram** is frequently normal but may demonstrate manifestations of long-standing hypertension, such as left ventricular hypertrophy and left atrial enlargement.

B. Chest radiography. Cardiomegaly, dilated ascending aorta, and prominent pulmonary vasculature are common. **Rib notching** usually develops by 4 to 12 years of age and is caused by enlarged intercostal collaterals. The **classic "3" or inverted-E sign is pathognomonic** for CoA and is created by a dilated left subclavian artery above the CoA, and poststenotic dilation of the aorta below the CoA.

C. **Echocardiography** is most useful in infants and children. In adults, the suprasternal notch view is most helpful; color Doppler can be used to localize the site of turbulence. Continuous-wave Doppler can assess the pressure gradient. If severe narrowing is present, persistence of flow in diastole (widening of the flow profile from systole into diastole) is seen by continuous-wave Doppler in the aorta below the coarctation such as in the abdominal aorta. This is useful method to ascertain the presence of coarctation, even if imaging the direct site of the obstruction is impossible. A complete study should measure left ventricular size and ascending aortic size, determine aortic valve anatomy and function, and identify any potential associated congenital anomalies. Transesophageal echocardiography can better define the anatomy if transthoracic echocardiography proves inadequate.

D. **Magnetic resonance Imaging (MRI)** provides excellent anatomic and hemodynamic information. MRI is increasingly used as a first-line investigation before catheterization, especially in adults. This enables the precise anatomy to be delineated and helps in the decision-making regarding surgery or catheterization as treatment options. Serial MRI scans may be used to follow results of therapeutic procedures. It is also useful in evaluating the intracranial vessels for associated berry aneurysms.

E. **Cardiac catheterization** provides excellent image data and pressure information, and is often more reliable than echocardiography in adults. An **aortic angiogram** in left anterior oblique or caudal and direct lateral projections usually best defines the lesion. Pressures should be obtained in the left ventricle and the ascending aorta, and the gradient across the lesion should be measured. A **pullback pressure of more than 20 mm Hg** signifies hemodynamic significance and usually warrants intervention if concomitant clinical factors allow. A **gradient of more than 50 mm Hg** generally mandates intervention. The presence of collateral vessels may falsely diminish the gradient.

XI. THERAPY.

Several factors need to be taken into account when deciding on optimal therapy for CoA, including the age of the patient, the anatomy of the coarctation, any prior CoA operations, and the local surgical expertise. Whatever the mode of treatment chosen, the presence of postprocedural upper extremity hypertension influences survival.

A. In general, **medical therapy** for CoA has limited utility, but it may be useful in a supportive role along with mechanical treatment. Hypertension should be medically treated, with the goal of controlling blood pressure and preventing end-organ damage.

B. **Percutaneous management**

1. **Percutaneous balloon angioplasty** is generally less effective than surgery for primary treatment of coarctation. Neonates and infants treated with angioplasty experience high rates of recurrent CoA (about 50% to 60%) and aneurysm formations (5% to 20%); therefore, surgical repair is preferred in this patient population. Likewise, balloon angioplasty of the unoperated coarctation in adults is controversial, with data suggesting higher rates of restenosis and aneurysm formation compared to surgical repair. Procedural complications can include acute aortic rupture (rare), aortic dissection, femoral artery trauma, recurrent coarctation (8%), and aneurysm formation (8% to 35%). The suspected mechanism for late aneurysm formation is intimal tear at the site of cystic medial necrosis within the coarctation site. It should be noted that the clinical impact of aneurysm formation is unclear, as most defects are small and have a low risk of rupture. Percutaneous angioplasty, however, is the preferred therapy for recurrent postsurgical coarctation. The procedure is successful in reducing the gradient to less than 20 mm Hg in approximately 80% of interventions, with a 1.5% incidence of late aneurysm formation.

2. **Stent implantation.** Theoretically, stent implantation may mitigate the development of aneurysm or dissection for a few reasons. By apposing the torn intima to the media and through disperson of force, stenting may limit vascular trauma. It can also oppose the vascular recoil of the coarcted segment and avoid overdilation. By allowing the use of smaller balloons and graded inflations in staged procedures, stents may also reduce rates of aneurysm formation. Early

and intermediate outcomes are promising with a good safety and efficacy profile as well as lower rates of restenosis and aneurysm formation compared to balloon angioplasty. Despite the lack of long-term outcome data, it has become the preferred treatment modality in adults and adult-sized adolescents with native CoA. For re-coarctation, balloon angioplasty with or without stenting is preferred in adults as well, if the anatomy is suitable.

C. **Surgery** remains the therapy of choice in neonates and infants. Three types of surgical repair have been used for correction of CoA: resection of the stenosed segment with end-to-end anastomosis, use of a subclavian flap, and patch aortoplasty. The approach with the best relief of obstruction and long-term outcome has been resection of the stenosed segment with end-to-end anastomosis. This approach carries with it the lowest risk of recurrent CoA (3%) and late aneurysm formation (rare). Paradoxical hypertension and bowel ischemia may occur in the postoperative period. Major surgical complications include paraplegia caused by perioperative spinal cord ischemia (0.4% to 1%), residual coarctation, aneurysm formation at the site of repair, and, rarely, death. Survival rates of more than 90% at 10 years and 84% at 20 years have been reported. Late deaths after surgical repair are related primarily to coronary artery disease, congestive heart failure, and aneurysm rupture. Young age favorably influences outcomes after surgery.

XII. **FOLLOW-UP.** Lifelong follow-up is indicated after the diagnosis of CoA is established, especially after any type of mechanical repair. Key issues to be cognizant of include the progression of hypertension either at rest or with exercise, development of CoA recurrence, aneurysm formation, left ventricular dysfunction, and associated aortic valve dysfunction when bicuspid valve is present. In older patients, hypertension commonly persists despite treatment by percutaneous intervention or surgery. Serial echocardiography is an important component of follow-up. Advanced imaging modalities such as computed tomography or MRI are used increasingly post-repair to screen for aortic wall complications. Therefore, these patients should be considered "treated" and not "cured" despite repair.

ACKNOWLEDGMENTS

The authors thank Drs. Michael S. Chen, J. Donald Moore, and Adrian W. Messerli for their contributions to earlier editions of this chapter.

Landmark Articles—PDA

Bermudez-Canete R, Santoro G, Bialkowsky J, et al. Patent ductus arteriosus occlusion using detachable coils. *Am J Cardiol* 1998;82:1547–1549.

Bilkis AA, Alwi M, Hasri S, et al. The Amplatzer duct occluder: experience in 209 patients. *J Am Coll Cardiol* 2001;37:258–261.

Eerola A, Jokinen E, Boldt T, et al. The influence of percutaneous closure of patent ductus arteriosus on left ventricular size and function: a prospective study using two- and three-dimensional echocardiography and measurements of serum natriuretic peptides. *J Am Coll Cardiol* 2006;47:1060–1066.

Fisher RG, Moodie DS, Sterba R, et al. Patent ductus arteriosus—long-term follow-up: nonsurgical versus surgical treatment. *J Am Coll Cardiol* 1986;8:280–284.

Harrison DA, Benson LN, Lazzam C, et al. Percutaneous catheter closure of the persistently patent ductus arteriosus in the adult. *Am J Cardiol* 1996;77:1094–1097.

Huggon IC, Qureshi SA. Is the prevention of infective endarteritis a valid reason for closure of the patent arterial duct? *Eur Heart J* 1997;18:364–366.

Ing FF, Mullins CE, Rose M, et al. Transcatheter closure of the patent ductus arteriosus in adults using the Gianturco coil. *Clin Cardiol* 1996;19:875–879.

Ing FF, Somner RJ. The snare-assisted technique for transcatheter coil occlusion of moderate to large patent ductus arteriosus: immediate and intermediate results. *J Am Coll Cardiol* 1999;33:1710–1718.

Janorkar S, Goh T, Wilkinson J. Transcatheter closure of patent ductus arteriosus with the use of Rashkind occluders and/or Gianturco coils: long-term follow-up in 123 patients and special reference to comparison, residual shunts, complications and technique. *Am Heart J* 1999;138:1176–1183.

Laborde F, Folliguet TA, Etienne PY, et al. Video-thoracoscopic surgical interruption of patent ductus arteriosus. Routine experience in 332 pediatric cases. *Eur J Cardiothorac Surg* 1997;11:1052–1055.

Pass RH, Hijazi Z, Hsu DT, et al. Multicenter USA Amplatzer patent ductus arteriosus occlusion device trial: initial and one-year results. *J Am Coll Cardiol* 2004;44:513–519.

Rao RP, Kim SH, Choi J-Y, et al. Follow-up results of transvenous occlusion of patent ductus arteriosus with the buttoned device. *J Am Coll Cardiol* 1999;33:820–826.

Schenck MH, O'Laughlin MP, Rokey R, et al. Transcatheter occlusion of patent ductus arteriosus in adults. *Am J Cardiol* 1993;72:591–595.

Shim D, Fedderly R, Beekman RH, et al. Follow-up coil occlusion of patent ductus arteriosus. *J Am Coll Cardiol* 1996;28:207–211.

Shyu KG, Lai LP, Lin SC, et al. Diagnostic accuracy of transesophageal echocardiography for detecting patent ductus arteriosus in adolescents and adults. *Chest* 1995;108:1201–1205.

Thanopoulos BD, Hakim FA, Hiari A, et al. Further experience with transcatheter closure of the patent ductus arteriosus using the Amplatzer duct occluder. *J Am Coll Cardiol* 2000;35:1016–1021.

Thilen U, Astrom-Olsson K. Does the risk of infective endarteritis justify routine patent ductus arteriosus closure? *Eur Heart J* 1997;18:503–506.

Wang J-K, Liau C-S, Huang J-J, et al. Transcatheter closure of patent ductus arteriosus using Gianturco coils in adolescents and adults. *Catheter Cardiovasc Interv* 2002;55:513–518.

Key Reviews—PDA

Brickner ME, Hillis LD, Lange RA. Medical progress: congenital heart disease in adults: first of two parts. *N Engl J Med* 2000;342:256–263.

Connelly MS, Webb GD, Sommerville J, et al. Canadian Consensus Conference on Adult Congenital Heart Disease, 1996. *Can J Cardiol* 1998;14:395–452.

Krasuski RA. Patent ductus arteriosus closure. *J Interv Cardiol* 2006;19:S60–S66.

Schneider DJ, Moore JW. Patent ductus arteriosus. *Circulation* 2006;114:1873–1882.

Book Chapters—PDA

Moore P, Brook MM, Heymann MA. Patent ductus arteriosus. In: Allen HD, Gutgesell HP, Clark EB, et al., eds. *Moss and Adams' heart disease in infants, children, and adolescents, including the fetus and young adult*, 6th ed. Philadelphia: Lippincott Williams & Wilkins, 2001:652–669.

Mullins CE, Pagotto L. PDA. In: Garson A, Bricker JT, Fisher DJ, et al., eds. *The science and practice of pediatric cardiology*, 2nd ed. Baltimore: Williams & Wilkins, 1998:1181–1197.

Perloff JL. *The clinical recognition of congenital heart disease*, 5th ed. Philadelphia: Saunders, 2003.

Topol EJ, ed. *Textbook of cardiovascular medicine*, 3rd ed.. Philadelphia: Lippincott Williams & Wilkins, 2006:506–507.

Landmark Articles—Coarctation

Blackford LM. Coarctation of the aorta. *Arch Intern Med* 1928;41:702–735.

Campbell M, Baylass JH. The course and prognosis of coarctation of the aorta. *Br Heart J* 1956;18:475–495.

Carr JA. The results of catheter-based therapy compared with surgical repair of adult aortic coarctation. *J Am Coll Cardiol* 2006;47:1101–1107.

Cowley CG, Orsmond GS, et al. Long-term, randomized comparison of balloon angioplasty and surgery for native coarctation of the aorta in childhood. *Circulation* 2005;111:3453–3456.

Fawzy ME, Awad M, et al. Long-term outcome (up to 15 years) of balloon angioplasty of discrete native coarctation of the aorta in adolescents and adults. *J Am Coll Cardiol* 2004;43:1062–1067.

Rao PS, Galal O, et al. Five- to nine-year follow-up results of balloon angioplasty of native aortic coarctation in infants and children. *J Am Coll Cardiol* 1996;27:462–470.

Walhout RJ, Lekkerkerker JC, et al. Comparison of surgical repair with balloon angioplasty for native coarctation in patients from 3 months to 16 years of age. *Eur J Cardiothorac Surg* 2004;25:722–727.

Key Reviews—Coarctation

Aboulhosn J, Child JS. Left ventricular outflow obstruction: subaortic stenosis, bicuspid aortic valve, supravalvar aortic stenosis, and coarctation of the aorta. *Circulation* 2006;114:2412–1422.

Inglessis I, Landzberg MJ. Interventional catheterization in adult congenital heart disease. *Circulation* 2007;115:1622–1633.

Relevant Book Chapters—Coarctation

Beekman III RH. Coarctation of the aorta. In: Allen HD, Gutgesell HP, Clark EB, et al., eds. *Moss and Adams' heart disease in infants, children, and adolescents, including the fetus and young adult*, 6th ed. Philadelphia: Lippincott Williams & Wilkins, 2001:988–1010.

Brickner JT, Fisher DJ, et al., eds. *The Science and Practice of Pediatric Cardiology*. 2nd ed. Baltimore: Lippincott Williams & Wilkins, 1998:1317–1346.

Morriss MJH, McNamara DG. Coarctation of the aorta and interrupted aortic arch. In: Garson A, Brickner JT, Fisher DJ, et al., eds. *The Science and practice of pediatric cardiology*, 2nd ed. Baltimore: Williams & Wilkins, 1998:1317–1346.

COMPLEX CONGENITAL HEART DISEASE

Yuli Y. Kim and Athar M. Qureshi

32

I. TETRALOGY OF FALLOT. Tetralogy of Fallot (TOF) is the most common form of cyanotic heart disease. It occurs in approximately 1 in 3000 live births and accounts for 10% of congenital heart disease in infants. It is also the most common congenital heart disease requiring surgical correction in the first year of life. The earliest description of TOF dates back to the 17th century; however, Fallot is credited with describing the classic features of the disease in 1888. Surgical treatment for TOF did not become available until well into the 20th century, and it dramatically improved life expectancy. The current reparative approach has shifted from palliative shunt procedures to primary surgical repair, usually performed in infancy. Without surgical intervention, only about 10% of patients survive beyond the age of 20 years. Adults with TOF usually have undergone surgical repair or palliation. A wide and complex spectrum of TOF exists including association with pulmonary atresia, absent pulmonary valve, and atrioventricular canal defects. Classic "simple" tetralogy of Fallot is discussed here.

A. Anatomy

1. **Anterocephalad deviation of the outlet septum** results in four defining features:
   - **a.** Right ventricular (RV) outflow tract obstruction
   - **b.** Nonrestrictive ventricular septal defect (VSD)
   - **c.** Aortic override of the ventricular septum
   - **d.** Right ventricular hypertrophy (RVH)
2. **Associated defects.** Anomalous origin of the left anterior descending coronary artery from the right coronary artery (5%), or a prominent conal branch from the right coronary artery can occur. These vessels cross the RV outflow tract. This anatomic feature is important to surgeons because infundibular resection or future conduit placement may be needed in this location. Right aortic arch occurs in 25% of cases. A secundum ASD occurs in 15% of cases, completing the pentalogy of Fallot. Left superior vena cava is found in 5% of patients. Among adult patients, aortic insufficiency can occur naturally from long-term dilation of the aortic root, after endocarditis, or as a postoperative sequela. Rarely supravalvular mitral stenosis and subaortic stenosis may occur. There is an association with deletion in the chromosome 22q11 region, and, hence, in association with DiGeorge syndrome and/or velocardiofacial syndrome.

B. Clinical presentation

1. **Patients who have not undergone surgical repair** have variable clinical features depending on the amount of RV outflow tract obstruction, degree of aortic override, and, to a lesser extent, systemic vascular resistance, all of which dictate the amount and direction of shunting across the VSD.
   - **a.** With severe RV outflow tract obstruction, patients have central cyanosis and clubbing by 6 months of age. Hypoxic "spells" may be seen and are characterized by tachypnea, dyspnea, cyanosis, or even loss of consciousness or death. If the obstruction is mild, however, the shunt through the VSD may be left-to-right resulting in "pink tet" and with minimal symptoms.
   - **b.** On physical examination, the patient is usually cyanotic and clubbed. A prominent RV impulse may be appreciated because of equalization of right and left ventricular pressures. A lift may be palpated under the right sternoclavicular junction with a right-sided arch. The first heart sound (S_1) is usually normal but

the second heart sound (S_2) is single because of an inaudible P_2. Auscultation is notable for a prominent systolic ejection murmur at the left upper sternal border, possibly with an associated thrill. The shorter the murmur, the more severe the infundibular pulmonic stenosis. The murmur of aortic insufficiency may be audible along with an aortic click resulting from a dilated overriding aorta. Continuous murmurs may be heard due to aortopulmonary collateral vessels. The presence of these vessels are more likely to be found in the setting of pulmonary atresia but can be acquired if progressive RV outflow tract stenosis develops.

2. Most adult congenital patients will have undergone surgical repair with or without a prior palliative procedure. The term "**palliation**" (as opposed to "repair") in these patients refers to a surgical procedure that consists of a **systemic-to-pulmonary artery shunt** (modified Blalock-Taussig shunt, classic Blalock-Taussig shunt, Potts shunt, or Waterston shunt); refer to Table 32.1. These procedures are initially performed to supplement the deficiency of antegrade pulmonary blood flow and are taken down at the time of complete repair. The latter two procedures have been abandoned owing to associated uncontrolled pulmonary blood flow and the development of pulmonary hypertension.
   a. Patients who have undergone palliative repair alone have variable clinical findings depending on the type of palliation performed. In those who have undergone a Blalock-Taussig shunt, the brachial pulse on that side may be diminished or absent. With time, the shunts may remain patent and produce a continuous murmur or may be silent if the shunt has occluded. Continuous murmurs from collateral formation may be audible. Branch pulmonary artery stenosis at prior shunt insertion sites can produce unilateral systolic or continuous murmurs. Systolic ejection murmurs may be audible depending on the degree of antegrade flow across the outflow tract.
3. **Complete (or total) repair** consists of patch closure of the VSD and variable degrees of RV outflow tract resection and reconstruction. It may involve pulmonary valvuloplasty or valvotomy, RV outflow tract patch augmentation, transannular patch enlargement, or placement of a right ventricle–to–pulmonary artery conduit (i.e., bioprosthetic or homograft). Distal branch pulmonary artery stenosis may have been repaired, or residual lesions may be present. These patients typically have first undergone a palliative shunt procedure, but the current surgical approach has shifted to primary complete repair in infancy.
   a. Patients are often asymptomatic. They may present with late symptoms such as dyspnea, exercise intolerance, palpitations, signs of right heart failure, or syncope.
   b. The jugular venous pressure is usually normal unless there is RV dysfunction, in which case elevated jugular venous pressure with a prominent *a* wave is seen. The brisk pulse of aortic insufficiency may be appreciated. On palpation, there may be an RV lift or a lift under the right sternoclavicular junction with a right-sided arch. Some degree of turbulence almost always remains across the RV outflow tract and produces a variable systolic ejection murmur at the left upper sternal border with radiation to the back and peripheral lung fields. Of importance is the presence of associated pulmonary insufficiency which, if severe, can occasionally be inaudible due to low pressure hemodynamics. It is appreciated also at the left upper sternal border, sometimes producing a to-and-fro murmur together with the outflow tract murmur. A high-frequency systolic murmur at the left lower sternal border suggests the presence of a residual VSD commonly caused by a small VSD patch leak. Continuous murmurs from collateral formation or prior shunts may be appreciated. The diastolic murmur of aortic insufficiency may be heard.

C. **Laboratory examination**
   1. **Chest radiographic** findings depend on the surgical history. The presence of a right aortic arch may be confirmed. A concave deficiency of the left heart border reflects various degrees of pulmonary arterial hypoplasia. Upturning of the apex from RVH causes the classic finding of a boot-shaped heart. Pulmonary vascular

TABLE 32.1 Index of Postoperative Anatomy Among Adult Patients with Congenital Heart Disease

Underlying pathology	Procedure	Notes
Single ventricle — hypoplastic left heart — tricuspid atresia — pulmonary atresia with intact ventricular septum — unbalanced complete AV canal defect	**1. Norwood**	— incorporation of native aorta and pulmonary artery (one of which may be hypoplastic or atretic) to produce a "**neoaorta**" for the single ventricle — main pulmonary artery is transected from the heart — pulmonary flow is maintained with placement of a **Blalock-Taussig shunt** — **atrial septectomy** is often performed to allow complete mixing at the atrial level
	2. Bidirectional Glenn	— usually performed at 4–6 months if pulmonary arterial anatomy, pressures, and resistance are adequate — anastomosis of the **superior vena cava to the pulmonary artery**, usually with takedown of a previously placed systemic to pulmonary artery shunt and repair of pulmonary arterial branch stenosis if necessary — term *bidirectional* is used in descriptions of this procedure because both right and left pulmonary arteries usually remain in continuity
	3. Fontan	— usually performed at 1–5 years depending on growth of vasculature and cyanosis — anastomosis of **inferior vena cava to the pulmonary artery** by intraatrial lateral tunnel or extracardiac conduit — pulmonary blood flow is achieved passively, without the assistance of a ventricular pumping chamber
D-Transposition of the great arteries (ventriculoarterial discordance)	**Rashkind**	— **atrial balloon septostomy** to create mixing of systemic and pulmonary circulation
	Blalock-Hanlon	— surgical atrial septectomy
	Mustard or Senning (atrial switch)	— baffle material (Mustard) or native atrial tissue (Senning) used to direct pulmonary venous blood → right ventricle → aorta; systemic venous blood → left ventricle → pulmonary artery
	Jatene (arterial switch)	— great arteries are transected and reanastomosed to the appropriate ventricle — coronary arteries are removed with a button of surrounding tissue and reimplanted to the appropriate sinuses
	Rastelli	— for D-TGA with VSD and pulmonary outflow tract obstruction — VSD patch closure that directs left ventricular blood across the VSD to the aorta — pulmonary valve is oversewn — valved conduit from the right ventricle to the pulmonary artery to create RV outflow
Deficient pulmonary artery or RV outflow tract — pulmonary atresia — tetralogy of Fallot with hypoplastic pulmonary arteries	**Classic Blalock-Taussig**	— native subclavian artery anastomosed to the right or left pulmonary artery
	Modified Blalock-Taussig	— expanded polytetrafluoroethylene (Gore-Tex) material connecting the subclavian or innominate artery to the pulmonary artery
	Waterston shunt	— anastomosis between the ascending aorta and right pulmonary artery
	Potts shunt	— anastomosis between the descending aorta and left pulmonary artery

markings may vary throughout the lung fields, depending on associated branch pulmonary artery stenosis and relative blood flow. Calcification or aneurysmal dilation of surgical conduits or RV outflow tract repair may be visible on plain radiographs.

2. An **electrocardiogram** usually demonstrates sinus rhythm with RVH. Both atrial and ventricular rhythm disturbances can be present. The QRS axis is usually normal or rightward. If left-axis deviation is present, an associated atrioventricular canal defect should be suspected. A patient who has undergone surgical repair typically has right bundle-branch block. A QRS duration of more than 180 ms is a predictor of sustained ventricular tachycardia and sudden cardiac death.

D. Diagnostic testing

1. Echocardiography

a. For a child or young adult, transthoracic echocardiography may be the only modality necessary for diagnosis. For adults or patients who have undergone surgical intervention, more information may be needed. The primary objectives in these cases are to **determine which residual lesions are present and their locations.**

i. Adequate views are obtained of the right heart, RV outflow tract, and proximal pulmonary arteries. Helpful views include the parasternal long-axis, parasternal short-axis, and apical four-chamber views. Further definition of residual lesions in the branch pulmonary arteries may be possible with a high parasternal short-axis view. Residual VSD and the presence of aortic insufficiency are sought on these views.

ii. Palliative shunts are often best visualized in the suprasternal notch view where the subclavian arteries course distally.

iii. Continuous flow is typically demonstrated with color Doppler techniques. Less common shunts may be difficult to image in adult patients. Aortopulmonary collateral vessels are difficult to visualize, but they may be seen in suprasternal notch views of the descending aorta.

b. **Transesophageal echocardiography** may allow improved imaging of the intracardiac anatomic structures in adults, but limitations often remain with regard to the distal pulmonary arteries, and additional testing frequently is necessary.

2. **Cardiac magnetic resonance (CMR) imaging** is considered the gold standard for evaluating the RV and quantitating pulmonary insufficiency in these patients. It can demonstrate the presence of scar, distal pulmonary arterial anatomy, and RV aneurysms, as well as other associated defects. It can also provide hemodynamic information about residual lesions. Previously placed shunts and possibly aortopulmonary collateral vessels can be identified. The anatomic information may be sufficient to proceed with surgical treatment or to guide the interventional cardiologist in planning a transcatheter procedure.

3. **Cardiopulmonary testing** should be performed as a baseline study and with progression of symptoms. It is useful in determining the timing for reintervention in the setting of RV volume overload secondary to free pulmonary insufficiency.

4. **Quantitative pulmonary flow scans** are useful to determine discrepancies in pulmonary flow that may be caused by branch pulmonary artery stenosis. These scans also provide an objective baseline clinical information when obtained after surgical or transcatheter intervention.

5. The role of **cardiac catheterization** is decreasing with the advent of other imaging modalities, but can be helpful in assessing residual shunts and pulmonary hypertension.

a. **Right heart catheterization.** Residual shunts are actively sought at the atrial and ventricular levels. The pulmonary arteries and branches are evaluated extensively in search of peripheral pulmonic stenosis. Findings at right heart catheterization and their clinical significance are as follows:

i. RV pressure is systemic in a patient who has not undergone surgical repair.

ii. After surgical repair, elevated RV pressure suggests the presence of residual obstructive lesions, the levels of which are to be documented.
iii. Careful pullback recordings are performed from the branch pulmonary arteries to the right ventricle because stenosis at each level is possible.
iv. The presence of stenosis at a prior shunt site is expected.
v. RV end-diastolic pressures may be elevated in the setting of pulmonary insufficiency.

b. **Left heart catheterization** is performed if noninvasive studies suggest residual VSDs.
   i. **Angiography** includes a cranialized right ventriculography and possibly selective pulmonary arterial injections if hemodynamic findings suggest stenosis.
   ii. **Left ventriculography** better demonstrates residual VSDs in the presence of subsystemic RV pressures.
   iii. **Aortic root injection** demonstrates the presence of aortic insufficiency, confirms the presence of grossly abnormal coronary artery origins or branching patterns, and reveals prior surgical shunts or aortopulmonary collateral vessels. If present, shunts and collateral vessels are best visualized in the posteroanterior and lateral projections after selective injection by hand.
   iv. **Selective coronary angiography** is recommended in the care of adult patients to exclude acquired coronary artery disease and to identify the path of any anomalous coronaries before surgical intervention.

E. Therapy and follow-up care

1. Medical treatment

a. If an adult has **not been surgically treated or has undergone palliative treatment**, a relatively well-balanced situation must exist. However, the following problems are to be expected.
   i. Long-term effects of RV outflow obstruction
   ii. Progressive infundibular pulmonary stenosis
   iii. Exposure of the pulmonary circulation to systemic shunt flow
   iv. Development of distal pulmonary arterial stenosis, typically at shunt sites
   v. Erythrocytosis
   vi. Chronic hypoxemia
   vii. Pulmonary hypertension
   viii. Paradoxical emboli
   ix. Atrial and ventricular arrhythmias
   x. Increased risk for aortic insufficiency over time
   xi. Endocarditis

b. Follow-up care increasingly involves **patients who have undergone surgical repair** and management of residual postoperative lesions.
   i. These patients are at increased risk of **sudden cardiac death**. Atrial and ventricular rhythm disturbances are common in the postoperative patient. Frequent Holter monitoring is warranted for this reason. Atrial tachyarrhythmias are found in up to one-third of patients and are predictive of morbidity and mortality. If patients are found to have nonsustained ventricular tachycardia, an electrophysiologic study and possible radiofrequency ablation or implantable cardioverter–defibrillator implantation are indicated. Atrial and ventricular arrhythmias may be the presenting problem for post-repair patients when a component of the repair is failing. There are no data to support prophylactic antiarrhythmic therapy to lower risk of sudden death in this patient population. An increased incidence of ventricular rhythm abnormalities has been associated with RV volume overload from pulmonary insufficiency and with QRS prolongation (>180 ms).
   ii. **Pulmonary insufficiency** can be tolerated for years, even decades, but chronic volume loading of the right ventricle can lead to diminished exercise tolerance, dysrhythmias, and **right heart failure**.
   iii. Residual VSD
   iv. Progressive dilation of the ascending aorta

v. Residual RV outflow tract gradient
vi. RV outflow tract aneurysm at previous patch site

c. Recent **infective endocarditis guidelines** have departed considerably from prior iterations such that antibiotic prophylaxis is recommended only for those who are at highest risk for adverse outcomes from endocarditis. Specifically, prophylaxis is still appropriate for patients with TOF who are unrepaired, including those who have undergone a palliative procedure. For patients with TOF who have undergone total repair, antibiotic prophylaxis is now only recommended 6 months after the placement of prosthetic material or device, or if there is a residual defect at, or adjacent to, the site of prosthetic material (VSD patch leak, for example). If the pulmonary valve has been replaced or repaired with prosthetic material, antibiotic prophylaxis is appropriate as well.

2. The primary therapeutic consideration for patients with TOF is **surgical intervention**—either repair or reintervention.

a. The goal of **total repair** is to relieve the outflow tract obstruction while maintaining competency of a preferably native pulmonary valve with closure of the VSD. Some younger patients need extensive reconstruction of the RV outflow tract with early placement of a bioprosthetic valved conduit or homograft. In time, these usually become restrictive to flow and insufficient. The result is progressive right heart hypertrophy, fibrosis, and failure if revision is not performed.

b. A common indication for **reintervention** is pulmonary valve replacement (PVR) for severe pulmonary valve insufficiency. Although free pulmonary insufficiency is generally well-tolerated for decades, on a long-term basis it can lead to structural changes in the right ventricle, the sequelae of which include right heart failure, arrhythmia, and sudden cardiac death. The exact timing for PVR, however, is controversial. Cardiac MRI may be helpful in determining optimal timing, and there is evidence to support pursuing pulmonic valve replacement before the RV end-diastolic volume reaches 170 mL/m^2.

c. Other indications for **reintervention** include the replacement or revision of conduits/homografts in the presence of symptoms, residual VSD with reasonable shunt (approximately 1.5:1), RV pressures greater than two-thirds of systemic pressures because of residual obstructive lesions, progressive aneurysmal dilation of RV outflow tract patch, residual systemic-pulmonary shunts with left ventricular volume overload, clinically signficant arrhythmias, symptomatic or progressive aortic insufficiency, and dilated aortic root greater than 5.5 cm.

3. Although the mainstay of therapy has been surgical, **transcatheter techniques** are increasingly used to treat patients in certain situations. For the most part, transcatheter therapies for adults with TOF are limited to patients who have undergone surgical treatment, with attention to residual obstructive lesions in the main pulmonary artery, right ventricle–to–pulmonary artery conduit, or distal pulmonary arteries. Prior shunt sites may become stenotic with time and necessitate balloon angioplasty and possibly stent placement. Residual VSD and ASD may be closed percutaneously in select situations. Percutaneous pulmonic valve replacement has been reported but is still considered experimental. Success has been reported in these transcatheter procedures but most residual lesions necessitate surgical reintervention.

II. **COMPLETE TRANSPOSITION OF THE GREAT ARTERIES (DTGA).** This is a relatively common congenital anomaly that occurs with a prevalence of 20 to 30 in 100,000 live births and is found more often in males (2:1). It is not associated with other syndromes and does not tend to cluster in families. Although it represents 5% to 8% of all congenital heart disease, it accounts for 25% of deaths in the first year of life. Adult patients almost invariably have undergone prior surgery and carry with them important morbidities that require ongoing surveillance and care.

A. **Anatomy**

1. The defining feature of this anomaly is **ventriculoarterial discordance** in which there is an abnormal alignment between the ventricles and great arteries. Hence, the aorta arises from the right ventricle and the pulmonary artery arises from the

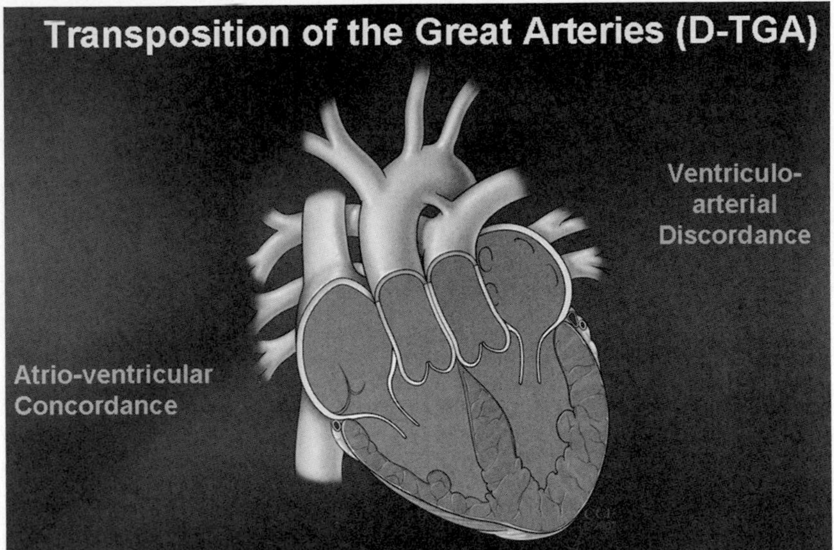

Figure 32.1. Complete transposition of the great arteries.

left ventricle, creating two parallel circuits instead of one in series. Deoxygenated blood flows from the right atrium across a tricuspid valve → right ventricle → aorta, whereas oxygenated blood flows from the left atrium across the mitral valve → left ventricle → pulmonary artery. Unless there is bidirectional shunting at the atrial (ASD), ventricular (VSD), or great artery level (patent ductus arteriosus) to allow mixing of blood, this anatomy is incompatible with life (Fig. 32.1).

2. There is an abnormal spatial relationship between the great arteries such that instead of the normal spiral configuration, they run parallel to one another. The aorta is rightward and anteriorly displaced, whereas the pulmonary artery occupies a position more leftward and posterior. This is the most common pattern, but other configurations can be seen such as side-by-side great arteries with the aorta to the right or an aorta directly anterior to the pulmonary artery.
3. Associated cardiac anomalies include VSD in 40% to 45% of cases (usually perimembranous but can involve any portion of the interventricular septum), left ventricular (or subpulmonary) outflow tract obstruction in 25%, aortic coarctation in 5%, patent foramen ovale, and patent ductus arteriosus.
4. This lesion is also referred to as "dTGA" in which the "d-"refers to the dextroposition of the bulboventricular loop, which is characterized by a right-sided RV.
5. The coronary anatomy in dTGA is variable. The aortic sinuses are described according to their relationship to the pulmonary artery (PA), such that the "facing sinuses" are closest to the PA. The most frequent coronary arrangement occurs in which the "left-facing" sinus gives rise to the left main coronary artery while the "right-facing" sinus gives off the right coronary artery.

B. Natural history and surgical repair

1. Without surgical intervention, survival beyond infancy is dismal, with 89% mortality by the first year of life and worse outcomes still for those without an associated lesion to allow for adequate mixing of blood. At birth, infants are treated with intravenous prostaglandin E to keep the ductus arteriosus open and some may undergo a **Rashkind procedure** (refer to Table 32.1) to improve oxygenation until definitive surgery can be performed.

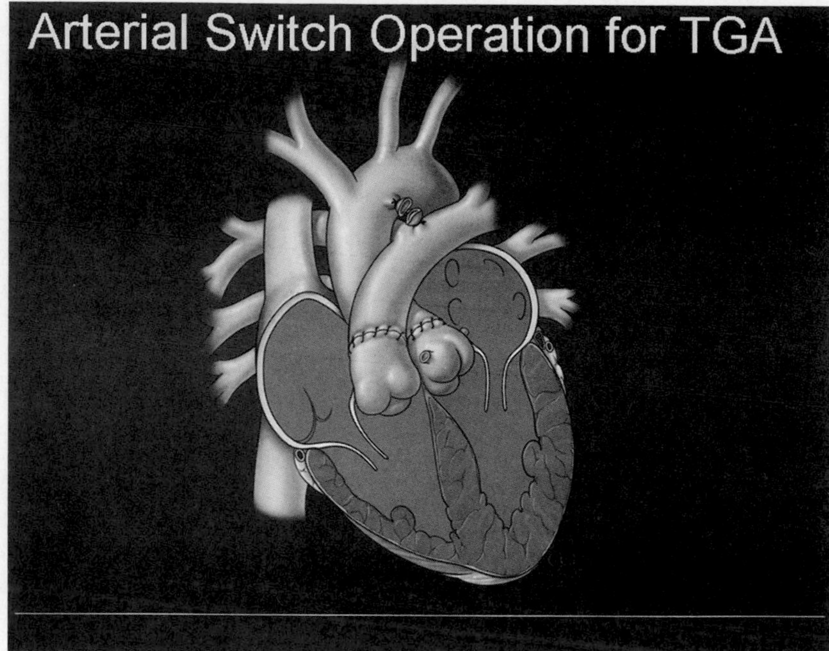

Figure 32.2. Arterial switch operation.

2. Adults invariably have undergone some type of cardiac surgery, although in rare cases may present with Eisenmenger physiology (see subsequent text) if a "balanced" situation exists with a concomitant large VSD and pulmonary vascular disease. These surgeries include the atrial switch procedure **(Senning or Mustard operation)**, the **arterial switch** procedure (Fig 32.2), or the **Rastelli operation**. Refer to Table 32.1.

C. Clinical presentation

1. The clinical presentation of the surgically repaired patient with dTGA depends on the type of surgery he/she has undergone. Although no longer cyanotic, these patients have a host of mid- to late-term morbidities that require life-long surveillance. Patients who have undergone an arterial switch procedure are only now approaching adulthood and presenting in adult congenital cardiology clinics.

2. **Atrial switch**

   a. Patients who have undergone an atrial switch operation usually report New York Heart Association (NYHA) functional class I–II symptoms but on exercise testing have significant exercise intolerance. They have a systemic right ventricle, which, over time, can develop systolic dysfunction and progressive tricuspid regurgitation. These patients may present with signs and symptoms of congestive heart failure—the most common cause of death. Arrhythmias are common and patients may present with palpitations, pre-syncope or syncope. Venous baffle obstruction can lead to peripheral edema, hepatomegaly, ascites, and fatigue due to low cardiac output. The obstruction of the superior limb can produce an SVC syndrome. Pulmonary venous baffle obstruction can lead to fatigue, exertional dyspnea, and chronic cough. Baffle leaks are often asymptomatic, but large leaks can lead to intracardiac shunting and cyanosis.

   b. On physical examination, focus should be on signs of atrioventricular regurgitation and heart failure. There may be an RV heave at the left sternal border on palpation. S_2 is loud at the second left intercostal space from an anterior aorta. Audible splitting of the S_2 may indicate the development of pulmonary hypertension.

3. Arterial switch

a. The majority of these patients are asymptomatic with NYHA functional class I symptoms. Arrhythmias are not a significant problem with this subset. Few will present with chest pain, and ischemia must be ruled out.

b. The physical examination is notable for turbulence across the RV outflow tract, which may be palpated as a thrill. The diastolic murmur of aortic insufficiency should be sought.

4. Rastelli operation

a. Both atrial and ventricular arrhythmias are mid- to late-term complications, and these patients may present with palpitations or syncope. Conduit obstruction may manifest as insidious exercise intolerance, dyspnea, or new-onset arrhythmias. On physical examination, the character of the pulmonic ejection murmur should be carefully noted to evaluate for conduit obstruction.

C. Laboratory examination

1. The **chest radiograph** of patients with dTGA displays a narrow mediastinum due to the parallel orientation of the great arteries. The cardiothoracic silhouette is normal. The pulmonary vasculature is normal in patients without pulmonary hypertension. The right ventricle to pulmonary artery conduit in patients who have undergone a Rastelli procedure may be visualized on plain radiograph due to calcification.
2. In patients who have undergone an atrial switch operation, the **electrocardiogram** may display an ectopic atrial or junctional rhythm due to loss of sinus node function. There is usually right-axis deviation and RVH as a result of the systemic position of the right ventricle. In patients who have undergone arterial switch, RVH is distinctly abnormal and suggests pulmonary outflow tract obstruction. After a Rastelli operation, the electrocardiogram is notable for a right bundle-branch block, and patients may develop complete heart block.

D. Diagnostic testing

1. **Transthoracic echocardiography** in atrial switch patients can assess the degree of tricuspid regurgitation and estimate RV function. Color Doppler is helpful in detecting baffle leaks or obstruction, although more detailed analysis may require transesophageal echocardiography. For those who have undergone arterial switch, transthoracic echocardiography can assess left ventricular function and help exclude supravalvar and pulmonary artery stenosis. Two-dimensional Doppler can be used to look for conduit stenosis after the Rastelli operation and estimate RV systolic pressures. It can also exclude any residual VSDs in these patients.
2. As in the TOF population, **CMR** imaging has emerged as an invaluable imaging modality for patients with repaired dTGA. For postatrial switch patients, CMR imaging is used to quantify the size and function of the right ventricle, assess tricuspid regurgitation, and evaluate the systemic and pulmonary venous limbs of the atrial baffle for potential obstruction or leaks. In patients who have undergone arterial repair, right and left ventricular function can be quantitated and both the right and left outflow tracts examined. Focus is placed on the great arteries to look for the presence of supravalvar and branch pulmonary artery stenosis as well as dilation of the neo-aorta. Conduit stenosis and gradients as well as RV size and function can be determined in those who have had a Rastelli operation.
3. **Cardiopulmonary testing** is very useful in detecting subtle clinical changes and decrease in functional capacity. As mentioned previously, frequently there is a discrepancy between self-reported symptoms and performance on metabolic exercise testing. Patients who have undergone atrial switch often have chronotropic incompetence and may benefit from pacemaker implantation. Stress testing may be useful in patients after arterial switch to detect coronary artery stenosis and resultant ischemia.

4. **Quantitative pulmonary flow scans** are an important part of the diagnostic work-up in patients with suspected pulmonary artery or branch pulmonary artery stenosis in those who have undergone arterial switch repair. It is useful to obtain these scans before and after potential intervention to assess for functional improvement.
5. **Cardiac catheterization** does not have a role in the routine management of these adult patients. It does have a role, however, in the diagnosis and treatment of baffle obstruction and leaks, pulmonary hypertension, pulmonary artery stenosis, coronary artery stenosis, conduit obstruction, and residual VSD.

E. Therapy and follow-up

1. Follow-up should focus on potential late complications after repair and depends on the type of surgery the patient has undergone.
   a. Atrial switch
      i. Arrhythmias including sinus node dysfunction and intra-atrial reentry tachycardia (frequent Holter monitoring is recommended)
      ii. Right ventricular dysfunction
      iii. Tricuspid regurgitation
      iv. Sudden cardiac death
      v. Baffle obstruction or leak
      vi. Pulmonary hypertension
      vii. Endocarditis
   b. Arterial switch
      i. Supravalvar or peripheral pulmonary artery stenosis
      ii. Pulmonary outflow tract obstruction
      iii. Neo-aortic regurgitation and aortic root dilatation
      iv. Coronary artery stenosis leading to ischemia, sudden death
      v. Left ventricular dysfunction
      vi. Endocarditis
   c. Rastelli operation
      i. Atrial and ventricular arrhythmias
      ii. Complete heart block
      iii. Sudden cardiac death
      iv. Left ventricular dysfunction
      v. Conduit stenosis
      vi. Endocarditis
2. **Medical management**
   a. In the treatment of systemic RV dysfunction, there are few data to show long-term benefit from drugs proven time and again in the acquired adult cardiology literature for left ventricular dysfunction. Despite this, angiotensin-converting enzyme inhibitors are often used for afterload reduction. β-Blockers should be used with caution in these patients after atrial switch repair that are prone to sinus node and atrioventricular conduction abnormalities.
   b. As mentioned previously, the latest **infective endocarditis** guidelines have changed such that in the absence of valve replacement or prosthetic material used to repair a valve, implantation of prosthetic material within the last 6 months, or prosthetic material accompanied by residual leaks, it is no longer officially recommended that dTGA patients post-repair receive antibiotic prophylaxis.
3. Late intervention options include both surgical and transcatheter procedures, and, again, depend on the type of repair. Systemic ventricular failure may ultimately require work-up for orthotopic heart transplantation.
   a. Atrial switch
      i. The procedure of choice in patients with baffle obstruction is transcatheter stent implantation, with good results especially in the systemic venous baffle. Although technically more challenging, transcatheter dilation of the pulmonary venous baffle can be performed but may require surgical revision. Clinically significant baffle leaks can be treated with catheter-based techniques as well as with septal occluder devices.

ii. Due to the high prevalence of atrial arrhythmias and sinus node dysfunction, these patients are referred for radiofrequency ablation procedures and pacemaker implantation.
iii. Conversion to an arterial switch for systemic RV dysfunction or left ventricular "training" by pulmonary artery banding has not been reliably successful in the adult population and has been largely supplanted by cardiac transplantation in many centers.

b. Arterial switch

i. Percutaneous balloon angioplasty with or without stent placement is an excellent option for those with pulmonary artery, supravalvar, or branch pulmonary artery stenosis if anatomy is appropriate. A safe procedure, there is an approximately 15% restenosis rate for balloon angioplasty and lower for stent implantation. The greatest success lies with branch pulmonary artery stenosis.
ii. Coronary artery stenosis can be treated with both stenting and coronary bypass surgery.
iii. Severe neo-aortic regurgitation is treated surgically with either valve repair or replacement.

c. Rastelli operation

i. All right ventricle to pulmonary artery conduits inevitably fail and eventually need replacement. There is a role for percutaneous stenting of conduit obstruction in some patients, which can delay the need for surgery. These transcatheter procedures have a risk of stent fracture as well as potential for coronary artery compression which can lead to catatrophic outcomes in the catheterization laboratory.
ii. Residual VSD leaks may be amenable to closure by percutaneous means but often require surgical revision. Clinically significant residual left ventricular outflow tract obstruction is also managed surgically.

III. CONGENITALLY CORRECTED TRANSPOSITION OF THE GREAT ARTERIES (ccTGA).

Ventricular inversion or ccTGA is a rare congenital anomaly that occurs in less than 1% of children with congenital cardiovascular defects. Among these patients, it is equally rare to have no other associated structural abnormalities. The natural history of ccTGA is gradual congestive failure caused by systemic atrioventricular (AV) valve insufficiency and systemic ventricular dysfunction, even in the absence of other associated malformations. The presence of associated defects and conduction abnormalities contributes to a further decrease in life expectancy without intervention. Life expectancy is generally good but does not reach normal.

A. Anatomy

1. The defining feature of this congenital abnormality of cardiac looping is **AV and ventriculoarterial discordance**. Blood flows from the right atrium across a mitral valve → right-sided, morphologic left ventricle → pulmonary artery → lungs → left atrium across a tricuspid valve → left-sided, morphologic right ventricle → aorta. (Fig. 32.3).
2. The great arteries are not in their normal configuration and often run parallel to one another instead of crossing. The pulmonary artery is more posterior and rightward than usual and the aorta is more anterior and leftward.
3. The anatomic coronary arteries, like the AV valves, follow their respective ventricles. The left-sided coronary artery resembles the anatomic right coronary artery as it courses in the AV groove and gives rise to infundibular and marginal branches. The right-sided coronary artery resembles the morphologic left coronary artery, which branches into the anterior descending and circumflex arteries (Fig. 32.4).
4. The conduction system likewise follows the respective ventricle as the right-sided, morphologic left ventricle depolarizes first. Accessory AV nodal tissue is located anteriorly with respect to normal, and the His bundle must traverse anterior to the pulmonary artery and along the superior margin of a ventricular septal defect (VSD) if present. There is increased risk for acquired **complete heart block** in this lesion because of the abnormally placed AV node and its extended course.

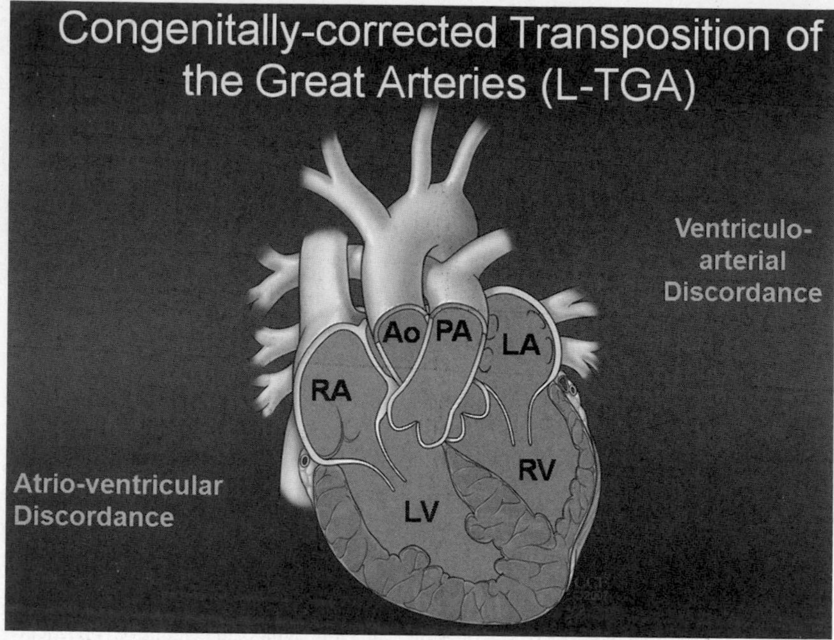

Figure 32.3. Congenitally corrected transposition of the great arteries.

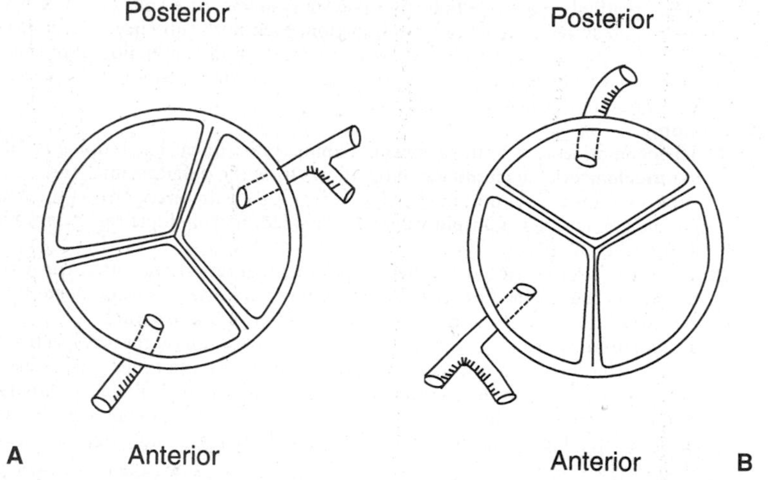

Figure 32.4. Schematic representation of coronary artery origins and branching in the normal heart **(A)** and in a congenitally corrected transposition **(B)**.

Approximately 30% of adolescents and adults develop complete heart block, the incidence of which is 2% per year without surgical intervention with the site of block being within or above the His bundle. Accessory pathways have been described and are typically left sided in the presence of an Ebstein anomaly–like malformation of the left-sided (tricuspid) AV valve.

5. Isolated ccTGA is the exception. **Associated lesions** are common and are considered in the diagnostic evaluation. They include VSD (70%), pulmonary outflow obstruction (~40% and usually subvalvular), or abnormalities of the left-sided, systemic tricuspid valve. Up to 90% of patients have some abnormality of the tricuspid valve in some form (i.e., dysplastic or Ebstein-like tricuspid valves).

B. Clinical presentation

1. Because physiologic blood flow is preserved, patients may have no symptoms through adulthood in the absence of other structural lesions or associated complications. This scenario is rare, however, because associated lesions commonly dictate the clinical features.
2. Without associated structural abnormalities, **failure of the systemic morphologic right ventricle** with various degrees of systemic AV valve (tricuspid) insufficiency is the norm. In this setting, the patient has nonspecific descriptions of fatigue, shortness of breath, and exercise intolerance or congestive failure. Patients may have **syncope or presyncope** caused by conduction abnormalities or complete heart block.
3. On physical examination, there is a loud A2 due to an anterior and leftward aorta. The murmurs of a VSD or pulmonic stenosis may also be appreciated. Tricuspid insufficiency can be heard with systemic ventricular failure.

C. Laboratory examination

1. In the usual anatomic configuration of ccTGA, the aorta is anterior and to the left, which produces a **chest radiograph** with a straight left heart border. The left pulmonary artery is not well defined and the ascending aorta is not visible on the right. The chest radiograph may appear normal or reflect the presence of associated lesions, such as increased pulmonary flow from a VSD or decreased pulmonary flow in the setting of pulmonary stenosis. Dextrocardia occurs in approximately 20% of these patients and the diagnosis should be suspected if seen with abdominal situs solitus.
2. The typical **electrocardiogram** shows a left-axis deviation. Among pediatric patients, there is loss of the usual Q waves in the precordial leads, with deep Q waves in leads II and aVF reflecting reverse septal activation. A variety of AV node conduction abnormalities may manifest with time and progress to complete heart block.

D. Diagnostic evaluation

1. In most instances, the diagnosis can be made with **echocardiography.** The essential findings of AV and ventriculoarterial discordance must be demonstrated. Imaging may be difficult in the presence of dextrocardia or mesocardia. Close attention must be paid to the morphologic details of each chamber.
   a. The morphologic **right ventricle** is identified on the basis of its triangular shape, the presence of trabeculations and moderator band, an inferiorly placed AV valve, and absence of AV valve attachments to the interventricular septum.
   b. The morphologic **left ventricle** is identified on the basis of its bullet shape, smooth wall, more superiorly positioned AV valve, and presence of AV valve attachments to the interventricular septum. In the case of ccTGA, these relationships are preserved but reversed.
   c. There is lack of anatomic continuity between the **left-sided (tricuspid) AV valve and aorta** but is present between the **right-sided (anatomic mitral) valve and pulmonary artery.** The left-sided AV valve is displaced inferiorly relative to the right-sided (mitral) valve and may appear malformed or have the characteristics of Ebstein anomaly.
   d. Apical four-chamber and subcostal images are particularly helpful. The suprasternal notch view is essential in evaluating for great vessels that lie in parallel to one another.

e. The **aortic arch** typically lies to the left of midline in the sagittal plane, and can often be visualized from the high left parasternal position. Because variations in great vessel position occur, the spatial orientation must be clarified.

f. **Associated defects** (e.g., systemic AV valve insufficiency, VSD, outflow tract obstruction) with ccTGA must be excluded or defined.

2. **Catheterization is unnecessary** for the diagnosis of ccTGA but may be helpful in preoperative planning with regard to the hemodynamic significance of associated lesions. In rare instances, ccTGA is diagnosed by catheterization that was not recognized during routine echocardiography. An unusual arterial catheter course is caused by the anterior and leftward position of the aorta in most instances. The left-sided coronary artery typically arises from the posterior sinus and assumes a right coronary branching distribution, whereas the right-sided coronary artery arises from the anterior and rightward sinus and assumes a typical left coronary branching distribution (Fig. 32.4). Because the ventricular septum often lies in the sagittal plane, ventriculography is usually best performed in the straight posteroanterior and lateral projections.

E. Therapy

1. **Medical management** is dictated primarily by the associated malformations.

   a. In the rare case of isolated ccTGA, the risk for development of conduction abnormalities is cumulative over time; therefore, periodic Holter monitoring is warranted. Permanent pacemaker placement often is needed.

   b. The systemic AV valve and ventricle may show signs of failure that necessitate initiation of anticongestive measures in the form of diuretics and afterload reduction, although data are lacking for the use of agents such as ACE inhibitors or β-blockers in systemic right ventricles.

   c. Associated lesions such as pulmonary stenosis or atresia, severe systemic AV valve regurgitation, or VSD may likewise contribute to the medical treatment of these patients, but often also necessitate surgical intervention.

   d. Recent American Heart Association (AHA) guidelines do not recommend routine antibiotic prophylaxis for these patients unless they have have had recent placement of prosthetic material within the preceding 6 months, or have a leak at, or adjacent to, the site of a previous prosthesis.

2. **Surgery**

   a. Infants and children who are brought to medical attention early often need surgical intervention in the form of relief of pulmonary outflow tract obstruction or placement of palliative shunts, depending on the associated lesions.

   b. For selected children, a **double switch** procedure may be performed. An **atrial switch** corrects the atrioventricular discordance by baffling atrial blood to the appropriate ventricle (i.e., oxygenated blood diverted from the left atrium rightward to the right-sided left ventricle and vice versa by the Mustard or Senning procedure). **Arterial switch** is performed in the same operation to restore anatomic ventriculoarterial concordance. The double switch operation may necessitate a period of "training" of the left ventricle by means of pulmonary artery banding. The results of this operation are generally less favorable in older patients in whom the right ventricle has been the systemic ventricle for a longer period. The intermediate-term results of this procedure are encouraging, but data for long-term results are limited. Those with a large VSD may undergo atrial baffling with a **Rastelli operation** (see Table 32.1).

   c. Adult patients with symptoms of progressive systemic AV valvular insufficiency may need valve repair or replacement. Most centers that have reported results with this procedure have found improved functional status after surgical treatment and acceptable risks. The timing of surgical intervention among patients with less severe symptoms is a topic of debate, but it is agreed that referral should be considered early before irreversible changes in ventricular function occur.

IV. EBSTEIN ANOMALY. This anomaly of the tricuspid valve represents 0.5% of congenital heart defects. The natural history of this lesion varies from early death to adult

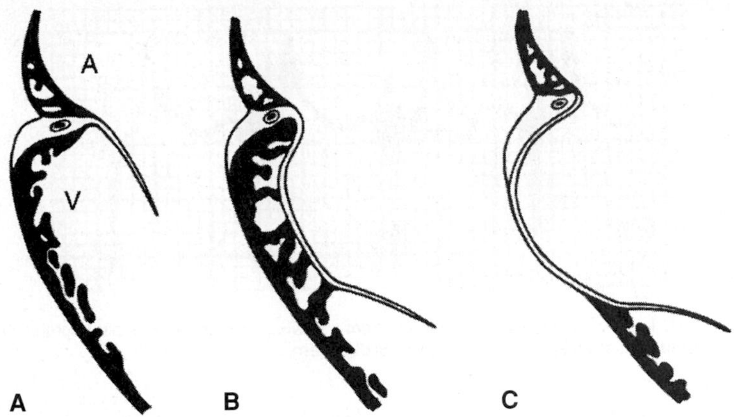

Figure 32.5. Section through the right atrioventricular junction. **A:** Normal heart, showing the right atrium (A) and right ventricle (V). **B:** Mild degree of Ebstein anomaly. **C:** Severe Ebstein anomaly. In **B** and **C**, there is apparent displacement of the tricuspid valve. (From Adams FH, Emmanouilides GC, Riemenschneider TA, eds. *Moss' heart disease in infants, children, and adolescents*, 4th ed. Baltimore: Williams & Wilkins, 1989, with permission.)

survival, depending on the degree of tricuspid valve involvement and the presence and type of arrhythmias. An increased risk for **sudden death** irrespective of functional class, presumably caused by arrhythmia, has been observed. Predictors of poor outcome include earlier age at presentation, cardiomegaly, severe RV outflow abnormalities, and disproportionate dilation of the right atrium relative to the other chambers. There is an association with maternal lithium administration but most cases are sporadic.

A. Anatomy

1. The **tricuspid valve** is morphologically and functionally abnormal. The basic features include adherence of the septal and posterior leaflet to the myocardium, which lowers the functional annulus toward the RV apex. This results in the classic atrialization of the right ventricle (Fig. 32.5) and dilation of the true tricuspid annulus. The anterior leaflet usually is not displaced but is redundant and may be fenestrated and tethered.
2. **Associated structural anomalies** include a patent foramen ovale or ASD (found in 80% to 94%), VSD, mitral valve prolapse, and pulmonary stenosis. Congenitally corrected transposition of the great arteries is associated with Ebstein-like anomaly of the tricuspid (systemic) valve.

B. Clinical presentation

1. **Signs and symptoms** are variable.
   a. The presence of a severely insufficient valve can be apparent at birth because of right-to-left shunting across a stretched patent foramen ovale (PFO) or ASD resulting in cyanosis. Pulmonary vacular resistance (PVR) is high in the neonate and worsens cyanosis, but as PVR falls, cyanosis may resolve. In adulthood, as tricuspid regurgitation becomes longstanding with associated decreased RV compliance, cyanosis can reappear. In subtle cases, the anomaly may not be evident until adulthood and then causes nonspecific descriptions of fatigue, shortness of breath, palpitations, near-syncope, or syncope. In the presence of an interatrial communication, patients may present with paradoxical embolization or brain abscess. Because the spectrum of involvement varies greatly, a high index of suspicion must be maintained.
   b. The downward displaced septal leaflet creates a substrate for accessory pathways and, clinical Wolff-Parkinson-White syndrome is found in 10% to 25% of patients. Arrhythmias include supraventricular tachycardia mediated by an accessory pathway or caused by atrial arrhythmias from progressive atrial

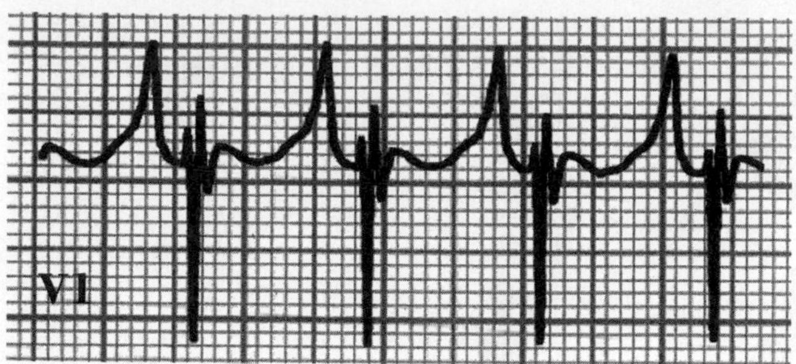

Figure 32.6. Lead V_1 of an electrocardiogram from a newborn infant with Ebstein anomaly demonstrates marked right atrial enlargement and an rSR8 pattern.

dilation. The combination of atrial fibrillation or flutter conducted rapidly across an accessory pathway is poorly tolerated.

2. Physical examination

a. General inspection usually reveals normal jugular venous pulsations despite severe tricuspid regurgitation, which is masked by a large compliant atrium. Cyanosis may be present as a result of right-to-left shunting at the atrial level. Digital clubbing will vary depending on the amount of cyanosis.

b. The most common auscultatory findings are the regurgitant murmur of tricuspid insufficiency, gallop rhythms, multiple systolic ejection sounds, and a widely split S_2.

C. Laboratory examination

1. Chest radiography may reveal cardiomegaly caused by right atrial enlargement from tricuspid insufficiency. Typically, it is described as a globe-shaped heart with a narrow waist.

2. The **ECG** can demonstrate PR prolongation, right atrial enlargement ("Himalayan" P waves), and superior axis with or without right bundle-branch block (Fig. 32.6). The QRS amplitude is characteristically low over the right precordial leads due to a diminuitive right ventricle. The preexcitation pattern, if present, is almost always type B (i.e., left bundle-branch pattern). Deep Q waves may be seen in leads II, III, and aVF from fibrotic thinning of the RV free wall and/or septal fibrosis.

D. Diagnostic evaluation

1. The diagnosis can be confirmed with transthoracic or transesophageal **echocardiography,** with the tricuspid valve readily visualized in the parasternal short-axis, apical four-chamber, and subcostal views.

a. Apical displacement of the septal leaflet from the insertion of the anterior mitral valve leaflet by at least 8 mm/m^2 body surface area is considered diagnostic. In less obvious cases, only tethering of the septal leaflet may be found, defined as at least three accessory attachments of the leaflet to the ventricular wall causing restricted motion. An imperforate valve may rarely occur.

b. The **anterior leaflet** may produce functional obstruction of the pulmonary outflow tract. The leaflet in this circumstance often is called "sail-like." The pulmonary outflow is carefully studied to discern functional obstruction from such a leaflet rather than true anatomic atresia of pulmonary outflow.

c. Views of the **atrial septum** are included in all studies to assess the size of the ASD and degree of shunting, if present.

d. The size of the **right ventricle** and true tricuspid annulus are assessed because size guides the feasibility of surgical intervention.

e. The size and function of the **left ventricle** are assessed. The shape of the left ventricle may be unusual because of extreme leftward bowing of the ventricular septum. Left ventricular function can be affected, and abnormalities may affect long-term outcome.

f. **Associated lesions** must be excluded, such as ASD, RV outflow tract obstruction, patent ductus arteriosus, and, in rare instances, mitral valve abnormalities with associated insufficiency.

2. **Cardiac catheterization is unnecessary** for the diagnostic evaluation of Ebstein anomaly, except to exclude coronary artery disease in adult patients with risk factors for whom surgical intervention is planned. Increased risk of cardiac arrest during catheterization has been reported. Diagnostic study may be indicated in the presence of associated hemodynamic abnormalities as part of preoperative planning.
3. Formal **electrophysiologic study** may be considered for patients with arrhythmias for or those being considered for surgical treatment. Radiofrequency ablation of accessory pathways is performed.

E. Therapy

1. A large number of adult patients may undergo **medical treatment,** which includes standard heart failure medications such as diuretics and digoxin. There are no good data to support ACE inhibitors in right heart failure due to Ebstein anomaly. Particular attention must be focused on the management of atrial dysrhythmias, which become more common with age. Permanent pacemaker therapy is required in 3.7% of patients, mostly for atrioventricular block and rarely for sinus node dysfunction. Endocarditis prophylaxis is no longer recommended for these patients unless they are cyanotic and unrepaired, have undergone placement of prosthetic material within the preceding 6 months (i.e., ASD occluder device), have a leak adjacent to or at the site of prosthetic material, or have had tricuspid valve replacement.
2. **Surgical correction** usually is recommended for patients with NYHA functional class III–IV symptoms despite medical therapy. The tricuspid valve may be repaired primarily, or complete replacement may be necessary and an interatrial communication, if present, is closed. Patients with symptomatic cardiomegaly, cyanosis, or arrhythmias are considered for surgical intervention. Favorable results have been achieved at centers experienced in the care of adult patients, and functional class has improved after therapy.
3. **Transcatheter closure** of an interatrial shunt can be considered in select patients with cyanosis on exercise, only in the setting of mild or moderate tricuspid regurgitation. Patient selection must be carefully evaluated, as closure of an ASD may lead to worsening RV dysfunction. In the case of paradoxic embolic events, that is, stroke, consideration of ASD closure should be entertained with the same caveat in mind.

V. EISENMENGER SYNDROME is the clinical phenotype of an extreme form of pulmonary arterial hypertension associated with congenital heart disease. Over the last few decades, rapid advances in the modalities of diagnosis and treatment of congenital heart disease have resulted in the ability to repair defects at a much younger age. Pulmonary vascular injury is prevented in many of these children. However, Eisenmenger syndrome is still seen in older patients and occasionally in younger patients, particularly in those from developing countries, where these therapies are not readily available. The natural history of Eisenmenger syndrome is variable, and although a cause of significant morbidity, many patients survive 30 years or more after the onset of the syndrome.

A. Physiology. Patients with a systemic–to–pulmonary circulation connection will initially have left-to-right shunting of blood due to the lower pulmonary vascular resistance compared with systemic vascular resistance. Over time, because of excessive flow to the pulmonary vasculature, pulmonary vascular resistance increases, which eventually results in reversal of the shunt, creating right-to-left flow. Although the classic form of the disease was initially used to describe the long-term consequences of a VSD, it can occur with any congenital defect with an initial left-to-right shunt such as ASD, AV canal defect, patent ductus arteriosus, aortopulmonary window, surgically created systemic-to-pulmonary artery shunts, or other complex congenital heart lesions. It is important to note, however, that the physiology and clinical presentation differ depending on the level of shunt. In contrast to patients with nonrestrictive shunts at the ventricular or arterial level, most patients with ASDs do not develop Eisenmenger syndrome, and, if they do, they present much later in life. In this case, atrial level shunting is determined by the compliance of the ventricles and not due to systemic or supra-systemic pulmonary artery pressures.

B. Clinical presentation of Eisenmenger syndrome has multi-organ involvement.

1. Symptoms. Pulmonary congestion (from the left-to-right shunt) in early childhood may be evident from the history but improves as the shunt reverses with ensuing cyanosis. Exercise intolerance is very common. Hypoxemia can lead to erythrocytosis and symptoms of hyperviscosity (e.g., headache, dizziness, fatigue, and cerebrovascular accidents). These patients can have a bleeding diathesis due to thrombocytopenia and inadequate clotting factors. This can complicate the management of intrapulmonary thrombosis, which occurs in up to one-third of patients. Hemoptysis is a common symptom—alone or due to pulmonary infarction. Infectious complications include bacterial endocarditis and cerebral abscesses. Atrial arrhythmias and symptoms of congestive heart failure are usually a late sign and are associated with increased risk of sudden cardiac death.

2. Physical examination. The initial murmur of the associated lesion goes away with reversal of the shunt. Cyanosis and digital clubbing are present, and arterial pulses may be diminished. The cardiac examination reveals signs of elevated right heart pressure such as jugular venous distention with a prominent *v* wave, a right parasternal heave, a loud pulmonary component of S_2 (sometimes palpable), a right-sided S_4, a holosystolic murmur of tricuspid regurgitation, and a diastolic decrescendo murmur of pulmonary regurgitation. Signs of congestive heart failure such as peripheral edema, ascites, and hepatosplenomegaly are seen later in the disease course.

C. Laboratory examination

1. Chest radiography is variable. It may show dilated, even calcified, central pulmonary arteries. Reduced peripheral lung markings are not commonly seen. Patients with ASDs tend to have cardiomegaly due to RV enlargement.

2. The **electrocardiogram** shows evidence of right atrial enlargement and RV hypertrophy. Atrial arrhythmias should be sought.

D. Diagnostic evaluation

1. Echocardiography. Two-dimensional echocardiography helps in a detailed assessment of the level of the defect, associated lesions, and ventricular function. Doppler measurements can demonstrate and assess the size of the shunt as well as RV pressure load and pulmonary hypertension.

2. Cardiac catheterization. Cardiac catheterization is often necessary in these patients to assess the pulmonary vascular resistance. Demonstration of pulmonary vasoreactivity to oxygen, nitric oxide, or other pulmonary vasodilators is prognostic for these patients and can help identify patients who may benefit from advanced therapies for pulmonary arterial hypertension.

E. Therapy

1. Medical management

a. Patients are counseled on keeping well-hydrated to maintain an optimal hemodynamic status, as the cardiac output in these patients is sensitive to changes in preload. Chronic nocturnal oxygen therapy has not been shown to be beneficial, although it may improve symptoms in some patients. Anticoagulation is controversial because it can also predispose to hemorrhage or hemoptysis, but it is helpful in preventing thromboembolic events. Hyperviscosity can be managed in *symptomatic* patients by performing phlebotomy with isovolumic replenishment, but routine phlebotomy is contraindicated due to its effect on iron stores, oxygen carrying capacity, and increased risk of stroke. Monitoring of iron levels and iron replacement, therefore, is paramount. The management of right-sided heart failure is problematic and the use of digoxin in these patients is controversial. Diuretics should be used cautiously because aggressive diuresis predisposes to hyperviscosity and decreases preload. Endocarditis prophylaxis is warranted.

b. Over the last few years, there has been a paradigm shift regarding the treatment of pulmonary hypertension in Eisenmenger syndrome with traditional therapy focused on preventive and palliative measures. There is accruing evidence to suggest that the disease is in fact modifiable and that selective pulmonary vasodilators are not only safe but likely beneficial in this population. These agents have been studied extensively in patients with pulmonary arterial hypertension and include bosentan, prostacyclin analogs, and phosphodiesterase-5 inhibitors. Despite a theoretical risk of some reduction in the systemic vascular resistance creating increased right-to-left shunting and worsened hypoxemia, safety studies have demonstrated no signficant drop in the systemic arterial oxygenation. Furthermore, these agents have been shown to improve hemodynamics in the pulmonary vascular bed, functional capacity, and 6-minute walking distance in select study patients with Eisenmeger syndrome, and are increasingly being offered as therapeutic options.

2. Surgical management. Selected patients may be candidates for combined heart–lung transplantation or preferably lung transplantation with concomitant repair of the intracardiac defect, if feasible. Timing of these interventions may be difficult because of the relatively long-term survival of these patients after the onset of the disease process.

F. Eisenmenger syndrome in special situations

1. Travel to areas of high altitude should be avoided because it may result in acute right heart failure. Air travel, however, is not contraindicated, as cabin pressures during commercial flights are generally well-tolerated.

2. Pregnancy in these patients is high risk to the fetus and mother and is contraindicated. Given the high risk of maternal and fetal mortality, contraceptive methods without the use of estrogen is critical. Elective abortion should be offered to pregnant women.

3. Noncardiac surgery is also associated with high risk and should be performed with supervision by anesthesiologists familiar with Eisenmenger syndrome.

ACKNOWLEDGMENTS

The authors thank Drs. Keith Ellis, J. Donald Moore, and Douglas S. Moodie for their contributions to earlier editions of this chapter.

Landmark Articles

Connelly MS, Liu PP, Williams WG, et al. Congenitally corrected transposition of the great arteries in the adult: functional status and complications. *J Am Coll Cardiol* 1996;27:1238–1243.

Cullen S, Celermajer DS, Franklin RCG, et al. Prognostic significance of ventricular arrhythmia after repair of tetralogy of Fallot: a 12-year prospective study. *J Am Coll Cardiol* 1994;23:1151–1155.

Diller GP, Dimopoulos K, Okonko D, et al. Exercise intolerance in adult congenital heart disease: comparative severity, correlates, and prognostic implication. *Circulation* 2005;112:828–835.

Dimas AP, Moodie DS, Sterba R, et al. Long-term function of the morphologic right ventricle in adult patients with corrected transposition of the great arteries. *Am Heart J* 1989;118:526–530.

Galie N, Beghetti M, Gatzoulis MA, et al. Bosentan therapy in patients with Eisenmenger syndrome: a multicenter, double-blind, randomized, placebo-controlled study. *Circulation* 2006;114:48–54.

Gatzoulis MA, Balaji S, Webber SA. Risk factors for arrhythmia and sudden cardiac death late after repair of tetralogy of Fallot: a multicentre study. *Lancet* 2000;356:975–981.

Gatzoulis MA, Till JA, Somerville JA, et al. Mechanoelectrical interaction in tetralogy of Fallot. QRS prolongation relates to RV size and predicts malignant ventricular arrhythmias and sudden death. *Circulation* 1995;92:231–237.

Karl TR, Weintraub RG, Brizard CP, et al. Senning plus arterial switch operation for discordant (congenitally corrected) transposition. *Ann Thorac Surg* 1997;64:495–502.

Liebman J, Cullum L, Belloc NB. Natural history of transposition of the great arteries: anatomy and birth and death characteristics. *Circulation* 1969;40:237–262.

Lundstrom U, Bull C, Wyse RKH, et al. The natural and unnatural history of congenitally corrected transposition. *Am J Cardiol* 1990;65:1222–1229.

Mukhopadhyay S, Sharma M, Ramakrishnan S, et al. Phosphodiesterase-5 inhibitor in Eisenmenger syndrome: a preliminary observational study. *Circulation* 2006;114:1807–1810.

Niwa K, Siu SC, Webb GD. Progressive aortic root dilation in adults late after repair of tetralogy of Fallot. *Circulation* 2002;106:1374–1378.

Nollert G, Fischlein T, Bouterwek S, et al. Long-term survival in patients with repair of tetralogy of Fallot: 36-year follow-up of 490 survivors of the first year after surgical repair. *J Am Coll Cardiol* 1997;30:1374–1383.

Penny DJ, Somerville J, Redington AN. Echocardiographic demonstration of important abnormalities of the mitral valve in congenitally corrected transposition. *Br Heart J* 1992;68:498–500.

Presbitero P, Somerville J, Rabajoli F, et al. Corrected transposition of the great arteries without associated defects in adult patients: clinical profile and follow up. *Br Heart J* 1995;74:57–59.

Rosezweig EB, Kerstein D, Barst RJ. Long-term prostacyclin for pulmonary hypertension with associated congenital heart defects. *Circulation* 1999;99:1858–1865.

Shin'oka T, Kurosawa H, Yasuharu I, et al. Outcomes of definitive surgical repair for congenitally corrected transposition of the great arteries or double outlet right ventricle with discordant atrioventricular connections: risk analysis in 189 patients. *J Thorac Cardiovasc Surg* 2007;133:1318–1328.

Therrien J, Provost Y, Merchant N, et al. Optimal timing for pulmonary valve replacement in adults after tetralogy of Fallot repair. *Am J Cardiol* 2005;95:779–782.

Therrien J, Siu SC, Harris L. Impact of pulmonary valve replacement on arrhythmia propensity late after repair of tetralogy of Fallot. *Circulation* 2001;103:2489.

Van Son JAM, Danielson GK, Huhta JC, et al. Late results of systemic atrioventricular valve replacement in corrected transposition. *J Thorac Cardiovasc Surg* 1995;109:642–653.

Wilson W, Taubert KA, Gewitz M, et al. Prevention of infective endocarditis: guidelines from the American Heart Association: a guideline from the American Heart Association Rheumatic Fever, Endocarditis, and Kawasaki Disease Committee, Council on Cardiovascular Disease in the Young, and the Council on Clinical Cardiology, Council on Cardiovascular Surgery and Anesthesia, and the Quality of Care and Outcomes Research Interdisciplinary Working Group. *Circulation.* 2007;116:1736–1754.

Key Reviews

Attenhofer Jost CH, Connolly HM, Dearani JA, et al. Ebstein's anomaly. *Circulation* 2007;115:277–285.

Bashore T. Right ventricular outflow tract lesions. *Circulation* 2007;115:1933–1947.

Brickner ME, Hillis LD, Lange RA. Medical progress: congenital heart disease in adults: Second of two parts. *N Engl J Med* 2000;342:334–342.

Connelly MS, Webb GD, Sommerville J, et al. Canadian Consensus Conference on Adult Congenital Heart Disease 1996. *Can J Cardiol* 1998;14:395–452.

Davos CH, Davlouros PA, Wensel R. Global impairment of cardiac autonomic nervous activity late after repair of tetralogy of Fallot. *Circulation* 2002;106:1–69.

Diller G, Gatzoulis MA. Pulmonary vascular disease in adults with congenital heart disease. *Circulation* 2007;115:1039–1050.

Edwards W. Embryology and pathologic features of Ebstein's anomaly. *Prog Pediatr Cardiol* 1993;2:5–15.

Harrison DA, Harris L, Siu SC, et al. Sustained ventricular tachycardia in adult patients late after repair of tetralogy of Fallot. *J Am Coll Cardiol* 1997;30:1368–1373.

Imai Y, Seo K, Aoki M, et al. Double-switch operation for congenitally corrected transposition. *Semin Thorac Cardiovasc Surg Pediatr Card Surg Annu* 2001;4:16–33.

Imamura M, Drummond-Webb JJ, Murphy DJ Jr, et al. Results of the double switch operation in the current era. *Ann Thorac Surg* 2000;70:100–105.

Inglessis I, Landzberg MJ. Interventional catheterization in adult congenital heart disease. *Circulation* 2007;115;1622–1633.

Khairy P, Marelli AJ. Clinical use of electrocardiography in adults with congenital heart disease. *Circulation* 2007;116:2734–2746.

Khairy P, Poirier N, Mercier L. Univentricular heart. *Circulation* 2007;115:800–812.

Kreindel MS, Moodie DS, Sterba R, et al. Total repair of tetralogy of Fallot in the adult: the Cleveland Clinic experience 1951–1981. *Cleve Clin Q* 1985;52:375–381.

Liao P, Feldt RH. Clinical profile of Ebstein's anomaly. *Prog Pediatr Cardiol* 1993;2:16–21.

Murphy JG, Gersh BJ, Mair DD, et al. Long-term outcome in patients undergoing surgical repair of tetralogy of Fallot. *N Engl J Med* 1993;329:593–599.

Olson TM, Porter CJ. Electrocardiographic and electrophysiologic findings in Ebstein's anomaly. *Prog Pediatr Cardiol* 1993;2:38–50.

Perloff JK, Warnes CA. Challenges posed by adults with repaired congenital heart disease. *Circulation* 2001;103:2637–2643.

Poirier NC, Mee RBB. Left ventricular reconditioning and anatomical correction for systemic right ventricular dysfunction. *Semin Thorac Cardiovasc Surg Pediatr Card Surg Annu* 2000;3:198–215.

Prieto LR, Hordof AJ, Secic M, et al. Progressive tricuspid valve disease in patients with congenitally corrected transposition of the great arteries. *Circulation* 1998;98:997–1005.

Rutledge JM, Nihill MR, Fraser CD, et al. Outcome of 121 patients with congenitally corrected transposition of the great arteries. *Pediatr Cardiol* 2002;23:137–145.

Therrien J, Webb G. Clinical update on adults with congenital heart disease. *Lancet* 2003;362:1305–1313.

Tuzcu EM, Moodie DS, Ghazi F, et al. Ebstein's anomaly: natural and unnatural history. *Cleve Clin J Med* 1989;56:614–618.

Warnes CA. Transposition of the great arteries. *Circulation* 2006;114:2699–2709.

Warnes CA. The adult with congenital heart disease: born to be bad? *J Am Coll Cardiol* 2005;46:1–8.

Warnes CA. Tetralogy of Fallot and pulmonary atresia/ventricular septal defect. *Cardiol Clin* 1993;11:643–650.

Wu JC, Child JS. Common congenital heart disorders in adults. *Curr Probl Cardiol* 2004;29:641–700.

Yemets IM, Williams WG, Webb GD, et al. Pulmonary valve replacement late after repair of tetralogy of Fallot. *Ann Thorac Surg* 1997;64:526–530.

Relevant Book Chapters

Bishop A. Corrected transposition of the great arteries. In: Redington A, Shore D, Oldershaw P, eds. *Congenital heart disease in adults: a practical guide.* London: WB Saunders, 1994:145–153.

Epstein ML. Congenital stenosis and insufficiency of the tricuspid valve. In: Allen HD, Gutgesell HP, Clark EB, et al., eds. *Moss and Adams' heart disease in infants, children, and adolescents, including the fetus and young adult*, 6th ed. Philadelphia: Lippincott Williams & Wilkins, 2001:810–819.

Freedom RM, Dyck JD. Congenitally corrected transposition of the great arteries. In: Allen HD, Gutgesell HP, Clark EB, et al., eds. *Moss and Adams' heart disease in infants, children, and adolescents, including the fetus and young adult*, 6th ed. Philadelphia: Lippincott Williams & Wilkins, 2001:1085–1101.

Freedom RM, Yoo SJ, Williams WG. Complete transposition of the great arteries: history of palliation and atrial repair. In: Freedom RM, Yoo SJ, Mikailian H, et al., eds. *The natural and modified history of congenital heart disease.* New York: Blackwell Publishing, 2004:306–322.

Freedom RM, Yoo SJ, Williams WG. Transposition of the great arteries: arterial repair. In: Freedom RM, Yoo SJ, Mikailian H, et al., eds. *The natural and modified history of congenital heart disease.* New York: Blackwell Publishing, 2004:323–347.

Gatzoulis MA. Tetralogy of Fallot. In: Gatzoulis MA, Webb GD, Daubeney PEF, eds. *Diagnosis and management of adult congenital heart disease.* Edinburgh, Scotland: Churchill Livingstone, 2003:315–326.

Hornung T. Transposition of the great arteries. In: Gatzoulis MA, Webb GD, Daubeney PEF, eds. *Diagnosis and management of adult congenital heart disease.* Edinburgh, Scotland: Churchill Livingstone, 2003:349–362.

MacLellan-Tobert SG, Porter CJ. Ebstein's anomaly of the tricuspid valve. In: Garson A, Bricker JT, Fisher DJ, et al., eds. *The science and practice of pediatric cardiology,* 2nd ed. Baltimore: Williams & Wilkins, 1998:1303–1315.

Mullins CE. Ventricular inversion. In: Garson A, Bricker JT, Fisher DJ, et al., eds. *The science and practice of pediatric cardiology,* 2nd ed. Baltimore: Williams & Wilkins, 1998:1525–1538.

Neches WH, Park S, Ettedgui JA. Tetralogy of Fallot and tetralogy of Fallot with pulmonary atresia. In: Garson A, Bricker JT, Fisher DJ, et al., eds. *The science and practice of pediatric cardiology,* 2nd ed. Baltimore: Williams & Wilkins, 1998:1383–1411.

Perloff JK. Survival patterns without cardiac surgery or interventional catheterization: a narrowing base. In: Perloff JK, Child JS, eds. *Congenital heart disease in adults,* 2nd ed. Philadelphia: WB Saunders, 1998:15–53.

Redington A, Shore D, Oldershaw P. Tetralogy of Fallot. In: Redington A, Shore D, Oldershaw P, eds. *Congenital heart disease in adults: a practical guide*, London: WB Saunders, 1994:57–67.

Snider AR, Serwer GA, Ritter SB. Abnormalities of ventriculoarterial connection. In: Snider AR, Serwer GA, Ritter SB, eds. *Echocardiography in pediatric heart disease,* 2nd ed. St. Louis: Mosby, 1997:317–323.

Snider AR, Serwer GA, Ritter SB. Defects in cardiac septation. In: Snider AR, Serwer GA, Ritter SB, eds. *Echocardiography in pediatric heart disease,* 2nd ed. St. Louis: Mosby, 1997:235–246.

Clinical Cardiology VII

SYNCOPE 33

Carlos Alves

I. INTRODUCTION

A. Syncope is a common medical problem that accounts for approximately 6% of medical admissions and 3% of emergency room visits. Syncope is defined as a **sudden translent loss of consciousness with associated loss of postural tone. Recovery is spontaneous, without neurologic deficit and without requiring electrical or chemical cardioversion.** Generally a fall in systolic blood pressure below 70 mm Hg or a mean arterial pressure of 40 mm Hg results in loss of consciousness. Cerebral blood flow usually decreases with aging, making the elderly at higher risk for syncope.

B. Syncope as a symptom can be caused by a **variety of medical diseases that produce a transient interruption of cerebral blood flow.**

1. A genuine effort should be made to **determine a specific cause of syncope**. Identifying a specific cause can help in the selection of therapy, prevent recurrences, minimize expensive evaluations, and decrease morbidity.
2. **Patients with cardiac syncope have higher rates of mortality and sudden death** at follow-up. Identifying and treating cardiac syncope can improve outcome (1).

II. CLINICAL PRESENTATION. Although a variety of diagnostic tests are available for evaluation of syncope, a thorough history and physical examination is crucial to determine the cause and the best diagnostic approach. A good history and physical examination can provide a clue to the diagnosis in up to 50% of cases.

A. Signs and symptoms. Accurately described symptoms can lead to specific diagnostic considerations, as illustrated in Tables 33.1 and 33.2.

1. **The most** important aspect of history-taking is to **determine the circumstances before syncope (i.e., the prodrome)**; whether there is association with any particular activity, exertion or change in position; and the frequency of occurrence.
2. The initial approach to any patient with syncope should include a **search for the presence of structural heart disease such as valvular stenosis, cardiomyopathy, or myocardial infarction.** Presence of any of these may suggest more malignant causes such as ventricular tachycardia.
3. **Symptoms of vasovagal syncope.** Calkins et al. (2) reported that a careful history could diagnose vasovagal syncope. They reported that **women (<55 years) with a postsyncopal recovery period that included fatigue** and patients with **clear**

TABLE 33.1 Cardiovascular Causes of Syncope
Neurally mediated (vasovagal)
Situational
Micturition
Defecation
Postprandial
Swallowing
Coughing
Sneezing
Glossopharyngeal neuralgia
Orthostatic syncope
Carotid sinus syncope
Cardioinhibitory
Vasodepressor
Mixed
Mechanical
Aortic stenosis
Hypertrophic cardiomyopathy
Atrial myxoma
Mitral stenosis
Pulmonic stenosis
Pulmonary hypertension or embolism
Myocardial infarction
Cardiac tamponade
Electrical
Second- and third-degree atrioventricular block
Sick sinus syndrome
Supraventricular tachycardia
Ventricular tachycardia
Torsade de pointes
Pacemaker malfunction

TABLE 33.2 Clinical Features Suggesting Specific Causes

Symptoms or finding	Diagnostic consideration
After sudden unexpected pain, unpleasant sight, sound, or smell	Vasovagal syncope
During or immediately after micturition, cough, swallow, or defecation	Situational syncope
With neuralgia (glossopharyngeal or trigeminal)	Bradycardia or vasodepressor
Upon standing	Orthostatic hypotension
Taking hypotensive medication	Drug-induced syncope
Symptoms within 1 hr after meals	Postprandial hypertension
Prolonged standing at attention	Vasovagal
Well-trained athlete after exertion	Vasovagal
Changing position (from sitting to lying, bending, turning over in bed)	Atrial myxoma, thrombus
Syncope with exertion	Aortic stenosis, pulmonary hypertension, mitral stenosis, HOCM, coronary artery disease
With head rotation, pressure on carotid sinus	Carotid sinus syncope
Associated with vertigo, dysarthria, diplopia	TIA, stroke
With arm exercise	Subclavian steal syndrome

HOCM, hypertrophic obstructive cardiomyopathy; TIA, transient ischemic attack.
Adapted from Kapoor WN, Smith M, Miller NL. Upright tilt testing in evaluating syncope: a comprehensive literature review. *Am J Med* 1994;97:78–88.

precipitating factors, diaphoresis, palpitations preceding syncope, and severe fatigue after syncope were more likely to have vasovagal syncope than ventricular tachycardia or complete heart block.

4. **Convulsive syncope.** Occasionally a syncopal episode is accompanied by **mild muscular jerking** as a result of cerebral anoxia. This phenomenon is not true epilepsy, and the physician must make every effort to distinguish between syncope and a seizure. Syncope typically occurs without an aura and has a more deliberate onset. Seizures are characterized by severe jerking motions, longer periods of unconsciousness, and severe fatigue after the event (i.e., postictal state). Seizures may occur without regard to patient positioning. In contrast, syncope rarely happens when a person is recumbent.
5. Other entities that make diagnosis difficult are **vertigo, transient ischemic events, somatization disorders (e.g., conversion, hysteria), cataplexy, epilepsy, and drop attacks.**
6. The examiner should always **carefully review the medications of a patient with syncope** for their potential role, directly or by interaction with other medications.

B. Physical findings

1. The **physical examination is especially important when the patient is unable to describe the event** and no witnesses are available, as certain findings on examination can direct the physician in the diagnostic evaluation.
2. The **comprehensive evaluation** should include a funduscopic examination of the eye for evidence of embolism. The evaluation should also search for the presence of carotid bruit and assessment of the carotid upstroke; subtle neurologic deficits that may result from a stroke or neuropathy; cardiac murmurs with attention given to valvular findings, and extra heart sounds (such as tumor plop); peripheral pulses for evidence of peripheral vascular disease and entities such as subclavian steal; and dermatologic clues that may suggest collagen vascular disease or vasculitis.

3. In examining a patient with syncope, it is important to check **blood pressure in both arms as well as orthostatic blood pressure**. Repeated orthostatic blood pressure measurements may be needed when there is a high level of clinical suspicion for orthostatic syncope (see **II.C.1.c**).
4. Syncope in the absence of underlying heart disease is not associated with increased mortality. The morbidity of such episodes are related to harm that may occur in association with a syncopal event.

C. Etiology and pathophysiology

1. **Neurally mediated syncope.** Vasovagal or neurally mediated syncope is the **most common cause of syncope**. Many situations can lead to vasovagal "fainting." Examples include unpleasant smell, sudden pain, acute blood loss, and sustained upright posture. Vasovagal reactions are often preceded by an increase in heart rate and blood pressure.
   a. **Neurocardiogenic syncope** is thought to be the result of **autonomic overactivity followed by a fall in peripheral vascular resistance, without a significant rise in cardiac output.** In susceptible individuals, the stimulation of mechanoreceptors located in the inferior and posterior wall of the left ventricle by stretch, cardiac distention, or rapid systolic contraction, leads to increased neural discharges through unmyelinated C fibers to the vasomotor center in the medulla, resulting in enhanced parasympathetic and decreased sympathetic activity. The withdrawal of the sympathetic nervous system results in sudden bradycardia or hypotension. Animal studies suggest that cardiac afferents may not be required to initiate a vasodepressor response, and that other potential mechanisms, such as release of endogenous opioids or nitric oxide inhibition of sympathetic nerve firing and primary central nervous system activation, may play a role in vasodepressor syncope.
   b. **Situational syncope.** Patients often recall situational syncopal episodes. **Micturition, defecation, cough, and trumpet playing** are examples. The action causes a reflex vasodilation (vagally mediated) that is exacerbated if the patient performs a Valsalva maneuver, which decreases the blood return to the right heart.
   c. **Orthostatic syncope. Postural hypotension** is reported in up to 24% of elderly people. Normally when a person stands, the systolic blood pressure drops only 5 to 15 mm Hg, and the diastolic pressure rises slightly. In orthostasis, the decrease in systolic blood pressure exceeds 20 mm Hg; frequently, the diastolic pressure drops by more than 10 mm Hg. This finding demands a search for a potential cause.
      (1) Common causes include **volume depletion, medications, diabetes, alcohol, infection, and varicose veins.**
      (2) **Dysautonomic syndromes** causing orthostatic hypotension are divided into two categories: primary and secondary. Primary autonomic failure is idiopathic and includes pure autonomic failure (i.e., Bradbury-Eggleston syndrome) and multisystem atrophy (i.e., Shy-Drager syndrome). Secondary causes include amyloidosis, tabes dorsalis, multiple sclerosis, spinal tumors, and familial dysautonomia.
   d. **Carotid sinus syncope.** Less than 1% of patients presenting with syncope have been given a diagnosis of carotid sinus syncope. This entity should be considered in patients with spontaneous symptoms while shaving, swimming, turning the head, or wearing a tight collar, as well as in older patients with recurrent syncope. A cardioinhibitory response (i.e., bradycardia) occurs in about 70%, and a vasodepressor response (i.e., hypotension) occurs in 10%. The remaining patients have a mixed response (i.e., bradycardia with hypotension). Carotid sinus syncope is elicited by manual pressure on the carotid sinus and can be blocked by atropine. Clinical presentation along with findings of carotid sinus hypersensitivity in the absence of other potential causes is enough to make the diagnosis. Symptom reproduction during carotid massage is not necessary for a diagnosis. A positive carotid test result is defined by cardiac asystole of 3 seconds or longer, a drop in systolic blood pressure of more than

50 mm Hg, or a drop of more than 30 mm Hg in blood pressure and symptoms. Carotid massage should be avoided in patients with a history of stroke or transient ischemic attack (TIA) within 3 months (unless they have had normal carotid Doppler results), or those patients who have carotid bruits heard on clinical examination.

2. Cardiac syncope

a. Mechanical causes

(1) Syncope or symptoms frequently occur with exertion and arise from left ventricular outflow obstruction, as seen in aortic stenosis or hypertrophic obstructive cardiomyopathy (HOCM). With exertion, peripheral vascular resistance falls, but the cardiac output is fixed, leading to hypotension. Arrhythmias and altered baroceptor response also play a role in syncope in patients with an obvious mechanical cause, such as aortic stenosis.

(2) Right ventricular outflow obstruction can also result in syncope. This condition can also trigger a vasodepressor component by mechanisms similar to neurocardiogenic syncope.

(3) Myocardial ischemia and infarction, pulmonary embolus, and cardiac tamponade should be kept in mind. **Syncope may be the initial complaint in 7% of patients older than 65 years presenting with myocardial infarction.**

(4) Hypertrophic obstructive cardiomyopathy (HOCM) patients have an annual risk of sudden death in nonselective populations of approximately 1% per year. Syncope increases the relative risk for sudden cardiac death by approximately fivefold. The presence or absence of other sudden death risk factors (family history of sudden cardiac death, nonsustained ventricular tachycardia, marked left ventricular hypertrophy, significant left ventricular outflow tract gradient) influences the risk of sudden cardiac death. Electrophysiological (EP) testing plays a minimal role in risk stratification, as at present does genotyping for specific mutations. Treatment in high-risk patients usually includes the use of β-blockers, calcium channel blockers, disopyramide and other antiarrhythmics, and frequently implantable cardioverter–defibrillator (ICD) placement.

(5) Arrythmogenic right ventricular dysplasia (ARVD) is a disorder in which syncope is caused by ventricular tachycardia originating in the right ventricle secondary to replacement of myocardium by adipose tissue and/or fibrosis. The imaging modality of choice is cardiac ([magnetic resonance imaging (MRI)] usually with fat supression), which usually shows thinning, aneurysms, and replacement of right ventricular myocardium with adiopse and fibrotic tissue. It is thought to be a common cause of sudden cardiac death in patients younger than 35 years of age, and may be familial in 30% to 50% of patients. It is usually diagnosed based upon the presenting electrocardiogram (ECG), suggested by the presence of premature ventricular contractions (PVCs) or sustained ventricular tachycardia with a left bundle-branch morphology. Treatment of syncope in this setting usually includes ICD implantation, and yearly ICD appropriate therapy rates are usually 15% to 20%.

(6) Ion Channel disorders

i. Long QT syndrome. Characterized by prolongation of the QT interval, with a measured QTc greater than 450 ms. The long QT sydromes are actually a heterogeneous group of disorders, and have been mapped to genetic defects in either cardiac potassium channels (LQT1 and LQT2) or sodium channels (LQT3). It is worthwhile mentioning that the potassium channel mutations involve a loss of function of the potassium channels, whereas sodium channel mutations involve a partial gain of function. The lifetime risk of syncope or sudden cardiac death increases with increasing QTc, reaching 50% for QTc greater than 500 milliseconds. Syncope is usually the result of an episode of torsade de pointes or self-terminating polymorphic ventricular tachycardia, and is an ominous finding. Treatment options include β-blockers and ICD implantation, as well as lifestyle modifications, including the restriction of strenuous or competitive exercise and avoidance of QT prolonging drugs.

ii. **Brugada syndrome** is a disorder of cardiac sodium channels that results in transient downsloping ST elevations in the anterior precordial leads, and leads to a susceptibility to polymorphic ventricular tachycardia. Patients with Brugada syndrome with syncope have a 2-year risk of sudden cardiac death of approximately 30%; therefore, treatment with an implantable defibrillator is recommended.

b. Electrical causes. Ventricular tachycardia, sick sinus syndrome, and atrioventricular block are the most common causes of syncope related to arrhythmias. One must also consider supraventricular tachycardia, Wolff-Parkinson-White syndrome, and torsade de pointes. Arrhythmic syncope carries the worst prognosis and must be thoroughly evaluated.

(1) **Primary cardiac arrhythmias are the most common cause of syncope in patients with known cardiac disease,** such as previous myocardial infarction, left ventricular dysfunction, or cardiomyopathy.

(2) **Medications that prolong the QT interval and electrolyte abnormalities** should also be considered as causes of arrhythmic syncope.

(3) **Patients with pacemakers** should have their pacemaker interrogated for possible malfunction. Possible causes include battery depletion, lead malfunction, or lead dislodgment. Individuals with pacemaker or implantable defibrillators should be educated about the devices and examined regularly. An observed phenomenon in patients with atrial fibrillation who undergo atrioventricular nodal ablation (and are subsequently pacemaker dependent) is the development of syncope secondary to ventricular tachycardia, presumably because of an R on T phenomenon. Because of this, such patients are usually programmed with a lower backup rate (at least 90 bpm) for the 4 to 6 weeks following atrioventricular nodal ablation.

3. Noncardiovascular syncope

a. Neurologic causes include stroke, transient ischemic attacks, normal pressure hydrocephalus, and seizures. Other causes include orthostatic hypotension from dysautonomia, and this diagnosis should be suggested based on history, screening neurologic examination, and orthostatic vital signs.

b. Metabolic causes include arrhythmias induced by hypoglycemia, hypoxia, and hypokalemia.

c. Psychogenic causes include anxiety disorder, panic disorder, hyperventilation, somatization, depression, hysterical syncope (i.e., no change in blood pressure or pulse), and conversion disorder.

d. Drugs that can cause syncope include **nitrates, angiotensin-converting enzyme inhibitors, calcium channel blockers, β-blockers, quinidine, procainamide, disopyramide, flecainide, amiodarone, diuretics, vincristine, insulin, cocaine, and digoxin. The α-blockers** (e.g., prazosin) are potent agents and commonly cause orthostatic hypotension, especially in the elderly. These agents should be initiated with careful instructions to the patient regarding orthostasis, and should be prescribed to be taken in the evening. Orthostatic hypotension can be induced by tricyclic antidepressants (TCAs) or antiparkinsonian agents as well.

4. Unknown or unexplained causes. Past studies indicated that 33% to 50% of patients with syncope had no identifiable cause. One study showed that these patients are still at a higher risk for subsequent death from any cause, with a multivariable-adjusted hazard ratio of death of 1.32 [95% confidence interval (CI), 1.09 to 1.60] (1). Other diagnostic tools such as tilt-table testing, loop recorders, signal-averaged electrocardiography (SAECG), and EP studies may assist physicians in identifying a previously unknown cause of syncope.

Stress testing, electroencephalography, computed tomography of the head, and cerebral angiography have a very low yield unless there is a history of trauma, stroke, or seizures.

III. DIAGNOSTIC TESTING. A single ECG offers the possible diagnosis in approximately 5% of cases. It can demonstrate sinus pause, high-degree atrioventricular block, prolonged QT interval, or Wolff-Parkinson-White syndrome. Echocardiography, Holter monitoring, loop recorders, SAECG, electrophysiologic testing, and tilt-table testing are major diagnostic tools. Their yield depends on the presence or absence of underlying structural heart disease.

A. In evaluating a patient with syncope, **it is important to differentiate patients with and without structural heart disease.** The goal of evaluation should be to obtain a correlation between symptoms and an abnormal finding during diagnostic testing. There are several key points:

1. Cardiac syncope carries a high mortality rate, and physicians should **admit any individual suspected of having cardiac syncope** for evaluation.
2. **Syncope in the elderly** is frequently multifactorial (e.g., drugs, structural heart disease, anemia, volume depletion, decreased baroreceptor sensitivity).
3. The **workup should be individualized** to be cost-effective and accurate, as suggested in Figure 33.1.

B. Echocardiography is routinely used for diagnosing patients with syncope who are suspected of having cardiac disease. The echocardiogram is useful in diagnosing valve pathology and myocardial processes that may contribute to syncope, such as aortic stenosis and cardiac tumors (i.e., myxomas). Some small studies and case reports suggest that echocardiographic data frequently aid in diagnosing a cardiac origin for syncope. However, larger studies have shown that the diagnostic yield of echocardiography is quite low in the absence of clinical, physical, or electrocardiographic findings, suggesting a cardiac abnormality. In patients with syncope or presyncope and a normal physical examination, mitral valve prolapse is the most common finding.

C. Holter monitoring. Holter or prolonged electrocardiographic monitoring is one of the most commonly used tests for the evaluation of syncope. However, symptomatic correlation of a cardiac arrhythmia with a syncopal spell occurs in only about 4% of cases. **A completely normal or negative Holter result may be just as helpful as a captured arrhythmia.** The sensitivity and specificity of electrocardiographic monitoring for arrhythmic syncope are not known because of the lack of criteria for abnormal results or a gold standard that is independent of arrhythmias diagnosed by monitoring. The difficulty is to establish a correlation between arrhythmia and a syncopal spell.

1. Gibson et al. (3) reviewed 1512 Holter recordings of patients referred for evaluation of syncope; a total of 255 (17%) patients reported syncope or related symptoms, of which only 30 (2%) were correlated with arrhythmias. Ventricular tachycardia was predominant in the syncope group, whereas supraventricular and sinus tachycardia were common in the presyncope group. There was an increasing incidence of supraventricular and ventricular tachycardia with age, but the correlation with syncope remained obscure.
2. Pratt et al. (4) studied 80 patients with structural heart disease by means of Holter monitors and follow-up EP study. The authors concluded that the combination of a clinical presentation of syncope, presence of coronary artery disease, and left ventricular ejection fraction less than 30% had a better positive predictive value in terms of inducibility of sustained ventricular tachycardia than any ambulatory electrocardiographic monitoring criteria.
3. Studies have shown that **sinus pauses longer than 2 seconds, second degree atrioventricular block (type II) or complete atrioventricular block, and runs of nonsustained ventricular tachycardia on Holter monitoring should be taken seriously.**
4. The duration of electrocardiographic monitoring is an important issue. It appears that **48 hours is optimal.**

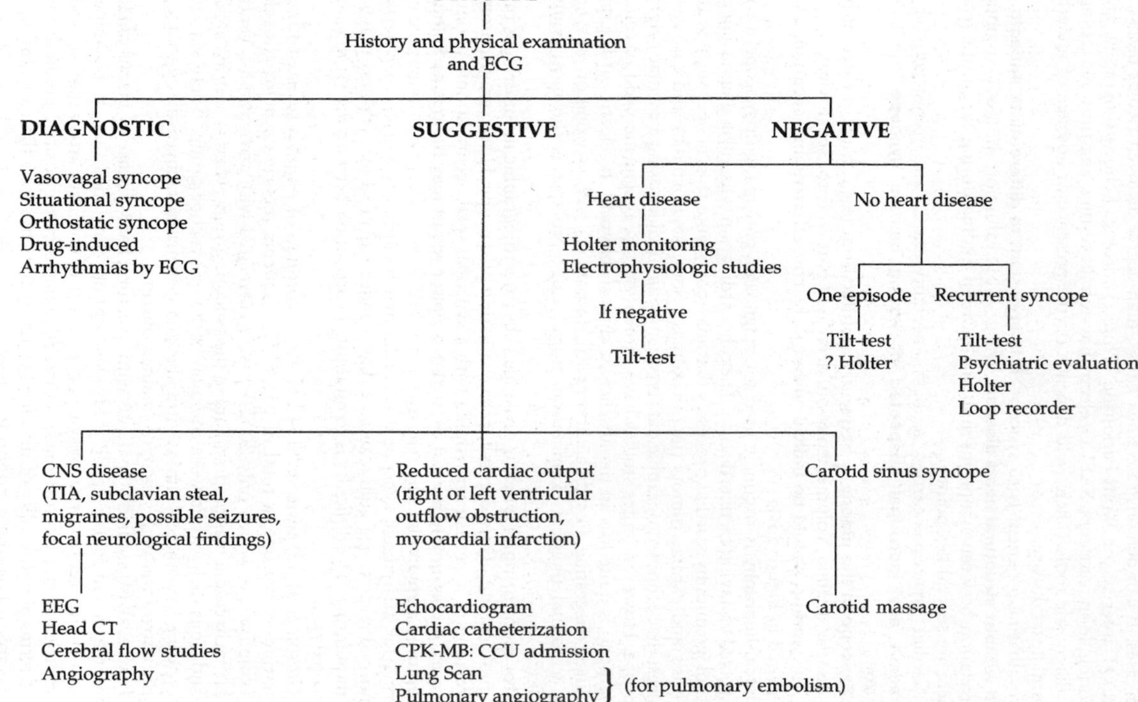

Figure 33.1. Schematic algorithm for the evaluation of patients presenting with syncope. (From Kapoor WN. Diagnostic evaluation of syncope. *Am J Med* 1991;90:91–106, with permission.)

D. Loop recorder. When used correctly, **loop recorders effectively couple arrhythmias and syncope.** Loop recorders are **useful in patients with recurrent frequent syncope**, who benefit from prolonged monitoring for weeks to months. When activated by the patient, loop recorders permanently record the previous 4 to 5 minutes of rhythm data. The recorder can capture arrhythmias during a syncopal episode if the patient activates it after regaining consciousness. The next-generation loop recorders (e.g., Medtronic-Reveal) are implantable devices similar to a pacemaker. They continuously record a single-lead ECG. These devices have the capability to store a 15-minute segment of cardiac rhythm when activated during or after a syncopal episode, and the physician can later retrieve this information for review. In patients with unexplained syncope for whom an arrhythmic origin is highly suspected, prolonged monitoring with an implantable loop recorder has been shown to be almost three times as likely to provide a diagnosis compared with standard testing, which included an external loop recorder, tilt testing, and EP testing (5).

E. Signal averaged electrocardiography (SAECG) is useful in predicting inducibility of ventricular arrhythmias by EP testing, especially in patients with ischemic heart disease. However, it is not helpful in diagnosing sinus pauses or atrioventricular block. Most patients with syncope in the setting of structural heart disease are likely to require an EP study or implantation of a defibrillator if left ventricular dysfunction or coronary artery disease is present. SAECG may, therefore, be more appropriately employed in patients with structurally normal hearts to predict whether an EP study is indicated. SAECG may also be helpful in identifying patients with arrhythmogenic right ventricular dysplasia or infiltrative cardiomyopathies.

1. **SAECG** is a collection of 100 to 300 single QRS complexes, which are amplified, filtered for noise, and averaged to determine the presence of late potentials. Late potential refers to the presence of low-amplitude, high-frequency signals in the terminal segment of the amplified QRS. The **late potentials seem to identify the presence of a reentrant substrate and may indicate an independent risk for the development of future life-threatening ventricular arrhythmias.**
2. When **combined with an ejection fraction of less than 40%, the presence of late potentials can be used to identify patients with an even higher risk for ventricular tachycardia.** Studies evaluating this profile of patients have demonstrated sensitivity of 90% and specificity of 95% to 100% in predicting inducible, sustained ventricular tachycardia.
3. Various commercially available devices use different filters, lead configurations, and processing algorithms; therefore, the **criteria for abnormal SAECG may vary among manufacturers.** Abnormal SAECG findings include total QRS duration greater than 114 milliseconds, root mean square voltage of the terminal 40 ms of the complex (RMS40) less than 20 μV, or duration of low-amplitude signals (LAS) in terminal QRS (LAS) greater than 38 milliseconds. The total duration of the QRS complex, including the late potential, is independent of other measures of cardiac risk. RMS40 is probably the most sensitive and specific of all three variables.
4. **A positive SAECG finding suggests the need for further EP testing,** especially in individuals with known heart disease.
5. The **absence of late potentials has a high negative predictive value** (94%). In patients with syncope and a negative SAECG result, electrophysiologic study is not absolutely indicated. A normal SAECG result is associated with a less than 5% risk of inducible ventricular tachycardia on EP testing.
6. **No satisfactory method of analysis is available to include patients with bundle-branch block,** because it is virtually impossible to distinguish between late activation due to the conduction defect and the reentrant substrate.

F. Electrophysiologic (EP) study. EP study should be considered in **patients with underlying structural heart disease or in elderly patients with recurrent syncope.** Similar to Holter monitoring, induced arrhythmias during EP study do not usually produce syncope in the laboratory; therefore, a cause-and-effect relationship often has to be assumed. Regardless, EP testing is useful in better delineating a cardiac cause of syncope, especially in people with baseline bundle-branch or bifascicular block.

1. **Indications** for EP study generally include the following:
   a. Known or suspected ventricular tachyarrhythmias, especially to guide therapy
   b. Uncertainty about the origin of wide QRS tachycardia
   c. Patients with unexplained syncope and history of heart disease
   d. Patients with nonsustained ventricular tachycardia, impaired left ventricular function, and late potentials on SAECG, used to stratify prognosis and guide therapy
   e. Patients with drug-refractory malignant ventricular arrhythmias who are candidates for ablative therapy
2. Some **EP findings** are considered important in the cause of syncope:
   a. Sustained monomorphic ventricular tachycardia
   b. Sinus node recovery time longer than 3 seconds
   c. Spontaneous or pacing-induced infranodal or infrahisian block
   d. Baseline His-ventricle (HV) interval greater than 100 milliseconds, or significant prolongation after procainamide challenge
   e. Paroxysmal supraventricular tachycardia with symptomatic hypotension
3. The sensitivity and specificity of induced, sustained monomorphic ventricular tachycardia is greater than 90%. However, the sensitivity of prolonged sinus node recovery time is low (69%), although the specificity is reported to be as high as 100% when EP studies are compared with results of Holter monitoring.
4. Patients with no known heart disease, ejection fraction greater than 40%, normal electrocardiographic and Holter results, and multiple syncopal episodes (more than five per year) often have **negative EP study results.** A 3-year follow-up of patients with negative EP test results revealed a 24% recurrence rate of syncope and a mortality rate of 15%; however, **a 3-year follow-up after positive EP study results and treatment revealed a 32% recurrence rate and higher mortality (61%)** (6).
5. For patients with coronary artery disease and syncope who have mild to moderate left ventricular dysfunction (left ventricular ejection fraction, 35% to 50%), inducible ventricular tachycardia during an EP study is unlikely, but the study is often appropriate given the significant implications of a positive test.
6. Patients with stable coronary artery disease and severe left ventricular dysfunction (<35%), have substantial benefits once treated with an ICD. Hence, an EP study is often not required.
7. Patients with severe nonischemic dilated cardiomyopathy (EF <40%) and New York Heart Association (NYHA) class II–III symptoms do not benefit from an EP study, and there is no evidence to support the use of antiarrhythmic medications in these patients. Evidence from the DEFINITE and SCD-HeFT trials supports the mortality benefit from ICD implantation in these patients with heart failure symptoms. Moreover, patients with wide QRS (>120 ms), and severe nonischemic cardiomyopathy with NYHA class III symptoms benefit symptomatically from cardiac resynchronization therapy (CRT), and have an improvement in mortality compared with antiarrhythmic medications by receiving a cardiac resynchronization therapy-defibrillator device.
8. The **limitations and disadvantages of EP testing** are high cost, invasive nature, lower specificity if a more aggressive electrical stimulation protocol is used, and poor prediction of bradyarrhythmias, and several other arrhythmias of unknown clinical significance without symptoms. A detailed discussion of EP studies is provided in Chapter 57.

G. Upright tilt-table testing

1. **Mechanism.** It is believed that a surge in catecholamines may paradoxically enhance the susceptibility to bradycardia and hypotension, resulting in syncope by activation of cardiac mechanoreceptors. Vasovagal syncope can be induced by keeping susceptible individuals upright on a tilt table with or without chemical stimulation. The mechanism is not completely understood, but it is believed to be similar to activation of the Bezold-Jarisch reflex.

2. The best candidate for a tilt-table study is a **person with unexplained recurrent syncope, with underlying heart disease and a negative EP study, or with no known structural heart disease.** In reviewing various tilt-table studies, Kapoor et al. (7) found that 49% of patients had a positive response during tilt-table testing, 66% had a positive response using isoproterenol with tilt-table testing, 65% had a cardioinhibitory response, and 30% had a vasodepressor response. The **number of positive responses increased with an increasing angle of tilt and longer duration**; however, there was no correlation between positive responses and maximum dose of isoproterenol. Although limited information is available on the sensitivity of upright tilt-table testing, it is reported to be about 70%. The specificity has ranged from 35% to 92% with isoproterenol. Kapoor et al. (7) reported higher false-positive rates with isoproterenol, especially at higher angle of tilt, indicating lower specificity.
3. It appears that **tilt-table testing, when used in the appropriate setting, is beneficial in diagnosing previously unexplained syncope,** preventing recurrences, and reducing morbidity. A detailed discussion of head-up tilt-table testing is provided in (7).

H. Adenosine triphosphate (ATP) test. The intravenous injection of ATP has been suggested to aid in the diagnosis of unexplained syncope. Patients are injected with a 20-mg bolus of ATP and are kept in a supine position with continuous electrocardiographic monitoring. Asystole lasting more than 6 seconds or atrioventricular block lasting longer than 10 seconds is considered abnormal. In patients with unexplained syncope, the ATP test may be able to diagnose syncope caused by transient atrioventricular block. However, it has not been able to reproduce sinus arrest. This test remains in the investigational phase, and outcome data are not yet available.

IV. TREATMENT. Treatment of syncope is individualized and depends on the underlying cause.

A. Medical therapy. The treatment of syncope hinges on preventing recurrent episodes and lowering mortality. The neurally mediated reflex syncopal syndromes can be treated in part by behavior modification. Initial measures aimed at reducing these syncopal events include advising patients to avoid precipitating triggers. Patients should also be counseled on the avoidance of volume depletion. Medication regimens such as chronic vasodilator therapy may predispose to syncope and should also be avoided. Moderate exercise training, tilt training, and increased intake of salt and electrolytes are some initial measures that help in reducing vasovagal syncope. Most long-term, randomized studies testing the utility of using medications to prevent syncope, including those of β-blockers, have failed to show any benefit over placebo. Table 33.3 addresses the various causes of syncope and potential medical treatment.

1. **Electrolyte abnormalities must be corrected** if they are suspected as the cause of arrhythmias (e.g., prolonged QT from hypomagnesemia or hypocalcemia).
2. **Particular attention should be given to the patient's medications,** since they may have drug–drug interactions or proarrhythmic potential that may cause orthostatic hypotension. Unnecessary medications should be discontinued.

B. Device therapy

1. **Symptomatic bradyarrhythmias and atrioventricular blocks require pacemaker implantation**
   a. Patients with an HV interval (i.e., impulse time from atrioventricular node to the ventricle) of more than 100 ms are at a high risk for **progression to heart block** and may benefit from a pacemaker.
   b. Although the mode of pacing is debated, in **patients with carotid sinus syncope,** a dual-chamber pacer with rate responsiveness is most desirable.
   c. Dual-chamber pacing has reduced the short- and long-term likelihood of syncope in highly selected patients with recurrent vasovagal syncope (8, 9). In patients with recurrent vasovagal syncope, dual pacing with hysteresis should be considered an option if other treatment modalities have been ineffective.
2. **Antiarrhythmic therapy** appears to decrease the frequency of syncope; however, it has not been shown to improve survival. In patients with malignant or

TABLE 33.3 Medical Therapy in Syncope

Cause	Treatment
Vasodepressor syncope	β-Blockers, disopyramide, fluoxetine, sertraline, dual-chamber pacing, theophylline, and scopolamine
Dysautonomic syncope	Elastic support hose, water exercise, increased sodium intake, fludrocortisone, ephedrine sulfate, midodrine, erythropoietin, and methylphenidate
Situational syncope	Stool softeners, urinating while sitting down
Carotid sinus syncope	Avoidance of tight collars, surgical removal of carotid sinus tumor, pacemaker in patients with predominantly cardioinhibitory syncope
Tachyarrhythmias	Implantable defibrillators or trial of antiarrhythmic agents

Adapted from Kapoor WN, Smith M, Miller NL. Upright tilt testing in evaluating syncope: a comprehensive literature review. *Am J Med* 1994;97:78–88.

life-threatening ventricular arrhythmias or inducible, sustained monomorphic ventricular tachycardia, **implantable defibrillators** are the best option based on study findings, especially in patients with unexplained syncope who have a history of coronary artery disease and severe left ventricular dysfunction.

C. Surgical therapy

1. **Patients who have exertional cardiac syncope** due to left or right heart outflow obstruction, such as HOCM, should be instructed to **avoid exertional activities** that precipitate syncope and **should be considered for surgical repair.**
2. Surgical septal myectomy is the procedure of choice in **patients with HOCM**; however, percutaneous septal ablation with alcohol is an alternative in patients who are considered at high surgical risk.
3. Coronary artery bypass grafting or percutaneous coronary intervention is strongly indicated in **patients with life-threatening arrhythmias (usually polymorphic ventricular tachycardias) due to myocardial ischemia.**

V. FOLLOW-UP. The follow-up of patients with syncope often depends on the cause and the therapy being instituted.

A. Patients with frequent spells of syncope without an identifiable cause should be considered for more extensive monitoring such as implantable loop recorders, because they may have an undiagnosed cardiac cause.

B. Patients with cardiac syncope require very close follow-up because their mortality rates are significantly higher than those of patients with other causes of syncope.

C. Elderly patients may require closer monitoring about their home situation, their need for assistance with activities of daily living, and changes in medications.

D. A consultant who diagnoses syncope should **communicate with the patient's primary physician about cause, therapy, and important warning signs** if devices such as pacemakers or defibrillators are implanted.

E. Hospitalization. The decision about which patients to hospitalize can be complex. Underlying heart disease has been found to be the most important factor in determining prognosis and risk stratification, and it mandates hospitalization for evaluation of syncope. Patients without evidence of structural heart disease who have a normal electrocardiogram and a high probability of having neurally mediated syncope are at low risk and generally have good long-term outcomes. Outpatient evaluation of syncope may be appropriate for these patients in many instances. Physicians should also consider hospitalization for patients with exertional syncope, syncope causing severe injury, and those with a strong family history of sudden death.

ACKNOWLEDGMENTS

The author thanks Drs. Keith Ellis and Vasant B. Patel for their contributions to earlier editions of this chapter.

Suggested Readings

Ammirati F, Colivicchi F, Santini M, for the Syncope Diagnosis and Treatment Study Investigators. Permanent cardiac pacing versus medical treatment for the prevention of recurrent vasovagal syncope: a multicenter, randomized, controlled trial. *Circulation* 2001;104:52–57.

Bardy GH, Lee KL, Mark DB, et al. for the Sudden Cardiac Death in Heart Failure Trial (SCD-HeFT) Investigators. Amiodarone or an implantable cardioverter-defibrillator for congestive heart failure. *N Engl J Med* 2005;352:225–237.

Bass EB, Elson JJ, Fogoros RN, et al. Long-term prognosis of patients undergoing electrophysiologic studies for syncope of unknown origin. *Am J Cardiol* 1988;62:1186–1191.

Calkins H, Shyr Y, Frumin H, et al. The value of the clinical history in the differentiation of syncope due to ventricular tachycardia, atrioventricular block, and neurocardiogenic syncope. *Am J Med* 1995;98:365–373.

Connolly S, Sheldon R, Roberts R, Gent M, for the Vasovagal pacemaker study investigators. The North American Vasovagal Pacemaker Study (VPS): a randomized trial of permanent cardiac pacing for the prevention of vasovagal syncope. *J Am Coll Cardiol* 1999;33:16–20.

Gibson TC, Heitzman MR. Diagnostic efficacy of 24-hour electrocardiographic monitoring for syncope. *Am J Cardiol* 1984;53:1013–1017.

Goldschlager N, Epstein AE, Grubb BP for the practice outline subcommittee, NASPE. Etiologic considerations in the patient with syncope and an apparently normal heart. *Arch Intern Med* 2003;163:151–162.

Kapoor WN, Smith M, Miller NL. Upright tilt testing in evaluating syncope: a comprehensive literature review. *Am J Med* 1994;97:78–88.

Krahn AD, Klein, GJ, Yee R, et al. Randomized Assessment of Syncope Trial: conventional diagnostic testing versus a prolonged monitoring strategy. *Circulation* 2001;104:46–51.

Moss AJ, Zareba W, Hall WJ, et al. for the MADIT II Investigators. Prophylactive implantation of a defibrillator in patients with myocardial infarction and reduced ejection fraction. *N Engl J Med* 2002;21:346:877–883.

Pratt CM, Thornton BC, Margo SA, et al. Spontaneous arrhythmia detected on ambulatory electrocardiographic recording lacks precision in predicting inducibility of ventricular tachycardia during electrophysiology study. *J Am Coll Cardiol* 1987;10:97–104.

Russo AM, Verdino R, Schorr C, et al. Occurrence of implantable defibrillator events in patients with syncope and nonischemic dilated cardiomyopathy. *Am J Cardiol* 2001;88:1444–1446.

Soteriades ES, Evans JC, Larson MG, et al. Incidence and prognosis of syncope. *N Engl J Med* 2002;347:878–885.

Landmark Articles

Kapoor WN. Diagnostic evaluation of syncope. *Am J Med* 1991;90:91–106.

Kapoor WN, Karpf M, Wieand S, et al. A prospective evaluation and follow-up of patients with syncope. *N Engl J Med* 1983;309:197–204.

Sra JS, Anderson AJ, Sheikh SH, et al. Unexplained syncope evaluated by electrophysiologic studies and head-up tilt testing. *Ann Intern Med* 1991;114:1013–1019.

Teichman SL, Felder SD, Matos JA, et al. The value of EPS in syncope of undetermined origin: report of 150 cases. *Am Heart J* 1985;110:469–479.

Key Reviews

Benditt G, Remole S, Milstein S, et al. Syncope: causes, clinical evaluation, and current therapy. *Annu Rev Med* 1992;43:283–300.

Brignole M, Alboni P, Bennitt L, et al. Guidelines on management (diagnosis and treatment) of syncope. *Eur Heart J* 2001;22:1256–306.

Kapoor WN, Smith M, Miller NL. Upright tilt testing in evaluating syncope: a comprehensive literature review. *Am J Med* 1994;97:78–88.

Kapoor WN. Current evaluation and management of syncope. *Circulation* 2002;106:1606–1609.

Relevant Book Chapter

Benditt DG. Syncope. In: Topol E, ed. *Textbook of cardiovascular medicine*, 3rd ed. Philadelphia: Lippincott-Raven Publishers, 2007:1137–1150.

Guidelines

Strickberger SA, et al. AHA/ACCF scientific statement on the evaluation of syncope. *Jb Am Coll Cardiol* 2006;47:473–484.

Benditt DG, et al. Tilt table testing for assessing syncope, ACC expert consensus document. *J Am Coll Cardiol* 1996;28;263–275.

34 ASSESSING AND MANAGING CARDIAC RISK IN NONCARDIAC SURGICAL PROCEDURES

Khaldoun G. Tarakji

I. INTRODUCTION

A. Background. Patients undergoing noncardiac surgeries can be at risk for major perioperative cardiac complications, particularly if they are elderly. Worldwide, it is estimated that approximately 500,000 to 900,000 patients per year undergoing noncardiac surgery suffer a perioperative cardiac death, nonfatal myocardial infarction (MI), or nonfatal cardiac arrest (1). Given the increasingly advanced age of patients undergoing surgeries, this risk is expected to remain substantial. The risk of death from a perioperative MI could be as high as 50%. The elevated risk of perioperative MI is multifactorial and could be due primarily to increased sympathetic tone, a proinflammatory state, hypercoagulability, and occasional hypoxia during the first few days after surgery. In 1977, Goldman et al. developed a multifactorial index of risk for cardiac morbidity and mortality. Extensive work has subsequently been done on various aspects of perioperative cardiac evaluation, including clinical factors and noninvasive testing. The variety of strategies and practices used has led to high costs associated with preoperative risk assessment. Many studies have recently challenged common practices in the area of perioperative care that were found to have no clear benefit. The American College of Cardiology/American Heart Association (ACC/AHA) task force committee developed practice guidelines aimed at providing a more efficient approach to preoperative evaluation. These guidelines were recently updated in 2007.

B. Objective. The purpose of preoperative evaluation is not to "clear" patients for an operation. The purpose is to **assess current medical status, assess cardiac risks posed by the planned operation**, and **recommend strategies that may influence short- and long-term outcomes.**

1. Although the preoperative assessment is a complex process, a few **basic questions and observations** by a physician with regard to the patient's general health, functional capacity, cardiac risk factors, comorbid medical illnesses, and type of anticipated operation can assist in evaluating cardiac risk.
2. It is not prudent to order noninvasive tests for every patient. The physician tries to obtain as much information as possible by means of **history and physical examination.** Noninvasive tests are requested only if the results are likely to influence treatment and outcome.
3. **As a general rule, preoperative intervention is rarely needed unless it is indicated irrespective of the preoperative context.** Patients with clinically stable heart disease may not need extensive preoperative testing.
4. Communication is vital among primary physicians, consulting physicians, anesthesiologists, and surgeons for short- and long-term care of patients.

II. CLINICAL PRESENTATION

A. History

1. The clinician needs to identify cardiac conditions that place a patient at increased risk, such as recent MI, decompensated congestive heart failure (CHF), unstable angina, significant arrhythmias, and valvular heart disease.
2. Attention is directed at serious **comorbid conditions** such as diabetes mellitus, peripheral vascular disease, history of stroke, renal disease, and pulmonary disease.
3. **Functional capacity** is determined on the basis of the patient's ability to perform certain daily tasks (Table 34.1).

TABLE 34.1	Estimated Energy Requirements for Various Activities
1 to 4 METs	
Eat, dress, or use the toilet	
Walk indoors around the house	
Walk on level ground at 2 mph (3.2 km/h)	
Do light housework such as washing dishes	
4 to 10 METs	
Climb a flight of stairs	
Walk on level ground at 4 mph (6.4 km/h)	
Run a short distance	
Heavy work such as vacuuming or lifting heavy furniture	
Play games such as golf or doubles tennis	
More than 10 METs	
Participate in strenuous activities such as swimming, singles tennis, basketball, or skiing	

MET, metabolic equivalent.

B. Physical findings. A thorough examination is crucial, and specific findings are addressed.

1. The physical examination includes blood pressure in both arms (supine and standing) and evaluation of carotid arterial pulse (character, volume, and upstroke), jugular venous pulsation, cardiac rhythm, heart sounds (murmurs, gallops, or rubs), and extremity pulses.
2. Lung fields are auscultated and the abdomen is palpated for a possible aneurysm.
3. **High risk findings** include severe aortic stenosis murmur, elevated jugular venous pressure, pulmonary edema, or S_3 gallop.

C. Indices to predict cardiac risk. Cardiac risk is a function of patient characteristics and the proposed operation.

1. **The Goldman index** was developed in 1977. The index is a score derived from nine independent variables that predict perioperative cardiac events, and each is assigned a point value (Table 34.2).
2. **Detsky et al.** developed a modified multifactorial index to address the severity of coronary artery disease (CAD) and heart failure (Table 34.3).
3. In 1999, **Lee et al. developed the Revised Cardiao Risk Index** to simplify the process using only six risk factors (Table 34.4). This is now the most widely used risk index and is the one incorporated in the ACC/AHA guidelines.

D. Clinical assessment of risk factors. Instead of dividing risk factors into major, intermediate, and minor groups, the new 2007 ACC/AHA guidelines adopted a more practical approach by recognizing the following conditions:

1. **Active cardiac conditions.** The presence of one or more of these conditions warrants intensive evaluation and management before proceeding with noncardiac surgery, and may result in delay or cancellation of the scheduled surgery (Table 34.5).
2. **Clinical risk factors.** With the exception of the type of surgery, these factors are the same risk factors identified by the Revised Cardiac Risk Index (Table 34.4), and they include the following:
   - **a.** History of ischemic heart disease
   - **b.** History of compensated or prior heart failure
   - **c.** History of cerebrovascular disease
   - **d.** Diabetes mellitus
   - **e.** Renal insufficiency
3. The original guidelines recognized a group of **minor** predictors that included advanced age, abnormal electrocardiogram (ECG), rhythm other than sinus, and uncontrolled hypertension. **Although the presence of many of these**

TABLE 34.2 Original Goldman Multifactorial Cardiac Risk Index

Criteria	Points
History	
Age older than 70 yr	5
MI in previous 6 months	10
Physical examination	
S_3 gallop or JVD	11
Significant AS	3
Electrocardiogram	
Rhythm other than sinus or PACs on last preoperative ECG	7
Greater than 5 PVCs/min documented at any time preoperatively	7
General status (one or more of the following)	
PO_2 <60 or PCO_2 >50 mm Hg, K <3.0 or HCO_3 <20 mEq/L, BUN >50 or Cr >3.0 mg/dL; abnormal AST, signs of chronic liver disease, or patient bedridden from noncardiac causes	3
Operation	
Intraperitoneal, intrathoracic, or aortic operation	3
Emergency operation	4
Total	53

Class	Points	Cardiac Deaths (%)
I	0–5	0.2
II	6–12	2.0
III	13–25	2.0
IV	≥ 26	56.0

AS, aortic stenosis; AST, aspartate aminotransferase; BUN, blood urea nitrogen; Cr, creatinine; ECG, electrocardiogram; JVD, jugular venous distention; MI, myocardial infarction; PAC, premature atrial contraction; PVC, premature ventricular contraction.
Adapted from Goldman L, Caldera DL, Nussbaum SR, et al. Multifactorial index of cardiac risk in noncardiac surgical procedures (2).

factors might lead to a *higher suspicion of CAD*, they have *not* been shown to increase perioperative risk independently and, therefore, they are no longer incorporated into the recommendations for treatment.

III. TYPE OF OPERATION. In addition to clinical markers and functional capacity, the proposed operation is an important factor, especially among patients with multiple clinical risk factors (Table 34.6). The consultant uses all the information available to estimate cardiac risk and provides recommendations to minimize perioperative risk. For surgical emergencies, the patient should proceed directly to the operating room; emphasis in these circumstances is on postoperative evaluation and management. For urgent surgical procedures, evaluation must be tailored to the underlying disease process. Elective procedures allow for more thorough evaluation, and all care should be taken to minimize risk. Testing is limited exclusively to those studies whose results might change management.

IV. SUPPLEMENTAL PREOPERATIVE EVALUATION

A. Routine laboratory tests such as serum creatinine, hemoglobin, platelets, potassium, liver profile, and oxygen saturation are important in determining whether a patient needs special attention. Such patients include those with bleeding risk, renal failure, or liver disease.

B. Patients with **pulmonary disease** (i.e., chronic obstructive pulmonary disease or pulmonary fibrosis) undergo a preoperative **arterial blood gas evaluation.**

C. A 12-lead **ECG** is recommended for patients with at least one clinical risk factor who are undergoing vascular surgery, and for patients with known history of

TABLE 34.3 **Detsky Modified Cardiac Risk Index**

Variable	Points
Coronary artery disease	
MI within 6 months earlier	10
MI more than 6 months earlier	5
Canadian class of angina	
Class 3	10
Class 4	20
Unstable angina within 3 months	10
Alveolar pulmonary edema	
Within 1 week	10
Ever	5
Valvular disease	
Suspected critical aortic stenosis	20
Arrhythmias	
Sinus plus atrial premature beats or rhythm other than sinus on last preoperative electrocardiogram	5
Greater than five ventricular premature beats at any time before operation	5
Poor general medical status[a]	5
Age older than 70 yr	5
Emergency operation	10
Total	120

[a]Defined as any of the following: PO_2 <60 mm Hg, PCO_2 >50 mm Hg, K+ <3.0, HCO_3 <20 mEq/L, BUN ≥18 mmol/L (>50 mg/dL), serum Cr >260 mmol/L (>2.9 mg/dL), abnormal AST, signs of chronic liver disease, or patient bed-ridden because of noncardiac causes. AST, aspartate aminotransferase; BUN, blood urea nitrogen; Cr, creatinine; MI, myocardial infarction. Adapted from Detsky AS, Abrams HB, McLaughlin JR, et al. Predicting cardiac complications in patients undergoing non-cardiac surgery (6).

CAD, peripheral vascular disease, or cerebrovascular disease who are undergoing an intermediate-risk surgical procedure. A 12-lead ECG also is reasonable in patients with no clinical risk factors undergoing vascular surgery, and possibly in patients with at least one clinical risk factor who are undergoing intermediate-risk surgery.

D. Echocardiography. Echocardiograms can provide information about certain pathologic conditions (left ventricular dysfunction, aortic stenosis) that predispose to increased perioperative cardiac risk. However, routine use of echocardiography is not helpful, and should be reserved for patients who meet ACC/AHA clinical guidelines, or for patients in whom the physical examination is suggestive of aortic stenosis, regardless of the planned surgery.

V. STEPWISE APPROACH TO PREOPERATIVE CARDIAC ASSESSMENT. The ACC/AHA task force developed an **algorithm for preoperative cardiac evaluation** to help physicians systematically identify clinical predictors and determine if noninvasive testing is indicated prior to the noncardiac surgery (Fig. 34.1).

VI. NONINVASIVE CARDIAC STRESS TESTING. The ability of noninvasive cardiac tests in predicting perioperative risk is uncertain. Recently there has been increasing evidence discouraging the need for their routine use in patients undergoing preoperative evaluation. This shift away from noninvasive testing was supported by the results of a recent randomized controlled trial of preoperative myocardial revascularization in vascular surgery patients that showed no improvement in perioperative or long-term outcomes associated with prophylactic revascularization. Another study challenged the old ACC/AHA guidelines by randomizing stable intermediate-risk patients undergoing major vascular surgery between cardiac stress testing strategy and no testing. By using excellent β-blocker therapy with tight heart rate control of 60 to 65 beats/min,

TABLE 34.4 Revised Cardiac Risk Index

Six independent predictors of major cardiac complications

High-risk surgery (intrathoracic, intraperitoneal, or suprainguinal vascular procedures)

History of ischemic heart disease (history of MI or a positive exercise stress test, current complaint of chest pain thought due to MI, use of nitrate therapy, or ECG with pathological Q waves; do not count prior coronary revascularization procedure unless one of the other criteria for ischemic heart disease is present)

History of heart failure

History of cerebrovascular disease

Diabetes mellitus requiring insulin therapy

Serum creatinine >2.0 mg/dL (177 μmol/L)

Rate of Cardiac death, nonfatal MI, and nonfatal cardiac arrest according to the number of predictors

No risk factors: 0.4 % (95% CI, 0.1–0.8%)

One risk factor: 1.0% (95% CI, 0.5–1.4%)

Two risk factors: 2.4% (95% CI, 1.3–3.5%)

Three or more risk factors: 5.4% (95% CI 2.8–7.9%)

Rate of cardiac death and nonfatal MI, cardiac arrest or ventricular fibrillation, pulmonary edema, and complete heart block according to the number of predictors and the nonuse or use of β-blockers

No risk factors: 0.4–1.0% versus <1% with β-blockers

One to two risk factors: 2.2–6.6% versus 0.8–1.6% with β-blockers

Three or more risk factors: >9% versus >3% with β-blockers

Adapted from Lee TH, Marcantonio ER, Mangione CM et al. Derivation and prospective validation of a simple index for prediction of cardiac risk of major noncardiac surgery (7).

TABLE 34.5 Active Cardiac Conditions that Warrant Evaluation and Treatment Before Noncardiac Surgery

Unstable coronary syndromes

Acute or recent myocardial infarction[a]

Unstable or severe[b] angina (Canadian class III or IV)[c]

Decompensated heart failure

Significant arrhythmias

High-grade atrioventricular block

Mobitz type II atrioventricular block

Third-degree atroventricular block

Symptomatic ventricular arrhythmias

Supraventricular arrhythmias (including atrial fibrillation) with uncontrolled ventricular rate

Symptomatic bradycardia

Newly recognized ventricular tachycardia

Severe valvular disease

Severe aortic stenosis (mean pressure gradient $\geq$40 mm Hg, aortic valve area $\leq$1.0 cm^2, or symptomatic)

Symptomatic mitral stenosis

[a]The American College of Cardiology National Database Library defines acute MI as within 7 days and recent MI as greater than 7 days and less than or equal to 1 month.
[b]May include stable angina among patients who are unusually sedentary.
[c]Data from Campeau L. Grading of angina pectoris. *Circulation* 1976;54:522–523.
Adapted from Fleisher LA, Beckman JA, Brown KA et al. ACC/AHA 2007 Guidelines on Perioperative Cardiovascular Evaluation and Care for Noncardiac Surgery: Executive Summary (5).

TABLE 34.6 Cardiac Risk Stratification by Type of Surgical Procedure

HIGH-RISK PROCEDURE (CARDIAC RISK >5%)
Aortic and other major vascular surgery (endovascular abdominal aortic aneurysm repair is considered intermediate risk) Peripheral vascular surgery (carotid endarterectomy is considered intermediate risk)
INTERMEDIATE-RISK PROCEDURE (CARDIAC RISK 1–5%)
Carotid endarterectomy, endovascular abdominal aortic aneurysm repair
Head and neck surgery
Intraperitoneal surgery
Intrathoracic surgery
Orthopedic surgery
Prostate surgery
LOW-RISK PROCEDURE (CARDIAC RISK <1%)
Breast surgery
Cataract surgery
Endoscopic procedures
Superficial procedures
Ambulatory surgery

Adapted from Fleisher LA, Beckman JA, Brown KA, et al. ACC/AHA 2007 Guidelines on Perioperative Cardiovascular Evaluation and Care for Noncardiac Surgery: Executive Summary (5).

there was no significant difference in the primary endpoint (composite postoperative cardiac death and/or nonfatal MI) between preoperative cardiac testing and no testing strategies. Therefore, **preoperative noninvasive cardiac testing should be reserved for patients who are candidates for these tests according to guidelines and who based on the results of these tests could potentially be considered for angiography and revascularization regardless of the planned surgery.**

These findings were reflected in the new ACC/AHA 2007 guidelines:

A. Patients with **active** cardiac conditions (Table 34.5) should be **evaluated and treated before noncardiac surgery** (class I).

B. In patients with **poor [<4 metabolic equivalents of the task (METs)] or unknown functional capacity**, who have **three or more clinical risk factors** and are undergoing **vascular surgery**, noninvasive **testing is reasonable if it will change management** (class IIa).

C. In patients with poor or unknown functional capacity, who have one to two clinical risk factors, and who are undergoing intermediate-risk surgery, noninvasive testing may be considered (class IIb).

D. In patients with good functional capacity who have one to two clinical risk factors and who are undergoing vascular surgeries, noninvasive testing may be considered (class IIb).

E. **Noninvasive testing** is **not** useful in patients *without* clinical risk factors who are undergoing **intermediate-risk surgery.**

F. **Noninvasive testing is not useful in patients who are undergoing low-risk surgery.**

There are **different modalities for stress testing** including exercise ECG, exercise or pharmacologic nuclear stress testing, and exercise or pharmacologic stress echocardiography. When ordering these tests **it is important to remember:**

A. When feasible, **exercise is the modality of choice** for stress testing because it provides an objective assessment of functional capacity. Pharmacologic stress testing (adenosine, dipyridamole, and dobutamine) should be reserved for patients who cannot exercise.

B. Exercise and pharmacologic stress testing have **excellent negative predictive values** (90% to 100%) but **poor positive predictive value** (6% to 67%), meaning that

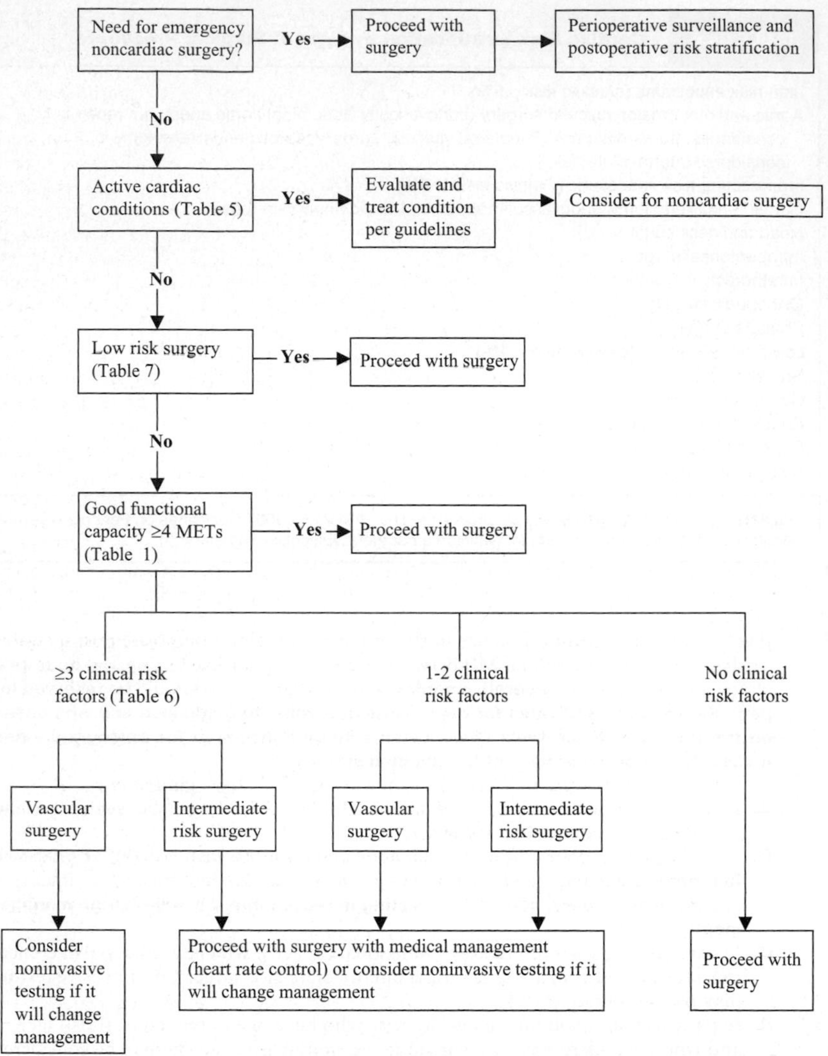

Figure 34.1. A stepwise approach to preoperative cardiac evaluation of a patient undergoing a noncardiac surgery. (Adapted from Fleisher LA, Beckman JA, Brown KA, et al. ACC/AHA 2007 Guidelines on Perioperative Cardiovascular Evaluation and Care for Noncardiac Surgery: Executive Summary [5]).

although a negative study is reassuring, a positive one is still a relatively weak predictor of a perioperative cardiac event.

C. Intravenous dipyridamole and adenosine should be avoided in patients with significant bronchospasm or critical carotid artery stenosis.

D. Dobutamine should be avoided in patients with significant arrhythmias, severe hypertension, or hypotension.

E. **Stress echocardiography** (exercise or dobutamine) offers the advantage of providing additional information about ventricular and valvular function.

VII. PREOPERATIVE CORONARY REVASCULARIZATION. The original ACC/AHA guidelines stated that the indications for revascularization before noncardiac surgery should be similar to those in the general population. In other words, there is no evidence to support the role of "prophylactic" preoperative revascularization, and the decision to pursue revascularization should be the same regardless of the planned surgery. However, these statements have been based on expert opinion, and there has been substantial variability among clinicians concerning general practice with cardiac revascularization preoperatively. **The Coronary Artery Revascularization Prophylaxis (CARP) trial** was the first large randomized trial that addressed this issue. It randomized 510 patients with established CAD, who were deemed to be at high risk for perioperative cardiac complications, to undergo either revascularization [percutaneous coronary intervention (PCI) or coronary artery bypass grafting (CABG)] or no revascularization before elective major vascular surgery. After a median follow-up of 2.7 years, the death rates were the same in both groups. Even among the subsets of patients who were considered to be at especially high risk according to imaging results or by the Revised Cardiac Risk Index, there were no differences in outcomes between the two groups. Although the study was not designed to test short-term benefit of prophylactic revascularization, there was also no reduction in early postoperative cardiac complications.

Patients who undergo **PCI** represent a clinical challenge in managing their antiplatelet therapy at the time of noncardiac surgery. Premature discontinuation of antiplatelet therapy (aspirin and clopidogrel) carries the risk of in-stent thrombosis. **Bare metal stent (BMS)** thrombosis is most common in the first 2 weeks after stent placement and is very rare after 4 weeks due to rapid endothelialization. On the other hand, there has been growing concern that the **DES** carrries greater risk for in-stent thrombosis compared to BMS. The optimal period to delay noncardiac surgery after the use of the DES remains unclear.

A. The **indications for revascularization (CABG or PCI) before noncardiac surgery should be similar to those in the general patient population irrespective of the planned surgery.**
   1. Stable angina with known left main disease.
   2. Stable angina with three-vessel disease [especially with ejection fraction (EF) <50%].
   3. Stable angina with two-vessel disease with siginificant proximal left anterior descending artery stenosis and either EF less than 50% or ischemia on nononvasive testing.
   4. High-risk unstable angina or non-ST-segment elevation MI.
   5. Acute ST-elevation MI.

B. Patients with **asymptomatic ischemia** (based on functional study) do not appear to benefit from preoperative revascularization prior to noncardiac surgeries.

C. Routine prophylactic revascularization should not be performed in patients with stable CAD before noncardiac surgery.

D. Small observational studies suggest that patients who undergo **CABG** should wait at least 4 weeks before proceeding with noncardiac surgery.

E. Patients who undergo **balloon angioplasty without stenting** should wait **at least 2 to 4 weeks** before proceeding with elective noncardiac surgery to allow adequate time for healing of the injured vessel. Daily aspirin should be continued whenever possible. The risk of stopping aspirin should be weighed against the benefit of reducing bleeding risk from surgery. Balloon angioplasty without the use of stent might provide a temporary bridge to go through noncardiac surgery with the intention of implanting stents after the surgery.

F. Among patients who undergo stenting with **BMS's**, it is safer to **wait 6 to 8 weeks** on dual antiplatelet therapy (aspirin and clopidogrel) before proceeding with surgery to avoid the risk of in-stent thrombosis with premature discontinuation of antiplatelet therapy. After 4 to 6 weeks, clopidogrel could be stopped preoperatively, ideally 5 to 7 days before the noncardiac surgery. Daily aspirin use should be continued unless the risk of bleeding outweighs the benefit of continuing aspirin therapy.

G. Among patients who undergo stenting with the **drug-eluting stent (DES),** the optimal duration for dual antiplatelet therapy is not well defined, but should be **at**

least 12 months. Elective noncardiac surgery that requires discontinuation of clopidogrel, or both clopidogrel and aspirin, should be delayed. In general, if noncardiac surgery is expected within the next 12 months, the physician should strongly consider avoiding the use of DES. BMS or balloon angioplasty might provide an alternative approach.

H. Perioperative management of patients with prior PCI undergoing unplanned surgery.

1. The waiting times before proceeding with noncardiac surgery should be at least
   a. 2 to 4 weeks for balloon angioplasty
   b. 4 to 6 weeks for BMS
   c. 12 months for DES
2. For patients who need noncardiac surgery that falls within the time frame that requires dual antiplatelet therapy and cannot be delayed, strong consideration should be given to continuation of dual antiplatelet therapy whenever possible.
3. If the risk of bleeding with dual antiplatelet therapy outweighs the benefit, serious consideration should be given to continuation of at least aspirin whenever possible. Clopidogrel should be resumed as soon as possible after surgery.

I. It is important to recognize that **the recommended time frames for dual antiplatelet therapy are arbitrary and based on expert opinion.** These cases should be addressed individually with good communication between the cardiologist, anesthesiologist, and the surgeon. **Certain conditions might require longer dual antiplatelet therapy** (e.g., left main stenting, history of stent thrombosis, multivessel stenting, and stenting of the only remaining coronary artery or bypass graft).

The use of short-acting intravenous glycoprotein IIb/IIIa inhibitor with or without heparin or low–molecular-weight heparin as a bridge around the time of surgery for patients who need dual antiplatelet therapy is still controversial and there is still no evidence to support its use.

VIII. MANAGEMENT OF SPECIFIC PREOPERATIVE CONDITIONS

A. Valvular heart disease. In general, the indications for evaluation and treatment of valvular heart disease are similar to those in the nonpreoperative setting. Symptomatic stenotic lesions are associated with increased perioperative morbidity, whereas symptomatic regurgitant valve diseases can usually be managed medically and with close monitoring perioperatively.

1. Critical **aortic stenosis** must be recognized promptly, and, if symptomatic, should be managed with valve replacement or, for selected patients, valvuloplasty as a short-term bridge through noncardiac surgery.
2. **Mitral stenosis** when mild and asymptomatic is managed medically with heart rate control. When mitral stenosis is severe and symptomatic, mitral valvuloplasty or valve replacement is considered before a high-risk operation is performed.
3. For patients with **aortic or mitral regurgitation,** the medical regimen is optimized with diuretics and afterload reduction.
4. Appropriate **prophylaxis for bacterial endocarditis** is administered for patients with valvular disorders according to the guidelines.
5. Patients with **prosthetic valves** who need **oral anticoagulation** can usually safely undergo minimally invasive procedures such as dental work or skin biopsy if the international normalized ratio (INR) is briefly reduced to a low or subtherapeutic range. Full anticoagulation is resumed after the procedure. For patients undergoing extensive surgical procedures with prosthetic valves, intravenous unfractionated heparin therapy is initiated. Heparin can be reserved for:
   a. Patients with recent thromboembolic events (<1year)
   b. Mechanical valve in the mitral position
   c. History of thromboembolism while not on anticoagulation
   d. Patients with Bjork-Shiley or Starr-Edwards valve
   e. Patients with three or more of the following risk factors (atrial fibrillation, previous thromboembolism, hypercoagulable condition, mechanical prosthesis and left ventricular ejection fraction <30%)

Mechanical valves in the mitral position are usually more thrombogenic, and, therefore, require a lower threshold for heparin conversion. The use of low-molecular-weight heparin may provide an alternative approach for anticoagulation, but is still controversial as valve thrombosis has been reported with its use. Oral anticoagulants are resumed after the procedure as soon as possible.

B. Arrhythmias. The ACC/AHA 2007 guidelines recognize **high-grade atrioventricular block, symptomatic bradycardia, symptomatic or newly recognized ventricular arrhythmias, supraventricular arrhythmias with uncontrolled ventricular rate, and symptomatic bradycardia as active cardiac conditions that require further evaluation before proceeding with noncardiac surgery.** The following points are important to remember while evaluating arrhythmias in the preoperative setting:

1. Identification of any **underlying cardiac disease, drug toxicity, or metabolic disturbances** that could be the cause of the arrhythmia is very important.
2. For symptomatic and hemodynamically significant arrhythmias, therapy should target the underlying cause and then the arrhythmia itself.
3. The indications for antiarrhythmic therapy and cardiac pacing are similar to those in nonoperative setting.
4. Frequent premature ventricular beats and asymptomatic nonsustained ventricular tachycardias are not associated with increased perioperative cardiac risk.

C. Permanent pacemakers and implantable cardioverter–defibrillators (ICDs). It is important to identify patients who have pacemakers or ICDs. Patients who are completely pacemaker-dependent should have their device checked within 3 to 6 months before surgery, and their device should be reprogrammed to an asynchronous mode during surgery (VOO or DOO); in certain models, a magnet can be placed over the device during surgery. Electrocautery should be used only briefly and with caution. Bipolar pacing minimizes the risk of electrocautery. After the operation, all pacemakers are interrogated to ensure that the settings are optimal and that no changes occurred during the operation or electrocautery. ICDs are programmed to *off* preoperatively and then reprogrammed to *on* after the procedure.

D. Hypertension. In general, patients with hypertension may be indirectly predisposed to perioperative myocardial ischemia, since CAD is more prevalent among these patients. In addition, because of the stiffness of the vascular system, they are predisposed to intraoperative hypotension; therefore, they should be **monitored closely during an operation.**

1. Patients with **mild or moderate** hypertension may undergo elective operations with continued medical therapy.
2. **Severe** hypertension (systolic blood pressure greater than or equal to 180 mm Hg and diastolic pressure greater than or equal to 110 mm Hg) should be controlled before the surgery. If possible, the operation is delayed until the pressure is consistently controlled. If urgent surgical intervention is needed, rapid-acting agents are used. β-Blockers are preferred, especially because they act as anti-ischemic agents as well.
3. Withdrawal of β-blockers and clonidine from patients undergoing long-term therapy with these agents **must be avoided** to prevent a rebound phenomenon.

E. Heart failure is associated with increased risk of perioperative morbidity. Identification of the etiology of heart failure is very important, since the treatment **depends on the cause** and overall clinical status.

1. Heart failure should be optimally controlled preoperatively with special attention to avoid over-diuresis, which can exacerbate postoperative hypotension.
2. Patients **with hypertrophic cardiomyopathy** need close monitoring of volume status, heart rate, and systemic vascular resistance to avoid intraoperative hypotension and hypovolemia that can lead to exacerbation of dynamic outflow obstruction.

IX. PERIOPERATIVE MEDICAL THERAPY

A. β-Blockers: Several trials and meta-analyses have examined the role of β-blockers in preventing perioperative cardiac complications. However, there remain multiple limitations in interpreting the data due to the paucity of randomized clinical trials, the lack of clear protocol for intitiation and titration of β-blockers, and the lack of comparison between different agents. These limitations were acknowledged in a recent update by the ACC/AHA regarding the use of β-blockers perioperatively and in the latest ACC/AHA 2007 guidelines. Despite these limitations, the weight of evidence is in favor of using perioperative β-blockers during noncardiac surgery, especially among high-risk patients. β-Blockers should be initiated before the surgery and titrated to a target heart rate of 50 to 60 bpm. Some data suggest that long-acting β-blockers may be superior than short-acting ones, but this has not yet been confirmed by randomized trials. In patients with indications for β-blockers, these agents can be continued indefinitely, and if there is no indication they should be continued for at least 7 days, and preferably 30 days after the noncardiac surgery.

1. β-Blockers should be continued in all patients undergoing surgery who are already receiving β-blockers for any class I guideline indication (to treat angina, arrhythmias, hypertension, etc.).
2. β-Blockers should be administered to all high-risk patients identified by myocardial ischemia on preoperative assessment undergoing vascular surgery.
3. β-Blockers are probably indicated for patients undergoing vascular or intermediate-risk surgery in whom preoperative evaluation reveals CAD.
4. β-Blockers are probably indicated for patients undergoing vascular or intermediate-risk surgery who have more than one clinical risk factor.
5. The usefulness of β-blockers is uncertain for patients undergoing vascular or intermediate-risk surgery who have only one or no clinical risk factor.
6. β-Blockers should not be administered in preoperative patients with absolute contraindications to the agents.

The POISE study, presented at the 2007 scientific sessions of the AHA, suggests that for every 1000 patients treated with metoprolol, 15 MIs would be prevented, but there would be an excess of 8 deaths and 5 strokes. β-Blockers should be continued if patients are already receiving them, but starting them routinely in all patient perioperatively is now open to question.

B. **α_2-Agonists** suppress the release of catecholamines and may decrease the incidence of cardiac events in patients with known CAD and at least one clinical risk factor who are undergoing noncardiac surgery.

C. The role of **calcium antagonists** is not well defined and requires further research.

D. **Statins.** There has been growing evidence suggesting an association between perioperative statin therapy and decreased perioperative cardiac complications. Definite indications for perioperative statin use awaits the results of ongoing and future clinical trials. However, it is important to note that perioperative evaluation represent an opportunity to identify patients who meet National Cholesterol Education Program criteria and impact their long-term outcome.

1. Statins should be continued in patients who are already on statin therapy and undergoing noncardiac surgery.
2. For patients undergoing vascular surgery it is reasonable to be on statin therapy.
3. Statins may be considered for patients with at least one clinical risk factor who are undergoing intermediate risk surgery.

X. ANESTHETIC AGENTS AND PERIOPERATIVE HEMODYNAMIC MONITORING

A. Several studies have evaluated the effect of **anesthetic agents and techniques** on cardiac morbidity. It appears that there is **no one best myocardial protective agent.** All inhalational agents cause depression of myocardial contractility and afterload reduction, which can lead to hypotension. Several studies have suggested that **neuroaxial (epidural, spinal)** may reduce pulmonary and thrombotic complications compared to general anesthesia. However, its role in lowering cardiac complications remains controversial. Decisions regarding anesthetic techiniques are best left to the anesthesiologist. Perioperative pain management is important because it reduces postoperative catecholamine response and cardiac stress.

B. **Pulmonary artery catheters** are occasionally used in high-risk patients (advanced heart failure, severe CAD) who are undergoing procedures associated with significant hemodynamic stress. The ACC/AHA guidelines advise to assess benefit versus risk when considering the use of pulmonary artery catheters. Catheter-guided volume optimization has no clear benefit perioperatively, and multicenter randomized trials have shown that pulmonary artery catheter use provides no benefit after noncardiac surgery or in the intensive care unit.

XI. POSTOPERATIVE MONITORING AND MANAGEMENT OF EVENTS

A. Postoperative MI. The pathophysiology of perioperative MI is not well defined and may be different than nonoperative MIs. Stress, inflammation, hypercoagulability, and hypoxia may all be contributing factors. The incidence of perioperative MI ranges from 2% to 6% in general. However, up to 50% of perioperative MIs may go unrecognized. The majority of perioperative MIs occur within the first 3 days after surgery, a period when the patients are receiving narcotics that could mask the pain, some patients are still intubated and sedated, and many of the clinical signs patients normally manifest are attributable to other causes (e.g., hypovolemia, bleeding, pain). Nonspecific findings, such as CHF, hypotension, nausea, or ST-segment depression, may be the only clues to postoperative ischemia. The prognosis of these unrecognized MIs is nevertheless similar to that of patients experiencing a recognized MI.

1. There are **no standard criteria for the diagnosis of perioperative MI in patients undergoing noncardiac surgery.**
2. **Troponin** is a more specific marker for perioperative MI than creatinine kinase-myocardial band (CK-MB), which could be falsely positive after surgery.
3. **ECG and troponin** should be checked postoperatively in **patients with signs and symptoms suggestive of ischemia, but based on the current literature, routine measurement of troponin is not recommened after noncardiac surgery.**
4. It is also important to rule out **other causes for positive troponin, such as pulmonary embolism.**
5. Although there is an increase in use of intraoperative **transesophageal echocardiography** to monitor myocardial ischemia through wall motion abnormalities, there is insufficient information to make firm recommendations.
6. There are **no clear guidelines for management of perioperative MIs. Identifying and treating correctible causes** is important (e.g., anemia and hypoxia). In general, primary PCI is preferred for **perioperative ST-elevation MI.** Although thrombolytics, antiplatelet, and anticoagulant therapies are beneficial in the treatment of non–ST-elevation MI or unstable angina in nonoperative setting, these therapies could potentially cause more harm than benefit in perioperative settings. Many drugs that are important in the long-term management of nonoperative MIs [e.g., aspirin, angiotensin-converting enzyme (ACE) inhibitors, β-blockers, and statins) may not carry the same positive effect in perioperative MI patients. Large randomized clinical trials are needed to answer these questions.
7. Nonfatal perioperative MI is an independent risk factor for cardiovascular death and nonfatal MI during the 6 months following the surgery. Therefore, close follow-up with aggressive risk-factor modification is important for these patients.

B. The management of **postoperative heart failure and pulmonary edema** is not much different than in nonoperative settings. ECG and troponin should be checked to rule out MI.

C. Arrhythmias. Perioperative arrhythmias are common, especially among elderly patients and after thoracic surgeries. For patients with arrhythmias, the metabolic profile and medications should be reviewed, and any underlying reversible conditions should be corrected including hypoxia, fever, bleeding, pain, and infection. β-Blockers and calcium channel blockers can reduce postoperative tachyarrhythmias.

1. Most **supraventricular tachycardias (SVTs)** necessitate rate control until the underlying cause is addressed. This can be achieved using β-blockers, calcium channel blockers, or digoxin). Adenosine can be effective in terminating certain reentrant tachycardias. New onset **atrial fibrillation (AF)** raises embolic risk. To avoid the increased bleeding risk with anticoagulation after surgery, restoring

sinus rhythm is often a preferred strategy. Rate control is advised and if the AF persists more than 24 hours antiarrhythmic drugs could be used. Most AF will resolve within 36 to 48 hours, but if it persists, then anticoagulation is warranted. At any time if the SVT causes hemodynamic compromise or ongoing myocardial ischemia, electrical cardioversion is the therapy of choice.

2. Symptomatic **bradyarrhythmias** are managed with temporary pacing, and a permanent pacemaker can be implanted if and when indicated.

XII. POSTOPERATIVE MANAGEMENT. In most cases, the results of the preoperative evaluation determine whether a patient is at substantial cardiac risk. For these patients, postoperative care is dictated by the findings before the operation. In a few urgent cases, or for patients who did not undergo preoperative evaluation, postoperative evaluation and care are individualized.

A. After a patient has successfully undergone a procedure, the physician **assesses and manages risk factors** for coronary and peripheral atherosclerosis.

B. Management of risk factors, including smoking cessation, control of labile hypertension, aggressive management of hyperlipidemia, and glycemic control for patients with diabetes are of paramount importance.

C. Particular attention is given to **patients who sustain perioperative MI or demonstrate perioperative ischemia** because these patients are at risk for recurrent MI or cardiac death in subsequent years. These patients should be followed closely and treated aggressively.

ACKNOWLEDGMENTS

The author thanks Drs. John H. Chiu and Vasant B. Patel for their contributions to earlier editions of this chapter.

Landmark Articles

Auerbach A, Goldman L. Assessing and reducing the cardiac risk of noncardiac surgery. *Circulation* 2006;113:1361–1376.

Devereaux PJ, Goldman L, Cook DJ, et al. Perioperative cardiac events in patients undergoing noncardiac surgery: a review of the magnitude of the problem, the pathophysiology of the events and methods to estimate and communicate risk. *Can Med Assoc J* 2005;173:627–634.

Devereaux PJ, Goldman L, Yusuf S, et al. Surveillance and prevention of major perioperative ischemic cardiac events in patients undergoing noncardiac surgery: a review. *Can Med Assoc J* 2005;173:779–788.

Key Reviews

Fleisher LA, Beckman JA, Brown KA, et al. ACC/AHA 2007 Guidelines on Perioperative Cardiovascular Evaluation and Care for Noncardiac Surgery: Executive Summary: A Report of the American College of Cardiology/American Heart Association Task Force on Practice Guidelines (Writing Committee to Revise the 2002 Guidelines on Perioperative Cardiovascular Evaluation for Noncardiac Surgery). Developed in Collaboration with the American Society of Echocardiography, American Society of Nuclear Cardiology, Heart Rhythm Society, Society of Cardiovascular Anesthesiologists, Society for Cardiovascular Angiography and Interventions, Society for Vascular Medicine and Biology, and Society for Vascular Surgery. *J Am Coll Cardiol* 2007;50:1707–1732.

Relevant Book Chapter

Roizen MF, Ellis J, Mantha S, et al. Perioperative anesthetic considerations in noncardiac surgery for those at high risk of cardiovascular disease. In: Topol EJ, *Textbook of cardiovascular medicine,* 3rd ed. Philadelphia: Lippincott Williams & Wilkins, 2007:721–735.

Suggested Readings

Auerbach A, Goldman L. Assessing and reducing the cardiac risk of noncardiac surgery. *Circulation* 2006;113:1361–1376.

Babapulle MN, Joseph L, Belisle P, et al. A hierarchical Bayesian meta-analysis of randomised clinical trials of drug-eluting stents. *Lancet* 2004;364:583–591.

Brady AR, Gibbs JS, Greenhalgh RM, et al. Perioperative beta-blockade (POBBLE) for patients undergoing infrarenal vascular surgery: results of a randomized double-blind controlled trial. *J Vasc Surg* 2005;41:602–609.

Breen P, Lee JW, Pomposelli F, et al. Timing of high-risk vascular surgery following coronary artery bypass surgery: a 10-year experience from an academic medical centre. *Anaesthesia* 2004;59:422–427.

Detsky AS, Abrams HB, McLaughlin JR, et al. Predicting cardiac complications in patients undergoing non-cardiac surgery. *J Gen Intern Med* 1986;1:211–219.

Devereaux PJ, Beattie WS, Choi PT, et al. How strong is the evidence for the use of perioperative beta blockers in non-cardiac surgery? Systematic review and meta-analysis of randomised controlled trials. *BMJ* 2005;331:313–321.

Devereaux PJ, Goldman L, Cook DJ, et al. Perioperative cardiac events in patients undergoing noncardiac surgery: a review of the magnitude of the problem, the pathophysiology of the events and methods to estimate and communicate risk. *Can Med Assoc J* 2005;173:627–634.

Devereaux PJ, Goldman L, Yusuf S, et al. Surveillance and prevention of major perioperative ischemic cardiac events in patients undergoing noncardiac surgery: a review. *Can Med Assoc J* 2005;173:779–788.

Durazzo AE, Machado FS, Ikeoka DT, et al. Reduction in cardiovascular events after vascular surgery with atorvastatin: a randomized trial. *J Vasc Surg* 2004;39:967–975; discussion 975–966.

Eagle KA, Berger PB, Calkins H, et al. ACC/AHA guideline update for perioperative cardiovascular evaluation for noncardiac surgery–executive summary: a report of the American College of Cardiology/American Heart Association Task Force on Practice Guidelines (Committee to Update the 1996 Guidelines on Perioperative Cardiovascular Evaluation for Noncardiac Surgery). *J Am Coll Cardiol* 2002;39:542–553.

Eltchaninoff H, Cribier A, Tron C, et al. Balloon aortic valvuloplasty in elderly patients at high risk for surgery, or inoperable. Immediate and mid-term results. *Eur Heart J* 1995;16:1079–1084.

Fleisher LA, Beckman JA, Brown KA, et al. ACC/AHA 2006 guideline update on perioperative cardiovascular evaluation for noncardiac surgery: focused update on perioperative beta-blocker therapy: a report of the American College of Cardiology/American Heart Association Task Force on Practice Guidelines (Writing Committee to Update the 2002 Guidelines on Perioperative Cardiovascular Evaluation for Noncardiac Surgery). Developed in collaboration with the American Society of Echocardiography, American Society of Nuclear Cardiology, Heart Rhythm Society, Society of Cardiovascular Anesthesiologists, Society for Cardiovascular Angiography and Interventions, and Society for Vascular Medicine and Biology. *J Am Coll Cardiol* 2006;47:2343–2355.

Fleisher LA, Beckman JA, Brown KA, et al. ACC/AHA 2007 Guidelines on Perioperative Cardiovascular Evaluation and Care for Noncardiac Surgery: Executive Summary: A Report of the American College of Cardiology/American Heart Association Task Force on Practice Guidelines (Writing Committee to Revise the 2002 Guidelines on Perioperative Cardiovascular Evaluation for Noncardiac Surgery). Developed in Collaboration with the American Society of Echocardiography, American Society of Nuclear Cardiology, Heart Rhythm Society, Society of Cardiovascular Anesthesiologists, Society for Cardiovascular Angiography and Interventions, Society for Vascular Medicine and Biology, and Society for Vascular Surgery. *J Am Coll Cardiol* 2007;50:1707–1732.

Goldman L, Caldera DL, Nussbaum SR, et al. Multifactorial index of cardiac risk in noncardiac surgical procedures. *N Engl J Med* 1977;297:845–850.

Harvey S, Harrison DA, Singer M, et al. Assessment of the clinical effectiveness of pulmonary artery catheters in management of patients in intensive care (PAC-Man): a randomised controlled trial. *Lancet* 2005;366:472–477.

Kaluza GL, Joseph J, Lee JR, et al. Catastrophic outcomes of noncardiac surgery soon after coronary stenting. *J Am Coll Cardiol* 2000;35:1288–1294.

Kertai MD, Boersma E, Westerhout CM, et al. A combination of statins and beta-blockers is independently associated with a reduction in the incidence of perioperative mortality and nonfatal myocardial infarction in patients undergoing abdominal aortic aneurysm surgery. *Eur J Vasc Endovasc Surg* 2004;28:343–352.

Kertai MD, Bountioukos M, Boersma E, et al. Aortic stenosis: an underestimated risk factor for perioperative complications in patients undergoing noncardiac surgery. *Am J Med* 2004;116:8–13.

Lee TH, Marcantonio ER, Mangione CM, et al. Derivation and prospective validation of a simple index for prediction of cardiac risk of major noncardiac surgery. *Circulation* 1999;100:1043–1049.

Lindenauer PK, Pekow P, Wang K, et al. Lipid-lowering therapy and in-hospital mortality following major noncardiac surgery. *JAMA* 2004;291:2092–2099.

Mangano DT, Layug EL, Wallace A, et al. Effect of atenolol on mortality and cardiovascular morbidity after noncardiac surgery. Multicenter Study of Perioperative Ischemia Research Group. *N Engl J Med* 1996;335:1713–1720.

McFalls EO, Ward HB, Moritz TE, et al. Coronary-artery revascularization before elective major vascular surgery. *N Engl J Med* 2004;351:2795–2804.

Oliver MF, Goldman L, Julian DG, et al. Effect of mivazerol on perioperative cardiac complications during non-cardiac surgery in patients with coronary heart disease: the European Mivazerol Trial (EMIT). *Anesthesiology* 1999;91: 951–961.

O'Neil-Callahan K, Katsimaglis G, Tepper MR, et al. Statins decrease perioperative cardiac complications in patients undergoing noncardiac vascular surgery: the Statins for Risk Reduction in Surgery (StaRRS) study. *J Am Coll Cardiol* 2005;45:336–342.

Pierpont GL, Moritz TE, Goldman S, et al. Disparate opinions regarding indications for coronary artery revascularization before elective vascular surgery. *Am J Cardiol* 2004;94:1124–1128.

Poldermans D, Bax JJ, Kertai MD, et al. Statins are associated with a reduced incidence of perioperative mortality in patients undergoing major noncardiac vascular surgery. *Circulation* 2003;107:1848–1851.

Poldermans D, Bax JJ, Schouten O, et al. Should major vascular surgery be delayed because of preoperative cardiac testing in intermediate-risk patients receiving beta-blocker therapy with tight heart rate control? *J Am Coll Cardiol* 2006;48:964–969.

Poldermans D, Boersma E, Bax JJ, et al. The effect of bisoprolol on perioperative mortality and myocardial infarction in high-risk patients undergoing vascular surgery. Dutch Echocardiographic Cardiac Risk Evaluation Applying Stress Echocardiography Study Group. *N Engl J Med* 1999;341:1789–1794.

Raby KE, Brull SJ, Timimi F, et al. The effect of heart rate control on myocardial ischemia among high-risk patients after vascular surgery. *Anesth Analg* 1999;88:477–482.

Rigg JR, Jamrozik K, Myles PS, et al. Epidural anaesthesia and analgesia and outcome of major surgery: a randomised trial. *Lancet* 2002;359:1276–1282.

Rohde LE, Polanczyk CA, Goldman L, et al. Usefulness of transthoracic echocardiography as a tool for risk stratification of patients undergoing major noncardiac surgery. *Am J Cardiol* 2001;87:505–509.

Sandham JD, Hull RD, Brant RF, et al. A randomized, controlled trial of the use of pulmonary-artery catheters in high-risk surgical patients. *N Engl J Med* 2003;348:5–14.

Sheifer SE, Manolio TA, Gersh BJ. Unrecognized myocardial infarction. *Ann Intern Med* 2001;135:801–811.

Stevens RD, Burri H, Tramer MR. Pharmacologic myocardial protection in patients undergoing noncardiac surgery: a quantitative systematic review. *Anesth Analg* 2003;97:623–633.

Stone JG, Foex P, Sear JW, et al. Myocardial ischemia in untreated hypertensive patients: effect of a single small oral dose of a beta-adrenergic blocking agent. *Anesthesiology* 1988;68:495–500.

Stuhmeier KD, Mainzer B, Cierpka J, et al. Small, oral dose of clonidine reduces the incidence of intraoperative myocardial ischemia in patients having vascular surgery. *Anesthesiology* 1996;85:706–712.

Theheart.org. POISEd to change the guidelines on perioperative use of beta blockers? Available at: http://www.theheart.org/article/826435.do.

Urban MK, Markowitz SM, Gordon MA, et al. Postoperative prophylactic administration of beta-adrenergic blockers in patients at risk for myocardial ischemia. *Anesth Analg* 2000;90:1257–1261.
Valentine RJ, Duke ML, Inman MH, et al. Effectiveness of pulmonary artery catheters in aortic surgery: a randomized trial. *J Vasc Surg* 1998;27:203–211; discussion 211–202.
Wallace AW, Galindez D, Salahieh A, et al. Effect of clonidine on cardiovascular morbidity and mortality after noncardiac surgery. *Anesthesiology* 2004;101:284–293.
Wallace A, Layug B, Tateo I, et al. Prophylactic atenolol reduces postoperative myocardial ischemia. McSPI Research Group. *Anesthesiology* 1998;88:7–17.
Wijeysundera DN, Beattie WS, Rao V, et al. Calcium antagonists reduce cardiovascular complications after cardiac surgery: a meta-analysis. *J Am Coll Cardiol* 2003;41:1496–1505.
Wijeysundera DN, Beattie WS. Calcium channel blockers for reducing cardiac morbidity after noncardiac surgery: a meta-analysis. *Anesth Analg* 2003;97:634–641.
Wijeysundera DN, Naik JS, Beattie WS. Alpha-2 adrenergic agonists to prevent perioperative cardiovascular complications: a meta-analysis. *Am J Med* 2003;114:742–752.
Wilson SH, Fasseas P, Orford JL, et al. Clinical outcome of patients undergoing non-cardiac surgery in the two months following coronary stenting. *J Am Coll Cardiol* 2003;42:234–240.
Zaugg M, Tagliente T, Lucchinetti E, et al. Beneficial effects from beta-adrenergic blockade in elderly patients undergoing noncardiac surgery. *Anesthesiology* 1999;91:1674–1686.
Ziegler DW, Wright JG, Choban PS, et al. A prospective randomized trial of preoperative "optimization" of cardiac function in patients undergoing elective peripheral vascular surgery. *Surgery* 1997;122:584–592.

35 HYPERTENSIVE CRISIS

Daniel J. Cantillon

I. INTRODUCTION

A. Epidemiology. More than 50 million persons in the United States are estimated to have systemic hypertension, many of whom are inadequately treated. Approximately 1% of these patients progress to a crisis phase, accounting for more than 50% of all cases of hypertensive crisis. Although the incidence is decreasing due to improved awareness, treatments, and public health measures, patients with untreated hypertension or suboptimal blood pressure control remain more susceptible to acute rises in blood pressure. Patients with secondary causes of hypertension are also at higher risk of hypertensive crises. Unless promptly recognized and treated, hypertensive crisis can lead to cardiovascular, renal, and central nervous system (CNS) organ disease and death. Effective and prompt antihypertensive treatment improves the prognosis.

B. Definitions. Hypertensive crisis includes **hypertensive emergency** and **urgency.** According to the Joint National Committee on Detection, Evaluation and Treatment of High Blood Pressure (JNC), and other authorities, normal blood pressure is defined as less than 120 mm Hg systolic and 80 mm Hg diastolic. Severe hypertension is defined as a systolic blood pressure greater than 180 mm Hg or diastolic pressure greater than 120 mm Hg. **Hypertensive emergency is defined as severe hypertension with evidence of acute end organ damage and is manifested in a variety of syndromes (Table 35.1).** Severe hypertension in the presence of chronic organ damage without associated symptoms does not constitute an emergency. Hypertensive urgency is generally defined as severe hypertension without significant acute end-organ damage (Table 35.2). Pseudoemergencies are acute rises in blood pressure attributed to a surge in sympathetic outflow from a physiologic trigger (i.e., pain, anxiety, a postictal state).

1. Hypertensive emergency. Severe hypertension with evidence of acute end-organ dysfunction implicates the need for immediate parenteral blood pressure

TABLE 35.1 Hypertensive Emergencies

Malignant hypertension with papilledema
Hypertensive encephalopathy
Severe hypertension in the setting of stroke, subarachnoid hemorrhage, head trauma
Acute aortic dissection[a]
Hypertension and left ventricular failure[a]
Hypertension and myocardial ischemia and infarction[a]
Hypertension after coronary artery bypass surgery
Heochromocytoma crisis[b]
Food or drug interactions with monoamine oxidase inhibitors[b]
Cocaine abuse[b]
Rebound hypertension after sudden drug withdrawal (clonidine)[b]
Idiosyncratic drug reactions (e.g., atropine)[b]
Eclampsia

[a]Exceptions include cardiovascular dysfunction in which low blood pressure may represent an emergency.
[b]Considered emergencies when associated with end-organ damage; otherwise treated as urgencies.

controlling therapy in a monitored setting (typically ICU) to minimize tissue damage and long-term complications. Delay may cause irreversible organ damage and death. **Accelerated or malignant hypertension** and **hypertensive encephalopathy** are the prototypical hypertensive emergencies.

a. **Accelerated or malignant hypertension** is a systemic disease characterized by an extreme elevation in blood pressure (mean arterial blood pressure [MAP] greater than 120 mm Hg), bilateral retinal hemorrhage, and exudates in the case of accelerated hypertension or papilledema in the case of malignant hypertension.
b. **Hypertensive encephalopathy** is characterized by headache, irritability, and an altered state of consciousness caused by a sudden marked increase in blood pressure. Hypertensive encephalopathy occurs when cerebral edema is induced by markedly elevated blood pressures that overwhelm the autoregulatory capabilities of the brain. This condition tends to affect previously normotensive patients who experience a rapid rise in blood pressure. Patients with chronic hypertension are relatively resistant to encephalopathy because their autoregulatory systems have adapted to the chronically elevated pressures. When encephalopathy does occur in these patients, it is usually in the setting of an extraordinarily elevated systemic pressures (i.e., diastolic blood pressures higher than 150 mm Hg). Mental status will classically revert to normal with the institution of antihypertensive therapy.

2. **Hypertensive urgency.** In the absence of symptoms or acute organ dysfunction, severe hypertension can be lowered over a period of hours to days. Patients can be

TABLE 35.2 Hypertensive Urgencies

Severe hypertension, accelerated hypertension
Pheochromocytoma crisis without end-organ dysfunction
Food or drug interactions with monoamine oxidase inhibitors
Rebound hypertension after sudden drug withdrawal
Idiosyncratic drug reactions
Preoperative hypertension
Postoperative hypertension

treated with oral medications, and even managed as outpatients. A poor response to initial therapy, and high risk patients (i.e., those with excessive medical and/or cardiac comorbidities) should be considered for admission.

3. **Pseudoemergencies.** These scenarios must be differentiated from true hypertensive emergencies because the treatments differ markedly. The increase in blood pressure in a pseudoemergency is caused by massive sympathetic outflow as the result of pain, hypoxia, hypercarbia, hypoglycemia, anxiety, or the postictal state. Treatment is directed at the underlying trigger.

II. CLINICAL PRESENTATION. If an emergency is suspected, appropriate arrangements for ICU admission and parenteral treatment should not be delayed by waiting for the results of further tests. Chest pain, shortness of breath, headache, blurred vision, signs of altered mental status, focal neurologic deficits, grade III or IV retinopathy, rales, an S_3 gallop, and pulse deficits all point toward an emergency.

A. History

1. **Constitutional symptoms** can occur such as nausea, vomiting, weight loss, or anorexia. Symptoms also can include shortness of breath, chest pain, headache, blurred vision, and abdominal pain. Patients with accelerated or malignant hypertension often have oliguria.
2. **Symptom chronology.** Among patients with hypertensive encephalopathy, the symptoms typically have progressed over a period of several days prior to presentation.
3. **History of hypertension.** Most patients with accelerated or malignant hypertension have an underlying history of chronic primary hypertension; however, a significant percentage do have secondary forms of hypertension.
4. **Contributory medication history** may include nonsteroidal anti-inflammatory drugs (NSAIDs), oral contraceptives, psychotropic agents, monoamine oxidase inhibitors, ephedrine, cyclosporine, over-the-counter cold remedies, and many other medications.
5. **Use of recreational drugs history** such as cocaine, amphetamines, and **nonprescription stimulants** including sympathomimetic weight loss pills, and performance enhancing substances for athletes are important to elicit.
6. **Smoking history.** Smokers are at increased risk for progression to malignant hypertension, perhaps due to endothelial dysfunction.

B. Physical findings

1. **Vital signs.** Blood pressure is measured in both upper and lower extremities to evaluate for stenosis or dissection of the aorta or great vessels. Severe hypertension is confirmed with two blood pressure measurements separated by 15 to 30 minutes. No absolute level of blood pressure differentiates an emergency from an urgency. The distinction is based upon the total clinical picture.
2. **Optic fundi** are examined for signs of retinopathy, including exudates, hemorrhages, or papilledema.
3. **Neurologic assessment** is performed to assess mental status and neurologic motor deficits. Patients with hypertensive encephalopathy may manifest neurologic signs of confusion or seizure activity.
4. **Heart and lungs** are examined for presence of an S_3, S_4, murmur or pulmonary edema.
5. **Vascular system** is examined by palpation of pulses and ausculatation for bruits.

III. ETIOLOGY. Table 35.3 lists underlying clinical conditions that can precipitate a hypertensive crisis. An evaluation for such secondary causes and precipitants is indicated in the evaluation of all patients with hypertensive crisis. Between 20% and 56% of patients have an identifiable underlying cause, compared with less than 5% of those with uncomplicated primary hypertension.

A. A common scenario is that of a patient inadequately treated for chronic hypertension, or one that is medically noncompliant.

B. Risk factors for progression to hypertensive crisis include male sex, black race, low socioeconomic status, cigarette smoking or other tobacco abuse, and oral contraceptive use. Unlike primary hypertension, the incidence of which increases with age, the peak incidence of hypertensive crisis occurs among persons 40 to 50 years old.

TABLE 35.3 Conditions that May Precipitate a Hypertensive Crisis

Essential hypertension (most common)
Preeclampsia (hypertension in pregnancy)
Renal diseases
Obstructive sleep apnea
Pheochromocytoma and other endocrine tumors
Head injuries and central nervous system events (e.g., stroke, hemorrhage)
Spinal cord injuries
Vasculitis
Collagen vascular disease (classically scleroderma)
Drug-induced (e.g., interactions, idiosyncratic reactions, exaggerated effects, abrupt withdrawal)

C. **Underlying pathology** that can precipitate hypertensive crisis include renal parenchymal disease, renovascular hypertension, collagen vascular disease, pheochromocytoma, vasculitis, preeclampsia, neurologic disorders, and head trauma.

D. A number of **medications and illicit drugs** can cause marked elevations in systemic blood pressure. The most common offenders are oral contraceptives, sympathomimetic agents (e.g., diet pills, amphetamines), cold remedies, nonsteroidal antiinflammatory drugs (NSAIDs), cocaine, tricyclic antidepressants, and monoamine oxidase inhibitors.

E. In rare instances, a hypertensive crisis is the first manifestation of disease. These patients tend to have secondary forms of hypertension, most commonly due to renovascular or renal parenchymal disease, medications or illicit drugs.

F. **Left ventricular failure or pulmonary edema.** Elevated blood pressure poses an enormous workload on a failing heart. Even patients with normal systolic function can have pulmonary edema in the setting of markedly elevated blood pressures (i.e., afterload mismatch).

G. **Myocardial ischemia.** Blood pressure, heart rate, and preload determine myocardial oxygen demand. Elevated blood pressure can induce ischemia or complicate myocardial infarction (MI).

H. Hypertensive crisis associated with **hypercatecholaminemla.** Hypercatecholamine states most commonly are induced by the exaggerated effects of medications, recreational drugs, or food–drug interactions. The common culprits include clonidine withdrawal, cocaine, amphetamines, alcohol withdrawl, LSD, and diet pills, as well as the interaction of certain foods with monoamine oxidase inhibitors. Pheochromocytoma can also cause marked blood pressure elevations.

I. **Postoperative hypertension.** Severe hypertension can complicate a patient's hospital course after coronary and peripheral vascular procedures. The elevated pressure threatens suture lines and promotes excessive bleeding.

IV. PATHOPHYSIOLOGY

A. Hypertensive emergencies are triggered by an **abrupt increase in systemic vascular resistance (SVR) caused by increases in circulating vasoconstrictors** (e.g., norepinephrine, angiotensin II). The resultant increase in blood pressure leads to **arteriolar fibrinoid necrosis** characterized by endothelial damage, platelet and fibrin deposition, and loss of autoregulatory function. Ensuing **ischemia and dysfunction** in the target organ cause further release of vasoactive substances, producing a cycle of increasing SVR, elevated systemic blood pressure, decreased cardiac output, vascular injury, and tissue damage. This is the vicious cycle that propagates a hypertensive emergency. Alternatively, the initially elevated blood pressure can be a complication of other another primary disease process such as aortic dissection, left ventricular failure, or stroke.

B. **Role of the renin–angiotension system.** Overproduction of renin stimulates the release of angiotensin II, which causes further vasoconstriction and elevated SVR. By the same vascular injury mechanism described previously, this amplifies the release of renin, which propagates the cycle of continually elevated blood pressure. The initial overproduction of renin is especially prominent when primary diseases of the renal vasculature or parenchyma are present, as classically occurs in the scleroderma renal crisis. Hence, angiotensin-converting enzyme (ACE) inhibition or angiotensin receptor blockade plays a central role in most treatment regimens. Some authors, in fact, advocate using plasma renin activity level (with a cutoff of $\geq$0.65 ng/mL per hour) in determining whether the therapy should primarily target the renin–angiotension system (i.e., beta-blocker, ACE inhibitor, angiotensin receptor blockade) or sodium/volume hypertension (i.e., calcium channel blockers, α-blockers).

C. Autoregulation

1. The kidney, brain, and heart all possess **autoregulatory mechanisms that maintain blood flow at near constant levels despite fluctuations in blood pressure.** Because the brain is encased in a finite space and because it maximally extracts oxygen at baseline, it is most vulnerable when its autoregulatory systems fail. Excess blood flow results in cerebral edema, elevated intracranial pressure (ICP), and ischemia.
2. Cerebral blood flow (CBF) is maintained at a near-constant level despite variations in cerebral perfusion pressure (CPP). The relationships among CBF, CPP, MAP, pulse pressure (PP), ICP, and diastolic blood pressure (DBB) are described in the following equations, which show that CBF varies with CPP:

$$\mathrm{CPP} = \mathrm{MAP} - \mathrm{ICP}$$
$$\mathrm{MAP} = \mathrm{DBP} + \tfrac{1}{3}\mathrm{PP}$$

3. An **elevated MAP causes an increase in CPP,** whereas a decreasing MAP causes decreased CPP. Despite changes in CPP, cerebral autoregulatory mechanisms maintain CBF; as MAP rises, vasoconstriction occurs, and as MAP decreases, vasodilation occurs. This system has upper and lower limits beyond which CBF can no longer be controlled.
   a. When **CPP decreases below the lower limits of autoregulation,** brain hypoxia ensues, and symptoms of hypoperfusion manifest: headache, nausea, dizziness, altered sensorium, and lethargy. If uncorrected or extreme, this may ultimately cause infarction.
   b. When **MAP exceeds autoregulatory capabilities,** hyperperfusion occurs, leading to an increase in ICP, cerebral edema, and progressive organ dysfunction.
4. Most patients with normal blood pressure maintain autoregulation of MAP between 50 and 80 mm Hg, although this is highly variable. These values generally increase among patients with chronic hypertension. These patients consequently may have cerebral hypoperfusion at a MAP that is considered normal. Elderly persons and patients who have had cerebrovascular accidents, subarachnoid hemorrhage, hypertensive encephalopathy, or accelerated or malignant hypertension have altered autoregulation.
5. Treatment must be tempered by the fact that **abrupt overzealous blood pressure reduction may lead to permanent neurologic damage.** Cerebrovascular accidents, blindness, paralysis, coma, MI, and death have been reported as consequences of overaggressive blood pressure reduction.

V. DIAGNOSTIC EVALUATION. The diagnostic evaluation should not delay treatment time in the setting of hypertensive emergency. Diagnostic imaging, if clinically indicated, can be performed after treatment has been instituted.

A. Complete blood count and blood smear. The presence of anemia with schistocytes should raise concerns for hemolysis and microangiopathic hemolytic anemia.

B. Blood chemistries to evaluate for renal dysfunction and associated electrolyte disturbances.

C. Urinalysis to look for proteinuria, hematuria, and casts. **Hematuria** and moderate to severe **proteinuria** are surrogate markers for renal dysfunction.

D. Finger-stick glucose test should be performed to exclude hypoglycemia as the cause of altered mental status in the setting of suspected hypertensive encephalopathy.

E. **Electrocardiogram** to evaluate for myocardial ischemia.

F. **Chest radiograph** to confirm pulmonary edema or other lung examination findings.

G. **Computed tomography (CT)** of the head may be indicated to evalaute neurologic deficits and altered mental status, especially in the setting of suspected primary stroke, hemorrhage or trauma.

VI. **THERAPY.** The presence of **acute or rapidly progressive end-organ damage, not the absolute blood pressure reading, determines whether the situation is an emergency or an urgency.** This determination dictates the type of treatment (i.e., parenteral or oral) and the setting (i.e., ICU, hospital ward, or outpatient) in which it is implemented. For example, a blood pressure of 120/80 mm Hg may represent a hypertensive emergency for a patient with aortic dissection, whereas a blood pressure of 200/120 mm Hg for a patient with asymptomatic chronic hypertension and organ dysfunction does not usually necessitate emergent parenteral therapy. The appropriate diagnostic evaluation and therapeutic plan also are dictated by the specific disease. For example, the specific pharmacologic regimen for a pregnant woman with preeclampsia differs from that for an elderly man who has had a stroke. **Regardless of drug regimen, the goal of treatment is to break the cycle of increasing SVR and blood pressure, preserve cardiac output and renal blood flow, and limit end-organ damage.**

A. **Neurologic emergencies.** Patients with neurologic findings and severe hypertension present a particular challenge. Neurologic emergencies can result from hypertensive emergencies or may themselves cause markedly elevated blood pressures, which may exacerbate neurologic damage. The key differentiating point is that **neurologic alterations caused by elevated blood pressure are reversed when blood pressure is controlled, whereas primary neurologic disorders are not.** The insidious progression of symptoms in hypertensive encephalopathy aids in differentiating hypertensive encephalopathy from cerebrovascular accidents, which usually manifest abruptly. Nevertheless, the diagnosis is one of exclusion because other hypertensive emergencies, such as cerebrovascular accident, subarachnoid hemorrhage, intraparenchymal bleeding, and primary seizure disorder, share many symptoms and signs. **Evaluation often necessitates further diagnostic imaging, such as CT, and consultation with a neurologist.** There is emerging controversy on blood pressure–lowering therapy in patients with acute stroke. Although all agree that abrupt "normalization" of blood pressure in such patients is imprudent, gradual lowering of the blood pressure after 24 to 48 hours with an angiotension receptor blocker may be considered.

B. **Hypertensive emergencies**

1. **Goals of therapy** include immmediate, but controlled reduction of the MAP. The pharmacologic characteristics and potential toxic side effects of antihypertensive agents must be understood and anticipated.

   a. Patients are **treated in an ICU,** where clinical status and vital signs can be constantly monitored with the aid of an arterial line.

   b. Attention is focused on the status of **airway, breathing, and circulation** (ABCs). Ancillary measures such as dialysis are often required.

   c. **Blood pressure is reduced in a controlled, predictable manner.** The lower limit of autoregulation among persons with normal blood pressure and those with hypertension is approximately 25% of MAP. It is recommended that **blood pressure be reduced initially by no more than 25% of MAP over minutes to hours,** and that further reductions occur over days to weeks to allow the autoregulatory mechanisms to reset. Exceptions include aortic dissection, left ventricular failure, and pulmonary edema, which demand more aggressive blood pressure reduction to limit tissue damage.

2. **Medical therapy.** A number of parenteral antihypertensive medications are available to manage hypertensive emergencies. The specific clinical scenario dictates the agents used. Characteristics of an ideal agent include rapid onset and cessation of action, a predictable dose-response curve, and minimal side effects. Table 35.4 lists parenteral antihypertensive agents, dosages, side-effect profiles, and specific indications.

TABLE 35.4 Parenteral Medications Used to Manage Hypertensive Emergencies

Drug	Dosage	Onset/duration	Indications	Side effects
Nitroprusside sodium (Nipride, Nitropress)	Infusion: 0.25–10 μg/kg/min	Immediate/3–5 min	Most emergencies	Nausea, vomiting, sweating, thiocyanate and cyanide poisoning
Glyceryl trinitrate (Nitro-Bid)	Infusion: 5–200 μg/min	Immediate/3–5 min	Myocardial ischemia, myocardial infarction, LV failure	Headache, methemoglobinemia, tolerance with prolonged infusion
Labetalol (Normodyne, Trandate)	Bolus: 20 mg/5 min until desired effect (max 80 mg) Infusion: 1–2 mg/min	5–10 min/1–8 h	Most emergencies except those complicated by LV failure	Heart block, orthostatic hypotension
Nicardipine (Cardene)	Infusion: 5–15 mg/h	5–10 min/1–4 h	Most emergencies except those complicated by LV failure	Reflex tachycardia, headache, nausea, flushing Avoid in heart failure
Enalapril (Vasotec)	1.25–5 mg every 6 h	15 min/6 h	LV failure, scleroderma crisis	Marked decreases in blood pressure in high-renin states, renal failure, hyperkalemia
Phentolamine (Regitine)	Bolus: 5–15 mg IV Infusion: 0.2–5.0 mg/min	1–2 min/3–10 min	Pheochromocytoma crisis Catecholamine crisis	Tachycardia, headache, flushing
Hydralazine (Apresoline)	Bolus: 10–20 mg IV every 30 min until desired effect achieved or side effects occur	10–20 min/3–8 h	Eclampsia	Marked hypotension, tachycardia, flushing Contraindicated in myocardial ischemia and aortic dissection
Fenoldopam (Corlopam)	Infusion: 0.1–0.3 μg/kg/min	<5 min/30 min	Most emergencies Renal insufficiency	Tachycardia, headache, nausea, flushing Caution with glaucoma

LV, left ventricular.

a. Sodium nitroprusside is the **drug of choice** for most hypertensive emergencies. Its favorable hemodynamic profile, rapid onset, and rapid cessation of action make it the preferred parenteral agent for most emergencies. A potent, direct vascular smooth muscle relaxant, sodium nitroprusside decreases afterload and preload by means of dilating arterioles and increasing venous capacitance. Hemodynamic effects include a decrease in MAP, afterload, and preload; renal blood flow and renal function may improve if cardiac output improves. Although the direct action of sodium nitroprusside on the cerebral vasculature may cause increased cerebral perfusion, this is counteracted by a potent effect on MAP. Most patients with neurologic crisis who need blood pressure control tolerate sodium nitroprusside without a worsening of neurologic status. Unlike intravenous nitroglycerin, nitroprusside does not raise intracranial pressure (ICP) or cause headaches. However, the possibility of a spontaneous increase in ICP and further clinical deterioration despite a decrease in MAP must be kept in mind as a potential problem.

1. **Administration.** Sodium nitroprusside must be administered by means of constant intravenous infusion in an intensive care setting with careful monitoring of arterial blood pressure. It has a rapid onset of action, and its effect ceases within 1 to 5 minutes of stopping the infusion.
2. **Side effects.** Red blood cells and muscle cells metabolize sodium nitroprusside to cyanide, which is converted to thiocyanate in the liver and excreted in the urine. **Thiocyanate levels rise in patients with renal insufficiency, and cyanide accumulates in patients with hepatic disease.** Signs of thiocyanate toxicity include nausea, vomiting, headache, fatigue, delirium, muscle spasms, tinnitus, and seizures. Monitoring for signs and symptoms of toxicity and maintaining thiocyanate levels less than 12 mg/dL allow safe use of sodium nitroprusside. Thiocyanate toxicity is extremely rare in the extensive experience with nitroprusside at the Cleveland Clinic.

b. Labetalol is useful in most hypertensive crises. The main disadvantage is its relatively long duration of action. Labetalol is an α-blocker and nonselective β-blocker with partial β_2-agonist activity. When given through continuous intravenous infusion, the relative β- to α-blocking effect of labetalol is 7:1.

1. The **hemodynamic effects** of labetalol include a decrease in SVR, MAP, and heart rate and a decrease or no change in cardiac output. Cardiac output often is spared because of the decrease in afterload. Labetalol has little direct effect on cerebral vasculature, does not increase ICP, and is **considered by some to be the drug of choice in situations characterized by markedly elevated ICP.** Labetalol begins to lower blood pressure within 5 minutes, and its effects can last 1 to 3 hours after cessation of the infusion.
2. **Contraindications.** Labetalol is contraindicated for patients with acutely decompensated heart failure, cardiogenic shock, bradycardia, heart block (more than first degree), and sometimes reactive airway disease.

c. Nitroglycerin is considered the drug of choice for managing hypertension in the setting of myocardial ischemia, acute MI, and congestive heart failure. It is primarily a venodilator and has modest effects on afterload at high doses. The decrease in preload and afterload decreases myocardial oxygen demand. Nitroglycerin also dilates the epicardial coronary arteries, inhibits vasospasm, and favorably redistributes blood flow to the endocardium. **Nitroglycerin directly increases CBF, raises ICP, and is not used in situations initially characterized by high ICP.**

d. Fenoldopam is a selective peripheral dopamine-1-receptor agonist approved for the management of severe hypertension. Fenoldopam is an arterial vasodilator with a rapid onset of action and a relatively short half-life when administered intravenously. It may be of particular benefit in patients with renal insufficiency, as it has been shown to improve renal perfusion. Fenoldopam may cause a reflex tachycardia, which can be blunted by the concomitant use of a β-blocker. Fenoldopam is contraindicated in patients with glaucoma because it can increase intraocular pressure. It is a potent systemic vasodilator and is used primarily by anesthesiologists to control blood pressure intraoperatively.

e. **Hydralazine.** The role of intravenous hydralazine is limited to the treatment of pregnant women with preeclampsia. Hydralazine is a direct arterial vasodilator with no effect on venous capacitance. It crosses the uteroplacental barrier but has minimal effects on the fetus. It is usually administered in intravenous boluses of 10 to 20 mg and has a long duration of action. Hydralazine decreases SVR, induces compensatory tachycardia, and increases ICP. It can exacerbate angina and is **contraindicated in the care of patients with ongoing coronary ischemia, aortic dissection, or increased ICP.**

f. **Nicardipine.** As a dihydropyridine calcium channel blocker, nicardipine inhibits vascular smooth muscle contraction but has little to no activity on the heart's atrioventricular or sinus nodes. It is particularly useful in the setting of postoperative hypertensive crises and neurological scenarios, as it does not raise intracranial pressure and directly reduces cerebral ischemia. It is contraindicated in heart block, acute myocardial infarction, and renal failure.

g. **Enalaprilat.** This is a short-acting intravenous ACE inhibitor that lowers blood pressure abruptly. It is not widely used in hypertensive emergencies, as it can precipitate hypotension, particularly in volume-depleted patients.

3. **Management of specific emergencies**

a. **Accelerated or malignant hypertension**

(1) In the **acute phase**, the pharmacologic agent of choice is **sodium nitroprusside.** Labetalol is an effective alternative.

(2) **Contraindications.** Because patients usually have marked elevations of SVR and volume depletion, diuretics are contraindicated.

b. **Hypertensive encephalopathy**

(1) The treatment of choice is **sodium nitroprusside or labetalol.** Agents that depress the sensorium or increase ICP (i.e., intravenous nitroglycerin) should be avoided.

(2) Management of markedly elevated blood pressure in the setting of hypertensive encephalopathy is tempered by **concerns about further reducing blood flow to underperfused areas of the brain.**

(3) Most patients with hypertensive encephalopathy improve within hours of blood pressure reduction; neurologic deficits persist in the other conditions. **If there is no improvement despite a decrease in blood pressure, the diagnosis must be reconsidered.**

c. **Neurologic complications** include cerebrovascular accident, embolic stroke, intraparenchymal hemorrhage, and subarachnoid hemorrhage.

(1) **Extreme caution** must be exercised when **lowering even markedly elevated blood pressures in the setting of a recent cerebrovascular accident.** Elevated ICP caused by cerebral edema or intraparenchymal hemorrhage increases the MAP needed to adequately perfuse the brain (CPP = MAP − ICP). Subarachnoid hemorrhage is characterized by intense vasospasm at and adjacent to the site of rupture. Reduction of blood pressure in these circumstances may cause global or, in the case of subarachnoid hemorrhage, focal hypoperfusion. Recently, however, this principle has been challenged. Although experts agree that abrupt lowering of high blood pressure in the setting of acute stroke remains contraindicated, gradual lowering of blood pressure after 24 to 48 hours may be indicated, with angiotension receptor blockers being the drug of choice.

(2) **Markedly elevated blood pressures, however, may increase risk for rebleeding** in subarachnoid hemorrhage or extend a hemorrhagic infarct.

(3) **Surgically treatable conditions** such as subarachnoid hemorrhage and neoplasms must be identified.

(4) Management of markedly elevated blood pressure in the setting of cerebrovascular accident or subarachnoid hemorrhage is tempered by

concerns about further reducing blood flow to underperfused areas of the brain.

(5) **Although specific treatment goals have been the subject of recent controversy, experts agree that precipitous blood pressure lowering to less than 140/90 mm Hg is dangerous, and lowering systolic blood pressure to less than 100 mm Hg has been clearly associated with adverse outcomes.** Maintaining systolic blood pressures in the stage I hypertensive range (systolic blood pressure 140 to 159 mm Hg) has long been thought to be cerebroprotective in the presence of intracranial stenosis. Data from two ongoing trials, the Continue or Stop Post-Stroke Antihypertensives Collaborative Study (COS-SACS) and Controlling Hypertension and Hypotension Immediately Post-Stroke (CHIPPS) remain pending at the publication of this book and are expected to add knowledge to this topic. Given the emerging data in this area, specific treatment decisions should be made in consultation with a neurologist trained in contemporary stroke management.

(6) When therapy is indicated, the drug of choice is **labetalol or sodium nitroprusside, whereas angiotension receptor blockers may be appropriate in the postischemic stroke setting after 24 to 48 hours.** Sublingual nifedipine has been associated with increased adverse cardiovascular outcomes.

(7) **Nimodipine,** a calcium channel blocker with modest antihypertensive effect, has been beneficial in the management of subarachnoid hemorrhage. If blood pressure remains higher than desired despite use of nimodipine, therapy with **sodium nitroprusside or labetalol** may be considered.

(8) Agents that directly increase CPP and, therefore, ICP are avoided.

d. **Aortic dissection.** Blood pressure must be lowered immediately. Patients with **type A dissection** have a mortality rate of 1% per hour in the first 48 hours unless medical therapy is instituted and the patient is referred for **emergency surgical intervention. Antihypertensive therapy** aimed at reducing vascular resistance and shear force on the vessel wall is the treatment of choice for **type B dissection.** Operative management is much less commonly required for a type B dissection. Decreased shear force is accomplished by means of reducing the inotropic state of the heart and the ratio of change in ventricular pressure to change in time (dP/dT). **Labetalol or the combination of sodium nitroprusside with a β-blocker** is the treatment of choice. **Aggressive blood pressure reduction** is indicated, even for patients with normal blood pressure, because shear force and afterload must be reduced to limit tissue damage. A reasonable goal is a MAP of approximately 70 mm Hg.

e. **Left ventricular failure or pulmonary edema.** Treatment is best accomplished with **sodium nitroprusside and intravenous diuretics. Nitroglycerin** is an effective alternative, especially if myocardial ischemia is present. Sodium nitroprusside and nitroglycerin are sometimes used concomitantly. β-Blockers and calcium channel blockers must be avoided in the decompensated state. However, amlodipine does not appear to worsen chronic heart failure, and may be useful in selected patients.

f. **Myocardial ischemia.** Blood pressure reduction with nitroglycerin and β-blockers are the treatments of choice. **Sodium nitroprusside** is added if further blood pressure reduction is required. **Reperfusion and antithrombotic therapy** are the mainstays of management of acute MI and unstable angina.

g. **Hypertensive crisis associated with hypercatecholaminemia.** The pharmacologic agents of choice include **sodium nitroprusside, labetalol, or calcium channel blockers. Phentolamine** can be useful in cases of pheochromocytoma. β-Blockers should not be used because they can cause a paradoxical increase in blood pressure because of the effects of unopposed α-receptor stimulation. However, they can be rationally combined with α-blockers such as phentolamine.

h. Postoperative hypertension. Parenteral treatment with **sodium nitroprusside, nicardipine, or labetalol** is preferred. **After coronary bypass grafting, nitroglycerin** is considered the initial drug of choice.

C. Hypertensive urgencies. Most patients diagnosed with hypertensive urgency actually have severe hypertension and **are not in any immediate danger of progressing to hypertensive emergency.** They are often persons with chronic hypertension who are suboptimally treated or noncompliant.

1. Goal of therapy

a. Hypertensive urgencies can often be managed with **oral medication without admission to the hospital.** End-organ damage is not imminent, and blood pressure can be lowered modestly over a period of hours as long as adequate follow-up care is ensured. **The great danger lies in overtreating these patients and inciting hypotensive complications.**

b. Lower initial doses of antihypertensive medications are used to treat patients with **cerebrovascular disease or coronary artery disease who are taking antihypertensive drugs or who are volume depleted.** These patients tend to have exaggerated responses to drug therapy. They also are especially vulnerable to **hypotension**. Monitoring for 4 to 6 hours is necessary to judge treatment effect and to look for complications. Urgent follow-up care is mandatory within 24 hours. Evaluation for secondary causes of hypertension is indicated.

2. Drug therapy. Oral agents used to manage hypertensive urgencies are listed in Table 35.5. The drugs of choice include captopril, clonidine, and oral labetalol.

a. Captopril. Considered by some to be the drug of choice, captopril is the **fastest-acting oral angiotensin-converting enzyme inhibitor.** At small doses, it rarely causes marked hypotension, although this potential exists in patients who are markedly volume depleted or who have renal artery stenosis. Captopril begins to work within 15 to 30 minutes of ingestion and has a 4- to 6-hour duration of activity. Caution is advised in the treatment of patients with marked renal insufficiency or volume depletion.

b. Clonidine acts through central α-agonist activity. It has been administered in repeated hourly doses and safely lowers blood pressure over a period of hours. Untoward effects include sedation and a proclivity for rebound hypertension if the drug is abruptly discontinued. Clonidine should not be administered to patients with altered sensorium or who may not comply with treatment as **abrupt clonidine withdrawl can provoke tachycardia and demand myocardial ischemia in patients with coronary artery disease.**

c. Labetalol. A combined α- and β-blocker, labetalol taken orally has a relative β- to α-blocking effect of approximately 3:1. Dosage begins at 100 mg (taken orally twice daily) and is titrated to the desired response. The onset of action is 30 minutes to 2 hours after administration; the duration of action is 8 to 12 hours.

TABLE 35.5 Oral Agents Used to Manage Hypertensive Urgencies

Drug	Dosage	Onset/duration	Indications	Side effects
Captopril	6.25–25 mg PO q6h	15–30 min/4 h	Well-tolerated in most instances	Can precipitate hypotension in high-renin states, cough, renal failure
Clonidine	0.1–0.2 mg PO q8–12h	30–60 min/6–12 h	Severe, uncomplicated hypertension	Sedation, bradycardia, dry mouth
Labetalol	100–200 mg PO q2–3h	30–120 min/2–8 h	Well-tolerated in most instances	Heart failure, heart block, bronchospasm

VII. PROGNOSIS. The prognosis of a patient with an untreated hypertensive crisis is poor. Before the introduction of effective antihypertensive agents, 1-year mortality exceeded 80% and 5-year mortality was 1%. In the modern era of effective antihypertensives, 10-year survival has improved to 70%. Therefore, appropriate recognition of these clinical syndromes and rapid treatment are strongly indicated.

ACKNOWLEDGMENTS

The author thanks Drs. John H. Chiu and Harpreet Bhalla for their contributions to earlier editions of this chapter.

Key Reviews

Aggarwal M, Khan IA. Hypertensive crisis: hypertensive emergencies and urgencies. *Cardiol Clin* 2006;24:135–146.

Blumenfeld JD, Laragh JH. Management of hypertensive crises: the scientific basis for treatment decisions. *Am J Hypertens* 2001;14:1154–1167.

Feldstein C. Management of hypertensive crisis. *Am J Therapeutics* 2007;14:135–139.

Messerli FH. Cerebroprotection by hypertension in ischemic stroke: the crumbling of a hypothesis. *Circulation* 2007;115:2907–2908.

Landmark Articles

Kaplan NM. Management of hypertensive emergencies. *Lancet* 1994;344:133–135.

McKindley DS, Boucher BA. Advances in pharmacotherapy: treatment of hypertensive crisis. *J Clin Pharm Ther* 1994;19:163–180.

Vaughan CJ, Delanty N. Hypertensive emergencies. *Lancet* 2000;356:411–417.

Relevant Book Chapters

Kaplan NM. Systemic hypertension: mechanisms and diagnosis. In: Braunwald E, ed. *Heart disease: a textbook of cardiovascular medicine,* 8th ed. Philadelphia: WB Saunders Company, 2008:1049–1070.

Rudd P, Osterberg LG. Hypertension: context, pathophysiology, and management. In: Topol EJ, ed. *Textbook of cardiovascular medicine,* 3rd ed. Philadelphia: Lippincott Williams & Wilkins, 2007:88–103.

EVALUATION OF CHEST PAIN IN THE EMERGENCY DEPARTMENT

36

Anthony A. Bavry and Samir R. Kapadia

I. INTRODUCTION. Chest pain is one of the most common problems evaluated in the emergency department (ED).

A. Each year, approximately 5 million persons who arrive at an ED with chest pain are admitted to the hospital, mainly to an intensive care unit; 1.2 million of these patients are ultimately diagnosed with acute myocardial infarction (MI). However, **2% to 4% of persons who arrive with chest discomfort and acute MI are inappropriately discharged** to home. This error in diagnosing MI is dangerous and costly. **Early recognition and treatment** are also important because time to treatment is the single most important factor in the management of ST-elevation MI.

B. Rapid evaluation and risk stratification of patients with chest pain is essential to identify life-threatening conditions and improve outcomes. Emergency treatment is initiated in the ED to minimize permanent myocardial damage and improve survival, especially in patients with MI. **The goal of treatment in ST-elevation myocardial infarction** is to achieve reperfusion as soon as possible, either by primary angioplasty or thrombolytic therapy. **Conversely, in patients with non–ST-elevation acute coronary syndrome (ACS), maintaining antegrade flow in the coronaries with prevention of**

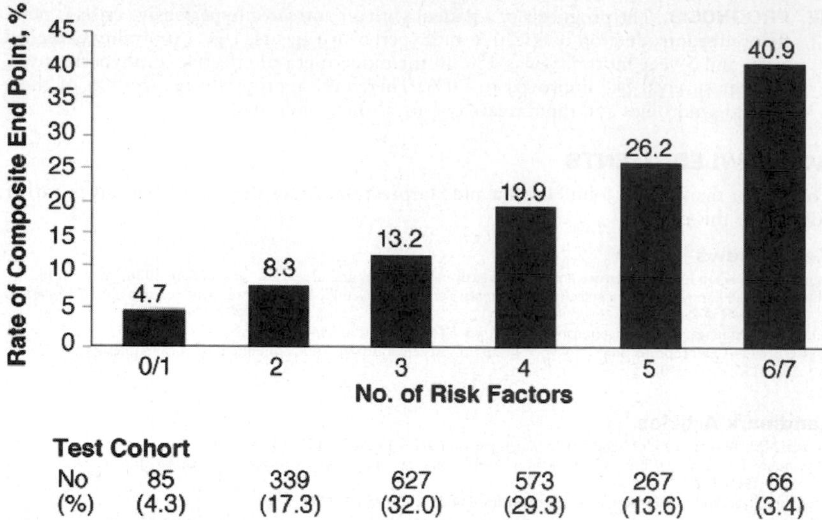

Figure 36.1. Incidence of all-cause mortality, myocardial infarction, and repeat revascularization at 14 days, based on the Thrombolysis In Myocardial Infarction (TIMI) risk score for non-ST-elevation acute coronary syndromes. (Reprinted with permission from Antman EM, Cohen M, Bernink PJ, et al. The TIMI risk score for unstable angina/non-ST elevation MI: A method for prognostication and therapeutic decision making. *JAMA* 2000;284:835–842.)

distal embolization is important. The Thrombolysis In Myocardial Infarction (TIMI) risk model is a validated mechanism to determine prognosis and guide therapy in patients with ACS. The model consists of seven variables with 1 point for each variable: age greater than 65 years, three or more risk factors for heart disease, known coronary stenosis, multiple anginal episodes in the last 24 hours, use of aspirin in the last week, electrocardiographic changes, and elevated cardiac biomarkers (Fig. 36.1). **High-risk patients** are typically admitted to a coronary care unit for management with antiplatelet and antithrombotic therapy. Urgent (within hours) cardiac catheterization and appropriate revascularization are recommended in these patients. **Intermediate-risk angina patients** are directed to a monitored telemetry unit and undergo further risk stratification such as stress testing and assessment of left ventricular function with possible cardiac catheterization. **The lowest risk patients** can be observed in a chest pain unit or discharged directely to home, depending on the clinical situation.

C. Assessment of chest pain in the ED involves careful patient **history, physical examination,** and **12-lead electrocardiogram (ECG).** Functional stress tests can supply additional data, but the data are not immediately available, and triage decisions are often made without them. With clinical history, physical examination, and initial ECG, 92% to 98% of cases of acute MI and approximately 90% of cases of unstable angina can be identified.

II. CLINICAL PRESENTATION

A. History

1. **Chest pain.** The initial history should accurately characterize the location and duration of the patient's discomfort, associated symptoms, and aggravating and alleviating factors (Table 36.1). Most patients with ischemic chest pain describe it as substernal pressure, squeezing feeling, or a sensation of suffocation. Some patients describe aching, burning, or tightness. The pain may radiate to the shoulder, neck, jaw, left or right arm, and the fingertips. Occasionally, the pain may be predominantly epigastric or interscapular.

TABLE 36.1 Differentiating Cardiac from Noncardiac Chest Pain

Favoring ischemic origin	Favoring non-ischemic origin
CHARACTER OF PAIN	
Squeezing Burning Heaviness	Sharp, knife-like Stabbing Aggravated by respiration
LOCATION OF PAIN	
Substernal Across mid-thorax Radiation to arms, shoulders, neck, head, forearms, interscapular region Associated with nausea, vomiting, diaphoresis	Left submammary area Left hemithorax Discomfort localized with one finger Back pain that suggests aortic dissection
FACTORS PROVOKING PAIN	
Exercise Excitement Stress Cold weather	Pain after completion of exercise Pain relieved by exercise Provoked by a specific body motion
DURATION OF CHEST PAIN	
Minutes	Seconds Hours without evidence of myocardial damage

From Selzer A. *Principles and practice of clinical cardiology,* 2nd ed. Philadelphia: WB Saunders, 1983:17, with permission.

2. **Atypical presentations.** Dyspnea is often associated with chest pain during an MI. **Dyspnea** may also be the only major presenting symptom in about 10% of patients with MI. Other atypical presentations include fatigue, syncope, altered sensorium, stroke, nausea or vomiting, and lethargy. **Atypical presentations of acute MI are more common in the elderly, in patients with diabetes, and in women**.
3. **Risk factors.** Although several clinical factors have been associated with an increased risk for cardiovascular disease, only the **age** of patient, **history of coronary artery disease,** and **male** sex are predictive of ACS among patients with chest pain. In some studies, diabetes and family history have been associated with ACS, but the overall power of these risk factors in predicting an ischemic event is low. The **absence of risk factors cannot be used to exclude cardiac ischemia.**

B. Physical examination

1. The physical examination helps to identify **signs of left ventricular dysfunction and occult valvular heart disease.** Presence of a third heart sound (S_3) gallop, rales, sinus tachycardia, hypotension, and increased jugular venous distention are associated with adverse outcome. The presence of these signs and symptoms indicates cardiac origin of the chest pain. A thorough physical examination also helps identify the cause of nonischemic chest pain. Chest wall tenderness, skin lesions, and pleural or pericardial rub can be useful in this regard.
2. **Response to treatment is not reliable** in unraveling the cause of chest pain. Pain relief after administration of nitroglycerin does not necessarily point to MI or unstable angina, as other etiologies for chest pain are relieved with nitroglycerin.

III. DIAGNOSTIC TESTING

A. The **ECG** is integral to the evaluation of chest pain and has important diagnostic and prognostic value. It is even more important in the evaluation of persons with diabetes and elderly persons who tend to have atypical symptoms.

1. Almost 50% of patients with MI have a normal or nondiagnostic ECG on presentation to the ED. **Sensitivity** depends on a number of factors, including

the time from symptom onset, coronary distribution of ischemia, baseline ECG abnormalities, and patient characteristics. Electrocardiographic findings should normalize rapidly after resolution of chest pain. The electrocardiographic findings of a patient who does not have active chest pain are difficult to interpret. **Circumflex distribution ischemia is notoriously silent on an ECG, as the posterolateral wall is underrepresented on a conventional 12-lead ECG.**

2. Among patients with the ischemic type of chest discomfort, ST-segment elevation on an ECG has a specificity of approximately 90% and a sensitivity of approximately 50% for the diagnosis of acute MI. Specificity decreases to 82% and sensitivity increases to 69% when ST-segment elevation or depression, Q waves, or left bundle-branch block (LBBB) is used to define abnormal electrocardiographic findings.
3. The ECG can be used to identify a population of patients at low risk for MI. A normal ECG indicates less than 3% risk for MI and less than 6% risk for death in the following year. However, approximately one-third of patients with unstable angina may have a normal or equivocal ECG. The **ECG cannot be used alone to exclude ACS.**
4. Preexisting abnormalities, including left ventricular hypertrophy, LBBB, Q waves, preexcitation, and paced ryhthms, make interpretation of the ECG difficult. Comparison of the initial ECG with a prior tracing often is helpful in this setting. Whether new or old, the presence of **LBBB is an adverse prognostic finding.** New LBBB suggests left anterior descending coronary artery ischemia or infarct. Preexisting LBBB alone defines a group of patients at high risk for cardiac morbidity and mortality. Although LBBB complicates the electrocardiographic diagnosis of acute MI, criteria have been proposed for ascertaining whether a patient has acute MI and LBBB from the Global Utilization of Streptokinase and Tissue Plasminogen Activator for Occluded Coronary Arteries (GUSTO I) database.

B. **Biochemical markers** of myocardial necrosis are used in conjunction with the clinical history and ECG to confirm the diagnosis of MI. Biochemical markers include cardiac **troponins, creatine kinase-myocardial band (CK-MB) isoenzyme, and myoglobin.** These markers, especially troponins, are sensitive and specific for myocardial injury and can provide important prognostic information.

1. **Serial blood samples** are collected over a 24-hour period to measure a temporal rise and fall for the diagnosis of MI. All biochemical markers follow a predictable pattern of release after the onset of myocardial injury.
2. An **ideal serum marker** is specific to myocardium, highly sensitive, and quantitative; the serum concentration is proportional to the amount of myocardial tissue injured. Furthermore, the levels have to increase rapidly to allow early diagnosis. None of the available markers are optimal for the diagnosis of ACS. In most cases, the combination of serial measurement of markers and interpretation of clinical data such as ischemic symptoms and ECG changes leads to the accurate diagnosis of ACS.
3. Enzymes such as aspartate aminotransferase (AST), lactate dehydrogenase (LDH), and total CK are released from dying myocytes but are relatively nonspecific for cardiac tissue.
   a. **CK-MB is released in the circulation after myocardial cell death.** There is some evidence in animal models that CK-MB can be released with reversible myocardial injury. However, this has not been shown in humans.
      - Most studies have confirmed that serial measurement of CK-MB for the diagnosis of acute MI has a sensitivity of approximately 92% with a specificity of 98%. The initial level of CK-MB, however, does not carry equal statistical weight and does not have sufficient negative predictive value to exclude MI when used in isolation. The CK-MB level can be increased with normal or minimally elevated total CK levels; however, the significance of this finding is debatable.

   b. **Myoglobin** is a small heme protein that is not specific to cardiac tissue. The use of myoglobin as a marker of myocardial necrosis does not carry the specificity of CK-MB measurement. The advantage of myoglobin as a marker lies in its release kinetics. Myoglobin is released rapidly after myocardial injury, and serum levels are detectable within 1 to 2 hours of the onset of symptoms. Peak serum levels are reached within 4 to 5 hours after MI. Within 1 to 3 hours of MI, serum myoglobin determination has a sensitivity of 62% to 100% in the detection of myocardial damage. Because of its short half-life, measurement of myoglobin may not help confirm the diagnosis for patients who seek treatment late after symptom onset. The specificity is low when there is a substantial release of skeletal muscle myoglobin and in the setting of renal failure.

c. Troponins

- Cardiac troponins are **proteins that regulate the calcium-dependent interactions between actin and myosin.** This interaction results in myocyte contraction and relaxation. **Troponin T** is a myofibrillary protein and is a constituent of the contractile apparatus of cardiac muscle. Cardiac troponins, like CK-MB, can be found in the serum soon after injury, but concentrations remain elevated for as long as 2 weeks. Cardiac troponin T and troponin I are useful in the diagnosis of ACS and have been shown to be very sensitive and specific markers of myocardial cell injury.
- A large, prospective analysis from the Global Use of Strategies to Open Occluded Coronary Arteries (GUSTO IIa) trial has provided important data on the **value of cardiac troponins for diagnosis and risk assessment.**
  - **i** Among patients who present within 12 hours of the onset of myocardial ischemia, elevated levels of **troponin T** (>0.1 mg/mL) are associated with significantly higher mortality within 30 days. This is true for all ECG subgroups examined, including those with ST depression, ST elevation, T-wave inversion, LBBB, and paced rhythms. A quantitative relation also has been demonstrated between levels of cardiac troponin T and long-term clinical outcome.
  - **ii** **Troponin I** also has similar prognostic value. Among patients with unstable angina and non–Q-wave MI, elevated cardiac troponin I levels (>0.4 ng/mL) are associated with significantly higher mortality.
  - **iii** **Bedside tests** for cardiac-specific troponins are **highly sensitive** for the early detection of myocardial cell injury in ACS. Qualitative and quantitative point-of-care tests for troponin T and troponin I are fast, yielding results within a few minutes that are reliable and accurate. **Negative test results have been associated with low risk** and allow rapid and safe discharge from the ED of patients with an episode of acute chest pain, as long as these tests are done at least 8 hours after the onset of chest pain.

d. Novel biomarkers. B-type natriuretic peptide (BNP), and C-reactive protein (CRP) are predictive of risk in patients with ACS. Measuring these markers in combination with troponin or CK-MB may improve the short- and long-term risk stratification of ACS patients. **Plasma myeloperoxidase** levels are elevated in persons with angiographically documented coronary disease and within culprit lesions prone to plaque rupture. Recent studies have shown that elevated myeloperoxidase levels predict cardiac risk in patients presenting to the ED with chest pain, independently of the level of CRP, troponin T, and other markers of inflammation. However, these novel biomarkers have yet to become incorporated into clinical practice guidelines for chest pain or ACS management.

C. Imaging studies. Although clinical history, initial electrocardiographic findings, and biochemical markers have been combined to diagnose ACS with high sensitivity and specificity, atypical presentations and equivocal electrocardiographic findings can make diagnosis challenging. Investigations aimed at overcoming these problems have focused on myocardial perfusion and functional imaging.

1. Echocardiography. Two-dimensional echocardiography provides valuable diagnostic data on ventricular function and regional wall-motion abnormalities.

a. Myocardial ischemia can cause abnormal segmental function of the myocardium manifested as impaired relaxation, hypokinesis, akinesis, or dyskinesia.

b. Although echocardiography alone has moderate sensitivity in the diagnosis of MI, it may be a useful adjunctive test, especially after reperfusion therapy. Echocardiography serves an important role in risk stratification after MI through assessment of left ventricular function.
c. Normal findings at echocardiography cannot be used reliably to rule out myocardial ischemia.
d. Echocardiography can be crucial in the evaluation of complications of MI, such as ruptured papillary muscle, free-wall rupture or ventricular septal defect.

2. **Radionuclide perfusion imaging** is useful to quantify myocardium at risk. It is rarely used for the diagnosis of ACS because of poor accessibility and cost.
   a. **Thallium-201 scintigraphy** has been used to detect areas of reduced or absent perfusion in AMI. Areas of myocardium with a negative scintigraphic image, indicating decreased myocardial uptake, can be demonstrated in ischemic or infarcted myocardium within 6 hours of symptom onset. The diagnostic utility of such imaging is limited by the so-called "moment-in-time problem"; perfusion defects may represent acutely ischemic myocardium or preexisting areas of scar tissue. Thallium-201 imaging has relatively poor specificity in women because of difficulties in distinguishing between breast attenuation and perfusion defects caused by coronary artery disease.
   b. **Technetium-99m sestamibi tomographic imaging** has the advantage that it does not redistribute after initial injection. This type of imaging allows definition of an initial ischemic zone that can be studied even after reperfusion. Technetium-derived image quality is also superior to that of thallium and allows quantification of regional and global ventricular function by gated-image acquisition. Perfusion imaging with technetium-99m appears to have a sensitivity equivalent to that of thallium-201 imaging in defining myocardium at risk.
3. **Triple Scan.** Recently, multi-slice detector computed tomography has been studied as a tool that can simultaneously assess for ACS, aortic dissection, and pulmonary embolism. This approach appears promising; however, its use in the ED cannot be advocated until its clinical utility has been validated.

D. **Early exercise stress testing.** In general, exercise stress testing can be safely performed to further risk-stratify patients who are considered to be at a low clinical risk for MI. Studies have shown that this approach is safe in patients who have a normal or nondiagnostic ECG and negative biochemical markers for myocardial necrosis assessed within 6 to 12 hours of presentation to the ED.

IV. **DIFFERENTIAL DIAGNOSIS.** Differentiating ischemic from nonischemic causes of chest pain can be difficult (Table 36.2). It has been estimated that more than 50% of patients

TABLE 36.2 Differential Diagnosis of the Causes of Acute Chest Pain

Cardiac	Aortic	Pumonary	Gastrointestinal	Miscellaneous
Acute coronary syndrome	Aortic dissection	Pulmonary embolus	Esophageal spasm/reflux	Costochondritis
Coronary spasm	Penetrating aortic ulcer	Pneumothorax	Esophagitis	Cervical spondylosis and other compression neuropathies
Syndrome X, microvascular disease	Aortic aneurysm	Pneumonia / Pleuritis	Esophageal rupture	Herpes zoster
Myopericarditis				Panic disorder
Aortic stenosis				Anxiety
Hypertrophic cardiomyopathy				

initially admitted to the hospital with a diagnosis of unstable angina are later discharged with a noncardiac diagnosis. Given that there is symptom overlap among a number of clinical entities, in most diagnostic strategies, it is assumed that **chest pain is cardiac in origin until proven otherwise.** It is important to understand the clinical characteristics that represent the leading noncardiac causes of chest pain. Life-threatening causes of chest pain that can be confused with ACS include aortic dissection, pericarditis with cardiac tamponade, and pulmonary embolus.

A. Pericarditis (see Chapter 26) often is accompanied by substernal chest pain, but the **pain** is more likely to be pleuritic in character and aggravated by recumbency, deep inspiration, and swallowing. **Physical examination** may reveal a three-component pericardial friction rub. The **ECG** often reveals ST elevation in multiple leads without reciprocal changes, whereas PR-segment depression in leads other than aVR and V_1 is a more specific sign of pericarditis. It is important to recognize that **pericarditis may be a late presentation of MI.**

B. Aortic dissection (see Chapter 25) requires **urgent** diagnosis because early surgical intervention reduces the high short-term mortality rate. The **chest pain** of aortic dissection is typically described as sudden, severe, and tearing pain that radiates to the back and interscapular areas, which is most intense at onset. **Examination** may reveal a difference in right and left arm blood pressures, pulse deficits, and focal neurologic deficits. Aortic dissection also may involve the aortic valve or coronary ostia. The latter may be associated with the diastolic murmur of aortic insufficiency, myocardial ischemia, and ST-segment elevation on **ECG.**

C. Pulmonary embolism is potentially life-threatening and can be associated with chest pain. The **chest pain** of pulmonary embolism is typically pleuritic in character and is associated with dyspnea and tachypnea. There is often a **history** of recent surgical intervention, malignant disease, or immobility. The cardinal **clinical findings** include hypoxia and tachycardia. An **ECG** may demonstrate right-axis deviation, right bundle-branch block, or occasionally the classic $S_1Q_3T_3$ pattern.

V. CONCLUSIONS. The ED is where life-saving therapy is initiated to patients with acute coronary syndromes. It is important to rapidly and accurately risk-stratify patients with suspected ACS. Many patients will present with noncardiac conditions for chest pain, some of which are life-threatening. It is important for the ED practitioner to have a working diagnosis of the varied causes of chest pain. There is a spectrum of ACS, which ranges from high to low risk. The highest risk patients require emergent reperfusion therapy, whereas lower risk patients can undergo urgent invasive therapy or further risk stratification. Such an understanding can help direct patient care most appropriately and improve important outcomes, including survival.

ACKNOWLEDGMENT

The authors thank Drs. Jason B. Wischmeyer and Michael Yen for contributions to this chapter.

Suggested Readings

Bavry AA, Kumbhani DJ, Rassi AN, et al. Benefit of early invasive therapy in acute coronary syndromes: a meta-analysis of contemporary randomized clinical trials. *J Am Coll Cardiol* 2006;48:1319–1325.

Brennan M, Penn MS, Van Lente F, et al. Prognostic value of myeloperoxidase in patients with chest pain. *N Engl J Med* 2003;349:1595–1604.

de Lemos JA, Morrow DA, Bentley JH, et al. The prognostic value of B-type natriuretic peptide in patients with acute coronary syndromes. *N Engl J Med* 2001;345:1014–1021.

Limkakeng AT, Halpern E, Takakuwa KM. Sixty-four-slice multidetector computed tomography: the future of ED cardiac care. *Am J Emerg Med* 2007;25:450–458.

Lindahl B, Toss H, Siegbahn A, et al, for the FRISC Study Group. Markers of myocardial damage and inflammation in relation to long-term mortality in unstable coronary disease. *N Engl J Med* 2000;343:1139–1147.

Sabatine MS, Morrow DA, de Lemos JA, et al. Multimarker approach to risk stratification in non-ST elevation acute coronary syndromes. *Circulation* 2002;105:1760–1763.

Landmark Articles

Antman EM, Tanasijevic MJ, Thompson B, et al. Cardiac-specific troponin I levels to predict the risk of mortality in patients with acute coronary syndromes. *N Engl J Med* 1996;335:1342–1349.

Hamm CW, Goldmann BU, Heeschen C, et al. Emergency room triage of patients with acute chest pain by means of rapid testing for cardiac troponin T or troponin I. *N Engl J Med* 1997;337:1648–1653.

Ohman EM, Armstrong PW, Christenson RH, et al. Cardiac troponin T levels for risk stratification in acute myocardial ischemia: GUSTO IIA investigators. *N Engl J Med* 1996;335:1333–1341.

Olatidoye AG, Wu AH, Feng YJ, et al. Prognostic role of troponin T versus troponin I in unstable angina pectoris for cardiac events with meta-analysis comparing published studies. *Am J Cardiol* 1998;81:1405–1410.

Puleo PR, Meyer D, Wathen C, et al. Use of a rapid assay of subforms of creatine kinase-MB to diagnose or rule out acute myocardial infarction. *N Engl J Med* 1994;331:561–556.

Sgarbossa EB, Pinski SL, Barbagelata A, et al. Electrocardiographic diagnosis of evolving acute myocardial infarction in the presence of left bundle-branch block: GUSTO-1 (Global Utilization of Streptokinase and Tissue Plasminogen Activator for Occluded Coronary Arteries) Investigators [correction appears in *N Engl J Med* 1996;334:931]. *N Engl J Med* 1996;334:481–487.

Key Reviews

Jesse RL, Kontos MC. Evaluation of chest pain in the emergency department. *Curr Probl Cardiol* 1997;22:149–236.

Koenig W. Cardiovascular biomarkers. Added value with an added approach. *Circulation* 2007;116:3–5.

Lee TH, Goldman L. Evaluation of the patient with acute chest pain. *N Engl J Med* 2000;342:1187–1195.

Relevant Book Chapter

Blomkalns AL, Gibler BW. Diagnosis of acute coronary syndromes in the emergency department: evolution of chest pain centers. In: Topol EJ, ed. *Acute coronary syndromes,* 3rd ed. New York: Marcel Dekker, 2001:233–246.

37 CARDIAC TRAUMA

Daniel J. Cantillon

I. INTRODUCTION. Trauma represents the leading cause of death in males younger than the age of 40 in the United States. Cardiothoracic injuries are a primary or contributing factor in up to 75% of all traumatic deaths. Cardiac trauma occurs most commonly in the setting of motor vehicle accidents, interpersonal violence, cardiopulmonary resuscitation, falls from great heights, as well as sporting and industrial accidents. **Cardiac trauma can be easily overlooked in the presence of distracting injuries, as it can occur in the absence of chest pain or visible wounds.** Emergency department physicians lead the initial management while contemporary trauma teams are typically led by surgical subspecialists. However, cardiologists play an important consultative role in the diagnosis and management of cardiac trauma.

A. Cardiac trauma is divided into **blunt trauma** (i.e., motor vehicle accidents and falls) and **penetrating trauma** (i.e., primarily, knife and gunshot wounds).

B. As many as 50% of people with cardiac injuries die in the field, but advances in diagnostic testing and surgical techniques have improved the prognosis of patients who reach emergency centers alive. Definitive management requires rapid mobilization of the surgical team and transport to the operating room.

C. Initial attention is focused on the airway, breathing, and circulation (ABCs), and the primary survey performed according to the published Advanced Trauma Life Support (ATLS) guidelines. The cardiac physical examination should assess vital signs, peripheral pulses, murmurs, signs of heart failure, distended neck veins, and the presence of pulsus paradoxus. Routine laboratory evaluation should include cardiac biomarkers, and a portable chest radiograph should be performed rapidly. **Transthoracic echocardiography (TTE) at the bedside is the preferred modality for the initial assessment of cardiac trauma.** Focused assessment with sonography for trauma (FAST) is a widely applied technique using bedside ultrasound to rapidly asses blunt trauma at multiple body sites, including the heart. An electrocardiogram (ECG) is indicated to evaluate for suspected coronary dissection or traumatic coronary thrombosis. The role for cardiac computerized tomography (CCT) using intravenous contrast is expanding, and it remains the diagnostic study of choice to evaluate suspected trauma and/or dissection of the aorta and great vessels, along with transesophageal echocardiography (TEE).

II. BLUNT TRAUMA

A. Blunt cardiac trauma generally occurs in the setting of motor vehicle accidents, but may also be related to falls, blows from blunt objects, or cardiopulmonary resuscitation.

B. Blunt trauma may injure the **pericardium, myocardium, valves or subvalvular apparatus, coronary arteries**, or the **great vessels**. The clinical presentation is generally one of **tamponade** or **hemorrhage**, depending on whether the pericardium is intact. Although hypotension and tachycardia are seen in both scenarios, tamponade is suggested by elevated neck veins, muffled heart sounds, pulsus paradoxus, and is easily confirmed by a bedside echocardiogram. A new murmur coupled with signs of heart failure should raise clinical suspicion for injury to the valves or subvalvular apparatus.

1. **Pericardium.** Increased shear forces during blunt trauma may lead to lacerations or tears in the pericardium. Clinically, the patient may experience pleuritic chest pain, and an ECG may reveal the typical findings of pericarditis. Management is with analgesics, although late cases of constriction occasionally develop after traumatic injury to the pericardium.
2. **Myocardium**
   a. **Myocardial rupture.** The myocardium can be injured by several mechanisms in sudden deceleration injuries. Compression between the sternum and the spinal column, as well as sudden overdistention with blood after abdominal injuries, may lead to myocardial rupture. The thin walls and large diameter of the right atrium predispose it to rupture, and **more than 50% of cases of cardiac rupture involve the right atrium**. The left atrium may be involved in as many as 25% of cases, with the remainder involving the thicker-walled right and left ventricles. Most victims die immediately, but some series suggest that survival may approach 50% if patients arrive with intact vital signs. Management requires prompt thoracotomy and definitive surgical repair. Emergency pericardiocentesis is relatively contraindicated, as it can lead to reaccumulation and arrest, and is generally only considered as a desperate measure in an arresting patient when trained personnel are unavailable to perform a thoracotomy.

   b. **Myocardial contusion.** Blunt chest wall trauma may lead to focal injury and necrosis of cardiac myocytes, known as myocardial contusion. Definitive diagnosis is based on histology, and, therefore, the true incidence and clinical significance of myocardial contusion remain controversial. Patients may complain of precordial pain, but symptoms are usually difficult to interpret in the setting of chest wall trauma and associated injuries. A number of studies have investigated the use of ECG, cardiac enzymes, and transthoracic echocardiography (TTE) in diagnosing myocardial contusion, but none of these tests has been found to be sensitive or specific for the diagnosis. The ECG may be normal or show nonspecific ST-T-wave changes or findings consistent with pericarditis. Elevations in serum troponin levels, creatine kinase-myocardial band (CK-MB) isoenzymes, are observed in some patients, but CK-MB may be masked by skeletal muscle CK-MM release, especially when total CK is greater than 20,000 U/L. TTE may reveal a small effusion or focal wall-motion abnormalities. Patients with contusion are thought to be at increased risk of arrhythmic death during the recovery period as the injured, inflamed myocardium behaves much like scar tissue as a substrate for slowed conduction and unidirectional block in the development of reentry cycles. However, findings on ECG, TTE, or laboratory tests are insensitive in predicting outcomes. From a practical standpoint, the diagnosis of cardiac contusion does not generally alter management, as treatment is mostly supportive care, observation, and analgesia. However, making the diagnosis should alert physicians to the potential for arrhythmias. Most centers perform a baseline ECG and monitor patients with blunt chest wall trauma for at least 12 hours before discharge.

3. **Valvular insufficiency.** Injury to cardiac valves, papillary muscles, or chordae tendineae during blunt cardiac trauma may lead to acute valvular regurgitation. A review of 546 autopsies after blunt trauma suggested that valvular injury may occur in as many as 9% of cases, with a slight increase in frequency in patients with preexisting valvular heart disease. The **aortic valve is most commonly involved**, followed in decreasing frequency by the mitral and tricuspid valves. A new murmur, hypotension, and fulminant pulmonary edema should suggest the diagnosis. The differential diagnosis of a new holosystolic murmur (occasionally with a new right bundle-branch block or right-axis deviation on the ECG) should also include a traumatic ventricular septal defect. An emergency transthoracic echocardiogram and rapid transport to the operating room is generally required. Although less common, acute tricuspid regurgitation is generally well tolerated, with lower extremity edema and fatigue as the presenting symptoms.
4. **Coronary arteries.** Blunt trauma occasionally leads to **thrombosis** or **dissection** of a coronary artery and subsequent myocardial infarction. In general, the prognosis after a traumatic myocardial infarction is better than that of the usual acute coronary syndrome because patients tend to be younger and have less atherosclerotic burden and fewer comorbidities. Nevertheless, patients with infarctions related to trauma are at risk for all the mechanical complications associated with atherosclerotic disease, such as left ventricular aneurysm or pseudoaneurysm formation, ischemic mitral regurgitation, and ventricular septal defect. In rare cases, blunt trauma contributes to the formation of an arteriovenous fistula between the coronary artery and another structure, such as the coronary sinus, great cardiac vein, right atrium, or right ventricle. Clinically, the patient may have a loud, widely radiating murmur, and ligation of the coronary artery or bypass surgery may be necessary.
5. **Commotio cordis.** Case reports of sudden cardiac death in children and adolescents after relatively low-impact chest wall trauma (most commonly, a baseball or hockey puck striking the chest) have received significant media attention in the past. The mechanism is unclear, but it appears that a blow to the chest during an electrically vulnerable period of cardiac repolarization may induce ventricular tachycardia or ventricular fibrillation. Victims have been surprisingly refractory to cardiac defibrillation, and few survive. Autopsy reports consistently show no evidence of underlying structural heart disease.
6. **Great vessels.** The aorta may also be injured in motor vehicle accidents and falls when sudden deceleration leads to tears or disruption of the vessel. Not surprisingly, most patients with aortic rupture die immediately, but 10% to 20% may reach emergency centers alive if the bleeding is limited by clot or by the pleura. Aortic rupture typically occurs at the proximal portion of the descending aorta, where the aorta is tethered against the spine by intercostal arteries. Patients frequently present with chest or back pain and hypotension, but a high index of suspicion often is needed to make the diagnosis. Increased pulse pressure in the upper extremities and diminished pulse pressure in the lower extremities may be found on examination. The chest radiograph may reveal a widened mediastinum, large left pleural effusion, loss of the aortic knob contour, or deviation of the esophagus to the right. A normal chest radiograph does not rule out aortic pathology, and as many as 25% of patients will have a normal chest radiograph.

   Both CT scan with intravenous contrast and TEE are first-line imaging modalities for the diagnosis of ascending aortic dissection. The advantage of TEE is that it can be performed rapidly at the bedside in a critically ill patient who is not suitable for transport, but who requires sedation, and may not be feasible in patients with maxillofacial or cervical spine injures. Although TTE cannot be used to exclude the diagnosis of aortic dissection, a limited and focused study can be performed more rapidly at the bedside than any other test, and visualization of a flap in the aortic root or ascending aorta can clinch the diagnosis. Magnetic resonance angiography (MRA) is an alternative modality, but is not well-suited for unstable patients due to the time required to perform the study. CT can be performed rapidly, but requires the use of intravenous contrast dye. Aortography, once the gold standard, is now rarely performed out of concern for procedural complications in the setting of acute aortic dissection, when noninvasive tests perform very well. Definitive surgical repair is indicated for ascending aortic dissection.

III. PENETRATING TRAUMA

A. Gunshot wounds and stabbings are the most common types of penetrating trauma. The prognosis depends entirely on the extent of injury and the number of chambers involved. Overall mortality is estimated at 60% to 93% for gunshot wounds, 22% to 62% for knife injuries, and 25% for bolting instruments (i.e., nail guns). Less frequently, iatrogenic catheter-induced injury can occur in the setting of temporary or permanent pacemaker placement.

B. As with blunt cardiac trauma, the clinical presentation tends to be one of **tamponade** or exsanguinating **hemorrhage**, depending on the integrity of the pericardium. **However, unlike in the case of blunt trauma, tamponade carries a favorable pronosis in penetrating trauma.** One series described a survival rate of 73% among patients with penetrating trauma with tamponade versus 11% among those without. Thrombus within the pericardium is thought to stablize the rapid hemorrhagic shock associated with penetrating injuries. Pericardial lacerations may also seal spontaneously. Bleeding from the muscular, thicker walled left ventricle is also more likely to be self-limited, whereas injury to the relatively thin right ventricle or right atrium is more likely to be catastrophic and fatal. Knife wounds tend to be smaller and focal, whereas gunshot wounds tend to be larger, extensive, and more likely to present with frank hemorrhage.

C. The **right ventricle is the chamber most often involved in penetrating trauma** because of its anterior location in the chest. As described for blunt trauma, penetrating trauma may result in laceration of the pericardium or myocardium, valves, coronary arteries, or the aorta.

D. Diagnosis. In an unstable patient, a TTE should be obtained rapidly at the bedside. Although images may be suboptimal, both the sensitivity and specificity of transthoracic echocardiography for identifying cardiac abnormalities in this setting are 85% to 90%. A portable chest radiograph may reveal the presence of a pneumothorax or hemothorax.

E. Management. After the diagnosis of penetrating cardiac trauma has been made, the patient should be transported as rapidly as possible to the operating room for definitive surgical repair. The infusion of saline and blood products should be continued as needed. Warmed fluids are often needed to prevent hypotherma associated with massive volume resuscitation. There is no role for serial pericardiocenteses in patients with trauma and pericardial effusion, but emergency pericardiocentesis occasionally is necessary if there are delays in reaching the operating room.

IV. SPECIAL CONSIDERATIONS

A. Indwelling foreign bodies and missile embolization. Missile embolization from bullet fragments, air gun pellets, or shrapnel is an extremely rare complication from gunshot wounds or battlefield injuries. Data from the Vietnam conflict suggest that this phenomenon complicates 0.3% to 0.4% of all vascular missile injuries. Clinical suspicion for embolization should be raised in a scenario of multiple penetrating entrance wounds or a single penetrating entrance wound without a corresponding exit wound. The majority of patients with right heart or pulmonary embolization are asymptomatic, but up to 17.4% develop chest pain, dyspnea, or hemoptysis. Up to 4% of patients may exhibit cardiac arrhythmias. Patients with undiagnosed indwelling foreign bodies may also develop subacute bacterial endocarditis as a latent presentation. Metallic missile fragments are usually radiopaque and detected on plain x-rays or a noncontrast computerized tomography (CT) scan. Intracardiac indwelling foreign bodies should be evaluated by transesophageal echocardiography (TEE), especially when endocarditis is suspected. Ultimately, the decision to remove asymptomatic indwelling foreign bodies is made on a case-by-case clinical basis considering operative logistics and weighing risk against the potential benefit.

B. Device Implants. An awareness of device-related complications in the setting of cardiac trauma is important given the expanding patient population with pacemakers and/or implantable defibrillators. Common complications in the setting of blunt trauma would include pocket hematoma, lead dislodgement or fracture. Penetrating trauma could expose the generator and/or tunneled leads, and lead to bleeding or secondary infection. Lead perforation is an uncommon but life-threatening complication manifested as tamponade. Hypotension and bradycardia should prompt concern for lead fracture or dislodgement, especially if the patient is known to be pacemaker-dependent. Emergent transcutaneous or transvenous pacing is indicated if the underlying bradyarrhythmia is not hemodynamically tolerated. Device interrogation can also be performed at the bedside to assess pacer dependence and the functional status of all leads using computer equipment provided by the major manufacturers.

ACKNOWLEDGMENT

The author thanks Dr. John Hostetter for his contributions to this chapter.

Book Chapters

Braunwald E. Cardiac trauma. In: Braunwald E, ed. *Heart disease: a textbook of cardiovascular medicine*, 8th ed. Philadelphia: WB Saunders, 2008:1855–1862.

Ivatury RR. The injured heart. In: Moore EE, Feliciano DV, Mattox KL, eds. *Trauma*, 5th ed. New York: McGraw-Hill, 2004:555–569.

Kapadia SR, Topol EJ. Cardiac trauma. In: Topol EJ, ed. *Textbook of cardiovascular medicine*, 3rd ed. Philadelphia: Lippincott Williams & Wilkins, 2007:698–706.

Key Reviews

Karmy-Jones R. Jurkovich GJ. Blunt chest trauma *Curr Probl Surg* 2004;41:223–3080.

Khanna A, Drugas GT. Air gun pellet embolization to the right heart: case report and review of the literature. *J Trauma* 2003;54:1239–1241.

Meredith JW, Hoth JJ. Thoracic trauma: when and how to intervene. *Surg Clin North Am* 2007;87:95–118.

Sybrandy KC, Cramer MJ, Burgersdij C. Diagnosing cardiac contusion: old wisdom and new insights. *Heart* 2003;89:485–489.

Landmark Articles

Alexander RH, Proctor HJ. *Advanced trauma life support program for physicians: ATLS*, 6th ed. Chicago, IL: American College of Surgeons, 1997.

Asensio JA, Stewart BM, Murray J, et al. Penetrating cardiac injuries. *Surg Clin North Am* 1996;76:685–724.

Banning AP, Pillai R. Non-penetrating cardiac and aortic trauma. *Heart* 1997;78:226–229.

Kimura BJ, Bocchicchio M, Willis CL, et al. Screening cardiac ultrasonographic examination in patients with suspected cardiac disease in the emergency department. *Am Heart J* 2001;142:324–330.

38 PREGNANCY AND CARDIOVASCULAR DISEASE

Arti Choure, Brian P. Griffin, and Russell Raymond

I. INTRODUCTION. Maternal cardiac disease is a major risk factor for nonobstetric mortality and morbidity in pregnant women. Advances in congenital heart disease treatment have allowed more women with these problems to survive into childbearing age and, therefore, attempt pregnancy. Congenital heart disease now represents a common cause of heart disease complicating pregnancy in the United States. Advances in obstetrics have also allowed pregnancy in older mothers in whom hypertension and acquired heart disease are more prevalent and can pose challenges for the pregnancy. Rheumatic heart disease, although less common than in the past, is still prevalent, especially in immigrant populations in the United States, and may manifest clinically for the first time in pregnancy. Because cardiac disease has an important bearing on the health of the fetus and the mother during pregnancy, it is essential that cardiologists and internists have a working knowledge of the impact of various cardiac diseases on pregnancy and the peripartum period and how they may be appropriately managed.

II. NORMAL PHYSIOLOGIC CHANGES DURING PREGNANCY. A series of cardiocirculatory changes occur in pregnancy and peripartum. These changes **usually begin during the early first trimester** (5 to 8 weeks), peak in the late second trimester, and tend to plateau thereafter until the postpartum period. An understanding of these changes is essential to the management of pregnant women, especially those with heart disease.

A. Blood volume *increase* in pregnancy is attributed to estrogen-mediated stimulation of the renin–aldosterone system, leading to salt and water retention along with various other maternal and placental hormones. **The volume expansion varies from 20% to 100% and averages around 50%.** The relatively greater increase in plasma volume as compared to red blood cell mass leads to the physiologic anemia of pregnancy usually manifest around the 30th week.

B. Cardiac output, stroke volume, and heart rate. Table 38.1 summarizes the changes in heart rate, stroke volume, and cardiac output. The **cardiac output is estimated to increase by approximately 30% to 50% above baseline**. The increase is attributed to higher preload as a result of increased blood volume, decrease in systemic vascular resistance, and resulting afterload and increase in maternal heart rate by 10 to 15 beats/min. During the third trimester, stroke volume and cardiac output are dependent on body position and increase in the lateral position and decline in the supine position due to compression of the inferior vena cava by the gravid uterus.

C. Blood pressure and systemic vascular resistance. There is a decline in systemic vascular resistance and, therefore, blood pressure falls by about 10 mm of Hg during pregnancy. Blood pressure begins to fall in the first trimester, reaches a nadir in mid-pregnancy, and returns to baseline before term. The pulse pressure widens due to the greater fall in diastolic blood pressure than in systolic pressure. As many as 11% of women develop the **uterocaval syndrome** of pregnancy, with a significant and symptomatic drop in blood pressure when lying on their back due to vena caval compression from the gravid uterus. **A hypercoagulable state** with decreased protein S, increased stasis, and venous hypertension is also observed. **Weakening of**

TABLE 38.1 Normal Hemodynamic Changes During Pregnancy and Postpartum Period

	Changes during different phases of pregnancy				
Hemodynamic parameter	**First trimester**	**Second trimester**	**Third trimester**	**Labor and delivery**	**Postpartum**
Heart rate	↑5–10%	↑10–15%	↑15–20%	↑20–30%	↓
Stroke volume	↑5–30%	↑30–40%	↓20–30%	↑300–500 mL with each contraction	↓
Cardiac output	↑5–30%	↑30–40%	↑>40%	↑50%	Initial ↑ then ↓
Systolic BP	↔to ↓	↓	↔to ↑	↑	Baseline
Diastolic BP	↔to ↓	↓	↓to ↔	↑	Baseline
Systemic vascular resistance	↓10–30%	↓30–40%	↓30–40%	↑	Baseline

BP, blood pressure.

the vascular walls of the medium and large muscular arteries occurs because of a decreased collagen deposition as a result of estrogen release and the effects of circulating elastase and relaxin. This in turn makes pregnant women more susceptible to aortic dissection, most often in the third trimester, a risk that is especially increased in those with abnormally weak aorta tissue such as in Marfan's syndrome.

D. **Hemodynamic changes during labor and delivery.** Each uterine contraction results in displacement of about 300 to 500 mL of blood into the general circulation (autotransfusion). There is an increase in stroke volume, heart rate, and, therefore, cardiac output, blood pressure, and oxygen consumption also increase. However, these changes may be influenced by the type of delivery—vaginal versus cesarean section and also differ by type of anesthesia and analgesia.

E. **Hemodynamic changes in the postpartum period.** Despite the blood loss during delivery, there is a **temporary increase in effective venous return due to the relief of caval compression and autotransfusion.** This may lead to an increase in stroke volume, cardiac output and filling pressure. In women with preexisting cardiac disease, these hemodynamic changes may lead to profound clinical deterioration. The hemodynamic changes associated with pregnancy usually persist for a few weeks postpartum and may take up to 12–24 weeks to return to prepregnancy baseline.

III. CARDIOVASCULAR EVALUATION IN PREGNANCY

A. **Physical examination.** The hemodynamic changes in pregnancy manifest in various normal physical findings that are important to differentiate from pathologic findings. **Table 38.2** highlights the important cardiac findings in normal pregnancy.

TABLE 38.2 Findings in Normal Pregnancy
Symptoms
Fatigue
Dyspnea
Palpitations
Reduced exercise tolerance
Orthopnea
Lower extremity edema
Physical examination
Hyperventilation
Lower extremity edema
Distended neck veins with prominent *a* and *v* waves and brisk *x* and *y* descents
Increased heart rate and wide pulse pressure
Upward and leftward deviation of point of maximal impulse
"Flow" murmurs (pulmonic and aortic)
Mammary soufflé (left sternal border, continuous murmur)
Increased first heart sound and exaggerated splitting of second heart sound
Pulmonary basilar rales
Electrocardiographic findings
Sinus tachycardia
Leftward axis deviation
Increased R/S ratio in leads V_1 and V_2
Repolarization changes
Echocardiographic findings
Increased left ventricular diastolic dimension
Increased left ventricular wall thickness
Mild increase in contractility
Moderate increase in size of right atrium, right ventricle, and left atrium
Functional pulmonary, tricuspid, and mitral regurgitation
Small pericardial effusion

Symptoms of fatigue, dyspnea, and reduced exercise tolerance are very common as well as signs of jugular venous distention, displaced point of maximal impulse, and peripheral edema. A physiologic systolic murmur in the pulmonic area and continuous murmurs of "mammary soufflé" and cervical venous hum may also be heard.

B. Noninvasive testing with echocardiography is considered safe in pregnancy and findings are as outlined in **Table 38.2**. Chest radiography should be performed only when absolutely necessary and with shielding of the pelvic area with protective lead. Magnetic resonance imaging (MRI) is sometimes used for diagnosis of cardiac disorders; its safety profile in pregnancy is unknown, and it should be avoided if possible.

C. Invasive testing with pulmonary artery catheterization (without fluoroscopy) can be utilized during pregnancy, labor, delivery, and the postpartum period for hemodynamic monitoring. This is useful for patients with hemodynamic deterioration, especially during labor, delivery, and the early postpartum period when significant circulatory changes occur. Cardiac catheterization during pregnancy is rarely needed except in the setting of acute myocardial infarction or to allow balloon valvuloplasty. Fluoroscopy and cine time should be minimized and direct irradiation to the fetus avoided. Vascular access from the arm rather than the leg is preferred whenever feasible.

IV. RISK ASSESSMENT AND GENERAL PRINCIPLES OF MANAGEMENT. One of the most important steps in managing a patient with heart disease who is considering pregnancy is to establish the level of maternal and fetal risk. This involves a multidisciplinary approach with preconception counseling, contraception, and discussion of potential maternal and fetal acute and long-term morbidity and mortality. Baseline functional class, severity of cardiac disease, left ventricular function, and pulmonary pressures should guide the risk assessment. **Table 38.3** delineates a stepwise approach for management of women with preexisting cardiac disease, and **Table 38.4** lists high-risk predictors. **Maternal New York Heart Association (NYHA) class II or higher symptoms and left-sided obstruction** were predictive of neonatal complications including premature birth, intrauterine growth retardation, respiratory distress syndrome, and death in one study.

Management of the pregnant patient with heart disease is a team effort involving the patient's primary care physician, high-risk obstetric team, and cardiologist, and the active participation of the patients. **Prophylactic intervention for cardiac lesions that significantly increase the risk of pregnancy should be performed where appropriate and feasible *before* pregnancy is contemplated**. Most patients with relatively low-risk cardiac conditions are successfully managed throughout pregnancy, labor, and delivery with conservative medical measures designed to optimize intravascular volume and systemic loading conditions. Simple measures help, such as bed rest and avoidance of the supine position. Medications should be used judiciously and only when absolutely required during pregnancy. Medications that are contraindicated in pregnancy should be discontinued before conception if pregnancy is contemplated. **In certain conditions such as cyanotic congenital heart disease, Eisenmenger syndrome, or severe pulmonary hypertension, pregnancy should be strongly discouraged, as patients with these conditions do not tolerate the hemodynamic changes of pregnancy.**

Specific lesions and their management in pregnancy are described later. The list, although extensive, is not complete, as a detailed description of every lesion is beyond the scope of this chapter.

V. PREGNANCY IN WOMEN WITH CONGENITAL HEART DISEASE. In general, patients with noncyanotic congenital heart disease have a better outcome with pregnancy compared with patients with cyanotic disease. Where applicable, patients should be made aware of the potential inheritability of the congenital disease. The recently revised American Heart Association (AHA) endocarditis guidelines do not recommend the use of prophylactic antibiotics for vaginal delivery, even in high-risk patients, such as those with complex congenital heart disease or surgically constructed systemic-pulmonary shunts. However, owing to the difficulty in predicting

TABLE 38.3 Basic Management Principles for Pregnant Women with Valvular Heart Disease

Risk assessment
Preconception:
Thorough history of cardiac symptoms and arrhythmias
Baseline exercise tolerance and functional class
Baseline electrocardiogram and echocardiography with ventricular function and pulmonary pressures
Detailed discussion with the patient about the potential risks to self and fetus
During pregnancy:
Follow-up evaluation at least once per trimester
Close monitoring of new symptoms or change in functional class
Serial echocardiography for development of any new symptoms or signs
Treatment
Preconception:
Effective contraception until pregnancy is desired
Consider valve repair or replacement, correction of anomaly prior to conception if pregnancy poses significant risk of worsening clinical status
Adjust medications to prevent adverse fetal side-effects
During pregnancy:
Minimize medication use to only those absolutely required and discontinue or replace medications contraindicated in pregnancy
If symptoms worsen and if indicated consider correction of anomaly or valve repair or replacement
Labor and Delivery:
Invasive monitoring as needed
Cesarean section for obstetric indication
Monitor for decompensated heart failure and pulmonary edema, and treat accordingly
Postpartum:
Adjust and optimize medications
Consider correction of anomaly or valve repair or replacement if indicated
Treat postpartum anemia
Counseling and contraception for future pregnancies

Adapted from Stout KK, Otto CM. Pregnancy in women with valvular heart disease. *Heart* 2007;93:552–558.

TABLE 38.4 Risk Predictors of Adverse Maternal and Fetal Outcomes

Prior cardiac events
Prior arrhythmia
NYHA Class II or higher, or cyanosis
Ejection fraction <40%
Pulmonary hypertension (pulmonary artery systolic pressure >50% systemic pressure)
Severe aortic stenosis (valve area <1.5 cm^2, Doppler jet velocity >4 m/s
Symptomatic or severe mitral stenosis
Severe aortic or mitral regurgitation with NYHA class III or IV symptoms
Hypertrophic obstructive cardiomyopathy
Maternal anticoagulation

complicated deliveries and the potential complications of endocarditis, some authors still suggest antibiotic prophylaxis as reasonable for all patients with congenital heart disease, except in isolated secundum atrial septal defects and corrected patent ductus arteriosus.

1. **Atrial septal defect (ASD) and patent foramen ovale (PFO).** Isolated ASD or PFO is usually well tolerated in pregnancy and considered low risk in general. Paradoxical pulmonary embolism during pregnancy has been reported. Ideally, an ASD with a significant shunt (>1.5:1) should be corrected prior to pregnancy. Secundum ASD that is repaired prior to pregnancy is not associated with an increased risk of complications.
2. **Ventricular septal defect (VSD).** Isolated VSD without pulmonary hypertension is usually well tolerated during pregnancy, and correction of VSD prior to pregnancy and before development of pulmonary hypertension eliminates the risk. In pregnant patients with VSD and pulmonary hypertension, a drop in blood pressure during or after delivery can result in transient shunt reversal. This may be prevented by close monitoring of blood pressure, volume replacement, and the use of vasopressors, if necessary. VSD is commonly inheritable.
3. **Patent ductus arteriosus (PDA).** PDA without pulmonary hypertension usually has a favorable outcome. In patients with pulmonary hypertension, the management principles are similar to those with VSD.
4. **Coarctation of aorta (COA).** Coarctation, although usually associated with favorable outcomes, has been associated with severe hypertension, congestive heart failure, or aortic dissection in some cases. It is also associated with circle of Willis aneurysms, and cerebral hemorrhage from rupture of an aneurysm during pregnancy is possible. Limiting physical activity and controlling blood pressure may prevent complications such as cerebral hemorrhage and dissection. β-Blockers are usually the antihypertensive drugs of choice, and care should be taken not to lower the blood pressure unduly, as this may compromise uteroplacental circulation. Significant COA with evidence of systemic hypertension, heart failure, or a peak gradient of more than 20 mm Hg should be corrected prior to pregnancy. Women who had prior surgical repair of a coarctation remain at risk for dissection, as the aortic wall is still abnormally weak. Correction of COA during pregnancy is indicated in patients with severe uncontrollable hypertension or heart failure and may be performed percutaneously.
5. **Congenital aortic stenosis.** Congenitally bicuspid aortic valve is one of the most common causes of aortic stenosis. These patients should be screened for other cardiac malformations including COA. The details of management are described later in the section on valvular heart disease.
6. **Pulmonic stenosis.** Isolated pulmonic stenosis is usually well tolerated in pregnancy. It should be corrected prior to pregnancy if severe (peak gradient >60 mm Hg). Percutaneous balloon valvulotomy during pregnancy may be required in patients with severe right ventricular failure.
7. **Ebstein anomaly.** Noncyanotic Ebstein anomaly is usually well tolerated. Cyanotic patients are at very high risk of maternal heart failure and fetal prematurity or death. During labor and delivery, care should be taken to prevent a drop in blood pressure, and close hemodynamic monitoring is required along with rest, oxygen, antibiotic prophylaxis, and blood gas monitoring. It is sometimes associated with Wolff-Parkinson-White syndrome and pregnancy may precipitate supraventricular arrhythmias.
8. **Tetralogy of Fallot (TOF).** Women with TOF who have undergone successful repair during childhood with little or no residual outflow tract gradient, no pulmonary hypertension, and preserved ventricular function usually tolerate pregnancy well. In women with uncorrected or only partially corrected TOF, increased blood volume during pregnancy with increased venous return and decreased systemic vascular resistance may result in right to left shunt and cyanosis. A similar process may also occur with a fall in blood pressure during labor and delivery. **The outcome of pregnancy is very poor for both mother and fetus once cyanosis occurs**. It is

also associated with high rates of premature labor, spontaneous abortion, and fetal growth retardation. The risk of the fetus developing cardiac defects ranges from 3% to 17%. Patients with residual lesions after partial correction such as pulmonic regurgitation, right ventricular outflow obstruction, and right ventricular dysfunction are at risk for heart failure and arrhythmia during pregnancy. Poor prognostic signs include maternal hematocrit above 60%, arterial oxygen saturation below 80%, right ventricular hypertension, and syncopal episodes. Close hemodynamic and blood gas monitoring during labor and delivery and antibiotic prophylaxis is recommended. Patients with cyanotic disease should be strongly encouraged against pregnancy.

9. **Eisenmenger's syndrome. Pregnancy in women with Eisenmenger's syndrome is associated with a very high maternal mortality—in the range of 30% to 50%.** Maternal death occurs mostly between the first few days to first few weeks following delivery due to rapid hemodynamic deterioration. It is also associated with a high incidence of fetal loss. Therefore, patients with Eisenmenger's syndrome should be strongly discouraged against pregnancy. Early therapeutic abortion may be considered given the danger to the mother. If pregnancy is continued, close monitoring is necessary. Due to increased incidence of thromboembolism, anticoagulant therapy is recommended, starting from the third trimester until 4 weeks postpartum. Early elective hospitalization prior to delivery, high concentration of oxygen, and blood pressure, and blood gas monitoring is recommended. An attempt to shorten the second stage of labor by use of forceps or vacuum should be made. Antibiotic prophylaxis is recommended during delivery.

VI. VALVULAR HEART DISEASE AND PREGNANCY. The American College of Cardiology/American Heart Association (ACC/AHA) guidelines divide valvular heart lesions during pregnancy into lesions associated with high maternal and fetal risk and those associated with low maternal and fetal risk during pregnancy. **Lesions generally associated with high risk of maternal and/or fetal risks include symptomatic mitral stenosis, severe aortic stenosis (with or without symptoms), NYHA class III–IV symptoms with mitral or aortic regurgitation, valvular disease with severe pulmonary hypertension or left ventricular dysfunction, mechanical prosthetic valve requiring anticoagulation, Marfan's syndrome, and hypertrophic cardiomyopathy.** Those lesions generally associated with low maternal or fetal risk include asymptomatic aortic stenosis with normal ventricular function, MVP, mild mitral stenosis (MS), and NYHA functional class I or II mitral or aortic regurgitation. Some of the specific conditions are described later.

1. **Mitral stenosis (MS).** MS is one of the most common rheumatic valvular lesions seen in pregnancy. The physiologic changes in pregnancy with increased blood volume and heart rate can lead to increased pressure gradient across the valve and decreased filling time, respectively. This leads to increase in left atrial pressure and ensuing symptoms related to pulmonary edema with dyspnea, orthopnea, and paroxysmal nocturnal dyspnea and also predisposes to atrial arrhythmia and rapid ventricular rate. Patients with moderate to severe MS are more susceptible to these hemodynamic changes. The rapid increase in venous return during labor and delivery may cause significant decompensation and requires very close monitoring.

   Management depends upon the severity of stenosis, symptoms, and time of diagnosis. **If mitral stenosis is diagnosed prior to pregnancy, then patients with severe mitral stenosis (valve area <1 cm^2) or moderate symptomatic stenosis should be offered percutaneous mitral balloon valvuloplasty (PMBV) or valve repair if PMBV is not feasible, before pregnancy.** In patients with moderate asymptomatic stenosis, careful assessment of symptoms and exercise tolerance testing can help guide the decision for prepregnancy intervention. In patients with mild MS (valve area >1.5 cm^2), pregnancy is usually tolerated with a favorable outcome. **Optimal management of an already pregnant patient with MS is aimed at reducing heart rate and left atrial pressure.** β-Blockers are the drug of choice

TABLE 38.5 ACC/AHA Guidelines for Management for Atrial Fibrillation in Pregnancy
Class I (Benefits >>> Risk) Procedure/Treatment Should be Performed/Administered
Digoxin, a β-blocker, or a nondihydropyridine calcium channel antagonist is recommended to control the rate of ventricular response in pregnant patients with AF Direct-current cardioversion is recommended in pregnant patients who become hemodynamically unstable due to AF Protection against thromboembolism is recommended throughout pregnancy for all patients with AF (except for those with lone AF and/or low thromboembolic risk). Therapy (anticoagulant or aspirin) should be chosen according to the stage of pregnancy

and selective β-1-adrenergic drugs are preferred over nonselective β-blockers to avoid β-2-mediated uterine relaxation. Left atrial pressure may be controlled by salt restriction and very judicious use of diuretics (excessive use can lead to reduction in utero-placental circulation). In patients with fast atrial fibrillation (Table 38.5), digoxin may be used to control ventricular rate. Electrical cardioversion may be performed if necessary. In patients with symptoms and signs of clinical deterioration despite optimal medical therapy, PMBV may be necessary during pregnancy. This should be avoided in the first trimester if possible, and should be done with proper abdominal and pelvic shielding or under echocardiographic guidance by an experienced operator. In cases with severe mitral stenosis refractory to medical therapy and not amenable to PMBV, mitral valve repair or replacement may be considered.

Most patients with MS can safely undergo vaginal delivery. Patients with symptomatic moderate and severe MS should have hemodynamic monitoring and optimization with guidance of pulmonary artery catheterization during labor, delivery, and the immediate postpartum period (12–24 hours) when relief of uterocaval obstruction can cause increased venous return and pulmonary edema. Epidural anesthesia is usually better tolerated than general anesthesia, and cesarean section generally is performed for obstetric indications only.

Young pregnant women with a previous history of rheumatic carditis should continue to undergo penicillin prophylaxis as they did in the nonpregnant state.

2. **Mitral regurgitation (MR).** The most common cause of MR during pregnancy is either rheumatic heart disease or mitral valve prolapse. MR is usually well tolerated in pregnancy because the fall in systemic vascular resistance leads to a decreased left ventricular afterload. Atrial fibrillation and hypertension may sometimes cause acute symptomatic decompensation.

   Asymptomatic patients are managed conservatively without any therapy, and patients with left ventricular dysfunction and decompensated heart failure are managed with diuretics and digoxin. In the peripartum period, increased venous return and systemic vascular resistance sometimes lead to decompensation requiring diuretics and afterload reduction. Angiotensin-converting enzyme inhibitors (ACE-Is) are contraindicated in pregnancy because of their teratogenic effect. Hydralazine may be used in patients with MR and hypertension for afterload reduction. Acute MR due to ruptured chordae is rare in pregnancy and is usually not well tolerated. It may require intraaortic balloon pump placement and emergent surgery.
3. **Aortic stenosis (AS).** The most common etiology for AS in childbearing age is a congenitally bicuspid valve. Rheumatic AS is less common and may occur in conjunction with MS. Mild-to-moderate aortic stenosis with preserved left ventricular function usually is well tolerated during pregnancy. **Severe aortic stenosis (i.e.,**

aortic valve area <1.0 cm^2, mean gradient >50 mm Hg) significantly increases the risk of pregnancy and may lead to significant hemodynamic deterioration, heart failure, and premature delivery. Patients with severe AS should, therefore, undergo prompt intervention prior to surgery. Symptoms such as dyspnea, angina pectoris, or syncope usually become apparent late in the second trimester or early in the third trimester. Patients with bicuspid AV and aortic root dilation, especially those with coarctation of the aorta, are at increased risk for spontaneous aortic dissection, usually in the third trimester and during labor.

When severe symptomatic aortic stenosis is diagnosed during pregnancy, PABV should be performed before labor and delivery. Although PABV may reduce the risk of pregnancy in patients with severe aortic stenosis, it has limited durability and only suffices as a temporizing measure until the patient can safely undergo aortic valve replacement. Aortic insufficiency that occurs as a postprocedural complication of PABV usually is well tolerated during labor and delivery.

Close invasive hemodynamic monitoring, as in patients with MS, may be required. Spinal and epidural anesthesia are discouraged during labor and delivery because of their vasodilatory effects.

4. **Aortic regurgitation/aortic insufficiency (AI).** AI in young women can be caused by a congenitally bicuspid valve, infective endocarditis, connective tissue disease (e.g., systemic lupus erythematosus, rheumatoid arthritis), or a dilated aortic annulus. AI without left ventricular dysfunction is usually well tolerated in pregnancy owing to decreased systemic vascular resistance and increased heart rate causing a shorter diastole and, therefore, reducing regurgitation. In symptomatic patients with decompensated heart failure diuretics, digoxin and hydralazine for afterload reduction may be used.
5. **Hypertrophic cardiomyopathy (HOCM).** Most asymptomatic patients with HOCM have a favorable outcome during pregnancy. The overall morbidity and mortality with HOCM and pregnancy, however, is still higher than in the general population. Symptoms like chest pain, dizziness, palpitations, worsening shortness of breath, and syncope may occur, and are more common in women who were symptomatic prior to pregnancy. Various arrhythmias like supraventricular arrhythmias, atrial fibrillation with hemodynamic deterioration, and fetal distress requiring emergent cardioversion and ventricular fibrillation requiring defibrillation have also been reported. There is an increased risk of fetal prematurity, and the disease is inheritable.

   Women should receive genetic counseling before conception whenever possible; the risk of inheriting the disease may approach 50% in certain familial forms of HOCM.

   Management depends on the presence of symptoms and the severity of left ventricular outflow obstruction. Blood loss and vasodilators should be avoided, and medications should be reserved for symptoms of heart failure and arrhythmias. β-Blockers are usually the drug of choice for symptomatic patients. Patients with a history of syncope, life-threatening arrhythmias, or a family history of sudden cardiac death should be considered for prophylactic implantable defibrillators prior to pregnancy due to the potential arrhythmogenic effect of pregnancy.

   Vaginal delivery is considered safe, but tocolytics with β-adrenergic properties and prostaglandins should be avoided. Epidural anesthesia is used with caution because of the peripheral vasodilatory effect, and excessive blood loss should be promptly repleted with fluids or blood transfusion. The brisk diuresis immediately postpartum may lead to a rapid decrease in intravascular volume and, therefore, a symptomatic increase in outflow tract gradient. This can be avoided by gentle intravenous (IV) hydration decreasing over 24 to 48 hours postpartum to achieve a euvolemic state.
6. **Prosthetic heart valves.** The selection of an appropriate prosthetic valve in a woman of childbearing age is controversial. **Where possible, the patient's own valve should be conserved or repaired. When valve replacement is necessary, bioprosthetic and homograft valves are safer for mother and child, although their use is associated with an increased risk of degeneration in younger people**

that can be accelerated by pregnancy. Mechanical valves and their need for anticoagulation are associated with increased maternal mortality, morbidity, and fetal loss. A detailed discussion with the patient during preconception evaluation and consultation should include potential complications during pregnancy, potential harm to the fetus and mother with cardiac medications especially with anticoagulation, and recognition of the signs and symptoms of valve dysfunction or heart failure. The risk of complication during pregnancy depends on the type of valve, position of the valve, and prepregnancy cardiac function and functional capacity. Patients with NYHA class III or IV symptoms should be strongly advised against pregnancy. In pregnant patients with well-functioning bioprosthetic valves, the management is similar to that in patients with native valves. Patients should be made aware of the possibility of valve degeneration and should be monitored for signs and symptoms of this. Pregnancy should be discouraged in patients with mechanical heart valves. In pregnant patients with mechanical heart valves, management of anticoagulation is challenging. Pregnancy is a thrombogenic state, and thromboembolism has been reported in up to 10% to 15% of patients with mechanical prosthetic valves during pregnancy with a high incidence of valve thrombosis and death. The incidence is particularly high in patients with older generation valves (Björk-Shirley, Starr-Edwards) in the mitral position, but complications have also been reported in newer-generation valves in the aortic position. Patients with prosthetic valves and poor left ventricular function are also at risk for heart failure from volume overload during pregnancy and arrhythmias.

The management of anticoagulation during pregnancy is discussed in detail in a separate section of this chapter.

VII. OTHER CARDIOVASCULAR DISEASES AND PREGNANCY

1. **Hypertensive disorders in pregnancy.** Hypertensive disorders complicate 8% to 10% of pregnancies and are a major cause of maternal and perinatal morbidity and mortality. Hypertensive disorders can be broadly classified into chronic hypertension, gestational hypertension, and preeclampsia–eclampsia.

Chronic hypertension is defined as blood pressure of 140/90 mm Hg or greater before pregnancy, before 20 weeks of gestation, or persisting beyond postpartum day 42. It is associated with increased maternal and fetal morbidity. Therapy should be reserved for patients at high risk for preeclampsia and with evidence of end-organ damage such as left ventricular hypertrophy or renal insufficiency. **Drug therapy is initiated when systolic blood pressure exceeds 150 mm Hg or diastolic exceeds 100 to 110 mm Hg.** Frequent monitoring of blood chemistry and fetal growth is recommended.

Gestational hypertension is defined as hypertension induced by pregnancy and diagnosed after 20 weeks of gestation. It is not associated with proteinuria or other features of preeclampsia, and resolves by the 12th postpartum week. This condition may portend the development of future primary hypertension, but is otherwise associated with good maternal and fetal outcomes.

Preeclampsia occurs in 3% to 8% of pregnancies in the United States. Primigravid women younger than 20 years are at the highest risk for development of this disorder. Other risk factors include preeclampsia in a previous pregnancy, family history of preeclampsia, preexisting chronic hypertension, the antiphospholipid antibody syndrome, and a history of a connective tissue disorder. The classic clinical triad involves gradual onset of hypertension, proteinuria (>300 mg per 24 hours), and edema. Symptoms usually begin in the third trimester and resolve with delivery. The cause of preeclampsia remains unclear. **Eclampsia** is the development of grand mal seizures in a woman with preeclampsia. All patients with preeclampsia should be considered for delivery as soon as fetal maturity is verified or until after 37 weeks of gestation. When preeclampsia is accompanied by risk factors, including seizures, severe hypertension, **HELLP syndrome** (i.e., hemolysis, elevated liver enzyme levels, and low platelet levels), placental abruption, cerebral hemorrhage, pulmonary edema, renal failure, or liver failure, the fetus must be delivered immediately. Such patients should be treated aggressively with blood pressure

TABLE 38.6 Drug Therapy for Hypertension in Pregnancy

Drug	Mechanism of action	Dosing	Comments
Drugs for hypertensive urgency and emergencies			
Labetalol	Alpha-beta adrenergic blocker	20–80 mg IV Q10–20 min (up to 300 mg)	Appears efficacious; widely used, scant safety data
Hydralazine	Vasodilator	5–10 mg IV Q15–30 min	Efficacious and safe during pregnancy and lactation
Sodium nitroprusside	Arterial-veno dilator	0.5–5.0 μg/kg/min	Concern for fetal thiocyanate toxicity
Drugs for long term treatment of hypertension			
Drug	**Mechanism of action**	**Dosing**	**Comments**
Methyldopa	Central $alpha_2$-agonists	250 mg TID up to 4 g/day	Most commonly used; safety well established; drug of choice
Labetalol	Alpha-beta adrenergic blocker	100 mg TID up to 2400 mg/day	Appears efficacious; widely used, scant safety data
Nifedipine	Calcium channel blocker	10 mg QID up to 120 mg/day	Fetal distress from maternal hypotension is a concern

Adapted from Elkayam U. Pregnancy and cardiovascular disease. In: Braunwald E, ed. *Heart disease: a textbook of cardiovascular medicine*, 7th edition. Philadelphia: Elsevier Saunders, 2005:1965–1982.

control, IV magnesium sulfate to prevent seizures, bed rest, continued fetal monitoring for distress and corticosteroids for acceleration of fetal lung maturity. Because of the high risk of maternal and fetal mortality and morbidity, these patients should be managed at a tertiary care center with high risk obstetrics and neonatology.

Table 38.6 lists different drug therapies used to treat hypertension in pregnancy. Intravenous labetalol is the drug of choice for acute hypertensive urgency or emergency in pregnancy. Hydralazine may also be used as a vasodilator. Sodium nitroprusside is usually avoided, especially in later stages of pregnancy, due to concern for fetal cyanide toxicity if used for more than 4 hours, and should be used only as a last resort in cases where emergent control of blood pressure is required. **Methyldopa is the most commonly used agent for control of chronic hypertension in pregnancy and is considered the drug of choice.**

2. **Marfan's syndrome.** Marfan's syndrome is a connective tissue disorder resulting from mutations in the fibrillin gene. It is inherited in an autosomal-dominant fashion. The clinical manifestations include skeletal abnormalities, ectopia lentis, and cardiovascular abnormalities, such as aortic root dilation with or without aortic regurgitation, aortic dissection, and mitral valve prolapse. **Aortic dissection** and rupture are the most feared complications of pregnancy in patients with Marfan's syndrome and are more likely to occur during the **third trimester, including labor and delivery.**

   Screening echocardiography should be performed before pregnancy. **Enlargement of the aortic root to more than 4.0 cm increases the risk of aortic**

dissection and rupture from moderate risk to high risk. Elective repair of the aortic root before conception is advised with a root dimension of 4.5 cm or more. The aortic root should be monitored by serial echocardiography throughout pregnancy.

Medical management during pregnancy involves the use of **β-blockers** throughout pregnancy to reduce the risk of aortic rupture, careful control of blood pressure, adequate analgesia during labor and delivery and consideration of general anesthesia and cesarean section at the time of delivery to maximize hemodynamic control. Women with Marfan's syndrome who do not manifest any cardiac abnormalities have a low rate of complications and can usually tolerate normal vaginal delivery. In women with aortic dilation or evidence of dissection, cesarean section is preferred.

3. **Aortic dissection.** Aortic dissection has been reported in women with Marfan's syndrome, systemic hypertension, coarctation of the aorta, Turner's syndrome, and crack cocaine use. It occurs most commonly in the third trimester and the peripartum period. Transesophageal echocardiography is the most useful diagnostic tool, and a β-blocker is the preferred medication for management during pregnancy. Hydralazine and labetalol can also be used, as well as sodium nitroprusside in resistant cases, but the latter only in the postpartum period. Cesarean section is recommended in patients with dissection.
4. **Coronary artery disease (CAD). Myocardial infarction (MI) during pregnancy is rare**, occurring in 0.01% of pregnancies. The possibility of myocardial infarction should always be entertained in a pregnant or immediately postpartum woman, especially if her symptoms and electrocardiogram (ECG) are suspicious for coronary ischemia. **Most MIs occur during the third trimester in older women who have had multiple prior pregnancies.** Coronary spasm, in situ coronary thrombosis, and coronary dissection are more frequently the underlying precipitants of MI than is classic obstructive atherosclerosis. Acute MI may be the initial clinical manifestation of an underlying hypercoagulable state, such as the antiphospholipid antibody syndrome. The diagnosis and management of acute myocardial infarction in the pregnant patient should follow the guidelines established for the general population.

   Medical therapy for acute MI must be modified in the pregnant patient. Thrombolytic agents increase the risk of maternal hemorrhage substantially (8%). Low-dose aspirin, β-blockers, and nitrates are considered safe. Short-term heparin administration has not been associated with increased maternal or fetal adverse effects. ACE-Is and statins are contraindicated during pregnancy. Coronary angiography should be performed only when emergent angioplasty or coronary artery bypass grafting (CABG) is anticipated during pregnancy, and, if possible, avoided in first trimester.
5. **Arrhythmias.** The most frequent rhythm disturbances, premature atrial complexes (PACs) or premature ventricular complexes (PVCs), are not associated with adverse maternal or fetal outcomes and do not warrant antiarrhythmic drug therapy. Atrial fibrillation and atrial flutter are rare during pregnancy. Rate control may be achieved safely with digitalis and β-blockers. Direct-current cardioversion may be performed safely during any stage of pregnancy. Anticoagulation is recommended for chronic atrial fibrillation in the setting of underlying structural heart disease. **Atrioventricular nodal reentrant tachycardia (AVNRT)** is the most common supraventricular arrhythmia in pregnant and nonpregnant women. It can lead to hemodynamic deterioration in women with underlying heart disease owing to rapid rates. Adenosine may be administered safely to the pregnant patient for both diagnostic and therapeutic purposes.

   Ventricular tachycardia (VT) is rare during pregnancy. It may, however, be the presenting manifestation of peripartum cardiomyopathy (PPCM). VT has also been associated with thyrotoxicosis and hyperemesis gravidarum. Most antiarrhythmic medications used to treat VT are safe during pregnancy, **except** for **amiodarone**, which should be used with caution and only for arrhythmias not responding to other medications, as it may lead to **neonatal hypothyroidism**.

Bradyarrhythmias are uncommon during pregnancy. Complete heart block may be acquired or congenital. Pacemaker support is not usually required, unless the bradyarrhythmia is symptomatic, or there is hemodynamic deterioration.

6. **Peripartum cardiomyopathy (PPCM).** This is a type of dilated cardiomyopathy that is defined by development of heart failure in the last month of pregnancy or within 5 months of delivery, absence of any identifiable cause of heart failure or any recognizable heart disease prior to the last month of pregnancy, and echocardiographic evidence of left ventricular dysfunction with a low ejection fraction. The incidence of PPCM in the United States is estimated to be 1 in 3000 to 4000 live births, and is **more common in women older than 30 years**. The following risk factors for PPCM have been proposed: **multiparity, multiple fetuses, history of preeclampsia, eclampsia, or postpartum hypertension, African descent, history of maternal cocaine abuse, and selenium deficiency**. Symptoms become more apparent in the second trimester in women with preexisting cardiac dysfunction. Symptoms include fatigue, dyspnea on exertion, orthopnea, nonspecific chest pain, peripheral edema, and abdominal discomfort and distention.

    The prognosis after development of PPCM is variable. **Between 50% and 60% of women completely recover normal heart size and function, usually within 6 months of delivery**. The remainder either experience stable left ventricular dysfunction or continue to experience clinical deterioration. Estimated maternal mortality ranges from 10% to 50%. Women with PPCM and **persistent** left ventricular dysfunction who attempt subsequent pregnancy **face a high risk of complications**. They should be counseled to avoid further pregnancies.

    Patients presenting with decompensated heart failure should be treated vigorously with oxygen, diuretics, digitalis and vasodilators. ACE-Is are absolutely contraindicated in pregnancy. Vasopressors like dopamine, dobutamine, and milrinone have been used in pregnancy; however, the data regarding their use are very limited. Careful hemodynamic monitoring during labor and delivery may be necessary, and attempts should be made to minimize volume overload. Patients with severe cardiac dysfunction and decompensation should be evaluated for cardiac transplantation after pregnancy.

7. **Primary pulmonary hypertension. This is associated with very high maternal mortality (30% to 40%) and poor fetal outcomes**. Worsening of symptoms occurs in the second and third trimesters, and death is usually from right ventricular failure or arrhythmias. Pregnancy should be discouraged from becoming pregnant, and early therapeutic abortion should be considered for those who become pregnant. Anticoagulation throughout gestation or at least during the third trimester is recommended. Close hemodynamic monitoring during labor, delivery, and the early postpartum period is advised, and oxygen plus inhaled nitrous oxide or prostaglandins (inhaled or IV) may be used.

8. **Pregnancy after cardiac transplantation. Pregnancy after cardiac transplantation is considered high risk for mother and fetus.** Maternal morbidity is increased from hypertension, preeclampsia, renal failure, premature rupture of membranes, and infection. Fetal growth retardation and preterm labor is also a concern, along with potential adverse fetal effects of immunosuppressive medications. One study examined the outcomes of 47 pregnancies in 35 transplant recipients. There was no increase in maternal mortality in this study, but there were increased maternal morbidity, premature deliveries, and fetal growth retardation.

VIII. MEDICATION CONSIDERATIONS IN PREGNANCY

1. **Cardiovascular drugs.** The most commonly used cardiovascular drug classes and their potential adverse effects during pregnancy are shown in **Table 38.7.**
2. **Anticoagulation during pregnancy.** Conditions requiring anticoagulation during pregnancy include mechanical prosthetic heart valves, chronic atrial fibrillation, acute venous thromboembolism, Eisenmenger's syndrome, antiphospholipid antibody syndrome, and inherited deficiencies predisposing to thromboembolism (e.g., prothrombin gene mutation, factor V Leiden deficiency).

TABLE 38.7 Cardiovascular Drugs and Pregnancy

Drug	Indication	FDA category	Potential maternal or fetal side effects
Adenosine	Arrhythmia	C	Limited data on use
Amiodarone	Arrhythmia	C	Hyper/hypothyroidism, IUGR, congenital goiter
ACE-I/ARB	Hypertension	D/X	Contraindicated, IUGR, oligohydramnios, renal failure, fetal death
Aspirin	Coronary artery disease	C/D	IUGR and bleeding in mother and neonate
β-Blockers	Arrhythmia, Hypertension, MI, HOCM, Hyperthyroidism, Marfan's, mitral stenosis	C/D	Fetal bradycardia, hypoglycemia, IUGR
Calcium channel blockers	Hypertension	C	Maternal hypotension causing fetal distress reported
Digoxin	Arrhythmia, heart failure	C	No evidence of adverse effects, considered safe
Diuretics	Hypertension	C	Hypovolemia and reduced utero-placental blood flow
Flecainide	Arrhythmia	C	Limited data
Lidocaine	Arrhythmia	C	Neonatal CNS depression
Nitrates	Hypertension	C	Maternal hypotension causing fetal distress reported
Procainamide	Arrhythmia	C	No adverse effects reported
Propafenone	Arrhythmia	C	Limited data
Quinidine	Arrhythmia	C	Neonatal thrombocytopenia, oxytoxic effect
Sodium nitroprusside	Hypertension, aortic dissection	C	Fetal thiocyanate toxicity
Sotalol	Arrhythmia	B	Fetal bradycardia, IUGR, limited data

FDA category: A, Controlled studies show no risk; B, No evidence of risk in humans; C, Risk cannot be ruled out; D, Positive evidence of risk; X, Contraindicated in pregnancy; IUGR, Intrauterine growth retardation.

The three most common agents considered for use during pregnancy are **unfractionated heparin (UH), low-molecular-weight heparin (LMWH),** and **warfarin**. The Sixth American College of Chest Physicians (ACCP) Consensus Conference on Antithrombotic Therapy has recommended three potential strategies for anticoagulation during pregnancy (**Fig. 38.1, Table 38.8**).

The choice of anticoagulation regimens depends on the preferences of the patient and physician after consideration of the maternal and fetal risks associated with use of each drug.

a. Warfarin. Warfarin freely crosses the placental barrier and can adversely affect fetal development. It has been associated with a high incidence of spontaneous abortion, prematurity, still birth, and fetal bleeding. **The incidence of warfarin embryopathy (i.e., abnormalities of fetal bone and cartilage formation) has been estimated at 4% to 10%; the risk is highest when warfarin is administered during the 6th through the 12th weeks of gestation.** When administered

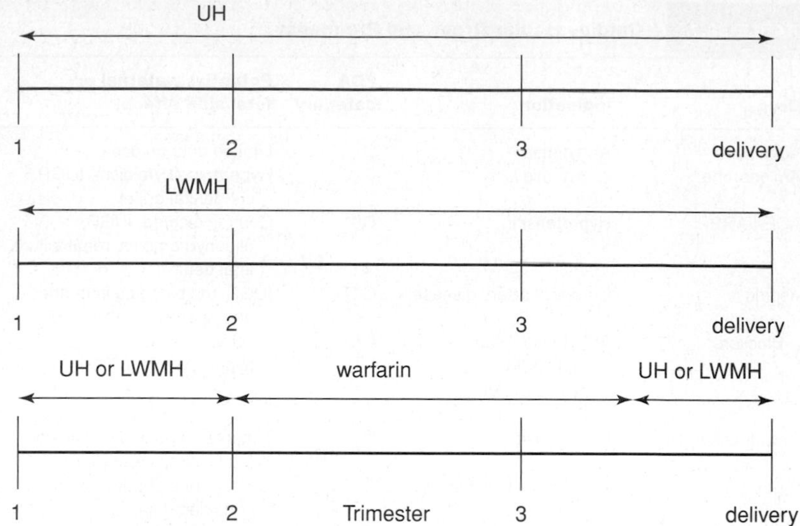

Figure 38.1. Anticoagulation options during pregnancy.

during the second and third trimesters, warfarin has been associated with fetal central nervous system abnormalities, such as optic atrophy, microencephaly, mental retardation, spasticity, and hypotonia. Warfarin is considered safe during breast-feeding.

Women taking warfarin prior to pregnancy should be counseled regarding the harmful effects, and if pregnancy is contemplated then frequent pregnancy tests or switching to unfractionated heparin or LMWH should be considered.

b. Unfractionated heparin (UFH). UFH does not cross the placenta, and unlike warfarin does not have the teratogenic effects and is, therefore, considered safer. **It is, however, associated with maternal osteoporosis, hemorrhage, thrombocytopenia or thrombosis (HITT syndrome), and a high incidence of thromboembolic events with older-generation mechanical valves.** UFH may be administered parenterally or subcutaneously throughout pregnancy. Subcutaneous heparin use in patients with mechanical valve carries an increased risk of valve thrombosis. The appropriate dose of UFH is based on an activated partial thromboplastin time (aPTT) of 2.0 to 3.0 times the control level. High doses of UFH are often required to achieve the goal aPTT because of the hypercoagulable state associated with pregnancy. Parenteral infusions should be stopped 4 hours before a cesarean section. In the event of preterm labor, spontaneous hemorrhage, or significant bleeding during delivery, UFH may be reversed with protamine sulfate.

c. Low–molecular-weight heparin (LMWH). The use of LMWH during pregnancy is still controversial as it has not been adequately studied. The manufacturer's label recommends caution for use in pregnant patients with mechanical heart valves. Its advantage over heparin include a more predictable anticoagulant response, less incidence of HITT, lower risk of heparin-associated osteoporosis, and lower risk of bleeding complications. It does not cross the placenta, and it may be safer to the fetus even though data in this regard are limited. With increased blood volume, especially during the later part of pregnancy, the volume of distribution for LMWH changes, and it is important to monitor anti-Xa level (goal = 0.7–1.2, 4 hours after morning dose). LMWH has been used successfully to treat venous thromboembolism in pregnancy, but

TABLE 38.8 **ACC/AHA Guidelines for Selection of Anticoagulation Regimen in Pregnant Patients with Mechanical Prosthetic Valves**

Class I (Benefits >>> Risk) Procedure/Treatment Should be Performed/Administered	**Level of evidence**
All pregnant patients with mechanical prosthetic valves must receive continuous therapeutic anticoagulation with frequent monitoring	B
For women requiring long-term warfarin therapy who are attempting pregnancy, pregnancy tests should be monitored with discussions about subsequent anticoagulation therapy, so that anticoagulation can be continued uninterrupted when pregnancy is achieved	C
Pregnant patients with mechanical prosthetic valves who elect to stop warfarin between weeks 6 and 12 of gestation should receive continuous intravenous UFH, dose-adjusted UFH, or dose-adjusted subcutaneous LMWH	C
For pregnant patients with mechanical prosthetic valves, up to 36 weeks of gestation, the therapeutic choice of continuous intravenous or dose-adjusted subcutaneous UFH, dose-adjusted LMWH, or warfarin should be discussed fully. If continuous intravenous UFH is used, the fetal risk is lower, but the maternal risks of prosthetic valve thrombosis, systemic embolization, infection, osteoporosis, and heparin-induced thrombocytopenia are relatively higher	C
In pregnant patients with mechanical prosthetic valves who receive dose-adjusted LMWH, the LMWH should be administered twice daily subcutaneously to maintain the anti-Xa level between 0.7 and 1.2 U per mL 4 h after administration.	C
In pregnant patients with mechanical prosthetic valves who receive dose-adjusted UFH, the aPTT should be at least twice control	C
In pregnant patients with mechanical prosthetic valves who receive warfarin, the INR goal should be 3.0 (range 2.5 to 3.5)	C
In pregnant patients with mechanical prosthetic valves, warfarin should be discontinued and continuous intravenous UFH given starting 2 to 3 weeks before planned delivery	C
Class IIa (Benefits >> Risk) It is Reasonable to Perform Procedure/ Administer Treatment	
In patients with mechanical prosthetic valves, it is reasonable to avoid warfarin between weeks 6 and 12 of gestation owing to the high risk of fetal defects	C
In patients with mechanical prosthetic valves, it is reasonable to resume UFH 4 to 6 h after delivery and begin oral warfarin in the absence of significant bleeding	C
In patients with mechanical prosthetic valves, it is reasonable to give low-dose aspirin (75 to 100 mg per day) in the second and third trimesters of pregnancy in addition to anticoagulation with warfarin or heparin.	C
Class III (Risk ≥ Benefits) Procedure/Treatment Should not be Performed/Administered	
LMWH should not be administered to pregnant patients with mechanical prosthetic valves unless anti-Xa levels are monitored 4 to 6 h after administration	C
Dipyridamole should not be used instead of aspirin as an alternative antiplatelet agent in pregnant patients with mechanical prosthetic valves because of its harmful effects on the fetus	B

Level of evidence: A, Multiple population risk strata evaluated; B, Limited population risk strata evaluated; C, Very limited population risk strata evaluated.
From: Benar R, et al. ACC/AHA Guidelines for Management of Patients with Valvular Heart Disease. *Circulation* 2006; 114:e84–e231.

data in patients with mechanical valves are limited, and there have been reports of valve thrombosis associated with its use.

- Therefore, anticoagulation in a pregnant patient can be challenging. The choice of anticoagulant should be made after detailed discussion with the patient. In the event of unplanned pregnancy in a patient on warfarin, it is advisable to change the warfarin to UH or LMWH until 12 weeks and then resume warfarin until the 35th week if the patient is willing to take it, and with careful monitoring of the international normalized ratio (INR).
- In patients with a **mechanical heart valve with high risk of thrombosis** (first-generation prosthesis; e.g., Starr-Edwards, Björk-Shiley in mitral position, atrial fibrillation, and history of thromboembolism) one of the following algorithms may be used:
- Continuous IV UFH (aPTT 2.5–3.5 times) for 12 weeks followed by Coumadin (INR 2.5–3.5) for up to 35 weeks followed by IV UFH (aPTT 2.5–3.5) until delivery **OR** subcutaneous (SC) LMWH (anti-Xa level ~0.7) for 12 weeks followed by Coumadin (INR 2.5–3.5) for up to 35 weeks followed by IV UFH (aPTT of 2.5–3.5 times) or SC LMWH (anti-Xa ~0.7).
- In patients with a **mechanical heart valve with relatively lower risk of thrombosis** (second-generation prosthesis; e.g., St. Jude Medical, Medtronic-Hall, and any mechanical prosthesis in aortic position) algorithm options include:
- Subcutaneous (SC) LMWH (anti-Xa ~0.6) or SC UFH (aPTT 2.0–3.0 times) for 12 weeks followed by Coumadin (INR 2.5–3.0) for up to 35 weeks followed by IV UFH (aPTT 2.0–3.0 times) or SC LMWH (anti-Xa ~0.6) **OR**
- SC UFH or SC LMWH throughout pregnancy (data supporting this algorithm are limited).

Suggested Readings

Autore C, Conte MR, Piccinirino M, et al. Risk associated with pregnancy in hypertrophic cardiomyopathy. *J Am Coll Cardiol* 2002;40:1864.

Bonow RO, Carabello BA, Chatterjee K, et al. ACC/AHA 2006 guidelines for the management of patients with valvular heart disease: a report of the American College of Cardiology/American Heart Association Task Force on Practice Guidelines. *Circulation* 2006;114:e84–e231.

Elkayam U, Bitar F. Valvular heart disease and pregnancy part II: prosthetic valves. *J Am Coll Cardiol* 2005;46:403–410.

Elkayam U, Tummala PP, Rao K, et al. Maternal and fetal outcomes of subsequent pregnancies in women with peripartum cardiomyopathy. *N Engl J Med* 2001;344:1567–1571. [Erratum in *N Engl J Med* 2001;345:552.]

Elkayam U, Singh H, Irani A, et al. Anticoagulation in pregnant women with prosthetic heart valves. *J Cardiovasc Pharmacol Ther* 2004;9:107–115.

Ginsberg JS, Greer I, Hirsh J. Use of antithrombotic agents during pregnancy. *Chest* 2001;119[Suppl]:122S–131S.

Stout KK, Otto CM. Pregnancy in women with valvular heart disease. *Heart* 2007;93:552–558.

Key Reviews

Branch KR, Wagoner LE, McGrory CH, et al. Risks of subsequent pregnancies on mother and newborn in female heart transplant recipient. *J Heart Lung Transplant* 1998;17:698.

Dajani AS, Taubert KA, Wilson W, et al. Prevention of bacterial endocarditis: recommendations by the American Heart Association. *Circulation* 1997;96:358–356.

Elkayam U, Ostrzega E, Shotan A, et al. Cardiovascular problems in pregnant women with the Marfan syndrome. *Ann Intern Med* 1995;123:117–122.

Siu SC, Sermer M, Harrison DA, et al. Risk and predictors for pregnancy-related complications in women with heart disease. *Circulation* 1997;96:2789–2794.

HEART DISEASE IN WOMEN

Kellan E. Ashley

39

I. INTRODUCTION. Cardiovascular disease (CVD) is the leading cause of death in the United States, regardless of gender. With advances in pharmacologic and interventional management and prevention over the last 20 years, the mortality rate in men has declined, but that has not been the case for women. CVD remains by far the leading cause of death for women in the United States and most developed countries, accounting for almost 39% of all female deaths in the United States. Despite this state of urgency, most women do not perceive the risk of CVD as a problem, and when polled still feel cancer, especially breast cancer, is the condition for which they are most at risk. **In reality, one in 2.6 women's deaths will be due to heart disease, stroke, or other CVD; in contrast, one in 30 women will die from breast cancer.** Coronary heart disease (CHD) claims the lives of 283,886 women annually, compared to 41,566 lives from breast cancer and 67,894 from lung cancer. Minority women are even less aware of their cardiovascular risk, although this risk is higher than for age-matched white women. Despite aggressive campaigns by the American Heart Association (AHA) and other organizations, only 46% of women spontaneously listed CHD as a woman's leading cause of death when surveyed, which was up from 30% in 1997. However, only 13% of the women surveyed identified CHD as a risk for them personally.

II. GENDER DIFFERENCES IN PATHOPHYSIOLOGY. Briefly, coronary artery disease (CAD) begins with **nascent atheroma**, the coalescence of small lipoprotein particles within the arterial intima. Over time, these lipoprotein particles become oxidized, inducing local cytokine elaboration. These inflammatory cytokines cause the increased expression of adhesion molecules for leukocytes, leading to leukocyte attraction and migration into the intimal layer. Blood monocytes become macrophages upon entering the intima and express scavenger receptors on their surface, owing to their interaction with certain cytokines present locally. These scavenger receptors promote the uptake of modified lipoprotein particles, leading to the formation of **foam cells**. Foam cells further elaborate inflammatory and attractant cytokines and other effector molecules. In response, smooth muscle cells migrate into the intima from the media, and they proliferate. Smooth muscle cell proliferation and extracellular matrix accumulation lead to the progression from a **fatty streak** to a **fibrofatty plaque**. Later stages are characterized by calcification and fibrosis, occasionally with smooth muscle cell death. This creates an acellular fibrous cap surrounding a lipid-rich core.

The process of atherosclerosis progresses slowly and patients often remain unaware and asymptomatic for many years. This is likely attributable to the capacity of the arteries to remodel—expanding outwardly as the intima expands, thereby preventing plaque encroachment on the lumen of the vessel. However, at some point the plaque burden exceeds the ability of the vessel to remodel, and narrowing of the lumen begins. Eventually, if unimpeded, atherosclerosis will progress until the degree of luminal narrowing impedes blood flow. Initially, this luminal narrowing is apparent mostly under conditions of stress, where arterial oxygen supply is unable to meet demand. Once this occurs, the patient begins to have symptoms, typically stable angina.

In some cases, however, the first manifestation of the underlying CAD is myocardial infarction (MI), unstable angina, or sudden death. In these instances, the underlying stenosis is usually less than 50% of the lumen diameter. The inciting event leading to symptoms in these cases is either physical disruption of the fibrous cap of the plaque or superficial erosion of the intima. Either setting exposes the underlying lipid-rich core to blood components and initiates thrombosis (see Chapters 1 and 2 for more detailed discussions). Women, **especially younger women, are twice as likely to have plaque erosion as the underlying cause of MI**, whereas men and older women more often have plaque rupture.

There appear to be other differences based on gender in the atherosclerotic process. For years it was noted that premenopausal women appeared to be protected from CAD, and estrogen emerged as the most likely reason. Hormones have been proven to influence many of the underlying pathophysiologic processes, including thrombosis and inflammation. Women have smaller coronary arteries than men and, interestingly, women taking androgens have much larger coronary arteries than their age-matched controls. The full spectrum of sex hormone effects on the heart and vascular system has yet to be fully determined.

In addition, there have been genetic links to the development of CAD noted to vary according to gender, with different single-nucleotide polymorphisms noted in men and others in women. Women tend to have more cellular and fibrous plaques. There are also differences in terms of endothelial function and hemostasis (women have higher levels of fibrinogen and factor VII). Some of these or other mechanisms may eventually be identified as the reason for gender differences in the development and progression of CAD.

In recent years, microvascular dysfunction has been postulated as the underlying process leading to symptoms of CHD in some women. This hypothesis was spurred by the fact that many women have minimal to no CAD when undergoing left heart catheterization (LHC) for chest pain, although they continue to have symptoms and often have abnormal stress tests. Further studies are needed to better define the populations at risk for microvascular dysfunction and determine potential therapeutic interventions.

III. GENDER DIFFERENCES IN RISK FACTORS

A. Diabetes mellitus. Diabetes affects more women than men after the age of 60. It is associated with a higher incremental risk for CAD (two to four times the risk of women without diabetes) and drastically increases the mortality of MI in women, much more so than in men. Type 2 diabetes is associated with other components of the metabolic syndrome, all of which increase risk for CAD. Diabetes is also strongly associated with the development of heart failure.

B. Hypertension (HTN). More than 73% of women 65 to 74 years of age have HTN. The risk of developing HTN increases for women if they are 20 pounds or more overweight, they have a family history of HTN, or they have reached menopause. Risk for CVD related to HTN rises steeply with age, although most studies show that treatment attenuates this risk.

C. Hyperlipidemia. Lipid fractions in women are affected by their menopausal status. Premenopausal women have lower low-density-lipoprotein cholesterol (LDL-C) levels and higher high-density-lipoprotein cholesterol (HDL-C) levels than age-matched men. With aging, LDL-C increases and HDL-C decreases, causing the risk for CAD to increase. Total cholesterol and LDL-C are less predictive in women, unlike HDL-C, which is inversely associated with risk. Non–HDL-C and total cholesterol to HDL-C ratio are more predictive in women than men. In addition, triglycerides are a more potent independent predictor of CAD, especially in older women.

D. Cigarette Smoking. This is the single most preventable risk factor. Smoking leads to more CVD deaths than any other risk factor, likely owing to its effects of increasing inflammation, thrombosis, and oxidation of LDL-C. Smoking also has an anti-estrogen effect, inducing unfavorable changes in lipid levels. There is a six- to ninefold increased risk of MI in female smokers compared to age-matched nonsmokers; in fact, the risk from smoking is equivalent to the risk of weighing about 42 kg more than a nonsmoking woman. However, with smoking cessation, risk is cut in half after one year without smoking and eventually declines back to baseline nonsmoker's risk.

E. Obesity and metabolic syndrome. More than 30% of American women are obese, and this number continues to climb. In women, obesity and body fat distribution (i.e., abdominal location) are independent risk factors for CAD. As shown by examination of a cohort of 115,195 women from the Nurses' Health Study, risk of death from CVD increased with increasing body mass index (BMI). Abdominal fat accumulation leads to the development of other components of the metabolic syndrome, such as HTN, diabetes, and hypertriglyceridemia. Obesity is also associated with elevated levels of C-reactive protein (CRP), more so in women.

Women with the metabolic syndrome more often have subclinical CAD than men. A substudy from the National Heart, Lung, and Blood Institute-sponsored WISE (Women's Ischemia Syndrome Evaluation) study revealed that women with the metabolic syndrome have twice the risk for CHD-related events compared to age-matched women without the metabolic syndrome. The metabolic syndrome is defined by the National Cholesterol Education Program Adult Treatment Panel-III in women as the presence of three or more of the following components:

1. Waist circumference >35 inches
2. Fasting triglycerides >150 mg/dL
3. HDL-C <50 mg/dL
4. HTN (systolic blood pressure ≥130 mm Hg, diastolic blood pressure ≥85 mm Hg, or use of antihypertensive drug therapy)
5. Fasting glucose ≥110 mg/dL

F. Estrogen/Menopause. Postmenopausal women have more CVD risk factors, such as obesity, HTN, and hyperlipidemia, likely owing to the changing hormonal environment (estrogen levels are one-tenth the premenopausal level). The predominant source of estrogen changes from estradiol in the premenopausal state to estrone (produced by the conversion of androgens in peripheral adipose tissue) during menopause. Animal studies have shown that estrogen can have favorable cardiovascular effects, reducing cellular hypertrophy, enhancing vessel wall elasticity, and providing antioxidative and antiinflammatory actions.

As part of the WISE study results, endogenous estrogen deficiency in young women was shown to be a strong risk factor for CHD, with a 7.4-fold increased risk. Because of the protection from CAD afforded premenopausal women, there was early enthusiasm for the use of hormone replacement therapy (HRT) to prevent CVD in postmenopausal women, sparked by data from observational studies. However, multiple randomized, placebo-controlled trials over recent years have shown evidence of increased risk of CVD with HRT, such that it is no longer recommended for primary or secondary prevention of CVD (see **VI.F**).

G. Physical inactivity. As women age, they become less physically active than their male counterparts. This contributes to weight gain and predisposes to the development of diabetes and HTN. In addition, with the cessation of estrogen production with menopause, there is increased abdominal fat deposition, further predisposing to CAD. There is a strong inverse association between activity level and incidence of CV events.

H. Novel risk factors. It has been increasingly realized that the traditional risk factors underestimate CHD risk in women. For this and other reasons research has been focused on identifying other novel biomarkers that can better define a person's risk. Multiple biomarkers have been investigated to various degrees [e.g., high-sensitivity C-reactive protein (hsCRP), brain natriuretic peptide, and fibrinogen], but the greatest promise appears to be with hsCRP. As part of the Women's Health Study, over 27,000 healthy American women had CRP and LDL-C levels measured. The women were then followed for a mean of 8 years for the occurrence of the primary endpoint (MI, ischemic stroke, coronary revascularization, or death from CVD). Although minimally correlated with each other, both CRP and LDL-C had strong linear relationships with CVD events, with CRP being the stronger predictor. Each biomarker tended to identify different high-risk groups, but better prognostic values were obtained when both were used together. These data suggest that CRP shows promise when added to traditional risk factors for prediction of long-term risk.

IV. GENDER DIFFERENCES IN CLINICAL MANIFESTATIONS. Women often present differently than men, potentially because of differences in underlying pathophysiology. This is particularly true for diabetic women. Women usually present at an older age, usually 5 to 10 years later than men, and have more comorbidities on presentation than men do. As such, once the diagnosis of CAD is made, women are at higher risk for adverse outcomes.

A. Like men, women can present with typical symptoms of angina, such as substernal **chest pain** and **dyspnea on exertion** that is relieved by rest. These symptoms more often occur in older women, who present more similarly to men.

B. Women can also present with **atypical chest pain**; **shortness of breath**; **neck, shoulder or arm pain**; **diaphoresis**; and **nausea/vomiting**.

C. However, women are more likely to have subtle symptoms that require detailed history-taking to elicit, such as chest "tightness," lightheadedness, palpitations, or fatigue. Women most often have symptoms that occur at rest, wake them from sleep, or occur in times of psychological stress.

D. Women more often present acutely without preexisting prodromes of symptoms or with **sudden cardiac death**.

V. GENDER DIFFERENCES IN ASSESSMENT

A. Exercise electrocardiography. Exercise electrocardiography, the most frequently employed diagnostic modality, is useful only in women with normal baseline electrocardiograms (ECGs) and the ability to undergo moderate or high levels of exercise (generally on the treadmill). An abnormality is identified if there is ≥1 mm of ST-segment depression or elevation. Generally, exercise ECG has lower sensitivity and specificity than other modalities, and this is even more prominent in women (sensitivity and specificity 60% to 70% in women vs. 80% in men). This difference is not well understood but has been attributed to several factors, such as lower overall prevalence of CAD in women or more submaximal stress tests, owing to the inability of women to exercise to sufficient levels to produce a diagnostic test. If women are unable to achieve at least 5 metabolic equivalents (METS), studies have shown that they are at increased risk for future CV events.

B. Stress myocardial perfusion scan. Because of the limited sensitivity and specificity of exercise ECG in women, other modalities are frequently employed to assess risk of CAD. The most frequently used test is the single-photon emission computed tomography (SPECT) scan, a nuclear-based technique. Because alterations in myocardial perfusion generally occur earlier than electrocardiographic changes or wall-motion abnormalities, this test is more sensitive than exercise ECG or echocardiography for estimating risk in either gender. For those individuals unable to exercise or attain target heart rates, adenosine or dipyridamole can be used as a pharmacologic stress. To increase specificity, the higher energy isotopes (technetium-99m) are recommended in women to reduce the soft tissue attenuation artifacts (influenced by both breast tissue and obesity) that tend to occur anteriorly and laterally. Other limitations with SPECT can be critical in women. Because women have smaller hearts, the limitations in spatial resolution of SPECT can lead to small areas of hypoperfusion being missed.

C. Stress echocardiography (TTE). Stress TTE tends to have higher specificity and lower sensitivity than stress perfusion imaging, as wall-motion abnormalities occur later than perfusion abnormalities. However, stress TTE has the advantages of eliminating radiation exposure, decreasing cost, and providing the ability to assess left ventricular (LV) function and cardiac structures. It has been shown to be a cost-effective initial strategy for determining cardiovascular risk in patients at intermediate risk as compared to stress electrocardiography, and we now use it as a first-line diagnostic test for CAD in women.

D. Magnetic resonance imaging (MRI). Although not as commonly used, this is an emerging modality, owing to its ability to evaluate for subendocardial ischemia, precisely assess LV function and mass, and evaluate the anatomy of the myocardium and vasculature. MRI provides the best spatial and temporal resolution, which is thought to be especially helpful when imaging women. Other benefits include the ability to detect ischemia by identifying altered metabolism.

This is achieved by magnetic resonance spectroscopy, which can detect alterations in high-energy phosphates and identify these areas of altered metabolism. Areas of altered metabolism have been shown in reports from the WISE study to be indicative of microvascular dysfunction, as women with nonobstructive CAD by LHC have altered high-energy phosphate ratios indicative of ischemia by spectroscopy.

E. Coronary angiography. Diagnostic coronary angiography is the gold standard for diagnosing CAD in both men and women. When evaluated by left heart catheterization, however, women more often have minimal to no obstructive CAD. For reasons not fully elucidated, women tend to experience vascular complications and renal failure related to diagnostic LHC more frequently than men do. The occurrence of a complication is thought to be related to older age at time of presentation, smaller body size, smaller vessel size, and higher prevalence of diabetes. There appears to be a selection-bias based on gender in terms of performing LHC. Studies in the past have been conflicting, but some have shown that men were up to six times more likely to be offered diagnostic LHC than women, even when both had a positive noninvasive test.

VI. GENDER DIFFERENCES IN THERAPIES. Most CVD in women, as in men, can be prevented if risk-factor modification occurs early and aggressively. Until recently, most of the clinical trial data, on which the guidelines for prevention and treatment of both genders are based, were derived from trials largely in men. This information had been extrapolated to women because gender-specific trial data were lacking. Because of this uncertainty, more recent clinical trials have offered insights into gender-specific results, allowing for evidence-based guidelines for disease prevention and treatment in women. However, with only several exceptions, the guidelines are the same for both men and women. The gender-specific results will be highlighted here; for full discussions, please see the appropriate sections of previous chapters.

A. Aspirin. Aspirin (ASA) is the principal antiplatelet agent in patients with CAD. Its benefit in secondary prevention as well as in acute coronary syndrome (ACS), ST-segment elevation MI, and after revascularization (coronary artery bypass grafting [CABG] or percutaneous coronary intervention [PCI]), are well known and discussed elsewhere. However, there are very few gender-specific data in these instances, so most recommendations are extrapolated from trials conducted largely in men.

The role of ASA in primary prevention of CAD in women is better defined. Despite early data that ASA may be protective as primary prevention for future CVD events in women, as it is in men, recent data prove otherwise. As part of the Women's Health Study, 39,876 healthy women older than age 45 were randomized to either ASA 100 mg on alternate days or placebo, and they were followed for the incidence of cardiovascular (CV) events (nonfatal MI, nonfatal stroke, or CV death) over 10 years. Despite a 24% reduction in ischemic stroke, ASA had no benefit over placebo in reducing MI or CV death. However, ASA did appear protective as primary prevention in those women 65 years of age or older, as it significantly decreased the risk of both MI and stroke in this age group. There was also an increased risk of bleeding observed, which highlights the need for an individualized approach to the use of ASA as primary prevention in older women.

The reason for the lack of benefit as primary prevention in younger women is not well understood but has been postulated to be related to baseline hyperresponsiveness of platelet function or more ASA-resistance in women. Further studies are needed to delineate these potential mechanisms.

B. Thienopyridines. The most commonly used agents in this class are clopidogrel and ticlopidine. The use of ticlopidine has decreased significantly with evidence of adverse effects, including neutropenia and thrombotic thrombocytopenic purpura. These agents have proven benefit, when given with ASA, to reduce the rate of stent thrombosis after PCI. Clopidogrel has also shown benefit in secondary prevention of CAD, ACS, and ST-segment elevation MI (discussed in detail elsewhere). Few of the clinical trials using clopidogrel have given gender-specific data, but there are some data available for specific settings.

In the substudy of the Clopidogrel in Unstable angina to prevent Recurrent Events (CURE) trial, in which the patients received PCI (PCI-CURE), 2658 patients with non–ST-segment elevation ACS undergoing PCI were randomly assigned to aspirin plus clopidogrel or placebo for 9 months. Of the study population, 30.2% were women. Clopidogrel plus aspirin long-term therapy improved outcomes in those patients that received PCI. This was more significant in men, but a definite trend toward benefit in women was evident as well. Similar results were seen for women in the Clopidogrel for the Reduction of Events During Observation (CREDO) trial, where 29% of the 2116 patients were women. The CREDO trial showed benefit in post-PCI therapy with ASA and clopidogrel out to 1 year of therapy, again with a trend toward benefit in women. CREDO also revealed, by subgroup analysis, equally beneficial effects of a loading dose of clopidogrel between men and women.

Newer, more potent agents, such as prasugrel, are still under investigation in phase 3 trials. In the recently released Trial to Assess Improvements in Therapeutic Outcomes by Optimizing Platelet Inhibition with Prasugrel—Thrombolysis in Myocardial Infarction 38 (TRITON-TIMI 38) trial, prasugrel had lower primary endpoints (CV death, nonfatal MI, or nonfatal stroke) than clopidogrel did in 13,608 patients (one-fourth of whom were women) with moderate-to-high-risk ACS with scheduled PCI (9.9% vs. 12.1%). However, the prasugrel group did have higher rates of bleeding particularly in patients with history of stroke or transient ischemic attack, patients 75 years of age or older, or patients weighing less than 60 kg. These data are especially important for women, as there was slightly less observed benefit with prasugrel therapy in women. In addition, women would likely be at higher risk for adverse effects than men, given their smaller body size and older age at presentation, placing them in the groups at risk for bleeding complications.

C. **Statins.** Prior to the last several years, almost 20,000 women participated in clinical trials of statin use, only about one-fourth of overall participants. Two exceptions to this were the Prospective Study of Pravastatin in the Elderly at Risk (PROSPER) trial (50% women) and the lipid-lowering therapy arm of the Antihypertensive and Lipid-Lowering treatment to prevent Heart Attack Trial (ALLHAT-LLT), which had 49% women. ALLHAT-LLT, a primary prevention trial, did not release gender-specific results; PROSPER, having patients with history of or at risk for CVD, did not show a statistically significant benefit in women.

Otherwise, the other major primary and secondary prevention trials of statin therapy have shown similar benefit with statin therapy on reduction of CV events in men and women. The largest number of women enrolled to date in a statin trial was in the Heart Protection Study. This gave encouraging evidence for the benefit of statin therapy in decreasing vascular events in both women and men, with a 20% reduction in women and a 25% reduction in men. In the Treating to New Targets (TNT) trial, patients treated with intensive lipid control with higher-dose atorvastatin (80 mg) was shown to significantly reduce the primary endpoint of a first major CV event (death from CHD, nonfatal MI, resuscitation after cardiac arrest, or fatal or nonfatal stroke) over those on lower dose therapy (atorvastatin 10 mg). Even more encouraging was that this benefit also extended to women. In women (19% of total population) from the TNT trial, the relative and absolute reductions in the primary endpoint were 27% and 2.7%, respectively; this was actually better than those observed in men, who had 21% and 2.2% reduction, respectively.

D. **β-Blockers.** There are no gender-specific data for the use of β-blockers in women for primary and secondary prevention, as previous studies have included insignificant numbers of women. However, a meta-analysis of 5474 patients (1121 women) enrolled in five randomized trials revealed similar reductions in CV death in men and women with metoprolol.

E. **Angiotensin-converting enzyme (ACE) inhibitors and angiotensin II receptor blockers (ARBs).** With respect to the use of ACE inhibitors in women with LV dysfunction, the data are lacking, because trials have included very few women.

Several trials have examined ACE inhibitors in primary and secondary prevention of CV events in patients without LV dysfunction, with conflicting results irrespective of gender. The Heart Outcomes Prevention Evaluation (HOPE) study showed that ACE inhibitors were associated with a mortality reduction in high-risk women that was similar to that in men. The EURopean trial On reduction of cardiac events with Perindopril in stable coronary Artery disease (EUROPA) could not confirm these beneficial findings in women, as the trial only included 14.5% women, but it did show benefit in men. To date, it appears that data for ACE inhibitors in women are not as favorable as for men; however, this needs to be further delineated.

In terms of ARBs for therapy after MI, only two trials have been reported—VALsartan in Acute myocardial iNfarcTion (VALIANT) and OPtimal Trial In Myocardial Infarction with Angiotensin II Antagonist Losartan (OPTIMAAL). Neither of these reported gender-specific data, as they included low numbers of women.

F. Hormone replacement therapy (HRT). Despite beneficial evidence from previous observational studies, recent data from randomized controlled trials have shown no benefit to HRT in postmenopausal women for preventing CV events. The first of these randomized trials was the Heart and Estrogen/progestin Replacement Study (HERS). In this study of secondary prevention, 2763 postmenopausal women with CAD were randomized to either 0.625 mg of conjugated equine estrogen plus 2.5 mg of medroxyprogesterone acetate, or placebo daily. After an average 4-year follow-up, there was no significant difference in the primary outcome of nonfatal MI or CHD death between the groups. Of interest, however, was the fact that the greatest numbers of CV events were noted within the first year in the HRT group. Not surprisingly, the HRT group had a greater incidence of venous thromboembolism and gallbladder disease.

Because of the high number of CV events in the first year, the investigators thought that beneficial effects of HRT might be observed after time, as it appeared HRT became more protective by 4 to 5 years of follow-up in the HERS population. With this in mind, the HERS II study followed 2321 of the original HERS patients, the majority of whom stayed on their original treatment in an open-label format, for an average of 6.8 years. After the longer follow-up, there was still no difference in nonfatal MI or CHD death between the groups. From that point forward, it was not recommended that women with CAD use HRT as secondary prevention to reduce CV risk.

To delineate the role of HRT in primary prevention of CV events, the Women's Health Initiative randomized 16,608 healthy, postmenopausal women to the same estrogen–progestin combination used in HERS or placebo. The primary endpoints were the same, nonfatal MI or death due to CHD. After a mean 5.2 year follow-up, the trial was stopped by the data and safety monitoring board due to untoward risks in the treatment arm. Estrogen and progestin therapy was associated with an increased risk for CV events, most impressively at one year. Despite some favorable effects on lipids, HRT should not be recommended for either the primary or secondary prevention of CVD in postmenopausal women.

G. Lifestyle modification. The good news for women is that initiating lifestyle modifications can reduce CV risk by reducing the risk of developing diabetes. As part of the Diabetes Prevention Program Research Group, 3234 patients (68% women) with impaired glucose tolerance were randomized to placebo, metformin (850 mg twice daily), or lifestyle modification (goal 7% weight loss and at least 150 minutes of physical activity per week). After almost 3 years of follow-up, the lifestyle modification group had a 58% reduction in the incidence of diabetes, compared to 31% in the group with metformin. This translates to decreased risk of CVD.

H. Folic acid and antioxidants. Despite previous recommendations to lower homocysteine levels with folic acid and vitamin B supplementation, there is now evidence to discourage this practice. Two randomized trials—the Norwegian Vitamin (NORVIT) study and the Heart Outcomes Prevention Evaluation (HOPE-2) trial—showed no benefit in reducing CV events. The NORVIT study included both men and women post-MI, and randomized the groups to one of four treatments: folic acid, B_{12}, and B_6; folic acid and B_{12}; B_6 alone; or placebo. Despite lowering of homocysteine levels, the treatment groups had no advantage in terms of reductions in the primary endpoint of recurrent MI, stroke, or sudden death attributed to CAD. In fact, the group that received all three therapies had a trend toward increased risk. Similar results were seen in the HOPE-2 trial. Therefore, these therapies should not be recommended. In addition, data from the Women's Health Study do not support the use of vitamin E in the primary prevention of CV events.

VII. EVIDENCE-BASED GUIDELINES FOR HEART DISEASE PREVENTION IN WOMEN. The American College of Cardiology/American Heart Association (ACC/AHA) guidelines emphasize the importance of recognizing the wide-ranging spectrum of CV disease in women. In general, a woman 20 years of age or older is first classified as at high risk, at risk, or at optimal risk based on the criteria in Table 39.1. Several factors should be evaluated, such as medical history, lifestyle, family history of premature CAD, Framingham risk score, and other genetic conditions, before decision regarding the aggressiveness of preventive therapy is finalized.

The guidelines are grouped into three main areas: lifestyle interventions, major risk factor interventions, and preventive drug interventions. Table 39.2 lists the class I and class IIa recommendations for primary or secondary prevention of CVD in women. These guidelines are suggested as a starting point, with therapy tailored to the needs of each individual patient.

In general, it is suggested that the initial evaluation begin with a complete history, specifically eliciting symptoms of CVD, as well as a complete physical examination, with particular attention to blood pressure, BMI, and waist size. Laboratory evaluation should follow, including fasting lipids and glucose levels. During the evaluation, assessment of Framingham risk should be performed, as well as depression screening in those women with known CVD. **All class I lifestyle interventions** should be employed in **all women**, regardless of risk level.

If the woman is **high risk** (established CAD, cerebrovascular disease, peripheral arterial disease, abdominal aortic aneurysm, diabetes, chronic kidney disease, or

TABLE 39.1 Risk Classification for CV Disease in Women

High risk	At risk	Optimal risk
■ Known CAD ■ Cerebrovascular disease ■ Peripheral arterial disease ■ End-stage renal or chronic kidney disease ■ Diabetes ■ 10-year Framingham global risk >20%	■ One or more major risk factors for CV disease: **A.** Cigarette smoking **B.** Poor diet **C.** Physical inactivity **D.** Obesity (especially abdominal location) **E.** Family history of premature CAD (<55 years in men, <65 in women) **F.** HTN **G.** Hyperlipidemia ■ Subclinical vascular disease (i.e., coronary calcification on cardiac CT) ■ Metabolic syndrome ■ Poor exercise capacity on exercise treadmill test and/or abnormal heart rate recovery after stopping exercise	■ Framingham global risk <10% ■ Healthy lifestyle ■ No risk factors

CAD, coronary artery disease; CT, computed tomography; CV, cardiovascular; HTN, hypertension.
Adapted from *ACC/AHA Guidelines 2007 Update. Circulation* 2007;115:1481–1501.

TABLE 39.2 Evidence-based Guidelines for Prevention of Heart Disease in Women

Lifestyle interventions	Major risk factor interventions	Preventive drug interventions
CLASS I RECOMMENDATIONS		
Smoking cessation	Maintain optimal BP (<120/80 mm Hg) with lifestyle modification	ASA in high-risk women (known CAD, cerebrovascular disease, PAD, AAA, ESRD, CKD, diabetes, and 10-year Framingham risk >20%)
Exercise 30 minutes of moderate intensity (i.e., brisk walking) exercise on most/all days of the week	Pharmacotherapy for BP when ≥140/90 mm Hg (≥130/80 mm Hg in CKD or diabetes)	Clopidogrel therapy for high-risk women intolerant of ASA
Weight loss to BMI <24.9 kg/m^2 and waist circumference ≤35 inches	Control of lipids through lifestyle modification (LDL-C <100 mg/dL, HDL-C >50 mg/dL, triglycerides <150 mg/dL, and non–HDL-C [total cholesterol–HDL-C] <130 mg/dL)	β-Blockers indefinitely in those women after MI, ACS, or LV dysfunction
Cardiovascular rehabilitation in those with recent ACS or PCI, angina, recent CVA, PAD, or CHF	Pharmacotherapy of lipids in those with CAD or diabetes to goal LDL-C <100 mg/dL	ACE inhibitors in those after MI or with clinical CHF, LV dysfunction (LVEF ≤40%), or diabetes. If intolerant of ACE inhibitor, ARB can be substituted
Diet counseling to promote intake of fruits and vegetables, whole-grain and high-fiber foods, and fish at least two times per week. Limit consumption of saturated fat, cholesterol, alcohol, sodium, and trans-fatty acids	Pharmacotherapy of lipids in those with LDL-C ≥130 mg/dL after lifestyle modification and presence of multiple risk factors (or if LDL-C ≥160 mg/dL in those with multiple risk factors, even if Framingham risk <10%)	Aldosterone blockade after MI in symptomatic women with LVEF ≤40% who are without renal dysfunction or hyperkalemia and who are already on an ACE inhibitor and β-blocker
	Pharmacotherapy of lipids in those with LDL-C ≥190 mg/dL regardless of other risk factors	
	Maintain HbA_{1C} <7% in diabetics	
CLASS IIA RECOMMENDATIONS		
Consider depression screening and therapy	Goal LDL-C <70 mg/dL is reasonable in the very high risk (known CAD + multiple major risk factors, severe and poorly controlled risk factors, or diabetes)	Low-dose ASA therapy (81 mg daily or 100 mg on alternate days) in women ≥65 years old if benefits outweigh risk of bleeding
	Pharmacotherapy with niacin or fibrates when HDL-C is low or non–HDL-C is elevated in high-risk women (after LDL-C goal reached)	

AAA, abdominal aortic aneurysm; ACE, angiotensin-converting enzyme; ACS, acute coronary syndrome; ARB, angiotensin II receptor blocker; ASA, aspirin; BMI, body mass index; BP, blood pressure; CAD, coronary artery disease; CHF, congestive heart failure; CKD, chronic kidney disease; CVA, cerebrovascular accident; ESRD, end-stage renal disease; HbA_{1C}, glycosylated hemoglobin; HDL-C, high-density-lipoprotein cholesterol; LDL-C, low-density-lipoprotein cholesterol; LV, left ventricular; LVEF, left ventricular ejection fraction; MI, myocardial infarction; mm Hg, millimeters of mercury; PAD, peripheral arterial disease; PCI, percutaneous coronary intervention.
Adapted from *ACC/AHA Guidelines 2007 Update. Circulation* 2007;115:1481–1501.

TABLE 39.3	Therapies Contraindicated in CV Disease Prevention in Women
Hormone replacement therapy or selective estrogen-receptor modulators Antioxidant vitamin supplementation (Vitamins E, C, and beta-carotene) Folic acid with or without vitamins B_6 or B_{12} ASA in healthy women <65 years old	

ASA, aspirin; CV, cardiovascular.
Adapted from *ACC/AHA Guidelines 2007 Update. Circulation 2007;115:1481–1501.*

Framingham risk greater than 20%), the **class I major risk factor and preventive drug interventions** should be initiated (see Table 39.2). Consideration should also be given to some of the class II recommendations, particularly the **LDL-C goal of less than 70 mg/dL.**

There are some interventions that should not be considered under any circumstances. Table 39.3 lists those therapies that are **contraindicated** based on the results of recent clinical trials.

Novel risk factors, such as CRP, as well as newer screening modalities may have a role in the future, but this role is not currently defined. Further research is needed in these areas before they can be incorporated into the guidelines.

VIII. CURRENT PROGRESS AND FUTURE INNOVATIONS. Despite clinical trial data that document the benefits of multiple therapeutic interventions, women are still inadequately treated. In fact, despite the vast amount of data on statins, the 1999–2000 National Health and Nutrition Examination Survey (NHANES) reported that only 10.2% of women with hyperlipidemia were receiving therapy, compared to 14% of men. Men, when treated, were also much more likely to reach their goal LDL-C. Strikingly, in a study of patients receiving care in an academic medical practice, women with diabetes were the group most likely to be inadequately treated for their modifiable CVD risk factors. Furthermore, even higher risk patients (women with ACS) have been shown to be less aggressively treated than their male counterparts.

Despite the aggressive campaigns of the AHA and other organizations, women are still not well informed regarding their personal risk for heart disease. In the 2003 AHA-sponsored survey of women, only 40% considered themselves either "very well" or "well" informed about heart disease, even fewer in the most at-risk minorities. Even more frightening is that a significant majority of the women surveyed received their information regarding heart disease from the mass media, with magazines and television the leading sources. Although nearly all of the women were comfortable discussing their risk for CHD with their physician, only 38% reported that their physician had actually discussed this risk with them. This highlights the need for healthcare providers to bridge this knowledge gap and seize the opportunities to discuss risks and risk factor modification with patients. Subsequently healthcare providers should aggressively treat the appropriate women based on guideline recommendations, in order to improve long-term outcomes.

The population is aging, and estimates are that by 2010 more than 80% of the population 85 years or older will be women. Therefore, the incidence of CVD is likely only to increase, unless we begin to institute preventive therapies earlier, and to aggressively continue them over a woman's lifespan. More attention should be paid by healthcare providers to promoting a woman's awareness of her risk for CVD as well as instituting therapies aggressively aimed at prevention that is tailored to a woman's specific needs.

Further research is needed in the area of gender-specific differences in CAD and all of its manifestations, as well as many of the pharmacologic and interventional therapies used in its treatment. Research that delves further into novel risk factors and the additional value that can be provided over traditional risk factors in terms of assessing risk for CVD, especially in women, is needed as well. Ongoing genetics research, as well as research related to sex hormones, could also provide useful information for tailoring gender-specific therapy. Novel imaging strategies are being studied and may provide important information. This may be especially important in women, given the difficulty with diagnosis of obstructive CAD in such a high percentage. Hopefully, once some of these data come to light, there will be appreciable changes in the occurrence and outcomes of CVD in women.

Key References/Suggested Readings

http://www.americanheart.org

1. The ALLHAT Officers and Coordinators for the ALLHAT Collaborative Research Group: major outcomes in moderately hypercholesterolemic, hypertensive patients randomized to pravastatin versus usual care: the Antihypertensive and Lipid-Lowering Treatment to Prevent Heart Attack Trial (ALLHAT). *JAMA* 2002;288:2998–3007.
2. Bairey Merz CN, Shaw LJ, Reis SE, et al. Insights from the NHLBI-sponsored Women's Ischemia Syndrome Evaluation (WISE) study. Part II: gender differences in presentation, diagnosis, and outcome with regard to gender-based pathophysiology of atherosclerosis and macrovascular and microvascular coronary disease. *J Am Coll Cardiol* 2006;47:21S–29S.
3. Bonaa KH, Njolstad I, Ueland PM, et al. Homocysteine lowering and cardiovascular events after acute myocardial infarction. *N Engl J Med* 2006;354:1578–1588.
4. Ford ES, Mokdad AH, Giles WH, et al. Serum total cholesterol concentrations and awareness, treatment, and control of hypercholesterolemia among US adults: findings from the National Health and Nutrition Examination Survey, 1999–2000. *Circulation* 2003;107:2185–2189.
5. Grady D, Herrington D, Bittner V, et al. Cardiovascular disease outcomes during 6.8 years of hormone therapy. Heart and Estrogen/progestin Replacement Study Follow-up (HERS II). *JAMA* 2002;288:49–57.
6. Hulley S, Grady D, Bush T, et al. Randomized trial of estrogen plus progestin for secondary prevention of coronary heart disease in postmenopausal women. *JAMA* 1998;280:605–613.
7. Jochmann N, Stangl K, Garbe E, et al. Female-specific aspects in the pharmacotherapy of chronic cardiovascular diseases. *Eur Heart J* 2005;26:1585–1595.
8. Knowler WC, Barrett-Connor E, Fowler SE, et al. Reduction in the incidence of type 2 diabetes with lifestyle intervention or metformin. *N Engl J Med* 2002;346:393–403.
9. Lee IM, Cook NR, Gaziano JM, et al. Vitamin E in the primary prevention of cardiovascular disease and cancer: The Women's Health Study: a randomized controlled trial. *JAMA* 2005;294:56–65.
10. Lonn E, Roccaforte R, Yi Q, et al. Effect of long-term therapy with ramipril in high-risk women. *J Am Coll Cardiol* 2002;40:693–702.
11. Manson JE, Hsia J, Johnson KC, et al. Estrogen plus progestin and the risk of coronary heart disease. *N Engl J Med* 2003;349:523–534.
12. Manson JE, Willett WC, Stampfer MJ, et al. Body weight and mortality among women. *N Engl J Med* 1995;333:677–685.
13. Mehta SR, Yusuf S, Peters RJ, et al. Effects of pretreatment with clopidogrel and aspirin followed by long-term therapy in patients undergoing percutaneous coronary intervention: the PCI-CURE study. *Lancet* 2001;358:527–533.
14. Mieres JH, Shaw LJ, Hendel RC, et al. American Society of Nuclear Cardiology consensus statement: task force on women and coronary artery disease—the role of myocardial perfusion imaging in the clinical evaluation of coronary artery disease in women. *J Nucl Cardiol* 2003;10:95–101.
15. Mosca L, Banka CL, Benjamin EJ, et al. Evidence-based guidelines for cardiovascular disease prevention in women: 2007 update. *Circulation* 2007;115:1481–1506.
16. Mosca L, Ferris A, Fabunmi R, et al. Tracking women's awareness of heart disease: an American Heart Association national study. *Circulation* 2004;109:573–579.
17. MRC/BHF Heart Protection Study of cholesterol lowering with simvastatin in 20,536 high-risk individuals: a randomized placebo-controlled trial. *Lancet* 2002;360:7–22.
18. Olsson G, Wikstrand J, Warnold I, et al. Metoprolol-induced reduction in postinfarction mortality: pooled results from five double-blind randomized trials. *Eur Heart J* 1992;13:28–32.
19. Ridker PM, Cook NR, Lee I, et al. A randomized trial of low-dose aspirin in the primary prevention of cardiovascular disease in women. *N Engl J Med* 2005;352:1293–1304.
20. Ridker PM, Rifai N, Rose L, et al. Comparison of c-reactive protein low-density lipoprotein cholesterol levels in the prediction of first cardiovascular events. *N Engl J Med* 2002;347:1557–1565.
21. Shaw LJ, Bairey Merz CN, Pepine CJ, et al. Insights from the NHLBI-sponsored Women's Ischemia Syndrome Evaluation (WISE) study. Part I: gender differences in traditional and novel risk factors, symptom evaluation, and gender optimized diagnostic strategies. *J Am Coll Cardiol* 2006;46:4S–20S.
22. Shepherd J, Blauw GJ, Murphy MB, et al. Pravastatin in elderly individuals at risk of vascular disease (PROSPER): a randomized controlled trial. *Lancet* 2002;360:1623–1630.
23. Visser M, Bonter LM, McQuillan GM, et al. Elevated c-reactive protein levels in overweight and obese adults. *JAMA* 1999;282:2131–2135.
24. Wenger NK. Preventing cardiovascular disease in women: an update. *Clin Cardiol* 2008;31:109–113.
25. Wenger NK, Lewis SJ, Welty FK, et al. Beneficial effects of aggressive low-density lipoprotein cholesterol lowering in women with stable coronary heart disease in the Treating to New Targets (TNT) study. *Heart* 2008;94:434–439.
26. Wexler DJ, Grant RW, Meiss JB, et al. Sex disparities in treatment of cardiac risk factors in patients with type 2 diabetes. *Diabetes Care* 2005;28:514–520.
27. Wiviott SD, Braunwald E, McCabe CH, et al. Prasugrel versus clopidogrel in patients with acute coronary syndromes. *N Engl J Med* 2007;357:2001–2015.

VIII Preventive Cardiology

40 DYSLIPIDEMIA

Matthew A. Kaminski

I. INTRODUCTION. Cardiovascular disease (CVD) is the leading cause of morbidity and mortality in the industrialized world. It is estimated that 30% of all deaths worldwide can be ascribed to cardiovascular causes, and this number is expected to rise further as the incidence of CVD in the developing world increases as a result of lifestyle changes.

A. Morbidity and mortality. CVD is the number one killer (1) in the United States, accounting for 36% of all deaths. CVD is responsible for one death every 36 seconds and claims more lives each year than cancer, accidents, chronic obstructive disease (COPD), and diabetets mellitus combined. One of every five deaths in the United States is caused by coronary heart disease (CHD). There are 15.8 million Americans with a history of myocardial infarction (MI) or angina pectoris. As many as 865,000 Americans have a new MI each year, and 164,000 are victims of sudden cardiac death. The average age at first MI is 65.8 years for men and 70.4 years for women. According to the Centers for Disease Control and Prevention (CDC), elimination of all forms of CVD would raise the overall life expectancy by 7 years.

B. Economic consequences of CVD. The economic burden of CVD and stroke in the United States was estimated to be $431.8 billion in 2007. In 2004, CVD was the leading cause of hospitalization, contributing to more than 6.4 million patient discharges and 4.2 million emergency department visits.

C. Prevention of coronary artery disease (CAD). Table 40.1 shows important targets for secondary prevention among patients with known coronary or non-coronary vascular disease. The goals for primary prevention are similar, but the cost-effectiveness of medical intervention is not so favorable in all populations. The consequences of modest population-wide risk reduction [e.g., reduction in fat intake (currently 33% of total calories) and cholesterol levels] and life-saving technologies (e.g., surgery, angioplasty, and coronary care units) have reduced the death rate and possibly contributed to reduced morbidity, but the burden of CVD remains a major challenge.

II. HYPERLIPIDEMIA. Dyslipidemia is an important **correctable predictive factor for CAD.** There is a strong, independent, continuous, and graded relation between total cholesterol (TC) or low-density-lipoprotein cholesterol (LDL-C) level and risk for CAD events. This relation has been clearly demonstrated in men and women in all age groups. More than one-half of U.S. adults (105 million) have TC levels greater than 200 mg/dL, and of these, 37 million have values greater than 240 mg/dL. In general, a 1% increase in LDL-C level leads to a 2% to 3% increase in risk for CAD.

A. Physiology

1. Lipoproteins are large molecular compounds that are essential to the transport of cholesterol and triglycerides within the blood. They contain a lipid core composed of triglycerides and cholesterol esters surrounded by phospholipids

TABLE 40.1 Goals for Secondary Prevention among Patients with Known Vascular Disease

Risk factor	Goal
Hypertension (mm Hg)	140/90 (130/80 if CKD or diabetes)
Dyslipidemia (mg/dL)	LDL <100 (<70 in high-risk patients)
	HDL ≥60
	Triglycerides <100
Physical activity	30 min, three or four times per week
Body mass index	≤24.9 kg/m^2
Diabetes mellitus	Near normal blood sugar (HbA1c <6.5%)
Smoking	Complete cessation

CKD, chronic kidney disease; HbA1c, hemoglobin A1c; HDL, high-density lipoprotein; LDL, low-density lipoprotein.

and specialized proteins known as **apolipoproteins.** The **five major families of lipoproteins** are **chylomicrons, very-low-density lipoproteins (VLDLs), intermediate-density lipoproteins (IDLs), low-density lipoproteins (LDL), and high-density lipoproteins (HDLs).**

2. **Apolipoproteins** are necessary for the structure and enzymatic processes of lipids. Apolipoprotein A1 (**apo A1**) is a major component of **HDL,** and apolipoprotein B (**apo B**) is the main apolipoprotein for the remaining **non-HDL** lipoproteins.

B. Lipid-lowering trials. Aggressive lipid-lowering drug treatment of persons at various risk levels reduces CAD morbidity and mortality rates and increases overall survival. Although the association between hyperlipidemia and CAD was established much earlier, the demonstration of a relationship between reduction in serum lipid levels and a reduction in all-cause mortality had to await the development of 3-hydroxy-3-methylglutaryl coenzyme A (HMG-CoA) reductase inhibitors, or "statins." Multiple randomized trials have provided overwhelming evidence of the benefit of statins in both primary and secondary prevention of cardiovascular events.

1. **Primary prevention trials**
   a. The **West of Scotland Coronary Prevention Study (WOSCOPS) (1995)** demonstrated that treatment of men at relatively high risk with profoundly elevated cholesterol levels significantly reduced risk for heart attack and death from heart disease. The double-blind study randomized 6600 healthy men with a baseline mean LDL cholesterol level of 193 mg/dL to pravastatin (40 mg/day) or to placebo, for an average of 5 years and demonstrated a 31% relative reduction in the incidence of nonfatal MI or CAD death. Recently published data (2007) showed that the statin group continued to experience lower rates of cardiovascular death after 10 years of additional follow-up, even though only one-third continued to take statins during the additional follow-up period.
   b. The **Air Force/Texas Coronary Atherosclerosis Prevention Study (AFCAPS/TexCAPS) (1998)** demonstrated benefit among patients with more typical risk profiles, including lower cholesterol values, than those in WOSCOPS. AFCAPS/TexCAPS patients had a baseline mean TC level of 220 mg/dL. The study randomized 6600 patients to lovastatin 20 to 40 mg daily or placebo, and demonstrated a 36% relative risk reduction for first acute major coronary events in the lovastatin group.
   c. The **Heart Protection Study (HPS) (2002)** randomized 20,536 subjects in a 2 × 2 factorial design to daily simvastatin (40 mg) or placebo and to antioxidants or placebo (the antioxidant arm did not show any benefit or harm). The study focused on patients who were deemed at high risk for cardiovascular

disease but not thought to merit treatment with statins based on the prevalent clinical practice at that time. Increased risk was defined as presence of or history of CAD, cerebrovascular disease, peripheral arterial disease, diabetes mellitus, or treated hypertension. Simvastatin therapy was associated with a 13% reduction in all-cause mortality, including an 18% reduction in coronary death rate. The beneficial impact of statin therapy was seen with respect to all cardiovascular endpoints, with significant reductions in risk for nonfatal MI, incidence of first stroke, and coronary and noncoronary revascularization. **Treating patients with LDL levels less than 100 mg/dL was also associated with a beneficial reduction in vascular events.** The benefit was maintained in patients receiving other cardioprotective medications, such as angiotensin-converting enzyme (ACE) inhibitors, β-blockers, and aspirin. Although not strictly a primary prevention trial, HPS provided evidence to support treatment of risk as endorsed by the National Cholesterol Education Program's (NCEP's) guidelines. However, the HPS results refuted the threshold LDL level (as proposed by NCEP III at that time) below which statins were not previously indicated.

d. **Pravastatin in Elderly Individuals at Risk of Vascular Disease (PROSPER) (2002)** randomized 5804 patients between the age of 70 and 82 years to placebo or pravastatin. These patients had preexisting coronary, cerebral, or peripheral vascular disease, or had a history of smoking, hypertension, or diabetes. The study demonstrated a 15% reduction in the composite of coronary death, nonfatal MI, and stroke over a period of 3 years. The study demonstrated efficacy of primary and secondary prevention in the elderly.

e. The **Antihypertensive and Lipid-Lowering Treatment to Prevent Heart Attack Trial (ALLHAT-LLT) (2002)** randomized 10,355 hypertensive patients with one other coronary risk factor and a baseline mean LDL-C level of 148 mg/dL to pravastatin 20 to 40 mg/day or usual care. The study did not demonstrate a mortality difference in the two arms after a follow-up period of 4.8 years. This lack of observable difference in outcome might have resulted from the relatively modest LDL reduction (17% with pravastatin vs. 8% in usual care) or the fact that 26% of the patients in the "usual care" group were taking a statin at the end of the trial.

f. The **Anglo-Scandinavian Cardiac Outcomes Trial—Lipid-Lowering Arm (ASCOT-LLA) (2003)** randomized 10,305 patients with hypertension and at least three other cardiovascular risk factors and a baseline mean LDL-C level of 133 mg/dL to atorvastatin, 10 mg/day, or placebo. The study was stopped prematurely after a median follow-up of 3.3 years by the safety monitoring committee because of a significantly higher incidence of the primary endpoint (non-fatal MI or fatal CHD) in the placebo group. The study demonstrated a relative risk reduction (RRR) in the primary endpoint of 36% in the atorvastatin group compared to the placebo group. Further analysis demonstrated that the benefit of statin therapy started after only 1 year of treatment. There was also a significant reduction (RRR of 27%) in the incidence of fatal and nonfatal stroke in the atorvastatin group. This study, like HPS, provided further evidence of the benefit of statins in patients at high risk for cardiovascular disease without regard for baseline TC or LDL levels.

g. The **Collaborative Atorvastatin Diabetes Study (CARDS) (2004)** randomized 2838 diabetic patients with one additional cardiovascular risk factor, no history of cardiovascular disease and an average baseline LDL-C of only 117 mg/dL to atorvastatin 10 mg/day or placebo. This study was also terminated prematurely owing to an excess incidence of the primary endpoint (a composite of acute coronary events, coronary revascularization, or stroke) in the placebo group after a median follow-up of 3.9 years. Overall, the atorvastatin group had a relative risk reduction of 37% for the primary endpoint and 27% for all-cause mortality. The importance of this trial was its demonstration of the clinical benefit of statin use in diabetic patients regardless of baseline LDL-C level, making a compelling case for statin use in all diabetic patients with at least one additional cardiovascular risk factor. According to NHANES-III data, 82% of diabetic patients in the United States would meet the entry criteria for the CARDS trial.

2. **Secondary prevention trials**
   a. The **Scandinavian Simvastatin Survival Study (4S) (1994)** was the first secondary prevention trial to demonstrate a clear reduction in total mortality. Simvastatin reduced total mortality among patients with CAD by 30%, largely because of a 42% reduction in deaths from CAD. The 4S treated 4444 men and women with CAD and mean baseline LDL of 188 mg/dL, with a range of 130 to 266 mg/dL.
   b. The randomized, controlled **Cholesterol and Recurrent Events Trial (CARE) (1996)** was designed to evaluate the effects of treatment with pravastatin on 4159 persons who had experienced acute MI, 3 to 20 months before randomization and had moderately elevated TC levels (mean, 209 mg/dL). The benefits of pravastatin therapy in preventing recurrent coronary events were similar in the subset analysis of age, sex, ejection fraction, hypertension, diabetes mellitus, and smoking.
   c. The **Long-Term Intervention with Pravastatin in Ischemic Disease Study (LIPID) (1998)** was the first to examine the use of a statin for patients with a history of unstable angina. The LIPID study provided new data on noncoronary mortality (i.e., stroke) and on other groups, such as women and patients with diabetes, who previously had been underrepresented in clinical trials. LIPID demonstrated improved CAD outcomes among all patients, including those with unstable angina.
   d. **Pravastatin or Atorvastatin Evaluation and Infection Therapy—TIMI 22 (PROVE-IT—TIMI-22) (2004).** This trial was designed to determine whether intensive lipid-lowering therapy in patients with acute coronary syndrome (ACS) reduced major coronary events and mortality more than "standard" lipid lowering. A total of 4162 patients who had been hospitalized for ACS within the preceeding 10 days were randomized to atorvastatin 80 mg/day or pravastatin 40 mg/day. After 2 years of follow-up, the composite endpoint (all-cause mortality, MI, unstable angina, coronary revascularization, and stroke) was significantly reduced by 16% with atorvastatin compared with pravastatin. High-dose atorvastatin was well tolerated, with no cases of rhabdomyolysis. Of importance to note, the LDL-C level attained on atorvastatin 80 mg/day was 33 mg/dL lower than on pravastatin with a mean of 62 mg/dL. These results suggested that the use of intensive lipid-lowering therapy to achieve very low LDL-C levels was of benefit in a group of patients at high risk for recurrent coronary events.
   e. The **Treating to New Targets (TNT) (2005)** trial sought to demonstrate the benefit of intensive lipid-lowering therapy in patients with stable coronary disease. The trial randomized 10,001 patients with clinically evident CHD and baseline LDL-C levels less than 130 mg/dL to atorvastatin 80 mg/day or atorvastatin 10 mg/day. After 4.9 years of follow-up, the group receiving atorvastatin 80 mg/day had a 22% relative risk reduction in the primary composite endpoint of death from CHD, nonfatal MI, resuscitation after cardiac arrest, or fatal or nonfatal stroke compared with the group receiving atorvastatin 10 mg/day. High-dose atorvastatin was remarkably safe, with a 1.2% incidence in elevation of alanine aminotransferase (ALT)/aspartate aminotransferase (AST) greater than three times the upper limit of normal, compared with a 0.2% incidence in the atorvastatin 10 mg group. Rates of myalgias and rhabodmyolysis were similar between the two groups. This study provided compelling evidence that the use of intensive statin therapy to reduce LDL-C to levels below 100 mg/dL had marked clinical benefit in patients with stable CHD.
   f. The **Incremental Decrease in End Points Through Aggressive Lipid Lowering (IDEAL) (2005)** trial randomized 8888 patients with a prior history of acute MI to atorvastatin 80 mg/day or simvastatin 20 mg/day. After 4.8 years

of follow-up, there was a nonsignificant difference in the risk of the composite endpoint of coronary death, acute MI, or cardiac arrest. However, if either stroke or revascularization was added to the primary endpoint, the results favored the atorvastatin group, and the associated hazard ratios were similar to the results of PROVE-IT and TNT. Despite the published negative result of this trial, it provided complementary evidence for the benefit of intensive LDL lowering in patients at high risk of coronary events.

3. **Meta-analyses**
   a. **CTT Collaborators (*Lancet*, 2005).** A large meta-analysis of 90,056 individuals from 14 radomized trials of statin drugs, this analysis demonstrated an impressive 12% reduction in all-cause mortality for each 1 mmol/L (39 mg/dL) reduction in LDL. There was a 19% reduction in coronary mortality and 21% reduction in MI, coronary revascularization, and stroke. Statin use showed benefit within the first year of use, but was greater in subsequent years. Statins were also remarkably safe, with no increase in cancer seen and a 5-year excess risk of rhabdomyolysis of 0.1%.
   b. **Cannon–Intensive Statin Therapy (*J Am Coll Cardiol*, 2006).** A meta-analysis of 27,548 patients from four trials that investigated intensive versus standard lipid-lowering therapy found a significant 16% odds reduction in coronary death or MI in the group who received intensive therapy. There was a nonsignificant trend toward decreased cardiovascular mortality.

C. **Management of lipids.** Despite overwhelming evidence supporting the treatment of dyslipidemia, a large number of patients remain untreated. The NCEP Adult Treatment Panel III (ATP III) has released guidelines for treatment of hyperlipidemia in adults. These guidelines focus on identification of risk of cardiovascular morbidity and appropriate targeting of therapy. The guidelines were most recently updated in 2004.

1. **Guidelines for primary prevention of CAD events** based on the NCEP ATP III (13)
   a. **TC, LDL-C, and HDL-C levels.** All adults 20 years of age or older and **without a history of CAD or other atherosclerotic disease** should have a fasting lipid panel (i.e., TC, LDL-C, HDL-C, and triglyceride levels) every 5 years. If a nonfasting lipid panel is obtained and the TC level is 200 mg/dL or the HDL-C is less than 40 mg/dL, a follow-up fasting lipid panel is recommended (Table 40.2).

TABLE 40.2 Lipid Classification According to the National Cholesterol Education Program III

Risk factor	Goal
LDL-C	
<100	Optimal
100–129	Near or above optimal
130–159	Borderline high
160–189	High
≥190	Very high
TOTAL CHOLESTEROL	
<200	Desirable
200–239	Borderline high
≥240	High
HDL-C	
<40	Low
≥60	High

HDL-C, high-density lipoprotein cholesterol; LDL-C, low-density lipoprotein cholesterol.

b. Determination of risk. The patient's risk of future events is based on the presence of known CAD or clinical atherosclerosis in a noncoronary bed, diabetes mellitus (i.e., CAD equivalent), and other risk factors. These include age (men 45 years or older and women 55 years or older) smoking, hypertension (>140/90 mm Hg or use of antihypertensive medication), family history of premature CAD (defined as CAD in first-degree male relatives before the age of 55 years and in a first-degree female relative before the age of 65 years), and low HDL-C (<40 mg/dL). An **HDL-C level 60 mg/dL or greater is considered a negative risk factor**. Patients are classified into three categories of risk based on these factors.

(1) CHD risk. Patients with highest risk of cardiovascular events are those with established CAD or evidence of atherosclerosis in noncoronary beds (i.e., abdominal aortic aneurysms, peripheral arterial disease, or symptomatic carotid disease), **diabetes mellitus**, or presence of multiple risk factors conferring a calculated 10-year risk of more than 20%. The risk is calculated according to the Framingham risk score. The target LDL-C level for this group is less than 100 mg/dL.

(2) The second category includes patients with multiple risk factors and an estimated 10-year risk of adverse events between 10% to 20%. The target LDL-C level for this group is less than 130 mg/dL.

(3) The third category includes those with no or one risk factor and an estimated 10-year risk of less than 10%. The target LDL-C level in this group is less than 160 mg/dL.

c. Treatment of dyslipidemia. The treatment of hyperlipidemia requires two approaches: therapeutic lifestyle changes (TLCs) and medications. To achieve target LDL levels, most patients need both approaches simultaneously.

(1) OHD risk equlvalent. These patients are at the highest risk of adverse events and, therefore, benefit the most from aggressive treatment. NCEP III, whose recommendations were published in 2001, had recommended therapy with a statin and TLCs if the LDL-C level was 130 mg/dL or greater. In patients with LDL-C levels between 100 and 130 mg/dL, it suggested that the clinician use judgement as to whether to begin treatment with a statin, TLCs, or another agent such as niacin or a fibrate. **The 2004 update, however, was more definitive and recommended starting a statin and TLCs for all patients with a CHD risk equivalent with LDL-C levels 100 to 130 mg/dL.** This was based on cited evidence from HPS and further supported by CARDS and ASCOT-LLA. In patients who have a baseline LDL-C concentration of less than 100 mg/dL, the 2004 update stopped short of recommending initial use of a statin, but acknowledged that there was evidence for statin use in this group regardless of the LDL-C level. It did, however, state that initiation of a statin drug in patients with an initial LDL-C <100 mg/dL who are at "very high risk" for future CVD events, with the goal of lowering the LDL-C to <70 mg/dL, was a "reasonable therapeutic option." The cited evidence included HPS and PROVE-IT—TIMI-22. The publication of TNT provided even more evidence for intensive lipid lowering in all patients with clinically evident CHD. **Given the balance of evidence in the most recently published trials and meta-analyses, a reasonable current approach for most clinicians would be to initiate statin therapy in all patients with CHD or a CHD risk equivalent, regardless of baseline LDL-C level, with a goal LDL-C of ≤70 mg/dL for patients with CHD or at high risk of future CVD events.**

(2) Ten-year risk of 10% to 20%. These are generally patients with two or more risk factors for CVD events. The target LDL-C level for this group is less than 130 mg/dL. The 2004 ATP III update stated that an LDL-C goal <100 mg/dL is a therapeutic option, and initiation of statin therapy along with TLCs for patients with baseline LDL-C level 100 to

130 mg/dL was reasonable. This recommendation was based on evidence from HPS and ASCOT-LLA.

(3) Ten-year risk less than 10% and zero or one risk factor. These patients should be treated with TLC to achieve a target LDL-C level of less than 160 mg/dL. If the LDL-C concentration remains above 160 mg/dL after 3 months of TLCs, drug therapy may be considered. Pharmacotherapy is recommended in those with LDL-C levels higher than 190 mg/dL. Factors favoring use of drugs include a 10-year risk close to 10% or the presence of a severe risk factor such as a strong family history of premature CAD, a very low HDL level, poorly controlled hypertension, or heavy smoking.

2. Types of therapy

a. TLCs encompass **increased physical activity, ideal weight maintenance, and a diet** that includes a reduced intake of saturated fat (<7% of total calories) and cholesterol (<200 mg/day). Other TLCs are listed in Table 40.3. Intake of *trans*-fatty acids should be kept to a minimum. For most patients, it is essential to reduce saturated fat intake over total fat intake; for patients with metabolic syndrome, a fat intake of 30% to 35% may be optimal for reducing lipid and nonlipid risk factors. High carbohydrate diets may worsen the lipid abnormalities in these patients. Dietary carbohydrates should be derived predominantly from foods rich in complex carbohydrates, such as whole grains, fruits, and vegetables. Daily intake of 5 to 10 g of viscous fiber reduces LDL levels by approximately 5%, and the use of plant stanols and sterols (2 to 3 g/day) by another 6% to 15%. **TLCs can achieve an almost 30% reduction in LDL-C level in highly motivated individuals and should form the cornerstone of all preventive activity**. LDL-C should be measured 6 weeks after initiating TLC diet, and if the goals are not met, intensification of TLCs and use of plant sterols or stanols should be considered. Referral to a dietitian for education and dietary counseling is often invaluable at this stage. If, after 3 months of TLCs, adequate control is not achieved, drug therapy should be considered.

TABLE 40.3 Components of Therapeutic Lifestyle

Component	Recommendation	Approximate LDL reduction
Diet		
Saturated fat	Less than 7% of total calories	8% to 10%
Dietary cholesterol	Less than 200 mg/day	3% to 5%
Polyunsaturated fat	Up to 10% of total calories	
Monounsaturated fat	Up to 20% of total calories	
Total fat	25% to 35% of total calories	
Carbohydrate	50% to 60% of total calories	
Dietary fiber	20 to 30 g/day	
Total protein	15% of total calories	
Therapeutic options for LDL lowering		
Plant stanols/sterols	2 g/day	6% to 15%
Increased viscous soluble fiber	5 to 10 g/day (consumption of 10 to 25 g/day may have added benefit)	3% to 5%
Physical activity	Enough moderate activity to expend at least 200 kcal/day	

LDL, low-density lipoprotein.

b. **Pharmacotherapy.** The high efficacy of statins in lowering LDL-C level and their demonstrated mortality benefits make them the agents of first choice for treatment of most forms of hyperlipidemia.

(1) **HMG-CoA reductase inhibitors.** The third report of the NCEP Adult Treatment Panel included **HMG-CoA reductase inhibitors** among the first-line alternatives in the management of hypercholesterolemia. The category includes six drugs: lovastatin, simvastatin, pravastatin, fluvastatin, atorvastatin, and rosuvastatin (see Appendix for dosages).

(a) **Effectiveness.** When dietary measures are inadequate, HMG-CoA reductase inhibitors effectively **lower TC and LDL-C levels in patients with mixed hyperlipidemias** (i.e., elevated cholesterol and triglyceride levels). HMG-CoA reductase inhibitors are **extremely effective in reducing LDL-C level in most patients with primary hypercholesterolemia.** HMG-CoA reductase inhibitors decrease TC by 15% to 60% and LDL-C by 20% to 59%, and increase HDL-C levels by 5% to 15%. Declines in apo B levels commensurate with reductions in LDL have been demonstrated. Statins also reduce triglyceride levels by 10% to 25%, but have minimal effects on apo A1, apo A2, and lipoprotein (a) [Lp (a)]. **All statin drugs at the starting dose and within one to two dose titrations are well-tolerated, efficacious,** and reasonably equivalent with respect to safety profiles.

(b) **Adverse effects.** Statins are remarkably safe drugs with a low incidence of side effects. However, they are contraindicated in pregnancy.

(i) **Minor side effects.** The most common side effects are **mild gastrointestinal disturbances** (e.g., nausea, abdominal pain, diarrhea, constipation, and flatulence). Headache, fatigue, pruritus, and myalgias are other minor side effects, but none of these complaints usually warrant discontinuation of therapy.

(ii) **Liver function test abnormalltles.** Mild, transient elevations in liver enzymes have been reported with all HMG-CoA reductase inhibitors. Marked elevation of transaminases is rare, but clinicians should avoid or use caution before starting statins in patients with acute or chronic liver disease. In HPS, only 0.5% of patients had to stop treatment because of elevated ALT levels. Even when taking the highest dose of atorvastatin (80 mg), patients in PROVE-IT and TNT had only a 3.3% and 1.1% incidence, respectively, of transaminase elevation more than three times above the upper limit of normal. In general, for each doubling of a statin dose, there is a 0.6% increase in risk for elevation of transaminase levels. **Current recommendations state that therapy should be discontinued when greater than threefold elevation occurs.** Enzyme levels typically return to normal within 2 weeks. Lower doses of the same medication can be reinstituted, or a different statin can be tried. **Monitoring of hepatic aminotransferase levels is recommended for those taking HMG-CoA reductase inhibitors, but the frequency of monitoring has been debated.** Current package inserts for most statins recommend obtaining a liver panel prior to initiation of statin therapy, prior to dose titration, and when "clinically indicated." More frequent monitoring is recommended for patients taking the highest dose of a statin. In recent clinical trials, the high-dose statin that appears to have the highest incidence of transaminase elevation is atorvastatin. A panel of hepatologists who examined the potential hepatotoxicity of statins made a recommendation to obtain a liver panel prior to initiating statins as a baseline measurement of hepatic transaminases and bilirubin. If the baseline measurements were within normal limits, the panel recommended follow-up measurement of transmainases, only if there was symptomatic or physical evidence of liver disease. An ACC/AHA/NHLBI clinical advisory panel on the safety and use of statins recommends measurement of transaminases at baseline, 12-weeks after starting therapy, then annually or more frequently if indicated.

(iii) Myopathy, a rare but potentially serious side effect of HMG-CoA reductase inhibitors, presents with muscle pain, stiffness, or aching, and elevations in serum creatine kinase (CK) level to more than 10 times the upper limit of normal. **CK measurements are not needed unless symptoms occur.** Statin-naïve patients should be warned to report symptoms of muscle pain or stiffness immediately if they occur after starting the drug. The risk of myopathy may be increased in the elderly, those with a low body mass index, those with multisystem disease such as chronic renal failure, in the perioperative period, and in those on multiple medications. Simvastatin 80 mg has been associated with a slightly higher incidence of myopathy and rhabdomyolysis compared with other statins, especially when combined with gemfibrozil. This could be due to the decreased rate of plasma clearance of simvastatin in older versus younger patients. Death from statin-induced rhabdomyolysis is exceedingly rare, with an incidence of 1.5 deaths per 10 million prescriptions. Statin-associated myalgias (muscle symptoms without elevations in serum CK) occur with somewhat higher frequency, about 1.4% to 1.5% in published clinical trials, and can appear at any time during statin therapy, even years after initiation of treatment. Muscle symptoms usually resolve with discontinuation of the statin. There is recent evidence that statin inhibition of mitochondrial coenzyme Q10 may be responsible for statin-induced myalgias, and there is evidence from small clinical trials that oral coenzyme Q10 supplementation may decrease symptoms of statin associated myalgias.

(iv) Drug interactions. When statins are used in combination with certain pharmaceutical agents, such as erythromycin, gemfibrozil, azole antifungals, cimetidine, methotrexate, or cyclosporine, the risks for CK elevation and myositis increase. These drug combinations should be avoided or used judiciously with interval measurements of CK levels and liver function. Pravastatin and fluvastatin are safer in combination with other drugs because these two drugs do not use the cytochrome P450 3A4 microsomal pathways for metabolism. Verapamil and amiodarone are two commonly used cardiovascular agents that inhibit this pathway, and the concurrent use of simvastatin, atorvastatin, or lovastatin may, therefore, predispose to an increased risk of myositis.

(2) Bile acid sequestrants lower LDL-C level by interfering with reabsorption of bile acids in the distal ileum, reducing the amount returned to the liver. They are safe and free of systemic side effects because they are not systemically absorbed; however, gastrointestinal side effects such as constipation are common, and compliance is poor as a result. The average LDL level decrease is approximately 20% to 22%, with a small rise seen in HDL level. Triglycerides show no change or may rise; therefore, these agents should be avoided in patients with elevated triglycerides. Two small angiographic trials, the NHLBI Type II Interventional Study and the St. Thomas Atherosclerosis Regression Study (STARS) have demonstrated reduced progression of CAD on serial angiograms in men with hypercholesterolemia who were taking cholestyramine. These agents may be of particular benefit in patients with minor elevation in LDL-C, for young patients, for women considering pregnancy, and in combination with a statin in those with very high LDL-C levels. In a pregnant patient, additional supplementation of iron and folate may be necessary because resins used over the long term can interfere with their absorption.

(3) **Nicotinic acid or niacin.** Niacin affects all lipid parameters favorably (i.e., LDL reduction of 5% to 25%, triglyceride reduction of 20% to 25%, HDL elevation of 15% to 30%). It is one of the only agents that reduces Lp(a) significantly (up to 30%). Unfortunately, compliance is poor because of frequent side effects. Flushing and pruritus, gastrointestinal discomfort, glucose intolerance, and hyperuricemia often accompany use of niacin. Hepatotoxicity is rare but is more commonly seen with the sustained-released preparation. It is often heralded by a dramatic reduction in lipid levels. There are limited data on long-term therapy with this agent. Niacin may be particularly useful for patients who do not have substantial elevations in their LDL-C levels, and low doses may be used to treat diabetic dyslipidemia. High doses should be avoided in diabetics, and the drug should be avoided in those with a history of gout, peptic ulcer disease, or active hepatic disease.

(4) **Fibrates** are **effective at lowering triglyceride levels** by 20% to 50% and raising HDL levels by 10% to 35%. The mechanism of action involves activation of the nuclear transcription factor peroxisome proliferator-activated receptor α (PPAR-α), with resultant increases in hepatic synthesis of apolipoproteins A-1 and A-2 (raising HDL) and increase in lipoprotein lipase-mediated lipolysis, thus lowering triglyceride levels. LDL level reduction varies with the agent used and may range from 5% to 20% in patients who are not hypertriglyceridemic. Fenofibrate appears to lower LDL more effectively than gemfibrozil. Although a higher mortality rate was seen in the clofibrate arm of the World Health Organization (WHO) clofibrate study, such a finding was not seen in subsequent studies of gemfibrozil or fenofibrate. These agents have been demonstrated to impart a reduction in risk of CAD events and are of use in patients with elevated triglycerides. VA-HIT (1999) found a reduction in fatal and nonfatal MI with gemfibrozil use in men with CAD who had low HDL levels (mean of 32 mg/dL), but the FIELD trial (2005) did not find a significant reduction in the primary endpoint of CAD death or MI in diabetic patients. Although fibrates are often used in combination with statin therapy to treat mixed dyslipidemia, there are no studies demonstrating reduction in clinical events with this approach. This combination increases the risk of myopathy. For patients with very high TG levels (>1000 mg/dL), fibrate therapy reduces the risk of pancreatitis.

(5) **Cholesterol absorption inhibitors** such as ezetimibe inhibit cholesterol absorption by the enterocyte. Ezetimibe reduces cholesterol absorption from the small bowel by 23% to 50% and reduces serum LDL level by 14% to 20% when used in combination with a statin. Reduction in clinical endpoints or surrogate endpoints has not been demonstrated for this group of drugs. The ENHANCE study failed to demonstrate any additional benefit of the use of ezetimibe added to statin over statin alone in slowing progression of carotid intimal thickness in a cohort of patients with famililial hyperlipidemia. However, a number of large-scale studies are currently in progress seeking to determine the utility of a statin ezetimibe combination on hard cardiovascular endpoints. The combination of a statin and ezetimibe is generally a well-tolerated and efficacious regimen.

(a) **Choice of an agent and combination therapy.** The use of statin therapy for treatment of hyperlipidemia should be guided by the expected change in LDL-C levels (Table 40.4). Most statins have a log-linear dose-response pattern, with each doubling of dose associated with a further 7% reduction in LDL-C levels. Adverse effects of statins are also dose dependent and rise with the use of higher doses.

(i) **HMG-CoA reductase inhibitors and bile acid resins.** In isolated forms of LDL elevation, this combination exhibits highly

TABLE 40.4 Average Reduction in LDL-C Associated with the Starting Dose of Statin Agents

Agent	Average LDL-C reduction
Lovastatin (20 mg)	24%
Pravastatin (20 mg)	24%
Simvastatin (20 mg)	35%
Fluvastatin (20 mg)	18%
Atorvastatin (10 mg)	37%
Rosuvastatin (10 mg)	47%

LDL-C, low-density lipoprotein cholesterol.

complementary mechanisms of action. The combination of a statin with a bile acid sequestrant is ideal, owing to the lack of potentiation of side effects. The sequestrant provides little added toxicity, and the LDL-C lowering needed may not necessitate a full sequestrant dosage. Unfortunately, patient compliance with the combination is poor because of the common side effects of resins. Although the combination may reduce **LDL level by as much as 70% in some patients**, there appears to be a ceiling effect, with no LDL lowering occurring beyond the original level with an increase in dose of either agent.

(ii) **Combining a statin with niacin** is attractive because it can favorably influence all lipid subfractions. The side effects of the combination are increased but not synergistic, and the risk of myopathy may be lower than previously believed. The main serious side effect of the combination is hepatotoxicity, which may be reduced by using extended-release niacin. In small studies using this combination, the risk of hepatotoxicity (i.e., persistent elevation of aspartate aminotransferase or ALT of more than three times the upper limit of normal) at niacin doses of 2 g/day was about 1%.

(iii) The combination of a statin plus fibrate is highly effective for treating mixed hyperlipidemias. Although theoretically appealing, no reduction in clinical events has been demonstrated with this approach. The combination is associated with an increased risk of myopathy. Although earlier work suggested a higher incidence, later studies suggest this complication may be seen in approximately 1% of patients with the currently used agents.

(iv) The combination of a statin plus ezetimibe has been studied in small studies and has proved to be highly safe and effective at lowering LDL-C levels. Given the small number of patients treated and short follow-up periods, it is suggested that this combination should be reserved for the patients who fail maximal statin doses or are intolerant of statins.

3. Therapy of specific lipid disorders

a. Very high LDL levels usually result from inherited disorders of lipoprotein metabolism and carry a high risk of premature atherosclerosis with its attendant morbidity and mortality. **Hypothyroidism** may be associated with markedly elevated LDL levels and should be ruled out in any patient presenting with elevated LDL level. Most of these patients respond to high-dose statin therapy in addition to dietary restrictions. The addition of a bile acid sequestrant with an additional third agent (i.e., niacin) often is warranted to achieve target levels. Ezetimibe is another agent that may prove useful in this group. Therapy should be initiated early, and family members should be screened for hyperlipidemia. Patients with homozygous familial hyperlipidemia are deficient in LDL receptors, and measures that reduce cholesterol absorption (e.g., diet, ileal exclusion, bile acid sequestrants, ezetimibe) or act by LDL receptor upregulation (e.g., statins) are largely ineffective. These patients are treated with LDL apheresis and should be managed in tertiary care centers only.

b. Elevated TG levels may be caused by many factors, and more than one cause may be active in a given patient. **Minor elevations in triglyceride levels (150 to 299 mg/dL)** usually are caused by obesity, sedentary lifestyle, smoking, excess alcohol intake, and high carbohydrate diets. In other patients, secondary causes such as diabetes, renal failure, Cushing's disease, nephrotic syndrome, or medications (e.g., protease inhibitors, corticosteroids, retinoids, oral estrogens) may be responsible. Genetic causes may be pertinent to others. The therapy for this group of patients involves identification and treatment of secondary causes (if present), change in medications, and lifestyle changes. These patients benefit from total caloric restriction and switching from a very high carbohydrate diet to a more balanced diet. Very high **triglyceride levels (≥500 mg/dL**) usually result from genetic defects of lipoprotein metabolism; in some patients, there is a combination of factors at play. These patients are at risk for acute pancreatitis (especially with triglyceride levels >1000 mg/dL), and treatment is directed to prevention of this condition. This is achieved with a combination of dietary measures [using very low fat diets (<15% calories from fat), and substituting medium-chain fatty acids in patients with triglyceride levels >1000 mg/dL], increasing physical activity, maintaining optimal weight, and initiating fibrates or niacin therapy. Fibrates are especially efficacious in this group. Statins are not especially effective agents for triglyceride reduction and should be considered only after the other two agents. Patients with an **intermediate rise in triglyceride levels (200 to 499 mg/dL)** are a more heterogenous group with a wide array of underlying pathogenetic mechanisms at play. This pattern often is a result of an intersection of poor lifestyle, secondary causes, and genetic factors. These patients often have other markers of increased atherogenic risk, such as increased small LDL, low HDL, or elevated VLDL remnants. They need to be treated aggressively to bring the LDL level to the target; statins, with their ability to lower non-HDL cholesterol, are the preferred agents. **After the LDL target has been achieved, the secondary goal is non–HDL-C (goal of 30 mg/dL higher than target LDL-C).** These patients also need aggressive TLCs. High-dose statins often suffice to achieve the LDL-C and non–HDL-C goals, but for most patients, a second agent becomes necessary. The choices are niacin or fibrates in addition to a statin; these combinations carry an increased risk for hepatotoxicity or myopathy, and careful monitoring for these is essential. Refractory cases may benefit from fish oil supplements (>3 g/day) which, by reducing VLDL production, can lower the serum triglyceride concentration by as much as 50% or more; however, many currently available over-the-counter fish oil supplements contain less than 50% active omega-3 fatty acids. The commercial preparation Omacor, which has been available for many years in Europe and is now also available in the United States, contains 90% omega-3 fatty acids. The U.S. food and Drug Administration (FDA) limited approval for Omacor to the treatment of severe hypertriglyceridemia (≥500 mg/dL) because of concerns that it appears to increase LDL-C levels. Weight loss by obese patients should be encouraged; it is associated with an improvement in the lipid profile and facilitates pharmacologic therapy if still necessary.

c. Low HDL cholesterol levels often accompany minor or modest elevations in triglyceride levels. Low HDL level has been shown in epidemiologic studies to be an independent risk factor for cardiovascular disease. However, despite a multitude of research on currently available therapies to raise HDL and recent investigation of several newer agents that raise HDL, there has been no conclusive evidence that raising serum HDL-C levels contributes to lower rates of CVD. Current guidelines specify that raising HDL should be a tertiary goal, after LDL and non–HDL-C goals have been reached. In patients who have isolated low HDL levels without any elevation in TG levels, the first goal is to identify and modify lifestyle factors (e.g., high carbohydrate diet, sedentary lifestyle, obesity, smoking) and medications (e.g., progestational agents, anabolic steroids). The next step encompasses calculation of 10-year risk and treating LDL-C with a statin when appropriate. The AFCAPS/TexCAPS study found a clear benefit for statin therapy in patients with low HDL-C levels. In patients who continue to have low HDL-C levels despite lifestyle modifications and who are at goal for LDL and triglycerides, either niacin or fibrate therapy is a reasonable choice to raise HDL-C.

d. Diabetic dyslipidemia. Patients with diabetes are at an increased risk for cardiovascular events and fare poorly after CAD manifests. Diabetes is associated with an increase in small LDL particles and often is associated with high triglyceride and low HDL levels. Hyperglycemia is an independent risk factor for CAD. Primary prevention is important in this group and was demonstrated to be efficacious in the HPS trial. **All diabetic patients (irrespective of LDL-C level) should be considered for statin therapy and TLCs.** Secondary goals include improved non–HDL-C levels and treatment for elevated triglyceride levels. Blood sugar control and insulin therapy often facilitate the former, but fibrates or low-dose niacin may be necessary in some patients. Patients with diabetes also often have coexisting hypertension. Blood pressure control and smoking cessation are essential because both interventions are highly effective at reducing cardiovascular events in this population.

ACKNOWLEDGMENTS

The author acknowledges the contributions of Drs. Hintinder S. Gurm and JoAnne Micale Foody to previous editions of this manuscript.

Suggested Readings

Baigent C, Keech A, Kearney PM, et al. Efficacy and safety of cholesterol-lowering treatment: prospective meta-analysis of data from 90,056 participants in 14 randomised trials of statins. *Lancet* 2005;366:1267–1278.

Cannon CP, Braunwald E, McCabe CH, et al. Intensive versus moderate lipid lowering with statins after acute coronary syndromes. *N Engl J Med* 2004;350:1495–1504.

Cannon CP, Steinberg BA, Murphy SA, et al. Meta-analysis of cardiovascular outcomes trials comparing intensive versus moderate statin therapy. *J Am Coll Cardiol* 2006;48:438–445.

Cohen DE, Anania FA, Chalasanin. An assessment of statin safety by hepatologists. *Am J Cardiol* 2006;97:77C–81C.

Colhoun HM, Betteridge DJ, Durrington PN, et al. Primary prevention of cardiovascular disease with atorvastatin in type 2 diabetes in the Collaborative Atorvastatin Diabetes Study (CARDS): multicentre randomised placebo-controlled trial. *Lancet* 2004;364:685–696.

Davidson MH, Robinson JG. Safety of aggressive lipid management. *J Am Coll Cardiol* 2007;49:1753–1762.

Executive Summary of The Third Report of The National Cholesterol Education Program (NCEP) Expert Panel on Detection, Evaluation, And Treatment of High Blood Cholesterol In Adults (Adult Treatment Panel III). *JAMA* 2001;285:2486–2497.

Fletcher GF, Bufalino V, Costa F, et al. Efficacy of drug therapy in the secondary prevention of cardiovascular disease and stroke. *Am J Cardiol* 2007;99:1E–35E.

Ford I, Murray H, Packard CJ, et al. Long-term follow-up of the West of Scotland Coronary Prevention Study. *N Engl J Med* 2007;357:1477–1486.

Graham DJ, Staffa JA, Shatin D, et al. Incidence of hospitalized rhabdomyolysis in patients treated with lipid-lowering drugs. *JAMA* 2004;292:2585–2590.

Grundy SM, Cleeman JI, Merz CN, et al. Implications of recent clinical trials for the National Cholesterol Education Program Adult Treatment Panel III guidelines. *Circulation* 2004;110:227–239.

Keech A, Simes RJ, Barter P, et al. Effects of long-term fenofibrate therapy on cardiovascular events in 9795 people with type 2 diabetes mellitus (the FIELD study): randomised controlled trial. *Lancet* 2005;366:1849–1861.

Knopp RH, Gitter H, Truitt T, et al. Effects of ezetimibe, a new cholesterol absorption inhibitor, on plasma lipids in patients with primary hypercholesterolemia. *Eur Heart J* 2003;24:729–741.

LaRosa JC, Grundy SM, Waters DD, et al. Intensive lipid lowering with atorvastatin in patients with stable coronary disease. *N Engl J Med* 2005;352:1425–1435.

Major outcomes in moderately hypercholesterolemic, hypertensive patients randomized to pravastatin vs usual care: The Antihypertensive and Lipid-Lowering Treatment to Prevent Heart Attack Trial (ALLHAT-LLT). *JAMA* 2002;288:2998–3007.

Marcoff L, Thompson PD. The role of coenzyme Q10 in statin-associated myopathy: a systematic review. *J Am Coll Cardiol* 2007;49:2231–2237.
McKenney J. New perspectives on the use of niacin in the treatment of lipid disorders. *Arch Intern Med* 2004;164:697–705.
MRC/BHF Heart Protection Study of cholesterol lowering with simvastatin in 20,536 high-risk individuals: a randomised placebo-controlled trial. *Lancet* 2002;360:7–22.
Pasternak RC, Smith SC Jr, Bairey-Merz CN, et al. ACC/AHA/NHLBI Clinical Advisory on the Use and Safety of Statins. *Stroke* 2002;33:2337–2341.
Pedersen TR, Faergeman O, Kastelein JJ, et al. High-dose atorvastatin vs usual-dose simvastatin for secondary prevention after myocardial infarction: the IDEAL study: a randomized controlled trial. *JAMA* 2005;294:2437–2445.
Prevention of cardiovascular events and death with pravastatin in patients with coronary heart disease and a broad range of initial cholesterol levels. The Long-Term Intervention with Pravastatin in Ischaemic Disease (LIPID) Study Group. *N Engl J Med* 1998;339:1349–1357.
Sever PS, Dahlof B, Poulter NR, et al. Prevention of coronary and stroke events with atorvastatin in hypertensive patients who have average or lower-than-average cholesterol concentrations, in the Anglo-Scandinavian Cardiac Outcomes Trial–Lipid Lowering Arm (ASCOT-LLA): a multicentre randomised controlled trial. *Lancet* 2003;361:1149–1158.
Shepherd J, Blauw GJ, Murphy MB, et al. Pravastatin in elderly individuals at risk of vascular disease (PROSPER): a randomised controlled trial. *Lancet* 2002;360:1623–1630.
Thompson PD, Clarkson PM, Rosenson RS. An assessment of statin safety by muscle experts. *Am J Cardiol* 2006;97: 69C–76C.

Landmark Articles

A co-operative trial in the primary prevention of ischaemic heart disease using clofibrate. Report from the Committee of Principal Investigators. *Br Heart J* 1978;40:1069–1118.
Brensike JF, Levy RI, Kelsey SF, et al. Effects of therapy with cholestyramine on progression of coronary arteriosclerosis: results of the NHLBI Type II Coronary Intervention Study. *Circulation* 1984;69:313–324.
Brown G, Albers JJ, Fisher LD, et al. Regression of coronary artery disease as a result of intensive lipid-lowering therapy in men with high levels of apolipoprotein B. *N Engl J Med* 1990;323:1289–1298.
Chen Z, Peto R, Collins R, et al. Serum cholesterol concentration and coronary heart disease in population with low cholesterol concentrations. *BMJ* 1991;303:276–282.
Downs JR, Clearfield M, Weis S, et al. Primary prevention of acute coronary events with lovastatin in men and women with average cholesterol levels: results of AFCAPS/TexCAPS. Air Force/Texas Coronary Atherosclerosis Prevention Study. *JAMA* 1998;279:1615–1622.
Harris WS, Connor WE, Illingworth DR, et al. Effects of fish oil on VLDL triglyceride kinetics in humans. *J Lipid Res* 1990;31:1549–1558.
Randomised trial of cholesterol lowering in 4444 patients with coronary heart disease: the Scandinavian Simvastatin Survival Study (4S). *Lancet* 1994;344:1383–1389.
Rubins HB, Robins SJ, Collins D, et al. Gemfibrozil for the secondary prevention of coronary heart disease in men with low levels of high-density lipoprotein cholesterol. Veterans Affairs High-Density Lipoprotein Cholesterol Intervention Trial Study Group. *N Engl J Med* 1999;341:410–418.
Sacks FM, Pfeffer MA, Moye LA, et al. The effect of pravastatin on coronary events after myocardial infarction in patients with average cholesterol levels. Cholesterol and Recurrent Events Trial investigators. *N Engl J Med* 1996;335:1001–1009.
Shepherd J, Cobbe SM, Ford I, et al. Prevention of coronary heart disease with pravastatin in men with hypercholesterolemia. West of Scotland Coronary Prevention Study Group. *N Engl J Med* 1995;333:1301–1307.
Stamler J, Wentworth D, Neaton JD. Is relationship between serum cholesterol and risk of premature death from coronary heart disease continuous and graded? Findings in 356,222 primary screenees of the Multiple Risk Factor Intervention Trial (MRFIT). *JAMA* 1986;256:2823–2828.
Watts GF, Lewis B, Brunt JN, et al. Effects on coronary artery disease of lipid-lowering diet, or diet plus cholestyramine, in the St Thomas' Atherosclerosis Regression Study (STARS). *Lancet* 1992;339:563–569.

Useful Internet Resources

1. NHLBI Guidelines based on NCEP/ATPIII: http://www.nhlbi.nih.gov/guidelines/cholesterol/atglance.htm
2. Framingham 10-year risk calculator: http://hp2010.nhlbihin.net/atpiii/calculator.asp?usertype=pub
3. NHLBI National Cholesterol Education Program: http://www.nhlbi.nih.gov/about/ncep/
4. Comprehensive Lipid News, Education and Discussion from Baylor: http://www.lipidsonline.org/

41 NONLIPID CARDIOVASCULAR RISK FACTORS

Adam W. Grasso

I. INTRODUCTION. Dyslipidemia constitutes a strong and well-described risk factor for the development of coronary artery disease (CAD). Nevertheless, almost one-half of myocardial infarctions (MIs) in the United States occur in individuals without overt lipid abnormalities (1). Additional risk factors must, therefore, be addressed to maximize preventive measures aimed at reducing the incidence of cardiovascular events. This chapter describes these additional cardiovascular risk factors, with special emphasis on prevalence, causes, evaluation, and treatment.

II. HYPERTENSION. Hypertension (HTN) contributes to the development of MI, stroke or cerebrovascular accident (CVA), systolic and diastolic heart failure, peripheral vascular disease (PVD), and increased total mortality among men and women of all ages and ethnic groups, with or without signs or symptoms of CAD. HTN, defined as a systolic blood pressure of ≥140 mm Hg or greater, **or** diastolic blood pressure of ≥90 mm Hg or greater, **or** the need for antihypertensive medication, is thought to be present in at least 25% of the U.S. adult population. This number probably underestimates the true prevalence, because an analysis of the Framingham Heart Study indicated that normotensive 55 year-old persons have a 90% residual lifetime risk of developing HTN.

A. Etiology. HTN is a complex disease modified by environmental and genetic determinants.

1. **In most cases, HTN does not follow classic Mendelian rules of inheritance** attributable to a single gene locus. The documented exceptions are a few rare forms, such as those related to a single mutation involving a chimeric 11-β-hydroxylase–aldosterone synthase gene, Liddle syndrome, and variants in the angiotensinogen locus, which cause primary HTN among white persons. Other potential candidate genes suggested by experimental data include those that affect various components of the renin–angiotensin–aldosterone system, the kallikrein–kinin system, and the sympathetic nervous system. Increased left ventricular (LV) mass, LV wall thickness, and altered peripheral vascular capacity and responsiveness occur more frequently among patients with a family history of HTN.
2. Potential contributors to HTN include variations in sodium intake, the renin–angiotensin system, renal function and natriuresis, the sympathetic nervous system, vascular function, cell membranes, hyperinsulinemia and insulin resistance, atrial natriuretic factor, and prostaglandins.

B. Pathophysiology

1. The **positive relationship between systolic and diastolic blood pressure and cardiovascular risk** has long been recognized. This relationship is strong, continuous, graded, consistent, independent, predictive, and etiologically significant for those with and without CAD.
   a. The **Multiple Risk Factor Intervention Trial (MRFIT)** (2), a prospective study (11.6 years average follow-up period) with more than 361,000 subjects, has provided the most data regarding the relationship between blood pressure and CAD. Baseline blood pressure was shown to be strongly and independently related to increased risk for CAD. The relationship was shown to be stronger for systolic than for diastolic blood pressure or pulse pressure, with the **risk for CAD progressively rising with increased systolic blood pressure.** The death rate for men with systolic blood pressures of 140 to 149 mm Hg (2.4 per

1000) and 150 to 159 mm Hg (3.1 per 1000) was 40% higher than the death rate for men with a baseline systolic blood pressure less than 120 mm Hg.

b. Data analysis has shown that the death rate in the follow-up period can be lowered 36% by means of primary prevention of HTN in the general population. A reduction in rates of stroke and CAD with antihypertensive therapy has been demonstrated even in the presence of isolated systolic HTN.

c. Subjects with systolic blood pressure less than <120 mm Hg **and** diastolic blood pressure less than <80 mm Hg (<120/<80 mm Hg) have the fewest cardiovascular events (2), and are said to have **normal blood pressure**. The guidelines recommend 140/90 mm Hg as the treatment cutoff point. There is, however, increasing evidence that blood pressure previously considered to be within the high-normal range (120 to 139 mm Hg systolic or 80 to 89 mm Hg diastolic) does confer some increased risk of cardiovascular disease, and is now referred to as **prehypertension**. Risk ratios of 2.5 for women and 1.6 for men have been reported. Patients with blood pressure in the prehypertensive range should undertake lifestyle modifications (e.g., diet, exercise, and weight loss) to help prevent the development of frank HTN in the future.

d. The gradual rise in blood pressure over a person's lifetime and the increased prevalence of **HTN among the elderly** are not benign occurrences, and should not to be viewed as normal, inevitable consequences of aging. In some epidemiologic studies involving elderly persons, the relationship between blood pressure and mortality appeared to be a U-shaped curve. After adjustment for confounding variables and exclusion of deaths within the first 3 years of the follow-up period, however, positive linear relationships between blood pressure and cardiovascular disease mortality, as well as between blood pressure and all-cause mortality, were demonstrated. Persons with isolated systolic HTN, the prevalence of which increases as the population ages, are at increased risk for morbidity and mortality related to cardiovascular disease.

(1) Data from the **Systolic Hypertension in the Elderly Program (SHEP)** (3) show that 8% of persons 60 to 69 years old have isolated systolic HTN, defined as systolic blood pressure greater than 160 mm Hg and diastolic blood pressure less than 90 mm Hg, as do 11% of those 70 to 79 years old and 22% of those 80 years or older.

(2) The relationship of systolic blood pressure and diastolic blood pressure to cardiovascular events is more pronounced among persons 65 years and older. The association is stronger and more consistent for systolic blood pressure than for diastolic blood pressure and is evident at levels considerably less than 140 mm Hg.

2. Elevations in diastolic or systolic values translate into significant increases in cardiovascular events. Generally, the yearly percent risk of cardiovascular events (i.e., risk of event by end of study, divided by duration of study) is between 0.5% and 2.5% at 40 years of age or older for hypertensive subjects. Beginning at 115/75 mm Hg, each increase in blood pressure of 20/10 mm Hg doubles the risk of cardiovascular disease.

3. Over the last few years, **greater emphasis has been placed on systolic pressure in characterizing cardiovascular risk.** The age-adjusted 10-year mortality in the MRFIT trial (2) revealed systolic blood pressure to be a stronger predictor of events from CAD than did diastolic blood pressure. High systolic blood pressure conferred a CAD risk regardless of diastolic blood pressure. A systolic blood pressure of 140 to 149 mm Hg confers greater CAD mortality risk than a diastolic blood pressure of 90 to 94 mm Hg. A systolic blood pressure of 150 to 159 mm Hg carries greater risk than a diastolic blood pressure of 95 to 100 mm Hg. According to the SHEP study (3), isolated systolic HTN, which accounts for 60% of cases of HTN among the elderly, is highly correlated with cardiovascular disease and is important to control.

C. Clinical presentation. Detection of HTN begins with proper **blood pressure measurements,** which should be obtained at each health care encounter.

1. Data for evaluation are acquired through the medical history, physical examination, laboratory tests, and other diagnostic procedures. Evaluation of patients with documented HTN has the following three objectives:
   a. To identify known causes of high blood pressure
   b. To assess the presence or absence of end-organ damage and cardiovascular disease, the extent of the disease, and response to therapy
   c. To identify other cardiovascular risk factors or concomitant disorders that may define prognosis and guide treatment
2. A **medical history** should focus on identifying important risk factors or symptoms of HTN.
3. Repeated **blood pressure measurements** determine whether initial elevations persist and necessitate prompt attention, or the blood pressure has returned to normal and the patient needs only periodic surveillance. Ambulatory blood pressure monitoring is clinically helpful and is most commonly used to evaluate patients with suspected "office" or "white-coat HTN." It is also helpful in the care of patients with apparent drug resistance, hypotensive symptoms with antihypertensive medications, episodic HTN, and autonomic dysfunction.
   a. **Office visits.** Clinicians should explain to patients the meaning of their blood pressure readings and advise them of the **need for periodic remeasurement.** Blood pressure is measured in a standardized manner with equipment that meets certification criteria.
      (1) The patient sits in a chair with her or his back supported and the arms bared and supported at heart level.
      (2) Patients should refrain from smoking or ingesting caffeine during the 30 minutes preceding the measurement.
      (3) Measurement should begin after at least 5 minutes of rest.
      (4) The appropriate cuff size must be used to ensure accurate measurement. The bladder within the cuff should encircle at least 80% of the arm. Many adults need a large adult cuff.
      (5) Measurements are taken preferably with a mercury sphygmomanometer; otherwise, a recently calibrated aneroid manometer or a validated electronic device can be used.
      (6) The systolic blood pressure and diastolic blood pressure are recorded. The first appearance of sound (phase 1) is used to define systolic blood pressure. The disappearance of sound (phase 5) is used to define diastolic blood pressure.
      (7) Two or more readings separated by 2 minutes should be averaged. If the first two readings differ by more than 5 mm Hg, additional readings should be obtained and averaged.
   b. **Ambulatory blood pressure monitoring.** A variety of commercially available monitors that are reliable, convenient, easy to use, and accurate are available. These monitors typically are programmed to take readings every 15 to 30 minutes throughout the day and night while patients go about their normal daily activities. The readings can be downloaded for computer analysis.
      (1) **Normal** ambulatory blood pressure values are **lower than clinical readings while patients are awake** (<135/<85 mm Hg) and are **even lower while patients are asleep** (<120/<75 mm Hg). The blood pressure of most persons falls by 10% to 20% during the night. This change is more closely related to patterns of sleep and wakefulness than to time of day, as illustrated by the blood pressure rhythm that follows the inverted cycle of activity of night-shift workers.
      (2) **Patients with HTN.** An extensive and consistent body of evidence indicates that **ambulatory blood pressure correlates more closely than clinical blood pressure with a variety of measures of end-organ damage,** such as left ventricular hypertrophy (LVH). Prospective data relating ambulatory blood pressure to prognosis are limited to two published studies, which suggest that among patients for whom an elevated clinic pressure is

the only abnormality, ambulatory monitoring may help identify a group at relatively low risk for morbidity.

4. **Physical examination** should include the following components:
   a. **Funduscopic examination** for hypertensive retinopathy (e.g., arteriolar narrowing, focal arteriolar constrictions, arteriovenous crossing changes, hemorrhages and exudates, and disk edema)
   b. Examination of the **neck** for carotid bruits, distended veins, or an enlarged thyroid gland
   c. Examination of the **heart** for abnormalities in rate and rhythm, increased size, precordial heave, clicks, murmurs, and S_3 and S_4
   d. Examination of the **lungs** for rales and evidence of bronchospasm
   e. Examination of the **abdomen** for bruits, enlarged kidneys, masses, and abnormal aortic pulsation. Abdominal bruits, particularly those that lateralize to the renal area or have a diastolic component, suggest renovascular disease. Abdominal or flank masses may be polycystic kidneys.
   f. Examination of the **extremities** for diminished or absent peripheral arterial pulsations, bruits, and edema. Delayed or absent femoral arterial pulses and decreased blood pressure in the lower extremities may indicate aortic coarctation.
   g. **Neurologic assessment**
   h. **Other assessments.** Labile HTN or paroxysms of HTN accompanied by any or all of the following symptoms and signs—chest discomfort ("**p**ressure"), headache ("**p**ain"), **p**alpitations, **p**allor, and diaphoresis ("**p**erspiration")—may indicate the presence of a pheochromocytoma. Truncal obesity with purple striae suggest Cushing's syndrome.

D. **Laboratory evaluation**
   1. It is recommended that the clinician request routine laboratory tests before initiating therapy to determine the presence of end-organ damage and other risk factors. These routine tests include **urinalysis, complete blood cell count, blood chemistry, and 12-lead electrocardiogram (ECG).**
   2. Additional diagnostic procedures may be indicated to seek causes of HTN, particularly for patients whose age, history, physical examination findings, severity of HTN, or initial laboratory findings suggest such causes; those whose blood pressures are responding poorly to drug therapy; those with well-controlled HTN whose blood pressures begin to increase; and those with sudden onset of HTN. **Optional tests** include creatinine clearance; microalbuminuria, 24-hour urinary protein, blood calcium, uric acid, fasting triglyceride (TG), low-density-lipoprotein cholesterol (LDL-C), glycosylated hemoglobin, and thyroid-stimulating hormone levels; and limited echocardiography to determine the presence of LVH.
      a. Examples of **clues from laboratory tests** include unprovoked hypokalemia (i.e., primary aldosteronism), hypercalcemia (i.e., hyperparathyroidism), and elevated creatinine or abnormal urinalysis (i.e., renal parenchymal disease).
      b. The **presence of LVH** as determined by ECG or echocardiography is an important risk factor for adverse cardiovascular events and an independent predictor of high risk for CAD, cardiovascular disease, and all-cause mortality. LVH, the consequence of chronic pressure or volume overload and obesity, seems to be a stronger predictor of MI and CAD death than the degree of HTN. LV mass, as assessed with echocardiography, is a powerful predictor of cardiovascular events, cardiovascular mortality, and all-cause mortality.
   3. **More complete assessment** of cardiac anatomy and function by means of conventional echocardiography, examination of structural alterations in arteries by means of ultrasonography, measurement of ankle-arm index, and plasma renin activity and urinary sodium determinations may be useful in assessing **cardiovascular status** in select patients.

E. **Risk stratification**
   1. Although classification of adult blood pressure is somewhat arbitrary, it is useful to clinicians who must make treatment decisions on the basis of a constellation

TABLE 41.1 Classification of Blood Pressure for Adults 18 Years and Older

Category	Systolic blood pressure (mm Hg)		Diastolic blood pressure (mm Hg)
Normal	<120	and	<80
Prehypertension	120–139	or	80–89
Stage 1 hypertension	140–159	or	90–99
Stage 2 hypertension	≥160	or	≥100

of factors. A classification of blood pressure is shown in Table 41.1. The criteria are limited to persons who are not taking antihypertensive medication and who have no acute illness. **Classification is based on the average of two or more blood pressure readings.** When systolic blood pressure and diastolic blood pressure fall into different categories, **the higher category should be selected** to classify the patient's blood pressure.

2. Risk for cardiovascular disease among patients with HTN is determined by the **level of blood pressure** and by the **presence or absence of end-organ damage or other risk factors** such as smoking, dyslipidemia, and diabetes. These factors independently modify risk for subsequent cardiovascular disease. The presence or absence of these factors is determined during the routine evaluation of patients with HTN (e.g., history, physical examination, laboratory tests). This empiric classification stratifies patients with HTN into risk groups for therapeutic decisions. The World Health Organization Expert Committee on Hypertension Control recommends a similar approach. Obesity and physical inactivity are also predictors of cardiovascular risk and interact with other risk factors, but they are of less importance in the selection of antihypertensive drugs.
   a. **Risk group A** includes patients with prehypertension or HTN at stage 1 or 2 (Table 41.1) who do not have clinical cardiovascular disease, end-organ damage, or other risk factors. Persons with stage 1 HTN in risk group A are candidates for a longer trial (up to 1 year) of vigorous lifestyle modification with vigilant blood pressure monitoring. If the desired blood pressure is not achieved, pharmacologic therapy is added. For those with stage 2 HTN, drug therapy is warranted.
   b. **Risk group B** includes patients with HTN who do not have clinical cardiovascular disease or end-organ damage, but who have one or more of the risk factors but not diabetes mellitus. This group includes most patients with high blood pressure. If multiple risk factors are present, clinicians consider antihypertensive drugs as initial therapy. Lifestyle modification and management of reversible risk factors are strongly recommended.
   c. **Risk group C** includes patients with HTN and clinically manifested cardiovascular disease or end-organ damage. According to Joint National Committee (JNC 7) criteria (4), some patients who fall into the prehypertensive category and have renal insufficiency or diabetes mellitus should be considered for prompt pharmacologic therapy. Appropriate lifestyle modifications always are recommended as adjunct treatment.
   d. **Therapy.** Antihypertensive treatment has proved **beneficial in the prevention and reduction of the progression of HTN, cerebrovascular accidents, congestive heart failure (CHF), renal insufficiency, and renal failure.** Among patients with mild to moderate HTN, antihypertensive therapy has not favorably influenced angina, MI, and other atherosclerotic diseases (e.g., PVD, aortic atherosclerosis). The lower-than-expected reduction in CAD risk in most trials of antihypertensive agents has been attributed to the choice of agents, such as thiazide diuretics and β-blockers, that might negatively influence risk for CAD, and to the short duration of the trials. Overall, antihypertensive

treatment markedly reduces the prevalence of CAD events: CAD mortality (by 16%), the rate of fatal stroke (by 40%), and the incidence of heart failure (by 50%), with similar numbers of deaths prevented.

1. **Nonpharmacologic therapy**
   a. **Weight reduction** reduces systolic and diastolic blood pressure. Most clinical trials have demonstrated that weight reduction is related directly to blood pressure reduction. A weight loss of approximately 10 lb (4.5 kg) may reduce both systolic and diastolic blood pressure 2 to 3 mm Hg. Among patients with high-normal blood pressure, the need for medical therapy may be averted for one-half of these patients through weight reduction by means of physical activity and calorie restriction.
   b. **Exercise** reduces blood pressure by means of decreasing resting heart rate and peripheral vascular resistance, and by modifying serum norepinephrine and insulin levels. After an increase in physical activity, both systolic and diastolic blood pressure have been demonstrated to fall 7 mm Hg with or without weight reduction. Moderate-intensity exercise is as effective as high-intensity exercise for reducing blood pressure.
   c. **Diet.** A modest, independent benefit of **salt reduction** has been demonstrated. HTN is rare in societies that consume low-salt, high-potassium diets. Although the theory that excessive salt intake produces HTN has been difficult to prove in large clinical trials, most data support the role of dietary salt excess for some persons. In general, low-salt diets such as the Dietary Approaches to Stop Hypertension (DASH) 2300-mg and 1500-mg sodium diets, are recommended to most patients with HTN. Pooled estimates have suggested that **salt restriction is most important for older persons, those with higher baseline levels of blood pressure, and particularly those who are salt sensitive.** Salt restriction reduces the need for combination antihypertensive medications.
   d. Tobacco and immoderate alcohol use (more than two daily drinks for men and more than one daily drink for women) increase blood pressure. **Cessation of smoking and excessive alcohol use** markedly reduces blood pressure and further reduces cardiovascular risk.
2. **Medical therapy.** Pharmacologic therapy should be initiated in the presence of severe blood pressure elevation, end-organ damage, clinical cardiovascular disease, or other risk factors.
   a. **Priority of therapy**
      (1) Therapy for most patients with **uncomplicated HTN** at stage 1 (Table 41.1) should **begin with the lowest dose** to prevent adverse effects. If blood pressure remains uncontrolled after 1 to 2 months, the next dose level may be prescribed. It may take months to adequately control HTN. Most antihypertensive agents may be taken once each day. To improve patient compliance, this regimen is used whenever possible.
      (2) For patients at **higher risk**, those in risk group 2, or those at particularly high risk for CAD or cerebrovascular accident event, drug therapy to **achieve maximum beneficial reductions** in blood pressure should **proceed without delay.** If blood pressure is elevated 20/10 mm Hg above the goal, guidelines recommend starting two agents simultaneously.
      (3) There is **no debate regarding the need for aggressive blood pressure reduction** in patients with **diastolic pressures greater than 115 mm Hg and systolic pressures greater than 160 mm Hg.** JNC 7 aggressively targets the 140/90 mm Hg cut-point and incorporates hypertensive therapy into an algorithm of overall risk.
      (4) In the setting of hypertensive emergency **(HTN with end-organ damage, often with neurologic symptoms),** patients with a systolic blood pressure greater than 200 mm Hg or a diastolic blood pressure greater than 120 mm Hg may need **hospitalization** for therapy.
      (5) Although some patients may respond to single therapy, **two or more drugs often are required.** The intervals between changes in regimen should not be prolonged, and the maximum dose of some drugs may be increased.

b. Selecting the medication. Special considerations include concomitant disease, demographic characteristics, quality of life, cost, and use of other drugs that may cause drug interactions.

(1) Concomitant diseases. Antihypertensive medications may worsen some diseases and improve others. Table 41.2 provides information on concomitant diseases and possible therapies. In selecting an agent, the physician considers coexisting disease in an attempt to increase overall patient benefit, simplify regimens, and reduce cost. Special emphasis should be given to diabetic patients and to those with chronic renal disease. Such patients should be aggressively treated to maintain a goal blood pressure of less than 130/ less than 80 mm Hg.

(a) When choosing a certain drug for its favorable effect on comorbidity, clinicians must be aware that **reduction of long-term cardiovascular morbidity and mortality** may or may not have yet been demonstrated. Diuretics and β-blockers were drug classes originally shown in randomized trials to reduce morbidity and mortality. From the Heart Outcomes Prevention Evaluation (HOPE) trial, angiotensin-converting enzyme (ACE) inhibitors reduced the risk of cardiovascular events in patients with vascular disease or diabetes plus one other cardiovascular risk factor (5). However, the fact that HOPE was a trial with placebo control rather than active control suggests that BP lowering, and not drug class effect, may have been responsible for the improved outcomes. The Losartan Intervention For Endpoint reduction in Hypertension (LIFE) study showed a preferential reduction in

TABLE 41.2 Management of Hypertension in Specific Clinical Syndromes

Condition	Treatment
Acute coronary syndromes	β-Blockers or nitrates; CCB
Hypertension among African Americans	Diuretic or CCB
Arrhythmia	
Sinus bradycardia, SSS, or AV block	Diuretic, ACE inhibitor, or α-blocker
Atrial fibrillation or flutter, SVT	β-Blocker, diltiazem, verapamil, or clonidine
Benign prostatic hypertrophy	α-Blocker
COPD with bronchospasm or asthma	CCB or ACE inhibitor
Diabetes	ACE inhibitor
Advanced age (>65 years)	Diuretic, CCB, or ACE inhibitor at lower doses to avoid postural hypotension
Gout	Any *except* diuretics
Congestive heart failure	
Systolic	ACE inhibitor, diuretic, β-blockers
Diastolic	CCB or β-blockers
HOCM	β-Blockers or verapamil
Liver dysfunction	Any *except* methyldopa and labetalol
Post–myocardial infarction	ACE inhibitor, β-blocker, or both
Osteoporosis	Thiazide diuretics
PVD	Vasodilator, ACE inhibitor, CCB or α-blocker
Renal insufficiency (creatinine >2 mg/dL)	Loop diuretics, ACE inhibitor, CCB, α-blocker, labetalol, or a combination of these
Diabetic nephropathy	ACE inhibitor
Smokers	α-Blockers, ACE inhibitors, or CCB
Isolated systolic hypertension	Diuretics, CCB, ACE, inhibitors

ACE, angiotensin-converting enzyme; AV, atrioventricular; CCB, calcium channel blocker; COPD, chronic obstructive pulmonary disease; HOCM, hypertrophic obstructive cardiomyopathy; PVD, peripheral vascular disease; SSS, sick sinus syndrome; SVT, supraventricular tachycardia.

cardiovascular events, with the angiotensin receptor blocker losartan compared with atenolol in hypertensive patients. This improvement was primarily driven by a reduction in the number of strokes in the losartan group (6).

(b) Regression of **LVH** has been associated with a reduction in risk for cardiovascular events. All commonly-used antihypertensive strategies, with the exceptions of direct vasodilators and weight loss, induce regression of LVH. Specifically, the ACE inhibitor ramipril has been shown to cause regression of electrocardiographic markers of LVH, with an associated reduction in death, MI, stroke, and CHF. The LIFE trial, in contrast, demonstrated superiority of the angiotensin II receptor blocker (ARB) losartan over the β-blocker atenolol in the absence of LVH regression, suggesting that LVH might not be as powerful a surrogate of risk as initially thought. Further study of this issue is needed.

(2) Dosage. For most patients, a **low dose of the initial drug** choice is initiated and then titrated to the desired effect. The optimal formulation provides 24-hour efficacy with a once-daily dose, with at least a 50% of the peak effect remaining at the end of 24 hours. Long-acting formulations increase adherence, incur lower cost for some patients, provide consistent blood pressure control, and protect against early-morning sudden death. Diurnal blood pressure control is reported to improve when long-acting medication is taken at night rather than in the morning.

(3) Special populations. Neither sex nor age usually affects responsiveness to various agents. In general, HTN among **African Americans** is more responsive to monotherapy with diuretics and calcium channel blockers than with β-blockers or ACE inhibitors. However, if a β-blocker is needed for other therapeutic benefits, differences in efficacy usually can be overcome with reduction of salt intake, higher doses of the drug, or addition of a diuretic.

(4) Drug interactions. Some drug interactions may be beneficial. For example, diuretics acting on different sites in the nephron may increase natriuresis and diuresis, and diltiazem may reduce the amount of cyclosporine needed in transplant recipients. Other interactions may be harmful. Nonsteroidal antiinflammatory drugs (NSAIDs) may blunt the action of diuretics, β-blockers, and ACE inhibitors.

c. Treatment of the elderly. The benefit of blood pressure lowering is evident in the elderly, with a marked **reduction in all-cause mortality and CAD mortality,** as shown in multiple trials and studies. SHEP (3) was the first study to show that antihypertensive treatment of the elderly can reduce these events. It is not clear, however, that all agents are equally effective in reducing the rate of cardiovascular events in the elderly.

d. Emerging evidence. The Antihypertensive and Lipid-Lowering Treatment to Prevent Heart Attack Trial (ALLHAT) compared the incidence of cardiovascular events in hypertensive patients treated with a thiazide-type diuretic (chlorthalidone), calcium channel blocker (amlodipine), or ACE inhibitor (lisinopril) who were followed over 5 years. A fourth arm of the trial consisting of treatment with the α-blocker doxazosin had been stopped prematurely because of increased cardiovascular events, specifically a doubling in the risk of CHF in the doxazosin arm compared with the chlorthalidone arm. The results indicated no difference in the three remaining groups regarding the primary outcome of combined fatal coronary heart disease or nonfatal MI. Chlorthalidone was superior to amlodipine in preventing heart failure and superior to lisinopril in preventing stroke and combined cardiovascular disease (7). Given their clear efficacy, relatively low cost and high tolerability, thiazide diuretics are therefore considered initial agents of choice for most patients with HTN, and core components of multidrug regimens.

III. DIABETES MELLITUS. Type 1 diabetes mellitus (DM1) and type 2 diabetes mellitus (DM2) are powerful, independent predictors of CAD. The leading cause of premature death among patients with either type of diabetes is CAD, accounting for almost 80% of all deaths (8) and hospital admissions in this population. An estimated 21 million persons in the United States have diabetes mellitus. DM2, a disease closely associated with overweight and obesity, is on the rise given the ongoing "epidemic of obesity" in the United States, with more than 10% of the population 65 years or older being diagnosed with DM2.

A. Etiology and pathophysiology

1. **Diabetes accelerates the natural process of atherosclerosis.** Accelerated atherosclerosis in a person with diabetes may be attributed to coexistent HTN, hyperlipidemia, obesity, and insulin resistance.
   a. At autopsy, most persons with diabetes are found to have a **greater number of affected coronary vessels, more diffuse distribution of atherosclerosis,** and **more severe narrowing of the left main coronary artery** than persons without diabetes. In an international study in which more than 7000 sets of coronary artery autopsy specimens were examined, diabetes was associated with an increase in the extent of lesions in the arteries whether the overall prevalence of CAD in the country was low or high (9).
   b. Younger persons with DM1 are not spared. Severe and extensive luminal narrowing of large coronary arteries has been found in persons who had an onset of DM1 before 15 years of age and died before the age of 40 years.
   c. Large angiographic trials have consistently demonstrated that patients with diabetes undergoing cardiac catheterization for MI, percutaneous coronary intervention (PCI), or planned coronary artery bypass grafting (CABG) have significantly more severe CAD. Although there is an increased plaque burden, persons with diabetes have decreased coronary collateral circulation. Multiple studies have demonstrated an increased risk of morbidity, mortality, and need for target-lesion and new-lesion revascularization in diabetic patients undergoing PCI or CABG. **Diabetes is a predictor for progression and occlusion of atherosclerotic lesions.**
2. Diabetes carries a greater burden of **additional cardiovascular risk.** Persons with diabetes in the Framingham study were nearly four times more likely to have additional cardiovascular risk factors than persons without diabetes. Men in the MRFIT study were three times more likely to die of CAD if they had three risk factors in addition to baseline diabetes alone.
3. **Tight glycemic control** of DM1 **decreases microvascular complications,** such as retinopathy, nephropathy, and neuropathy; there are similar data for patients with DM2. The increased incidence of hypoglycemia that frequently accompanies tight glucose control and the increase in body weight with insulin therapy must be viewed in the overall context of cardiovascular outcomes.
4. **Acute coronary syndrome** is the cause of death among a large percentage of patients with diabetes.
   a. Thirty percent of patients with acute coronary syndrome are persons with diabetes. Despite encouraging results from thrombolytic trials, the **in-hospital mortality rate among persons with diabetes with MI remains twice that of persons without diabetes.** Patients with diabetes who have survived MI have a higher late mortality than persons without diabetes.
   b. Survival and recurrent cardiovascular events among patients with diabetes after MI are closely related to post-MI ejection fraction, the presence of multivessel CAD, the prothrombotic state associated with diabetes, and increased risk for sudden death.
   c. **CHF and cardiogenic shock** are more common and more severe among patients with diabetes than among other patients. The high in-hospital mortality among persons with diabetes is related to the high incidence of CHF among this population and, to a lesser degree, to an increase in reinfarction rate and infarct extension.

B. Risk factors. In general, the prevalence of known major risk factors for CAD is amplified among persons with diabetes. The major risk factors for CAD of particular importance include alterations in lipoprotein concentration and composition (i.e., dyslipidemia), HTN, hyperinsulinemia, and central obesity, some of which have a genetic component.

1. **Dyslipidemia.** One of the most profound risk factors among persons with diabetes is hyperlipidemia. Diabetes is associated with metabolic abnormalities in the transport, composition, and metabolism of lipoproteins. These abnormalities are associated with the type of diabetes, glycemia control, obesity, insulin resistance, presence of diabetic nephropathy, and genetic factors. The dyslipidemia associated with diabetes includes high levels of triglycerides, low levels of high-density-lipoprotein cholesterol (HDL-C), alterations in LDL particle composition, and increased levels of apolipoprotein B (apoB) and apolipoprotein E (apoE). CAD among persons with diabetes is strongly associated with the dyslipidemia of diabetes: high triglyceride level; small, dense LDL particles (sdLDL); and low HDL-C level.
2. **Hypertriglyceridemia.** Elevated fasting plasma triglyceride levels are one hallmark of the diabetic lipid profile, which appears to contribute to an atherogenic vascular environment. Recent data have established high trigylceride levels as an independent CAD risk factor.
3. **Hypertension.** HTN is more **prevalent among persons with DM1 or DM2** than among persons without diabetes. The role of HTN as a risk factor for atherosclerosis is at least as strong among persons with diabetes as among persons without diabetes. HTN can be the result of diabetic nephropathy, although the frequency of HTN also appears to be higher among persons with diabetes without renal complications than among the general population. In DM2, HTN occurs as part of a syndrome in which it can coexist with central obesity, insulin resistance, and dyslipidemia. **In diabetic patients, HTN should be aggressively treated to maintain a goal blood pressure of less than 130/80 mm Hg.**
4. **Tobacco.** There is strong evidence that smoking markedly increases risk for MI and complications of PVD among those with diabetes, especially women. Smoking is believed to be associated with adverse changes in plasma lipids and lipoproteins, especially the lowering of HDL-C levels.
5. **Metabolic syndrome (MetS).** The **metabolic syndrome (MetS)**, alternatively termed the **insulin resistance syndrome,** is characterized by central obesity, hyperinsulinemia, glucose intolerance, low HDL-C level, increased production of atherogenic sdLDL, and an inflammatory, prothrombotic state. Such patients are at much higher risk than the general population for the development of frank diabetes. In addition, there is growing evidence that MetS patients are at increased risk for the development of CAD. The identification of these patients is important for health promotion and disease prevention programs. Criteria for the diagnosis of MetS, as defined by the National Cholesterol Education Program (NCEP) Adult Treatment Panel III (ATP III), are listed in Table 41.3. It is estimated that one in four American adults meets the criteria for the diagnosis of MetS.
   a. Cardiovascular risk factor status was documented for study subjects who initially did not have diabetes and later participated in a population-based study of diabetes and cardiovascular disease. Later evaluation of baseline values revealed that subjects with a prediabetic condition, compared with persons without diabetes, had higher levels of total cholesterol, LDL-C, triglycerides, fasting glucose and insulin, and 2-hour postload glucose; higher blood pressure and body mass index (BMI); and lower levels of HDL-C. The study results demonstrated that subjects with a **prediabetic condition have an atherogenic pattern of risk factors that may be induced by obesity, hyperglycemia, and hyperinsulinemia.** These factors may be present for a long time and may contribute to risk for CAD and clinical diabetes.
   b. Findings from the Paris Prospective Study support the hypothesis that a constellation of metabolic abnormalities, such as elevated triglyceride levels, insulin resistance, and obesity, may play a significant role in the elevation of CAD risk (10). In this long-term study of CAD risk factors in a sample

TABLE 41.3 Adult Treatment Panel III Criteria for Diagnosing Metabolic Syndrome

Factor[a]	Diagnostic level
Abdominal obesity (waist circumference)	
Men	>102 cm (40 in)
Women	>88 cm (35 in)
Triglycerides	≥150 mg/dL
HDL cholesterol	
Men	<40 mg/dL
Women	<50 mg/dL
Blood pressure	≥130/ ≥85 mm Hg
Fasting glucose	≥110 mg/dL

[a]Three or more of these criterla must be present.
HDL, high-density lipoprotein.

of 7028 men with a mean follow-up of 11 years, the leading independent predictors of CAD death were blood pressure, smoking, cholesterol level, and fasting and 2-hour postload plasma insulin levels. The strongest independent predictor of subsequent CAD death in this quintile was plasma triglyceride concentration, adding to the evidence that hyperinsulinemia and hypertriglyceridemia are related.

C. Therapies and risk interventions. Although our knowledge of the epidemiologic and pathophysiologic mechanisms of atherosclerosis associated with diabetes is incomplete, strategies aimed at prevention can be developed. The combination of HTN, hyperlipidemia, and tobacco use with diabetes greatly accelerates the development of CAD and diabetic complications. **Efforts to target all CAD risk factors among persons with diabetes must be undertaken.** With the exception of lipid-lowering therapies, strategies in the prevention of cardiovascular complications among persons with diabetes have not been studied extensively.

1. **Control of glucose levels.** Tight control of DM1 is indicated for the prevention of microvascular events and possibly macrovascular events. Whether tight control of glucose in persons with DM2 reduces the risk of major cardiovascular events is unknown. The ongoing Action to Control Cardiovascular Risk in Diabetes (ACCORD) trial is testing the hypothesis that tight glycemic control (treatment targeted to HgbA1C <6.0%) will provide a greater reduction in major cardiovascular events compared with looser glycemic control (HbA1c 7.0% to 7.9%).
2. **Lipid-lowering therapy** is considered critical in the management of DM2. In the Scandinavian Simvastatin Survival Study (4S), there was a 55% reduction in CAD among persons with diabetes, and in the Cholesterol and Recurrent Events (CARE) trial, there was a 25% reduction. In the NCEP ATP III recommendations, diabetes is considered a **CAD risk equivalent.** In other words, given their striking predilection for the development of symptomatic CAD, patients with diabetes are treated as aggressively as those with established CAD. As of the 2004 ATP III Update, a **target LDL-C level of <70 mg/dL** is recommended for primary prevention of CAD in these patients.
   a. The 20-year follow-up results of the Seven Countries Study (11) indicate that **decreased intake of saturated fatty acids** and **high vegetable consumption** are associated with a lower incidence of glucose intolerance and a decrease in lipid levels.
   b. The American Dietary Association recommends **mild or moderate weight loss** (10 to 20 lb [4.5 to 9 kg]), which improves diabetes control even if ideal body weight is not achieved.

c. **Lipid-lowering pharmacologic agents** that can be used by patients with diabetes include fibric acid derivatives and HMG-CoA reductase inhibitors.

(1) **Nicotinic acid** has been demonstrated to increase insulin resistance and adversely affect blood glucose levels.

(2) **Bile acid–binding resins** may cause gastrointestinal autonomic neuropathy, increase constipation, and increase already elevated triglyceride levels, a characteristic of most patients with DM2. They are used with **caution.**

(3) The use of β-blockers, diuretics, estrogens, or glucocorticoids may increase triglyceride levels and should be closely monitored.

3. **Management of hyperinsulinemia**

a. Patients are monitored closely for metabolic and physiologic derangements associated with hyperinsulinemia. Although it is not feasible in most instances to check insulin levels, a **hgA1c level greater than 6.5% is a useful clinical marker** for glucose intolerance and is managed aggressively for all patients at risk.

b. Therapy focused at **reducing insulin levels** whether through diet or drug therapy is considered in the care of patients at high risk.

IV. OBESITY.

IV. OBESITY. Obesity is established as a leading predictor of CAD and is associated with several cardiovascular risk factors—cholesterol, HTN, and glucose intolerance—which may increase all-cause mortality and cardiovascular mortality. Currently, 64% of U.S. adults are overweight, defined as having a BMI of greater than 25. Moreover, 30% of Americans are classified as obese, with a BMI of 30 or more. This has come to be a critical problem for African American women, among whom the prevalence of obesity is more than 50%. The percentage of children and adolescents with obesity has doubled over the last 20 years.

A. Pathophysiology

1. A positive association between BMI, increased total cholesterol and triglyceride levels, and a decreased HDL-C levels has been documented in various age groups.

2. **Distribution of fat appears to be a more important predictor of CAD than total amount of fat** because android fat patterns are more metabolically active and highly associated with dyslipidemia. Although BMI and waist-to-hip ratios have indicated a linear association between obesity and CAD, the **waist-to-hip ratio,** which accounts for abdominal adiposity, is viewed as a more **accurate predictor of CAD.** Among obese persons, those with central adiposity are at particularly high risk. In a cohort of 1500 women observed for 20 years, the waist-to-hip ratio, but not BMI, was highly predictive of the occurrence of fatal MI.

3. The **National Center for Health Statistics still uses BMI,** defined as **weight (kg)/height (m)^2, as the recognized measurement of obesity.** Their guidelines define obesity as a BMI of 27.8 or more for men and 27.3 or more for women. Morbid obesity has been defined as a BMI of 31.1 for men and 32.3 for women. The Nurses Health Study showed that women with a BMI of 25 to 29 had an age-adjusted relative risk for CAD of 1.8 compared with the leanest women. Women with a BMI greater than 29 had a relative risk for CAD of 3.3.

4. Obesity among adults is associated with **increased LV mass,** a powerful independent predictor of mortality and morbidity from cardiovascular disease. LV mass in persons with obesity but without diabetes probably depends, at least in part, on the degree of insulin resistance and hyperinsulinemia and not BMI and blood pressure.

5. Central obesity is part of the **metabolic syndrome,** which appears to be associated with increased risk for CAD in both sexes. This condition is characterized by elevated plasma triglyceride and low plasma HDL-C levels.

a. An essential feature is the presence of **dense, atherogenic LDL.**

b. Other features are HTN, impaired glucose intolerance with hyperinsulinemia, and decreased sensitivity to the action of insulin on peripheral tissues.

c. Hyperinsulinemia is associated with **lipid derangements, increased production of plasminogen activator inhibitor, and enhanced proliferation**

of cells in atherosclerotic plaque. Among patients with hyperinsulinemia, an increased prevalence of CAD and a relationship among abnormal insulin levels, glucose metabolism, and severity of CAD have been reported. The physiologic response to insulin resistance is increased secretion of insulin, which may lead to glucose intolerance or frank diabetes mellitus.

B. Therapy

1. **Calorie restriction, behavior modification, and exercise** are the main treatment modalities for weight loss. The greatest weight losses have occurred with a combined regimen of diet and exercise rather than diet or exercise alone.
2. Several **medications** can be used for temporary management of obesity. Although pharmacologic agents temporarily aid in the struggle against obesity, the National Task Force on Obesity **cautions against the use of these agents for long-term maintenance because of the potential for unknown side effects.**
   a. **Noradrenergic drugs** influence weight loss through stimulation of the hypothalamus.
   b. **Orlistat,** a pancreatic lipase inhibitor, reduces weight through inhibition of fat absorption.
   c. **Serotonin reuptake inhibitors (SSRIs),** including sibutramine, fluoxetine, and sertraline, promote weight loss with various degrees of side effects.
   d. Use of dexfenfluramine and fenfluramine, already of concern because of rare instances of pulmonary HTN, has been discontinued because of associated acquired valvular heart disease.
3. In the most extreme cases, **surgical therapy** can be provided. Among morbidly obese patients (BMI >40) and obese patients (BMI between 35 and 40) with coexisting conditions, jejunoileal shunts and gastroplasty often aid in the maintenance of weight loss. About 10 years after surgical intervention, 80% of patients maintain a weight 10% less than preoperative weight.
4. **Risk of weight loss.** Even if weight is lost, weight loss maintenance fails in most instances. Health risks that accompany weight cycling are increases in cardiovascular morbidity and mortality, abdominal fat, blood pressure, and insulin resistance.

V. TOBACCO. Smoking, the single most preventable cause of death in the United States, is a leading risk factor for CAD, CVA, and PVD. Second-hand smoke has been shown to increase the risk for CAD. The causal role of smoking in cardiovascular disease has been derived from more than 20 million person-years of follow-up study (NHLBI, 1996). Twenty-eight percent of white men and 25% of white women smoke, as do 34% of African-American men, 22% of African-American women, 24% of Hispanic men, and 15% of Hispanic women. It is estimated that 37% of the population is exposed to second-hand smoke. Exposure to second-hand smoke increases by 30% the risk of death by CAD. More than 90% of current smokers began their habit before they were 21 years of age.

A. Pathophysiology. Cigarette use activates platelets, increases circulating fibrinogen, increases heart rate, and elevates blood pressure. It appears to promote plaque disruption. A strong dose–response relationship exists between smoking and CAD. Duration of smoking and the daily amount markedly influence risk for CAD. The number of cigarettes smoked per day is directly proportional to risk for MI. The adverse effect of smoking is present among men and women (but may be stronger among women) of all ages and ethnic groups with or without prior CAD. Data suggest that risk for cardiac death is two to four times greater among current smokers than nonsmokers.

B. Risk reduction and therapy. Risk for cardiovascular disease begins to decline soon after smoking cessation, irrespective of age and sex. There is a 50% reduction in cardiovascular events within the first 2 to 4 years of cigarette cessation; however, increased cardiovascular risk still exists 10 years after cessation. It is thought to take as long as 20 years to regain baseline risk.

1. **Behavioral and psychosocial treatment.** Several techniques have been developed to help patients stop smoking and maintain cessation.

2. Pharmacotherapy

a. Nicotine replacement therapy (NRT). Approximately 50% to 70% of patients discontinue cigarette use after a major cardiac event, such as MI or CABG. Cessation for another 10% to 20% can be accomplished with cigarette cessation programs, which often incorporate nicotine patches or the somewhat less efficacious nicotine gum. Programs that incorporate a nurse clinician increase cessation beyond 30%. Eight-week treatment appears to be as effective as longer periods of use.

(1) The patch. Clinical practice guidelines support the use of the transdermal nicotine patch as the **primary pharmacologic agent for all patients who smoke.** The risk of use of the patch among patients with CAD is now considered to have been overstated. Use of the patch is contraindicated for persons who continue to smoke because it leads to nausea. **Side effects** of NRT include itching and skin rash among as many as 50% of patients. NRT approximately doubles cessation rate. One-year follow-up evaluations of patch-cessation therapy indicated cessation rates of 20% to 25%, compared with 5% to 10% for a placebo.

(a) Standard dosages (Nicoderm, Prostep, Nicotrol) include the maximum for 4 weeks and lesser doses for another 4 weeks.

(b) Because baseline nicotine levels (i.e., the number of cigarettes smoked per day) are inversely associated with cessation rates, **patients who smoke less than 1 pack per day** may be adequately treated with **submaximal nicotine doses.**

(2) Nicotine gum. Use of gum for NRT appears to delay postcessation weight gain, a typical deterrent to cigarette cessation. Multipack users should use 4 mg gum, whereas patients who smoke less than 1 pack per day may need only 2 mg.

(3) Nicotine nasal spray has been approved as a smoking cessation treatment. Nasal spray provides a more rapid rise in nicotine level than that with gum or patch, with peak levels occurring in less than 10 minutes. Nicotine nasal spray has markedly more severe **side effects** and appears to be best suited for patients who have not had success with other forms of NRT.

b. Other pharmacologic agents. For select patients, supplementation with agents other than NRT may be useful, even though NRT is the only strategy recommended in standard smoking cessation guidelines.

(1) Bupropion, which is approved for smoking cessation, has dopaminergic and noradrenergic properties. Clinical trials have demonstrated the efficacy of bupropion sustained release (SR) with or without transdermal nicotine for smoking cessation. The recommended dosage of bupropion is 150 mg two times per day. In clinical trials, the medication was typically started 1 to 2 weeks before cessation and was continued for 7 to 12 weeks after cessation. Abstinence rates at 12 months were 30% for patients treated with bupropion for 9 weeks in one study, and combination therapy with bupropion and a nicotine patch resulted in a 35.5% abstinence rate (12).

Bupropion must be **avoided by patients with a seizure disorder or who are at risk for seizures** (i.e., patients with head injury, those who abuse alcohol, or patients who have alcohol dependence) because the medication lowers seizure threshold. Common **side effects** of bupropion include headache, nausea, and restlessness. Bupropion has no serious adverse effects on the cardiovascular system.

(2) Clonidine, an α_2-agonist, **dampens the sympathetic activity associated with withdrawal.** Dosages used for smoking cessation typically range from 0.1 to 0.4 mg/day for 2 to 6 weeks in the oral or the transdermal preparation. The most common **side effects** are dry mouth, constipation, postural hypotension, and sedation. Clonidine is **recommended for patients who prefer not to take nicotine or who have not had success with NRT.** Nasal spray clonidine has been effective among nicotine-dependent women who are intolerant of the patch.

(3) **Varenicline,** the most recent U.S. Food and Drug Administration (FDA)–approved medication for smoking cessation, is a partial agonist of the nicotinic acetylcholine receptor, in particular, the $\alpha_4\beta_2$subtype. Several trials have demonstrated improved efficacy in achieving smoking cessation when compared to NRT and buproprion SR. However, because of case reports of adverse psychiatric behavior occurring during varenicline administration, including suicidal ideation, suicidal behavior, and erratic behavior, practitioners are encouraged to monitor their patients closely for signs of psychiatric changes.

VI. SEDENTARY LIFESTYLE

A. Pathophysiology. A sedentary lifestyle is associated with increased risk for CAD. Sedentary persons have almost double the risk for CAD death of active persons. In five prospective exercise studies, persons at the lowest levels of exercise conditioning had an age-adjusted CAD mortality risk 2 to 10 times that of the best-conditioned participants. Meta-analyses of epidemiologic studies suggest a nearly twofold increase in risk among sedentary persons for development of CAD and for CAD death. A sedentary lifestyle also is associated with obesity, HTN, DM2, and hypercholesterolemia, which point to the need for changes in exercise patterns. More than 50% of the U.S. population does not exercise at least 20 minutes three times a week, and 40% of adults are classified as sedentary. Only 22% of U.S. adults partake in 30 or more minutes of exercise five times a week; 25% report no leisure-time physical activity.

B. Risk reduction. Even moderate physical activity provides a reduction of risk. Regular physical activity prevents obesity, may reduce weight, and promotes positive effects on blood pressure, LDL-C, HDL-C, and triglyceride levels. Independent of other risk factors, physical fitness has a direct protective effect from CAD events. Among patients who have had MI, controlled cardiac rehabilitation programs significantly reduce cardiovascular mortality by 20% to 25%. The American Heart Association (AHA) currently recommends that adults accumulate 30 minutes or more of moderate-intensity physical activity on most (preferably all) days of the week.

1. Mechanism

a. Exercise **improves glucose tolerance and insulin sensitivity, increases fibrinolysis, increases HDL-C levels, improves oxygen uptake** in the heart, and **increases coronary artery diameter.** Exercise reduces the sensitivity of the myocardium to the effects of catecholamines and reduces risk for ventricular arrhythmias, important factors in sudden cardiovascular death. Exercise is commonly believed to increase HDL-C and lower LDL-C levels, and, as such, reduce cardiac events. Exercise can alter the progression of coronary atherosclerosis. Among patients with angiographically documented CAD, exercise training may increase regression and reduce the progression of coronary lesions.

b. Studies on the effect of exercise have been difficult to conduct and are known to have difficulties in quantification of exercise. Reviews on the effects of cardiac rehabilitation on morbidity and mortality demonstrated reductions in all-cause mortality of 20% to 24% and in CAD mortality of 23% to 25%. The data support a reduction in anginal episodes and mortality, although the reduction in mortality is no better than 15%. A direct relationship has been shown between exercise intensity and angiographic modifications: 1533 kcal/week is necessary to stabilize coronary lesions, and 2200 kcal/week is needed to induce coronary regression.

2. Fitness (measured in metabolic equivalents or METs achieved) and **physical activity** (measured in caloric expenditure per time period) appear to be closely linked, although it remains unclear which of the two is the better predictor of cardiovascular morbidity and mortality.

a. Several studies have shown that **higher degrees of physical activity** are associated with decreased risk for death of CAD. There is an inverse association between increasing physical activity (measured in MET-hours/week) and the risk of cardiovascular events. These studies suggest that **changes in fitness**

from low to high levels and level of current activity are the best predictors of reduction in risk for CAD.

b. **The death rate decreased 50% among men** 60 years or older who changed from unfit to fit status over an 18-year follow-up period. The age-adjusted cardiovascular disease mortality rate decreased 52%.

c. An important measurement of fitness among **older postmenopausal women** is leisure-time physical activity; it can reduce risk of MI substantially. Even moderate-intensity exercise has been shown to confer substantial benefits for postmenopausal women. Such women who walk or exercise vigorously at least 2.5 hours each week have been shown to have a cardiovascular risk reduction of approximately 30%.

3. **Problems with compliance.** Only 50% of persons who begin an exercise program adhere to it for more than 6 months.

a. Physicians may need to help **tailor exercise programs for individual patients** to participate in activity that is sustained in the long term.

b. As for healthy persons, **precautions** must be taken to **prevent injury.** The current guidelines may be **slightly modified for elderly exercisers** to emphasize a longer warm-up period to enable musculoskeletal and cardiorespiratory readiness for exercise and an adequate cool-down period to help dissipate heat.

VII. NOVEL RISK FACTORS.

Screening studies have shown that HTN, hyperlipidemia, tobacco use, family history, and diabetes are predictive of less than half of all future cardiovascular events. Among patients with premature atherosclerosis, the predictive value of these traditional cardiovascular risk factors is limited. Many patients with few traditional risk factors experience life-threatening acute coronary syndromes without prior symptoms of disease. Several potential risk factors have been identified that may enhance risk for CAD. These are levels of C-reactive protein (CRP), lipoprotein(a) or Lp(a), homocysteine, fibrinogen, and myeloperoxidase (MPO), and genetic mutations and single-nucleotide polymorphisms in a number of candidate genes.

A. **CRP** is a marker of systemic inflammation. As the role of **inflammation** in the initiation and progression of atherosclerosis becomes better understood, CRP has gained prominence as an important player in the assessment of cardiovascular risk.

1. **Pathophysiology**

a. CRP has been shown to be an independent risk factor for the development of cardiovascular events in both apparently healthy individuals and in patients with established coronary heart disease. The exact role CRP plays in this association has not yet been well characterized. Initially, it was believed that CRP provided an indirect measurement of the inflammatory milieu in at-risk individuals. Emerging evidence, however, indicates that CRP itself may have a direct causal influence on the development of atherosclerosis. CRP binds to oxidized LDL, promoting the uptake of LDL by macrophage scavenger cells in the arterial wall, and possibly enhancing the atherosclerotic process.

b. The degree of associated risk throughout various levels of CRP, often measured as high-sensitivity CRP (hsCRP), has been evaluated in several studies.

(1) Men in the Physicians' Health Study with the highest quartile CRP had **three times the risk of MI** and **twice the risk of ischemic stroke** compared with men in the lowest quartile (13).

(2) For women, the difference is even more pronounced. The relative risk of cardiovascular events in the highest compared with the lowest quartile of CRP in women is **4.4** (14).

(3) An increased risk of sudden cardiac death has also been seen in patients with elevated CRP levels.

2. **Clinical use**

a. Standard CRP assays are not sufficiently sensitive to discriminate within the narrow range of CRP values associated with an increase in cardiovascular events. The development of hsCRP assays, however, has made this possible. AHA/Centers for Disease Control and Prevention (CDC) guidelines have established cut-points of risk for hsCRP: a level of less than 1 mg/L is considered low, 1.0 to 3.0 mg/L is average, and more than 3.0 mg/L is high and associated with increased cardiovascular risk (15). Higher levels (>10 mg/L) suggest an alternative cause for inflammation, such as infection or underlying rheumatologic illness.

b. When deciding whether to initiate statin therapy for the primary prevention of coronary events, hsCRP measurement may prove helpful in patients with a moderate level of cardiovascular risk (calculated 10-year major cardiac event risk of 10% to 20%). If found to have an elevated hsCRP level, these patients may benefit from more intensified therapy, including dietary modifications, and, perhaps, statin therapy. In the Air Force/Texas Coronary Atherosclerosis Prevention Study (AFCAPS/TexCAPS), lovastatin reduced the incidence of cardiovascular events in patients with low lipid levels **if** CRP levels were elevated. No improvement was seen in the cohort of patients with low lipid levels and normal CRP values.

c. The AHA/CDC panel recommends against widespread screening of the general population. In secondary prevention, hsCRP assessment can be performed, but proven intensified therapy (including statins) should not be withheld based on the level of hsCRP attained. Serial hsCRP measurements should not be used to monitor the effects of lipid treatment.

3. Risk reduction and therapy. Weight loss by caloric-restriction diets has been shown to decrease plasma CRP levels. Additional data indicate that women who exercise regularly have lower CRP levels compared with sedentary women. In primary prevention trials, pravastatin has been shown to reduce CRP levels by about 17%, in a manner independent of LDL lowering. Evidence suggests that simvastatin lowers CRP within the first 2 weeks of therapy, before any LDL-lowering effect is seen. What is not known, however, is whether reducing CRP by any such means confers an independent benefit in regard to lowering cardiovascular morbidity and mortality.

B. Lipoprotein (a) or Lp(a) is identical to LDL, except for the addition of apolipoprotein A (apoA), a highly glycosylated protein. Although it is a lipoprotein, Lp(a) often is considered a **marker of thrombosis.**

1. Pathophysiology

a. There is a striking amino acid sequence homology between apoA and plasminogen, suggesting that Lp(a) may play an important role in the connection between atherosclerosis and thrombosis. **Lp(a) may be atherogenic;** it accumulates in atherosclerotic lesions, binds to apoB-containing lipoproteins and proteoglycans, and can be taken up by foam cell precursors. It also may promote thrombosis when it binds to fibrin and blocks the fibrinolytic action of plasmin.

b. Lp(a) may be more predictive of CAD among younger men, women, and in persons with hyperlipidemia.

c. Studies have had mixed results

(1) Cross-sectional and retrospective case-control studies usually have supported the role of Lp(a) in CAD. Lp(a) is a marker among patients at particular risk for poor outcomes, in terms of severity and progression of cardiovascular disease.

(2) Several prospective studies have correlated baseline Lp(a) levels with vascular disease in general.

(3) Other prospective studies have found little or no association between Lp(a) and CAD risk.

d. Few studies have been conducted on the role of Lp(a) in **women.** Cardiovascular risk tends to increase with an Lp(a) value greater than 30 mg/dL.

2. Therapy. Niacin is the only agent currently available that reduces Lp(a). However, the multiplicity of lipid effects exerted by niacin therapy, it is unknown if reduction in Lp(a) levels is beneficial. In addition, the atherogenicity of Lp(a) may be modified through **substantial reductions in LDL-C levels.**

C. **Homocysteine** is a product of folate metabolism. It is derived from the sulfur-containing amino acid methionine and is metabolized through pathways associated with folic acid, vitamin B_6, and vitamin B_{12} as cofactors.

1. **Etiology and pathophysiology**
   a. Elevated plasma homocysteine levels (>15 μ/L) confer an **independent risk for vascular disease,** according to cross-sectional and prospective case-control studies. The risk was first identified because of increased thromboembolic events, including MI and stroke, in patients with **homocystinuria,** a rare inherited deficiency of cystathionine β-synthase characterized by very high serum homocysteine levels (>100 μmol/L).
   b. Elevated homocysteine levels are found among more than 20% of patients with atherosclerotic disease, including PVD. In PVD, there may be direct endothelial toxicity, smooth muscle cell proliferation, enhanced LDL oxidation, abnormalities in platelet function, or increased thrombotic risk because of abnormal clotting factors (e.g., factor V, factor VII), or altered secretion of von Willebrand's factor.
   c. The **relative risk for stroke and MI is approximately 2.0 for homocysteine levels greater than 15 μmol/L** compared with those less than 10 μmol/L. The relative risk for PVD is much greater than 3.0. Risk enhancement is continuous over the spectrum of homocysteine values.
   d. A meta-analysis of case-control observational studies is less compelling. This study examined patients with a genetic polymorphism of an enzyme involved in folate metabolism; this alteration resulted in elevated homocysteine levels. Individuals with this mutation had only a 16% higher risk of developing CHD compared with normal controls (16).
   e. **Secondary causes** of increased homocysteine levels include age, male sex, menopause, renal function, and some medications (e.g., niacin, oral contraceptives with estrogen, phenytoin, methotrexate, theophylline). Thyroid function also is relevant.
   f. The mechanism by which homocysteine appears to promote vascular disease is **unclear.** Elevated homocysteine levels seem to play a role in the production of arterial lesions, but deficiencies of other factors, such as vitamin B_{12} and folic acid, also may be involved, especially in the elderly.
   g. **Possible mechanisms** of increased risk are that hyperhomocystinemia may impair release of nitric oxide from endothelial cells, stimulate proliferation of atherogenic smooth muscle cells, and contribute to thrombogenesis through activation of protein C.
      (1) **Deficiencies in the cofactors** lead to elevated serum concentrations of homocysteine, although profound deficiencies are rare among persons with high-homocysteine CAD.
      (2) Rare defects in the genes for 5,10-methylene tetrahydrofolate reductase, cystathionine β-synthase (0.5% prevalence), methylene tetrahydrofolate homocysteine methyltransferase (rare), and methionine synthases (rare) can lead to increases in homocysteine.
2. **Laboratory examination.** For patients with abnormal homocysteine values, further evaluation includes thyroid-stimulating hormone, B_{12}, B_6, folate, and creatinine.
3. **Trials of homocysteine lowering.** The results of three such large, prospective, randomized trials of have been reported in recent years. In the Vitamin Intervention for Stroke Prevention (VISP) trial, patients with a history of stroke were treated with two different doses of folic acid, vitamin B_6, and vitamin B_{12} (17). Although a dose-dependent reduction in homocysteine levels was observed, no difference in vascular events were observed between the two groups. The Norwegian Vitamin Trial (NORVIT) randomized patients with history of MI to four treatment different groups: folic acid, vitamin B_6, and vitamin B_{12}; folic acid and vitamin B_{12}; vitamin B_6 alone; or placebo. After a mean 40 months of therapy, homocysteine levels were decreased by 27% in the group treated with folic acid and vitamin B_{12}. However, these subjects had no difference in the development of the

primary endpoint (recurrent MI, stroke, or sudden death from CAD) compared to the placebo group. In the group treated with all three supplements, there was a marginally significant trend toward fewer strokes, but also a near-significant trend toward more myocardial infarctions. Finally, the Heart Outcomes Prevention Evaluation 2 (HOPE-2) trial was a mixed primary and secondary prevention trial, treating vascular disease or diabetic patients with either a combination of folic acid, vitamin B_6, and vitamin B_{12}; or placebo (18). Despite a significant decrease in homocysteine levels with active treatment, there was no significant difference in the primary outcome (MI, stroke, or death from cardiovascular causes) when compared to placebo treatment. There was a marginally significant decrease in stroke with vitamin administration (19). It is unknown whether the negative results of these studies result from incorrectness of the homocysteine atherosclerotic hypothesis, or from pathologic effects of vitamin therapy offsetting possible benefit of homocysteine reduction. Regardless, given the lack of benefit (and in some cases, suggestion of harm) provided by folic acid with or without B vitamins, such therapy cannot be recommended for the prevention of cardiovascular disease.

D. Fibrinogen, a large hepatically synthesized glycoprotein, is a clotting factor that activates thrombin, induces platelet aggregation through the glycoprotein IIb/IIIa receptor, and stimulates smooth muscle proliferation.

1. Etiology and pathophysiology. There is increasing evidence that **fibrinogen is important in the development of premature atherosclerosis.** The link is likely and plausible.

a. Several prospective studies, including the Framingham study, have shown an **impressive relationship between plasma fibrinogen level and the occurrence of CAD and stroke.** Plasma fibrinogen levels higher than 350 mg/dL are powerful independent risk factors for stroke and MI. A high fibrinogen level is an independent risk factor for CAD with a twofold to threefold increase in risk, and markedly enhances risk for hypercholesterolemia.

b. Clinical findings suggest that a **high fibrinogen level also may be a risk factor for the sequelae of CAD.** In the Northwick Park Heart Study, a fibrinogen level in the upper third for the population was associated with risk for cardiovascular disease three times higher than that among patients with a plasma level in the lower third. In the Göteburg study, baseline fibrinogen level was significantly related to the incidence of MI and ischemic stroke.

2. Cofactors. Determinants of high fibrinogen levels include age, female sex, menopause, African American race, smoking, obesity, stress, use of oral contraceptives, pregnancy, and a consumption of large amounts of dietary fat.

3. Risk reduction and therapy

a. Factors associated with a decrease in fibrinogen level include smoking cessation, physical activity, moderate alcohol intake, normalization of body weight, and postmenopausal hormone replacement.

b. Although no clinical trial has identified a drug that reduces fibrinogen level safely and selectively, the following medications have been shown to decrease fibrinogen level in various clinical settings: fibrates, pentoxifylline, ticlopidine, *n*-3 polyunsaturated fatty acids, and anabolic steroids.

E. Myeloperoxidase (MPO). As discussed previously, inflammation plays a major role in the pathogenesis of CAD and the development of MI. MPO is a protein with enzymatic activity that is released during activation and degranulation of neutrophils and monocytes. For patients in the emergency department with chest pain, serum levels of MPO have been shown to predict risk of MI at 30 days and 6 months, even in the absence of myocardial necrosis (20). In patients with non–ST-elevation MI, MPO levels have recently been shown to predict 30-day risk of recurrent nonfatal MI or hospitalization for acute coronary syndrome.

F. Nonlipid genetic factors. Although a familial predisposition for CAD has been well-documented, little is known about the causative factors leading to premature events in such kindreds. In one family, a seven amino acid deletion in the gene encoding the MEF2A transcription factor was found to confer autosomal dominant susceptibility to CAD and MI (21). The thrombospondins are a family of glycoproteins that play a pivotal role in cell adhesion, vascular integrity, and thrombosis. Single nucleotide polymorphisms (SNPs) in thrombospondin genes have been linked to premature atherosclerosis and MI, providing another example of how genetic variations may contribute to the development of coronary disease. Recently, the general excitement regarding genetics of CAD has been somewhat tempered by publications of negative findings (22,23). Nevertheless, the identification of genetic risk factors for cardiovascular disease, and the elucidation of their mechanism of risk elevation, is still one of the newest and most promising areas of translational cardiology research.

ACKNOWLEDGMENTS

The author thanks Drs. J. Christopher Merritt and JoAnne Micale Foody for their contributions to earlier editions of this chapter.

References

1. Rubins HB, Robins SJ, Collins D, et al. Distribution of lipids in 8500 men with coronary artery disease. Department of Veterans Affairs HDL Intervention Trial Study Group. *Am J Cardiol* 1995;75:1196–1201.
2. Multiple risk factor intervention trial: multiple risk factor changes and mortality results—Multiple Risk Factor Intervention Trial Research Group. *JAMA* 1982;248:1465–1477.
3. Kostis JB, Davis BR, Cutler J, et al. Prevention of heart failure by antihypertensive drug treatment in older persons with isolated systolic hypertension: SHEP Cooperative Research Group. *JAMA* 1997;278:212–216.
4. Chobanian AV, Bakris GL, Black HR, et al. The Seventh Report of the Joint National Committee on Prevention, Detection, Evaluation, and Treatment of High Blood Pressure: the JNC 7 Report. *JAMA* 2003;289:2560–2572.
5. The HOPE Investigators. Effects of an angiotensin-converting-enzyme inhibitor, ramipril, on cardiovascular events in high-risk patients. *N Engl J Med* 2000;342:145–152.
6. Dahlof B, Devereux RB, Kjeldsen SE, et al. Cardiovascular morbidity and mortality in the Losartan Intervention for Endpoint Reduction in Hypertension study (LIFE): a randomized trial against atenolol. *Lancet* 2002;359:995–1003.
7. The ALLHAT Collaborative Research Group. Major outcomes in high-risk hypertensive patients randomized to angiotensin-converting enzyme inhibitor or calcium channel blocker vs diuretic: the Antihypertensive and Lipid-Lowering Treatment to Prevent Heart Attack Trial (ALLHAT). *JAMA* 2002;288;2981–2997.
8. Kannel WB. Lipids, diabetes, and coronary heart disease: insights from the Framingham Study. *Am Heart J* 1985;110:1100–1107.
9. Burchfiel CM, Reed DM, Marcus EB, et al. Association of diabetes mellitus with coronary atherosclerosis and myocardial lesions: an autopsy study from the Honolulu Heart Program. *Am J Epidemiol* 1993;137:1328–1340.
10. Charles MA, Fontbonne A, Thebult N, et al. Risk factors for NIDDM in white population. *Diabetes* 1991;40:796–799.
11. Farchi G, Fidanza F, Mariotti S, et al. Is diet an independent risk factor for mortality: 20 year mortality in the Italian rural cohorts of the 7 country study. *Eur J Clin Nutr* 1994;48:19–29.
12. Jorenby DE, Leischow SJ, Nides MA, et al. A controlled trial of sustained-released bupropion, a nicotine patch, or both for smoking cessation. *N Engl J Med* 1999;340:685–691.
13. Ridker PM, Cushman M, Stampfer MJ, et al. Inflammation, aspirin, and the risk of cardiovascular disease in apparently healthy men. *N Engl J Med* 1997;336:973–979.
14. Ridker PM, Hennekens CH, Buring JE, et al. C-reactive protein and other markers of inflammation in the prediction of cardiovascular disease in women. *N Engl J Med* 2000;342:836–843.
15. Pearson TA, Mensah GA, Alexander RW, et al. Markers of inflammation and cardiovascular disease: application to clinical and public health practice; a statement for healthcare professionals from the Centers for Disease Control and Prevention and the American Heart Association. *Circulation* 2003;107:499–511.
16. Klerk M, Verhoef P, Clarke R, et al. MTHFR 677C T polymorphism and risk of coronary heart disease: a meta-analysis. *JAMA* 2002;288:2023–2031.
17. Toole JF, Malinow MR, Chambless LE, et al. Lowering homocysteine in patients with ischemic stroke, myocardial infarction, and death: the Vitamin Intervention for Stroke Prevention (VISP) randomized controlled trial. *JAMA* 2004;291:565–575.
18. Bønaa KH, Njølstad I, Ueland PM, et al. Homocysteine lowering and cardiovascular events after acute myocardial infarction. *N Engl J Med* 2006;354:1578–1588.
19. The Heart Outcomes Prevention Evaluation (HOPE) 2 Investigators. Homocysteine lowering with folic acid and B vitamins in vascular disease. *N Engl J Med* 2006;354:1567–1577.
20. Brennan ML, Penn MS, Van Lente F, et al. Prognostic value of myeloperoxidase in patients with chest pain. *N Engl J Med* 2003;349:1595–1604.
21. Wang L, Fan C, Topol SE, et al. Mutation of MEF2A in an inherited disorder with features of coronary artery disease. *Science* 2003;302:1578–1581.
22. Morgan TM, Krumholz HM, Lifton RP, et al. Nonvalidation of reported genetic risk factors for acute coronary syndrome in a large-scale replication study. *JAMA* 2007;297:1151–1161.
23. Lieb W, Mayer B, König IR, et al. Lack of association between the MEF2A gene and myocardial infarction. *Circulation* 2008;117:185–191.

IX Noninvasive Assessment

42 EXERCISE ELECTROCARDIOGRAPHIC TESTING

Eiran Z. Gorodeski

I. INTRODUCTION

A. Exercise electrocardiographic testing is a field in flux. In the last decade it has become clear that ST-segment changes during exercise have low sensitivity and specificity in the evaluation of coronary artery disease (CAD), and are poor predictors of risk. This may be partially due to the fact that stable obstructive plaques, which typically result in exercise-mediated ischemia, are less relevant to myocardial infarction (MI) and sudden cardiac death (SCD) than unstable non-obstructive plaques. Although the bulk of obstructive CAD screening has now shifted to echocardiographic or nuclear assessment immediately following pharmacologic or exercise testing, evaluation of functional capacity, heart rate changes, burden of ectopy, and dynamic electrocardiographic changes during and after exercise have emerged as powerful prognostic indicators. As such, the main uses of exercise electrocardiographic testing should be *evaluation of prognosis* and as *a gateway to other imaging modalities*. Stand-alone testing for CAD diagnosis is reserved for patients with *intermediate risk for CAD*, and should be ordered with a careful understanding of the limitations of the test for this purpose.

1. The **advantages** of exercise electrocardiographic testing are its ability to assess a variety of prognostic markers, most importantly **functional capacity**, which is a powerful predictor of mortality, widespread availability, safety, ease of administration, and relatively low cost.
2. **Disadvantages.** As a screening test for CAD in persons without symptoms, exercise electrocardiography is not helpful. It has a **low sensitivity and specificity,** which can be improved with careful selection of the patient population undergoing testing.

B. Submaximal exercise electrocardiographic testing (i.e., testing at submaximal heart rate, which is discussed later) is a useful assessment before hospital discharge for **patients who have had MI.** The advantages are as follows:

1. It assists in setting **safe levels** of exercise (exercise prescription) and reassuring patients and families.
2. It is beneficial in **optimizing medical therapy,** in triage for intensity of follow-up testing and care, and in recognition of exercise-induced ischemia and arrhythmias.
3. For patients with uncomplicated MI who have received reperfusion therapy, submaximal exercise testing may be safely **performed as early as 3 days after MI,** with maximal exercise testing 3 to 6 weeks later.

II. INDICATIONS.

The indications for exercise electrocardiographic testing are divided into three classes on the basis of degree of likelihood of disease or severity of diagnosed disease (Table 42.1).

III. CONTRAINDICATIONS.

Contraindications to exercise testing are divided into absolute and relative categories (Table 42.2).

TABLE 42.1 ACC/AHA Guidelines for Exercise Testing

Exercise testing in diagnosis of obstructive coronary artery disease

Class 1[a]

- Adult patients (including those with complete right bundle-branch block or less than 1 mm of resting ST depression) with an intermediate pretest probability of coronary artery disease (CAD) on the basis of sex, age, and symptoms

Class 2a

- Patients with vasospastic angina

Class 2b

- Patients with a high pretest probability of CAD on the basis of age, symptoms, and sex
- Patients with a low pretest probability of CAD on the basis of age, symptoms, and sex
- Patients with less than 1 mm of baseline ST depression and taking digoxin
- Patients with electrocardiographic criteria of left ventricular hypertrophy and less than 1 mm of baseline ST depression

Class 3

- Patients with baseline electrocardiographic abnormalities
  - Preexcitation (Wolff-Parkinson-White) syndrome
  - Electronically paced ventricular rhythm
  - Greater than 1 mm of resting ST depression
  - Complete left bundle-branch block
- Patients with a documented myocardial infarction or prior coronary angiographic findings of disease and an established diagnosis of CAD (ischemia and risk can be determined with testing)

Risk assessment and prognosis among patients with symptoms or a history of coronary artery disease

Class 1

- Patients undergoing initial evaluation with suspected or known CAD (exceptions in class 2b), including those with complete right bundle-branch block or less than 1 mm of resting ST depression
- Patients with suspected or known CAD previously evaluated, now presenting with marked change in clinical status
- Low-risk, unstable angina patients 8 to 12 hours after presentation who have been free of active ischemic or heart failure symptoms
- Intermediate-risk unstable angina patients 2 to 3 days after presentation who have been free of active ischemic or heart failure symptoms

Class 2a

- Intermediate-risk unstable angina patients with initial cardiac markers that are normal, a repeat electrocardiographic study without significant change, cardiac markers 6 to 12 hours after symptom onset that are normal, and no other evidence of ischemia during observation

Class 2b

- Patients with baseline electrocardiographic abnormalities
  - Preexcitation (Wolff-Parkinson-White) syndrome
  - Electronically paced ventricular rhythm
  - 1 mm or more of resting ST depression
- Complete left bundle branch block or any interventricular conduction defect with QRS duration greater than 120 msec
- Patients with a stable clinical course who undergo periodic monitoring to guide treatment

Class 3

- Patients with severe comorbidity likely to limit life expectancy and/or candidacy for revascularization
- High-risk unstable angina patients

(*continued*)

TABLE 42.1 ACC/AHA Guidelines for Exercise Testing (*Continued*)

After acute myocardial infarction

Class 1

- Before discharge for prognostic assessment, activity prescription, or evaluation of medical therapy (submaximal at about 4 to 6 d)
- Early after discharge for prognostic assessment and cardiac rehabilitation if the predischarge exercise test was not performed (symptom limited, about 14 to 21 d)
- Late after discharge for prognostic assessment, activity prescription, evaluation of medical therapy, and cardiac rehabilitation if the early exercise test was submaximal (symptom limited, about 3 to 6 wk)

Class 2a

- After discharge for activity counseling or exercise training as part of cardiac rehabilitation of patients who have undergone coronary revascularization

Class 2b

- Patients with electrocardiographic abnormalities
  - Complete left bundle-branch block
  - Preexcitation (Wolff-Parkinson-White) syndrome
  - Left ventricular hypertrophy
  - Digoxin therapy
  - Electronically paced ventricular rhythm
  - Greater than 1 mm of resting ST depression
- Periodic monitoring for patients who continue to participate in exercise training or cardiac rehabilitation

Class 3

- Severe comorbidity likely to limit life expectancy or candidacy for revascularization
- Patients with acute myocardial infarction and uncompensated congestive heart failure, cardiac arrhythmia, or noncardiac conditions that severely limit exercise ability
- Before discharge, patients who have been selected for or have undergone cardiac catheterization (stress imaging tests are recommended)

Exercise testing for persons without symptoms or known coronary artery disease

Class 1

- None

Class 2a

- Asymptomatic persons with diabetes mellitus to start vigorous exercise

Class 2b

- Persons with multiple risk factors
- Men older than 45 years and women older than 55 years without symptoms
  - Who plan to start vigorous exercise (especially if sedentary)
  - Who are involved in occupations in which impairment might affect public safety
  - Who are at high risk for CAD because of other diseases

Class 3

- Routine screening of men or women without symptoms

[a] *Class 1,* Conditions for which there is evidence or agreement that a given procedure or treatment is useful and effective; *Class 2,* conditions for which there is conflicting evidence or a divergence of opinion about the usefulness or efficacy of a procedure or treatment; *Class 2a,* weight of evidence or opinion is in favor of usefulness and efficacy; *Class 2b,* usefulness or efficacy is less well established on the basis of evidence and opinion; *Class 3,* conditions for which there is evidence or general agreement that the procedure or treatment is not useful or effective and in some cases may be harmful.

From Gibbons RJ, Balady GJ, Bricker JT, et al. ACC/AHA 2002 Guideline update for exercise testing: a report of the American College of Cardiology/American Heart Association Task Force on Practice Guideline (Committee on Exercise Testing). *J Am Coll Cardiol* 2002;40:1531–1540, with permission.

TABLE 42.2 Contraindications to Exercise Testing
Absolute contraindications
Acute myocardial infarction (within 2 days)
High-risk unstable angina
Uncontrolled cardiac arrhythmias causing symptoms or hemodynamic compromise
Symptomatic, severe aortic stenosis
Uncontrolled symptomatic heart failure
Acute pulmonary embolus or pulmonary infarction
Suspected or known dissecting aneurysm
Active or suspected myocarditis, pericarditis, or endocarditis
Acute noncardiac disorder that may affect exercise performance or be aggravated by exercise (e.g., infection, renal failure, or thyrotoxicosis)
Considerable emotional distress (psychosis)
Relative contraindications
Left main coronary stenosis or its equivalent
Moderate stenotic valvular heart disease
Resting diastolic blood pressure >110 mm Hg or resting systolic blood pressure >200 mm Hg
Electrolyte abnormalities (e.g., hypokalemia, hypomagnesemia)
Fixed-rate pacemaker
High-degree atrioventricular block
Frequent or complex ventricular ectopy
Ventricular aneurysm
Uncontrolled metabolic disease (e.g., diabetes, thyrotoxicosis, myxedema)
Chronic infectious disease (e.g., mononucleosis, hepatitis, acquired immunodeficiency syndrome)
Neuromuscular, musculoskeletal, or rheumatoid disorders exacerbated by exercise
Advanced or complicated pregnancy
Hypertrophic cardiomyopathy and other forms of outflow tract obstruction
Mental impairment leading to inability to cooperate

Adapted from Kenney WL, Humphrey RH, Bryant CX, eds. *ACSM's guidelines for exercise testing and prescription.* Baltimore: Williams & Wilkins, 1995; from Fletcher GF, Fletcher GF, Blair SN, Blumenthal J, et al. Statement on exercise. Benefits and recommendations for physical activity programs for all Americans. A statement for health professionals by the Committee on Exercise and Cardiac Rehabilitation of the Council on Clinical Cardiology, American Heart Association. *Circulation* 1992;86:340–344; and from Gibbons RJ, Balady GJ, Bricker JT, et al. ACC/AHA 2002 Guideline update for exercise testing: a report of the American College of Cardiology/American Heart Association Task Force on Practice Guideline (Committee on Exercise Testing). *J Am Coll Cardiol* 2002;40:1531–1540.

IV. LIMITATIONS OF EXERCISE ELECTROCARDIOGRAPHIC TESTING. Before ordering an exercise electrocardiography test, the physician should have an understanding of Bayes' theorem and the limitations of the test.

A. Bayes' theorem states that the probability of a positive test result is affected by the likelihood (i.e., conditional probability) of a positive test result among the population that has undergone the test (i.e., pretest probability). The higher the probability that a disease is present in a given individual before a test is ordered, the higher is the probability that a positive test result is a true-positive test result. Pretest probability is determined on the basis of symptoms, age, sex, and risk factors, and can be divided into very low, low, intermediate, and high (Table 42.3).

B. Sensitivity and specificity. The likelihood that an abnormal electrocardiographic finding indicates CAD is much higher for an older person with multiple risk factors than for a young person with no risk factors. Sensitivity and specificity vary with the population being tested.

TABLE 42.3 Pretest Probability of Coronary Artery Disease According to Age, Sex, and Symptoms

Age (y)	Sex	Typical/ definite angina pectoris	Atypical/ probable angina pectoris	Nonanginal chest pain	Asymptomatic
30–39	Men	Intermediate	Intermediate	Low	Very Low
	Women	Intermediate	Very low	Very low	Very low
40–49	Men	High	Intermediate	Intermediate	Low
	Women	Intermediate	Low	Very low	Very low
50–59	Men	High	Intermediate	Intermediate	Low
	Women	Intermediate	Intermediate	Low	Very low
60–69	Men	High	Intermediate	Intermediate	Low
	Women	High	Intermediate	Intermediate	Low

Reproduced with permission from Gibbons RJ, Balady GJ, Bricker JT, et al. ACC/AHA 2002 Guideline update for exercise testing: a report of the American College of Cardiology/American Heart Association Task Force on Practice Guideline (Committee on Exercise Testing). *J Am Coll Cardiol* 2002;40:1531–1540.

1. Exercise electrocardiographic testing is **best used** in the evaluation of a patient at intermediate risk with an atypical history or a patient at low risk with a typical history.
2. For the general population, the sensitivity is 68%, and the specificity is 70%. Values are lower for persons at low risk.
3. Exercise electrocardiographic testing has a higher sensitivity and specificity for **persons at high risk.** For most of these patients, however, invasive testing is preferred for a more definitive diagnosis and possible intervention. Excluding patients with left ventricular hypertrophy or resting ST depression and those taking digoxin also improves sensitivity and specificity.

C. Positive predictive value (PPV). After pretest probability and the sensitivity and specificity are known, PPV can be calculated. PPV is a measure of the likelihood that an abnormal test finding represents a true-positive result. It is highly dependent on pretest probability (i.e., prevalence of disease) in the population being tested. For example, in a population at low risk, the PPV of electrocardiographic exercise testing is only 21%, but in a population at high risk, PPV rises to 83%.

V. PATIENT PREPARATION

A. Instructions. Table 42.4 provides a list of directions to give to patients before testing.

B. Medications

1. Before diagnostic testing, **cardiovascular drugs are withheld** at the discretion of and under the guidance of the supervising physician. This greatly increases the sensitivity of the test.
   a. **β-Blockers** pose a special problem. Patients taking β-blockers often do not have an adequate increase in heart rate to achieve the level of stress needed for the test. Abrupt withdrawal of β-blockers is to be discouraged because of reflex tachycardia. The best possible solution is to withdraw the β-blocker over several days before an exercise test, if the test is for diagnostic purposes. This is not always possible, however, because of time constraints or the necessity of drug therapy. In these cases, the clinician records that β-blockers were in use at the time of the test.
   b. **Digoxin** may cause problems in test interpretation. To avoid a reading that cannot be used to confirm a diagnosis, digoxin should be withheld for 2 weeks before testing.

TABLE 42.4 Patient Preparation

Patients should refrain from ingesting food, alcohol, or caffeine or using tobacco products within 3 hours of testing.
Patients should be rested for the assessment, avoiding significant exertion or exercise on the day of the assessment.
Patients should wear clothing that allows freedom of movement, including walking or running shoes, and a loose-fitting shirt with short sleeves that buttons down the front. They should not wear restrictive undergarments during the test.
Outpatients should be warned that the evaluation may be fatiguing and that they may wish to have someone available to drive them home afterward.
If the test is for diagnostic purposes, it may be helpful for patients to discontinue prescribed cardiovascular medication after discussion with their physician. Antianginal agents alter the hemodynamic response to exercise and significantly reduce the sensitivity of electrocardiographic changes for ischemia. Patients taking intermediate or high-dose beta-blockers should taper their medication over a 2- to 4-day period to minimize hyperadrenergic withdrawal responses.
If the test is for functional purposes, patients should continue their medication regimen on their usual schedule, so that the exercise responses will be consistent with responses expected during exercise training.
Patients should bring a list of their medications with them to the assessment.

Reproduced with permission from Kenney WL, Humphrey RH, Bryant CX, eds. *ACSM's Guidelines for exercise testing and prescription.* Baltimore: Williams & Wilkins, 1995.

2. Patients undergoing diagnostic testing take their **other usual medications** on the day of the test to reproduce more closely the conditions outside the exercise laboratory.

VI. EXERCISE PROTOCOLS. There are advantages and disadvantages to each exercise protocol (Table 42.5). Selection depends on patient characteristics, the equipment available, and the familiarity and comfort of the testing personnel with the protocol.

A. An **optimal protocol** achieves peak workload and maximizes the sensitivity and specificity of the test.

1. **Workload.** An optimal protocol incorporates a **gradual increase** in the level of work, so that the patient's true peak workload can be determined. If there are large increases in workload, maximum oxygen consumption (Mvo_2 max) may fall between two levels. The test also is more comfortable for the patient if the increases in workload are not large.
2. **Duration.** The optimal duration for an exercise test is **8 to 12 minutes.** Periods longer than this measure muscular endurance rather than cardiovascular fitness. Periods shorter than this do not allow adequate time for the patient to warm up and achieve maximum workloads.
3. **Stage length.** Steady-state oxygen consumption is reached after about 2 minutes of exercise at a given workload. The optimal protocol would have stage lengths of **2 to 3 minutes.**
4. **Exercise method.** Although **bicycle riding** is a better method for testing, **treadmill testing** is more common in the United States.
   a. The primary physiologic **advantage of bicycle riding** is the ability to take **direct measurements** of workload in watts, which has direct linear relation to Mvo_2. With a **treadmill**, the examiner can only **estimate workload** because workload depends on the efficiency of walking, the weight of the patient, and the change in energy expenditure between walking and running. Other advantages of a bicycle are the stable platform that it provides for electrocardiographic and blood pressure recordings, the smaller amount of space it occupies, quieter use, and a lower initial cost of equipment.

TABLE 42.5 Common Exercise Protocols

Functional class	O_2 Cost mL/kg per min	MET	Treadmill protocol: Bruce (3-min stages mph/grade)		Cornell (2-min stages mph/grade)		Balke (2-min stages mph/grade)		Naughton (2-min stages mph/grade)		Jogger (2-min stages mph/grade)	
World-class athlete	70.0	20	—	—	—	—	—	—	—	—	—	—
	66.5	19	6.0	22	—	—	—	—	—	—	—	—
	63.0	18	—	—	—	—	—	—	—	—	6.0	20.0
	59.5	17	5.5	20	—	—	—	—	—	—	6.0	17.5
Athlete	56.0	16	5.0	18	5.0	18	—	—	—	—	6.0	15.0
	52.5	15	—	—	—	—	4.0	20	—	—	6.0	12.5
	49.0	14	—	—	4.6	17	—	—	—	—	6.0	10.0
Fit	45.5	13	4.2	16	4.2	16	3.5	20	—	—	6.0	7.5
	42.0	12	—	—	—	—	—	—	—	—	6.0	5.0
	38.5	11	—	—	3.8	15	3.0	20.0	—	—	5.5	2.5
Normal and 1	35.0	10	3.4	14	3.4	14	3.0	17.5	—	—	5.0	2.5
	31.5	9	—	—	—	—	3.0	15.0	—	—	—	—
	28.0	8	—	—	3.0	13	3.0	12.5	2.0	21.0	—	—
	24.5	7	2.5	12	2.5	12	3.0	10.0	—	7.5	—	—
2	21.0	6	—	—	2.1	11	3.0	7.5	2.0	14.0	—	—
	17.5	5	1.7	10	1.7	10	3.0	5.0	2.0	10.5	—	—
	14.0	4	—	—	—	—	3.0	2.5	2.0	7.0	—	—
3	10.5	3	1.7	5	1.7	5	3.0	0	2.0	3.5	—	—
	7.0	2	1.7	0	1.7	0	—	—	2.0	0	—	—
4	3.5	1	—	—	—	—	—	—	1.0	0	—	—

MET, metabolic equivalent; mph, miles per hour.

b. Treadmill testing is used more commonly in the United States because most Americans do not regularly ride bicycles and, therefore, have less training and a subsequent (falsely) lower peak workload than that achieved on a treadmill.

B. Protocol options

1. Bruce protocol

a. Advantages. The Bruce protocol has been widely used in the past and often is the basis of older studies; therefore, **comparisons are easier.** Because the Bruce protocol has a final stage that cannot be completed, it is a good protocol for a highly fit person.

b. Disadvantages

(1) The main disadvantage of the Bruce protocol is the **large increments of change in workload between stages.** These large increases mean that peak workload falls somewhere between stages for many people. This is a problem in evaluating functional capacity and may result in a lower sensitivity for the test.

(2) The fourth stage of the Bruce protocol is an awkward stage that can be run or walked, resulting in divergent oxygen costs and workloads.

2. Modified Bruce protocol. Developed for less-fit persons, the modified Bruce protocol adds additional stages 0 and 1/2. These stages, at 1.7 mph (2.7 km/hour) with, respectively, 0% and 5% grades, provide a **lower workload for persons with poor cardiovascular fitness.** However, even these workloads may be too great for some debilitated patients and may result in premature fatigue.

3. Other protocols. Protocols superior to the Bruce protocol have been developed. These protocols have more gradual increases in workload and can be modified to suit the individual.

a. The **Naughton protocol** is good for older or debilitated persons and allows a gradual increase in workload.

b. The **Balke protocol** is good for younger, fit persons. It maintains a speed of 3, 3.5, or 4 mph (4.8, 5.6, or 6.4 km/hour) and increases the grade every 2 minutes.

c. The **Cornell protocol** is good for a wider range of fitness levels depending on starting grade. It allows for a gradual increase in grade and speed and may be started at 0%, 5%, or 10% grade, depending on fitness level.

d. Ramp protocols are computer-driven protocols that continuously increase workload until maximum exertion is reached. This is the ultimate in continuous advancement; but steady state may not be reached at any given workload.

VII. POTENTIAL COMPLICATIONS. Complications of exercise electrocardiographic testing are rare, but they do occur (Table 42.6). Exercise testing of healthy persons without CAD rarely results in cardiac complications, which are most likely to occur among persons with underlying CAD. Several researchers have looked at large numbers of unselected persons involved in various activities to determine risk.

A. Cardiac arrest

1. For the **general population,** there is approximately one cardiac arrest per 565,000 person-hours of exercise.

2. Among **persons with known CAD,** there is an estimated one arrest per 59,000 person-hours of vigorous activity. Exercise testing may precipitate acute coronary symptoms. Acute MI has been reported in approximately 1.4 per 10,000 exercise tests.

3. Among **persons at low risk** for CAD, however, the risk for cardiac arrest during exercise testing is much lower. In one study, no complications occurred in 380,000 exercise tests of young persons with presumably no heart disease.

B. Arrhythmic complications are a potential hazard of exercise testing (Table 42.7). Arrhythmias are more likely among persons with a history of arrhythmia. In this population, they occur in 9% of tests compared with an overall incidence of 0.1%.

1. Atrial fibrillation is the most common arrhythmia that occurs during testing, occurring in 9.5 per 10,000 tests.

2. Ventricular tachycardia is less common, occurring in 5.8 per 10,000 tests.

TABLE 42.6 Potential Medical Complications of Exercise Electrocardiographic Testing

Cardiovascular complications
Cardiac arrest
Ischemia
  Angina
  Myocardial infarction
Arrhythmias
  Superventricular tachycardia
  Atrial fibrillation
  Ventricular tachycardia
  Ventricular fibrillation
Bradyarrhythmias
  Bundle-branch blocks
  Atrioventricular nodal blocks
Congestive heart failure
Hypertension
Hypotension
Aneurysm rupture

Underlying medical conditions predisposing to increased complications
Hypertrophic cardiomyopathy
Coronary artery anomalies
Idiopathic left ventricular hypertrophy
Marfan's syndrome
Aortic stenosis
Right ventricular dysplasia
Congenital heart defects
Myocarditis
Pericarditis
Amyloidosis
Sarcoidosis
Long QT syndrome
Sickle cell trait
Sudden death

Pulmonary complications
Exercise-induced asthma
Bronchospasm
Pneumothorax
Exercise-induced anaphylaxis
Exacerbation of underlying pulmonary disease

Gastrointestinal complications
Vomiting
Cramps
Diarrhea

Neurologic complications
Dizziness
Syncope (fainting)
Cerebrovascular accident (stroke)

Musculoskeletal complications
Mechanical injuries
Back injuries
Joint pain or injury
Muscle cramps or spasms
Exacerbation of musculoskeletal disease

TABLE 42.7 Absolute and Relative Indications for Termination of an Exercise Test

Absolute indications
Acute myocardial infarction or suspicion of myocardial infarction
Onset of moderate to severe angina or increasing anginal pain
Drop in systolic blood pressure with increasing workload accompanied by signs or symptoms or drop below resting pressure
Serious arrhythmias (e.g., second- or third-degree atrioventricular block, sustained ventricular tachycardia or increasing premature ventricular contractions, atrial fibrillation with fast ventricular response)
Signs of poor perfusion, including pallor, cyanosis, or cold and clammy skin
Unusual or severe shortness of breath
Central nervous system symptoms, including ataxia, vertigo, visual or gait problems, or confusion
Technical inability to monitor the electrocardiogram
Patient's request
Relative indications
Pronounced electrocardiographic changes from baseline >2 mm of horizontal or downsloping ST-segment depression, or >2 mm of ST-segment elevation except in aVR
Any chest pain that is increasing
Physical or oral manifestations of severe fatigue or shortness of breath
Wheezing
Leg cramps or intermittent claudication (grade 3 on 4-point scale)
Hypertensive response (systolic blood pressure >260 mm Hg, diastolic blood pressure >115 mm Hg
Less serious arrhythmias such as supraventricular tachycardia
Exercise-induced bundle branch block that cannot be differentiated from ventricular tachycardia
General appearance

Adapted from Kenney WL, Humphrey RH, Bryant CX, eds. *ACSM's guidelines for exercise testing and prescription.* Baltimore: Williams & Wilkins, 1995; and from Fletcher GF, Blair SN, Blumenthal J, et al. Statement on exercise. Benefits and recommendations for physical activity programs for all Americans. A statement for health professionals by the Committee on Exercise and Cardiac Rehabilitation of the Council on Clinical Cardiology, American Heart association. *Circulation* 1992;86:340–344; and from Gibbons RJ, Balady GJ, Bricker JT, et al. ACC/AHA 2002 Guideline update for exercise testing: a report of the American College of Cardiology/American Heart Association Task Force on Practice Guideline (Committee on Exercise Testing). *J Am Coll Cardiol* 2002;40:1531–1540.

3. **Ventricular fibrillation** is even less common, occurring 0.67 times per 10,000 tests.

C. Deaths during exercise testing are exceedingly rare among well-monitored patients, but may occur in 1 of 25,000 tests. If death occurs, it is usually caused by sudden cardiac death or MI.

VIII. DATA

A. Electrocardiographic data. Although not the only data that should be examined, electrocardiographic changes garner the most attention (Table 42.8). The **portion of the electrocardiogram (ECG) most sensitive to ischemia** is the ST segment. The pathophysiologic mechanism of the ST change is net depression caused by a current of ischemia from the affected myocardial cells. The TP segment may be useful at rest and should be used when possible; however, it shortens or disappears with exercise. Baseline electrocardiographic abnormalities that can obscure the correct diagnosis of ST changes are listed in Table 42.9.

1. ST-segment changes

a. Measurement of the ST segment. There is no clear consensus as to where to measure the ST segment. Traditionally, it is measured 80 milliseconds past the J point, but some investigators suggest measuring at the J point or at the

TABLE 42.8 Baseline Abnormalities that May Obscure Electrocardiographic Changes During Exercise

Left bundle-branch block
Left ventricular hypertrophy with repolarization abnormality
Digitalis therapy
Ventricular paced rhythm
Wolff-Parkinson-White syndrome
ST abnormality associated with supraventricular tachycardia or atrial fibrillation
ST abnormalities with mitral valve prolapse and severe anemia

midpoint of the ST segment (using the end of the T wave or the peak of the T wave to determine the end of the segment) (Fig. 42.1A).

b. ST-segment changes are measured from the isoelectric baseline, which can be determined from the PR interval. If the ST segment is elevated at rest, any depression that occurs with exercise still is measured from the isoelectric line; early repolarization of the ST segment at rest is normal. If, however, the ST segment is depressed at rest, any further depression should be measured from the baseline ST segment (Fig. 42.1B).

c. Normal response. During exercise, there is depression of the J junction that is maximal at peak exercise and returns to baseline during recovery. This normal depression is upsloping and typically less than 1 mm below the isoelectric line 80 milliseconds after the J point.

d. ST depression does not localize the area of ischemia.

(1) ST depression of at least 1 mm that is horizontal or downsloping is abnormal, as is upsloping ST depression of at least 2.0 mm.

(2) Baseline ST abnormalities are less likely to represent exercise-induced myocardial ischemia, and the baseline ST depression should be subtracted from the peak ST depression.

(3) **Criteria that increase the probability of ischemia** are the **number of leads** involved (i.e., more leads increase the probability of ischemia), the **workload** at which the ST depression occurs (i.e., lower workload increases probability), the **angle of the slope** (i.e., a downsloping angle has a higher probability than a horizontal one), **ST-segment adjustment relative to**

TABLE 42.9 Functional Capacity Classifications by Age and Sex

Age (y)	Low[a]	Fair	Average	Good	High
Women					
20–29	<7.5	8–10.3	10.3–12.5	12.5–16	>16
30–39	<7	7–9	9–11	11–15	>15
40–49	<6	6–8	8–10	10–14	>14
50–59	<5	5–7	7–9	9–13	>13
60–69	<4.5	4.5–6	6–8	8–11.5	>11.5
Men					
20–29	<8	8–11	11–14	14–17	>17
30–39	<7.5	7.5–10	10–12.5	12.5–16	>16
40–49	<7	7–8.5	8.5–11.5	11.5–15	>15
50–59	<6	6–8	8–11	11–14	>14
60–69	<5.5	5.5–7	7–9.5	9.5–13	>13

[a]Functional capacities are given in metabolic equivalents (METs).

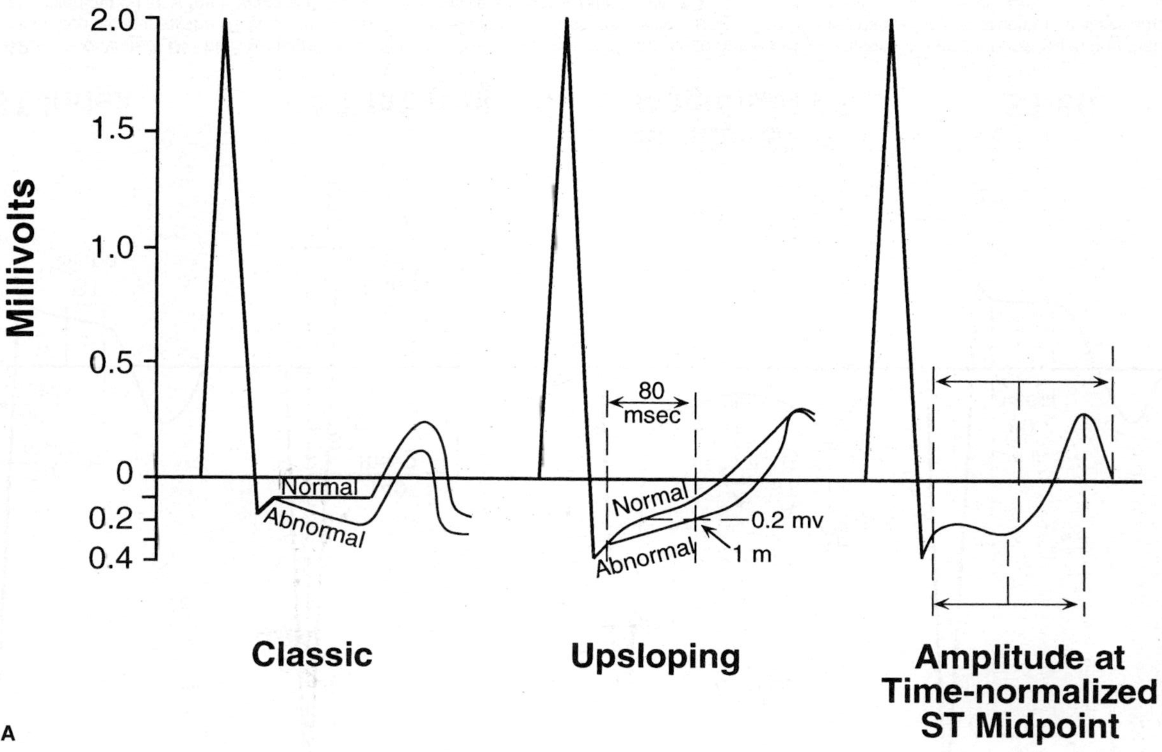

Figure 42.1. **A:** Blomqvist recommended using the end of the T wave for measuring the midpoint of the ST segement, but Simons used the peak of the T wave. This change was made to have a more stable endpoint, because the end of the T wave is much more difficult to find than the peak of the T wave. (*continued*)

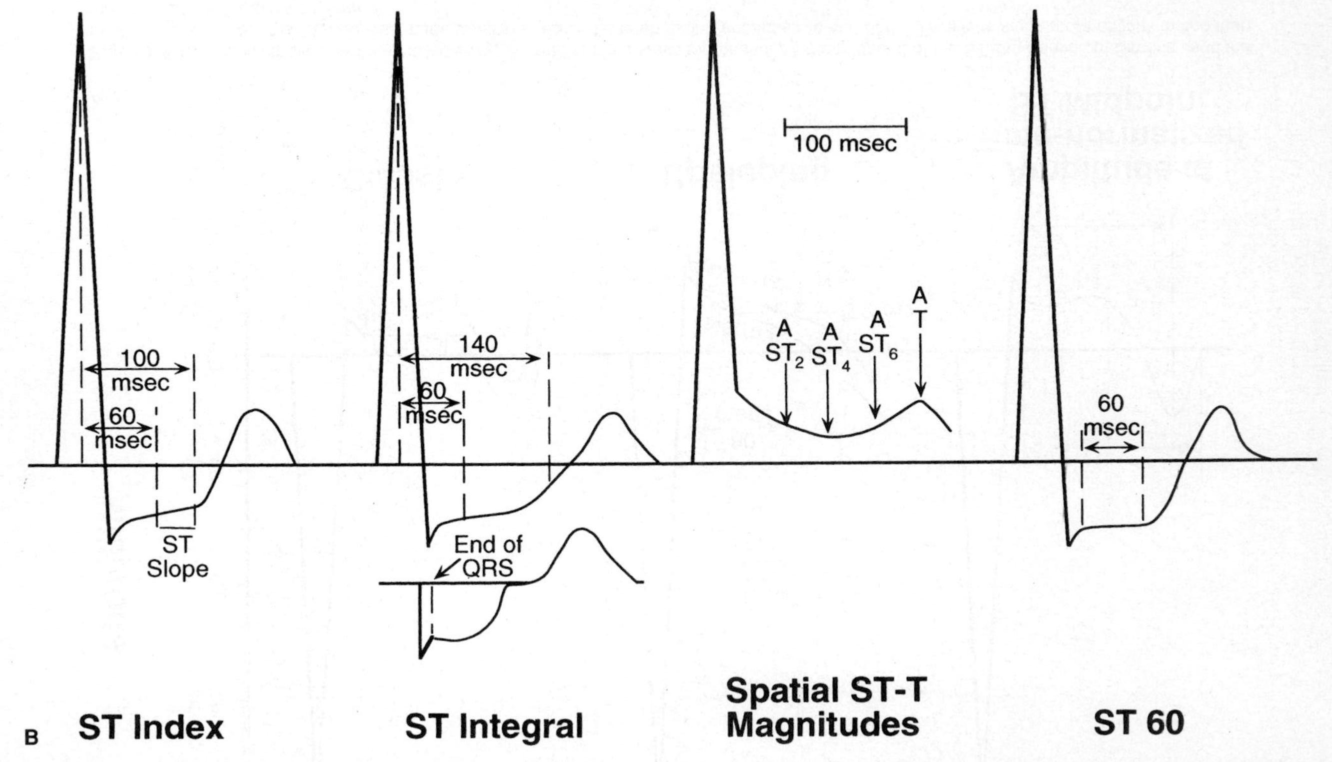

Figure 42.1. (*Continued*) **B:** The ST integral, as defined by Sheffield, required that the end of the QRS complex, or J junction, be found and that the area measurement stop as soon as the ST segment crossed the isoelectric line or as the T wave began. The ST integral used by most commercial systems initiates the area at a fixed period after the R wave and then ends 80 milliseconds thereafter.

heart rate (ST/HR index), amount of time in recovery before normalization of the ST segment (i.e., longer recovery increases the probability), and possibly the **magnitude of the depression.** Changes in the lateral leads, particularly V_5, are more specific than in any of the other leads. Changes in the inferior leads alone are likely to be a false-positive result.

e. The **meaning of ST elevation** depends on the presence or absence of Q waves of prior MI.

(1) ST-segment elevation **with Q waves of prior MI** is a common finding among patients who have had MI. It occurs among up to 50% of patients with anterior MI and 15% of patients with previous inferior MI, and it is not caused by ischemia. The mechanism is thought to be dyskinetic myocardium or ventricular aneurysms. There may even be reciprocal ST-segment depression. Patients with more extensive Q waves have more pronounced ST elevation. These patients typically have a lower ejection fraction than those without elevated ST segment with a Q wave. These changes do not imply ischemia (although they may imply viability) and should be interpreted as normal.

(2) ST-segment elevation **without Q waves of prior MI** represents marked transmural myocardial ischemia. ST elevation also may indicate the location of the ischemia. This finding should be interpreted as abnormal.

f. ST normalization, or the lack of ST changes during exercise, **may be a sign of ischemia.** This phenomenon occurs when ischemic ST depression and ST elevation cancel one another. This effect is rare but should be considered in tests of patients with no electrocardiographic changes but with a high likelihood of CAD.

2. R waves may change in amplitude during exercise. There is no diagnostic value in these changes.

3. T wave and U wave changes

a. The **T wave** normally decreases gradually in early exercise and begins to increase in amplitude at maximal exercise. One minute into recovery, the T wave should be back to baseline. T-wave **inversion is not a specific marker of ischemia** and may occur normally.

b. If the U wave is upright at baseline, **U-wave inversion** may be associated with ischemia, left ventricular hypertrophy, and valvular disease.

4. Arrhythmias. Table 42.7 lists abnormal arrhythmias that may occur during exercise. Ectopic atrial and ventricular beats during exercise are not predictive of outcome, but ventricular ectopy during recovery may be associated with worse outcome. Sustained ventricular tachycardia and ventricular fibrillation are abnormal but rarely occur.

5. Time to resolution of changes. The longer into recovery that it takes for electrocardiographic changes to resolve, the higher is the probability that they are important. Rapid recovery (<1 min) indicates less likelihood of disease and that disease if present is less severe.

6. Bundle-branch block or conduction delay. Exercise-induced left bundle-branch block is predictive of a worse outcome.

B. Age-predicted maximum heart rate (APMHR). Many formulas have been developed to predict maximum heart rate (MHR). These formulas are generated by measuring MHR in a sample population and plotting a regression line against various factors that may affect heart rate. There is a great deal of scatter on either side on the regression line, and the fit of the line seldom reaches an *r* value greater than 0.9. It is well known that MHR decreases with age, and most equations incorporate age. The two most common formulas are as follows:

$$\text{APMHR} = 220 - \text{age}$$
$$\text{APMHR} = 200 - 1/2\ \text{age}$$

The APMHR may be much lower or much higher than a person's actual measured MHR. **Heart rate should not be used as an indicator of maximal exertion or in**

the decision to terminate testing, except in a submaximal test. If MHR does not exceed 85% of APMHR during testing and there are no substantial electrocardiographic changes, the test is usually read as nondiagnostic. If there are substantial electrocardiographic changes, the test is read as abnormal, regardless of the heart rate achieved.

C. Rating of perceived exertion (RPE) is a better marker of maximal level of exertion.

1. A useful indicator of percentage of maximum workload achieved is the **RPE scale.** This is a subjective scale used to rate how hard much effort the subject feels they are expending during an exercise test. The subject should be advised to rate how he or she feels overall and not according to an individual element such as leg fatigue. Although subjective, the scale has been shown to be reproducible, and maximum ratings correspond well with maximum exertion.
   a. The **Borg scale** is used most often. The original scale ranges from 6 to 20, which is meant to correspond to a heart rate increase from 60 to 200 beats/min during exercise.
   b. The **modified Borg scale** is 0 to 10. The scale includes word anchors, which are important for accurate assessment of work level. The scales are not linear, and at higher workloads, the changes in RPE are closer together.
2. A maximal level of exertion is marked by a score greater than 18 (Borg scale) or 9 (modified Borg scale), respiratory quotient (RQ) greater than 1.1 (if carbon dioxide exchange is monitored), and overall patient appearance.

D. In addition to electrocardiographic monitoring, **blood pressure monitoring** is an important aspect of the exercise test for safety and for the diagnosis of CAD. It should be checked in each walking stage. It may not be practical to check blood pressure while the subject is running.

1. **Systolic blood pressure** (SBP) normally rises during exercise. A **failure of SBP to rise** with increasing workload or a drop in SBP usually indicates the presence of CAD and is an indication to **terminate testing.**
2. **Diastolic blood pressure** decreases with exercise and may be audible down to zero during vigorous activity. Unlike SBP, diastolic blood pressure is not useful in diagnosis or safety monitoring.

E. Symptoms. The presence or absence of symptoms and their change over time are included in the final report.

F. Functional capacity. Functional testing is a powerful marker for prognosis. Persons who achieve more than 6 metabolic equivalents (METs) of workload have a significantly lower mortality rate than those who do not achieve this workload, regardless of electrocardiographic changes. On the basis of age and workload achieved, functional capacity can be divided into five classifications (Table 42.9). Among 3400 patients with no history of diagnosed CAD undergoing exercise testing at the Cleveland Clinic, those with average or better classifications had a 2.5-year mortality of less than 2%, compared with 6% and 14% for those who were in the fair and poor groups. The adjusted relative risk for fair or poor functional capacity in this population was almost 4.

IX. TERMINATION OF EXERCISE TESTING. The American Heart Association (AHA) and American College of Sports Medicine (ACSM) have developed very similar indications for exercise termination (Table 42.7). The decision when to terminate a test ultimately relies on the expertise and judgment of those performing the test.

A. Absolute indications are all serious findings. A drop in SBP with increasing workload is a particularly ominous sign and usually, but not always, indicates the presence of severe CAD.

B. Relative indications for termination of testing are findings that should increase the level of concern and vigilance among those administering the test and possibly cause cessation of testing. Relative indications for termination rely heavily on the judgment of the personnel performing the test, and the decision to continue the test should not be made lightly (Table 42.7).

C. Indications for termination of submaximal exercise testing include any one of the following endpoints:

1. Signs or symptoms of ischemia
2. Achievement of a workload of 6 METs
3. Eighty-five percent of the APMHR
4. Heart rate of 110 beats/min for a patient taking β-blockers
5. A score on the Borg RPE of 17 or modified Borg RPE of 7

D. Postexercise recovery

1. In **all routine exercise tests, a cool-down period** adds safety to the test. The length of the cool-down period may vary from 30 seconds to several minutes, depending on the person. A general rule is to allow enough time for the heart rate to drop to less than 110 beats/min. A shorter cool-down period increases the sensitivity of exercise ECG because of increased venous return; resuming the supine position leads to increased wall stress. This same mechanism also increases the risk of testing.
2. The exception to observing a cool-down period may be made for exercise echocardiography, in which it is important to image the subject when he or she is as close as possible to maximum heart rate.

X. INTERPRETATION OF DATA. An experienced clinician must interpret an exercise electrocardiographic test. Although the terms *positive* and *negative* often are used, these terms do not accurately describe the results of an exercise electrocardiographic test and should be avoided. The information to include in an exercise electrocardiographic report is listed in Table 42.10.

A. Exercise electrocardiographic test results can be normal, abnormal, normal except for, or nondiagnostic (Table 42.11). Nondiagnostic tests are those in which the subject does not achieve 85% of APMHR and has no abnormal electrocardiographic changes or in which baseline electrocardiographic changes are present that obscure ST changes (Table 42.8).

B. Prognosis.

1. The **Duke nomogram** (Fig. 42.2) is a simple chart that factors in ST-segment deviation, amount of angina during exercise, and exercise capacity to give an

TABLE 42.10 Elements of Conclusion Section of a Modern Exercise Test Report

Exercise protocol used, duration of exercise, peak treadmill speed and grade, maximum heart rate and percentage of age-predicted maximum heart rate achieved, resting and peak blood pressure, and symptoms
(Negative/positive/equivocal) standard ST-segment response to exercise
The ST/HR index of ≤1.6 μV/bpm is consistent with the absence of obsturctive coronary disease and makes anatomically, functionally, and prognostically important coronary disease unlikely"; "The ST/HR index >1.6 μV/bpm is consistent with the presence of obsturctive coronary disease and predicts increased cardiovascular risk
The estimated functional capacity of (X METs) predicts (high/low) risk of all-cause mortality
The Duke treadmill score of (X) predicts a cardiac mortality of (X%) per year over the next 5 years. This implies a (low/intermediate/high) risk
The chronotropic response index of (0.XX) predicts an (increased/decreased) risk of death compared with the Duke treadmill score. For patients not on β-blockers, a value ≤0.80 raises concerns; for patients on β-blockers, a value ≤0.62 is abnormal
The heart rate recovery of (X bpm) further predicts an (increased/decreased) risk of death
The (presence/absence) of frequent ventricular ectopy during recovery further (increases/decreases) predicted risk of death

Adapted from: Kligfield P, Lauer MS. Exercise electrocardiogram testing: beyond the ST segment. *Circulation* 2006;114;2070–2082.

TABLE 42.11 Guidelines for Interpretation of Results of Exercise Electrocardiography

Variable	Normal	Normal except for	Abnormal
Symptoms	Neuromuscular chest pain	Angina as an isolated finding	Syncope
	Fatigue, shortness of breath, leg or joint pain	Atypical angina	Angina when associated with ST- or T-wave changes, including borderline
		Chest discomfort of questionable causation	Angina when associated with exercise hypotension
		Claudication	
		Dizziness, lightheadedness	
		Other noteworthy symptoms	
Blood pressure response (mm Hg)	SBP increases >10 but is <230 at peak	SBP ≥ 230 at peak exercise	Any drop in SBP as exercise intensity increases
	DBP increases ≤ 10 but is <120 at peak	DBP ≥ 120 at peak exercise	
	DBP stays the same or decreases	DBP ≥ 12 increase from rest if peak is ≥ 100	
	DBP increases ≥ 12 from rest but peak is <100		
Arrhythmias	Occasional PVCs	Paroxysmal SVT	Sustained SVTs, AFIB, atrial flutter, or junctional rhythm
	PACs	Increased frequency of PVCs or couplets during exercise	Nonsustained VT
	Frequent PACs or PVCs at rest that abate during exercise	Isolated run of nonsustained VT	Second- or third-degree AV block
	Chronic AFIB, atrial flutter	Ventricular couplets	AV dissociation
		Paroxysmal escape rhythms	Exercise induced before excitation
			Idioventricular rhythm
			Very abnormal
			Sustained VT (≥ 30 s)
			VF/cardiac arrest
			Asystole

ST segments	<1.0 mm ST depression or elevation	Borderline ST changes (0.5–0.9 mm ST depression) ST elevation in leads in area of prior MI T-wave inversion Pseudonormalization of resting T-wave abnormalities	≥1.0 mm H or D ST depression ≥1.5 mm upsloping ST depression ≥1.0 mm U ST depression if associated with anginal symptoms ≥1.0 mm ST elevation in leads without q waves or not over a prior MI *Very abnormal* ≥2.0 mm H or D ST depression ≥2.5 mm upsloping ST depression ≥2.0 mm ST elevation in leads without Q waves or not over a prior MI
Functional capacity	Normal or mildly impaired exercise tolerance	Low exercise tolerance	Inability to achieve 3 MET workload

AFIB, atrial fibrillation; AV, atrioventricular; D, downsloping; DBP, diastolic blood pressure; H, horizontal; MET, metabolic equivalent; MI, myocardial infarction; PAC, premature atrial contraction; PVC, premature ventricular contraction; SBP, systolic blood pressure; SVT, supraventricular tachycardia; U, upsloping; VF, ventricular fibrillation; VT, ventricular tachycardia.

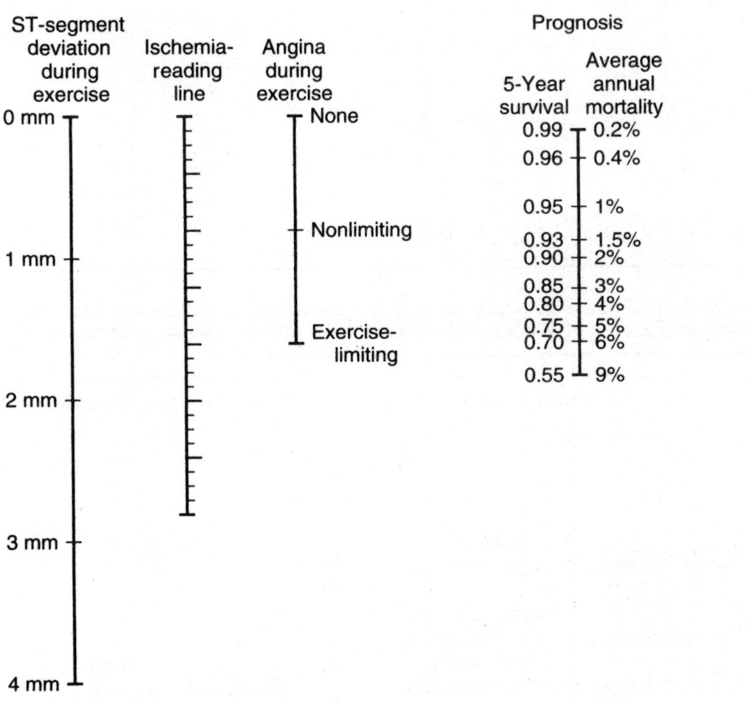

Figure 42.2. Duke nomogram for estimation of the prognosis.

estimate of 5-year survival and average annual mortality. This nomogram was derived by means of regression analysis and can be a useful tool in determining prognosis and the degree of aggressiveness needed in treating a patient. The **Duke treadmill score (DTS)** is a numeric form of the nomogram and has been validated in several studies as an important predictor of mortality.

$$\text{DTS} = \text{the duration of exercise (in minutes)}$$

$$-(5 \times \text{maximal ST-segment deviation}) - (4 \times \text{angina score})$$

In the previous equation, 0 = no angina, 1 = non–test-limiting angina, and 2 = exercise-limiting angina.
Low risk: DTS $\geq +5$
Intermediate risk: DTS – 10 to $<+5$
High risk: DTS <-10

2. The **heart rate recovery**, defined as the decrease in heart rate from peak exercise to 1 minute after cessation of exercise, has important prognostic significance. A heart rate recovery of 12 beats/min or less is considered abnormal during an upright cool-down period. For patients assuming an immediate supine position, such as during exercise echocardiography, a value of less than 18 beats/min is considered abnormal.
3. The **chronotropic response index (CRI)** is a measure of maximal heart rate in relation to chronotropic reserve. A normal response is defined as a CRI of more than 0.8 (0.62 for patients on β-blockers).

   $$\text{CRI} = (\text{peak HR} - \text{resting HR})/(\text{age} - \text{predicted maximum HR} - \text{resting HR})$$

4. **Ventricular ectopy in recovery** from exercise, including frequent ventricular ectopics (>7 per minute), couplets, bigeminy, trigeminy, ventricular tachycardia, and ventricular fibrillation have been shown to be predictive of all-cause mortality. These findings in recovery are a better predictor of death than ventricular ectopy during exercise.
5. A recently published **nomogram (Lauer et al.,** ***Ann Intern Med,*** **2007;147:821–828)** for patients with suspected CAD and a normal ECG undergoing exercise treadmill testing demonstrates how a simple combination of clinical and stress-testing variables can be used to predict mortality.

ACKNOWLEDGMENTS

The author thanks Drs. Christopher Cole and Judy Huang for their contributions to earlier editions of this chapter.

Key Reviews

Kligfield P, Lauer MS. Exercise electrocardiogram testing: beyond the ST-segment. *Circulation* 2006;114:2070–2082.

Lauer MS, Sivarajan Froelicher E, Williams M, et al. Exercise Testing in Asymptomatic Adults: A Statement for Professionals From the American Heart Association Council on Clinical Cardiology, Subcommittee on Exercise, Cardiac Rehabilitation, and Prevention. Circulation 2005;112:771–776.

Gibbons RJ, Balady GJ, Bricker JT, et al. ACC/AHA 2002 Guideline update for exercise testing: a report of the American College of Cardiology/American Heart Association Task Force on Practice Guideline (Committee on Exercise Testing). *J Am Coll Cardiol* 2002;40:1531–1540.

Books

Wasserman K, Hansen JE, Sue DY, et al., eds. *Principles of exercise testing and interpretation,* 4th ed. Philadelphia: Lippincott, 2005.

43 NUCLEAR IMAGING

Gregory G. Bashian

I. INTRODUCTION. Nuclear cardiology has an integral role in the noninvasive detection of coronary artery disease (CAD), assessment of myocardial viability, and stratification of risk. It imparts improved sensitivity and specificity over standard exercise stress testing. The average sensitivity of single photon emission computed tomography (SPECT) with technetium 99m is reported to be 90%, and the average specificity is 74%. Nuclear imaging can provide functional and prognostic information, is quantifiable and reproducible, and is readily obtainable in diverse patient populations.

II. INDICATIONS (Table 43.1)

A. Diagnosis of CAD. Nuclear perfusion studies are performed to establish noninvasively the diagnosis of CAD in the following situations: history of **stable angina; chest pain of unclear causation; unstable angina** after stabilization; **abnormal exercise test result** without symptoms; **screening** for risk factors; scheduled standard exercise testing in the setting of an **abnormal electrocardiogram (ECG);** and previously **nondiagnostic graded exercise test.**

B. Assessment of the physiologic importance of known CAD. Perfusion imaging is utilized in the care of patients with borderline coronary stenosis (40% to 70%) and small-vessel stenosis in a distal branch. It is also useful to evaluate a specific coronary lesion before percutaneous intervention.

C. Assessment after therapeutic intervention. Perfusion imaging is often performed as a routine follow-up procedure after percutaneous intervention, coronary artery bypass grafting, or medical therapy, and for evaluation of recurrent symptoms.

D. Risk stratification. With nuclear imaging, it is possible to stratify risk among patients with stable angina or unstable angina, those who have had myocardial infarction (MI), and those about to undergo noncardiac operations.

E. Identification of MI among patients with angiographically normal coronary arteries is afforded by nuclear imaging.

III. CONTRAINDICATIONS. In addition to standard contraindications to exercise stress testing, specific considerations apply uniquely to nuclear imaging in general and the subgroup of dipyridamole stress perfusion studies.

A. General contraindications to nuclear studies. Nuclear imaging is contraindicated for patients who have had **iodine 131 therapy** within 12 weeks; **technetium 99m studies** within 48 hours, including bone, lung, multigated acquisition (MUGA), liver, tagged red blood cell (to evaluate gastrointestinal bleeding), and renal scans; **indium 111 scans** within 30 days; **gallium 67 scans** within 30 days; **oral intake** within 4 hours (except for water); and **caffeine** consumption within 4 hours.

B. Contraindications to dipyridamole and adenosine administration include allergy to dipyridamole or adenosine, allergy to aminophylline, ongoing theophylline therapy (must be discontinued for 36 hours), history of asthma or reactive airway disease, significant AV nodal block, and caffeine consumption within 12 to 24 hours.

IV. EQUIPMENT. The most basic tool in nuclear imaging is the **gamma or scintillation camera,** which is used to detect gamma rays (i.e., x-ray photons) produced by the chosen radionuclide. Three types of gamma camera exist.

A. A single-crystal camera consists of one large sodium iodide crystal. Other essential elements of this camera include the **collimator**, a lead device that screens out

TABLE 43.1 Indications for Nuclear Imaging Based on ACC/AHA/ASNC Guidelines (Class I indications only)

Disease state	Class	Test	Specific indication
Suspected ACS in emergency department	I A	Rest MPI	Assessment of myocardial risk when ECG and initial serum enzymes and markers are nondiagnostic
	I B	Stress/Rest MPI	Diagnosis of CAD in patients with chest pain, nondiagnostic ECG and negative serum markers/enzymes or normal resting scan
Risk assessment, prognosis, and assessment of therapy in STEMI	I B	ECG-gated SPECT MPI	Assess resting LV function
	I B	ECG-gated SPECT MPI with stress	Detection of inducible ischemia and myocardium at risk in patients treated with thrombolytic therapy without catheterization
	I B	ECG-gated SPECT MPI with stress and rest	Assessment of infarct size and and residual viable myocardium
Risk assessment, prognosis, and assessment of therapy in NSTEMI and UA	I B	ECG-gated SPECT MPI with stress	Identification of inducible ischemia in the distribution of the 'culprit lesion' or in remote areas in patients with intermediate or low risk of major adverse cardiac events
	I A	ECG-gated SPECT MPI with stress	Identfication of severity/extent of inducible ischemia in patients whose angina is satisfactorily stabilized with medical therapy or in whom diagnosis is uncertain
	I B	Stress MPI	Identification of hemodynamic significance of coronary stenosis after coronary angiography
	I B	ECG-gated SPECT MPI	Measurement of baseline LV function

(*continued*)

TABLE 43.1 Indications for Nuclear Imaging Based on ACC/AHA/ASNC Guidelines (Class I indications only) (*Continued*)

Disease state	Class	Test	Specific indication
Diagnosis or risk stratification in patients with intermediate or high likelihood of CAD and who *are able* to exercise	I B	Exercise SPECT MPI	Evaluate extent, severity and location of ischemia in patients without LBBB or ventricular pacemaker but do have a baseline ECG abnormality (which interferes with ETT)
	I B	Adenosine/dipyrid-amole SPECT	Patients with LBBB or ventricular paced rhythm
	I B	Exercise SPECT MPI	Assess the functional significance of intermediate coronary lesions
	I B	Exercise SPECT MPI	Intermediate Duke treadmill score
Diagnosis or risk stratification in patients with intermediate or high likelihood of CAD and who *are unable* to exercise	I B	Adenosine/dipyrid-amole SPECT	Identify extent, severity and location of ischemia
	I B	Adenosine/dipyrid-amole SPECT	Assess functional significance intermediate coronary lesions
Risk assessment prior to noncardiac surgery	I B	ECG-gated SPECT MPI with stress	Initial diagnosis of CAD with intermediate pretest probability of disease and abnormal baseline ECG or inability to exercise
	I B	ECG-gated SPECT MPI with stress	Evaluation of patients after change in clinical status (e.g., ACS) with abnormal baseline ECG or inability to exercise
	I B	Adenosine/dipyrid-amole SPECT	Initial diagnosis of CAD in patients with LBBB with intermediate pretest probability of disease
	I C	Adenosine/dipyrid-amole SPECT	Assessment of patients with intermediate clinical risk predictors and poor functional capacity (<4 METS) who require high-risk noncardiac surgery
	I C	ECG-gated SPECT MPI with stress	Assessment of patients with intermediate clinical risk predictors, abnormal ECG and moderate or higher functional capacity (>4 METS) who require high-risk noncardiac surgery

Adapted from the 2003 ACC/AHA/ASNC Guidelines for the Clinical Use of Cardiac Radionuclide Imaging.

background or scattered photons, and the **photomultiplier**, an electronic processor that translates photon interactions with the crystal into electric energy.

1. Electric signals from the photomultiplier are processed by the **pulse height analyzer** before reaching a final form. Only signals in a specified energy range are incorporated into the interpreted images. The range recognized by the pulse height analyzer is adjustable and is established on the basis of the radiopharmaceutical used.
2. **Digitalization** of the single-crystal camera has greatly enhanced its performance.

B. A **multicrystal camera** works with an array of crystals with increased count-detection capability. Because of the availability of an individual crystal to detect scintillation at any given time, this type of camera can be used to detect many more counts than a single-crystal camera can (up to 600,000 counts/s, compared with 200,000 to 400,000 counts/s for a single-crystal camera).

C. A **positron camera** is a gamma camera used to detect the photon products of positron annihilation. Interaction between a positron and an electron causes annihilation with the generation of two high-energy photons (511 keV) that travel in opposite directions.

1. An array of multiple concentric rings of crystals constitute a positron camera. Each crystal is linked optically to multiple photomultipliers. The crystals are oriented in diametric pairs in such a way that each pair of crystals must be struck simultaneously by annihilation photons to record activity. Background interference and stray photon energy are automatically accounted for, and artifact is limited.
2. Most positron cameras contain **bismuth germanite** for annihilation photon detection. The clinical utility and radiopharmaceuticals for positron emission tomography (PET) are discussed in section X.

V. MECHANICS AND TECHNIQUES

A. Image acquisition. Basic perfusion imaging can be performed by means of **planar** and **tomographic** techniques.

1. **Planar images** are acquired in three views: **anterior, left anterior oblique (LAO)**, and **steep LAO** or **left lateral orientation (LLAT)** (Fig. 43.1). The patient is supine for anterior and LAO views, but is placed in the lateral decubitus position for LLAT image acquisition. Although it allows examination of specific myocardial segments, planar imaging superimposes vascular distributions and therefore can compromise the ability to implicate a specific vascular supply when a defect is present. For example, normally perfused myocardial segments may overlap perfusion defects in a separate distribution.
2. Using SPECT, a series of planar images usually are obtained over a 180-degree arc to reconstruct a three-dimensional representation of the heart. The arc typically extends from the 45-degree right anterior oblique plane to the 45-degree left posterior oblique plane with the patient in the supine position.
   a. Three orientations are analyzed in the final representation: **short axis, vertical long axis**, and **horizontal long axis.** A computer-generated display, the **polar map**, also is analyzed as a quantifiable representation of count density.
   b. Unlike planar imaging, **SPECT** can be used to **separate vascular territories** and improve image interpretation. SPECT, however, also **increases the time needed** for image acquisition and requires close attention to quality-control issues.

B. Radiopharmaceuticals available for nuclear imaging include thallium 201, technetium 99m, and several positron imaging agents. Each possesses specific energy characteristics, kinetic profiles, and biodistribution (Tables 43.2 and 43.3).

1. **Thallium 201**
   a. **General characteristics.** Thallium 201 (i.e., thallous chloride) is a metallic element in group IIIA of the periodic table; it is produced in a cyclotron. Thallium emits gamma-rays at an energy range of 69 to 83 keV, and has a **half-life of 73 hours.** The biologic activity of this element is very similar to that of potassium; the ionic radii of the two elements are virtually identical. Thallium

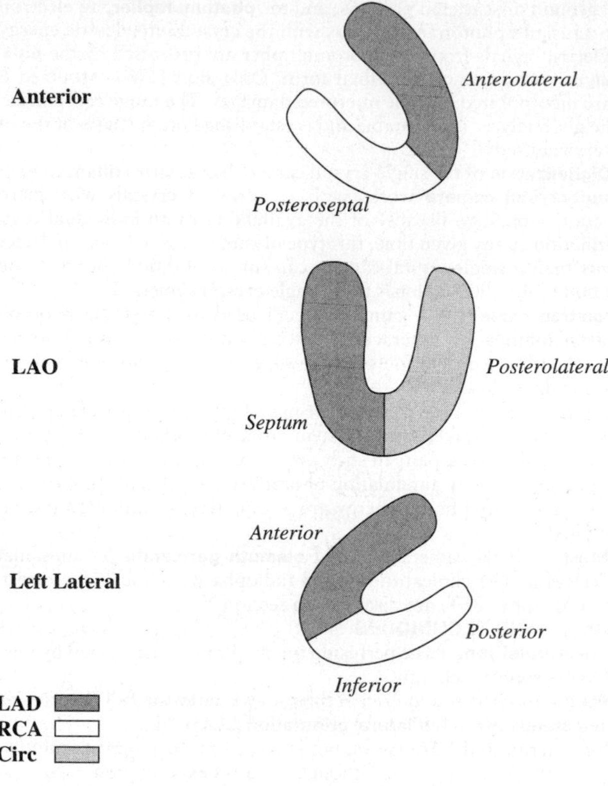

Figure 43.1. Standard planar views and vascular territories.

is actively transported into cells by the sodium-potassium–adenosine triphosphatase (Na-K–ATPase) pump.

b. Kinetics. Approximately 5% of the administered dose of thallium 201 is distributed to the myocardium, proportionate to the blood flow delivered to the coronary circulation. Almost 85% of the thallium 201 is extracted by myocytes in the first pass.

(1) The **initial uptake** of thallium 201 by myocardium is directly related to regional blood flow. The myocardial extraction of thallium 201, however, increases at low flow rates (<10% of basal) and decreases at high flow rates (more than twice basal rate).

(2) Washout. After initial uptake into myocytes, a state of continuous exchange across the cell membrane occurs. The distribution of this radiotracer changes after administration, and thallium 201 washes out from the myocytes, a process called **redistribution.** Thallium 201 washout generally approaches 30% at 2 to 2.5 hours after injection.

(3) Ischemic myocardium. Uptake of thallium 201 in ischemic myocardium is lower than uptake in nonischemic segments. Washout time from ischemic zones is slower than that from nonischemic zones.

(4) Over time, counts become equal in the ischemic and nonischemic regions (or thallium 201 concentration may increase in ischemic regions) so that thallium 201 concentrations in these disparate areas approach one

TABLE 43.2 Characteristics of Common Perfusion Agents

Attribute	Thallium 201	Technetium 99m sestamibi	Technetium 99m tetrofosmin	Technetium 99m teboroxime
Energy (keV)	69–83	140	140	140
Dose (mCi)	2.5–3.5	20–30	20–30	20–30
Half-life (h)	74	6	6	6
Cyclotron required	Yes	No	No	No
Perfusion imaging	Yes	Yes	Yes	Yes
Viability evaluation	Yes	Yes	Yes?	No
Redistribution	Yes	Yes (minimal)	Yes (minimal)	Yes
Gating (electrocardiogram)	No	Yes	Yes	No

another. This disparity is taken advantage of during thallium 201 viability imaging (described below).

2. **Technetium 99m–labeled agents**
   a. **General characteristics.** Technetium 99m is a radiopharmaceutical that can be produced on site in molybdenum 99–technetium 99m generators. It possesses several ideal imaging characteristics.
      (1) Technetium-99m has a **half-life of 6 hours** and emits gamma rays with a single photopeak of 140 keV.
      (2) Technetium-99m–labeled **perfusion agents** include ^{99m}**Tc-sestamibi,** ^{99m}**Tc-tetrofosmin,** and ^{99m}**Tc-teboroxime**. Although ^{99m}Tc-sestamibi

TABLE 43.3 Radiopharmaceuticals Useful In Single Photon Emission Computed Tomography

Myocardial perfusion
- Thallium 201
- [^{99m}Tc]isonitriles (sestamibi)
- [^{99m}Tc]tetrofosmin
- Thallium 201 (reinjection)

Myocardial metabolism
- [^{123}I]hexadecanoic acid
- [^{123}I]heptadecanoic acid
- [^{123}I]iodophenylpentadecanoic acid

Myocardial infarction
- [^{99m}Tc]pyrophosphate
- [^{99m}Tc]tetracycline
- [^{99m}Tc]glucoheptonate
- ^{111}In-labeled antimyosin antibody
- ^{131}I-labeled antimyosin antibody

Myocardial innervation and receptor
- [^{123}I]metaiodobenzylguanidine (MIBG)
- [^{123}I]3-quinuclidinyl-4-iodobenzylate (QNB)

Coronary thrombosis
- ^{111}In-labeled antifibrin antibody
- ^{111}In-labeled antiplatelet antibody
- ^{131}I-labeled antiplatelet antibody
- ^{111}In-labeled tissue plasminogen activator

Adapted from Saha GB, Go RT, MacIntyre WJ. Radiopharmaceuticals for cardiovascular imaging. *Nucl Med Biol* 1992;19:1–20.

and ^{99m}Tc-tetrofosmin have similar properties, ^{99m}Tc-tetrofosmin may be less sensitive at detecting ischemic changes and its use for viability detection is less well validated.

b. Kinetics. After administration of ^{99m}Tc-sestamibi, approximately 40% to 60% of the agent is extracted by the myocardium. Initial uptake of the agent is proportional to regional myocardial blood flow, and it is bound to the inner mitochondrial membrane. ^{99m}Tc-tetrofosmin has similar pharmacokinetics to ^{99m}Tc-sestamibi.

(1) Myocardial washout of ^{99m}Tc-sestamibi and ^{99m}Tc-tetrofosmin is very slow, and little redistribution occurs. The absence of redistribution requires two separate injections of the agent, at **rest** and at **peak exercise** (or with pharmacologic stress).

(2) The **utility of technetium 99m** in the evaluation of viability remains **controversial.** Although redistribution is minimal, increased uptake of technetium 99m over time after rest injection is observed and suggests the presence of viable myocardium. Areas that have diminished counts but retain at least 60% of the highest count density exhibit improved wall motion after revascularization.

VI. IMAGING PROTOCOLS

A. Thallium 201

1. General features. Stress imaging with thallium 201 involves **injection at peak exercise** (or with pharmacologic stress) and **immediate imaging,** followed by **redistribution images** 3 to 4 hours after injection.

a. Because of the long half-life of thallium 201 (i.e., 73 hours), to reduce the total radiation exposure to the patient, limited amounts are administered. Although a single injection typically is used because of the redistribution phenomenon, a second injection may be given to enhance the filling of reversible defects.

b. The low energy range of thallium 201 is marginal for imaging with the gamma camera because of scatter and diminished spatial resolution.

2. Variations from standard protocol. Exact imaging techniques vary among institutions. Initial thallium 201 doses range from 2 to 3.5 mCi, acquisition times vary from 20 to 40 seconds per image, and the number of images varies from 32 to 64 depending on whether 180-degree or 360-degree image acquisition is used.

a. The use of **360-degree versus 180-degree imaging** has been the subject of debate. With 180-degree tomography, contrast is better, there is less artifact, and imaging times are shorter. Slight variations also exist depending on the use of exercise stress testing or pharmacologic stress protocols.

b. When **exercise thallium 201 scintigraphy** is performed, the radionuclide (2 to 3.5 mCi) usually is injected approximately 1 minute before peak exercise to allow time for distribution. Initial images are obtained within 5 to 10 minutes of injection. Redistribution images are obtained 2.5 to 4 hours after the initial images.

c. In some cases, **persistent defects** that would ordinarily be **interpreted as myocardial scar represent viable myocardium.**

(1) For this reason, some advocate **delayed (late redistribution) imaging** 18 to 24 hours after injection. Some studies indicate that up to 40% of persistent defects exhibit radiotracer uptake after revascularization. Delayed imaging has resulted in further redistribution in as many as 45% of patients.

(2) Alternative approaches in **differentiating viable tissue from scar** include **rest reinjection** of thallium 201, in effect to boost fill-in of perfusion defects. As many as 50% of persistent defects have been shown to exhibit improved thallium 201 uptake after rest injection of 1 mCi of thallium 201, suggesting viability.

d. Minor changes in imaging protocol may be observed with **pharmacologic stress testing** with adenosine, dipyridamole, or dobutamine.

B. Technetium 99m. The relative lack of redistribution requires **two injections** of technetium 99m to obtain rest and stress images.

1. **Basic protocols**
   a. **Same-day protocol.** At peak exercise, 25 to 30 mCi of technetium 99m is injected. Rest images are obtained first, and stress imaging follows to minimize residual scintigraphic activity caused by the higher-dose stress injection.
      (1) **Rest images** are obtained with injection of 7 to 10 mCi of technetium 99m and image acquisition up to 1 to 1.5 hours later. Imaging is delayed because of slower liver clearance with rest injection.
      (2) **Stress images** are obtained approximately 45 to 60 minutes after injection. Hepatic uptake of technetium 99m occurs within 15 to 30 minutes of injection, and the tracer is excreted into the gastrointestinal tract through the biliary system. Appearance of the tracer in the gastrointestinal tract can interfere with imaging of the inferior wall of the left ventricle.
   b. The **separate-day protocol** allows time for decay of activity. Larger doses of technetium 99m can be administered for rest and stress images, and there is minimal interference between the images.
      (1) Between 22 and 30 mCi of technetium 99m is injected for stress and rest imaging, separated by 1 to 2 days.
      (2) The higher doses possible with the 2-day protocol produce increased count density and better image quality at the cost of inconvenience.
2. **Factors that affect image quality.** Consumption of a **fatty meal** can enhance biliary excretion of technetium 99m and improve image quality. Because of possible interference from noncardiac uptake, image processing with technetium 99m relies on normalization to the brightest cardiac pixel.

C. Dual isotope imaging. Use of both thallium 201 and technetium 99m substantially reduces the time required to obtain stress and rest images.

1. The patient receives thallium 201 at rest (3.5 mCi) and, immediately after rest imaging, undergoes stress. At peak stress, the patient is given an injection of 25 mCi of technetium 99m. Stress images are obtained 15 minutes later.
2. This technique makes use of the dissimilar energy levels of the two radionuclides to shorten the protocol while still allowing acquisition of ECG-gated images (because of the use of technetium 99m).
3. The sensitivity (91%) and specificity (75%) of this combination protocol are comparable with the values for conventional technetium 99m SPECT.

VII. STRESS PROTOCOLS

A. Exercise stress testing. Standard exercise testing (see Chapter 44) is frequently complemented with nuclear imaging. The radioisotope is injected at peak exercise, and time is allowed for circulation of the agents (usually at least 1 minute before termination of exercise).

B. For patients who are unable to exercise, **pharmacologic testing** is used in concert with nuclear imaging. Adenosine and Dipyridamole are indirect vasodilators that are useful in noninvasive testing because of differences in coronary flow reserve. In the presence of marked coronary stenosis, the distal vessel is maximally dilated and therefore possesses little flow reserve. Dipyridamole substantially enhances coronary flow in normal beds (ie, normal flow reserve), although much less so in distributions supplied by a stenotic artery. The resultant disproportionate flow is the basis for heterogenous radiotracer uptake.

1. **Administration.** Dipyridamole is infused over a 4-minute period (0.142 mg/kg/min). Maximum vasodilatory effect is achieved 4 minutes after completion of the infusion, and the radiotracer is injected at this point. A slight increase in heart rate (10 beats/min) and decrease in blood pressure (10 mm Hg) frequently are observed.
2. **Side effects.** Headache, nausea, chest pain, hypotension, dizziness, and flushing have been reported. Severe side effects may necessitate reversal of the dipyridamole effect with aminophylline, given as a 50- to 100-mg intravenous bolus.

C. Adenosine is the vasoactive end product of dipyridamole infusion and acts similarly although with a substantially shorter half-life.

1. **Administration.** Adenosine is infused at 140 μg/kg/min for 6 minutes. The radiotracer is injected after 3 minutes of infusion.
2. **Side effects** include chest pain, headache, nausea, flushing, dyspnea, and atrioventricular block.

D. Dobutamine

1. **Administration.** Infusion is begun at 5 μg/kg/min and increased every 3 minutes to a maximum dose of 40 μg/kg/min. The radiotracer is injected at maximum dose (or at 85% of age-predicted maximum heart rate), and the infusion is continued for 2 to 3 minutes.
2. **Side effects** associated with dobutamine include ectopy, headache, flushing, dyspnea, paresthesias, and hypotension.

VIII. IMAGE INTERPRETATION

A. Standard view of normal anatomy. Uptake of radiotracer is homogeneous in persons with normal myocardial perfusion. The predominance of tracer is distributed to the left ventricle; the right ventricle usually appears as a faint, thin structure. Understanding and interpreting these images, however, requires an understanding of standard planar and SPECT views of left ventricular (LV) anatomic features.

1. **Planar images** are represented as LAO, anterior, and LLAT views.
2. Standard **SPECT views** include the short axis, vertical long axis, and horizontal long axis. The short-axis view is further divided into apical, midventricular, and basal views.
   a. As with planar views, SPECT images in various projections **correspond with specific myocardial segments** (Fig. 43.2).
   b. In addition to the standard SPECT sections, short-axis sections can be compiled into a so-called **bull's eye display** (i.e., **polar map**). This computer-generated polar map (i.e., "bull's eye" image) arranges short-axis tomographic images such that the center portion represents apical slices and the periphery consists of the basal segments.

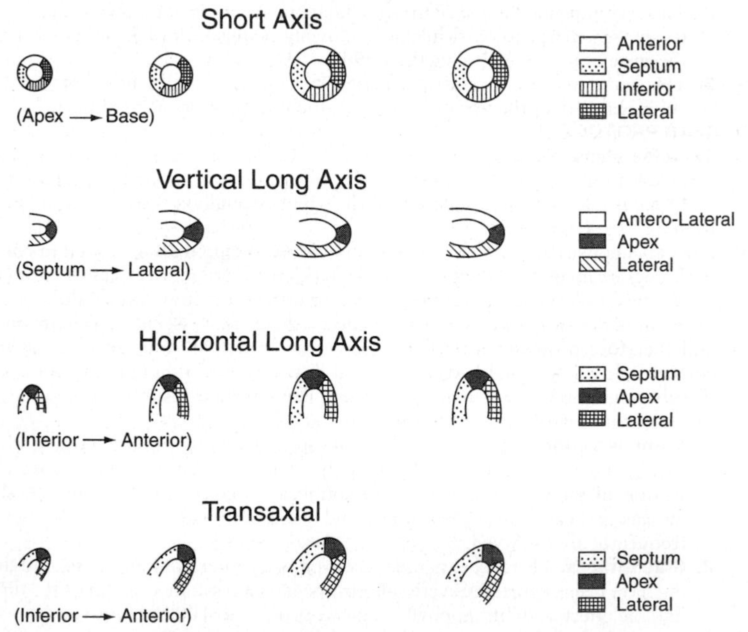

Figure 43.2. Standard tomographic projections and myocardial segments.

B. Reviewing sequence. Review of nuclear images follows an organized sequence:

1. **Examine unprocessed images** for artifact, extracardiac uptake, and evidence of increased lung uptake.
2. **Compare rest and stress images** for enlargement of the LV cavity.
3. **Examine rest images.** Document fixed defects and the number of segments involved.
4. **Examine stress images.** Document defects and segments.
5. **Evaluate the polar map** in comparison with pooled normal images (derived from a database of patients with low probability of having CAD).
6. **Incorporate the gated SPECT images** to establish overall ventricular function and evaluate wall function in areas of questionable artifact. Segmental defects that demonstrate normal motion on gated SPECT images likely represent artifact.

C. Characterization of defects. Given that initial perfusion images represent regional myocardial blood flow, defects in these images represent an area of myocardium with relatively less uptake and diminished regional blood flow. Defects can be characterized as **fixed, reversible, or partially reversible** or as displaying **reverse redistribution.** (The term *redistribution* is not appropriately used in context with technetium 99m imaging.)

1. **Fixed defects.** Nonreversible or fixed defects are areas of absent tracer uptake that appear unchanged on both rest and stress images. Fixed defects can **represent scar or viable myocardium.** With thallium 201 imaging, nonreversibility suggests similar rates of clearance from the two regions.
   a. **Differentiating scar from viable myocardium** in the setting of a nonreversible defect can be accomplished through the use of **metabolic radiopharmaceuticals and PET, delayed imaging, or rest reinjection** with thallium 201. The level of tracer activity reflects viability. Severe deficits (<50% of normal counts) are less predictive of viability than are milder count deficits.
   b. Differentiating viable myocardium from scar is paramount, because there is clinical and experimental evidence of improved LV function after revascularization of such hibernating regions. As methods of revascularization become increasingly applicable in an arena of increasingly complex patient problems, fully defining the so-called fixed defect through metabolic imaging assumes greater importance (see Chapter 43).
2. **Reversible defects** are present on initial stress images but resolve on rest or delayed images. This pattern is consistent with the presence of **ischemic myocardium** in the region of reversibility.
   a. In the setting of **thallium 201 imaging,** resolution of the defect is a function of variable tracer concentrations in ischemic and nonischemic segments, which approach one another as redistribution occurs, along with continuous exchange of myocyte and blood pool thallium 201. **Fill-in** of reversible defects on thallium 201 images can be enhanced by means of delayed imaging or rest reinjection.
   b. **Technetium 99m imaging,** which lacks redistribution, demonstrates reversibility on the basis of differential uptake during stress compared with rest.
3. **Partially reversible defects** are present on stress images and partially resolve on rest images but do not fill in completely. This type of defect is thought to reflect a **mixture of scar and ischemic myocardium.** Nonetheless, reversibility may be incomplete even in the absence of nonviable tissue and represent purely ischemic myocardium.
4. A pattern of **reverse redistribution** occurs when a defect appears larger on rest images or is absent on stress images but present on rest images.
   a. Such a pattern is seen in the presence of **acute MI** when the infarct artery has been rendered patent through thrombolysis, primary angioplasty, autolysis, or another form of revascularization.
   b. The pattern is thought to reflect post-MI hyperemia with excess radiotracer uptake in a region of reperfused myocardium followed by accelerated myocardial washout of radiotracer in the defect region.

c. The regions in question may demonstrate viability on PET imaging and do not indicate ischemia.

5. **Artifacts.** Apparent perfusion defects can be attributed to soft tissue attenuation, a problem that occurs more often with thallium 201 imaging than when a higher-energy agent (technetium 99m) is used.
   a. Common causes of the presence of artifacts include **breast attenuation** (affecting the anterolateral, septal, anteroseptal, and posterolateral walls of the ventricle) and **diaphragmatic attenuation** (predominantly altering the inferior and posterior walls).
   b. Planar images with perfusion defects seen in only a single view are suspect, and the presence of artifact must be considered.
   c. SPECT artifacts may be more elusive because of processing and reconstruction of tomographic images. However, with good technique most are avoidable.
6. **High-risk perfusion scan.** Specific patterns of perfusion imaging that suggest high-risk coronary anatomic features include **perfusion defects in more than one vascular distribution, increased lung thallium uptake, and transient LV dilatation.**

D. **Quantitative analysis.** The principles of image analysis rely on visual inspection, which is fraught with observer variability.

1. **Computer-aided analysis** of planar data involves comparison of regional radionuclide activity on stress and rest images; count discordance coincides with reversibility. **SPECT** data are quantitatively analyzed by means of comparing count densities on short-axis images (displayed as a polar map) with normal count profiles. Although they improve sensitivity, these methods are **used in concert with visual analysis.**
2. **PET imaging**, although evaluated in large part in a visual manner, also possesses great clinical utility with the application of **quantitative analysis** (similar in principle to that used with SPECT) **of coronary flow reserve.** On the basis of comparison of baseline blood flow and hyperemia induced by pharmacologic agents, this analysis may have great clinical utility in ascertaining whether a patient needs revascularization and in evaluating the success of revascularization. The administration of adenosine or dipyridamole has demonstrated at least a twofold to threefold increase in coronary blood flow over baseline. Quantitative analysis of coronary flow reserve may prove useful in overcoming the Achilles heel of the angiographically present but clinically enigmatic coronary lesion.

IX. CLINICAL APPLICATIONS

A. Perfusion analysis

1. Detection of CAD

a. **Sensitivity and specificity.** Since the introduction of thallium 201 imaging in 1975, the utility of perfusion agents in the diagnosis of CAD has been well established. Quantitative planar imaging and SPECT demonstrate 90% or greater sensitivity.
   (1) **Sensitivity** is affected by the number of vessels involved. Single-vessel disease is the most likely to produce a false-negative finding. Multivessel CAD rarely produces a normal perfusion scan result. The **specificity** of planar imaging is 83%, and that of SPECT is 60% to 70%.
   (2) In general, radionuclide imaging is best used to evaluate a population at intermediate risk for CAD. The choice of radionuclide agent seemingly has little effect on the accuracy of these techniques.
   (3) The introduction of **PET**, however, has brought with it **advanced diagnostic accuracy,** with approximately 10% to 15% improvement over SPECT. The ability to detect CAD in a noninvasive manner offers numerous additional applications in risk stratification, prognosis, and imaging of acute infarction.

b. Causes of **false-positive** perfusion study results include attenuation defect, technical inadequacies, coronary vasospasm, anomalous coronary circulation, cardiomyopathy, conduction defects such as left bundle branch block, and recanalization of a thrombosed coronary artery.

c. Causes of **false-negative** perfusion study results include a submaximal exercise stress test, antiischemic medical therapy, presence of nonobstructive CAD, collateral or overlap circulation, inaccurate interpretation of perfusion images or angiograms, acquisition of suboptimal images, presence of balanced coronary stenoses, and delay in stress imaging.

2. Risk stratification. In addition to indicators of higher risk taken from perfusion images, such as increased lung uptake, determinants in the assessment of risk are as follows:

a. Presence of reversible as opposed to fixed defects is associated with greater likelihood of cardiac events at follow-up evaluation. This relation has clinical utility in a number of settings, including risk stratification after MI or in the preoperative setting. In one study involving patients who had had MI without complications, patients with single, fixed defects on thallium 201 images had a 6% cardiac event rate, compared with a rate of 51% for those with thallium 201 scans that indicated high risk of such an event.

b. Radionuclide **imaging abnormalities** have been identified as **independent predictors of subsequent infarction or death.** In general, the number of abnormal segments identified on nuclear images can be seen as inversely proportional to survival rate. Normal findings on a nuclear perfusion study, however, suggest an excellent prognosis, with a yearly mortality rate less than 1%. The application of such prognostic information to the care of patients preparing for noncardiac operations reflects significantly on the patient's surgical risk and has an established role in preoperative evaluation and clearance. For this population, evidence of ischemia on perfusion images portends higher risk for a perioperative cardiac event.

3. Myocardial perfusion imaging may aid in diagnosis and risk stratification for patients with **acute coronary syndromes.**

a. Patients with **chest pain of ill-defined origin** can be given an injection at rest of thallium 201 or technetium 99m. In the presence of true ischemia (ie, without infarction), **reversible defects** are documented, and insight into **regional distribution of ischemia** and extent of myocardium involved is gained. The **absence of any perfusion defect with ongoing chest pain makes a diagnosis of angina unlikely.**

b. Injection of thallium 201 or technetium 99m within 6 hours of the onset of **chest pain in acute infarction** allows imaging of non-ST-elevation and ST-elevation events. As the time from onset of pain to injection increases, perfusion defects tend to normalize, probably as a result of autolysis or administration of thrombolytic therapy.

c. In the setting of **thrombolysis,** imaging with technetium 99m can provide important information about reperfusion or lack thereof. Injection of technetium 99m before initiation of thrombolysis captures a picture of hypoperfusion, which can, because of the extensive half-life, be imaged at a later time. Subsequent injections reveal the status of perfusion as the period after thrombolysis proceeds (i.e., persistent, large defect that represents failed reperfusion). Such applications in the setting of thrombolysis and in acute coronary syndromes have limited clinical utility because of the logistics of staffing and availability of radiopharmaceuticals.

d. A further application that affects the arena of revascularization and management of ischemic syndromes involves **assessment of myocardial viability.**

B. Assessment of ventricular function. In addition to its use in perfusion analysis, radionuclide imaging can establish cardiac performance. Radionuclide-based assessment of ventricular function includes first-pass radionuclide angiocardiography and gated blood pool imaging.

1. First-pass radionuclide angiocardiography involves injection of a radionuclide and analysis as the agent passes through the central circulation.

a. Technetium 99m–labeled agents typically are administered in bolus form, and scintigraphic data are recorded for 15 to 30 seconds after injection. Multicrystal cameras oriented in a straight anterior projection are used for detection of high count rates.

b. This method of ventricular function analysis is more useful in evaluating **right ventricular function** than is gated blood imaging. In patients with **severe LV dysfunction,** the radiotracer may be dispersed, and proximal venous access and rapid administration may be necessary.

2. **Gated blood pool imaging**, or multigated acquisition (MUGA), relies on ECG gating to correlate multiple individual images of the cardiac blood pool to specific phases of the cardiac cycle.

a. The blood pool is labeled by means of removing a 2- to 3-mL sample of the patient's blood after the intravenous administration of stannous pyrophosphate. The sample is labeled with technetium 99m.

b. A single-crystal gamma camera is used in the LAO, anterior, LLAT, and left posterior oblique projections to obtain serial static images of the cardiac blood pool gated to the R-R interval.

c. Because multiple cardiac cycles are averaged to obtain the final images, this technique is not optimal for evaluating regional wall motion.

3. **ECG-gated perfusion imaging.** Perfusion imaging with technetium 99m–labeled tracers produces sufficient count densities on individual images to allow ECG gating. The standard injection of 20 to 30 mCi of technetium 99m allows evaluation of **perfusion and function in a single study.** Comparison of this method with two-dimensional echocardiography in the evaluation of regional wall motion has shown good correlation between the two. This correlation is not applicable to stress echocardiography, however, because of the time lag from the period of stress to the acquisition of nuclear images. The greatest utility of ECG-gated perfusion imaging may be in elucidating perceived artifacts on perfusion images. For example, if a region has a perceived fixed perfusion defect, yet wall motion is normal in the same region, artifact becomes a more likely consideration as the cause of the filling defect.

X. **PET** in the evaluation of CAD allows blood flow imaging and evaluation of metabolic activity. Positron imaging agents can be considered blood flow tracers and metabolic radiopharmaceuticals.

A. **Blood flow tracers.** A number of radiopharmaceuticals exist for the assessment of myocardial blood flow. They can be produced by a cyclotron or generator.

1. **Rubidium 82,** the most readily used blood flow tracer, can be generated on site without the use of a cyclotron. Much like thallium 201, rubidium 82 is a potassium analogue that is actively transported into myocytes through the Na-K pump. **Uptake into myocardium** is proportionate to regional blood flow. Approximately 65% of the radiotracer is extracted at first pass. Because of a short half-life (76 seconds), rubidium 82–based imaging protocols can be used to assess myocardial blood flow rapidly (within 1 hour).

2. Other perfusion agents include the cyclotron-produced: Copper 62 pyruvaldehyde bis (*N*-4-methyl-thiosemicarbazone) copper (II) **([^{62}Cu] PTSM), nitrogen 13 ammonia** and **oxygen 15 water.** Image quality with **oxygen 15 water** is poor and requires extensive processing to subtract the blood pool. **Nitrogen 13 ammonia** image quality is excellent, although the impracticality of cyclotron production is a limiting factor for both agents.

B. **Metabolic radiopharmaceuticals.** Metabolic imaging with PET depends on the use of radiolabeled substrates of cardiac metabolism, largely in the form of [^{18}F] fluoro-2-deoxyglucose (FDG), carbon 11 palmitate, and carbon 11 acetate.

1. **FDG** is a glucose analogue used by ischemic myocardium because of a transition to alternative fuel sources in the hypoxic state. Ischemic myocardium diminishes the oxidation of long-chain fatty acids and increases the use of glucose as a secondary fuel source. FDG is phosphorylated to FDG-6-phosphate after transport across the cell membrane. FDG imaging therefore reflects myocardial use of exogenous glucose, and FDG is a widely used metabolic radiopharmaceutical.

2. [^{11}C]Palmitate is taken up by myocytes, converted to acyl-CoA, and relegated to triglyceride stores or β-oxidized to produce [^{11}C]carbon dioxide. The release of this product of β-oxidation is reflective of long-chain fatty acid oxidation in myocardium.
3. [^{11}C]Acetate is metabolized to [^{11}C]carbon dioxide after entering the tricarboxylic acid cycle. Measuring the production of [^{11}C]carbon dioxide in this setting correlates with myocardial oxygen consumption.

C. **Metabolic imaging with SPECT.** Although infrequently performed, metabolic imaging with SPECT cameras allows application of higher-energy photons even when PET is unavailable.

1. FDG has been imaged with SPECT when outfitted with a high-energy collimator. Various fatty-acid radiopharmaceuticals now are available that are SPECT compatible.
2. These techniques allow **perfusion, ischemia, and viability assessment** with standard SPECT equipment.

D. **Protocols.** Image acquisition with PET is similar to that with SPECT in that tomographic images are obtained in short-axis, horizontal long-axis (sagittal), and vertical long-axis (coronal) views. A positron camera consists of an array of crystals arranged in a circle. Unlike in SPECT, the camera remains stationary in PET.

1. The heart is localized with the patient's arms extended above the head. An **attenuation scan** is performed that allows the density of the surrounding thorax to be subtracted to leave only cardiac count activity. This performance of attenuation correction which makes **allowance for noncardiac interference** adds a great deal to the accuracy of PET.
2. After the attenuation scan, the positron **radiopharmaceutical is injected,** and **images are obtained** 2 to 5 minutes later.
3. Metabolic imaging can be undertaken after flow imaging with the administration of 5 to 10 mCi of FDG. Tomographic images are typically obtained 30 to 50 minutes after FDG injection.

E. **Patterns of perfusion and metabolic imaging.** Specific patterns of perfusion and metabolic imaging are identifiable. For example, **normal flow–normal FDG (match)** indicates normal perfusion and normal metabolic activity. **Reduced flow–normal or increased FDG (mismatch)** demonstrates viability (ie, hibernating myocardium). **Reduced flow–reduced FDG** identifies scar tissue.

F. **Clinical applications**

1. **Diagnosis of CAD.** Flow imaging with PET is highly sensitive and highly specific for the detection of coronary stenosis, approaching 93% for both.
   a. Certain perfusion agents allow for quantitative analysis of coronary flow reserve (oxygen 15 water) and aid greatly in assessment of the functional significance of a stenotic lesion.
   b. Higher-energy photons (511 keV), higher count densities, shorter half-life, and the ability to correct for attenuation place PET substantially ahead of SPECT in the accurate detection of CAD.
2. **Assessment of myocardial viability.** The use of **PET with metabolic radiotracers is the standard for identifying viable myocardium.** The presence of a flow-metabolism mismatch, which indicates underperfusion in the presence of metabolically active myocytes, indicates a hibernating myocardium. Revascularization of these zones as identified with PET has been shown to result in improvement in wall motion. This utility of nuclear imaging finds increasing application as the ever-growing population of patients with heart failure and increasingly complex CAD demands better methods of viability assessment.

ACKNOWLEDGMENT

The author would like to thank Dr. Jeffrey A. Skiles for his contributions to earlier editions of this chapter.

Landmark Articles

Beller GA, Watson DD, Ackell P, et al. Time course of thallium-201 redistribution after transient myocardial ischemia. *Circulation* 1980;61:791–797.

Marshall RC, Tillisch JH, Phelps ME, et al. Identification and differentiation of resting myocardial blood flow in man with positron emission tomography, ^{18}F-labeled fluorodeoxyglucose and N-13 ammonia. *Circulation* 1983;67:766–778.

Strauss HW, Harrison K, Langan JK, et al. Thallium-201 for myocardial imaging: relation of thallium-201 to regional myocardial perfusion. *Circulation* 1975;51:641.

Wackers FJ, Berman DS, Maddahi J, et al. Technetium-99m hexakis 2-methoxyisobutyl isonitrile: human biodistribution, dosimetry, safety, and preliminary comparison to thallium-201 for myocardial perfusion imaging. *J Nucl Med* 1989:30:301–311.

Relevant Book Chapters

Iskandrian AE, Verani MS. Chapter 53—Imaging Techniques in Nuclear Cardiology. In: *The Topol Solution: Textbook of Cardiovascular Medicine, Third Edition with DVD, Plus Integrated Content Website* Lippincott Williams & Wilkins, 2006.

Udelson JE, Dilsizian V, Bonow RO. Nuclear cardiology. In: *Braunwald's Heart disease: a textbook of cardiovascular medicine*, 8th ed. Philadelphia: WB Saunders, 2007.

44 STRESS ECHOCARDIOGRAPHY

Ryan P. Daly

I. INTRODUCTION. Stress echocardiography (SE) is an **effective method of evaluating for myocardial ischemia,** by the detection of **stress-induced systolic regional wall-motion abnormalities (RWMAs).** Stressors include exercise, pharmacologic agents, and pacing. SE is used to **screen for coronary artery disease (CAD)** and can help **identify the coronary vessels involved.** The accuracy of SE for the detection of significant coronary artery stenosis is 80% to 90%, which is superior to that of exercise electrocardiographic testing and comparable to that of nuclear stress imaging. In patients with left ventricular (LV) dysfunction and documented CAD, SE can **differentiate viable from scarred myocardium,** which may help predict whether LV function will improve after revascularization. As a diagnostic test for CAD, **SE is safe, relatively inexpensive, and can be rapidly performed in experienced hands.** However, interpretation of SE images remains primarily subjective and requires a considerable learning curve. Stress echocardiography also can be used to assess the severity of valvular disease, hypertrophic cardiomyopathy, and exercise-induced pulmonary hypertension. In addition, it provides important prognostic information after myocardial infarction (MI) and prior to noncardiac surgery.

II. PATHOPHYSIOLOGY

A. Exercise stress testing. Myocardial ischemia results from a mismatch between nutrient supply and demand. The ischemic cascade is illustrated in Figure 44.1. Echocardiography detects ischemia by identifying new or worsening wall-motion abnormalities earlier in the cascade than detected by the electrocardiogram (ECG) or before the onset of symptoms, but usually after the onset of worsening diastolic function. Exercise can be done with a treadmill, upright bicycle, or supine bicycle ergometry.

B. Pharmacologic stress testing. In patients who cannot exercise, pharmacologic stressors can be used. These drugs are sympathomimetic agents or vasodilators.

1. **Sympathomimetic agents** produce stress through **an increase in myocardial oxygen demand,** inotropic effects, increased heart rate (chronotropic), and increased blood pressure. Although a number of agents have been evaluated in combination with echocardiography, **dobutamine** is most widely used.

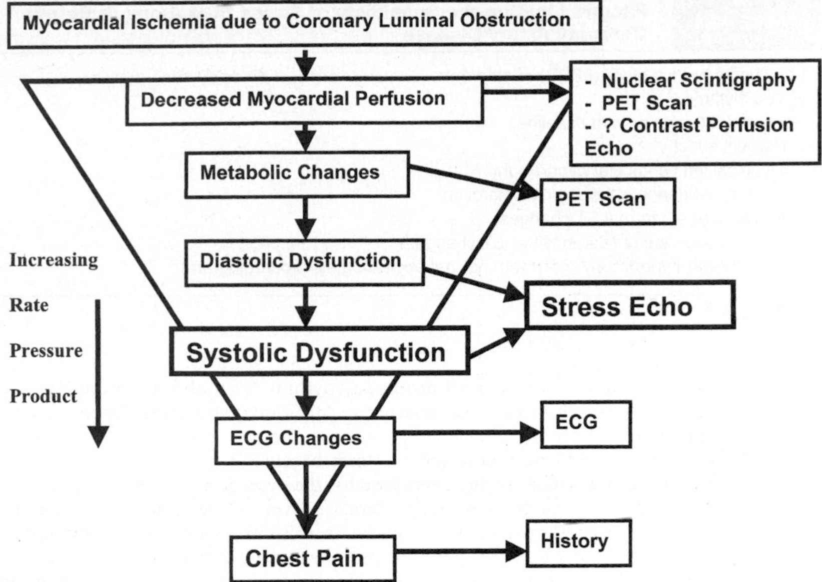

Figure 44.1. Ischemic cascade. PET, positron emission tomography.

Low-dose dobutamine has positive inotropic effects mediated through cardiac α_1 and β_1 receptors. At higher doses, dobutamine has positive chronotropic effects mediated through β_2 receptors. The plasma half-life is 2 to 3 minutes. The normal response to dobutamine involves an increase in heart rate and hyperdynamic wall motion, with only minimal effect on end-diastolic LV volume. It can be **combined with atropine** to achieve the usual target of at least 85% of age-predicted maximum heart rate (APMHR).

2. A **vasodilator stress** test is performed with **dipyridamole** or **adenosine** infusion. These agents cause perfusion abnormalities when blood is preferentially shunted away from myocardial segments supplied by stenotic coronary arteries (i.e., coronary steal). These agents are less commonly used for SE. Adenosine has fewer side effects than dypyridamole, owing to the former's shorter half-life. However, because of the shorter duration of action of adenosine, the echocardiographic findings tend to be less pronounced and of shorter duration, resulting in a lower sensitivity.
3. **Atrial pacing** with a transvenous or transesophageal approach has been used to achieve stress. This method is often poorly tolerated and produces smaller increments in rate-pressure product than other modalities; it is rarely used now.

III. INDICATIONS AND CHOICE OF STRESSOR

A. The **indications and contraindications** for SE testing are the same as for electrocardiographic stress testing (see Chapter 42). The addition of an imaging modality improves the sensitivity and specificity of exercise electrocardiographic testing. Table 44.1 lists groups of patients for whom an imaging modality such as SE may be be required.

Additional **contraindications** to SE occur with pharmacologic stress and depend on the underlying pharmacologic stressor. Patients with severe bronchospastic obstructive lung disease or high grade atrioventricular (AV) block should avoid adenosine. Patients with unstable ventricular arrhythmias should avoid dobutamine infusion. **Relative contraindications** include unstable angina, severe baseline

TABLE 44.1 Factors Limiting the Sensitivity of Stress ECG Alone to Detect Coronary Artery Disease

Left bundle-branch block (LBBB) or other intraventricular conduction delay abnormalities
Paced rhythms
Abnormal ST segments at baseline:
Digitalis effect
Electrical left ventricular hypertrophy
Previous evidence of myocardial infarction
Nonspecific, abnormal ST changes
Women (higher rate of false-positive ST changes)
Left ventricular hypertrophy (even with normal-appearing electrocardiogram)

hypertension (uncontrolled), uncontrolled arrhythmias, a mobile LV thrombus, critical aortic stenosis, hypertrophic obstructive cardiomyopathy, and decompensated heart failure.

B. Exercise is preferred over nonexercise stress because it more closely reproduces daily activity and is slightly more sensitive for the detection of ischemia, providing that the patient is able to achieve an adequate level of stress. No single **exercise modality** has been shown to have superior sensitivity, although the **treadmill** is more widely accepted among patients and physicians. **Bicycle ergometry** can be performed in the upright and supine positions. Images with treadmill stress testing must be obtained after exercise, whereas images may be obtained at peak exercise with bicycle ergometry while the patient continues to exercise. The sensitivity of treadmill testing to detect ischemia is reduced if images are not rapidly obtained (<90 seconds) after exercise. However, the treadmill usually results in a greater level of stress than is associated with bicycle ergometry, which is more dependent on patient effort.

C. Up to 30% of patients referred for exercise echocardiography may **not be able to achieve an adequate level of exercise stress** because of peripheral vascular disease, chronic obstructive pulmonary disease, or musculoskeletal problems. **Pharmacologic stress testing is usually indicated** in these patients. When myocardial viability is sought, dobutamine is the most appropriate stressor.

IV. METHODOLOGY

A. Patient preparation

1. Patients should avoid heavy food intake for 4 hours before the test.
2. Rate-slowing agents (particularly β-blockers) blunt the normal heart rate response to exercise and may limit the ability of the patient to achieve at least 85% of the APMHR. This may reduce the sensitivity of the test results. If possible, these agents should be withheld before the stress test, unless the aim of the test is to evaluate their effectiveness in preventing exercise-induced ischemia.
3. The **standard connections for a 12-lead ECG** may be used with minor modifications to allow imaging in the parasternal and apical windows without affecting the accuracy of the exercise electrocardiographic testing results.

B. Equipment. All SE studies are conducted with **exercise electrocardiographic testing and standard hemodynamic monitoring equipment.** An SE software package on the echocardiographic machine is necessary to acquire digital images and allow side by side comparison of prestress images with peak or post–peak stress images. Resuscitation equipment and a defibrillator should be readily available.

C. Performing the test

1. **Exercise stress echocardiography.** Regardless of the exercise modality, a quick, complete **baseline** echocardiographic scan is obtained for all patients. Resting images are obtained in the parasternal long- and short-axis and apical two- and four-chamber views and stored digitally and on videotape. An apical long-axis view may be substituted for a parasternal long-axis view if the

parasternal images are suboptimal. If endocardial definition is suboptimal, intravenous ultrasound contrast should be given to optimize the images according to current guidelines.

a. **Treadmill exercise** is performed with standard protocols according to the functional status of the patient. Exercise is continued until at least 85% of the APMHR is reached, but it is preferably continued to the level of maximum exertion (to maximize test sensitivity). **Post–peak stress images** are obtained as quickly as possible (in the left lateral decubitus position) after the patient transfers from the treadmill to the imaging table. Stress images in the same views as the baseline study are stored digitally and recorded on videotape. All post–peak stress images should be **obtained within 90 seconds of completing exercise** to maximize test sensitivity.

b. During **upright bicycle echocardiography, baseline images** are obtained in the standard left lateral position and are repeated with the patient in the upright position on the cycle ergometer. Adequate parasternal images may be recorded by having the patient lean forward on the cycle ergometer. These images are recorded and digitized to allow comparable windows for the rest and peak-stress images. Cycle ergometry is started at a workload of 25 watts and increased by 25 to 50 watts every 2 to 3 minutes until the patient reaches his or her level of perceived maximal effort. During upright bicycle echocardiography, **images are obtained and digitized at rest, before peak, at peak, and after peak exercise.**

c. With **supine bicycle exercise,** the entire study is performed in the left lateral decubitus position, and images are obtained and digitized **at rest, before peak, at peak, and after exercise.** This exercise modality is not widely used.

2. **Pharmacologic stress echocardiography**

a. **Dobutamine stress echocardiography (DSE)**

(1) Dobutamine **infusion** is started at 10 μg/kg per minute and increased every 3 minutes to 20, 30, and 40 μg/kg per minute. If the patient has not reached 85% of APMHR by the end of the 40 μg/kg per minute dose, a 3-minute dosage of 50 μg/kg per minute may be used. Infusion is begun at lower doses (5 μg/kg per minute) if baseline LV function is abnormal and myocardial viability is being sought. Images are digitized at rest and at low dosage (5 to 10 μg/kg per minute), pre–peak dosage (30 μg/kg per minute), and peak dosage. Dobutamine increases myocardial oxygen demand in a manner analogous to exercise, increasing heart rate, systolic blood pressure, and contactility.

(2) **Atropine** is used as needed to reach target heart rate (>85% of APMHR) if dobutamine alone is not effective. Atropine 0.25 to 0.5 mg is given intravenously every minute, starting at the 40 μg/kg per minute dobutamine dose level and continuing until an endpoint is reached or a total dose of 2.0 mg is given. Atropine should be avoided in patients with glaucoma and obstructive prostatic symptoms. Isometric handgrip may be performed at the peak infusion rate to help achieve target heart rate. **Endpoints** include 85% of APMHR (target heart rate), intolerable chest pain (angina), hypertension [systolic blood pressure(SBP) >220 mm Hg], hypotension, [blood pressure (BP) <90 mm Hg, or a fall in SBP >30 mm Hg from baseline], sustained ventricular tachycardia, the development of a new wall-motion abnormality (WMA) of more than segments. If 85% APMHR has been achieved without any other endpoints, it is preferable to complete the protocol to the end of 40 μg/kg per minute to increase the sensitivity of the test. **If angina develops**, the effects of dobutamine may be reversed more rapidly with intravenous β-blockade [0.5 mg/kg of esmolol given over 1 minute or 5 mg intravenous (IV) metoprolol]. Like dobutamine, esmolol has a very short half-life and, therefore, may be preferable.

(3) **Side effects.** The most serious potential side effect of dobutamine is arrhythmia provocation. However, serious complications (e.g., arrhythmia,

MI, cardiac arrest) are rare, occurring in about 0.3% of studies in a large series of more than 5000 patients. Less serious side effects include tremor, nervousness, and marked hypertensive and hypotensive responses. The most common minor complication is hypotension, requiring termination of the test (3.8%), which usually responds to supportive methods, including intravenous fluids. A hypotensive response with dobutamine may be caused by ischemia, dynamic outflow tract obstruction, or may result from the vasodilatory effect of dobutamine in combination with a small hyperdynamic left ventricle and a low stroke volume.

b. Dipyridamole or adenosine stress echocardiography

(1) Patients with hypotension, substantial atrioventricular block, or a history of severe bronchospasm **should not undergo** testing with this method.

(2) Different **protocols** of dipyridamole infusion have been studied. The protocol recommended by the American Society of Echocardiography is a low-dose two-stage infusion. The first stage begins at 0.56 mg/kg dipyridimole over 4 minutes, If no adverse effect or clinical endpoint is reached, an additional 0.28 mg/kg is infused over 2 minutes. **A high-dose** regimen of 0.84 mg/kg given over 10 minutes has been developed to improve the sensitivity of the test relative to low-dose protocols. As with dobutamine, atropine may used to increase heart rate. Adenosine is given as a continuous infusion because of its very short half-life. A typical protocol starts at low dose of 80 μg/kg per minute and is increased every 3 minutes by 30 μg/kg per minute to a peak dose of 170 to 200 μg/kg per minute.

(3) End points include substantial ST-segment depression, third-degree AV block, severe hypotension, and intolerable side effects. In the event of an ischemic endpoint or severe hypotension, aminophylline (25 to 50 mg given intravenously over 1 to 2 minutes) may be given to counteract the effects of dipyridamole. Symptoms usually start to resolve within 60 seconds. Symptoms caused by adenosine resolve promptly because of its very short half-life.

D. Imaging techniques. It remains standard clinical practice **to obtain images digitally and on videotape**. Digital cine loops allow side-by-side comparison in a split-screen display, enabling easy comparison of regional wall motion at rest and peak stress, or after stress. Detailed frame-by-frame evaluation of wall thickening or excursion is possible, which helps in the evaluation of regional myocardial function. The main limitation is that only single cardiac cycles are recorded, and it is customary practice to review the videotape images, especially if there is some concern about specific segments. Videotape enables the recording of nonstandard views and multiple cardiac cycles. Obesity and lung disease remain the primary reasons for poor quality images. **Harmonic imaging** has improved endocardial definition, which can be further optimized with **ultrasound contrast injection**.

V. INTERPRETATION (Table 44.2)

A. Qualitative approach. Interpretation of SE findings is predominately subjective and qualitative. Each myocardial segment is visually assesed for wall thickening, rather than just wall-motion, which may be influenced by myocardial tethering and translation. Normal, ischemic, and viable responses to stress are summarized in Table 44.3. Regional wall motion is assessed with the 16-segment model outlined by the American Society of Echocardiography (Fig. 44.2), with results being graphically reported in a bull's eye form (Fig. 44.3). A new American Heart Association (AHA) LV segmentation model (17 segment) has been proposed, and is intended to be commonly applied to echocardiography, nuclear medicine, and magnetic resonance imaging (MRI), although it has not been widely used. Coronary artery territories are conventionally outlined as in Figure 44.2. This approach makes a number of assumptions that are not always correct, especially that the left anterior descending always supplies the entire apex and that the posterior wall is always supplied by the left circumflex artery. In general, **the number of coronary arteries with marked stenosis is directly related to the number of myocardial segments found to be ischemic.**

TABLE 44.2 Suggestions to Optimize Interpretation of Stress Echocardiographic Images

1. Ensure that pre- and post-stress images are comparable views
2. Ensure that the apex is not foreshortened, especially in two-chamber views
3. True two-chamber view should not show any of the right ventricle
4. Use ultrasound contrast whenever resting images are suboptimal in accordance with current guidelines
5. Check that digital images are timed to begin in systole. If digital clips include diastole, there is an increased likelihood of calling a false-positive wall-motion abnormality
6. Check the heart rate for each post-stress image. If images are obtained after the heart rate has returned toward normal, the sensitivity of the test will be reduced
7. Compare the wall motion of individual segments from rest to stress in the four-screen display to define ischemia and infarction. Then compare segments in the post-stress images to identify differences in contraction and the development of "hinge points"
8. Confirm any wall-motion abnormalities in a second view if possible
9. Avoid overcalling ischemia in the basal inferior or basal septal segments
10. Avoid calling a new wall-motion abnormality if it is limited to only one myocardial segment; the abnormality should involve at least two contiguous segments

Wall motion is subjectively graded as normal, mildly hypokinetic, severely hypokinetic, akinetic, or dyskinetic, and may be assigned a wall motion score of one to four (normal, hypokinetic, akinetic, dyskinetic respectively). Each myocardial segment in the rest and stress images is graded in this manner.

Quantitative techniques are under investigation but have not yet seen widespread clinical use. The American Society of Echocardiography recommends further validation and simplification of analysis techniques before quantitative methods become routine. Tissue Doppler imaging and strain rate imaging have recently been applied to stress echo for quantifying regional longitudinal and radial myocardial functioning. Strain rate is a measure of the speed or velocity of regional myocardial contraction. During dobutamine stress echocardiography, strain rate increases in normal hearts and is reduced in areas of myocardial ischemia. The optimal cut-off for strain rate that gives the best sensitivity and specificity was recently reported to be an increment of <0.6 per second. **Strain rate imaging** has been found to be a reliable predictor of detecting significant coronary stenosis, is

TABLE 44.3 Stress Echocardiographic Responses and Interpretation

Interpretation	Resting or baseline function	Response to low-dose pharmacologic stress	Peak and post-stress function
Normal	Normal	Normal	Hyperdynamic
Ischemic	Normal	Normal; in severe ischemia (new WMA)	Decreased (new WMA); left ventricular dilation (severe ischemia)
Scar	Resting WMA	No change	No change
Viable and ischemic (hibernating)	Resting WMA	Improved	Decreased (biphasic response)
Viable and not ischemic (stunned)	Resting WMA	Improved	Improved
Nonspecific	Resting WMA	No change	Improved

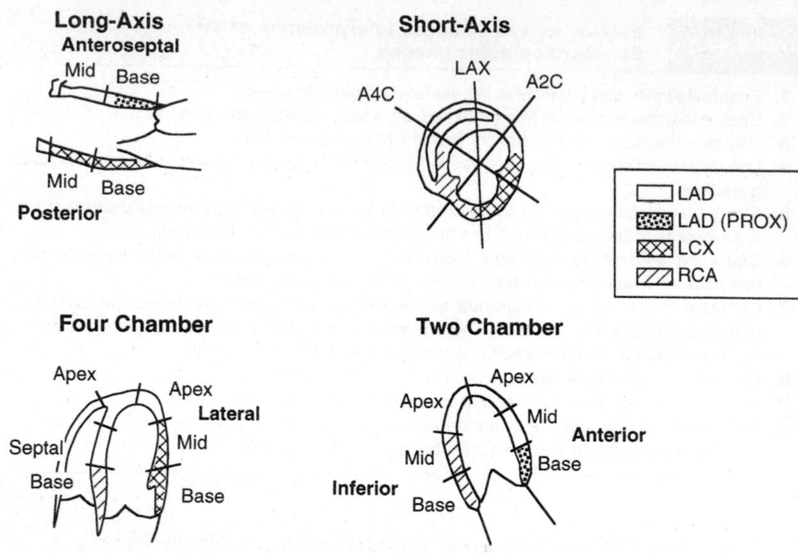

Figure 44.2. The relationships among the 16 myocardial segments and their coronary artery supply in the American Society of Echocardiography (ASE) classification system. The four standard views are used to delineate the associations between coronary artery distribution and the segments. The new American Heart Association (AHA) segmentation uses similar segments, with an additional distal apical segment.

more specific than visually assessed wall-motion scoring, and may allow readers to detect intermediate severe coronary stenosis that produced only subtle wall-motion abnormalities.

Strain rate imaging does not need to be performed in all DSE. Visual inspection is excellent in detecting wall-motion synchronicity, which is highly predictive of a normal study. When a regional radial wall-motion abnormality is visually identified, the quantitative assessment of regional long-axis velocity and long-axis strain and strain-rate responses during DSE can be used. It has been proposed that strain and strain-rate imaging should be used first line in hearts that have abnormal rhythms or resting wall-motion abnormalities.

Reading beyond wall motion. Important prognostic information may be obtained beyond traditional wall-motion analysis. Ischemic heart disease may cause sub-clinical diastolic dysfunction. **Left atrial enlargement** has been shown to correlate with the chronicity and severity of diastolic dysfunction. A normal resting left atrial volume index (LAVI) (28 mL/m^2) has been shown to be strongly predictive of a normal stress echocardiogram (ECG). An **abnormal right ventricle** has also been shown to be a significant predictor of events, independent of LV ischemia or ejection fraction.

B. Exercise stress echocardiography

1. A **normal response** to exercise stress involves a global increase in contractility, development of hyperdynamic wall motion, and a gradual rise in heart rate. This is manifested by increased wall thickness and increased endocardial excursion with stress.
2. **Resting WMAs** usually indicate prior MI, although regional variability may be seen in diffuse myopathic processes. Resting regional WMAs may be defined as hypokinetic, akinetic, or dyskinetic. Akinesia and dyskinesia usually indicate transmural infarction, whereas hypokinetic segments may be partially infarcted or viable.

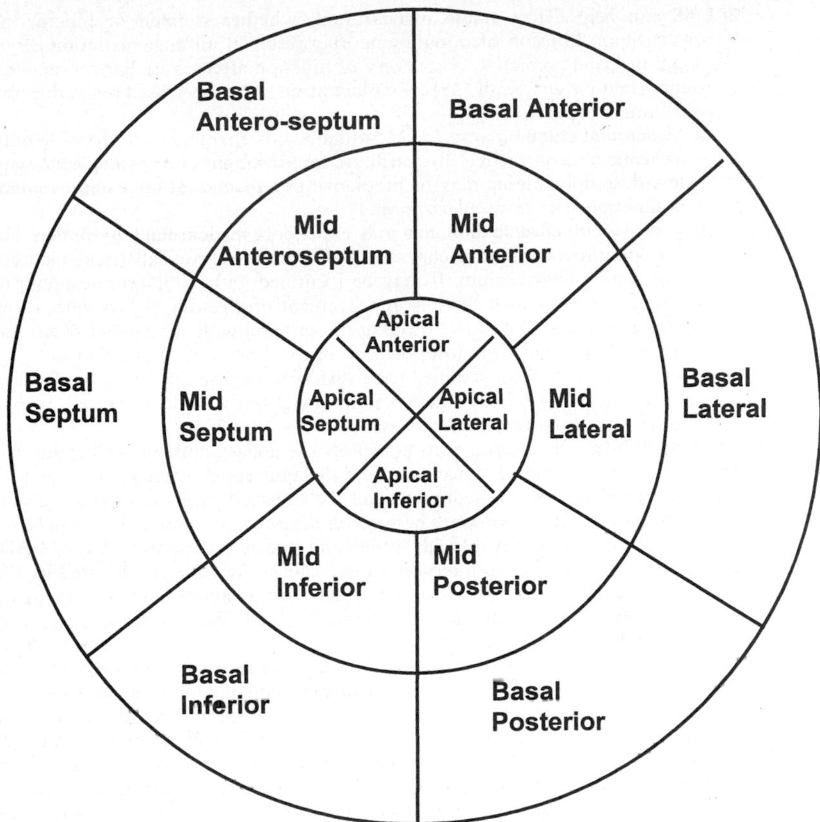

Figure 44.3. Typical bull's eye representation used for reporting the modes of the 16 myocardial segments.

3. An **abnormal** response to exercise may be defined as the **development or worsening of regional myocardial function with or without a decrease or lack of increase in the LV ejection fraction (LVEF). Regional myocardial dysfunction,** as manifested by decreases in endocardial excursion and wall thickening, is **specific for myocardial ischemia. Decreased excursion** alone is less specific and can occur with conduction abnormalities, paced rhythms, and in the normal basal inferior myocardial segment. A decrease or failure to augment LVEF is also a less specific finding and can represent multivessel CAD, a hypertensive response to exercise, medications (e.g., β-blockers), and valvular heart disease (e.g., severe mitral regurgitation).

C. Pharmacologic stress echocardiography. With only a few exceptions, the principles of interpretation of DSE findings are the same as those for exercise echocardiography.

1. The **typical ischemic response** is characterized by normal resting wall motion and an initial hyperdynamic response with low-dose dobutamine followed by a decline in function at higher doses. Ischemia also may be identified on the basis of deterioration of normal wall motion without any transient hyperdynamic response.

2. DSE can help detect **viable** myocardium, whether stunned or hibernating myocardium. Infusion of dobutamine may result in an augementation of regional function predictive of recovery of function after revascularization. This is important prognostically as revascularization of hypoperfused but viable myocardium improves survival.
   a. **Myocardial stunning** after MI is common. It is characterized by viable nonischemic noncontracting myocardium. **Improvement of a resting WMA** with low-dose dobutamine may be predictive of **subsequent later improvement in function** after revascularization.
   b. Patients with **chronic ischemia** may experience **myocardial hibernation.** Hibernating myocardium is characterized by viable chronically ischemic noncontracting myocardium. It may be identified with a biphasic response to dobutamine in which there is improvement of a resting WMA with a low dose of dobutamine (5 to 10 μg/kg per minute) with subsequent deterioration in function at high doses because of the development of ischemia.
3. Interpretation of results obtained with vasodilators requires detection of a new or worsening RWMA during the infusion. There is only a mild increase in cardiac contractility during vasodilator stress.

D. **Reproducibility.** The person who interprets the images must be well trained to develop an acceptable level of accuracy, and must interpret an adequate number of studies on a regular basis to maintain accuracy. Concordance within centers generally is good; however, concordance between different centers may be less than 80%, particularly with technically difficult studies and studies of patients with mild CAD.

E. **Limitations.** The ability to interpret stress echocardiograms is mitigated by the image quality, the presence of arrhythmias, conduction abnormalities, respiratory interference from hyperventilation, and difficulty in allowing for translational and rotational motion of the heart.

VI. DIAGNOSIS OF CAD.

The **diagnostic accuracy of SE is superior to exercise electrocardiographic testing alone, and equivalent to that obtained with radionuclide perfusion techniques** (Table 44.4). Reported sensitivities and specificities (using coronary arteriography as the gold standard) vary between studies, depending on the prevalence of disease in the study population, the angiographic definition of significant disease, and the criteria used for a positive test. Clinical factors such as age, cardiac risk factors, and symptoms that influence the pretest likelihood of CAD also influence sensitivity and specificity. For the overall detection of patients with CAD, **sensitivity ranges from 75% to 92%, depending on lesion severity,** and **specificity ranges from 64% to 100%.** As with other imaging methods, the sensitivity is less for the detection of single-vessel disease and greater for the detection of multivessel disease.

A. Exercise stress echocardiography

1. **Comparison with exercise electrocardiographic testing.** Exercise electrocardiographic testing remains the first-line diagnostic test for CAD. However, **SE has greater diagnostic sensitivity and specificity**, which is predictable on the basis of the earlier occurrence of a systolic WMA before electrocardiographic changes or symptoms in the ischemic cascade (Fig. 44.1). Many factors limit the sensitivity of electrocardiographic testing alone to detect CAD (Table 44.1), and these subgroups should be considered for exercise electrocardiographic testing with an imaging modality.
2. **Comparison with nuclear imaging.** Myocardial perfusion scintigraphy is based on detection of a perfusion defect during maximal hyperemia, with reduced perfusion of areas subtended by significant coronary artery stenosis (>50% stenosis). Perfusion abnormalities occur at an earlier stage in the ischemic cascade than do systolic WMAs, and nuclear scintigraphy theoretically should have a higher sensitivity than SE for CAD. Studies using **single photon emission computed tomography (SPECT) myocardial perfusion scintigraphy have demonstrated a sensitivity of greater than 90%, slightly higher than that for SE.** The **specificity of SE is superior to that of nuclear scintigraphy**, especially in cases with left ventricular hypertrophy (LVH) or left bundle-branch block (LBBB). The overall accuracy of SPECT and SE has been found to be

TABLE 44.4 Causes of False-Positive and False-Negative Stress Echocardiographic Test Results

Causes of false-positive stress echocardiographic results	Factors reducing specificity or sensitivity
FALSE-POSITIVE RESULTS	
Abnormal septal motion (LBBB, after cardiac surgery)	Reduced or abnormal septal excursion with normal septal thickness
Nonischemic cardiomyopathy	May develop regional WMAs (exact cause unknown)
Hypertensive response to exercise (SBP >230 mm Hg, DBP >120 mm Hg)	Nonischemic WMAs or LV dilation
Poor image quality	
Overinterpretation	Observer bias may result in a lower threshold for calling a positive study; important to be blinded
Basal inferior or septal wall segments	Areas most likely to be overcalled; reduced excursion due to annular tethering effects
FALSE-NEGATIVE RESULTS	
Single-vessel disease	More likely to have subtle, rapidly resolving WMA than multivessel disease
Inadequate level of stress (more likely with β-blockers)	Important to stress maximally; reach at least 85% of age-predicted maximum heart rate
V cavity obliteration (more likely to occur with dobutamine)	Makes segmental wall-motion analysis difficult
Poor image quality	
Left circumflex disease	Lateral wall drop-out; more likely to miss ischemia

DBP, diastolic blood pressure; LBBB, left bundle-branch block; LV, left ventricular; SBP, systolic blood pressure; WMAs, wall-motion abnormalities.

similar in meta-analyses; the superior sensitivity of SPECT is balanced by SE's superior specificity. The exception may be in women, where SE may be more accurate than SPECT, owing to less artifact from breast attenuation.

SE is convenient, can provide **information on cardiac structure and function** and results can be interpreted immediately, with rapid feedback to the patient and referring physician. SE also avoids exposure to radioactive tracers and is substantially less expensive.

Nuclear stress testing allows more objective interpretation, with quantification of perfusion abnormalities. Nuclear scintigraphy may be slightly superior for patients on antianginal therapy when it is unnecessary to induce ischemia. Nuclear scintigraphy also appears to be more sensitive for the detection of single-vessel disease and may be superior in the detection of ischemia in the setting of resting wall-motion abnormalities, in which the recognition of worsening wall motion may be difficult. SPECT may also be superior in patients that have poor acoustic windows, for example, chronic obstructive pulmonary disease (COPD). **Local expertise, cost, exposure to radiation, and patient selection are all important factors in determining which imaging modality to use.**

B. Pharmacologic stress echocardiography

1. Dobutamine echocardiography has been found to have a **sensitivity ranging from 68% to 96% and a specificity of 80% to 85%**, similar to values for exercise echocardiography. **Vasodilator echocardiography** has been found to have a sensitivity of 52% to 92% and a specificity of 80% to 100%. In general, the specificity of vasodilator SE is superior to that of other echocardiographic stress techniques. However, single-vessel disease is more difficult to detect with this technique.

2. **Perfusion scintigraphy.** Compared with dipyridamole thallium scintigraphy, dipyridamole echocardiography is believed to be less sensitive but more specific; however, few studies have compared the two tests in the same patients. As with exercise echocardiography, DSE appears to be slightly more specific and less sensitive than perfusion scintigraphy.

VII. **ASSESSMENT OF CORONARY ARTERY DISEASE SIGNIFICANCE.** In patients with known CAD, SE can be useful to **demonstrate the physiologic significance of a lesion or localize the "culprit" lesion.** However, its use to identify the culprit lesion may be constrained by the assumptions inherent in allocating territories of the heart to individual coronary vessels, especially the assumption that the entire apex is supplied by the left anterior descending artery and that the posterior wall is part of the left circumflex territory. This is also problematic if multivessel disease is present, in which case the territory with the most ischemia is identified and less severe lesions may not be apparent.

VIII. **ROLE OF DSE FOR ASSESSMENT OF VIABILITY.** Demonstration of a **biphasic response** to dobutamine strongly suggests viable myocardium. A biphasic response is present when a resting wall-motion abnormality improves in response to low-dose dobutamine, and decreases in function at peak or post stress. This response predicts eventual functional recovery of the myocardium after revascularization. A uniphasic response is less predictive of recovery, and a classic ischemic response is not predictive of the recovery of resting function. Because the biphasic response is the most reliable finding, the preference is to induce ischemia whenever possible by proceeding to maximal stress (40 μg/kg per minute). Myocardial thickness is also an important marker of myocardial viability. When the wall is thin <6 mm, there is low likelihood of recovery of function. The use of DSE for assessment of viability has declined with the wider availability of PET and MRI.

IX. **PROGNOSTIC ROLE OF SE**

A. **Patients with suspected or known chronic CAD.** The **major determinants of prognosis** in patients with chronic CAD are **overall LV function and the presence and severity of myocardial ischemia**. SE is an excellent modality for the evaluation of both.

1. **Negative test result.** Perhaps the most important aspect of the prognostic literature is that a **negative test result portends an extremely low risk of subsequent cardiovascular events, as evidenced by an event rate of less than 1% per year for the subsequent 4 to 5 years.** However, the risk is slightly higher in patients with diabetes or chronic kidney disease.

2. **Presence of ischemia.** Abnormal findings at SE indicate high risk for future cardiac events. Patients at medium risk for CAD who have abnormal SE findings have been reported to have a 1-year cardiac event (i.e., MI, percutaneous transluminal coronary angioplasty, coronary artery bypass grafting, or death) rate of 10% to 30%. However, this information needs to be integrated with other stress data (i.e., exercise capacity, hemodynamic responses to exercise and ST-segment response to exercise, ischemic threshold and the type and extent of abnormal wall motion). Electrocardiographic changes and hypotension are relatively insensitive measures of ischemia during DSE. However, from the prognostic standpoint, the development of echocardiographic evidence of ischemia with dobutamine is analogous to its development during exercise.

3. **Presence of nonviable myocardium.** In patients with the same pretest probability of disease, patients with evidence of nonviable myocardium only during SE have higher rates of cardiac events than patients with normal SE findings, but they have fewer events than patients with evidence of ischemia at SE. Heart failure is a more common endpoint among the group of patients with nonviable myocardium.

B. **Patients post myocardial infarction.** High-risk patients after acute MI are routinely identified by age, recurrent angina, heart failure, and shock. In addition, echocardiographic features predicting outcome after MI include ejection fraction, the extent of resting WMAs, inducible ischemia (detected as stress induced WMA), and the amount of viable myocardium. All of these may be identified using SE, and several large studies (most with pharmacologic stressors) have gathered prognostic data using SE in patients post MI. In contrast to patients with chronic stable coronary disease, cardiac events more commonly occur in patients without evidence of ischemia or low ejection fraction.

C. Patients undergoing major noncardiac surgery. Preoperative evaluation studies have been predominantly conducted with pharmacologic stress, mainly dobutamine, but if the patient can exercise, SE should be considered. Preoperative risk assessment should be considered in patients who are at high risk for perioperative MI or cardiac death, including patients with previous infarct, angina, heart failure, diabetes, or chronic kidney disease. A low ischemic threshold during stress (ischemia at heart rate <70% APMHR) is the strongest predictor of perioperative cardiac events.

AHA guidelines state that, for DSE, the predictive value of a positive test ranges from 7% to 25% for hard events (i.e., MI or death). The negative predictive value ranged from 93% to 100%. Only a few studies have compared SE and SPECT for the prediction of perioperative cardiac events. A meta-analysis concluded that the tests had comparable levels of accuracy, but the cost features weighted in favor of echocardiography.

D. SE in cardiac transplantation. Surveillance for CAD is important in patients after cardiac transplantation, for whom accelerated coronary vasculopathy of the allograft remains a major source of mortality after transplantation. DSE appears to be a useful alternative to screening with serial coronary angiography.

X. SE AND OTHER NONISCHEMIC CARDIAC DISEASE. SE can be used to evaluate the functional significance of a variety of valvular lesions as well as hypertrophic cardiomyopathy. SE can be especially helpful when there is a discrepancy between clinical symptoms and assessment of severity of the valve at rest.

A. Aortic stenosis. Exercise testing in asymptomatic patients with severe aortic stenosis may be clinically useful and is strongly recommended by the European guidelines; however, currently it is a IIb ACC/AHA recommendation. Development of symptoms duing exercise, a fall in systolic blood pressure, ST depression, or ventricular arrhythmias or decreased functional capacity would consititute an abnormal stress test and predict increased risk of future cardiac events.

Dobutamine stress echocardiography can be used in patients with aortic stenosis and LV dysfunction ("low flow, low gradient aortic stenosis") to help differentiate true aortic stenosis where decreased cardiac output ("low flow") is caused by a fixed severe stenotic aortic valve versus low flow from cardiomyopathy with low stroke volume (pseudostenosis). In severe aortic stenosis, dobutamine infusion during a DSE results in increased cardiac output with a parallel rise in the mean transvalvular gradient. Provided the calculated aortic valve area remains less than 1.2 cm^2, an increase in the mean transvalvular gradient rise above 30 mm Hg at any time during dobutamine indusion is consistent with severe aortic stenosis. In patients with pseudostenosis, the cardiac output also increases with dobutamine infusion, but the mean gradient increases only slightly or not at all, leading to a large increase in caclulated valve area. Finally, dobutamine stress echocardiography can be used to identify patients with aortic stenosis and reduced systolic function who have "contractile reserve" defined as >20% increase in stroke volume [equating to a 20% increase in the LV outflow tract (LVOT) pulse-wave Doppler velocity time intergral (VTI) with dobutamine infusion. Although low flow, low gradient aortic stenosis has a poor prognosis, patients with contractile reserve have a better prognosis with surgery than without.

B. Mitral regurgitation. Stress echocardiography is a class IIa, level C recommendation in asymptomatic patients with severe MR to assess functional capacity and the effect of exercise on pulmonary atery pressures and the severity of MR. SE can help predict latent LV dysfunction in patients with normal baseline LV systolic function, severe mitral regurgitation, and minimal or no symptoms. An increase in the LV cavity size or decrease in ejection fraction at peak stress suggests latent LV dysfunction and an increased risk of LV dysfunction post valve repair.

C. **Mitral stenosis.** In patients with symptoms but echocardiographic evidence of only moderate mitral stenosis, or in those who are asymptomatic despite anatomically severe stenosis, SE can evaluate the patient's exercise tolerance and functional response to exercise. Elevation in pulmonary pressures, as estimated from the tricuspid regurgitant jet, is useful additional information for deciding optimal timing of surgical intervention. A mean trasmitral gradient of >18 mm Hg across the mitral valve during the stress test predicts clinical events such as risk of hospitalization with 90% accuracy. A more aggressive interventional approach may be warranted in this patient population. Stress testing in this patient population is a class IIb, level C recommendation.

D. **Hypertrophic cardiomyopathy.** In patients with hypertrophic cardiomyopathy and high resting LVOT gradients, routine exercise testing is not performed, owing to increased risks of arrhythmias and hypotension. Stress echocardiography does provide valuable information, including exercise hemodynamics and the inducibility of LV outflow obstruction, worsening of mitral regurgitation, and provocable gradients in those patients who are asymptomatic at rest. Although these patients may have only mild to moderately elevated resting LVOT gradients, using SE to identify elevated provocable gradients may help to explain their exertional symptoms and quantify their exercise tolerance.

XI. NEW TECHNIQUES

A. **Ultrasound contrast for LV opacification.** Addition of ultrasound contrast can be used in SE studies when baseline images are suboptimal. These agents should be administered slowly and in small aliquots to prevent attenuation artifacts (especially the posterior wall and basal myocardial segments) caused by an injection that is too rapid. These agents are well tolerated and have a low complication rate. On the basis of current data, it is not advisable to administer them to patients with known intracardiac shunts, active myocardial ischemia, decompensated heart failure, or advanced pulmonary vascular disease.

B. **Myocardial contrast echocardiography.** Myocardial contrast echocardiography (MCE) allows for the assessment of the myocardial microcirculation. Inert gas-filled bubbles are injected intravenously and may be visualized in the vascular space and in the myocardium as they eventually reach a steady state. Using ultrasound energy, these microbubbles can then be destroyed. The rate of microbubble replenishment is measured and represents mean red blood cell velocity. This modality has shown great promise in research studies; recently the extent of residual myocardial viability predicted by MCE has been shown to be a powerful and independent predictor of hard cardiac events in patients after AMI. There are numerous on-going clinical trials that may provide important insights into this modality's clinical role.

C. **Real-time three-dimensional 3-D imaging.** Recently 3-D echocardiography has seen increasing use in research labs, although its role in SE remains limited due to limited image quality. The transducer has a large "footprint," which can cause difficulty in obtaining adequate windows to visualize the anterior and sometimes the lateral segments of the myocardium, resulting in reduced sensitivity in detecting anterior ischemia. Most studies have demonstrated the need to use intravenouus contrast for adequate endocardiual visualization with this technology.

ACKNOWLEDGMENTS

The authors thank Drs. Matthew Deedy and Patrick Nash for their contributions to earlier editions of this chapter.

Landmark Articles

Armstrong WF, O'Donnell J, Dillon JC, et al. Complementary value of two-dimensional exercise echocardiography to routine treadmill exercise testing. *Ann Intern Med* 1986;105:829–835.

Cerqueira MD, Weissman NJ, Dilsizian V, et al. Standardized myocardial segmentation and nomenclature for tomographic imaging of the heart: a statement for healthcare professionals from the Cardiac Imaging Committee of the Council on Clinical Cardiology of the American Heart Association. *Circulation* 2002;105:539–542.

Fleischmann KE, Hunink MG, Kuntz KM, et al. Exercise echocardiography or exercise SPECT imaging? A meta-analysis of diagnostic test performance. *JAMA* 1998;280:913–920.
Picano E, Lattanzi F, Orlandini A, et al. Stress echocardiography and the human factor: the importance of being expert. *J Am Coll Cardiol* 1991;17:666–669.
Secknus MA, Marwick TH. Evolution of dobutamine echocardiography protocols and indications: safety and side effects in 3,011 studies over 5 years. *J Am Coll Cardiol* 1997;29:1234–1240.
Spes CH, Klauss V, Mudra H, et al. Diagnostic and prognostic value of serial dobutamine stress echocardiography for noninvasive assessment of cardiac allograft vasculopathy: a comparison with coronary angiography and intravascular ultrasound. *Circulation* 1999;100:509–515.
Takeuchi M, Otani S, Weinert M, et al. Comparison of contrast-enhanced real-time live 3-dimensional dobutamine stress echocardiography with contrast 2-dimensional echocardiography for detecting stress-induced wall-motion abnormalities. *J Am Soc Echocardiogr* 2006;19;294–299.
Weidemann F, Jung P, Hoyer C, et al. Assessment of the contractile reserve in patients with intermediate coronary lesions: a strain rate imaging study validated by invasive myocardial fractional flow reserve. *Eur Heart J* 2007;28:1425–1432.

Guidelines

Cheitlin MA, Armstrong WF, Aurigemma GP, et al. ACC/AHA/ASE Guideline Update for the Clinical Application of Echocardiography. *J Am Coll Cardiol* 2003;42:954–970.
Fleisher LA, Beckman JA, Brown KA, et al. ACC/AHA 2007 Guidelines on Perioperative Cardiovascular Evaluation and Care for Noncardiac Surgery: A Report of the American College of Cardiology/American Heart Association Task Force on Practice Guidelines (Writing Committee to Revise the 2002 Guidelines on Perioperative Cardiovascular Evaluation for Noncardiac Surgery). *J Am Coll Cardiol* 2007;50:159–241.
Pellikka PA, Naguch SF, Elhendy AA, et al. American Society of Echocardiography Recommendations for Performance, Interpretation, and Application of Stress Echocardiography. *J Am Soc Echocardiogr* 2007;20:1021–1041.

Key Reviews

Armstrong WF, Zoghbi WA. Stress echocardiography: current methodology and clinical applications. *J Am Coll Cardiol* 2005;45:1739–1747.
Marwick TH. Stress echocardiography *Heart* 2003;89:113–118.
Merli E, Sutherland G. Can we quantify ischemia in stress echocardiography in clinical practice. *Eur Heart J* 2004;25:1477–1479.
Pierard LA , Lancellotti P. Stress testing in valve disease. *Heart* 2007;93:766–772.
Senior R, Monaghan M, et al. Stress echocardiography for the diagnosis and risk stratification of patients with suspected or known coronary artery disease: a critical appraisal. *Heart* 2005;91:427–436.

TESTING FOR VIABLE MYOCARDIUM 45

Anne Kanderian

I. INTRODUCTION. Patients with left ventricular (LV) dysfunction secondary to coronary artery disease (CAD) have significant morbidity and mortality. Given the prognostic implications of poor ventricular function, it is imperative to identify any reversible myocardial dysfunction that may improve with revascularization.

II. DEFINITIONS

A. Viability is defined as myocardium that demonstrates abnormal function at rest and improves with revascularization.

1. From a pathophysiologic standpoint, chronically reduced perfusion leads to cellular changes that ultimately cause irreversible myocyte dysfunction.
2. Biopsies of myocardium reveal a spectrum of fibrosis and sarcomere loss that correlates with the likelihood of recovery of function. Several studies have found that once fibrosis is found in more than 35% of the myocardium, the likelihood of recovery of function is low.
3. **Stunning** refers to transient myocardial dysfunction, which is often caused by abrupt cessation of flow typical of an acute coronary occlusion.

4. Myocardial **scar** from cellular necrosis is irreversible and does not improve with revascularization.

B. **Hibernation** occurs when viable myocardium has reduced its function as a metabolic mechanism to cope with chronically inadequate blood supply (chronic stable angina) or repetitive ischemic injury.

III. **CLINICAL PRESENTATION.** Ischemia, stunning, hibernation, scarring, and normal myocardium may coexist in the same patient. Unfortunately, clinical symptoms are unreliable in determining if a patient has viable myocardium, as often patients experience no symptoms in the face of considerable LV dysfunction and ischemia.

IV. **TREATMENT OPTIONS.** It has been demonstrated that revascularization of viable myocardium improves quality of life and survival. As medical and surgical technology improve in the field of cardiovascular medicine, it is important to accurately identify patients who will benefit from revascularization.

A. **Thrombolytic therapy or emergency percutaneous revascularization** is used in the setting of an acute thrombotic occlusion to restore normal blood flow and hopefully to minimize cellular damage.

B. **Revascularization procedures**, such as coronary artery bypass grafting and percutaneous transluminal coronary angioplasty, may improve regional and global LV systolic function caused by significant coronary artery disease. The presence and extent of viable myocardium has been demonstrated as a marker for patients who will do significantly better with revascularization than with conventional medical care.

C. **It is notable that patients with nonviable myocardium have similar outcomes with medical therapy as compared with revascularization.**

D. Because not all patients benefit from revascularization procedures, the identification and referral of patients who will derive benefit is important to reduce costs and morbidity with the associated procedures. The goal, therefore, is to reliably identify patients who will benefit from revascularization and subsequently refer these patients for appropriate intervention.

V. **TECHNIQUES TO ASSESS VIABILITY** (Fig. 45.1). Assessment of myocardial viability is indicated in patients with CAD and resting LV dysfunction who are eligible for revascularization. Coronary angiograms provide information about anatomy and feasibility of revascularization, but do not predict recovery of function. Resting echocardiography provides information regarding overall LV function and segmental wall-motion abnormalities, but does not address recovery of function with revascularization techniques. Single photon nuclear imaging techniques (single photon emission computed tomography, SPECT), positron emission tomography (PET) with a metabolic agent, dobutamine echocardiography, contrast echocardiography, and, more recently, delayed-enhancement magnetic resonance imaging (MRI) have been identified as techniques that can distinguish viable from nonviable myocardium. Each technique exploits a separate property of dysfunctional myocardium in order to determine the potential for recovery of function after revascularization. The test that is used often depends on the strengths and preference of each medical center, although an approach based on the individual patient would be preferable.

A. **SPECT.** SPECT is the most common technique used in the United States to identify viable myocardium. This technique has been successful because thallium-201 and technetium-99m radiopharmaceuticals act as perfusion agents that are only taken up by viable tissue. The long half-lives of these agents allow for regional distribution, which makes them feasible to use in medical centers without a generator or cyclotron. In addition, stress SPECT protocols (exercise or pharmacologic) are frequently used to assess for ischemia, which makes this technique cost-effective in a busy clinical center. Routine studies also include gated imaging analyses that provide further information regarding LV function and wall-motion assessment, which are important in the evaluation of viability.

1. **Thallium-201** is a potassium analog that utilizes the Na^+/K^+-ATPase active cellular transport system for concentration in cells, and relies on intact cells. This characteristic of thallium makes it useful for identification of viable as opposed to necrotic cells. Uptake of thallium is also dependent on regional myocardial perfusion.

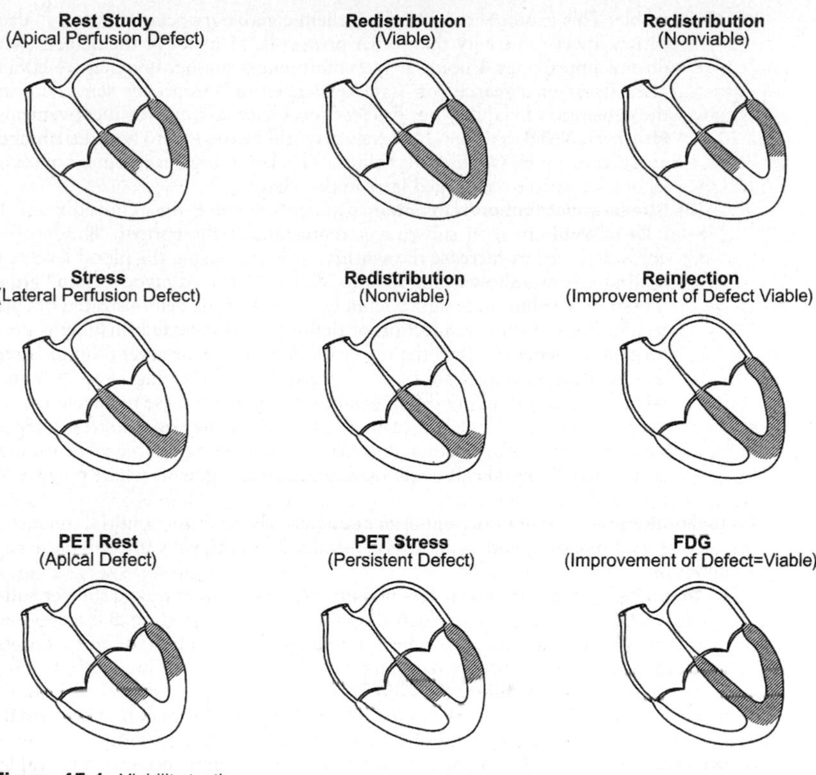

Figure 45.1. Viability testing.

a. Thallium-201 has a relatively long half-life (73 hours), which means that a small dose (2 to 4 mCi) must be used. It emits x-rays from 68 to 80 keV (94% abundant) and γ-rays at 135 and 167 keV (10% abundant). There is a linear relationship between blood flow and uptake of the thallium at rest, which is maintained with exercise enhancement of its use as a reliable indicator of perfusion.

b. Redistribution of thallium between the intracellular and intravascular space begins to occur after the first pass of thallium. It is recognized that with time, initial defects on thallium imaging improve. This is thought to be related to the accumulation of tracer in hypoperfused areas over time as well as rapid washout in normally perfused areas. On the basis of these principles, several protocols have been used to identify viable myocardium.

(1) Rest/redistribution thallium imaging involves imaging 30 to 60 minutes after an initial injection followed by reimaging 4 hours later. Defects on the initial images that improve in 4 hours are considered to represent areas of viable myocardium. This protocol does not address ischemia and has been proven to be less sensitive for detecting viable myocardium than other protocols using thallium or PET with 18-fluorodeoxyglucose (FDG).

(2) Stress/redistribution imaging uses pharmacologic or exercise-induced stress with subsequent thallium injection and imaging, immediately followed by reimaging 4 hours later. Myocardium that is not perfused with stress or rest is considered to be scar. Myocardium that has a defect with stress but that improves on rest images is considered to be ischemic and viable. This protocol can identify ischemic viable myocardium, but it also shows lower sensitivity than other protocols, as many of the defects that do not improve at 4 hours may contain viable tissue. Imaging 24 hours after stress in a search for "late redistribution" improves sensitivity in the detection of viability but has low specificity and may be inconvenient. However, blood thallium-201 levels may still be too low to be redistributed and picked up by viable myocardium. This led to the development of reinjection protocols mentioned later in this chapter.

(3) **Stress/redistribution/reinjection** protocols involve the reinjection of 1 mCi of thallium with subsequent reimaging of the patient. This protocol is designed to increase the sensitivity by increasing the blood levels of thallium. It was shown that 50% to 70% of "scarred myocardium" after 4 hour redistribution imaging actually was viable, as demonstrated by this technique. Typically, reinjection of thallium and repeated imaging is performed immediately after the redistribution images or several hours after the initial stress images, followed by redistribution imaging 18 to 24 hours later. Sensitivity does not differ significantly between these two techniques. Scar is considered to be myocardium that has a defect on the stress images and does not improve upon reinjection and reimaging. Viable myocardium is indicated by uptake of tracer on reinjection in segments where no uptake occurred with stress.

2. **Technetium-99m–labeled radiopharmaceuticals** rely on mitochondrial function, sarcolemmal integrity, and intact energy production pathways for cellular accumulation.
   a. **Technetium characteristics.** Technetium-99m compounds have a shorter half-life (6 hours) than thallium, which allows for the administration of larger doses (10 to 30 mCi) depending on the compound. Technetium-99m emits γ-rays at 140 keV. Commonly used agents include ^{99m}Tc-sestamibi, -tetrofosmin, -teboroxime, -furifosmin, and -NOET.
   b. Redistribution of technetium compounds is significantly less than that for thallium, making it relatively unhelpful as an aid in detecting viability.
3. **Quantitation** of SPECT imaging has been found to be a more accurate method to identify high- and low-risk populations than qualitative analysis. Quantification of perfusion has been proven to be an accurate predictor of recovery of function and superior to qualitative measurements at providing clinically useful information about future risk.
4. **Diagnostic accuracy**
   a. Multiple studies have been performed comparing the various thallium protocols versus PET with FDG as the gold standard. Typically sensitivity improves as one goes from redistribution to reinjection/redistribution and finally quantitative analysis of reinjection/redistribution. Semiquantitative analysis of stress/redistribution/reinjection has good concordance with PET.
   b. In the prediction of functional improvement after revascularization, rest/redistribution thallium scans (sensitivity 90%, specificity 54%) and stress/redistribution/reinjection thallium scans (sensitivity 86%, specificity 47%) have been found to be less reliable. Regions that demonstrate less than 60% regional thallium uptake on redistribution have a very low chance of recovery.
   c. Unfortunately, attenuation and patient artifact frequently make SPECT thallium images difficult to interpret. In addition, methods for quantification have not been standardized across medical centers.
   d. **Quantification** of sestamibi has compared favorably to that of thallium, with redistribution in the prediction of recovery of function after revascularization. Several other technetium compounds used for assessment of viability have been tested (^{99m}Tc-tetrofosmin, -teboroxime, -furifosmin, -NOET). None of these other agents has had significant use except for ^{99m}Tc-NOET, which has similar redistribution kinetics to that of thallium and may be a useful agent in the future. Sestamibi has a limited role in viability assessment owing to its cost.

B. PET in conjunction with a metabolic agent, usually FDG, has been considered the gold standard for assessment of myocardial viability. PET uses positron-emitting isotopes capable of releasing two high-energy (511 keV) photons at 180 degrees from each other. The PET camera can detect these higher-energy rays through coincidence counting. As a result, PET provides higher temporal and spatial resolution than SPECT, which translates into a higher-quality image. Additional features of PET include quantification of

1. Practical issues, including the cost of a PET camera and the short half-life of the several of the cyclotron-produced radiotracers, limit the use of PET to specialized medical centers.
2. Unlike SPECT, PET uses separate agents to measure perfusion and viability.
3. **Perfusion** agents commonly used in PET imaging include nitrogen-13 ammonia, rubidium-82, and oxygen-15 water.
   a. **Rubidium-82** is a generator-produced potassium analog that relies on intact cellular functioning for its uptake and distribution. Hence, rubidium-82 is washed out of necrotic cells and trapped in viable cells.
   b. **Nitrogen-13 ammonia** is cyclotron produced and also relies on intact cellular functioning for its uptake and distribution. The most commonly used perfusion agent in PET, it can be used to quantify blood flow and assess for myocardial viability.
   c. **Oxygen-15 water** is a freely diffusable agent that has been used to quantify blood flow. Blood flow of less than 0.25 mL/g per minute within a region of myocardium is correlated with regions of scar. Unfortunately, intermediate blood flow ranges have not been reliable in predicting recovery of function, which makes this technology less useful for quantifying viability. Oxygen-15 water has also been used to create a perfusible tissue index that has been shown to improve the accuracy in the assessment of viable myocardium but has not been utilized by many centers.
4. **Metabolic** agents used in PET include FDG, carbon-11 acetate, and carbon-11 palmitate. **FDG** (cyclotron produced) has the most clinical data to support its use. It has a long half-life, which makes its transportation to regional medical centers more practical. FDG is taken up by viable cells and then phosphorylated so that it cannot be metabolized further. This effectively traps FDG in the myocardium. In normal myocardium, free fatty acids are preferentially used. During periods of ischemia, metabolism is altered so that primarily glucose is utilized. The limitation of FDG has been in diabetics with impaired cellular uptake of glucose, where approximately 10% of studies are difficult to interpret owing to poor tracer uptake.
5. The combination of perfusion and metabolic tracers gives three possible interpretations:
   a. Normal perfusion is indicative of viability on its own and does not require specific assessment of metabolism.
   b. Reduced perfusion in myocardial segments with intact metabolic function as evidenced by the uptake of FDG is termed flow–metabolism mismatch and is indicative of hibernating, viable myocardium.
   c. Impaired FDG uptake combined with reduced perfusion (flow–metabolism match) is indicative of myocardial scar.
6. **Diagnostic accuracy.** PET-FDG and cardiac MRI are considered the most reliable tests of myocardial viability. Image quality with PET is better than that with SPECT, and myocardial metabolism may be assessed directly with FDG. The sensitivity and specificity of PET in predicting functional improvement in myocardial segments after revascularization are 71% to 100% and 38% to 91%, respectively. PET has been shown to predict low surgical risk in patients with LV dysfunction and viability, improvement in exercise capacity with revascularization, and benefit from revascularization over medical therapy.

C. Dobutamine echocardiography has proven to be a reliable predictor of recovery of function after myocardial revascularization.

1. **Protocol.** Viability studies with dobutamine echocardiography use low doses of dobutamine starting as low as at 5 μg/kg per minute and slowly increasing the dose at 3-minute intervals up to 40 μg/kg per minute or the development of other endpoints, such as target heart rate or symptoms. Imaging is performed throughout the study at each level of dobutamine infusion. Accurate, consistent results are contingent on the acquisition of excellent images for interpretation and an experienced reader to interpret the study.
2. **Pathophysiology.** Dobutamine echocardiography exploits the inotropic effect of dobutamine at low doses on viable myocardium. This improvement in function and wall thickening is referred to as contractile reserve. In viable myocardium, with increasing doses of dobutamine, myocardial oxygen consumption increases, and ischemia develops with worsening of wall motion abnormalities. Therefore, in viable myocardium a segment with reduction in wall thickening at rest demonstrates an improvement or even normalization of wall thickening upon infusion of low-dose dobutamine. At higher doses of dobutamine, wall thickening deteriorates and may revert to the baseline level or may be even more severely reduced than at baseline. This **biphasic response** during dobutamine echocardiography is thought to be the most specific sign of dobutamine echocardiography for predicting improvement in function in myocardial segments with revascularization and indicates segments with underperfused but viable tissue. Myocardial segments with impaired contraction at rest that do not improve upon infusion of dobutamine are considered to be scarred (nonviable). Those segments with impaired thickening at rest that show improvement in thickening upon dobutamine infusion but that do not show deterioration in thickening at higher doses of dobutamine infusion are considered to have a uniphasic response. A uniphasic response is seen in the setting of myocardial damage with subsequent reperfusion (i.e., an open artery without a flow-limiting stenosis) and is much less predictive of improvement after revascularization.
3. **Diagnostic accuracy.** Dobutamine echocardiography has good specificity for detection of viability. Part of the high specificity is derived from the fact that echocardiography is the most common method of assessing postoperative improvement. In addition, improvement of hypocontractile myocardium in response to low-dose dobutamine is the defined endpoint that revascularization is trying to achieve, although it is less sensitive than cellular metabolic function as a marker of viability. Sensitivity and specificity for recovery of function are 84% and 81%, respectively.
4. **Limitations** of dobutamine echocardiography include difficulty in obtaining images in patients with poor ultrasound windows, interobserver variability, even among expert readers, provocation of ventricular arrhythmias with testing, and reduced sensitivity in comparison with nuclear imaging.

D. Cardiac MRI. Delayed-enhancement MRI using gadolinium-based agents given intravenously (0.2 mmol/kg) has been shown to reliably distinguish infarcted from viable myocardium. Unlike SPECT-based techniques, MRI poses no risk of ionizing radiation exposure.

1. **Pathophysiology.** Gadolinium-based contrast agents are extracellular compounds which, when injected intravenously, pass quickly through normal areas of myocardium. In scarred tissue, the interstitial space between collagen fibers is larger than in normal myocardium, causing a delayed "wash in" of gadolinium contrast. The gadolinium then remains trapped in the scarred tissue, causing a longer "wash out" of gadolinium from the infarcted or fibrotic myocardium. Delayed-enhancement MRI takes advantage of this delayed wash in and wash out of gadolinium to detect fibrotic or scarred myocardium, which appear as hyperenhanced (bright) areas of myocardium on images taken 10 to 20 minutes after contrast injection.
2. In patients with ischemic heart disease, scarred or nonviable myocardium occurs in a coronary artery distribution. Scarring typically begins at the subendocardial surface and extends outward at a variable distance toward the epicardium. The **transmural extent of hyperenhancement** on delayed-enhancement images

is then used to determine the viability of each myocardial segment. Segments with 0% to 25% transmural extent of hyperenhancement represent viable tissue with mostly normal myocardium and minimal fibrosis. Segments with 75% to 100% transmural extent of hyperenhancement represent scarred, nonviable myocardium. Segments with 25% to 75% transmural extent are said to have intermediate viability, although in clinical practice the amount of viable tissue in adjacent myocardium is often taken into account when classifying these intermediate segments. Finally, the amount of hyperenhancement within a region can be correlated with segmental wall function and rest/stress perfusion to determine ischemia and viability.

3. The absence of significant hyperenhancement has been shown to correlate well with improvement in function, whereas hyperenhancement of more than 75% has been correlated with irreversible injury. Of interest to note, the mean transmural extent of hyperenhancement that predicted irreversibility was 41 ± 14% by MRI, which correlates with a biopsy series wherein 35% fibrosis predicted similar lack of improvement after revascularization.
4. **Diagnostic accuracy.** Studies comparing different imaging modalities for viability have shown superior sensitivity and specificity for MRI compared to SPECT, and similar sensitivity with slightly improved specificity compared to PET. The main advantage of MRI is its ability to delineate the transmural extent of infarction, owing to its better spatial and contrast resolution. The pattern of hyperenhancement on MRI can also be used to identify nonischemic causes of cardiomyopathy.
5. **Limitations.** MRI is generally contraindicated in patients with implanted ferromagnetic objects [e.g., pacemakers, implantable cardioverter–defibrillators (ICDs), ferromagnetic cerebral aneurysm clips], although some centers will image selected patients with permanent pacemakers/ICDs under careful electrophysiologic evaluation. Gadolinium is contraindicated in patients with chronic kidney disease [glomerular filtration rate (GFR) <30 mL/min], particularly in those undergoing dialysis, owing to a small but important risk of nephrogenic systemic fibrosis (see Chapter 46). Finally, image quality may be compromised in patients unable to comply with breath holding for the study (10 to 12 seconds each) and severe claustrophobia, as well as in patients with arrhythmias or frequent ectopy.

VI. CHOICE OF TECHNIQUE. Cost, clinical expertise, and access to radioisotopes are all issues that affect the appropriateness of each imaging technique. SPECT thallium and dobutamine echocardiography are significantly less expensive than PET and MRI, but they require significant clinical experience for appropriate data collection and interpretation. Both PET and cardiac MRI are robust techniques for assessment of viability, but their use may be limited due to cost, availability, and, for MRI, the presence of patient contraindications to MR imaging. The choice of technique is ultimately determined by local expertise and access to the appropriate technology.

ACKNOWLEDGMENTS

The author thanks Drs. Benjamin Atkeson and C. Patrick Green for their contributions to earlier editions of this chapter.

Landmark Articles

Allman KC, Shaw LJ, Hachamovitch R, et al. Myocardial viability testing and impact of revascularization on prognosis in patients with coronary artery disease and left ventricular dysfunction: a meta-analysis. *J Am Coll Cardiol* 2002;39:1151–1158.

Bax JJ, Wijns W, Cornel JH, et al. Accuracy of currently available techniques for prediction of functional recovery after revascularization in patients with left ventricular dysfunction due to chronic coronary artery disease: comparison of pooled data. *J Am Coll Cardiol* 1997;30:1451–1460.

Brunken RC, Mody FV, Hawkins RA, et al. Positron emission tomography detects metabolic viability in myocardium with persistent 24-hour single-photon emission computed tomography 201Tl defects. *Circulation* 1992;86:1357–1369.

Chaudhry FA, Tauke JT, Alessandrini RS, et al. Prognostic implications of myocardial contractile reserve in patients with coronary artery disease and left ventricular dysfunction. *J Am Coll Cardiol* 1999;34:730–738.

Di Carli MF, Asgarzadie F, Schelbert HR, et al. Quantitative relation between myocardial viability and improvement in heart failure symptoms after revascularization in patients with ischemic cardiomyopathy. *Circulation* 1995;92:3436–3444.

Haas F, Haehnel CJ, Picker W, et al. Preoperative positron emission tomographic viability assessment and perioperative and postoperative risk in patients with advanced ischemic heart disease. *J Am Coll Cardiol* 1997;30:1693–700.

Kim RJ, Wu E, Rafael A, et al. The use of contrast-enhanced magnetic resonance imaging to identify reversible myocardial dysfunction. *N Engl J Med* 2000;343:1445–1453.

Klein C, Nekolla SG, Bengel FM, et al. Assessment of myocardial viability with contrast-enhanced magnetic resonance imaging: comparison with positron emission tomography. *Circulation* 2002;105:162–167.

Marwick TH, Nemec JJ, Lafont A, et al. Prediction by postexercise fluoro-18 deoxyglucose positron emission tomography of improvement in exercise capacity after revascularization. *Am J Cardiol* 1992;69:854–859.

Samady H, Elefteriades JA, Abbott BG, et al. Failure to improve left ventricular function after coronary revascularization for ischemic cardiomyopathy is not associated with worse outcome. *Circulation* 1999;100:1298–1304.

Schinkel AF, Poldermans D, Elhendy A et al. Assessment of myocardial viability in patients with heart failure. *J Nucl Med* 2007;48:1135–1146.

Review Articles and Book Chapters

Iskandrian AE, Verani MS. Nuclear imaging techniques. In: Topol EJ, ed. *Textbook of cardiovascular medicine*, 2nd ed. Philadelphia: Lippincott Williams & Wilkins, 2002:1191–1212.

Pohost GM, Berman DS, Shah PM. *Imaging in cardiovascular disease*. Philadelphia: Lippincott Williams & Williams, 2000.

Schvartzman PR, White RD. Magnetic resonance imaging. In: Topol EJ, ed. *Textbook of cardiovascular medicine*, 2nd ed. Philadelphia: Lippincott Williams & Wilkins, 2002:1213–1256.

Schwaiger M, Ziegler SI. Positron emission tomography. In: Topol EJ, ed. *Textbook of cardiovascular medicine*, 2nd ed. Philadelphia: Lippincott Williams & Wilkins, 2002:1257–1281.

Vanoverschelde JL, Melin JA. The pathophysiology of myocardial hibernation: current controversies and future directions. *Prog Cardiovasc Dis* 2001;43:387–398.

46 CARDIOVASCULAR MAGNETIC RESONANCE IMAGING

Ronan Curtin

I. INTRODUCTION. Cardiovascular magnetic resonance imaging (CMRI) has undergone rapid development over the last two decades and is now an important technique for imaging of the heart and great vessels. Advantages of CMRI include its large field of view, high spatial and temporal resolution, and ability to characterize different tissue types. In contrast to nuclear imaging and cardiac computed tomography (CT), magnetic resonance imaging (MRI) does not involve exposure to ionizing radiation. Applications of CMRI include acquisition of anatomic-quality still and cine images of the heart and great vessels in multiple planes, precise measurement of cardiac chamber volume and function, assessment of myocardial perfusion and fibrosis, quantification of blood velocity and flow, and noninvasive magnetic resonance angiography (MRA). CMRI is not a "push button" technique. It requires skilled operators to protocol, perform, and interpret the multitude of potential pulse sequences and imaging planes that comprise a single examination. It is important to clearly communicate the reason for performing the CMRI examination and to adequately screen patients before the procedure.

II. INDICATIONS. Common indications and components of the CMRI evaluation are listed in Table 46.1.

III. CONTRAINDICATIONS. Contraindications to CMRI are listed in Table 46.2.

IV. BASICS OF CARDIAC MRI

A. MRI Physics. Atoms behave like tiny bar magnets and will align parallel to an external magnetic field. Application of a weak radiofrequency (RF) pulse with the same natural frequency as that of the atomic nucleus will cause excitation or resonance of the nucleus, temporarily changing its alignment within the magnetic field. The atomic nucleus generates an RF signal as it returns to its original alignment,

TABLE 46.1 Cardiovascular MRI Indications and Applications

Indication(s)	Applications
Aortic disease	Aortic aneurysm morphology and size; acute aortic pathology (dissection, intramural hematoma, penetrating ulcer); coarctation of the aorta; branch vessel disease; evidence of vasculitis; postoperative graft stenosis, infection or leak; assessment for aortic regurgitation or other associated pathologies
Ischemic heart disease	Ventricular volumes and function; myocardial scar and viability; quantification of mitral regurgitation; assessment for LV aneurysm, thrombus, VSD and other complications
Nonischemic cardiomyopathies	Ventricular volumes and function; myocardial wall thickness; LV outflow tract obstruction in hypertrophic cardiomyopathy; presence and patterns of myocardial scar/fibrosis; assessment for myocardial iron deposition in suspected hemochromatosis; quantification of mitral regurgitation; evaluation for ARVD in patients with ventricular arrhythmias or syncope
Pericardial disease	Pericardial effusion; pericardial thickening with or without calcification; pericardial tethering; signs of constrictive physiology including conical/tubular deformity of the ventricles, diastolic septal bounce, early cessation of diastolic filling, and dilated IVC
Congenital heart disease	Anatomic definition; ventricular volume and function; valve morphology and function; shunt calculation; assessment for anomalous origin of the coronary arteries; anomalies of the aorta, pulmonary arteries, and systemic and pulmonary veins
Valvular heart disease	Valve morphology; regurgitation and/or stenosis etiology and severity; ventricular size and function
Cardiac masses	Size and extent of mass; tissue characterization
Pulmonary veins	Pulmonary vein anatomy and stenosis; cardiac anatomy and function

IVC, inferior vena cava; LV, left ventricular; RV, right ventricular; ARVD, arrhythmogenic RV dysplasia; VSD, ventricular septal defect.

which can be readily measured. Hydrogen is the most abundant atom in the body, and it is the excitation of hydrogen nuclei, often referred to as protons, that forms the basis for clinical MRI. The signal generated by an excited proton is dependent on its molecular environment, such that the MR signal from a hydrogen atom in blood can be discriminated from the MR signal from a hydrogen atom in fat or other tissue types. An MRI machine, therefore, includes a strong magnet that creates a continuous magnetic field and RF coils for transmitting the excitation pulses and receiving the radio signals generated by the excited protons. Application of predictable variations or "gradients" in the magnetic field using gradient coils within the magnetic bore allow three-dimensional (3-D) spatial localization of each signal. The raw data are initially mapped in "k-space" before a Fourier transform of the data creates the final MRI image.

B. Image contrast. The rate of relaxation of an excited proton in the longitudinal axis (i.e., along the direction of the external magnetic field) is described by its T1 time and in the transverse axis by its T2 time. T1 and T2 times depend on the tissue type or molecular environment of the proton and the magnetic field strength. T1 and T2 relaxation times of different tissues are important determinants of image contrast, and although not measured directly, images can be either T1 or T2 "weighted" to facilitate tissue characterization.

C. Issues specific to CMRI. Cardiac and respiratory motion poses significant challenges to CMRI. In contrast to echocardiography, which is based on real time

TABLE 46.2 Contraindications to CMRI

Specific devices	Special issues
Cerebral aneurysm clips	Certain cerebral aneurysm clips pose a danger due to potential for displacement when exposed to a magnetic field. Aneurysm clips classified as "nonferromagnetic" or "weakly ferromagnetic" are safe.
Cardiac pacemakers and ICDs	The presence of a pacemaker/defibrillator is a strong relative contraindication to MRI owing to several potential problems, including (1) movement, (2) malfunction, (3) heating induced in the leads, and (4) current induced in the leads. In addition, artifact from the leads will often cause significant image degradation.
Cardiovascular catheters	Catheters with conductive metallic components (e.g., pulmonary artery catheters) have the potential for excessive heating. Hence patients with such devices should not undergo MRI.
Cochlear implants and hearing aids	Most types of implants employ a strong magnet or are electronically activated. Consequently, MRI is contraindicated because of potential injury or damage to the function of these implants. External hearing aids can and should be removed before the MRI procedure.
Intravascular coils, stents, and filters	These devices typically become incorporated securely into the vessel wall within 6–8 wk after implantation; hence most are considered MRI safe. However, specific information on the type of device should be obtained before MRI is planned. Intracoronary stents have been shown to be safe during MRI, even when performed on the day of implantation, although many stent manufacturers recommend waiting 6–8 wk.
ECG electrodes	MR-safe ECG electrodes are strongly recommended to ensure patient safety and proper ECG recording.
Foley catheters	Certain Foley catheters with temperature sensors have the potential for excessive heating. They are generally safe if positioned properly and disconnected from the temperature monitor during MRI.
Heart valve prostheses	All types of heart valve prostheses have been shown to be safe during MRI. However, prosthetic material may lead to image artifacts.
Metallic foreign bodies	All patients with a history of injury with metallic foreign bodies such as a bullet or shrapnel should be thoroughly evaluated, as serious injury may result from movement or dislodgement of the foreign body.
Metallic cardiac occluders (e.g., management of PDA, ASD, or VSD)	MRI is safe for nonferromagnetic devices immediately after implant. Weakly ferromagnetic devices are safe from approximately 6–8 wk after placement, unless there is concern about retention of the device.
Retained epicardial pacing wires	MRI in patients with retained epicardial pacing wires after cardiac surgery appears safe. Retained transvenous pacing wires are a contraindication to MRI.

ASD, Atrial septal defect; ECG, electrocardiogram; ICD, implantable cardioverter–defibrillator; MRI, magnetic resonance imaging; PDA, patent ductus arteriosus; VSD, ventricular septal defect.

imaging, CMRI sequences usually acquire a single image over several heart beats to optimize the spatial and temporal resolution. It is, therefore, necessary to gate images to the cardiac cycle with either an electrocardiographic or pulse signal. Electrocardiographic gating is usually retrospective, although prospective gating is sometimes useful, particularly in patients with arrhythmias. Respiratory motion is typically negated by performing breath-holds during the examination. In patients who are unable to maintain a breath-hold, averaging multiple MR signals may help to decrease the noise created by respiratory motion, at the expense of increasing the examination time by a factor of the *number of signals averaged* (NSA). Respiratory navigator sequences that coordinate imaging with a particular phase of diaphragmatic and hence respiratory motion are also effective, and they are typically used for pulse sequences that are too long for a single breath-hold, such as 3-D coronary MRA sequences. Finally, real-time imaging using newer ultra-fast pulse sequences can be used in the absence of electrocardiographic or respiratory gating at the expense of a significant decrease in temporal and spatial resolution.

D. CMRI Pulse sequences and applications

1. **Spin echo.** Spin-echo sequences are characterized by a refocusing RF pulse after delivery of the initial excitation pulse. Rapidly flowing blood appears dark, hence they are also known as "black blood" sequences. Spin-echo sequences provide still images, which are typically used for anatomic delineation of the heart and great vessels owing to their excellent tissue contrast and high signal to noise ratio (SNR). They are relatively insensitive to magnetic field inhomogeneities and artifacts related to ferromagnetic objects such as sternal wires and prosthetic heart valves. Turbo spin echo is a newer technique that provides faster acquisition times than standard spin echo does. The main disadvantage of spin-echo sequences is the relatively long time it takes to acquire an image, making them more susceptible to motion artifacts and unsuitable for cine imaging.
2. **Gradient echo.** Gradient echo sequences are characterized by the use of refocusing gradients after the delivery of the initial excitation pulse. Rapidly flowing blood appears bright, hence they are also known as "bright blood" sequences. Gradient echo is a fast imaging technique that is relatively insensitive to motion artifacts, making it ideal for cine imaging. However, it has less tissue contrast and increased sensitivity to magnetic-field inhomogeneities and ferromagnetic-related artifacts than spin-echo imaging. A variety of gradient echo sequences are used widely in CMRI for cine imaging, myocardial perfusion and scar assessment, coronary imaging, and MRA.
3. **Cine imaging.** The most widely used pulse sequence for cine imaging is a gradient echo sequence called balanced steady-state free precession (B-SSFP), which is characterized by high SNR, high contrast between blood and myocardium, and low sensitivity to motion artifact. B-SSFP is relatively insensitive to blood flow and, therefore, is not ideal for imaging of valve dysfunction or intracardiac shunts, which can usually be better illustrated using other gradient echo pulse sequences, such as echo planar imaging (EPI) or phase velocity mapping.
4. **Myocardial tagging.** RF pulses can be applied before the excitation pulse to generate dark saturation lines or grids on cine images, which are then distorted by myocardial motion. The tags can be used to help qualitatively assess myocardial motion and pericardial tethering or to quantitatively measure myocardial strain.
5. **Perfusion imaging.** Very fast gradient echo sequences are used for dynamic imaging of left ventricular (LV) myocardial perfusion during the first pass of a gadolinium contrast agent during rest and stress states. Fast gradient echo techniques are commonly used, such as fast low-angle shot (FLASH) or B-SSFP with a pre-pulse to null or darken the myocardium. Normally perfused myocardium shows an increase in signal intensity due to gadolinium contrast, whereas abnormally perfused areas remain dark or hypoperfused.
6. **Delayed imaging.** Delayed hyperenhancement imaging for myocardial scar or fibrosis is performed 10 to 30 minutes after injection of gadolinium contrast using gradient echo sequences with an inversion recovery prepulse to null signal from the myocardium. Areas of myocardial scar or fibrosis have a larger

extracellular space with a greater accumulation and slower washout of gadolinium and, therefore, appear bright compared to dark, normal myocardium on delayed imaging.

7. **Phase velocity mapping.** The phase difference in the spin of protons in moving blood compared to nonmoving protons within a magnetic gradient is called the "spin phase shift" and is proportional to the velocity of the moving protons. A phase-encoded image is constructed with the gray level of each pixel coded for velocity. Phase velocity mapping is analogous to Doppler echocardiography and can be used to accurately measure blood velocity and hence quantify cardiac output, shunts, and valve dysfunction.
8. **Magnetic resonance angiography.** MRA of the great vessels typically involves a 3-D fast gradient–echo acquisition after injection of gadolinium contrast. The image resolution is characteristically 2 × 2 × 3 mm, making MRA an excellent option for imaging of large to intermediate size arteries, but less optimal for imaging of smaller vessels.
9. **Parallel Imaging.** A number of parallel imaging techniques make use of multiple receiving body coils to acquire extra data after each excitation pulse. This helps to decrease the imaging time and improve temporal resolution, but at the cost of a small relative decrease in the SNR.

E. Contrast agents. A number of gadolinium chelates are used as contrast agents in clinical MRI. Gadolinium significantly shortens the relaxation time of nearby protons, thereby increasing their signal intensity. These contrast agents are extremely safe, with a low side-effect profile. Prevalence of adverse reactions is approximately 2% and includes transient headache, nausea, vomiting, local burning or cool sensation, and hives. Anaphylactoid reactions are extremely rare. Recently, gadolinium has been linked to a severe and rapidly progressive form of systemic sclerosis called **nephrogenic systemic fibrosis (NSF)**, which appears to be related to extracellular accumulation of gadolinium after its administration in patients with end-stage renal disease. The U.S. Food and Drug Administration (FDA) has advised that gadolinium contrast agents should not be administered to patients with a glomerular filtration rate (GFR) of less than 15 mL/min. Caution should be exercised in patients with moderate or severe renal impairment. Dialysis is only partly effective at filtering gadolinium and may not prevent development of NSF.

V. PRACTICAL CONSIDERATIONS

A. Safety

1. **Magnetic force.** Cardiac MRI scanners typically utilize powerful magnets of 1.5 to 3.0 Tesla, several tens of thousands times stronger than the earth's magnetic field (0.00005 Tesla). Large or small ferromagnetic objects in the vicinity of the MRI magnet bore can become fast moving projectiles, which may cause severe injury to patients and/or damage the MRI scanner. A number of fatalities related to such events have been reported. Health-care professionals working in the vicinity of an MRI scanner require MRI safety training and should be vigilant to risk posed by patients and health-care professionals not familiar with the danger.
2. **Magnetic field gradients.** Switching of magnetic field gradients during a CMRI study produces high acoustic noise levels (up to 115 dB) and can also lead to peripheral nerve stimulation. The FDA has determined limits to the power of magnetic field gradients and noise exposure. Headphones and earplugs are recommended to prevent discomfort and hearing loss to patients and MRI staff in the vicinity of the scanner.
3. **Bioeffects of radiofrequency energy.** The majority of RF energy to the patient is dissipated as heat and is recorded as the specific absorption rate (SAR). 1 SAR equals 1 joule of RF energy per second per kilogram of body weight (i.e., watts/kg). The recommended SAR limit for the whole body is 4 watts/kg.

B. Patient preparation

1. **Screening.** All patients should be screened for contraindications to MRI before the procedure (Table 46.2). Proper screening technique involves the use of a printed sheet and review of the completed form with the patient by an MR safety trained health-care worker to verify the information.

2. **Patient size.** Because of the fixed internal diameter of the magnet bore, very large patients may not fit within the MRI magnet. Typically patients with a torso circumference of greater than 60 cm cannot be imaged. Discussion with the MRI technologist before scanning is recommended for specific recommendations related to your unit.
3. **Claustrophobia.** The enclosed space of the magnet poses problems for many patients, even those who do not have a history of claustrophobia. The study can usually be successfully completed with the help of clear communication with the patient before and during the procedure, presence of a friend or relative at the head of the MRI scanner, or light oral sedation (e.g., lorazepam 0.25 to 0.5 mg) 30 to 60 minutes before the procedure.
4. **Attire.** Patients should wear a cotton hospital gown with no metal snaps. All metal items, jewelry, and nylon undergarments should be removed for reasons of safety and possible image degradation.
5. **Body coil.** Phased array body coils are placed on the patient's torso over the imaging area of interest. These use several smaller coils to acquire RF signals simultaneously, thereby optimizing the SNR and facilitating parallel imaging.
6. **Electrocardiogram (ECG) monitoring.** A good electrocardiographic tracing is essential for CMRI. Three or four MRI-safe, nonmetallic electrodes are placed on the patient's chest, and a single lead signal is used to trigger or gate the MRI images. The magnetic field affects the electrocardiographic tracing (magnetohydric effect), which limits its use for detection of ischemia.
7. **Emergencies.** MRI is not appropriate in patients who are clinically unstable because of difficulties monitoring and treating patients within the magnet bore. Although MRI-safe equipment is available, it is safer to remove a patient who becomes clinically unstable during an MRI examination from the room on an MRI-safe trolley.
8. **Pregnancy.** There is insufficient evidence regarding the safety of MRI in pregnant patients. Current guidelines state that MRI may be used in pregnant patients where other forms of nonionizing imaging are inadequate or if the examination provides important information that would otherwise require exposure to ionizing radiation.
9. **Children.** CMRI may be necessary in pediatric patients with congenital and acquired cardiovascular disease. Typically children younger than 8 years of age will require general anesthesia.

VI. CLINICAL APPLICATIONS

A. Diseases of the aorta

1. **Aortic aneurysm.** MRI can clearly visualize both the aortic vessel wall and lumen. It is a reliable method for the identification, characterization, and follow-up of thoracic and abdominal aortic aneurysms with accuracy comparable to that of CT. A combination of spin-echo sequences for characterization of the vessel wall, gradient echo cine sequences for dynamic imaging of the aorta and aortic valve, and contrast-enhanced MRA (CE-MRA) for aortic and branch vessel luminography are characteristically used. The aorta may be highly tortuous and should be imaged in multiple planes with measurements performed from true short-axis cuts.
2. **Aortic dissection.** MRI is a highly sensitive and specific technique for the detection of aortic dissection (sensitivity 98% to 100%, specificity 98% to 100%). Spin echo, gradient echo, and CE-MRA are used to identify the intimal flap, true and false lumens, and involvement of aortic branch vessels, including the coronary arteries. Administration of contrast is not critical to the examination, so that MRI may be particularly helpful in patients where there is concern for significant renal impairment. In addition, potential complications of aortic dissection (e.g., pleural effusion, pericardial tamponade, and aortic regurgitation) are easily evaluated. However, the longer study acquisition time with MRI compared to CT and its unsuitability for imaging of unstable patients limits its application in the acute setting.

3. **Intramural hematoma and penetrating aortic ulcer.** Intramural hematoma appears as a smooth crescentic to circumferential area of thickened aortic wall without evidence of blood flow in the false channel. The intramural hematoma may be isointense (acute) or hyperintense (subacute) relative to skeletal muscle on spin-echo imaging. Penetrating aortic ulcers appear as deep ulcerations of an atheroma that extend through the intima to disrupt the underlying media and cause bulging of the outer aortic contour. They commonly appear in the isthmus beyond the left subclavian artery and in the distal descending thoracic aorta near the diaphragm. If acute, there may be evidence of intramural bleeding in the rim adjacent to the ulcer.
4. **Atherosclerotic disease.** MRI can clearly show irregular thickening of the aorta in atherosclerotic disease. CE-MRA has good accuracy for detecting significant peripheral stenoses and occlusions. Recent research has focused on the ability of MRI to accurately identify and characterize atherosclerotic plaques in the aorta and carotid arteries, as well as the development of novel contrast agents that target atherosclerotic plaques.
5. **Trauma to the aorta.** MRI may detect chronic or missed aortic tears, usually related to a previous motor vehicle accident. Tears are usually found in the area of the ligamentum arteriosus and are characterized by a localized saccular aneurysm, with or without an associated periaortic hematoma.
6. **Aortitis.** In patients with inflammatory disorders affecting the aorta such as Takayasu's disease or giant cell arteritis, MRI can accurately detect diffuse wall thickening of the thoracic and abdominal aorta as well as stenosis and occlusion of the aortic branch vessels.
7. **Aortic stents and stent grafts.** Aortic stents and stent grafts can be safely imaged using MRI; however, gradient echo sequences are prone to ferromagnetic artifacts. Spin-echo imaging can be used successfully to evaluate stent graft morphology. Artifacts may limit assessment for graft leaks using CE-MRA.

B. Ischemic heart disease

1. **Assessment of global ventricular function.** CMRI is now the gold standard for the assessment of ventricular volumes and systolic function. A typical approach is to perform a short-axis stack of B-SSFP cine sequences through the left and right ventricles. Manual or semi-automated tracing of the endocardial borders at end-diastole and end-systole is later performed off line, and ventricular volumes and ejection fraction are calculated using Simpson's method of discs.
2. **Assessment of regional ventricular function.** CMRI is superior to echocardiography for precise assessment of regional wall motion. B-SSFP cine sequences provide good spatial and temporal resolution in addition to excellent blood-myocardial contrast that permits clear definition of the endocardial border.
3. **Myocardial ischemia.** CMRI stress testing can detect myocardial ischemia with either wall motion or perfusion analysis. The use of dobutamine stress CMRI for wall motion analysis is more established than stress perfusion imaging with adenosine or dipyridamole. Studies of stress CMRI with dobutamine have revealed good sensitivity (83% to 92%) and specificity (86%) for detection of significant coronary artery disease (CAD). Stress perfusion imaging by CMRI appears to have slightly higher accuracy to that of thallium single positron emission computed tomography (SPECT), with a sensitivity of 91% and specificity of 81% for detection of significant CAD reported in a recent meta-analysis. The absence of ionizing radiation with MRI is an important consideration, particularly in younger patients.
4. **Myocardial infarction and viability.** T2-weighted spin-echo sequences with fat suppression may show areas of increased signal intensity consistent with tissue edema in the acute or subacute phase of a myocardial infarction (MI). The current state-of-the-art technique for myocardial scar detection is delayed-enhancement imaging with an inversion recovery gradient echo sequence 10 to 30 minutes after injection of gadolinium contrast agent. This method shows areas of myocardial scarring as bright and normal myocardium as dark, and has shown

excellent correlation with the location and extent of scar on histopathologic analysis. The superior spatial resolution of CMRI makes it more sensitive for the detection of myocardial scar, and in particular subendocardial scar, than SPECT or positron emission tomography (PET). The transmural extent of scar is associated with myocardial viability. Transmural or near transmural scar (>50%) suggests nonviable myocardium, whereas the absence of myocardial scar suggests functional recovery is very likely post revascularization.

5. **LV thrombus.** CMR is more sensitive than echocardiography for the detection of LV thrombus. Delayed enhancement imaging has the greatest sensitivity for detection of thrombus, where it appears as a dark filling defect on the endocardial surface of the left ventricle.

C. Nonischemic cardiomyopathies

1. **Dilated cardiomyopathy.** CMRI is useful for precise assessment of cardiac morphology and function in patients with dilated cardiomyopathy (DCM). Delayed-enhancement imaging typically shows focal or diffuse enhancement in a mid-myocardial distribution, with a predilection for involvement of the lateral LV wall. Delayed enhancement during the acute presentation of DCM has been shown to correlate with areas of active myocarditis. Thus CMRI may help guide myocardial biopsy and improve its sensitivity. The extent of delayed enhancement tends to improve over time, but patchy areas often remain and may represent areas of ongoing inflammation or fibrosis.
2. **Hypertrophic cardiomyopathy.** MRI is accurate for evaluation of the pattern and extent of hypertrophy, systolic anterior motion of the mitral valve, resting LV outflow tract (LVOT) obstruction, and secondary mitral regurgitation. Because of the precise anatomic definition provided by CMRI, it is particularly helpful in planning for surgical myectomy or alcohol septal ablation. CMRI can also help identify abnormal chordal or papillary muscle attachments, which may contribute to LVOT obstruction, and have been reported in up to 20% of patients with hypertrophic cardiomyopathy (HCM). Delayed enhancement is frequently seen in patients with HCM and corresponds to areas of interstitial fibrosis. It is typically seen in areas of increased wall thickness as well as the right ventricular (RV) insertion points in the interventricular septum. The extent of delayed enhancement in patients with HCM is associated with the presence of risk factors for sudden cardiac death, but further research is needed to establish a role for myocardial fibrosis detection in risk prediction in patients with HCM.
3. **Restrictive cardiomyopathy.** Infiltration of the myocardium may lead to restrictive cardiomyopathy (RCM), which is characterized by normal ventricular size and systolic function, severe diastolic dysfunction, and biatrial enlargement. LV and RV wall thickness may or may not be increased. CMRI can clearly visualize the typical findings of RCM and simultaneously distinguish it from constrictive pericarditis, the main differential diagnosis. In addition, specific causes of RCM may be diagnosed by CMRI. Amyloidosis is associated with thickening of the interatrial septum and atrial free walls, as well as increased LV and RV wall thickness. Delayed-enhancement imaging shows a typical pattern of diffuse subendocardial enhancement in patients with cardiac amyloidosis. Several findings have been noted in patients with cardiac sarcoidosis, including areas of increased or decreased signal intensity on T2-weighted images and patchy areas of delayed hyperenhancement. Hemochromatosis is characterized by extensive signal loss on T2-weighted images, resulting from iron deposition in the myocardium. Measurement of the T2 relaxation time of the myocardium (T2* technique) allows more precise detection of iron overload.
4. **Arrhythmogenic right ventricular dysplasia.** CMRI is the primary imaging test for patients with suspected arrhythmogenic right ventricular dysplasia (ARVD), although nonimaging criteria are also required to confirm the diagnosis. CMRI identifies typical features of ARVD including RV wall thinning and fibrofatty replacement, RV dilation, global RV dysfunction, focal RV wall aneurysms, and regional hypokinesia. Fibrofatty replacement of the RV myocardium on

CMRI is not a diagnostic criterion for ARVD. It must be confirmed by histopathology. The CMRI examination for ARVD is different than that for other cardiomyopathies. Axial and short-axis stacks of high-resolution T1-weighted spin-echo images are acquired through the right ventricle for anatomic definition of the RV and LV myocardium. The spin-echo pulse sequences may be repeated with fat saturation prepulses to facilitate detection of fatty infiltration of the RV free wall. B-SSFP cines are performed in the same axial and short-axis imaging planes for identification of RV wall-motion abnormalities. Finally, delayed-enhancement imaging is performed for identification of myocardial fibrosis. ARVD must be differentiated from RV outflow tract (RVOT) tachycardia, which is associated with less dramatic findings on CMRI, including focal wall thinning and regional hypokinesis above the level of the crista terminalis in the right ventricle and in the RVOT.

D. Diseases of the pericardium. Normal pericardium appears on MRI as a thin (≤2 mm) curvilinear line situated between the epicardial and pericardial fat. The normal pericardium is low intensity on both T1- and T2-weighted imaging sequences.

1. **Pericardial effusions** are typically low intensity on T1-weighted spin-echo images and high intensity on gradient echo images. The exception is hemorrhagic effusion, which is high intensity on T1-weighted spin-echo images and low intensity on gradient echo images.
2. **Pericarditis and constriction.** MRI can readily define the presence and extent of pericardial thickening (≥4 mm), which may be present in acute pericarditis as well as constrictive pericarditis. In **inflammatory pericarditis,** the pericardium may have increased signal intensity on delayed-enhancement imaging. CMRI is now the imaging technique of choice in the diagnosis and management of **constrictive pericarditis.** Typical features include pericardial thickening and tethering associated with conical or tubular deformity of the ventricles. Secondary changes include atrial enlargement, systemic and pulmonary vein dilation, hepatomegaly, ascites, and pleural effusions. Cine sequences can demonstrate features of constrictive physiology, including diastolic septal bounce and abrupt limitation of late diastolic filling of the ventricles, which is distinguishable from the more generally delayed diastolic filling patterns seen with restrictive cardiomyopathies. MRI is of limited value compared with CT in the evaluation of calcification of the pericardium because of its inability to reliably distinguish between fibrous tissue and calcification.
3. **Congenital absence of the pericardium**, which may be complete or partial and often left sided, can be demonstrated on CMRI, and is typically associated with a leftward orientation and "teardrop" appearance of the heart. Insinuation of lung tissue between the aorta and pulmonary artery and between the inferior surface of the heart and left hemidiaphragm is also characteristically seen.
4. **Pericardial cysts.** These are benign developmental lesions formed when a portion of the pericardium is pinched off during embryogenesis. Pericardial cysts are classically seen at the right cardiophrenic angle. They typically contain fluid and are well marginated. Spin-echo images demonstrate round or ovoid lesions that are often contiguous with the normal pericardium. Simple cysts demonstrate low signal intensity on T1-weighted and high signal intensity on T2-weighted images. Hemorrhagic or proteinaceous filled cysts show high signal intensity on T1-weighted images.

E. Congenital heart disease. CMRI is now an essential tool in the management of patients with congenital heart disease. Scans can be performed safely and reliably from infancy through adulthood. CMRI provides excellent anatomic definition of simple and complex heart defects and precise, noninvasive quantification of cardiac function and shunts. Because of the complex morphology and physiology in a given patient, MRI examinations are tailored to the individual, with frequent adjustments made during the examination. Consequently, the supervising radiologist or cardiologist should have a thorough understanding of congenital heart disease and be ready to attend at the scanner during the test. Common applications of CMRI in adult congenital heart disease include noninvasive quantification of intracardiac shunts; evaluation of pulmonary regurgitation severity, ventricular volumes and function, and pulmonary artery branch vessel stenosis in patients post tetralogy of Fallot repair; identification of RVOT or branch pulmonary artery obstruction in patients who are post arterial switch for dextro transposition of the great arteries (D-TGA); evaluation of baffle stenosis or leak and RV dysfunction in patients post Mustard or Senning procedure for D-TGA; and assessment for dysfunction of the systemic ventricle in patients with congenitally corrected or levo transposition of the great arteries (L-TGA).

F. Valvular heart disease. Although echocardiography remains the primary imaging modality for the diagnosis and management of valvular heart disease, CMRI may provide additional important information in select cases. Particular strengths of CMRI in the evaluation of valve dysfunction include an often clearer visualization of valve morphology, valve planimetry, precise quantification of regurgitant volumes, accurate and reproducible measurement of ventricular volumes and function, and assessment of associated abnormalities (e.g., bicuspid aortic valve and ascending aortic dilation).

G. Cardiac masses. CMRI plays a major role in the evaluation of cardiac and paracardiac masses, because in addition to providing excellent anatomic detail, it also has the ability to perform tissue characterization. Thrombus is the most common intracardiac mass. Fresh thrombus has higher signal intensity than myocardium on T1-weighted images. Older thrombi may have increased signal intensity on T1-weighted and decreased signal intensity on T2-weighted images. Thrombi usually have low signal intensity on delayed-enhancement imaging. Myxomas are the most common intracardiac tumor and in addition to a variegated and irregular appearance, typically have higher signal intensity than myocardium on T2-weighted spin-echo imaging. Lipomas have a distinctive short T1 and, therefore, high signal intensity on T1-weighted images. Fat saturation sequences that null lipomatous tissue confirm the diagnosis. Fibromas are an uncommon cardiac tumor and are typically seen in the ventricular myocardium in pediatric or young adult patients. They have decreased signal intensity relative to myocardium on T2-weighted images and show rim enhancement on delayed-hyperenhancement imaging.

Primary malignant tumors of the heart are rare. The most common is angiosarcoma, and, next, rhabdomyosarcoma. Angiosarcomas are most commonly seen in the right side of the heart and have a heterogenous appearance with hyperintense areas on T1-weighted images. Delayed hyperenhancement shows heterogenous enhancement, most marked in the periphery of the tumor. Metastatic disease of the heart is more common and typically involves the myocardium or pericardium. It is not always possible to differentiate benign from malignant cardiac tumors. Features of malignant tumors are local invasion, pericardial involvement, and increased signal intensity relative to myocardium after injection of gadolinium suggestive of increased vascularity. One limitation of CMRI is its reduced sensitivity for the detection of calcification in cardiac masses.

H. Pulmonary veins. With the growth of percutaneous RF ablation procedures for atrial fibrillation, imaging of the pulmonary veins is being increasingly performed. CMRI with spin and gradient echo sequences complemented by CE-MRA is effective in assessing pulmonary vein anatomy and stenoses before and after the procedure.

VII. FUTURE APPLICATIONS

A. Coronary artery assessment. Although CMRI can be used reliably for detection of coronary artery anomalies, it has not yet fulfilled its early promise for noninvasive imaging of coronary atherosclerotic disease. The coronary arteries provide significant challenges to imaging by MRI because of cardiac and respiratory motion, their small size and tortuosity, normal cyclic variations in coronary flow, and competing signal from neighboring blood pools. Coronary imaging is usually performed with 2-D or 3-D gradient echo sequences, with either fat-saturation or T2 prepulses to enhance the signal difference between the coronary lumen and surrounding myocardium. 2-D sequences are performed with a breath-hold and 3-D sequences use a navigator sequence for respiratory gating.

B. Molecular imaging. MRI shows significant promise for the selective imaging of target tissue or cells using novel molecular contrast agents. Magnetically labeled mesenchymal stems cells have been successfully tracked by MRI in a pig model of stem cell therapy for myocardial injury. Supermagnetic nanoparticles have also been used to detect atherosclerotic plaque in both animal and human studies.

C. Interventional CMRI. MRI is appealing for use in interventional procedures because it does not entail exposure to ionizing radiation. MRI has been used successfully to guide a variety of interventional procedures including balloon angioplasty and interatrial septal puncture in animals. In addition, the first human MRI-guided stenting of the iliac arteries has been reported in a study of 13 patients.

ACKNOWLEDGMENTS

The author thanks Drs. Monvadi B. Srichai and Richard D. White for their contributions to earlier editions of this chapter.

Articles

Constantine G, Shan K, Flamm SD, et al. Role of MRI in clinical cardiology. *Lancet* 2004;363:2162–2171.

Grizzard JD, Ang GB. Magnetic resonance imaging of pericardial disease and cardiac masses. *Cardiol Clin* 2007;25:111–140.

Hendel RC, Patel MR, Kramer CM. et al. ACCF/ACR/SCCT/SCMR/ASNC/NASCI/SCAI/SIR 2006 Appropriateness Criteria for Cardiac Computed Tomography and Cardiac Magnetic Resonance Imaging: a report of the American College of Cardiology Foundation Quality Strategic Directions Committee Appropriateness Criteria Working Group, American College of Radiology, Society of Cardiovascular Computed Tomography, Society for Cardiovascular Magnetic Resonance, American Society of Nuclear Cardiology, North American Society for Cardiac Imaging, Society for Cardiovascular Angiography and Interventions, and Society of Interventional Radiology. *J Am Coll Cardiol* 2006;48:1475–1497.

Maceira AM, Joshi J, Prasad SK, et al. Cardiovascular magnetic resonance in cardiac amyloidosis. *Circulation* 2005;111:186–193.

Nandalur KR, Dwamena BA, Choudhri AF, et al. Diagnostic performance of stress cardiac magnetic resonance imaging in the detection of coronary artery disease: a meta-analysis. *J Am Coll Cardiol* 2007;50:1343–1353.

Rickers C, Wilke NM, Jerosch-Herold M, et al. Utility of cardiac magnetic resonance imaging in the diagnosis of hypertrophic cardiomyopathy. *Circulation* 2005;112:855–861.

Sakuma H, Ichikawa Y, Chino S, et al. Detection of coronary artery stenosis with whole-heart coronary magnetic resonance angiography. *J Am Coll Cardiol* 2006;48:1946–1950.

Tandri H, Castillo E, Ferrari VA, et al. Magnetic resonance imaging of arrhythmogenic right ventricular dysplasia: sensitivity, specificity, and observer variability of fat detection versus functional analysis of the right ventricle. *J Am Coll Cardiol* 2006;48:2277–2284.

Thomson LE, Kim RJ, Judd RM. Magnetic resonance imaging for the assessment of myocardial viability. *J Magn Reson Imaging* 2004;19:771–788.

Weber OM, Higgins CB. MR evaluation of cardiovascular physiology in congenital heart disease: flow and function. *J Cardiovasc Magn Reson* 2006;8:607–617.

Wood JC. Anatomical assessment of congenital heart disease. *J Cardiovasc Magn Reson* 2006;8:595–606.

Woodard PK, Bluemke DA, Cascade PN, et al. ACR Practice Guideline for the Performance and Interpretation of Cardiac Magnetic Resonance Imaging (MRI). *J Am Coll Radiol* 2006;3:665–676.

Book Chapters

Desai MY, White RD, Bluemke DA, et al. Cardiovascular magnetic resonance imaging. In: Topol EJ, ed. *Textbook of cardiovascular medicine*, 3rd ed. Philadelphia: Lippincott Williams & Wilkins, 2007:897–931.

Gerber BL, Rosen BD, Mahesh M, et al. Physical principles of cardiovascular imaging. In: St. John Sutton MG, Rutherford JD, eds. *Clinical cardiovascular imaging. A companion to Braunwald's heart disease.* Philadelphia: Elsevier, 2004:1–77.

Recommended Texts

Bogaert J, Dymarkowski, Taylor AM, eds. *Clinical cardiac MRI,* Berlin: Springer-Verlag, 2005.

Mitchell DG, Cohen MS, eds. *MRI Principles,* 2nd ed. Philadelphia: Saunders, 2004.

Shellock FG, ed. *The reference manual for magnetic resonance safety, implants and devices: 2007 Edition,* Los Angeles: Biomedical Research Publishing Group, 2007.

Websites

http://www.scmr.org
http://www.mrisafety.com

CARDIOVASCULAR CT

Deepu Nair

47

I. INTRODUCTION. Cardiovascular computed tomography (CT) has evolved rapidly over the past decade, gaining new and expanded indications for noninvasive assessment of the heart, great vessels, and peripheral vasculature. Technological improvements, including increasing numbers of detectors, improved temporal and spatial resolution, and advanced postprocessing have broadened the clinical utility of this imaging modality. Advanced multidetector computed tomography (MDCT) scanners and new scanning protocols may significantly reduce radiation and contrast dose. Numerous considerations are involved in the proper selection of cardiovascular CT protocols, and skilled operators are required to plan and interpret these exams.

II. BASICS OF CARDIAC CT

A. CT physics. Images are created in CT by rotating an x-ray source emitting a fan-shaped beam of x-rays, which then passes through the body. Some x-rays are absorbed or scattered, but others are transmitted and subsequently sensed by detectors located directly across from the x-ray source. In MDCT, the x-ray tube and detectors are mounted on a gantry that rotates rapidly around the patient as he or she passes through the scanner. As in traditional x-ray radiography, different structures **attenuate** the x-ray beam to differing extents depending on their atomic composition and density, as well as the energy of the incident photons. The data collected by the detectors then go through a complex set of mathematical reconstruction algorithms that create a set of axial images through the technique of **back projection**.

Each voxel in the resulting axial image is ascribed a specific attenuation value, which is expressed in **Hounsfield units (H.U.)**. Using a reference of 0 H.U. for water and −1000 H.U. for air, different points are assigned their respective attenuation values. This information is then converted into a grayscale image that can be manipulated by the interpreting physician.

B. Technical challenges for cardiac imaging

1. The fast cyclical motion of the heart requires high **temporal resolution** to avoid blurring or degradation of images due to cardiac motion artifact. In cardiac CT, image acquisition is referenced, or **gated,** to the cardiac cycle. Although data can be acquired throughout the cardiac cycle, most image datasets are reconstructed during periods of minimal cardiac motion, typically a brief 100- to 300-millisecond interval in late diastole (60% to 75% of the R-R interval).
2. High **spatial resolution** is required to image relatively small vessels such as the coronary arteries. Current MDCT scanners provide a spatial resolution of 0.4 mm, compared to approximately 0.2 mm for invasive angiography, the gold standard.
3. Respiratory motion artifact can be minimized by having the patient hold his/her breath during image acquisition. Most clinically available scanners can cover the entire heart in 10 to 12 seconds, whereas the newest 256-slice MDCT scanners can cover this area in just one or two heartbeats.

C. Current CT hardware

1. **MDCT** involves using an x-ray tube mounted opposite multiple detector rows on a gantry, which is then rotated around the patient at a rapid rate (220 to 400 milliseconds/rotation). The patient is moved at either a fixed or variable speed, or **pitch**, through the scanner. An increasing number of detectors allows

for an increased z-axis (cranial–caudal) coverage, permitting faster scans with improved image quality due to less cardiac and respiratory motion artifact. Temporal resolution is improved by faster gantry rotation; the use of two x-ray tubes and detector arrays mounted at 90-degree angles to each other (dual-source MDCT); and special reconstruction techniques. The fastest scanners provide a temporal resolution of 83 to 105 milliseconds. Spatial resolution is largely determined by detector architecture (typically 0.4 mm isotropic resolution), although thicker slices (1 to 5 mm) can be acquired to reduce radiation dose according to the study indication. MDCT can be used for both cardiac and noncardiac studies, and it is now the most widely used type of CT hardware for cardiac imaging.

2. **Electron beam CT (EBCT)**, although rarely used today, was specifically developed for cardiac imaging. It involves the use of a rapidly oscillating electron beam reflected onto a stationary tungsten target. Because there is no mechanical motion within the gantry, EBCT is capable of very high temporal resolution (50 to 100 milliseconds). EBCT is used primarily for quantitative detection of coronary artery calcification (CAC).

D. Image acquisition techniques

1. **Acquisition modes.** Most current MDCT scanners use spiral, retrospectively gated acquistion techniques for cardiac imaging, as this mode provides the greatest flexibility in image selection during different phases of the cardiac cycle and the ability to edit the image data set for artifacts due to ectopic beats. Recently introduced software has made the older axial prospectively gated acquisition mode possible for cardiac imaging in selected patients, and this has resulted in a 60% to 70% reduction in radiation dose.
   a. **Sequential (axial, "step-and-shoot") mode.** Single transaxial slices are sequentially acquired while the patient table is incrementally advanced between successive rotations of the gantry.
   b. **Spiral (helical) mode.** Data is continuously acquired during constant rotation of the gantry with simultaneous, constant movement of the patient through the scanner. As the tube does not perform a complete rotation in any plane, x-ray data is interpolated from a series of sequential frames to create a single tomographic image.
2. **ECG gating**
   a. **Prospective triggering.** The trigger signal is derived from the patient's ECG based on a prospective estimation of the RR interval. The scan is usually triggered to begin at a defined point after the R wave, usually allowing image acquisition to occur during diastole. Prospective ECG triggering is one of the most dose-efficient ways of cardiac scanning, as only the very minimum scan data needed for image reconstruction is acquired. Limitations of prospective triggering (or "**gating**") include the fact that the acquired data set will be of a limited portion (or phase) of the cardiac cycle only, limiting the opportunity for evaluating image data sets from other cardiac phases. In addition, prospective triggering depends greatly on the regularity of the patient's heart rate and can result in serious misregistration artifact in the setting of arrhythmia.
   b. **Retrospective gating.** Unlike prospective triggering, retrospective ECG gating collects data during the entire cardiac cycle. Once the scan is complete, data from specific periods of the cardiac cycle are used for image reconstruction by retrospective referencing to the ECG signal. This approach allows reconstructions to be made from multiple segments of the cardiac cycle and allows some assessment of cardiac function via four-dimensional reconstruction. However, retrospective gating requires higher radiation dose exposure, although this can be somewhat mitigated by **dose modulation** (see subsequent text).
3. **Other imaging considerations**
   a. **Segmented reconstruction** refers to image acquisition algorithms that use scan data from more than one cardiac cycle for image reconstruction. This can reduce the effective temporal resolution of the scan at the cost of a slight increase in radiation dose.

b. **Dose (or tube current) modulation.** MDCT scanners may operate with fluctuating tube currents that increase radiation dose during portions of diastole (when diagnostic images are most likely to be obtained) and reduce it during systole. Dose modulation typically reduces effective radiation dose by approximately 33%, and it is most effective at lower heart rates.

4. **Image reconstruction and interpretation.** Images are most frequently viewed from axial and double oblique planes, in which the three-dimensional data set is manipulated by the interpreting physician so that multiple planes can be viewed to assess cardiac morphology and coronary anatomy. Additional post-processing techniques can be performed to provide additional diagnostic information or, more frequently, to present to the referring physician.
   a. **Multiplanar reformation (MPR)** involves creating straight or curved image planes by cutting orthogonally or obliquely through the three-dimensional acquisition. This aids in evaluating complex three-dimensional structures, such as the coronary arteries.
   b. **Maximal-intensity projections (MIP)** are created by compressing a predetermined volume of image data into a two-dimensional projection of the brightest voxels. This is similar in principle to the two-dimensional images created by typical invasive angiography.
   c. **3-D or volume rendering** is an advanced image processing approach that uses semitransparent visualization of the outer contours of volumetric data, giving the appearance of a three-dimensional structure. Although often not as useful for assessing smaller structures, these reconstructions can be very helpful for understanding complex spatial relationships between major intrathoracic structures.
   d. **4-D or cine imaging** from spiral retrospectively gated images generate cine images of the CT data for evaluating cardiac and valvular function.

E. **Contrast-enhanced imaging.** Administration of iodinated contrast media increases the attenuation of the blood pool, improving vessel delineation and tissue characterization. When using contrast, image acquisition must be timed such that images are acquired when the blood pool enhancement in the target structure is maximal. Various techniques exist to time the arrival of the contrast bolus in the arterial tree and initiate imaging. The specific risks of contrast media are discussed separately below.

III. **INDICATIONS.** The role of cardiac CT in evaluating patients with cardiovascular disease continues to evolve. Generally accepted indications for cardiac CT are listed in Table 47.1 and are discussed in the context of specific clinical situations later in this chapter (see section VI). The following is a brief listing of the more common indications for MDCT:

A. **Evaluation of chest pain** in patients at low to intermediate pretest probability of disease and persistent chest pain after an equivocal stress test.

B. **Suspicion of coronary artery anomalies.** Due to high spatial resolution and the ability to create three-dimensional reconstructions of the vasculature, MDCT has very high sensitivity and specificity for coronary anomalies.

C. **Pulmonary vein evaluation** can be performed, often before or after pulmonary vein isolation for atrial fibrillation.

D. **Evaluation of cardiac masses** when other modalities such as TTE, TEE, or MRI are unrevealing.

E. **Evaluation of pericardial disease** when other modalities such as TTE, TEE, or MRI are unrevealing.

F. **Assessment of anatomy in complex congenital heart disease.**

G. **Presurgical evaluation, particularly before redo open heart surgery.** MDCT can aid in describing prior bypass graft location, identifying safe sites for surgical approach.

H. **Assessing graft patency after prior bypass surgery** is feasible in many cases, though sometimes limited by artifacts related to calcium and surgical clips.

I. **Evaluation of aortic disease.** MDCT is the test of choice for evaluating aortic aneurysm and suspected aortic dissection. It can be useful in the long-term

TABLE 47.1 Appropriate Indications for Cardiac CT

Category	Specific appropriate indications
Suspected CAD with symptoms	Intermediate pre-test probability of CAD with uninterpretable ECG or unable to exercise Acute chest pain with intermediate pre-test probability of CAD and no ECG changes and negative serial enzymes Evaluation of coronary artery anomalies Chest pain syndrome with uninterpretable or equivocal stress test (exercise, perfusion, or stress echo)
Evaluation of intra- and extra-cardiac structures	Evaluation of cardiac mass in patients with limited images from TTE, MRI, or TEE
Pericardial disease	Evaluation of pericardial conditions (pericardial mass, constrictive pericarditis, or complications of cardiac surgery) in patients with limited images from TTE, MRI, or TEE
Congenital heart disease	Assessment of complex congenital heart disease including anomalies of coronary circulation, great vessels, and cardiac chambers and valves
Pulmonary vein anatomy	Evaluation of pulmonary vein anatomy prior to invasive radiofrequency ablation for atrial fibrillation
Biventricular pacing	Noninvasive coronary vein mapping prior to placement of biventricular pacemaker
Aortic disease	Evaluation of suspected aortic dissection or thoracic aortic aneurysm
Pulmonary disease	Evaluation of suspected pulmonary embolism
Surgical planning	Noninvasive coronary arterial mapping, including internal mammary artery, prior to repeat cardiac surgical revascularization

CAD, coronary artery disease; ECG, electrocardiogram; MRI, magnetic resonance imaging; TEE, transesophageal echocardiography; TTE, transthoracic echocardiography.
Adapted from the ACCF/ACR/SCCT/SCMR/ASNC/NASCI/SCAI/SIR 2006 appropriateness criteria for cardiac computed tomography and cardiac magnetic resonance imaging. *J Am Coll Cardiol* 2006;48:1475–1497.

follow-up of patients who have undergone prior aortic surgery or endovascular stenting.

J. Evaluation of suspected pulmonary embolism

IV. CONTRAINDICATIONS. Unlike with cardiac MRI, few absolute contraindications exist for cardiac CT. However, there are important risks associated with radiation and/or contrast exposure that must be weighed against the benefits of the scan. **Relative contraindications** to CT scanning are listed below.

A. Renal insufficiency. Given the potential for contrast nephropathy, patients with significant renal insufficiency (i.e., Cr >1.6 mg/dL) should not undergo contrast-enhanced CT unless the information from the scan is critical and the risks/benefits are thoroughly discussed with the patient.

B. Contrast (iodine) allergy. Patients with allergic reactions to contrast should be pretreated with diphenhydramine and steroids before contrast administration. A prior anaphylactic response to contrast is generally felt to be an absolute contraindication to intravenous iodinated contrast administration at many institutions.

C. Recent intravenous iodinated contrast administration. Patients who have received an intravenous dose of iodinated contrast should avoid contrast-enhanced CT scanning for 24 hours to reduce the risk of contrast nephropathy. For younger patients with normal renal function without risk factors for contrast nephropathy, contrast doses of up to 150 to 200 mL per 24 hours are generally well tolerated.

D. Hyperthyroidism. Iodinated contrast is contraindicated in the setting of uncontrolled hyperthyroidism due to possible precipitation of thyrotoxicosis.

E. Atrial fibrillation, or any irregular heart rhythm, is a contraindication to coronary CT angiography due to image degradation from suboptimal ECG gating.

F. Inability to breath hold for at least 10 seconds. Image quality will be significantly reduced due to respiratory motion artifact if the patient cannot comply with breath hold instructions.

V. SAFETY

A. Radiation exposure is recognized as an important risk of various cardiac imaging modalities, including CT. Radiation doses of cardiac CT scans vary greatly depending on the scan parameter settings, scan range (cranial-caudal length of the scan), gender (women receive more radiation due to breast tissue), and patient body habitus (obesity increases exposure).

1. **Estimates of radiation dose from MDCT** have varied widely in the literature. **Effective dose** is an estimate of the dose to patients during an ionizing radiation procedure and is expressed in **millisieverts (mSv)**. For reference, the estimated dose from a chest x-ray is 0.04 to 0.10 mSv, and the average annual background radiation in the United States is 3 to 3.6 mSv. Invasive diagnostic coronary angiography provides effective doses of 2.1 to 4 mSv. In comparison, coronary CT angiography studies have reported doses ranging from 3.6 mSv to as high as 18 mSv, depending on the scan parameters, with most estimates ranging from roughly 4 to 11 mSv. Table 47.2 lists radiation dose ranges for the most commonly used cardiac imaging modalities.
2. **Feasibility of low-dose CT coronary angiography.** With use of prospective-ECG triggering, axial imaging modes, and software adaptations, recent studies have reported the feasibility of CT coronary angiography with comparable image quality and substantially reduced radiation doses (i.e., 1.1 to 3.0 mSv). This remains an area of active investigation.

B. Contrast nephropathy. Iodinated contrast media can cause renal ischemia by reducing renal blood flow or increasing oxygen demand and may also have a direct toxic effect on tubular epithelial cells. If a contrast-enhanced CT study is necessary in patients with significant renal insufficiency, prophylactic measures should be taken

TABLE 47.2 Estimated Radiation Exposure from Cardiac Imaging Procedures

Diagnostic procedure	Typical effective dose (mSv)	Equivalent period of natural background radiation
Natural background radiation	3–4 (range 1.5–7.5)	1 year
Chest x-ray (PA and lateral)	0.04	6 days
Transatlantic flight	0.03	5 days
Lung ventilation (81 mKR)	0.1	2–4 weeks
Lung perfusion study (99m-Tc)	1	4–6 months
Calcium scoring	0.8–2	3–6 months
CT head	2	8 months
Cardiac catheterization (diagnostic)	3–4	1 year
64-slice MDCT (with dose modulation)	8–12	2–3 years
Myocardial perfusion (Tl-201)	15–18	4–5 years
CT abdomen/pelvis	10–20	3–6 years
Cardiac PET	14–20	4–6 years

PA, posterolateral; mKR, author to define; MDCT, multi-detector computed tomographyl mSv, millisievert; PET, positron emission tomography;

to reduce risk of renal damage. Most cardiac CT studies require between 80 and 100 cc of contrast dye.

1. **Risk factors.**
   a. Preexisting renal insufficiency
   b. Diabetes mellitus
   c. Volume of contrast media
2. **Prophylactic measures** include saline hydration, n-acetylcysteine, use of low-osmolar agents, and sodium bicarbonate infusion, though the data for each of these measures remains somewhat controversial.

VI. CLINICAL APPLICATIONS

A. Coronary calcium scoring uses the observation that coronary calcium is a surrogate marker for coronary atherosclerotic plaque. Studies have shown that the complete absence of coronary artery calcium makes the presence of significant coronary luminal obstruction highly unlikely and indicates a very low risk of future coronary events. Men tend to have higher calcium scores, and individuals of either gender with renal insufficiency or diabetes tend to have higher coronary calcium scores.

1. Either noncontrast EBCT or MDCT can be used (typically with 3.0-mm slice thickness). Contrast is not necessary because calcium is readily identified secondary to its very high x-ray attenuation coefficient (high Hounsfield unit score).
2. The **Agatston coronary artery calcium (CAC) volume score** is the most frequently used scoring system. It is derived by measuring the area of each calcified coronary lesion and multiplying it by a coefficient of 1 to 4, depending on the maximum CT attenuation within that lesion. It is important to realize the reproducibility of the Agatston score before applying the recommended guidelines for cut points. Importantly, the variability in score has very little meaning at the very high and very low scores. Inter-reader variability can be as high as 3%.
   a. The **CAC score** can be classified into five groups: 1) zero, no coronary calcification; 2) 100, mild coronary calcification; 3) >100 to 399, moderate calcification; 4) >400 to 999, severe calcification; 5) >1000, extensive calcification.
   b. The CAC score is age and gender specific. Therefore, there has to be a comparison of the individual data to a "normal" cohort in order to produce meaningful data, usually presented as the percentile distribution. In general, CAC develops 10 to 15 years later in life in women than in men. Similarly, CAC is generally 5 to 7 times lower at any given age in women than in men.
   c. In a typical cohort of CAD patients, the median CAC score is 975 for men and 370 for women. In comparison with a CAC score of zero, the presence of any CAC is associated with a fourfold risk of coronary events over 3 to 5 years.
   d. In patients at intermediate clinical risk for coronary events (e.g., by Framingham score), the CAC score can help to reclassify patients to a higher or lower risk group. For instance, a CAC score of zero confirms low risk of events. Conversely, a CAC score of greater than 400 is observed with a significant cardiac event rate (greater than 2%/year) in patients who appear to be intermediate risk by Framingham score.
   e. Because statins have no documented effect on CAC progression, there is no value in repeating CAC in persons with a score of greater than 100 or the 75th percentile.
3. However, not every atherosclerotic plaque is calcified, and even the detection of a large amount of calcium does not imply the presence of significant stenoses. Therefore, it adds only incrementally to traditional risk assessment and should not be used in isolation. The test is most useful in intermediate risk populations, in which a high or low score may reclassify individuals to a higher or lower risk group. Unselected screening is not recommended.

B. Coronary CT angiography has been shown to be an accurate noninvasive modality for visualizing the coronary arteries, with high sensitivity (85% to 95%) and specificity (95% to 98%) compared with invasive angiography as the gold standard.

1. Coronary CT angiography for evaluating CAD is most useful in low- to intermediate-risk patients with angina or anginal equivalent. The **negative**

predictive value of coronary CT angiography is uniformly high in studies, approaching 93% to 100%; in other words, coronary CT angiography is an excellent modality for ruling ***out*** coronary disease.

2. Patients who are generally poor candidates for coronary CT angiography include those who are likely to have heavily calcified coronary arteries (older than 75, end-stage renal disease, Paget's disease), atrial fibrillation/flutter, frequent ventricular ectopic beats, or uncontrolled tachycardia. Quantification of stenosis severity is often impossible in densely calcified arteries, whereas image quality is significantly degraded in patients with arrhythmias or tachycardia.
3. Known severe CAD is generally a contraindication to coronary CT angiography. However, cardiac CT has been shown to have high sensitivity and specificity for assessment of bypass graft patency in patients with previous coronary artery bypass grafting (CABG) (see subsequent text).
4. **Stent patency**. Patients with prior coronary artery stents are generally poor candidates for CAD, although selected patients with proximal LAD or left main stents may be successfully imaged. Current CT technology does not allow for the accurate quantification of in-stent stenosis severity.
5. When assessing the coronaries, **noncalcified plaque** appears as a low to intermediate attenuation irregularity in the vessel wall. **Calcified plaques** are bright, high-attenuation lesions in the vessel wall and may be associated with positive remodeling of the vessel. Densely calcified plaques are often associated with **calcium blooming artifact**, which can lead to overestimation of luminal stenosis severity.
6. The accuracy of coronary CT angiography is highest in the larger proximal to medium vessels, which are more likely to benefit from an invasive management strategy. Coronary stenoses are generally categorized as mild (less than 50% diameter stenosis), moderate (50% to70% stenosis), or severe (greater than 70% stenosis).

C. Bypass graft imaging.

1. **Graft location.** MDCT can accurately characterize the origin, course, and touchdown of prior bypass grafts, using intermediate slice thickness (e.g., 1.5 mm). This can be important for surgical planning (see details in subsequent text of this chapter).
2. **Graft patency**. Using a protocol similar to that used for coronary artery assessment (less than 1 mm slice thickness), patency of both arterial and venous bypass grafts can be assessed. Recent studies have suggested that the sensitivity and specificity of MDCT for detecting stenosis or occlusion of bypass grafts, when compared with invasive angiography, is 97% and 97%, respectively. Occasionally, artifacts related to metallic clips can interfere with assessment of the distal anastomosis of an arterial graft (internal mammary or radial artery graft).

D. Coronary artery anomalies. Due to the three-dimensional data acquisition, MDCT is an excellent modality for assessing patients with known or suspected coronary artery anomalies. MDCT can accurately assess the origin and course of anomalous coronaries, and can describe the relationship of the coronary artery to neighboring structures. Although MRI can also be used to assess anomalous coronaries without the need for radiation exposure, the spatial resolution, ease of data acquisition, and reliable image quality of MDCT make it a reasonable first choice. Intramyocardial **bridging** can also be detected with high sensitivity, though the clinical significance of this relatively common finding is uncertain.

E. Cardiac morphology/function. Contrast-enhanced MDCT can provide high-resolution morphologic images of the cardiac chambers as well as accurate assessment of right and left ventricular systolic function. However, other imaging modalities such as echocardiography or MRI, which do not require radiation exposure, are generally preferred initially for assessing cardiac morphology.

1. Patients with prior **myocardial infarction** can have fibrous replacement of myocardium with or without calcification, ventricular wall thinning, aneurysm formation, and cavitary thrombus.

2. **Ventricular dysplasia** is characterized by: fibrous and/or fatty replacement of myocardium, ventricular wall thinning and/or focal aneurysm formation, and ventricular cavity dilation with regional or global wall motion abnormalities.
3. **Mass.** CT provides somewhat less information about tissue type than cardiac MRI, though the attenuation of a mass (in HU) can be helpful. For instance, lipomas have low CT numbers, cysts have water density (i.e., 0 to 10 H.U.), and thrombi have low to intermediate CT numbers. Atrial myxoma can be visualized easily in the left atrium, though right atrial masses may be difficult to visualize due to contrast mixing at the junction of the right atrium and inferior vena cava (IVC).

F. **Pericardial diseases.** The pericardium appears as a thin line (1 to 2 mm) surrounding the heart, usually visible with a small amount of adjacent pericardial fat. The pericardium normally enhances with contrast administration; hyperenhancement of the pericardium in the appropriate clinical setting is characteristic of pericarditis.
1. By CT, **congenital absence of the pericardium** is easily diagnosed.
2. Findings of pericardial **constriction** on CT include irregular pericardial thickening and calcification, conical or tubular compression of one or both ventricles, enlargement of one or both atria, dilation of the IVC, and a characteristic diastolic bounce of the interventricular septum.
3. Pericardial effusions can be reliably detected by CT, and a small amount of fluid is normal even in healthy subjects. Pericardial tamponade is better evaluated by echocardiography, however, due to its ability to provide hemodynamic information.
4. A pericardial **cyst** will appear as a well circumscribed paracardiac mass with characteristic water attenuation (H.U. = 0), usually in the right costophrenic angle.
5. Both primary **neoplasms** and, more commonly, metastatic neoplasms can be visualized in the pericardium.

G. **Congenital heart disease.** MDCT may be used in selected patients in whom echocardiography is non-diagnostic or inadequate and MRI is not available. The ability to evaluate cardiovascular anatomy in multiple planes is often helpful for delineating cardiac morphology in congenital heart disease, particularly with regard to the relationship of the great vessels, pulmonary veins, and coronary arteries. Specific situations in which MDCT is helpful include "hard-to-find" adult shunt detection (sinus venosus atrial septal defect, patent ductus arteriosus); visualization of pulmonary arteries in cyanotic congenital heart disease; precise definition of aortic anatomy in Marfan's syndrome or coarctation; and definition of partial or total anomalous pulmonary venous drainage. Additionally, CT can be useful for follow-up imaging in patients with congenital heart disease who have had prior pacemaker or ICD implantation, such as L-transposition of the great arteries.

H. **Diseases of the aorta** constitute a common and important indication for CT examinations. Contrast-enhanced MDCT is nearly 100% sensitive and specific for evaluating acute aortic syndromes. ECG gating is critically important for studies of the aortic root and ascending aorta, given the propensity for motion artifacts to appear similar to dissection flaps on non-gated studies.
1. **Acute aortic dissection** (see Chapter 25) is characterized on CT by visualization of a dissection flap (i.e., separation of the intima from the media) that forms true and false lumens. The CT study can characterize the origin and extent of the dissection, classify it as Type A or B, assess for concomitant aneurysmal aortic dilatation, and identify branch vessels involvement.
2. **Aortic intramural hematomas** are believed to be caused by spontaneous hemorrhage of the vaso vasorum into the medial layer. They appear as crescent-shaped areas of increased attenuation with eccentric aortic wall thickening. Unlike dissections, hematomas do not spiral around the aorta.
3. **Aortic aneurysm** is a permanent dilation of 150% of the normal aortic caliber (usually greater than 5 cm in the thoracic aorta and greater than 3 cm in the abdominal aorta). Given the often tortuous course of a dilated aorta, it is important that these measurements be made in the true short axis of the aorta, as oblique

cuts can result in erroneous overestimation of the aortic diameter. Quantitative measurements of an aortic aneurysm can be made for planning endovascular repair with a **stent graft.**

4. **Penetrating atherosclerotic ulcer.** These tend to be focal lesions of the descending thoracic aorta that appear as contrast-filled irregular outpouchings of the aortic wall.

I. **Evaluation of pulmonary veins.** In the context of electrophysiology interventions such as pulmonary vein isolation (PVI), preprocedural MDCT can be used to define pulmonary venous anatomy and identify supernumerary veins, and postprocedural MDCT can be used to evaluate for pulmonary vein stenosis. Additionally, in the setting of congenital heart disease, CT can be used to identify anomalous pulmonary venous return.

J. **Evaluation of pulmonary embolism (PE).** MDCT is highly accurate in detecting PE, which appear as a filling defect in the pulmonary arteries. This modality is most sensitive for proximal (main through segmental branches) thrombi, and small, distal emboli may be missed.

K. **Valvular heart disease.** Visualization of the valve leaflets, particularly the aortic valve, is feasible with newer-generation scanners due to their improved temporal resolution. Nonenhanced MDCT is also useful for assessing prosthetic mechanical valve leaflet motion.

L. **Surgical planning.** The utility of MDCT in surgical planning before cardiothoracic surgery, particularly for reoperations, is increasingly recognized. Preoperative scans can evaluate the proximity of mediastinal structures to the sternum (i.e., aorta, right ventricle, bypass grafts); the degree of aortic calcification (i.e., to guide cannulation sites); and concomitantly provide information about cardiac morphology (e.g., presence of a ventricular aneurysm). Ongoing studies are evaluating whether this added information might reduce intraoperative and perioperative complications.

M. **Peripheral arteries.** MDCT can also be used to evaluate peripheral arteries, including the carotid, renal, visceral, and lower-extremity vessels. Indeed, imaging these vessels is generally more straightforward than coronary imaging, due to their large caliber and minimal motion. CT can be used for planning and follow-up of vascular disease in these peripheral vascular beds. Given the larger caliber of these vessels, assessment of stent patency is often quite feasible.

ACKNOWLEDGMENT

The authors thank Drs. Paul Schoenhagen, Richard D. White, Sandra S. Halliburton, and Stacie A. Kuzmiak, for their contributions to earlier editions of this chapter.

Key Articles

Achenbach S, Moshage W, Ropers D, et al. Value of electron-beam computed tomography for the noninvasive detection of high-grade coronary-artery stenoses and occlusions. *N Engl J Med* 1998;339:1964–1971.

Achenbach S, Moselewski F, Ropers D, et al. Detection of calcified and noncalcified coronary atherosclerotic plaque by contrast-enhanced, submillimeter multidetector spiral computed tomography: a segment-based comparison with intravascular ultrasound. *Circulation* 2004;109:14–17.

Bae KT, Hong C, Whiting BR. Radiation dose in multidetector row computed tomography cardiac imaging. *J Magn Reson Imaging* 2004;19:859–863.

Fayad ZA, Fuster V, Nikolaou K, et al. Computed tomography and magnetic resonance imaging for noninvasive coronary angiography and plaque imaging: current and potential future concepts. *Circulation* 2002;106:2026–2034.

Feuchtner GM, Schachner T, Bonatti J, et al. Diagnostic performance of 64-slice computed tomography in evaluation of coronary artery bypass grafts. *AJR Am J Roentgenol* 2007;189:574–580.

Hunold P, Vogt FM, Schmermund A, et al. Radiation exposure during cardiac CT: effective doses at multi-detector row CT and electron-beam CT. *Radiology* 2003;226:145–152.

Leber AW, Becker A, Knez A, et al. Accuracy of 64-slice computed tomography to classify and quantify plaque volumes in the proximal coronary system: a comparative study using intravascular ultrasound. *J Am Coll Cardiol* 2006;47:672–677.

Leber AW, Knez A, Becker A, et al. Accuracy of multidetector spiral computed tomography in identifying and differentiating the composition of coronary atherosclerotic plaques: a comparative study with intracoronary ultrasound. *J Am Coll Cardiol* 2004;43:1241–1247.

Meyer TS, Martinoff S, Hadamitzky M, et al. Improved noninvasive assessment of coronary artery bypass grafts with 64-slice computed tomographic angiography in an unselected patient population. *J Am Coll Cardiol* 2007;49:946–950.

Pundziute G, Schuijf JD, Jukema JW, et al. Prognostic value of multislice computed tomography coronary angiography in patients with known or suspected coronary artery disease. *J Am Coll Cardiol* 2007;49:62–70.

Raff GL, Gallagher MJ, O'Neill WW, Goldstein JA. Diagnostic accuracy of noninvasive coronary angiography using 64-slice spiral computed tomography. *J Am Coll Cardiol* 2005;46:552–557.

Rudnick MR, Kesselheim A, Goldfarb S. Contrast-induced nephropathy: how it develops, how to prevent it. *Cleve Clin J Med* 2006;73:75–80, 83–87.

Schroeder S, Kopp AF, Baumbach A, et al. Noninvasive detection and evaluation of atherosclerotic coronary plaques with multislice computed tomography. *J Am Coll Cardiol* 2001;37:1430–1435.

Smith AD, Schoenhagen P. CT imaging for acute aortic syndrome. *Cleve Clin J Med* 2008;75:7–9, 12, 15–17.

Relevant Book Chapters

Achenbach SA, Daniel WG. Computed Tomography of the Heart. In: Libby P, Bonow RO, Mann DL, Zipes DP, ed. *Braunwald's Heart Disease: A Textbook of Cardiovascular Medicine,* 8th ed. Philadelphia: WB Saunders, 2008:415–438.

Hubbard C, Sola S. Cardiac MRI and CT. In: Griffin BP, Rimmerman CM, Topol EJ, ed. *The Cleveland Clinic Cardiology Board Review*. Philadelphia: Lippincott Williams & Wilkins, 2007:421–438.

Murphy RT, Garcia MJ. In: Topol EJ, ed. *Textbook of cardiovascular medicine,* 3rd ed. Philadelphia: Lippincott Williams & Wilkins, 2007:941–960.

Relevent Guidelines and Appropriateness Criteria

Hendel RC, Patel MR, Kramer CM, et al. ACCF/ACR/SCCT/SCMR/ASNC/NASCI/SCAI/SIR 2006 appropriateness criteria for cardiac computed tomography and cardiac magnetic resonance imaging: a report of the American College of Cardiology Foundation Quality Strategic Directions Committee Appropriateness Criteria Working Group, American College of Radiology, Society of Cardiovascular Computed Tomography, Society for Cardiovascular Magnetic Resonance, American Society of Nuclear Cardiology, North American Society for Cardiac Imaging, Society for Cardiovascular Angiography and Interventions, and Society of Interventional Radiology. *J Am Coll Cardiol* 2006;48:1475–1497.

Greenland P, Bonow RO, Brundage BH, et al. ACCF/AHA 2007 clinical expert consensus document on coronary artery calcium scoring by computed tomography in global cardiovascular risk assessment and in evaluation of patients with chest pain: a report of the American College of Cardiology Foundation Clinical Expert Consensus Task Force (ACCF/AHA Writing Committee to Update the 2000 Expert Consensus Document on Electron Beam Computed Tomography) developed in collaboration with the Society of Atherosclerosis Imaging and Prevention and the Society of Cardiovascular Computed Tomography. *J Am Coll Cardiol* 2007;49:378–402.

ELECTROPHYSIOLOGIC PROCEDURES

X

ELECTROPHYSIOLOGIC STUDIES

48

Carlos Alves

I. INTRODUCTION. Electrophysiologic studies (EPS) are a specialized form of cardiac catheterization that help identify, characterize, and manage cardiac arrhythmias. Over the past 25 to 30 years, EPS have advanced our knowledge of mechanisms of cardiac arrhythmias and revolutionized the way these arrhythmias are managed. The studies should be performed by trained clinicians with the help of skilled laboratory personnel in appropriately equipped laboratories. A joint task force of the American College of Cardiology and the American Heart Association in collaboration with the North American Society of Pacing and Electrophysiology has published guidelines outlining the accepted indications and the required training for personnel performing EPS.

II. INDICATIONS for EPS can be divided into three broad categories: bradyarrhythmias, tachyarrhythmias, and syncope.

A. Bradyarrhythmias can be caused by sinus node dysfunction, atrioventricular (AV) nodal disease, or infranodal conduction system disease. EPS for bradyarrhythmias are rarely necessary because the decision to implant a pacemaker depends primarily on correlation between symptoms and documented bradycardia or demonstration of severe bradycardia or prolonged pauses. EPS should complement the clinical evaluation, conventional 12-lead electrocardiogram (ECG), and Holter or event monitoring. EPS can be of value in identifying disorders associated with adverse outcome, such as severe infranodal conduction system disease.

B. More often, EPS may suggest bradycardia as the underlying disorder among patients with **syncope** of unknown cause. Thus, patients with syncope of uncertain cause may benefit from EPS.

C. EPS are of tremendous value in evaluating **tachyarrhythmias.** They are generally more successful in reproducing re-entrant cardiac rhythms than those caused by triggered activity or enhanced automaticity. Among patients with re-entrant tachyarrhythmias, EPS are useful in documenting the presence of the anatomic or physiologic substrate responsible for the arrhythmia, defining electrical mechanism of the arrhythmia and its associated hemodynamic response, as well as guiding therapy. The response of the tachyarrhythmia during an EPS to various drugs or maneuvers may also be helpful in further defining the underlying substrate and prognosis.

III. EQUIPMENT AND SETTING

A. The most important element in the performance of safe and useful EPS is the presence of **well-trained personnel.** The presence of at least one trained physician and well-trained laboratory support personnel, including a nurse, as well as engineering assistance to maintain and repair the laboratory equipment is necessary. Personnel involved should be familiar with basic electrophysiologic and electropharmacologic principles, the indications for EPS, and the various diagnostic and therapeutic modalities that can be used in the laboratory.

B. It is important that the laboratory be equipped with appropriate high-quality **radiographic equipment.**

C. Appropriate selection of **tools** is a very important aspect of the performance of safe and cost-effective EPS. The minimum instrumentation required for a complete study is a stimulator, an amplifier, display monitors, reliable recording devices, and an external defibrillator.

1. The **stimulator** must be capable of burst pacing, delivery of at least three or four extra stimuli, synchronization of the stimulator to appropriate electric events during intrinsic or paced rhythms, and an adjustable current output. An appropriate unit should have a constant current source and minimal current leakage. It also should be relatively easy to manipulate.
2. The **junction box** connects electrode catheters to the recording apparatus and to the stimulator.
3. **Recording** is best achieved on solid media (e.g., CD or other optical media).
4. The presence of at least two functioning **external defibrillators** is extremely important, particularly during studies in which ventricular arrhythmias may be induced. Biphasic defibrillators should be the equipment of choice due to their superior defibrillation capacity.
5. The presence of a cardiac surgical team in the same institution is not mandatory for routine EPS or simple radiofrequency (RF) ablation procedures. However, for more complex RF ablation procedures where full heparinization is used and where cardiac perforation is a potential complication, the presence of a cardiac surgical team in the institution provides an added safety factor to the performance of these procedures.

D. Intracardiac signals are recorded using various **electrode catheters.**

1. The most common catheters used are **quadripolar woven Dacron polyester** or **polyurethane.** The distal poles of these catheters can be used for pacing.
2. For general-purpose sensing and pacing in the atrium or ventricle, a **nondeflectable catheter** usually is sufficient. Deflectable catheters facilitate mapping and ablation by allowing more precise movement.
3. Some catheters have a lumen through which a guidewire can be inserted and dye can be injected.
4. Interelectrode distance varies from 2 to 10 mm. Smaller interelectrode distance is useful for precise mapping and timing.
5. For most EPS, **bipolar recording** is used. However, in some situations, especially during mapping of tachyarrhythmias, unipolar recording can be of value in localizing the earliest sites of activity.

IV. TECHNIQUES AND PROCEDURES

A. Preprocedure preparation

1. Before the patient is taken to the EPS laboratory, a **discussion** of the indications and proposed procedure is conducted with the patient, and informed consent is obtained.
2. For most indications, EPS is an **elective** procedure. The patient's condition should be clinically **stable** at the time of the study. EPS on patients whose condition is unstable, including those with active, recent, or untreated coronary disease or in those with clinical heart failure, carry much higher risk for complications.
3. **Electrolytes, serum digoxin level, and bleeding measurements** are checked and verified as being within the acceptable range.
4. A mild **sedative** is administered (e.g., a benzodiazepine).
5. The patient is attached to continuous ECG and blood pressure **monitoring** devices.

B. Access and catheter placement

1. The usual approach to inserting electrode catheters is through the **femoral veins under local anesthesia** unless there is a clear contraindication to this approach, such as the presence of deep venous thrombosis or an inferior vena caval filter. In the latter situations or when a coronary sinus catheter is difficult to insert, a superior vein approach is used. At times, when a single catheter insertion is appropriate, an antecubital vein may be used to avoid a central vein access.

2. Up to three **introducers** are placed in each femoral vein depending on the planned procedure. For patients with **left-sided bypass tracks or left ventricular (LV) tachycardia,** access to the left side of the heart is necessary. This can be achieved through the retrograde transaortic approach via an arterial access or by transseptal puncture via a femoral vein access. Systemic heparin is used for all left-sided procedures.
3. **For a complete EPS, three catheters are needed**
   a. One catheter is placed in the **high right atrium,** preferably in the appendage or against the high lateral wall. Another is placed in the **right ventricular (RV) apex,** and the third is placed across the **tricuspid valve** to obtain a His electrogram.
   b. To obtain a **His electrogram,** the electrode catheter is advanced into the right ventricle across the anterior septal portion of the tricuspid valve. Under gentle clockwise torque, the catheter is then slowly withdrawn to straddle the tricuspid valve. A high-frequency sharp deflection that precedes ventricular activation and follows septal atrial activation represents a **His** or **proximal right bundle potential.** If the catheter is drawn further, this sharp signal occurs slightly earlier. A satisfactory position of the His catheter is achieved when an atrial signal is recorded followed by the His potential and, finally, the ventricular potential is recorded via the same pair of electrodes. A catheter with 1-cm interelectrode spacing is preferable for this purpose.
4. In **supraventricular tachycardia (SVT)** studies when a left-sided accessory pathway or left atrial origin is suspected, an octapolar or decapolar catheter may be placed in the coronary sinus (CS) rather than in the high right atrium. This more stable catheter position allows mapping of the left AV groove. Although the coronary sinus is easily entered from the superior venous approach, successful catheterization is expected in most attempts through the femoral approach as well. The catheter is placed in the CS with the proximal electrodes just inside the CS ostium.

C. Baseline assessment

1. When all the catheters are in place, a baseline ECG (generally leads I, aVF, V_1, and V_6) and intracardiac electrogram are obtained (Fig. 48.1).

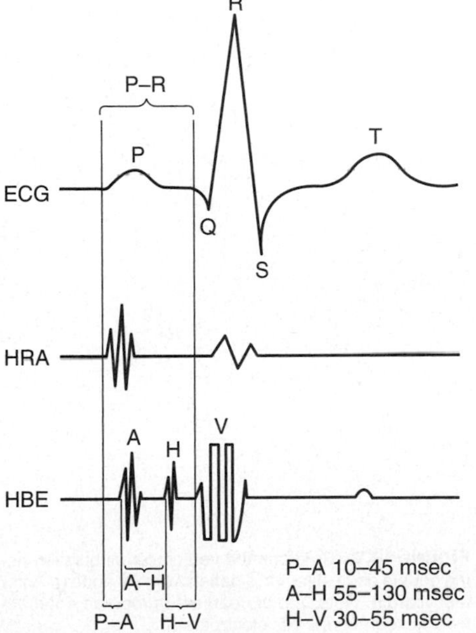

Figure 48.1. Normal baseline intervals. Typically, up to four surface ECGs (I, aVF, V_1, and V_6) are displayed along with atrial (CS), His (HBE), and ventricular (RVA) electrograms. CS 7–8 refers to the proximal bipolar CS electrogram. Fast sweep speeds are used, ranging from 100 to 400 mm/second. On the time scale, each large division is 100 milliseconds, and each minor division is 10 milliseconds. In addition to intervals, pattern of atrial and ventricular activation should be evaluated. If the CS catheter is placed correctly (see text), the earliest A in sinus rhythm is seen on the HRA electrogram (not shown), then on the His electrogram, and progressively later along the CS electrograms. In the absence of bundle branch block or left-sided accessory pathway, the earliest ventricular activity is seen on right-sided electrograms (His and RV electrograms). (Adapted from *Dorland's Illustrated Medical Dictionary.*)

2. In general, **cycle lengths** rather than beats per minute are measured. The following measurements are made at baseline: sinus cycle length and PR, QRS, QT, AH, and HV intervals. To convert an arrhythmia's rate from cycle length to beats per minute, divide 60,000 by the cycle length to obtain the arrhythmia rate in beats per minute.
   a. The **AH interval** is measured from the onset of the local A deflection to the H deflection on the His electrogram.
   b. The **HV interval** is measured from the H deflection on the His electrogram to the earliest ventricular activity in any lead.
3. When measurements are made during pacing, it is important to **measure from the resulting deflection** rather than from the pacing artifact to avoid errors caused by latency (delay between the pacing artifact and activation at the recording site).
4. All measurements are recorded in **milliseconds.** Interpretation of baseline intervals is shown in Figure 48.2.

D. Programmed stimulation

1. After baseline measurements are made, programmed stimulation is performed. The protocol used depends on the indication for the study and varies among

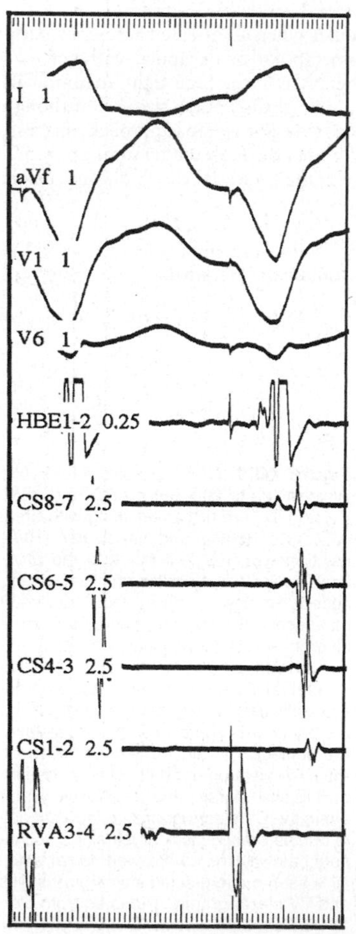

Figure 48.2. Programmed ventricular stimulation using double extra stimuli in a patient with AV node re-entry tachycardia. Note that the earliest retrograde atrial activity is seen on the His electrogram.

institutions. During programmed stimulation, the **hemodynamic response** of the patient to pacing and induced tachycardia is closely monitored.

2. **Pacing stimuli** are usually delivered at 1- or 2-millisecond pulse width and at twice diastolic pacing thresholds. This is important during ventricular stimulation because pacing at higher outputs increases the risk for inducing nonclinical rhythms. There are two main types of programmed stimulation: burst pacing and the extra stimulus technique.
   a. **Burst pacing** involves continuous pacing at rates faster than the patient's intrinsic rate.
   b. In the **extra stimulus technique,** premature beats are introduced either during intrinsic rhythm (sensed extra stimuli) or after a paced drive train (paced extra stimuli). Extra stimulus techniques are useful in evaluating refractory periods of the AV node, atrial tissue, ventricular tissue, and accessory pathways. It is possible to evaluate infranodal conduction system refractory periods with atrial or ventricular stimulation. Extra stimulus techniques also are useful in inducing, terminating, and identifying re-entrant arrhythmias.
      (1) In the **sensed extra stimulus** technique, a single extra stimulus (S_2) is introduced initially with a coupling just below the intrinsic rate. The coupling interval is reduced progressively by 10 to 20 milliseconds until the premature stimulus no longer captures. A pause of 2 to 5 seconds is allowed between stimulation sequences. Multiple extra stimuli (S_3, S_4) can be added if necessary and the sequence repeated.
      (2) In the **paced extra stimulus** technique, a drive train of 6 to 10 beats at a fixed cycle length is followed by the premature beat. The drive train cycle length (S_1S_1) usually ranges from 350 to 800 milliseconds (most frequently 400 to 600 milliseconds) but depends on the resting heart rate. When this technique is used, testing at two drive-train cycle lengths is recommended. The premature stimulus (S_2) is introduced with a coupling interval just below S_1S_1 cycle length. The coupling interval of the premature stimulus is decreased progressively by 10 to 20 milliseconds until it no longer captures. The longest coupling interval (S_1S_2) that does not capture the myocardium is the absolute refractory period. S_3 and S_4 are added if necessary. This protocol can be varied depending on the indication and operator preference.

3. **Continuous monitoring** and recording of external and intracardiac electrograms is maintained throughout programmed stimulation. When a particular event such as a tachycardia occurs, stimulation is stopped and the event evaluated. The operator should be ready to respond to the event appropriately depending on the effect that the event has on the patient. For example, induction of a sustained tachycardia may result in severe hypotension, angina, or loss of consciousness. In such circumstances, expeditious termination of the tachycardia is indicated through overdrive pacing or cardioversion. The operator should also be ready to perform pacing or other maneuvers to further assess the mechanisms and re-entrant circuit of the induced tachycardia.

V. ATRIAL STIMULATION

A. An atrial study is an integral part of EPS. The only time an atrial study is not performed is in the presence of persistent atrial fibrillation.

1. **Burst atrial pacing** at incremental rates causes slowing of AV nodal conduction (a process known as decremental conduction), and can induce tachycardia, including AV node re-entry tachycardia and AV re-entrant tachycardia. Other forms of tachycardia unrelated to AV nodal conduction can also be induced, such as atrial flutter, atrial fibrillation, atrial tachycardia, and certain forms of idiopathic ventricular tachycardia.
2. Burst pacing is performed by means of **continuous pacing** (e.g., 10 to 20 stimuli) at a fixed cycle length starting at 100 milliseconds below the baseline cycle length. Repeat burst pacing is performed at progressively shorter cycle lengths until 1:1 conduction through the AV node is no longer maintained. The shortest cycle length showing consistent 1:1 conduction through the AV node is recorded.

This is related to the **effective refractory period (ERP)** of the AV node, which is the longest A1-A2 interval that fails to be conducted to the His bundle. Another interval that can be measured is the **functional refractory period (FRP)** of the AV node: it is defined as being the shortest output interval from the AV node to the His bundle, given any input signal.

3. If a patient is believed to have **atrial flutter** or **atrial tachycardia,** repeat burst pacing at even shorter cycle lengths is performed until 1:1 atrial capture is no longer maintained.

B. Another form of atrial stimulation that is performed is paced extra stimulus

1. The **effect of atrial premature beats** on the AH interval is assessed. Normal response of the AH interval is to progressively prolong with shorter A_1A_2 coupling. This is a direct demonstration of the normal decremental conduction properties of the AV node.
2. At a critical A_1A_2, the AV node fails to conduct, and on the His electrogram an atrial signal is seen without a His or ventricular deflection. This indicates that **block has occurred in the AV node.** It is important to continue stimulation until the atrial refractory period is reached because a gap phenomenon may occasionally exist as a result of dual AV nodal pathways.
3. The **gap phenomenon** is demonstrated by apparent achievement of the AV nodal refractory period followed by resumption of conduction at shorter A_1A_2 coupling intervals. It reflects functional differences in conduction velocity or refractoriness in several regions of the AV junction.
4. If **narrow complex tachycardia** is induced, it is evaluated with regard to type, mechanism, response to maneuvers, and method of termination (see **IX.B.3**).

C. Sinus node evaluation. For patients who may have underlying sinus node dysfunction, sinus node tests are sometimes performed.

1. **Sinus node recovery time (SNRT)** is evaluated through burst pacing at various cycle lengths in the atrium for 30 to 60 seconds, followed by abrupt termination of pacing. SNRT is the escape interval between the last paced atrial beat and the first atrial recovery beat. A **corrected SNRT (CSNRT)** is calculated by means of subtracting baseline sinus cycle length from SNRT. A normal value for CSNRT is less than 550 milliseconds. SNRT is used to evaluate the automaticity mechanism of the sinus node.
2. **Sinoatrial conduction time (SACT)** is a combined measure of conduction in the atrial tissue that includes the area of the sinus node and sinus node automaticity. The assumptions are first that the conduction times into and out of the sinus node are equal, second that the pacing train does not alter the automaticity of the sinus node, and third that the pacemaking site does not change after premature stimulation. The SACT is measured with one of two methods.
   a. In the **Strauss method,** a sensed premature atrial beat is used to reset the sinus node, and the return cycle length after the premature beat is measured. Basic cycle length is subtracted from return cycle length, leaving the time necessary to penetrate and leave the sinus nodal tissue. SACT is one half this interval.
   b. In the **method proposed by Narula,** the same measurements are obtained after pacing for eight beats at a rate slightly faster than the sinus rate. The upper range of SACT is 100 to 120 milliseconds.

   The sensitivity of each individual (SACT and SNRT) test in diagnosing sinus node dysfunction is approximately 50% when used alone and 65% when combined. The specificity of the two combined tests is 88%, which gives the test a high positive predictive value. However, because of its low sensitivity, a normal test does not exclude sinus node disease.

VI. VENTRICULAR STIMULATION

A. Ventricular stimulation is performed in evaluations of suspected SVTs or ventricular tachyarrhythmias. Some SVTs, such as unusual forms of AV nodal re-entry, may be more easily induced with ventricular stimulation. To further characterize the tachycardia, the response of the tachycardia to premature ventricular beats can be assessed.

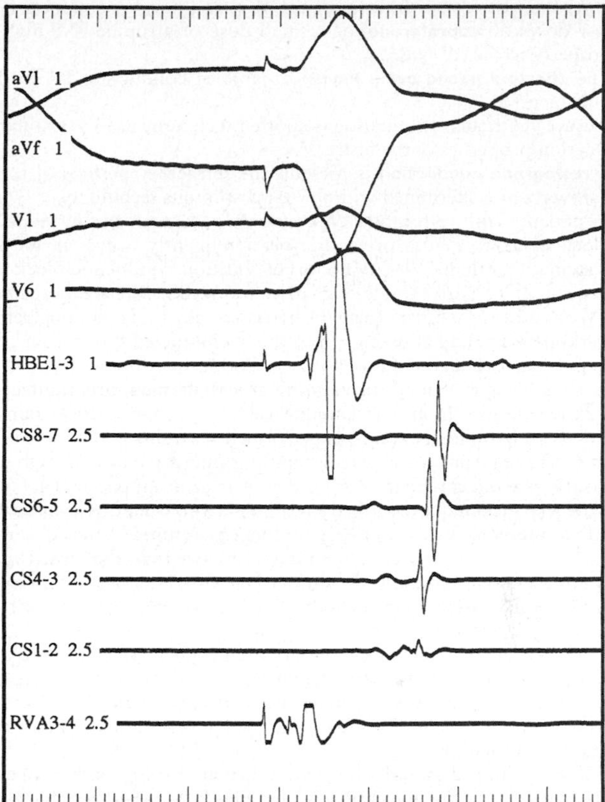

Figure 48.3. This is an example from a 17-year-old patient with left lateral manifest pathway. Ventricular stimulation results in retrograde atrial activation with the earliest A seen in CS 1–2 (eccentric atrial activation).

1. When ventricular stimulation is performed for the evaluation of ventricular or wide complex tachyarrhythmias, **pacing at two sites** is necessary. These sites typically are the RV apex and the RV outflow tract.
2. Before programmed stimulation is begun, pacing thresholds are determined, and the output of the pacing stimulus is set to twice the diastolic capture threshold. Higher outputs or coupling intervals shorter than 200 milliseconds may cause induction of nonclinical arrhythmias.

B. Burst pacing in the right ventricle is one of two techniques used when assessing retrograde ventriculoatrial (VA) conduction in the evaluation of SVT.

1. The presence of **retrograde atrial activation** is documented, and a sequence or pattern of atrial activation is evaluated.
2. The **earliest atrial activity** during retrograde conduction via the AV node typically is recorded on the His electrogram (see Fig. 48.2). This indicates that retrograde conduction has proceeded through the AV node fast pathway. **Absence of VA conduction,** with rare exceptions (e.g., the Mahaim type of accessory pathway), excludes the presence of a bypass track. The **presence of eccentric atrial activation** (late atrial activation on the His electrogram; see Fig. 48.3) suggests the presence of a retrogradely conducting bypass track.

3. For some patients with no evidence of retrograde VA conduction, infusion of low doses of **isoproterenol** or a small dose of atropine (0.5 mg) restores this property to the AV node.
4. The **shortest paced cycle length** capable of conducting 1:1 to the atrium is documented.

C. Premature ventricular stimulation is another technique used to evaluate retrograde conduction properties of the heart.

1. If **retrograde conduction** is present, the refractory periods of the conducting pathways are determined with the extra stimulus technique.
2. In patients with **retrograde VA conduction through the AV node,** conduction block of a ventricular premature beat frequently occurs in the His-Purkinje system rather than in the AV node. His-Purkinje conduction block is more likely to occur at long drive trains. Such drive trains therefore are more likely to induce AV re-entry tachycardia (using a bypass track) by facilitating retrograde His-Purkinje block and allowing a retrograde conducted beat through the pathway to propagate antegrade through the AV node.

D. In patients being evaluated for **ventricular arrhythmias,** programmed stimulation with extra stimuli is the initial technique used. Pacing at two drive-train cycle lengths (e.g., 600 and 400 milliseconds) is performed with single, double, and triple extra stimuli. Simultaneous atrial pacing at the same drive-cycle length sometimes is necessary to avoid competition from the intrinsic atrial pacemaker.

E. Like the A_1A_2 technique described earlier, **V_2 is introduced at progressively shorter coupling intervals** (V_1V_2) until V_2 no longer captures (ventricular refractory period). Then V_2 is set at a coupling interval longer than the refractory period and **V_3 is introduced** at progressively shorter coupling intervals until it no longer captures. The use of **triple extra stimuli** (V_3V_4) is usually reserved for patients being evaluated for ventricular arrhythmias.

A pause of 4 to 5 seconds is allowed after each cycle to assess response and for the patient to recover after ventricular pacing. An increase in number of extra stimuli increases sensitivity of the study in reproducing clinical arrhythmias, but at the cost of a lower specificity due to initiation of polymorphic ventricular tachycardia or ventricular fibrillation.

If programmed stimulation with ventricular extra stimuli does not induce ventricular tachycardia in a patient at very high risk, other techniques may be used. One is **burst pacing in the ventricle.** A series of 10 paced ventricular beats are introduced at a constant cycle length. The paced cycle length is then decreased by 50 to 100 milliseconds in successive bursts until reaching within 50 milliseconds of the predicted refractory period of the right ventricle, when the decrements proceed at 10-millisecond intervals until 1:1 capture is no longer maintained. Burst pacing in the atrium can at times induce idiopathic LV tachycardia in susceptible persons.

F. In some patients, particularly those with underlying dilated cardiomyopathy, **bundle branch re-entry (BBR) tachycardia** (see Fig. 48.4) may be induced.

1. This type of tachycardia usually involves the right bundle branch as the antegrade limb and the left bundle branch as the retrograde limb of the re-entrant circuit. It usually is a rapid and hemodynamically unstable tachycardia.
2. Because His bundle refractoriness increases after a pause, a short–long–short stimulation sequence can be used to cause retrograde block in the right bundle so that the paced stimulus can conduct retrograde up the left bundle branch and possibly initiate tachycardia if the right bundle branch is no longer refractory for antegrade conduction.
3. The sequence most commonly used consists of a 6-beat drive train at 400 milliseconds followed by V_2 coupled at 600 to 700 milliseconds. V_3 is then introduced at a coupling interval 100 milliseconds longer than the refractory period of the ventricle. V_2V_3 is progressively decreased until V_3 no longer captures. V_4 can be introduced if necessary.

VII. INDUCTION OF VENTRICULAR FIBRILLATION. Under certain circumstances, the operator may decide that induction of ventricular fibrillation is necessary. This is of value when testing implantable defibrillators for detection of arrhythmias and during

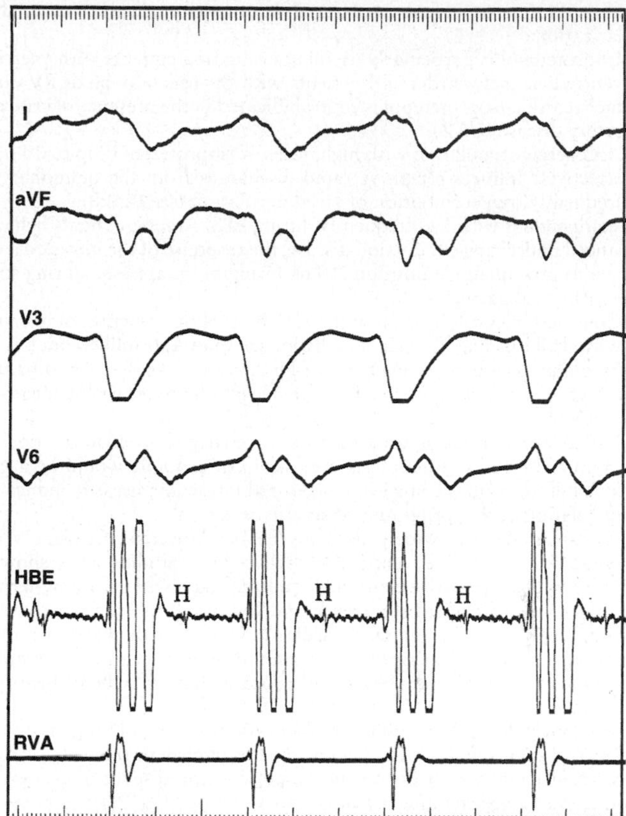

Figure 48.4. Bundle branch re-entry tachycardia. This example is from a 52-year-old man with dilated cardiomyopathy who presented with syncope. This ventricular tachycardia exhibits left bundle branch block morphology, and there is an H deflection preceding every V on the His electrogram. To be absolutely certain of this diagnosis (as opposed to myocardial ventricular tachycardia with retrograde His), one has to look for cycle length variation and document that changes in the H-H interval precede changes in the V-V interval.

assessment of defibrillation thresholds. Ventricular fibrillation can be induced by means of direct application of alternating current or rapid ventricular pacing at high output. The current can be delivered through a catheter electrode or through the **implantable cardioverter defibrillator (ICD)** lead. Another means of inducing ventricular fibrillation is to deliver a low-energy shock (around 1 J) via the intracardiac leads at the peak of the T wave.

VIII. USE OF CARDIOACTIVE DRUGS DURING EPS. Cardioactive drugs can be used during EPS as diagnostic or therapeutic agents. The drugs most commonly used are isoproterenol, procainamide, atropine, and adenosine.

A. Isoproterenol in doses ranging from 0.5 to 5 μg/kg per minute is used during EPS to facilitate induction of SVTs and ventricular tachyarrhythmias.

1. For patients with SVTs that are AV node dependent, isoproterenol facilitates conduction through the AV node by means of shortening its refractoriness.
2. It is not absolutely certain how isoproterenol facilitates induction of ventricular tachycardia, but possible mechanisms include enhanced conduction,

altered refractoriness, and enhanced automaticity related to delayed afterdepolarization.

3. Isoproterenol is particularly useful in evaluating patients with exercise-induced ventricular tachycardia and patients with the special type of RV outflow tract tachycardia. Isoproterenol is contraindicated in the presence of critical coronary artery disease (CAD).
4. Adrenergic stimulation with high doses of isoproterenol (up to 20 μg/min) also effectively induces repetitive rapid discharges from the pulmonary veins that frequently trigger initiation of atrial fibrillation (see **IX.B.3**).

B. **Procainamide** is used less frequently during EPS. Among patients believed to have advanced underlying conduction disease, the response of the infranodal conduction system to procainamide infusion (10 to 15 mg/kg) is assessed during sinus rhythm and with atrial pacing.

1. Considerable prolongation of the HV interval or induction of infranodal block with atrial pacing at cycle lengths longer than 400 milliseconds is considered by many experts to be evidence of His-Purkinje disease. Procainamide can facilitate the induction of atrial and ventricular arrhythmias by means of slowing conduction.
2. Procainamide often is used to prevent recurrent atrial fibrillation when programmed atrial stimulation is necessary. An example would be a patient with atrial flutter who is being evaluated for ablation and is easily induced into atrial fibrillation during programmed stimulation.
3. Procainamide was widely used in the past for risk assessment among patients with inducible ventricular tachycardia. Studies have shown that patients with suppressible ventricular tachycardia have better long-term prognosis (lower rate of clinical recurrence and lower mortality) than those with nonsuppressible ventricular tachycardia. However, with wider use of ICDs and evidence of their superiority even among persons with suppressible ventricular tachycardia, this application of procainamide may be of historical interest only.

C. **Adenosine,** in doses that produce transient AV block (6 to 18 mg), is used frequently in EPS of patients with SVTs to define the mechanism of the tachycardia, establish AV node dependence, or document the presence or absence of accessory pathway conduction before and after RF ablation.

IX. INTERPRETATION OF FINDINGS IN EPS

A. **Bradyarrhythmia evaluation.** EPS are *not* indicated when symptomatic bradycardia is documented. Among patients who have a clear indication for implantation of a permanent pacemaker, findings of EPS are unlikely to alter that decision. However, EPS are more helpful to patients believed to have underlying **sinus node or conduction system disease and symptoms** but for whom noninvasive monitoring has failed to document a correlation between bradycardia and symptoms. EPS also are helpful in assessing patients who continue to have symptoms after permanent pacemaker implantation.

1. **Baseline evaluation.** Sinus bradycardia, sinus arrest with junctional or ventricular escape, various degrees of heart block, and intraventricular conduction delay, isolated or in various combinations, may occur among patients with bradycardia and can be further evaluated by examining the intracardiac recordings.
   a. **Conduction intervals** are measured and evaluated. Disease in the AV node often produces prolongation in the AH interval, whereas disease in the infranodal conduction system produces prolongation in the HV interval.
   b. A long HV interval is suggestive but not diagnostic of an underlying bradyarrhythmia. It is commonly associated with wide QRS on surface ECG. A long HV interval at rest can be considered an indication for prophylactic pacemaker implantation (class IIa) if it exceeds 100 milliseconds (3).
   c. Documentation of intermittent spontaneous infranodal block or infranodal block in response to atrial pacing (see Fig. 48.5) or upon administration of procainamide is an indication for implanting a permanent pacemaker.

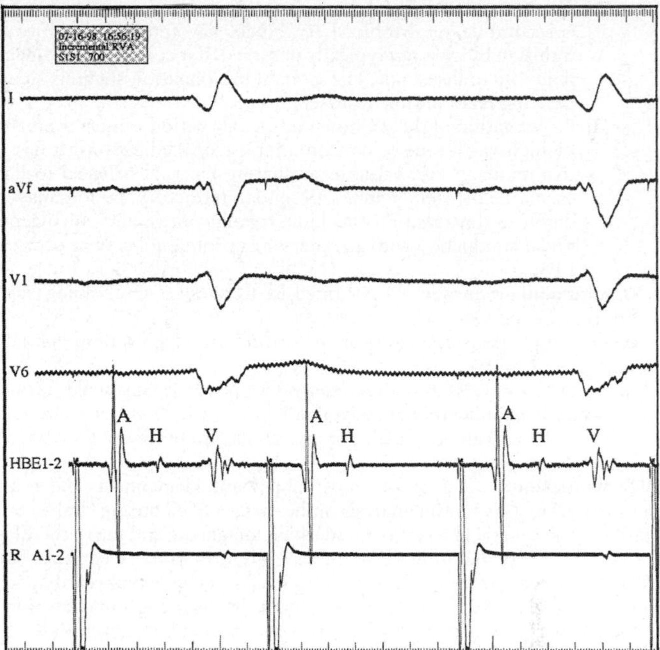

Figure 48.5. Infrahisian block in response to slow atrial pacing. This tracing is from a 70-year-old man who presented with syncope. Baseline H-V was 110 milliseconds. As shown in this tracing, burst pacing in the right atrium at cycle length of 700 milliseconds resulted in intermittent infrahisian block (H deflections not followed by V). This patient had a dual-chamber pacemaker implanted.

2. Programmed stimulation

a. After baseline intervals are measured, **SNRT and SACT** are determined. SNRT is used to evaluate automaticity of the sinoatrial node.

b. Rapid pacing causes overdrive suppression of the sinus node. Among patients with sinus node dysfunction, recovery time after cessation of pacing is prolonged. The situation is similar to sudden termination of atrial fibrillation, which can be followed by a prolonged pause.

c. After cessation of pacing, the **longest SNRT following pacing at varying cycle lengths and secondary pauses** are documented. Secondary pauses are those intervals related to the sinus beats that occur after the first escape beat. CSNRT, which is calculated by means of subtracting baseline cycle length from SNRT, is considered abnormal if it exceeds 550 milliseconds.

d. SACT is used to evaluate conduction velocities in the atrium and in tissues surrounding the sinoatrial node. SACT is performed with the methods described earlier. A normal SACT is between 50 and 125 milliseconds. When both CSNRT and SACT are normal, symptoms are uncommon. The sensitivities of CSNRT (54%) and SACT (51%) combined are higher (64%), and the specificity is approximately 88%. The low sensitivity of these tests limits their value in predicting development of symptoms in asymptomatic patients.

e. AV node and infranodal conduction system integrity is tested with atrial stimulation techniques. Attention is paid to the AH and HV intervals during atrial pacing.

(1) The refractory period of the AV node is determined at two cycle lengths. The shortest cycle length with 1:1 AV conduction is also determined.

(2) The normal AV nodal response to burst pacing at short cycle lengths is second-degree Mobitz I AV block. HV interval prolongation or infrahisian block is not typically observed. If it occurs at cycle lengths longer than 400 milliseconds, HV interval prolongation suggests significant underlying His-Purkinje disease.

(3) Prolongation of the AV nodal refractory period is most frequently caused by high vagal tone or concomitant use of medications. It has no predictive or diagnostic value in evaluating patients believed to have bradycardia. However, a long AV nodal refractory period may mask underlying abnormal His-Purkinje refractoriness, and enhancement of AV nodal conduction with atropine or isoproterenol may be necessary during EPS.

3. **Carotid sinus massage** is performed in all patients undergoing evaluation of bradycardia or syncope.
   a. Firm pressure is applied over the carotid artery pulsation, behind the angle of the mandible.
   b. A **positive cardioinhibitory response** is present if pauses of 3 seconds or more occur. A **vasodepressor response** is present if blood pressure decreases by more than 50 mm Hg in the absence of marked bradycardia. Mixed responses are common.

B. SVT evaluation. One of the most important elements in the evaluation of tachyarrhythmias is careful analysis of the surface ECG during clinical tachycardia. This can give several clues to the underlying diagnosis and make the EPS more focused. Most SVTs that induced in the EPS laboratory are re-entrant. They include AV nodal re-entry tachycardia, orthodromic AV re-entry tachycardia, atrial flutter, and re-entrant atrial tachycardia. Automatic tachyarrhythmias are relatively uncommon except in acutely ill patients. They characteristically exhibit a warm-up phenomenon, are difficult to induce with extra stimulus techniques, but may be induced with drugs such as isoproterenol.

1. **Baseline evaluation**
   a. Resting ECG and intracardiac recordings can provide important information about a possible cause even before any tachycardia is induced. The presence of a short PR interval on the ECG and wide QRS complex suggests preexcitation.
   b. Absence of preexcitation at rest does not rule out the presence of an accessory pathway. For the diagnosis of SVT, an atrial and a ventricular study have to be performed.
   c. If tachycardia is not induced at the baseline study, programmed stimulation in the atrium and ventricle is repeated with isoproterenol.
   d. Some SVTs, particularly those involving AV re-entry using a bypass tract, can be induced with ventricular stimulation, whereas atrial flutter and, to a lesser extent, atrial tachycardia rarely are induced by means of ventricular stimulation.
2. **Programmed stimulation** begins with burst pacing in the ventricle to document and characterize VA conduction. Absence of VA conduction practically excludes a concealed bypass tract, and ventricular extra stimulus technique may not need to be performed unless ventricular tachycardia is suspected.
   a. **Earliest retrograde atrial activity** usually is seen on the His electrogram during normal retrograde atrial activation through the AV node. Early retrograde atrial activity on the distal coronary sinus electrogram, if the position of the coronary sinus catheter is correct, suggests the presence of a left-sided accessory pathway (see Fig. 48.4). Early atrial activity in the proximal coronary sinus electrodes suggests a posteroseptal pathway or AV node slow-pathway conduction.

(1) Eccentric atrial activation is any atrial activation that does not activate the AV node and the area around the AV node first. This is frequently seen with retrograde ventricular stimulation, when the retrograde impulse finds the AV node refractory. The site of earliest atrial

activation is then in the distal CS catheter and not in the proximal area closest to the AV node/His bundle. Evidence of eccentric atrial activation may not be clear during burst pacing when there is fusion of retrograde impulses, arriving both through the AV node and the accessory pathway.

(2) The retrograde 1:1 cycle length should be documented.

(3) Programmed ventricular stimulation is performed with single premature beats at two drive-train cycle lengths (e.g., 600 and 400 milliseconds). During programmed stimulation the following are recorded:

(a) Retrograde refractory periods

(b) The pattern and any changes in retrograde atrial activation

(c) The site of retrograde VA block

(d) The presence of dual retrograde AV node function

(4) If an accessory pathway is found, its retrograde 1:1 conduction cycle length and refractory period are documented.

b. During atrial stimulation, particular attention is paid to the **AH and HV intervals.**

(1) Sudden prolongation of A_2H_2 of more than 50 milliseconds in response to a decrement of 10 milliseconds in A_1A_2 is called a **jump** (see Fig. 48.6) and has been classically described as a sign of dual AV physiology. **However, more recent reports have demonstrated that the normal AV node has dual pathways even if this "jump" is not demonstrated.** Furthermore, initiation of AV nodal re-entrant tachycardia does not require the presence of such a jump in the AV nodal conduction curve.

(2) Induction of re-entrant tachycardias generally depends on the occurrence of **unidirectional block and conduction delay.** In the case of AV nodal re-entry, antegrade block in the fast pathway combined with critical delay in the slow pathway allows the impulse to conduct retrograde on the fast pathway and excite the atrium. This first retrograde-conducted atrial depolarization is called an **echo beat** (see Fig. 48.6). If this echo beat succeeds in conducting antegrade down the slow pathway again and retrograde up the fast pathway, sustained AV nodal re-entry occurs.

(3) **Induction of AV node re-entry** is facilitated by use of shorter drive-train cycle lengths and, if necessary, use of more than one extra stimulus or rapid burst atrial pacing. Occasionally, initiation of AV nodal re-entry requires ventricular pacing or premature beats.

(4) In the presence of an accessory pathway, the site of critical delay is also in the AV node. However, to induce orthodromic AV re-entry tachycardia, antegrade block of an atrial impulse has to occur in the accessory pathway so that it is excitable by the time the same impulse propagates through the AV node and ventricle and arrives to conduct retrogradely through the accessory pathway to the atrium (see Fig. 48.7).

3. Evaluation of induced tachycardia

a. If a tachycardia is induced, the first assessment is its **hemodynamic consequences.** Hemodynamically unstable tachycardia should be immediately terminated. Only if the tachycardia is hemodynamically stable can further evaluations during tachycardia be conducted.

(1) Whether the QRS is narrow or wide, the relation between atrial rate and ventricular rate is noted (AV association or dissociation).

(2) Lack of a 1:1 AV relation excludes AV re-entry tachycardia and, for practical purposes, AV nodal re-entry. In rare instances AV node re-entry tachycardia can exhibit 2:1 AV block.

(3) If the atrial rate is faster than the ventricular rate, the diagnosis is **atrial tachycardia or atrial flutter,** depending on the rate and pattern of atrial activation.

(4) If the ventricular rate is faster than the atrial rate, the diagnosis is ventricular tachycardia.

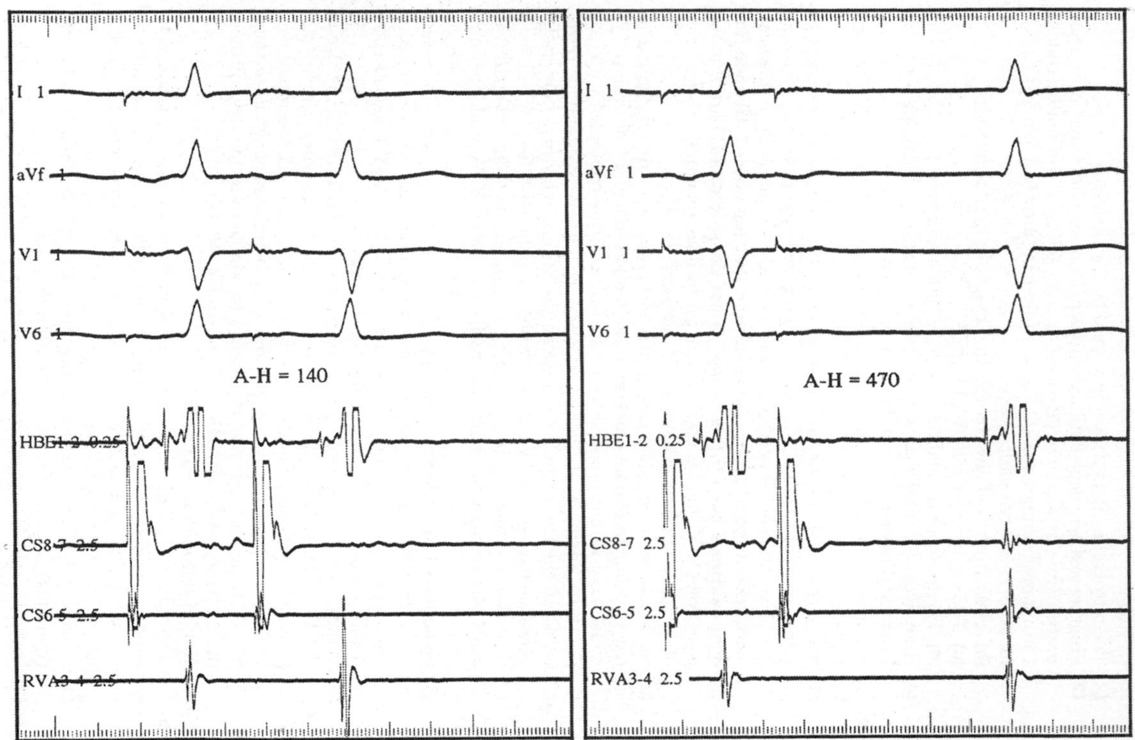

Figure 48.6. AV nodal jump and echo. A 10-millisecond decrement in S_1S_2 resulted in marked prolongation of A_2H_2 by more than 300 milliseconds. In addition, an echo beat with a short H-A is seen on the CS electrogram, a definite evidence of dual AV node physiology. The atrial premature beat, blocked antegrade in the fast pathway, was conducted with sufficient delay in the slow pathway to encounter a nonrefractory retrograde fast pathway.

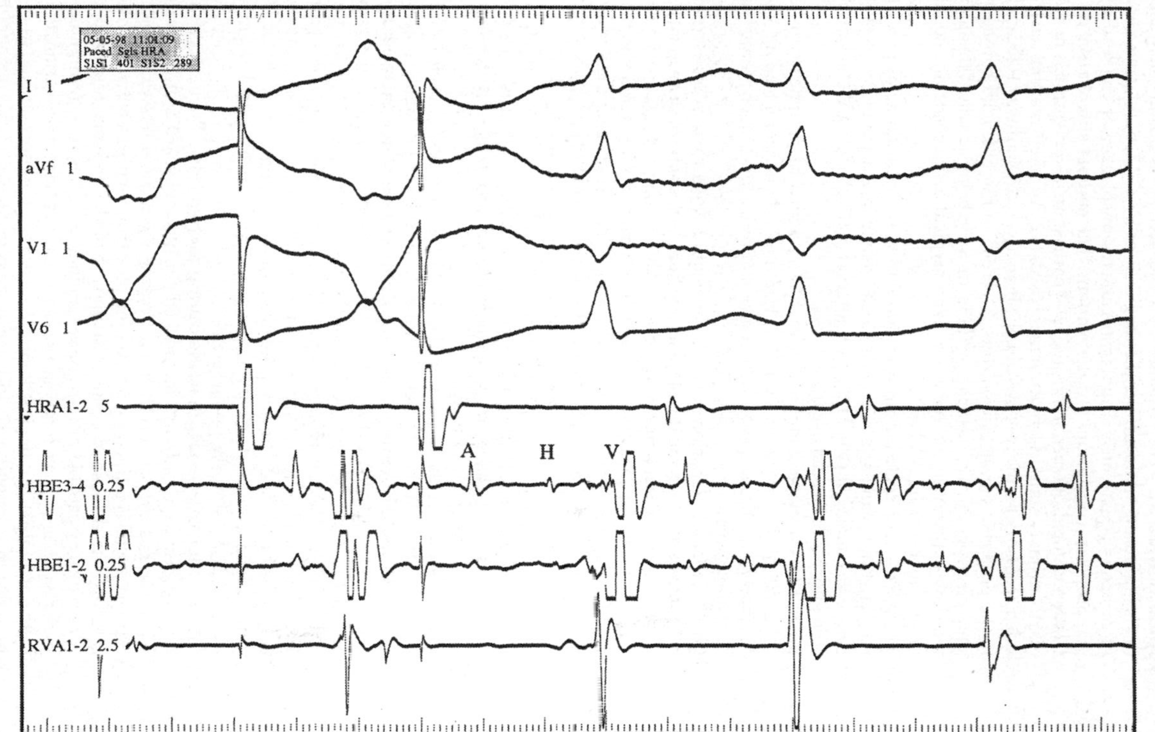

Figure 48.7. Orthodromic AV re-entry tachycardia. In this example from a patient with a manifest right-sided accessory pathway, premature atrial stimulation (S) blocks in the accessory pathway (resulting in a narrow QRS complex), conducts with a longer A-V, and re-excites the atrium. The tachycardia is narrow complex, with an H-A interval of 180 milliseconds. The earliest A is seen on the HRA catheter.

b. When a **1:1 AV relation** exists, **further evaluation** is needed. The following observations and techniques are helpful in arriving at the most likely mechanism:

(1) Atrial activation. The sequence of atrial activation during tachycardia is important in the differential diagnosis of SVT. Accurate placement of catheters is extremely important; catheter misplacement can lead to inappropriate conclusions or interventions. The **earliest site of atrial activation** is noted. As mentioned above, if earliest atrial activation is in the distal coronary sinus, a left atrial tachycardia or AV re-entry using a left-sided accessory pathway is most likely. If an accessory pathway is located in the posterior septum, the earliest A is seen in the proximal coronary sinus electrogram. This also is true if the atria are being activated through the slow pathway of the AV node, as in atypical atrioventricular nodal reentry tachycardia (AVNRT).

(2) The presence of **cycle length variation** during tachycardia helps predict the activation sequence. For example, a change in AA coupling interval before an equal change in HH or VV interval (with changing VA) suggests a diagnosis of atrial tachycardia.

(a) In cases of wide complex tachycardia in which there appears to be a 1:1 relation between H and V, HH interval change preceding VV interval change suggests supraventricular or bundle branch re-entrant tachycardia.

(b) Cycle length variation may also be helpful when there is **slowing of tachycardia with the development of bundle branch block and acceleration with resolution of the block.** This finding is suggestive of AV re-entry using an accessory pathway ipsilateral to the bundle branch block as the retrograde limb. This can be appreciated on the surface ECG. In fact, prolongation in tachycardia cycle length in association with a bundle branch block is caused by prolongation of the VA interval. The activation wavefront must travel down the contralateral bundle and across the intraventricular septum before it reaches the pathway. The change in cycle length is more pronounced with lateral than with septal pathways.

(3) HA and VA intervals. A constant HA or VA relation despite cycle length variation (even in the absence of bundle branch block) is highly suggestive of **AV node re-entry or accessory pathway–mediated tachycardia.** The change in tachycardia cycle length is caused by varying antegrade conduction time through the AV node. The VA time can also be used to differentiate AV nodal re-entry from AV re-entry. A VA interval less than 70 milliseconds is rarely seen with AV re-entry and strongly suggests the diagnosis of AV nodal re-entry (see Fig. 48.8). VA times in excess of 70 milliseconds are seen with AV re-entry and atypical AV nodal re-entry (so-called fast–slow AV nodal re-entry).

(4) Introduction of premature beats during tachycardia. Premature ventricular beats typically are introduced during tachycardia at intervals when the His bundle is refractory. Because the normal retrograde path (His-AV node) is refractory, preexciting the atrium with a premature ventricular beat at those intervals is diagnostic of the presence of an accessory pathway capable of retrograde conduction. Consistent termination of tachycardia with such premature beats without retrograde conduction to the atrium is also diagnostic of AV re-entry. An important clue to the presence of a second accessory pathway is a change in the retrograde atrial activation sequence with a premature ventricular beat when the His bundle is refractory.

(5) Initiation and termination of tachycardia. To understand the mechanism of tachycardia, it is important to know the mechanism of initiation. For re-entry to occur, block in one limb of the re-entrant circuit and slow conduction in the other limb must take place. It is important to review

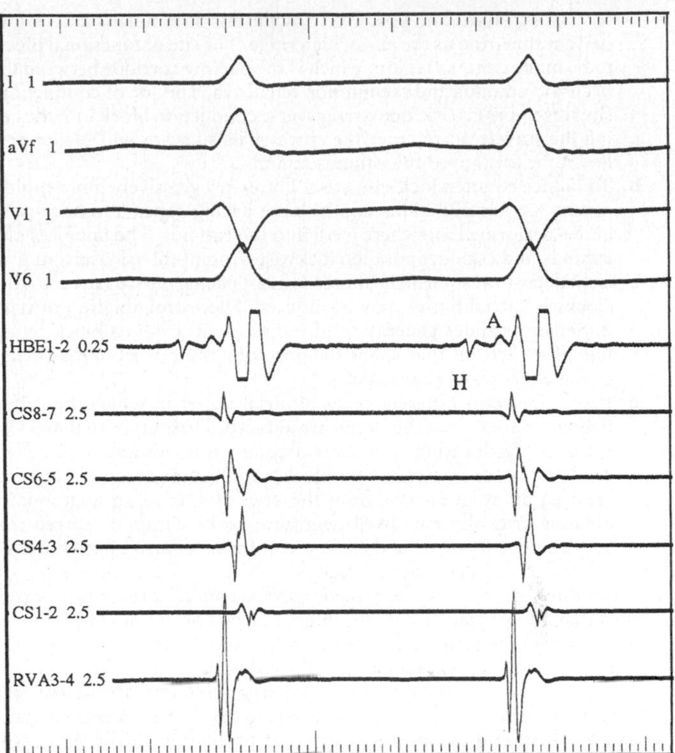

Figure 48.8. AV node re-entry tachycardia. Tachycardia is narrow complex, and characterized by very short V-A interval and an H-A interval of less than 70 milliseconds.

the stimulation sequences that did not induce tachycardia and compare them with those that did. A sudden jump in the AH interval suggests, but is not diagnostic of, AV nodal re-entry. Orthodromic AV re-entry tachycardia develops during atrial stimulation after antegrade block in the accessory pathway takes place in combination with a critical delay in the AV node. With ventricular stimulation, AV re-entry tachycardia develops after block in the AV node or His-Purkinje system occurs. Termination of the tachycardia simultaneous with AV node block (A with no H) suggests AV node dependence and is helpful in excluding AV node–independent tachycardias (atrial tachycardia and flutter).

4. **Significance of induced tachycardia.** With the exception of atrial fibrillation, induced re-entrant SVTs signify the presence of an established anatomic circuit. Comparison with the clinical arrhythmia is important and, unless significant differences exist, it can safely be assumed that the induced tachycardia is clinically significant. If a wide complex tachycardia with a supraventricular mechanism is induced, the recording is compared with a clinical recording. If the QRS morphology is different from that of the clinical arrhythmia, a search for ventricular arrhythmia may be warranted.
5. **Atrial flutter,** a special type of atrial tachycardia that involves a well-defined anatomic circuit, and is amenable to curative catheter ablation techniques.
   a. In the typical variety of atrial flutter, the waveform travels counterclockwise around the tricuspid annulus. The circuit is bounded anteriorly by the

tricuspid annulus and posteriorly by the crista terminalis and its inferior medial continuation as the eustachian ridge. The site of functional block appears to be in the isthmus region, which is the narrow corridor between the inferior tricuspid annulus and the inferior vena cava. The site of conduction delay or slowing appears to be due to transverse conduction block into the crista, forcing the wavefront to enter the crista at its superior end before propagating down the crista into the isthmus region.

b. To induce counterclockwise atrial flutter, progressively more rapid (approximately 250 to 200 milliseconds) burst pacing appears to be most successful and is performed anywhere medial to the isthmus. The impulses block in the isthmus and conduct counterclockwise around the tricuspid ring with sufficient delay to sustain atrial flutter. If burst pacing is used lateral to the isthmus, clockwise atrial flutter may be induced. Successful ablation of typical atrial flutter necessitates generation of bidirectional isthmus block by applying a line of RF lesions that spans the posterior isthmus from the tricuspid valve to the inferior vena cava (IVC).

c. Less commonly, different types of atrial flutter in which the subeustachian isthmus is not part of the circuit are induced. These atypical flutters have many varieties and locations but share a common re-entrant circuit that revolves around an area of conduction block, usually scar tissue. Treatment involves creating an ablation line from the area of scar to an anatomic barrier or ablating critically narrowed re-entrant paths within a scarred region. The success rates in ablating these atypical forms of atrial flutter are not as high as for isthmus-dependent flutters.

6. Atrial fibrillation. Previous evidence favored multiple re-entrant wavelets as the predominant mechanism responsible for atrial fibrillation. However, it has been recently demonstrated that atrial fibrillation is frequently initiated by rapidly firing foci located predominantly in the pulmonary veins, where sleeves of atrial muscle with abnormal automaticity or perhaps re-entry are present. Our current concept of atrial fibrillation revolves around two factors: a triggering mechanism and a substrate that can maintain atrial fibrillation. Most atria, especially in relatively normal hearts, are quite resistant to initiation of atrial fibrillation. Thus, the concept of focal initiation of atrial fibrillation by rapid bursts of focal atrial tachycardia emerged as a triggering mechanism, making it possible to map and target these sites for catheter ablation. The current understanding is that a vast majority of these triggering sites are near the os of the pulmonary veins in the left atrium.

a. Ectopic beats emanating from the left pulmonary veins will produce broad and notched p waves with a left-to-right activation sequence (negative in aVL). This is confirmed by inversion of normal activation in the coronary sinus recording.

b. The right pulmonary veins are close to the interatrial septum and to the right of midline. The os of the superior right pulmonary vein is quite close to the sinus node. Thus, p-wave and intracardiac recordings of atrial premature beats emanating from the right pulmonary veins are compatible with a right-to-left activation sequence and often very similar to sinus p waves.

c. An esophageal recording can be helpful in localizing the right pulmonary veins as the source of premature atrial beats because it records activation of the posterior left atrium. Early activation in that recording is good evidence of right pulmonary vein involvement.

d. Ablation of these triggering foci requires left atrial access by transseptal puncture. Following transseptal puncture, a decapolar mapping catheter with a ring configuration is used to record electrical activity around the circumference of the pulmonary vein ostia. It displays a far-field atrial signal and a near-field pulmonary vein potential. This is characterized as a very sharp spike following the atrial deflection during sinus rhythm. However, discharges from the vein will invert this activation sequence; the pulmonary vein potential will precede the atrial activation.

e. RF ablation delivered around the circular catheter to abolish the pulmonary vein potentials is the most common method used to electrically isolate the pulmonary veins from the left atrium. In that manner, abnormal firing would be confined to the veins and no atrial fibrillation would be induced.

f. Rarely, atrial fibrillation may be induced by rapid discharges originating from nonpulmonary vein foci, most commonly from the superior vena cava. Circumferential catheter ablation can be performed in the same fashion, aiming at abolition of all venous potentials (electrical isolation).

C. Evaluation of accessory pathways

1. The **most common locations** for accessory pathways in decreasing order of frequency are left free wall, posterior region, posteroseptal region, right free wall, and anteroseptal region. Concealed accessory pathways (no evidence of antegrade conduction) with only retrograde conduction are more common than manifest pathways, which have antegrade conduction manifested by delta waves on the surface ECG.

a. Right-sided accessory pathways are more likely than left-sided accessory pathways to be associated with **congenital heart disease.** An unusual type of right-sided accessory pathway is the atriofascicular accessory pathways, which originate in the right atrium, traverse the right anterior region of the tricuspid valve annulus, and insert in the region of the right bundle or the right-sided Purkinje network. These accessory pathways have unidirectional antegrade conduction with decremental conduction properties similar to an AV node. These pathways are frequently referred to as Mahaim pathways.

b. Multiple accessory pathways are more frequently encountered on the right side and in survivors of sudden death. In these patients the most common combination is posteroseptal and right free wall pathways.

c. Antidromic and orthodromic AV re-entrant tachycardia both require participation of the accessory pathway. In rare instances, antidromic tachycardia can involve one accessory pathway in the antegrade direction and a second pathway in the retrograde direction.

2. Evidence of preexcitation is supported by the presence of **short HV interval** (less than 35 milliseconds) **at rest** or with atrial pacing and the appearance of increasing preexcitation either with atrial pacing or with administration of drugs that cause AV nodal conduction slowing, or with autonomic maneuvers. The electrophysiologic properties of the accessory pathway are examined, including its antegrade and retrograde conduction and refractory periods. If tachycardia is induced during atrial or ventricular stimulation, its mechanism is defined according to the techniques discussed earlier. This depends on whether the tachycardia is narrow or wide complex.

3. Orthodromic AV re-entry tachycardia is commonly initiated by a ventricular premature stimulus that blocks in the His-Purkinje system or, rarely, in the AV node, but conducts in a retrograde direction over the accessory pathway. It also can be induced by an atrial premature stimulus (echo beat) that blocks the accessory pathway and conducts slowly over the AV conducting system. Induction is facilitated by the presence of a relatively **long accessory pathway antegrade refractory period** or a **long His-Purkinje system retrograde refractory period.**

4. Antidromic AV re-entry tachycardia (see Fig. 48.9) can be initiated with burst pacing in the atrium or with a premature atrial stimulus that **blocks in the AV node** and **conducts over the accessory pathway.** Less often it can be induced with a premature ventricular stimulus that blocks the accessory pathway in a retrograde manner and conducts over the AV node. Induction of antidromic tachycardia necessitates excellent retrograde conduction over the His-Purkinje system–AV node; it almost always involves a free wall accessory pathway as the antegrade limb, and is frequently associated with the presence of multiple accessory pathways.

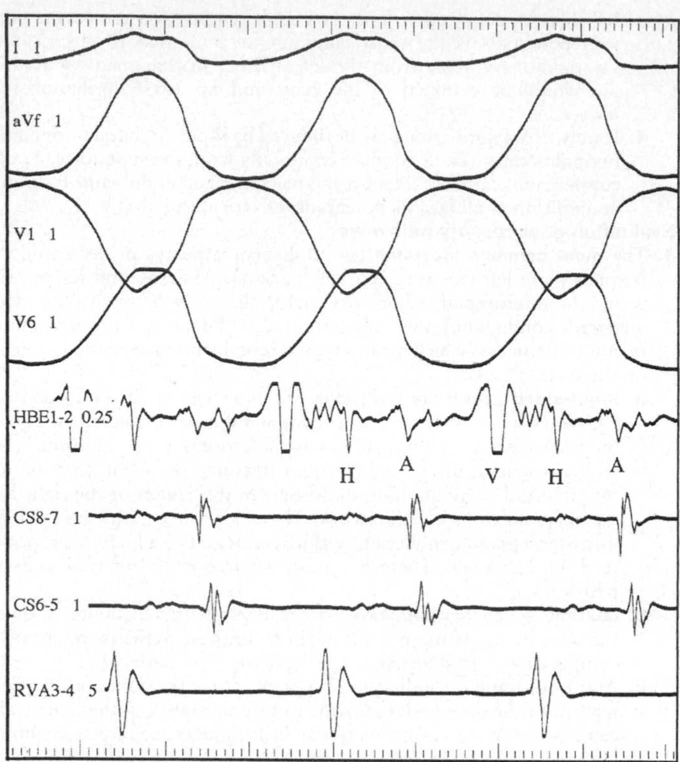

Figure 48.9. Antidromic AV re-entry tachycardia. This tachycardia was induced with atrial burst pacing in a young patient with two right-sided manifest accessory pathways. The tachycardia is rapid, wide complex, with the earliest retrograde A seen in HBEI-2, consistent with retrograde activation through the AV node. AV node re-entry with antegrade activation using the accessory pathway (bystander accessory pathway) was excluded by lack of evidence of dual AV node physiology.

5. Localizing accessory pathways

a. Surface electrocardiographic localization

(1) Delta wave vectors

(a) Left lateral: Negative in I and aVL, Positive II, III, aVF, and V_1–V_6

(b) Left posterior wall: Positive I, aVL, Negative II, III, aVF, Positive V_1–V_3/V_4

(c) Posteroseptal: Positive I, aVL, Negative II, III, aVF, R/S <1 in V_1

(d) Right free wall: Positive I, aVL, II Negative III, biphasic V_1 and V_2

(e) Anteroseptal: Positive I, aVL, Positive II > III, Negative V_1–V_6

(2) P-wave morphology during orthodromic tachycardia

(a) Left lateral: Negative I and aVL, Positive III > aVF > II, Negative V_5 and V_6

(b) Posteroseptal: Positive aVR, >aVL, Negative II, III, aVF

(c) Right free wall: Positive I, aVL, II, Negative III, biphasic V_1 and V_2

b. Localization during EPS

(1) Pacing from multiple atrial sites: shortest A-delta occurs with pacing close to the atrial insertion site of AP and results in maximal preexcitation.

(2) Retrograde atrial activation during orthodromic tachycardia and V pacing
(a) Atrial activation sequence
(i) Left and right free wall: eccentric
(ii) Posteroseptal: A_{CSos} earlier than A_{His}
(iii) Anteroseptal: A_{CSos} later than A_{His}
(b) Atrial activation sequence when a ventricular premature stimulus is delivered during tachycardia at the time when His is refractory
(c) The earliest site of atrial activation identifies the site of atrial insertion of an accessory pathway
(3) Relation of local ventricular electrogram to delta: earliest V correlates with ventricular insertion site
(4) Effects of bundle branch block
(a) Bundle branch block increasing the VA interval and tachycardia cycle length by more than 35 milliseconds; ipsilateral free wall accessory pathway
(b) With septal accessory pathways the increase in VA times is less than 25 milliseconds
(c) Left anterior fascicular block can increase VA times 15 to 35 milliseconds with left free wall accessory pathway, particularly with an anterolateral left-sided accessory pathway
(5) Recording of accessory pathway potential: sharp spike 10 to 30 milliseconds before the onset of the delta wave

6. Identifying the presence of multiple accessory pathways
a. Changing antegrade delta waves during sinus rhythm, atrial pacing, atrial fibrillation, and with antiarrhythmic drugs
b. Evidence of multiple routes of retrograde atrial activation
(1) Changing VA time or activation sequence
(2) Failure to prolong VA time with ipsilateral bundle branch block
c. Orthodromic tachycardia with antegrade fusion
d. Preexcited tachycardia
(1) Antegrade conduction over septal accessory pathway
(2) Antidromic tachycardia faster than orthodromic tachycardia
e. Atypical patterns of preexcitation
f. Mismatch of site of antegrade preexcitation and retrograde atrial activation during AV re-entry tachycardia

D. Ventricular tachycardia evaluation

1. Most patients referred for evaluation of ventricular arrhythmia have underlying **coronary artery disease (CAD) or dilated cardiomyopathy.** The most common reason for performing EPS on these patients is documentation of inducible tachycardia, drug testing, testing the effect and response to antitachycardia pacing, and endocardial mapping to direct attempts at ablation. In rare patients, there is underlying normal LV function, and those patients typically have special types of ventricular arrhythmia. However, in general, the most common underlying mechanism is re-entry.

2. An **atrial study** is considered for all patients undergoing evaluation of ventricular tachycardia. This serves three main purposes: diagnosis of underlying advanced conduction system disease, documentation of coexisting SVT, and induction of rare forms of ventricular tachycardia that may be inducible only with atrial pacing.

3. Programmed ventricular stimulation is performed as described earlier. If ventricular tachycardia is not induced despite program stimulation from two RV sites (RV apex and outflow tract), repeat stimulation can be performed after isoproterenol infusion. However, isoproterenol should not be given to patients with active ischemic heart disease. It is primarily of value to those with exercise- or catecholamine-dependent ventricular tachycardia. LV stimulation is not necessary because RV stimulation techniques have adequate sensitivity and specificity, and the risk of left heart catheterization is avoided. If no ventricular tachycardia is induced with any of these techniques, the arrhythmia is deemed noninducible.

4. **Techniques for terminating induced ventricular tachycardia.** Pacing terminates as many as 85% of induced ventricular tachycardias in the laboratory. Success is more likely to be achieved with slower tachycardia rates (less than 200 beats/minute) and in hemodynamically tolerated tachycardias. Other factors predictive of success of pacing include the site of stimulation in relation to the tachycardia zone, ventricular conduction properties, and refractoriness. Pacing also can accelerate tachycardia, an important consideration when antitachycardia pacing is being considered.
5. **Techniques for terminating tachycardia with pacing.** One technique entails use of one or more **progressively earlier premature ventricular stimuli.** The other technique uses **burst pacing** to overdrive the tachycardia, but there is a greater risk for accelerating the tachycardia into a hemodynamically unstable arrhythmia. Techniques that can be used if pacing fails include delivery of ultrarapid train stimulation and synchronized direct current cardioversion.
6. There are a variety of **responses to programmed stimulation.** What is important is the correlation between these responses in different populations of patients and future risk for adverse outcome. For example, induction of single or double bundle branch re-entrant beats has no bearing on long-term outcome among persons with normal LV function and is not considered an abnormal finding. Induction of sustained monomorphic ventricular tachycardia, particularly among persons with poor LV function, identifies a subset of patients at high risk for sudden death.

   a. Sustained monomorphic ventricular tachycardia

   (1) Induction of sustained monomorphic ventricular tachycardia is the **most important response** and has the highest predictive value. This is particularly true if the induced tachycardia is similar to the clinical arrhythmia in both rate and structure. Patients with easily induced ventricular tachycardia (e.g., with single premature beats) have worse outcome than those in whom tachycardia is more difficult to induce. It is important to document reproducibility of ventricular tachycardia during programmed stimulation. Slow, sustained tachycardia, particularly in patients with ischemic substrate, is more reproducible than more rapid tachycardia and among those with nonischemic etiologic factors. Sustained tachycardia has clearly worse prognostic implications than nonsustained tachycardia. There is no agreement on what constitutes an abnormal response among patients with nonsustained tachycardia or whether any therapeutic intervention should be pursued for these patients.

   The Multicenter Unsustained Tachycardia Trial (MUSTT) randomized 2022 patients with nonsustained ventricular tachycardia, ischemic cardiomyopathy with an EF <40%, and all of whom had an EP study to determine whether they had inducible sustained ventricular tachycardia. If they had inducible ventricular tachycardia, they were randomized to either conservative treatment (with an ACE inhibitor and/or beta-blocker) or EP-guided treatment using a pre-specified drug sequence, which included Class Ia, Ic, and III agents or ICDs. Patients proceeded to the next round if a repeat electrophysiology test induced ventricular tachycardia, until ventricular tachycardia could not be induced. An EP study revealed 767 subjects with inducible ventricular tachycardia, from which 704 patients were randomized to the conservative group (n = 353) and antiarrhythmic therapy group (n = 351). In the antiarrhythmic therapy group, 45% of patients received antiarrhythmic drugs, 46% received an ICD, and 7% received no therapy. The mortality rate in the antiarrhythmic therapy group (12% and 25%, at 24 and 60 months, respectively) was significantly lower than that of the conservative group (18% and 32%, respectively, P = 0.043). In subgroup analysis, the patients who received an ICD clearly performed better than any other group, with

92% being alive at 60 months. In fact, when the ICD patients were removed from the antiarrhythmic therapy group, there was no significant difference between the conservative group and the antiarrhythmic drug group. This trial, coupled with others, has decreased the usefulness of EPS in patients at high risk for ventricular arrhythmias, for risk stratification in the decision to implant ICDs or initiate antiarrhythmic medications.

(2) Among patients with ischemic substrate, programmed stimulation induces sustained monomorphic ventricular tachycardia in as many as 95% of patients with history of clinical sustained ventricular tachycardia, approximately 60% of those with nonsustained ventricular tachycardia, and approximately 50% of patients experiencing sudden cardiac death. Induction of sustained monomorphic ventricular tachycardia in any of the above subsets has very high specificity (more than 90%) for spontaneous clinical ventricular tachycardia and sudden death. Testing at two RV sites increases sensitivity without sacrificing specificity. The Multicenter Automatic Defibrillator Implantation (MADIT I) trial randomized patients with coronary artery disease, EF *less than* 35%, at high risk for life-threatening arrhythmias, who had an ischemic event greater than 20 days before randomization. The two groups were randomized to ICD therapy versus medical therapy that included amiodarone (74% of patients in the nondevice arm), digitalis, disopyramide, mexiletine, procainamide, tocainide, beta-blockers, and sotalol; few patients received type IA agents and no patients received type IC agents. The trial showed a 56% reduction in total mortality in the ICD arm versus the medical therapy arm. The MADIT II trial prospectively followed 1232 patients with ischemic cardiomyopathy and EF *less than* 30%, at least 29 days post myocardial infarction (MI). It randomized patients to medical therapy or medical therapy plus ICD implantation. It showed a 31% relative reduction in all cause mortality, with curves separating out at 9 months. Unlike the MADIT I trial, which required an EPS to be performed, this trial took into account only the patient's EF requirement, and hence has influenced the current practice guiding ICD implantation.

(3) Patients with **nonischemic substrate** are more challenging to evaluate because EPS are less sensitive and specific. Although inducible sustained monomorphic ventricular tachycardia has a worse prognosis than the noninducible type, the positive predictive value of abnormal results of EPS is at best 70%. Patients with negative results of EPS are still at high risk for sudden death, even if they have no prior clinical events. The prognosis may be more favorable if inducible tachycardia is suppressed by drugs, but the risk of future events continues to be high. One can never be reassured about the outcome among patients with nonischemic cardiomyopathy using results of EPS. The Sudden Cardiac Death in Heart Failure (SCD-HeFT) trial enrolled patients with New York Heart Association (NYHA) class II and III congestive heart failure (CHF) and reduced left ventricular ejection fraction (LVEF) less than or equal to 35%, and its goal was to evaluate the effectiveness of amiodarone therapy or an implantable cardioverter defibrillator (ICD). The results of the trial showed no difference in all-cause mortality between the amiodarone and placebo arm (28% vs. 29%), but mortality was lower in the ICD arm compared with placebo (22% vs. 29%, HR 0.77, 97.5% CI 0.62–0.96, $p = 0.007$). The Defibrillators in Nonischemic Cardiomyopathy Treatment Evaluation (DEFINITE) trial included patients with nonischemic cardiomyopathy and EF less than 35% (mean EF 21%) with PVCs or nonsustained ventricular arrhythmias. It compared standard medical therapy to treatment with ICDs in addition to medical therapy. It showed a non-statistically significant decrease in all cause mortality in the ICD and medical therapy compared to the standard medical therapy arm, but a statistically significant reduction in arrhythmic deaths (14.1% vs. 7.9% at 29 months). A subset analysis of this trial showed a statistically significant decrease in all cause mortality in patients with EF less than 40% and NYHA class III symptoms.

(4) Bundle Branch Re-entry (BBR) tachycardia is a type of ventricular tachycardia with a well-defined macro re-entrant circuit. It occurs most often among patients with dilated cardiomyopathy and is frequently symptomatic.

(a) In the **typical pattern,** the impulse travels antegrade down the right bundle branch, across the interventricular septum, and retrograde up the left bundle branch. The tachycardia exhibits a left bundle branch block pattern with a **His deflection preceding every QRS complex**. In sinus rhythm, the **HV interval is abnormally long,** and during tachycardia it is at least equal and frequently longer than the baseline HV.

(b) In rare instances it is difficult to differentiate BBR tachycardia from an SVT with aberration or from a myocardial ventricular tachycardia with retrograde His deflections.

(c) BBR tachycardia frequently is rapid and exhibits AV dissociation. If cycle length variation takes place, it is important to assess the order of changes in the HH and VV intervals. If HH changes take place before VV changes, BBR is likely. A VV change that occurs before HH change and is also associated with a variation in the HV interval suggests myocardial ventricular tachycardia.

(d) Treatment with **antiarrhythmic agents,** including amiodarone, is not helpful and may lead to stabilization of the re-entrant circuit. BBR tachycardia is curable with RF ablation of the right bundle.

b. Polymorphic ventricular tachycardia frequently occurs with high-output stimulation. It also is more likely to occur with increasing numbers of extra stimuli.

(1) Interpretation of the induction of polymorphic ventricular tachycardia depends on the clinical situation. For example, inducible polymorphic ventricular tachycardia in a survivor of sudden cardiac death is considered significant. In a patient with ventricular ectopy and normal ventricular function, inducible polymorphic ventricular tachycardia is a nonspecific response.

(2) Similar interpretation applies to **induced ventricular fibrillation.** If the patient has never had clinical ventricular tachycardia or ventricular fibrillation and has no underlying heart disease, the induced ventricular fibrillation is considered a nonspecific finding that does not warrant therapy.

c. Patients with **hypertrophic cardiomyopathy** represent another subset for whom the predictive value of EPS is problematic. Induction of sustained monomorphic ventricular tachycardia, induction of ventricular fibrillation without aggressive stimulation protocols, and induction of ventricular arrhythmias with atrial pacing or as a result of atrial fibrillation are generally considered to be **poor prognostic signs.**

d. Summary. It is important to have a thorough understanding of the underlying clinical problem and anatomic substrate to assess the appropriateness of any EPS findings for an individual patient.

(1) Repetitive responses caused by BBR usually are physiologic, whereas intramyocardial repetitive ventricular responses are abnormal. However, neither of these responses should be used to guide therapy.

(2) Induced polymorphic ventricular tachycardia and ventricular fibrillation can be considered nonspecific findings or clinically significant depending on the clinical circumstances. However, they should not be used to guide drug therapy in any situation.

(3) Induced sustained monomorphic ventricular tachycardia identical to the clinical arrhythmia has the highest sensitivity and specificity and has greater importance in predicting outcome.

(4) Suppression of ventricular tachycardia with drugs constitutes a desirable end point. Changing the clinical features of ventricular tachycardia to a hemodynamically tolerated slower arrhythmia is also desirable. However, implantation of an ICD may still be indicated due to persistent risk of sudden death. In the **Antiarrhythmics Versus Implantable Defibrillators (AVID)** trial, 1016 survivors of sudden cardiac death either from ventricular tachycardia or fibrillation were randomized to antiarrhythmic medications or ICDs. The results showed statistically significant 30% reduction in 1- and 2-year cardiac mortality, driven entirely by a decrease in arrhythmic deaths, in the ICD arm versus empirically chosen amiodarone or sotalol. The **Cardiac Arrest Study Hamburg (CASH)** trial confirmed these findings in a similar set of patients. It showed that ICDs reduce both sudden death and total mortality compared to a class Ic drug (propafenone), amiodarone, or metoprolol.

(5) The importance of nonsustained ventricular tachycardia remains controversial. Noninducibility in patients with nonischemic cardiomyopathy or survivors of sudden cardiac death may not provide prediction as accurate as that for patients with underlying ischemic substrate and documented nonsustained ventricular tachycardia. Therapeutic decisions therefore have been individualized.

7. Mapping of ventricular tachycardia. Mapping of ventricular tachycardia involves identification of the **earliest sites of activation** during tachycardia and detailed outlining of the **tachycardia circuit.** Endocardial mapping has aided in the evaluation of mechanisms of tachycardia. More recently, mapping has been coupled with RF ablation with high rates of success.

a. Mapping can be performed with steerable electrode catheters during EPS or can involve introduction of specialized catheters with various configurations designed to compare several simultaneously acquired endocardial electrograms.

b. For the most part, mapping of ventricular arrhythmias takes place in the left ventricle. However, several types of ventricular tachycardia that originate from the RV, including those from the outflow tract, have been successfully mapped and ablated.

c. Activation mapping takes place during the tachycardia. The objective is to identify the site of earliest endocardial activation. Because this lengthy process has to take place during tachycardia, it must be hemodynamically tolerable. The earliest activation site corresponds to the exit site of the circuit.

d. Sites of origin of tachycardia in patients with ischemic heart disease usually are found in the periinfarction zone or in the border of an LV aneurysm. To confirm the site, entrainment from that site is performed. Entrainment involves transient overdrive pacing without terminating the tachycardia. When entrainment is achieved within the re-entrant circuit inside the slowly conducting scarred regions of the heart, pacing produces QRS morphologic match on all 12 surface ECG leads. The return cycle length of activation at the site of pacing after cessation of pacing equals the tachycardia cycle length (see Fig. 48.10). These two observations imply that depolarization caused by pacing have the same exit from the scar as the tachycardia and that the pacing site is within the circuit.

e. Pace mapping can be used in evaluations of patients with hemodynamically intolerable tachycardia. Ventricular pacing is performed at various sites at rates that do not cause hemodynamic instability. The site where pacing results in QRS match with clinical tachycardia corresponds to the exit sites of the tachycardia circuit.

f. Recently, delineation of tissue voltage became possible with the use of an electroanatomic mapping system, providing accurate delineation of scar tissue

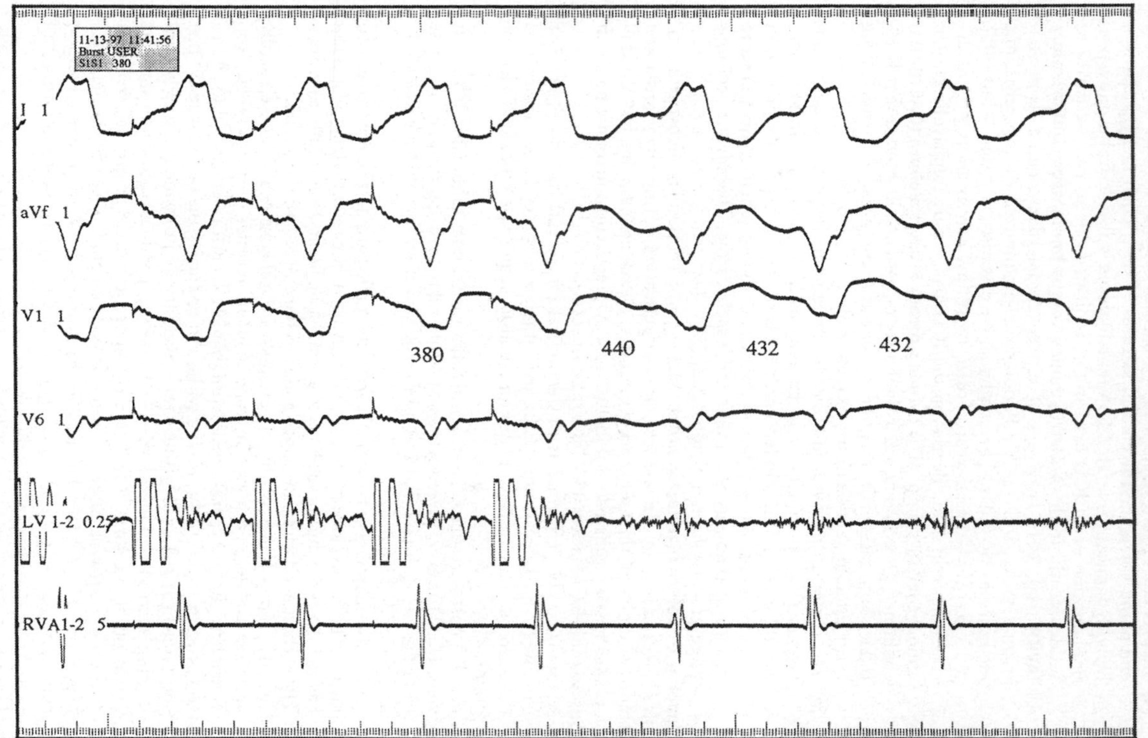

Figure 48.10. Entrainment of ventricular tachycardia. Pacing at a rate slightly faster (380 milliseconds) than tachycardia cycle length at a site believed to be the isthmus of the tachycardia resulted in QRS morphology very similar to the native ventricular tachycardia (concealed entrainment) in all 12 leads (only 4 leads shown). In addition, the post-pacing interval is very close to the tachycardia cycle length, suggesting that the pacing site is within the tachycardia circuit. Application of radiofrequency energy at this site resulted in successful ablation of this tachycardia.

and its boundaries. Thus, mapping in sinus rhythm allows for delimitation of the scar and areas of the scar border that are likely sites of tachycardia exit. Pace mapping can be used to identify those sites around the scar that correspond to tachycardia exits. Linear lesions, performed to interrupt these exit sites responsible for re-entrant circuits, can be undertaken, allowing successful ablation of tachycardias that would not be otherwise mapped due to patient intolerance of any sustained tachycardia. Another method of mapping a hemodynamically unstable ventricular tachycardia is to use a mapping system that can acquire the map of the entire endocardium in a single beat. This requires insertion of a "balloon" catheter into the LV that acquires the electrograms from 64 points on the balloon and calculates the virtual activation on the endocardial surface.

g. Mapping can also be performed intraoperatively when endocardial resection is considered. Although this approach can still be used, it is infrequently recommended, as other approaches described above in combination with implantable defibrillators have yielded good patient survival and excellent success in eliminating problematic ventricular tachycardias.

ACKNOWLEDGMENT

The author thanks Dr. Eduardo B. Saad for his contributions to prior editions of this chapter.

Suggested Readings

AVID investigators. A Comparison of Antiarrhythmic-Drug Therapy with Implantable Defibrillators in Patients Resuscitated from Near-Fatal Ventricular Arrhythmias; Antiarrhythmics Versus Implantable Defibrillators (AVID). *New Engl J Med* 1997;337:1576–1583.

Bardy GH, Lee KL, Mark DB, et al. Amiodarone or an implantable cardioverter-defibrillator for congestive heart failure. *N Engl J Med* 2005;352:225–237.

Buxton AE, Lee KL, Fisher JD, et al. A randomized study of the prevention of sudden death in patients with coronary artery disease. Multicenter Unsustained Tachycardia Trial Investigators. *N Engl J Med* 1999;341:1882–1890.

Gregoratos G, Abrams J, Epstein AE, et al. ACC/AHA/NASPE 2002 guideline update for implantation of cardiac pacemakers and antiarrhythmia devices—summary article: a report of the American College of Cardiology/American Heart Association Task Force on Practice Guidelines (ACC/AHA/NASPE Committee to Update the 1998 Pacemaker Guidelines). *Circulation* 2002;106:2145–2161.

Josephson ME, Maloney JD, Barold SS, et al. ACC Core Cardiology Training Symposium (COCATS): guidelines for training in adult cardiovascular medicine—training in specialized electrophysiology, cardiac pacing and arrhythmia management. *J Am Coll Cardiol* 1995;25:23–26.

Kadish A, et al. Prophylactic Defibrillator Implantation in Patients with Nonischemic Dilated Cardiomyopathy (DEFINITE). *N Engl J Med* 2004;350:2151–2158.

Moss AJ, Hall WJ, Cannom DS, et al. Improved survival with an implanted defibrillator in patients with coronary disease at high risk for ventricular arrhythmia. Multicenter Automatic Defibrillator Implantation Trial Investigators. *N Engl J Med* 1996;335:1933–1940.

Moss AJ, Hall WJ, Cannom DS, et al. Improved survival with an implanted defibrillator in patients with coronary disease at high risk for ventricular arrhythmia. (MADIT.) *N Engl J Med* 1996;335:1933–1940.

Moss AJ, Zareba W, Hall WJ, et al. Prophylactic implantation of a defibrillator in patients with myocardial infarction and reduced ejection fraction. (MADIT II.) *N Engl J Med* 2002;346:877–883.

Zipes DP, DiMarco JP, Gillette PC, et al. Guidelines for clinical intracardiac electrophysiological and catheter ablation procedures: a report of the American College of Cardiology/American Heart Association Task Force on Practice Guidelines (Committee on Clinical Intracardiac Electrophysiological and Catheter Ablation Procedures). *J Am Coll Cardiol* 1995;26:555–573.

Relevant Book Chapters

Josephson ME. Electrophysiologic investigation: general concepts. In: Josephson ME, ed. *Clinical cardiac electrophysiology: techniques and interpretations*. Philadelphia: Lippincott Williams and Wilkins, 2001.

Medina EO, Wilde AM. Sinus bradycardia, sinus arrest and sinoatrial exit block: pathophysiological, electrocardiographic and clinical considerations. In: Zipes DP, Jalife J, eds. *Cardiac electrophysiology: from cell to bedside*. Philadelphia: WB Saunders, 2000.

Miller JM, Zipes DP. Therapy for cardiac arrhythmias. In: Braunwald E, Zipes DP, Libby P, et al, eds. *Braunwald's Heart Disease: a textbook of cardiovascular medicine*, 8th ed. Philadelphia: Saunders Elsevier, 2008.

Singer I. Catheterization and electrogram recordings. In: Singer I, ed. *Interventional electrophysiology*. Philadelphia: Lippincott Williams and Wilkins, 2001.

49 CARDIAC PACING

Timothy H. Mahoney and Patrick Tchou

I. INTRODUCTION. The indications and technology of cardiac pacing continue to evolve, leading to a rapid increase in the number of pacemakers implanted. Pacemaker implantation rates have increased from 329 implants per million population in 1990 to 612 per million population in 2002. It is imperative that the physician caring for the pacemaker patient understand the basic physiology and technology of cardiac pacing and be able to apply these principles to effectively manage the unique problems with which these patients may present.

II. BASIC COMPONENTS OF CARDIAC PACEMAKERS

A. Pulse generator (PG)

1. **Power source (battery).** Lithium iodine is the most common chemical compound used. Lithium batteries deplete over a more predictable time course than other types of compounds, such as zinc mercuric oxide, that were used in prior generations of devices.
2. **Circuitry**
    a. **Output circuits.** These circuits control programmable features of the output pulse, including amplitude and pulse width.
    b. **Sensing circuits.** These circuits process the intracardiac electrogram, including amplification and filtering of the signal, and also provide other functions such as management of external electromagnetic interference (EMI). A bandpass filter allows signals of a certain frequency range to be passed while signals of other frequency ranges are blocked or attenuated. Pacemakers use a bandpass filter to distinguish between cardiac depolarization signals and repolarization or extracardiac signals, such as myopotentials from the chest wall musculature. Some appropriate signals that pass through the filter are small in amplitude, and a sense amplifier increases the appropriate signal for the device to process.
    c. **Timing circuits.** These circuits control the pacing intervals and sensing/refractory periods. They may be altered by input from the sensing circuits.
    d. **Telemetry circuit.** These circuits allow communication between an external programmer and the pulse generator for pacemaker programming or retrieval of information.
    e. **Microprocessor.** Some pacemakers have computer chips with memory (ROM and RAM) and therefore have enhanced capabilities, such as downloading of new features via telemetry and increased storage of diagnostic data.
    f. **Sensor circuit for rate-adaptive pacing.** See below.

B. Lead system

1. **Terminal pin.** The male portion of the proximal lead that connects to the pulse generator.
2. **Lead body.** Consists of conductor(s) and insulation. The conducting wire connects the stimulating and sensing electrodes to the terminal pin. The lead insulation is most commonly silicone rubber or a polyurethane material.
3. **Stimulating/sensing electrode(s).** Distal end of the lead that connects via a fixation mechanism to atrial or ventricular myocardium.
4. **Fixation device.** Passive fixation represents an attachment mechanism (e.g., "fins" or "tines") that anchors electrodes to the endocardial trabeculae. These

types of leads have a higher rate of early dislodgement, but lower chronic capture threshold than active fixation leads. Active fixation leads are secured to the endocardium using a "screw-in" mechanism. These types of leads have a lower rate of early dislodgement and higher chronic capture threshold than passive-fixation leads. Threshold is higher in active fixation leads secondary to fibrosis and scar formation around the lead tip after implant.

C. Polarity. This refers to the electrode configuration of the pacing lead or the configuration of the pulse generator. Polarity may be unipolar or bipolar; however, some pacemakers can be programmed to pace in one polarity and sense in another (only if a bipolar lead is present).

1. **Unipolar.** Configuration in which the cathode (negative) is on the lead, usually the lead tip, and the anode (positive) is the pacemaker's can. This results in a large sensing "antenna" and produces large pacemaker artifact (spikes) on the electrocardiogram (ECG) due to proximity of circuit to electrocardiography (ECG) electrodes.
   - **a.** Advantages. Better sensing of premature ventricular contractions (PVC), low-amplitude signals, and shifted axis.
   - **b.** Disadvantages. Oversensing of extraneous signals, especially pectoralis muscle activity (myopotentials), and inadvertent skeletal muscle stimulation may occur. Moreover, large pacemaker artifacts on the ECG may obscure native electrical activity.
2. **Bipolar.** Both electrodes are at the end of the lead—the cathode (negative) at the distal tip, and the anode (positive) at the proximal ring. This results in a smaller sensing "antenna" with smaller pacemaker artifact (spikes) on the ECG. Myocardial stimulation occurs as electrons from the cathode travel through the myocardium and back to the anode.
   - **a.** Advantages. Less myopotential oversensing and skeletal muscle stimulation, and the smaller pacemaker artifact on the ECG, do not obscure native wave morphology.
   - **b.** Disadvantages. More complex lead design is more susceptible to malfunction/failure. Small pacemaker artifact on the ECG may be difficult to see.

D. Lead–heart Interface. This is equivalent to the site of energy transfer (pacing) and sensing functions.

III. PACEMAKER CLASSIFICATION. The Revised NASPE/BPEG Guidelines were published in 2002 and are the accepted nomenclature for pacemaker therapy (see Table 49.1). This is a five-position code developed by the North American Society of Pacing and Electrophysiology (NASPE) and the British Pacing and Electrophysiology Group (BPEG).

IV. INDICATIONS FOR PACEMAKER IMPLANTATION. The American College of Cardiology (ACC)/American Heart Association (AHA)/NASPE Task Force on Practice Guidelines has published revised guidelines for pacemaker implantation (see Table 49.2).

V. PHYSIOLOGY OF CARDIAC PACING

A. Pulse generator output. This is determined by the output voltage and duration of the stimulating pulse (pulse width). Most implanted cardiac pacemakers use constant-voltage output (as opposed to most temporary cardiac pacemakers, which use constant-current output).

B. Strength–duration relation. There is an exponential relationship between the stimulus amplitude for myocardial stimulation and the pulse width, such that there is a rapidly rising strength–duration curve at pulse widths less than 0.25 millisecond and a flatter curve at pulse widths greater than 1.0 millisecond (see Fig. 49.1).

1. **Rheobase.** The flattened portion of the strength–duration curve indicating the point at which increasing pulse width is no longer associated with a progressive decrease in stimulus amplitude (voltage) required for myocardial stimulation. In general, the rheobase voltage is determined by assessing the threshold stimulus voltage at a pulse width of 2.0 milliseconds.

TABLE 49.1 Revised NASPE/BPEG Generic (NBG) Code for Antibradycardia, Adaptive Rate, and Multisite Pacing

Position	I	II	III	IV	V
Category	Chamber(s) paced	Chamber(s) sensed	Response to sensing	Programmability, rate modulation	Multisite pacing
Letters	0 = none	0 = none	0 = none	0 = none	0 = none
	A = atrium	A = atrium	T = triggered	R = rate modulation	A= atrium
	V = ventricle	V = ventricle	I = inhibited		V= Ventricle
	D = dual (A + V)	D = dual (A + V)	D = dual (T + I)		D = dual (A + V)
Manufacturers' designation only	>S = single (A or V)	S = single (A or V)			

BPEG, British Pacing and Electrophysiology Group; NASPE, North American Society of Pacing and Electrophysiology. *Pacing Clin Electrophysiol* 2002;25:260–264.

TABLE 49.2 Indications for Cardiac Pacing

	Class I	Class II	Class III
SND	SND documented in association with symptomatic bradycardia, and due to factors that are irreversible, or due to essential drug therapy Symptomatic chronotropic incompetence	IIa: No clear association between SND (with heart rate <40 bpm) and symptoms can be documented IIb: In minimally symptomatic patients, chronic heart rate <40 bpm while awake	SND with marked sinus bradycardia or pauses, but no associated symptoms including that due to long-term drug therapy SND in patients with symptoms suggestive of bradycardia that are clearly documented as not associated with a slow heart rate SND with symptomatic bradycardia due to nonessential drug therapy
Acquired AV block	3° and advanced 2° AV block at any level with any of the following conditions: Bradycardia with symptoms presumed to be due to AV block Arrhythmias and other medical conditions that require drugs that result in symptomatic bradycardia Documented periods of asystole ≥3.0 s or any escape rate <40 bpm in awake symptom-free individuals After catheter ablation of the AV junction	IIa: Asymptomatic 3° AV block at any anatomic site with average awake ventricular rates ≥40 bpm Asymptomatic type II 2° AV block; if associated with wide QRS it becomes a class I indication Asymptomatic type I 2° AV block at intra- or infra-His levels found incidentally at (EP) study performed for other indications 1° AV block with symptoms suggestive of pacemaker syndrome	Asymptomatic 1° AV block Asymptomatic type I 2° AV block at the supra-His (AV node) level or not known to be Intra- or infra-Hisian AV block expected to resolve and unlikely to recur (e.g., drug toxicity, Lyme disease)

(continued)

TABLE 49.2 Indications for Cardiac Pacing (*Continued*)

	Class I	Class II	Class III
	Postoperative AV block that is not expected to resolve Neuromuscular diseases with AV block such as myotonic muscular dystrophy, Kearns-Sayre syndrome, Erb's dystrophy (limb girdle), and peroneal muscular dystrophy	IIb: Marked 1° AV block (>0.30 s) in patients with LV dysfunction and symptoms of congestive heart failure in whom shorter AV interval results in hemodynamic improvement, presumably by decreasing left atrial filling pressure	
	2° AV block regardless of type or site of block, with associated symptomatic bradycardia	Neuromuscular diseases with any AV block regardless of symptoms, because progression is unpredictable	
Post myocardial infarction (MI)	Persistent 2° AV block in the His-Purkinje system with bilateral bundle-branch block or 3° AV block within or below the His-Purkinje system after acute myocardial infarction (MI) Transient advanced (2° or 3°) infranodal AV block and associated bundle-branch block. If the site of block is uncertain, an EP study may be necessary Persistent and symptomatic 2° or 3° AV block	IIa: None IIb: Persistent 2° or 3° AV block at the AV node level	Transient AV block without intraventricular conduction defect Transient AV block in the presence of isolated left anterior fascicular block Acquired left anterior fascicular block in the absence of AV block Persistent 1° AV block in the presence of bundle-branch block that is old or age indeterminate
Chronic bifascicular and trifascicular block	Intermittent 3° AV block Type II 2° AV block Alternating bundle-branch block	IIa: Syncope not proved to be due to AV block when other likely causes have been excluded, specifically ventricular tachycardia HV interval >100 ms found at EP study	Fascicular block without AV block or symptoms Fascicular block with 1° AV block without symptoms

(*continued*)

TABLE 49.2 Indications for Cardiac Pacing (*Continued*)

	Class I	Class II	Class III
		Pacing-induced block below the His that is not physiologic IIb: Neuromuscular diseases with any degree of fasicular block, with or without symptoms secondary to unpredictibility of disease progression	
Carotid sinus hyper-sensitivity (carotid sinus irritability) and neurally mediated syncope	Recurrent syncope caused by carotid sinus stimulation; minimal carotid sinus pressure induces ventricular asystole of >3 s duration in the absence of any medication that depresses the sinus node or AV conduction	IIa: Recurrent syncope without clear, provocative events and with a hypersensitive cardioinhibitory response Significantly symptomatic and recurrent neurocardiogenic syncope associated with bradycardia documented spontaneously at the time of tilt table testing. IIb: None	A hyperactive cardioinhibitory response to carotid sinus stimulation in the absence of symptoms or in the presence of vague symptoms such as dizziness, lightheadedness, or both Recurrent syncope, lightheadedness, or dizziness in the absence of a hyperactive cardioinhibitory response Situational vasovagal syncope in which avoidance behavior is effective
Termination of tachy-arrhythmias		IIa: Symptomatic recurrent SVT that is reproducibly terminated by pacing after drugs and catheter ablation fail to control the arrhythmia or produce intolerable side effects IIb: Recurrent SVT or atrial flutter that is reproducibly terminated by pacing as an alternative to drug therapy or ablation	Tachycardias frequently accelerated or converted to fibrillation by pacing The presence of accessory pathways with the capacity for rapid anterograde conduction whether or not the pathways participate in the mechanism of the tachycardia

(*continued*)

TABLE 49.2 **Indications for Cardiac Pacing (*Continued*)**

	Class I	Class II	Class III
Prevention of tachycardia	Sustained pause-dependent VT, with or without prolonged QT, in which the efficacy of pacing is thoroughly documented	IIa: High-risk patients with congenital long QT syndrome IIb: AV re-entrant or AV node re-entrant SVT not responsive to medical or ablative therapy Prevention of symptomatic, drug-refractory, recurrent atrial fibrillation	Frequent or complex ventricular ectopic activity without sustained VT in the absence of the long QT syndrome Long QT syndrome due to reversible causes

AV, atrioventricular; EP, electrophysiologic; LV, left ventricular; SND, sinus node dysfunction; SVT, sustained ventricular tachycardia; VT, ventricular tachycardia.
Class I: Conditions for which there is evidence and/or general agreement that pacing is beneficial, useful, and effective.
Class II: Conditions for which there is conflicting evidence and/or a divergence of opinion about the usefulness/efficacy of pacing.
IIa: Weight of evidence/opinion is in favor of usefulness/efficacy.
IIb: Usefulness/efficacy is less well established by evidence/opinion.
Class III: Conditions for which there is evidence and/or general agreement that pacing is not useful/effective and in some cases may be harmful.
From Gregoratos G, Abrams J, Epstein AE, et al. ACC/AHA/NASPE 2002 guideline update for implantation of cardiac pacemakers and antiarrhythmia devices: summary article. A report of the American College of Cardiology/American Heart Association Task Force on Practice Guidelines. *Circulation* 2002;106:2145–2161.

2. **Chronaxie.** This corresponds to the threshold pulse width at twice the rheobase voltage. The chronaxie pulse duration approximates the point of minimal threshold energy on the strength–duration curve.

C. **Safety margins**

1. **Voltage.** The voltage output should be programmed to a level that is approximately twice the capture (stimulation) threshold for a 2:1 output safety margin.
2. **Pulse width.** The pulse duration should be programmed to a level approximately three times the pulse width capture threshold for a 3:1 output safety margin. The typical range for pulse width is 0.2 to 1.0 millisecond.

D. **Temporal changes in stimulation threshold.** Typically, the stimulation threshold rises within 24 hours following implantation of a permanent pacemaker lead. The threshold peaks at 1 to 2 weeks, then gradually declines and plateaus at approximately 6 weeks at a level less than the acute peak, but greater than that measured at implantation. The absolute value of the temporal changes in stimulation thresholds varies between individuals and also between various types of electrodes.

VI. PACEMAKER TIMING CYCLES AND INTERVALS

A. **Timing circuits.** A pacemaker can be thought of as a series of timing circuits. An understanding of how these timing circuits interact can facilitate the analysis of pacemaker rhythms. The timing circuit runs until the cycle is completed or until it is reset. Completion of a timing cycle results in the release of a pacing output or the initiation of another timing cycle. Figure 49.2 illustrates the basic timing cycles

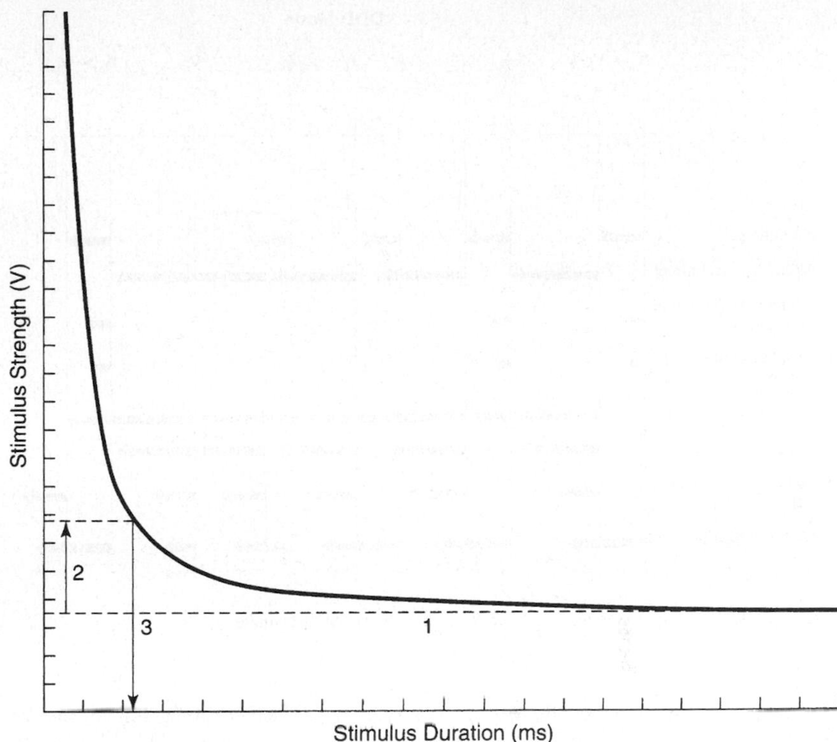

Figure 49.1. Strength–duration curve.

and intervals for a dual-chamber pacemaker. The basic terms and abbreviations used for the pacemaker timing cycles and refractory periods are defined in the glossary.

B. Base rate behavior

1. Single-chamber pacemakers have a timing circuit that either is inhibited (reset) by a sensed native heartbeat or completes its cycle with a stimulus output. Dual-chamber pacemakers are more complex and incorporate more timing circuits. Figure 49.2 illustrates the timing cycles of a dual-chamber pacemaker in DDD mode. In general, base rate (lower rate) pacing for dual-chamber pacemakers involves two timing circuits:
   - **a.** The first timing circuit is the interval from a ventricular sensed or paced event to an atrial paced event (atrial escape interval, or AEI).
   - **b.** The second timing circuit is the interval from an atrial sensed or paced event to a ventricular paced event (AV interval, or AVI). An atrial sensed event that occurs before the completion of the AEI results in termination of that interval and initiation of the AVI.
2. The response of a dual-chamber pacemaker to a sensed ventricular signal varies among manufacturers. Some pacemakers use a ventricular-based timing system, and others use an atrial-based timing system.
   - **a. Ventricular-based timing.** In this type of pacemaker timing system, the AEI is fixed. A ventricular sensed event during the AEI will reset the timing circuit. A ventricular sensed event during the AVI terminates that interval and initiates the AEI.

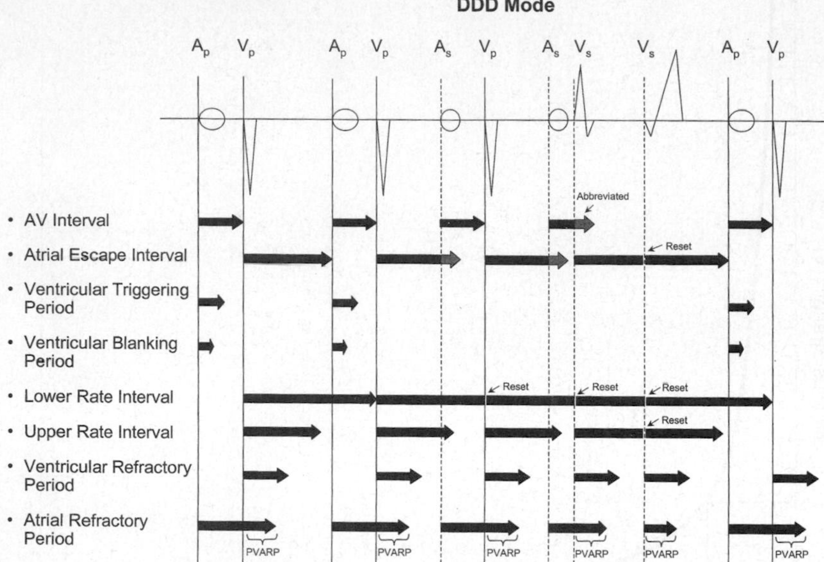

Figure 49.2. Timing cycles and intervals for a dual-chamber pacemaker.

b. **Atrial-based timing.** In this type of pacemaker timing system, the AA interval is fixed. A ventricular sensed event during the AEI will reset the AA timing circuit and add the programmed AVI. A ventricular sensed event during the AVI will inhibit a ventricular output, but will not alter the AA interval.

3. Interpretation of pacemaker rhythm that has ventricular sensed beats requires knowledge of the type of timing system the pacemaker uses. Both the ventricular-based and atrial-based timing systems should be analyzed by measuring backward from an atrial-paced event. The point of ventricular sensing for a ventricular-based timing system will be found at the point before the atrial-paced event that is equal to the AEI. For an atrial-based timing system, the measurement before the atrial-paced event should be to the point that is equal to the AA interval. Knowledge of these principles allows one to evaluate the ventricular sensing for a given pacemaker. Be aware that some pacemakers have incorporated modifications of these systems that take advantage of features from both timing systems. For example, a pacemaker with an atrial-based timing system may behave as a ventricular-based timing system.
4. **Hysteresis** is a pacing feature that attempts to allow the heart's native conduction system to predominate and therefore modifies base rate behavior. This feature works by using a longer escape interval after a sensed beat than after a paced beat. For example, the device sets the hysteresis rate at 50 bpm while the basal rate is 60 bpm. Therefore, if the patient's intrinsic rate is greater than 50 bpm, the device will not pace. However, if the patient's rate falls below 50 bpm, the pacer will pace at 60 bpm. As hysteresis can appear as an unusually long delay on the ECG strip, it can be misinterpreted as failure to pace or as inappropriate sensing.

C. **Upper rate behavior**

1. As the sinus rate accelerates, the sensed atrial events terminate the AEI and initiate the AVI. The result is P-wave synchronous ventricular pacing (unless

the PR interval is shorter than the PV interval, in which case pacing will be fully inhibited).

2. The maximal atrial rate that a dual-chamber pacemaker can sense is determined by the total atrial refractory period (TARP). As defined earlier in this chapter, the TARP is composed of the AVI and postventricular atrial refractory period (PVARP). PVARP is an interval during which the atrial channel can see incoming signals, but will not respond to them. However, because signals are seen in PVARP, the pacer can use advanced features to assess whether high atrial rates are occurring. As the sinus rate accelerates, the native atrial intervals become shorter than the TARP, and some atrial events will not be sensed. An abrupt, fixed block occurs as the pacemaker only intermittently senses the P-waves, which may result in symptoms as the rate drops precipitously.
3. Maximal tracking rate interval (MTRI) or upper-rate limit (URL) is an additional timing circuit designed to avoid abrupt blocks at upper pacing rates. It works in conjunction with the AVI to determine the highest ventricular pacing rate that can be achieved in response to atrial sensed events. A sensed atrial event initiates the AVI and the MTRI.
   - **a.** If the AVI completes its cycle and the MTRI has also completed its cycle, then a ventricular output occurs at the programmed AV interval.
   - **b.** If the AVI completes its cycle and the MTRI has not completed its cycle, then the ventricular output is delayed until the MTRI has timed out. This prolongs the PV interval and allows continued tracking of the atrial rate. However, the longer PV interval also places the ventricular output closer to the following P-wave.
   - **c.** If the sinus rate accelerates to a sufficient rate, the delayed ventricular output may cause the following P-wave to fall within the PVARP and not be sensed. The result is an intermittent "dropped" beat and a pause similar to Wenckebach behavior. However, abrupt block is less likely. More modern pacemakers may incorporate features designed to limit the degree of fixed block at the upper rate limit, such as rate smoothing (adjustment of the AEI as the PV interval changes) and rate-responsive AV delay. However, fixed block at the upper rate limit may still occur, particularly if the device is suboptimally programmed.

VII. RATE-ADAPTIVE PACING. The primary purpose of rate-adaptive pacing is to emulate the function of the sinus node for patients with chronotropic incompetence or atrial arrhythmias that preclude reliable sensing of native sinoatrial rhythm. This function is expressed with the letter "R" in the fourth position (AAIR, VVIR, DDDR, and so on).

A. Primary components of a rate-adaptive pacemaker system

1. A sensor located in the pacing lead or pacemaker itself detects a physical or physiologic parameter that is directly or indirectly related to metabolic demand.
2. Rate-modulating circuitry within the pacemaker contains an algorithm that translates a change in the sensed parameter to a change in pacing rate.
3. Algorithm programmability such that a physician can make adjustments to accommodate the heart rate requirements of the individual patient.
4. Pacemakers can set the sensor to on or off. Some pacemakers can be put in a passive mode in which they store information in order to predict how the pacer would act if set to rate-responsive behavior.

B. Basic technical categories of pacemaker sensors (see Table 49.3). Motion sensors are the most commonly used due to their simplicity, speed of response, and compatibility with standard unipolar and bipolar pacing leads. Other sensors are more physiologic but may require technically complex pacing leads. Of the physiologic sensors, only the minute ventilation type is widely available. Minute ventilation sensors are prone to interference from electromagnetic sources, coughing, hyperventilation, and arm swinging.

TABLE 49.3 Sensors in Rate-Responsive Pacing

Methods	Physiologic parameters	Mechanism	Advantages	Disadvantages
Impedance sensing	Respiratory rate Minute ventilation Stroke volume	Impedance plethysmography	Highly physiologic Highly proportional to metabolic demand	Delayed response Susceptible to electrode motion artifact
Ventricular evoked response	Evoked QT interval (stim-T interval)	Reflects catecholamines	More physiologic	Requires ventricular pacing
Vibration, acceleration, gravitation, motion sensing	Body movement	Piezoelectric element	Rapid response No special lead needed	Nonphysiologic and nonspecific Late plateau response
Special sensors on pacing electrode	Central venous temperature[a] *dP*/*dt*[b] Mixed venous oxygen saturation[b]	Thermistor Piezoelectric element Optical sensor	More physiologic	Complex lead

[a]No longer produced, although still in use in Japan.
[b]Presently available only in clinical trials.
From Lau, 1995.

VIII. AUTOMATIC MODE SWITCHING. Automatic mode switching is a programmable response of a dual-chamber pacemaker during an atrial tachyarrhythmia (atrial tachycardia, atrial fibrillation, or atrial flutter) designed to avoid nonphysiologic ventricular pacing due to atrial tracking. Generally the device switches from DDD mode to a VVI mode, usually with a gradual reduction of the pacing rate. The device switches back to the DDD mode after the atrial tachyarrhythmia resolves. Mode switch information can also be helpful in documenting atrial arrhythmia burden in order to help dictate medical therapy for arrhythmias.

IX. BASIC PACING MODES. The choice of pacemaker generator and the mode of pacing depend mainly on the underlying rhythm disturbance, and whether AV synchrony and rate response are desired (see Table 49.4).

A. Ventricular demand pacing (VVI). This remains the most commonly used pacing mode worldwide. Although VVI pacing protects the patient from lethal bradycardias, AV synchrony is not restored or maintained, nor does it provide rate responsiveness in the patient with chronotropic incompetence. Because AV synchrony is absent, the rate of pacemaker syndrome is high (up to 83% in randomized trials).

B. AAI (atrial demand pacing). This mode is appropriate for patients with sinus node dysfunction who have intact AV conduction. A sensed atrial event will inhibit atrial pacing, and expiration of a preset AA interval will pace the atrium at a preset rate. Because there will be no ventricular support if AV block should occur, careful

TABLE 49.4 Guidelines for Choice of Pacemaker Generator in Selected Indications for Pacing

	Sinus node dysfunction	AV block	Neurally mediated syncope or carotid sinus hyperreactivity
Single-chamber atrial pacemaker	No suspected abnormality of AV conduction and not at increased risk for future AV block Maintenance of AV synchrony during pacing if desired RR if desired	Not appropriate	Not appropriate (unless AV block systematically excluded)
Single-chamber ventricular pacemaker	Maintenance of AVS during pacing not necessary RR available if desired	Chronic AF or other atrial tachyarrhythmia or maintenance of AVS not necessary RR available if desired	Chronic AF or other atrial tachyarrhythmia RR available if desired
Dual-chamber pacemaker	AVS during pacing desired Suspected abnormality of AV conduction or increased risk of AV block	AVS during pacing desired Atrial pacing desired RR available if desired	Sinus mechanism present RR available if desired
Single-lead, atrial-sensing ventricular pacemaker	Not appropriate	Normal sinus function and no need for atrial pacing Desire to limit the number of pacemaker leads	Not appropriate

AV, atrioventricular; AF, atrial fibrillation; RR, rate response; AVS, atrioventricular synchrony.

testing of AV conduction is necessary at the time of pacemaker implantation (incremental atrial pacing). This mode is infrequently used in the United States.

C. AV sequential pacing

1. DDI. There is both atrial and ventricular sensing and pacing, but no atrial tracking can occur, because mode is by inhibition only. The pacemaker rate is therefore fixed, and this mode is rarely used.

2. VDD. In this mode ventricular stimulation can either be inhibited by a spontaneous ventricular beat or be initiated by an atrially tracked beat, and it can therefore be used in patients with normal sinus function but impaired AV conduction. This modality uses a "floating" sensing electrode on the atrial portion of the ventricular lead, but it is altogether rarely used.

3. DDD. This system provides the most physiologic pacing mode. The pacer can be totally inhibited with normal sinus rhythm, can pace the atrium with spontaneous ventricular depolarization, can pace the ventricle in response to a spontaneous P-wave, and can sequentially pace both atrium and ventricle. This system is most appropriate in patients who have impaired AV conduction with either an intact or dysfunctional sinus node.

X. BIVENTRICULAR PACING. Because patients with systolic left ventricular dysfunction and wide QRS complexes have dyssynergic contractility, the use of multisite atrial, right ventricular, and left ventricular pacing strategies has been proposed. For this purpose, an additional pacemaker lead is placed transvenously into the coronary sinus, or epicardially during open-chest surgery for simultaneous stimulation of the left ventricle.

A. Biventricular cardiac resynchronization pacing for heart failure has been accepted as standard therapy for patients with a depressed ejection fraction (EF less than 35%), QRS duration greater than 120 milliseconds, and NYHA class III or IV symptoms despite appropriate medical therapy. Several randomized studies, including MUSTIC, MIRACLE, MIRACLE-ICD, PATH-CHF, and VENTAK-CHF/CONTACT-CD, have demonstrated improved functional status, exercise capacity, and quality of life with biventricular pacing. CARE-HF demonstrated a decrease in the primary endpoint of death and hospitalization with biventricular pacing (see Chapter 51) in heart failure patients with depressed systolic function, class III/IV symptoms, and wide QRS.

B. Although the overall rate of clinical improvement with biventricular pacing is high in these trials (about 70% of patients), it is not entirely clear how to identify patients who will respond ahead of time. Multiple echocardiographic and electrocardiographic measures have been investigated to help predict an individual patient's likelihood of clinical response, but so far no single modality has proven entirely reliable.

XI. PACEMAKER IMPLANTATION: PERTINENT ISSUES FOR THE PHYSICIAN

A. Preoperative issues. Several issues must be addressed for the patient scheduled for routine pacemaker implantation.

1. History and physical examination. Attention should be given to any findings that may affect the site and approach for pacemaker implantation, such as patient handedness (pacemakers are generally implanted on the contralateral side), history of mastectomy, presence of congenital abnormalities (e.g., anomalous venous drainage), current central venous lines, or tricuspid valve disease or surgery.

2. Informed consent (risks, benefits, and alternatives)

3. Tests

a. Posteroanterior (PA) and lateral chest radiograph

b. Twelve-lead ECG should be obtained.

c. Blood tests may include serum electrolytes, complete blood count, creatinine, prothrombin/INR, and partial thromboplastin times.

4. Medications

a. Most physicians prefer warfarin to be discontinued at least 3 days before the procedure. In some cases, such as primary implants, or generator changes, coumadin can be kept close to therapeutic with INR at approximately 2.0.

Consider admission to hospital for intravenous heparin if the risk of discontinuation of anticoagulation is high. Heparin may be discontinued 4 to 6 hours before the procedure.

b. The dosage of oral hypoglycemics or insulin may have to be adjusted.

5. Patient preparation

a. The patient should have nothing by mouth for at least 6 to 8 hours before the procedure. IV hydration should be initiated upon arrival to the laboratory to prevent hypovolemia, which may make venous cannulation more difficult.

b. An intravenous catheter is particularly helpful if placed in the arm ipsilateral to the proposed pacemaker site. This allows the ability to perform a venogram if there is difficulty in obtaining venous access during pacemaker implantation.

c. The patient should be shaved and cleansed (e.g., with povidone iodine) in the area from above the nipple line to the angle of the jaw and from the sternum to axillary line on the side of the implantation site.

d. Antibiotic prophylaxis before pacemaker implantation is a controversial issue, and various prospective studies have provided conflicting information. Some centers have advocated antibiotic prophylaxis with an agent active against staphylococci for patients at high risk for endocarditis, such as those with prosthetic valves or complex congenital heart disease, or for redo procedures or for prolonged or potentially contaminating procedures. Other centers use antibiotic prophylaxis routinely (systemically and/or locally).

B. Postoperative issues

1. General recommendations. Patients are usually admitted for overnight observation on telemetry after pacemaker implantation.

2. Postoperative testing. PA and lateral chest radiograph should be obtained to document proper position of the pacemaker leads and connection of the terminal pins to the pulse generator. The radiograph should also be examined for evidence of pneumothorax, pericardial effusion, or pleural effusion.

3. Resuming anticoagulation. Intravenous heparin may be resumed 8 to 12 hours after the procedure with avoidance of a heparin bolus. A pressure dressing should be applied to the site of pacemaker implantation to prevent hematoma formation in those patients. Warfarin may be reinstituted as early as the evening after the procedure. Anticoagulation should not be aggressive in the early postimplantation period due to the risk of pacemaker pocket hematoma, which has been associated with increased risk of complications such as reoperation and infection.

4. Pacemaker evaluation

a. Evaluation in the pacemaker clinic before discharge includes assessment of pacing and sensing thresholds and lead impedance. The pacemaker is programmed to optimize patient hemodynamics and minimize battery expenditure.

b. Capture thresholds are expected to rise over the first 2 to 6 weeks after implantation. Therefore, the pacemaker should be programmed with an adequate safety margin to account for these changes.

c. Rate adaptation for activity-sensing pacemakers may be programmed according to informal (e.g., hallway walking) or formal (e.g., treadmill) exercise testing.

5. Discharge planning

a. Discharge instructions. Usually includes patient education regarding the recognition of pacemaker pocket complications, such as signs of infections, bleeding, or hematoma. The patient is generally advised to avoid heavy lifting or vigorous activity (especially forceful abduction) with the arm ipsilateral to the implant site.

b. The patient should be provided with information regarding his or her pacemaker, including a wallet card identifying the pacemaker and lead(s) manufacturer, model numbers, and serial numbers.

c. The patient may be provided with and instructed in the use of a trans-telephonic monitoring system for remote evaluation of the pacemaker.
d. Endocarditis prophylaxis is generally *not* recommended routinely for patients with pacemakers, according to updated AHA guidelines.

XII. COMMON PACEMAKER PROBLEMS

A. Acute complications of pacemaker implantation

1. Pneumothorax/Hemothorax

a. This complication may be asymptomatic and detected only by chest radiograph. The diagnosis should be considered in a patient with dyspnea and/or pleuritic chest pain after implantation.
b. A small pneumothorax may resolve without intervention. However, presence of severe symptoms, a pneumothorax greater than 10%, or an expanding or persistent pneumothorax often necessitates placement of a chest tube.

2. Pacemaker pocket hematoma

a. This is one of the most common complications of pacemaker implantation and is often due to small vessel venous bleeding inside the pacemaker pocket. Bleeding may also arise from arterial vessels or retrograde flow of venous blood along the pacemaker leads into the pocket.
b. Signs and symptoms may include pain, swelling, and sometimes bleeding at the pocket site.
c. Small hematomas may be managed conservatively with elevation (head of bed at least 45°) and analgesics. Larger or expanding hematomas may require pressure dressings. The patient should be positioned on his or her side contralateral to the pacemaker site. Large hematomas may compromise the integrity of the incision site and result in dehiscence. The patient may require urgent surgical exploration and hematoma evacuation in the electrophysiology lab or operating room.
d. Percutaneous insertion of a needle to drain a hematoma increases the risk of infection and should be avoided.

3. Cardiac or central venous perforation. Perforation may lead to pericardial effusion and cardiac tamponade and should be suspected in the patient with chest pain, pericardial friction rub, or hypotension after pacemaker implantation. A chest radiograph may reveal an enlarged cardiac silhouette or an extracardiac lead tip. A change in the paced ventricular morphology, particularly a right bundle-branch pattern, may indicate ventricular lead migration. The hemodynamically unstable patient with tamponade may require urgent pericardiocentesis and drainage of the effusion.

4. Diaphragmatic stimulation. Stimulation of the left diaphragm may occur with a pacing lead at the right ventricular apex, particularly at high pacing outputs. The possibility of cardiac perforation should be considered. Stimulation of the right diaphragm may occur due to stimulation of the right phrenic nerve by a displaced atrial lead. Reduction in the pacemaker output voltage or lead repositioning may be necessary.

5. Local muscular stimulation

a. This may occur with a unipolar pacemaker configuration, particularly if the pulse generator is positioned upside down within the pocket (a node directly in contact with the pectoralis muscle).
b. A pacing lead fracture may result in leakage of current into the surrounding tissue, resulting in local muscle stimulation.

6. Pacemaker malfunction

a. The pulse generator may be defective or may have been damaged at the time of implantation (e.g., by electrocautery or direct-current defibrillation).
b. Improper fixation of the terminal pins of the pacing leads into the pulse generator (e.g., loose-set screws) may result in complete or intermittent pacemaker malfunction.

7. Lead dislodgement or damage

a. Pacing leads may become dislodged soon after implantation before the lead has a chance to become more fixed in place through clotting and fibrosis. Lead dislodgement may be suspected by noncapture, undersensing, or oversensing on telemetry or ECG, and confirmed by chest radiography or formal pacemaker testing.

b. The lead may be damaged at the time of implantation by forceful handling or excessively tight retention sutures.

c. Interrogation of a device with a damaged lead may reveal changes in impedance. A break in the insulation of the lead results in low impedance, and a contained fracture of the lead conductor results in high impedance.

B. Chronic complications of pacemaker implantation

1. Pacemaker system infection

a. The reported incidence of pacemaker infection is 0% to 19%. The infection may involve only the pacemaker pocket or the entire system with subsequent life-threatening sepsis. There is a higher incidence with repeat operations (e.g., pulse generator replacement). Causative organisms tend to be skin flora such as *Staphylococcus* species.

b. Treatment should include intravenous antibiotics; however, antibiotic therapy rarely eradicates the infection unless the pacemaker system is removed. In the largest study to date (2), mortality rates for device-related endocarditis range from 31% to 66% without device removal. Mortality improves to 18% or less with a combined approach of medical therapy and complete device removal.

c. The timing of system removal depends on the clinical status of the patient; however, prolonged delays should be avoided.

2. Intravascular thrombosis or obstruction

a. Vascular complications are common with device therapy. They range from asymptomatic venous occlusion to extremity edema. Mortality from vasular complications is rare. Initial treatments may include heat and upper-extremity elevation. Symptomatic thrombosis of the subclavian or axillary veins may require anticoagulation or systemic thrombolytic therapy. It is recommended that documented deep venous thrombosis (DVT) be treated with anticoagulation with warfarin for at least 6 months, unless contraindicated.

b. Superior vena cava stenosis or occlusion may require percutaneous balloon dilatation or surgical consultation for consideration of repair.

3. Twiddler's syndrome. A situation in which the pacemaker is turned (usually unintentionally) upside down within the pacemaker pocket. The leads may become twisted, resulting in excessive traction on the leads and dislodgement.

XIII. PACEMAKER SYSTEM MALFUNCTION

A. In assessing the patient with suspected pacemaker malfunction, it is important to interpret the ECG carefully. Ideally, intracardiac tracings obtained by pacemaker interrogation should be interpreted. Pacing artifacts or spikes are high-frequency signals and are often filtered out by newer digital surface ECG machines. Furthermore, pacing artifacts from bipolar leads are smaller and more difficult to see than artifacts from unipolar leads. It may be necessary to record multiple leads or use an older analog recorder to clearly visualize the pacing artifact. Pseudomalfunction occurs when recording and digital artifacts are misinterpreted. Approaching the paced patient's ECG systematically will help to determine the appropriateness of pacing.

B. General evaluation for possible pacemaker malfunction

1. If a recent pacemaker interrogation is available, review the programmed parameters for the pacemaker, particularly the mode, base rate, upper rate limit, intervals, and the presence of other features such as automatic mode switching, hysteresis, rate adaptive features, or managed ventricular pacing.

2. Obtain a 12-lead ECG and evaluate the following:

a. Determine whether pacing stimulus artifacts are present and whether the appropriate chamber is captured.

b. If no pacing stimulus artifact can be seen, native depolarization should be adequate.

c. Evaluate whether native beats are appropriately sensed in relation to paced complexes.

d. Evaluate the timing cycles of a dual-chamber pacemaker by measuring backward from an atrially paced event, as described in the section in this chapter that discusses ventricular- and atrial-based timing systems.

C. Patients with pacemaker system malfunction generally demonstrate absence of a pacing stimulus artifact, failure to capture, or failure to sense.

1. **Failure of pacemaker stimulus output.** A differential diagnosis of the more common causes of pauses during a paced rhythm is listed later in this chapter. Application of a magnet over the pacemaker should result in asynchronous pacing. If the pauses resolve when the magnet is applied, then the diagnosis of oversensing is most likely. If the pauses do not resolve, then one of the other causes should be considered.

   a. **Pulse generator failure.** The pulse generator may be at the end of life, which may easily be detected with a pacemaker check.

   b. **Lead failure.** This can be due to loose-set screw or terminal pin disconnection, lead conductor failure, or lead insulation failure. Suspicion of lead malfunction should prompt the clinician to obtain a chest radiograph. This may reveal the terminal pin not situated properly within the header of the pulse generator, or it may demonstrate a defect in the lead insulation or conductor coil. A significant increase in the lead impedance suggests lead conductor failure, and a significant decrease in the lead impedance suggests lead insulation failure.

   c. **Oversensing.** EMI, myopotentials, crosstalk, or T-wave oversensing can lead to falsely interpreted signals.

   d. **Pseudomalfunction.** Pacemaker malfunction can be mistakenly diagnosed if the small spikes from a bipolar system are not appreciated on the surface ECG. Malfunction can also be diagnosed mistakenly if attention is not paid to additional features that allow the heart rate to fall below or above the set base rate. It is important to remember additional features such as hysteresis, sleep settings, rate adaptive behaviors, or automatic mode switch, which can each be mistaken for pacemaker malfunction.

2. **Failure to capture**

   a. **Elevated capture threshold.** Electrolyte disturbance (e.g., hyperkalemia, acidemia), antiarrhythmic drugs (particularly class Ic agents such as flecainide), and myocardial fibrosis (e.g., cardiomyopathy, myocardial infarction [MI]) can increase the capture threshold.

   b. **Lead malfunction**

      (1) Lead fracture.

      (2) Lead dislodgement or perforation may result in a change in the paced morphology, especially a change from left to right bundle-branch morphology.

   c. **Exit block.** Exit block is defined as failure of the pacing output at the distal electrode to stimulate adjacent myocardium. This is often caused by the inflammatory reaction that occurs at the pacemaker lead tip at the time of implantation. It occurs in approximately 5% of cases and may be managed with systemic steroids. Some pacing leads have steroid-eluting electrodes designed to minimize the degree of inflammation at the electrode tip and decrease the incidence of exit block.

   d. **Latency.** Defined as the delay between the delivery of an output pulse and the onset of electrical systole, such as occurs with severe electrolyte disturbances.

   e. **Pseudomalfunction.** Artifact with small spikes on the surface ECG, such as occurs when the patient's refractory periods interfere with pacer function.

3. **Failure to sense**

   a. Lead dislodgement is usually accompanied by failure to capture (see discussion earlier in this chapter)

   b. Lead insulation failure (see discussion earlier in this chapter)

c. Inadequate endocardial signal
d. Change in electrogram. Transient changes may occur due to electrolyte or acid-base disturbance, and permanent changes may occur due to MI or cardiomyopathy
e. Ectopic beats
f. Pulse generator failure (sensing circuits)
g. Functional undersensing. Defined as undersensing that occurs due to normal pacemaker function, such as refractory periods, blanking periods, or safety pacing.

D. Other pacemaker malfunctions

1. **Pacemaker syndrome.** Defined as the signs and symptoms that occur in the pacemaker patient because of inadequate timing of atrial and ventricular contractions. Pacemaker syndrome is commonly caused by retrograde ventriculoatrial (VA) conduction, which causes atrial contraction against closed mitral and tricuspid valves. Pacemaker syndrome may also occur during an exercise-induced atrial arrhythmia due to loss of AV synchrony when a device with an automatic mode-switching feature converts to VVI pacing.
2. **Pacemaker-mediated tachycardia (PMT).** This is defined as a paced tachycardia that is sustained by the continued active participation of the pacemaker in the rhythm. At first glance, the resultant wide-complex (paced) tachycardia may appear to be ventricular tachycardia, especially for pacemakers with bipolar leads where the pacing artifact may be difficult to discern on ECG.
   a. One form of PMT is the rapid ventricular pacing that occurs as a dual-chamber pacemaker attempts to track the rapid atrial rate during an atrial tachyarrhythmic episode.
   b. Another form of PMT occurs when there is oversensing in the atrial channel, such as myopotentials.
   c. Endless-loop tachycardia (ELT). Another form of PMT in which a repetitive sequence of sensing of retrograde atrial activity results in triggering of a ventricular paced beat at the end of the MTRI. ELT requires a trigger for initiation, which may be any event that results in AV dissociation and allows retrograde (VA) conduction to occur after a native or paced ventricular beat. The trigger may be a premature ventricular contraction, atrial undersensing, atrial oversensing, or atrial noncapture. ELT is sustained until there is VA block. Application of a magnet over the pacemaker will terminate ELT. The most reliable way to prevent ELT is to program the PVARP to a value that exceeds the VA conduction interval. Some of the more modern pacemakers have PMT or ELT recognition and termination algorithms designed to prevent and/or terminate PMT and ELT.

XIV. COMMON ISSUES FOR THE PATIENT WITH A PACEMAKER

A. Perioperative patient

1. **Preoperative assessment.** Review of pertinent history and a physical examination should be performed. The patient should undergo a pacemaker evaluation to assess the programmed parameters, pacing and sensing thresholds, and lead impedance.
2. The degree of pacemaker dependence should be determined. A patient who is pacemaker dependent should have temporary pacing equipment readily available.
3. If the operative field is in the area near the pacemaker, the rate response feature of the pacemaker should be deactivated to avoid inappropriate rapid pacing due to vibrations or pressure transmitted to the pulse generator.
4. Electrocautery may result in temporary inhibition of pacemaker output due to oversensing of the EMI. Electrocautery should be used sparingly and in short bursts, and the cautery electrode should be placed at a distance from the pacemaker site.
5. Postoperatively, the pacemaker should be reevaluated for any sign of malfunction, the presence of a reset mode, and any change in lead threshold or

impedance values. A chest radiograph should be obtained after cardiac surgery to evaluate for lead damage or dislodgement.

B. EMI in the hospital environment

1. **Magnetic resonance imaging (MRI).** The magnetic field generated by the electromagnet and the radiofrequency signal produced to modulate the magnetic field for MRI may cause torque forces or malfunction for cardiac pacemakers. More modern pacemakers contain fewer ferromagnetic components than previous pacemakers, so that torque forces are less common. The magnetic forces may close the pacemaker reed switch and result in asynchronous pacing. The radiofrequency signal may result in inhibition of pacing, rapid pacing, or reversion to reset mode. Unipolar pacemakers are more susceptible to interference from MRI. In general, MRI should be avoided in pacemaker patients unless absolutely necessary. There are new "MRI-safe" pacers currently in development and testing.
2. **Extracorporeal shock-wave lithotripsy (ESWL)**
   - **a.** ESWL is a treatment for renal calculi that involves the production of focused hydraulic shock waves from an underwater spark gap. Interference or damage to a pacemaker may occur due to the spark gap or the shock waves. Activity-based rate adaptation pacemakers with piezoelectric crystals may be damaged by the shock waves, and the shock waves may cause oversensing and subsequent nonphysiologic rapid pacing rates. Such pacemakers should be reprogrammed with the rate-adaptive feature deactivated before the procedure. If the pacemaker with a piezoelectric crystal is located in the abdomen, then ESWL should not be performed.
   - **b.** The shock waves may be misinterpreted as atrial activity; therefore, dual-chamber pacemakers should be programmed to VVI mode to avoid rapid ventricular pacing.
   - **c.** A patient with a pacemaker may undergo ESWL; however, the pulse generator should be as far as possible from the focal point of the lithotripsy shock waves, and a cardiologist who is experienced in pacemaker management should be available nearby during the procedure.
3. **Radiation therapy**
   - **a.** Diagnostic irradiation does not interfere with cardiac pacemakers. Therapeutic radiation therapy to the thorax such as that used for breast or lung malignancies may result in interference and/or cumulative damage. The damage to the integrated circuitry of the pacemaker results from leakage currents between the insulated parts. This damage is directly related to the cumulative radiation dose.
   - **b.** The pacemaker should be assessed before and after a treatment session. ECG monitoring is recommended for patients who are pacemaker-dependent. The pulse generator should be shielded from the ionizing radiation or moved to another site if necessary.
4. **Cardiac monitors.** Cardiac monitors that inject current into the patient's body in order to measure minute ventilation may interfere with pacemakers that use minute ventilation for rate adaptation.
5. **Transcutaneous electric nerve stimulation (TENS)** is considered safe for patients with bipolar pacemakers. Patients with unipolar pacemakers may require a reduction in sensitivity.
6. **Dental equipment.** Some types of dental equipment may cause pacemaker inhibition, particularly for unipolar pacemakers. Vibrations may increase the pacing rate of activity-sensing rate-adaptive pacemakers.
7. **Cardioversion/defibrillation.** The shock from a direct current (DC) cardioversion or defibrillation may cause damage to the pulse generator or result in the device being reset. If DC cardioversion or defibrillation is necessary, the patch electrodes should be positioned as far from the pulse generator as possible. A pacemaker evaluation should be performed after the procedure.
8. **Electroconvulsive therapy (ECT)** generally does not interfere with pacemaker function. The patient should have a pacemaker evaluation before and after each

session. ECG monitoring during the session is prudent. Seizure activity during the procedure may produce myopotential inhibition of unipolar pacemakers.

9. **Diathermy** may result in pacemaker interference or damage if applied to the region near the pulse generator.
10. **Electrocautery** (discussed earlier in this chapter)

C. Environmental EMI

1. **Cellular telephones.** These devices may interfere with cardiac pacemakers while transmitting or receiving calls. Analog cellular phones seem to be safer than digital ones. A pacemaker patient should not carry a cellular telephone near the pacemaker site (i.e., shirt pocket) and should hold the telephone to the contralateral ear during use.
2. **Electronic article surveillance (EAS)** is a type of antitheft system consisting of a gate that produces an electromagnetic field through which individuals must walk. The field may result in pacemaker interference, primarily inhibition of pacemaker output. Patients with unipolar dual-chamber pacemakers are particularly susceptible to interference from EAS systems.
3. **Industrial electrical equipment.** This includes devices, such as arc welders, that may generate strong electrical fields. The strength of the electrical field varies among types of equipment and if sufficiently strong may interfere with unipolar pacemakers. Patients may require individual environmental testing to ensure safety.
4. **Microwave ovens.** Due to better sealing of microwave ovens and improved shielding of pulse generators, interference with pacemakers by microwave ovens is no longer considered a significant problem.
5. **Metal detectors.** Although the metal detectors in public places such as airports may alarm due to detection of a pacemaker, there is generally no significant interference with pacemaker function. Patients should avoid lingering around these devices and pass through them at a normal speed.
6. **High-voltage power lines and electrical substations.** These areas may cause inhibition or asynchronous pacing in unipolar pacemakers if the patient is quite close to the electrical field. At usual public distances from such areas, there should be no pacemaker interference.

D. Pacemaker response to electromagnetic interference

1. **Pacing inhibition.** For obvious reasons, this may be catastrophic. The majority of pacemakers used today contain protective alogorithms that make prolonged inhibition uncommon.
2. **Rapid pacing.** Oversensing of EMI by the atria channel in a device set to DDD can cause the pacer to trigger ventricular pacing at or near the upper tracking limit. This response is usually well tolerated, but in certain individuals when sustained, it may cause palpitations, hypotension, or angina. Rapid pacing may also occur via activation of minute ventilation sensors.
3. **Reversion to asynchronous pacing.** Most pacers have algorithms that protect against prolonged inhibition from noise. Algorithms are based upon the principle that detected rapid frequency signals are unlikely to represent myocardial activation. The pacemaker is programmed to have a noise sampling window during the ventricular refractory period. In most devices, repetitive signaling detected in the noise sampling window reverts the device to asynchronous pacing. Asynchronous pacing is generally safe, but it is not without the risks of losing AV synchrony. Also, pacing may rarely occur during the ventricular vulnerable period and may initiate ventricular arrhythmias.

XV. CARDIAC PACING: CLINICAL TRIALS

A. Conventional pacing trials

1. Numerous clinical trials, mostly small and nonrandomized, have been performed with regard to exercise capacity and quality of life for various pacemaker modes, chamber(s) paced, rate-adaptive pacing, and types of sensors.
2. Clinical trials have firmly established the superiority of rate-adaptive (VVIR) over fixed-rate ventricular pacing (VVI) with regard to quality of life and exercise performance.

3. Numerous clinical trials have been undertaken to prove the benefit of dual-chamber/atrial-based pacing in patients undergoing PPM implantation for sinus node dysfunction or high-degree AV block.
4. There are conflicting data regarding the benefit of dual-chamber pacing over rate-adaptive ventricular pacing. Early nonrandomized trials demonstrated mortality benefit with DDD pacing over VVI in patients with CHB. However, in randomized prospective trials, atrial pacing has not been shown to decrease rates of death or heart failure in patients treated for sinus node dysfunction and high-degree AV block. However, there are several randomized trials demonstrating that atrial-based pacing does, in fact, lead to a reduction in both atrial fibrillation and stroke. However, this benefit may be limited to patients with sinus node dysfunction. The one clear benefit that dual-chamber/atrial-based pacing provides is the avoidance of pacemaker syndrome, which can be seen in up to 10% of patients with VVI pacing.
5. The following paragraphs summarize some of the larger-scale, randomized studies of ventricular- versus atrial-based cardiac pacing modes:
   a. **Pacemaker Selection in the Elderly (PASE) trial.** A single blind, randomized, controlled trial of ventricular pacing versus dual-chamber pacing in 407 patients older than 65 years. The primary end point was quality of life with up to 30 months follow-up. Quality of life improved with pacemaker implantation. Patients with sinus node dysfunction, but not AV block, had significantly better quality of life with dual-chamber pacing than ventricular pacing (3).
   b. **Canadian Trial of Physiologic Pacing (CTOPP).** In this trial, 1,474 patients were assigned to ventricular pacing and 1,094 patients to physiologic pacing. During a mean follow-up period of 3 years, there was no significant effect on the risk of death, stroke, or hospitalization for congestive heart failure (CHF) according to the type of pacemaker used. However, the annual rate of AF was significantly lower in the atrial pacing group, although there was a 2-year delay before this beneficial effect emerged. There was a 50% reduction in perioperative complications with the implant of ventricular pacing systems, but in the ventricular pacing group there was a 5% incidence of pacemaker syndrome that required upgrade to a dual-chamber device. (4).
   c. **Mode Selection Trial in Sinus Node Dysfunction (MOST).** Randomized trial that attempted to compare dual-chamber with single-chamber ventricular pacing in 2,010 patients with sinus node dysfunction. There was no advantage for dual-chamber pacing over single-chamber ventricular pacing in terms of the trial's primary end point: death from any cause, or nonfatal stroke over 33.1 months of follow-up. However, some advantages were seen with the dual-chamber modality in secondary end points, including reductions in AF and symptoms of heart failure, and improvement in quality of life (5). There was no difference in heart failure admission rates between the two groups.
   d. **Pacemaker Atrial Tachycardia (Pac-A-Tach) trial.** This was a mode randomization study in 198 patients (median age 72 years), all of whom received dual-chamber rate-adaptive pacemakers programmed to either VVIR or DDDR pacing. Intention-to-treat analysis showed no significant difference in atrial tachyarrhythmia recurrence rates at 1 year (VVIR 43%; DDDR 48%; $p = 0.09$) (6).
   e. **UK Pacing and Cardiovascular Events (UK PACE) trial.** Trial comparing VVI(R) and DDD pacing in 2,021 elderly patients (mean age of 80 years) with high-grade AV block. Patients randomized to DDD (50%), VVI (25%), and VVIR (25%). No difference was detected in rates of stroke, atrial fibrillation, or heart failure hospitalizations (7).
   f. **Meta-analysis of trials comparing atrial- and ventricular-based pacing.** Healey, et al. in 2006 completed a large meta-analysis of all randomized control trials comparing ventricular and atrial-based pacing modes.

A total of 35,000 patient-years of follow-up were reviewed (8). There was no significant reduction in mortality or heart failure with atrial-based pacing. However, there was a significant reduction in atrial fibrillation (hazard ratio 0.80, 95% CI 0.77 to 0.89) and a borderline reduction in stroke (hazard ratio 0.81, 95% CI 0.67 to 0.99).

6. The practice of RV apical pacing as the preferred method remains controversial. It provides a reliable and stable position for long-term ventricular pacing. However, RV pacing creates ventricular desynchronization and leads to several adverse effects, including LV systolic and diastolic dysfunction. Retrospective and prospective analysis have linked increased numbers of RV paced beats with increased incidence of atrial fibrillation and heart failure. Current forms of pacemaker technology that minimize RV pacing are preferred to older pacemaker technologies. The following are landmark trials that have associated RV pacing with deleterious outcomes.

a. DAVID. The DAVID Trial was the first study of ventricular pacing strategies in ICD patients. The trial hypothesized that dual-chamber pacing would result in a lower rate of HF in these patients with EF less than 40% (9). At 1 year, rates of death and first hospitalization for HF were significantly increased in the dual-chamber group. The authors noted an increased rate of RV apex pacing in the DDD-70 group (60%) versus the VVI-40 group (3%). The authors concluded that the greater exposure to the deleterious effects of RV pacing in the DDD group led to worse outcomes.

b. SAVE PACe. This trial examined whether the application of newer technologies to limit frequency of ventricular pacing could lead to a decrease in atrial fibrillation in patients with dual-chamber pacemakers. Patients with sinus node disease, intact AV conduction, and a normal QRS interval were randomly assigned to receive convential dual-chamber pacing or dual-chamber minimal ventricular pacing with the use of features to promote AV conduction and reduce ventricular dyssynchrony (10). Persistent atrial fibrillation was found to occur less frequently in the dual-chamber minimal ventricular pacing group (hazard ratio 0.60, 95% CI, 0.41 to 0.88) than in the conventional dual chamber group

c. Recommendations. The most recent recommendations for cardiac pacing and resynchronization released by the European Society of Cardiology in 2007 are the first recommendations to specifically address the implications of apical versus RVOT/septal pacing. The recommendations mention that small trials have demonstrated septal pacing preserved LV function over the mid to long term and that HIS bundle pacing also appears to be beneficial. However, the guidelines note that it is too early to propose a recommendation concerning the optimal location of the right ventricular pacing lead.

XVI. EVOLVING INDICATIONS FOR PACEMAKER THERAPY

A. Hypertrophic Cardiomyopathy

1. Presumed mechanism of benefit. The idea of RV pacing to treat hypertrophic cardiomyopathy is based on the effective increase in LVOT diameter caused by altered septal activation.

2. Recommendations. Pacing is a class IIb recommendation in the 2002 ACC/AHA/NAPE guidelines and is reserved for drug refractory patients who have contraindications for septal ablation or myectomy (see Chapter 9).

B. Long QT syndrome

1. Presumed mechanism of benefit. In patients with long QT syndrome, life-threatening episodes of polymorphic VT and Torsades are typically preceded by pauses or severe bradycardia. By preventing these episodes, pacing may decrease the likelihood of events.

2. Recommendations: The 2002 ACC/AHA/NAPE guidelines do not comment on the use of pacing in long QT syndrome. There are no randomized trials to support use, but benefit was reported in several observational studies, especially in patients with acquired long QT syndrome.

XVII. FUTURE DIRECTIONS

A. Sensor technology. Advances in physiologic sensors and rate adaptation algorithms include the following:

1. **Multiple sensors for more physiologic pacing.** For example, a desirable sensor combination is an activity sensor, which typically has a more rapid response, and another sensor such as minute ventilation, which typically has a more delayed but workload-proportional response.
2. **Sensor blending** refers to the relative contribution of each sensor during each phase of activity and may be programmable.
3. **Sensor "cross-checking"** is done to determine if an increase in the intrinsic atrial rate is appropriate. If the sensor does not confirm activity while the pacemaker senses an increased atrial rate, the pacemaker will use the sensor to dictate the appropriate heart rate. Also, pacemakers with multiple sensors are able to detect intersensor disagreement and thereby avoid inappropriately rapid pacing due to a false-positive response of one sensor.

XVIII. GLOSSARY

A. Cardiac pacing: basic terminology

1. **"60,000 rule":** Converts rate (beats per minute) to interval (milliseconds) and vice versa, as there are 60,000 milliseconds in 1 minute. Note the formula: 60,000/interval (milliseconds) = rate (beats/minute).
2. **Anode:** Refers to the positive pole. The anode of a unipolar pacing system is the pulse generator case. The anode of a bipolar pacing system is the proximal ring electrode of the pacing lead.
3. **Capture:** The effective cardiac depolarization resulting from a pacing stimulus.
4. **Cardiac stimulation threshold (mA):** The minimal electrical energy required to consistently depolarize cardiac tissue through a given electrode. This threshold changes with time after implantation (acute, subacute, and chronic).
5. **Cathode:** Refers to the negative pole. The cathode of a unipolar pacing system is the electrode at the distal portion of the pacing lead. The cathode of a bipolar pacing system is the distal tip electrode of the pacing lead.
6. **Cross-talk:** In dual-chamber pacing systems, the inappropriate detection (sensing) of an event or signal in one chamber by the sense amplifier of the other chamber (usually inhibition of a ventricular output pulse due to ventricular channel detection of an atrial output pulse).
7. **Current (*I*):** The rate of transfer or the flow of electricity, measured in milliamperes (mA).
8. **Elective replacement interval (ERI), also known as elective replacement time (ERT) or recommended replacement time (RRT).** Terms indicating the pulse generator has reached a point in its service life where system failure will likely occur within 3 to 6 months. The ERI indicator for a pacemaker varies between models and manufacturers, but is usually indicated by a change in pacing rate, mode, or function. Pacemaker manufacturers generally recommend pulse generator replacement when the ERI is identified. ERI/ERT indicators for various pacemaker models are published in a handbook that should be available in the pacemaker clinic.
9. **External electromagnetic interference (EMI):** Electrical signals from noncardiac or nonphysiologic sources that may affect pacemaker function. Sources of EMI are discussed below.
10. **End of life (EOL):** Term indicating the depletion of battery power for the pulse generator. The end-of-life indicator for a pacemaker varies between models and manufacturers, but it is usually indicated by a decrease in the magnet-related pacing rate to a certain percentage of the beginning-of-life rate. There may also be a change in pacemaker mode (e.g., from DDD to VVI). Telemetry of the cell impedance of the pulse generator also provides information regarding the status of battery power for those pacemakers with such a feature. Pacemaker manufacturers generally recommend urgent pulse generator replacement if EOL of a device is identified. EOL indicators for various pacemaker models are published in a handbook that should be available in the pacemaker clinic.

11. **Fusion:** Results when the pacemaker output occurs at the same time as an intrinsic event, and both contribute to cardiac depolarization. The morphology of the fused beat has characteristics of both the paced and intrinsic events.
12. **Impedance (*Z*):** Total resistance to the flow of current through a conductor. For pacemaker systems, this includes resistance produced by electronic components and body tissues. Temporal changes in pacing impedance usually include a decreasing impedance over the first 1 to 2 weeks following implantation, then increasing impedance to a level that is somewhat higher than the impedance at the time of implantation. Serial measurements of pacing impedance may be useful for assessing lead integrity, as discussed later in this chapter.
13. **Magnet mode:** The response of a pacemaker when a magnetic field of sufficient strength is applied and closes the pulse generator's reed switch. The pulse generator paces at a predetermined rate and mode, which varies among pacemaker models and manufacturers. Generally, the mode is asynchronous pacing. Magnet mode can be used to assess pacemaker function and battery status (see discussion on ERI and EOL later in this chapter).
14. **Noncapture:** The absence of cardiac depolarization following a pacing stimulus.
15. **Ohm's law:** $V = I \times R$ *(voltage = current x resistance)*
16. **Output:** The output of a pacemaker is determined by the voltage and pulse width.
17. **Oversensing:** The sensing of inappropriate cardiac or extracardiac signals and responding to them as if they were appropriate native sensed events. "Oversensing results in underpacing."
18. **Pacemaker-mediated tachycardia (PMT):** Sudden onset of a sustained ventricular paced rhythm at the maximum tracking rate of the pacemaker. PMT is sustained by continued active participation of the pacemaker in the tachycardia circuit. PMT is discussed in more detail below.
19. **Pacing interval (milliseconds):** The interval between two consecutive paced events.
20. **Pseudofusion:** Results when an intrinsic event occurs before the pacemaker output is delivered. When this happens, the pacemaker output does not contribute to cardiac depolarization. The morphology of the pseudofusion beat resembles the intrinsic event.
21. **Pseudo-pseudofusion:** Results when a PVC that resembles the ventricular paced complex follows an atrial output spike.
22. **Pulse width:** The measurement in milliseconds of the pacemaker output spike (also known as pulse duration).
23. **Reed switch:** A switch within the pulse generator that closes when a magnetic field of sufficient strength is applied to it (such as a ring or donut magnet, or a programming head). The pacemaker will convert to magnet mode.
24. **Resistance (*R*):** The opposition to the flow of electrical current through a material, measured in ohms (O).
25. **Sensing:** The ability of a pacemaker to recognize native cardiac signals. Refers to the amplitude of the signal (millivolts) required for the pacemaker to detect the signal. Higher numbers reflect less sensitivity; lower numbers reflect more sensitivity.
26. **Undersensing:** The failure to recognize and respond appropriately to cardiac signals. "Undersensing results in overpacing."
27. **Voltage (*V*):** The difference in potential energy between two points, measured in millivolts.

B. Cardiac pacing: timing cycles and refractory periods

1. A = atrial paced event
2. Absolute refractory period: The period following a sensed or paced event during which the sense amplifier is unresponsive to incoming signals.
3. AEI = atrial escape interval: For atrial single-chamber pacing systems, the period from a sensed atrial event to the next atrial paced event. For

dual-chamber pacing systems, the period initiated by a ventricular sensed or paced event and ending with the next atrial paced event.

4. ARP = atrial refractory period, which is the atrial timing cycle during which the atrial sense amplifier is unresponsive to incoming signals. For single-chamber atrial pacing modes, the atrial refractory period is initiated by an atrial sensed or paced event. For dual-chamber pacing modes, the AV interval and the postventricular atrial refractory period (PVARP) determine the total atrial refractory period (TARP). TARP = AVI + PVARP.
5. AV = atrioventricular sequential pacing
6. AVI = atrioventricular pacing interval (also known as AV delay): In dual-chamber pacing, the period between an atrial sensed or paced event and a ventricular paced event (usually programmable).
7. Blanking period: An interval (usually 12 to 125 milliseconds) initiated by an output pulse during which the sense amplifier is temporarily disabled. In dual-chamber pacing, the blanking period is designed to prevent the inappropriate detection of signals from the other chamber (crosstalk). For example, an atrial sensed or paced event initiates a ventricular blanking period during which the ventricular sense amplifier is temporarily disabled.
8. CDW = crosstalk detection window. In dual-chamber pacing, a timing cycle (usually 51 to 150 milliseconds) immediately following the ventricular blanking period during which a ventricular sensed event is considered to be crosstalk but results in a triggered ventricular output at the end of an abbreviated AV interval (safety pacing).
9. LRL = lower rate limit (also known as base rate or minimum rate): The rate at which the pacemaker paces in the absence of sensed intrinsic events (generally programmable in most pacemakers).
10. MSR = maximal sensor rate: A programmable value in rate-adaptive pacemaker systems that designates the highest pacing rate that can be achieved in response to a sensor input. The MSR may be programmed independently of the MTR.
11. MTR = maximal tracking rate (also known as upper rate limit, URL): A programmable value for dual-chamber pacemaker sensing and tracking modes that designates the highest ventricular pacing rate that can be achieved in response to atrial sensed events with 1:1 AV synchrony at the programmed AV delay.
12. P = native atrial depolarization
13. R = native ventricular depolarization
14. Relative refractory period: A "noise sampling" period following the absolute refractory period during which some incoming signals (generally those signals in the frequency range of interference) are monitored by the sense amplifier. Sensed signals during this period may result in the initiation of a new refractory period but do not reset the timing circuit.
15. RRAVD = rate-responsive atrioventricular delay. A programmable feature of some dual-chamber pacing systems that progressively shortens the PV or AV interval as the sinus or sensor-driven atrial rate increases. This is designed to provide a more physiologic AVI at higher heart rates, and to allow tracking of higher atrial rates (a shorter AVI decreases the TARP), thereby lessening the chance of a fixed-block upper-rate response.
16. V = ventricular paced event
17. VRP = ventricular refractory period. The timing cycle initiated by a ventricular sensed or paced event during which the ventricular sense amplifier is unresponsive to incoming signals. This is not the same as the ventricular blanking period (see information regarding this later in this chapter).

ACKNOWLEDGMENT

The authors thank Drs. Barbara Hesse and Matthew Hook for their contributions to earlier editions of this chapter.

References

1. Birnie D, Williams K, Guo A, et al. Reasons for escalating pacemaker implants. *Am J Cardiol* 2006;98:93–97.
2. Sohail MR, Uslan DZ, Khan AH, et al. Management and outcomes of permanent pacemaker and implantable cardioverter-defibrillator infections. *J Am Coll Cardiol* 2007; 49:1851–1859.
3. Lamas GA, Orar EJ, Stambler BS, et al. Quality of life and clinical outcomes in elderly patients treated with ventricular pacing as compared with dual-chamber pacing, Pacemaker Selection in the Elderly Investigators. *N Engl J Med* 1998;338:1097–1104.
4. Skanes AC, et al. Progression to chronic atrial fibrillation after pacing: the Canadian Trial of Physiologic Pacing. CTOPP Investigators. *J Am Coll Cardiol* 2001;38:167–172.
5. Lamas GA, Lee KL, Sweeney MO, et al. Ventricular pacing or dual-chamber pacing for sinus-node dysfunction Trial (MOST). *N Engl J Med* 2002;346:1854–1862.
6. Healey JS, Toff WD, Lamas GA, et al. Cardiovascular outcomes with atrial-based pacing compared with ventricular pacing: Meta-analysis randomized trials, using individual patient data. *Circulation* 2006;114:11–17.
7. Wilkoff BL, Cook JR, Epstein AE, et al. Dual Chamber and VVI Implantable Defibrillator Trial Investigators: Dual-chamber pacing or ventricular backup in patients with an implantable defibrillator: The Dual Chamber and VVI Implantable Defibrillator (DAVID) Trial. *JAMA* 2002;288:3115–3123.
8. Sweeney MO, Blank AJ, Koullick M, et al. Minimizing ventricular pacing to reduce atrial fibrillation in sinus node disease. *N Engl J Med* 2007;357:1000–1008.

Landmark Articles

Toff WD, Skeehan JD, De Bono DP, et al. The United Kingdom pacing and cardiovascular events (UKPACE) trial. United Kingdom Pacing and Cardiovascular Events. *Heart* 1997;78:221–223.

Wharton J, Sorrentino RA, Campbell P, et al. Effect of pacing modality on atrial tachyarrhythmias recurrence in the tachycardia-bradycardia syndrome. Preliminary results of the Pacemaker Atrial Tachycardia Trial. *Circulation* 1998;98:494.

Key Reviews

Gregoratos G, Abrams J, Epstein AE, et al. ACC/AHA guidelines for implantation of cardiac pacemakers and antiarrhythmia devices: Summary article: A report of the American College of Cardiology/American Heart Association Task Force on Practice Guidelines (ACC/AHA/NASPE Committee to update the 1998 pacemaker guidelines). *Circulation* 2002;106:2145–2161.

Gregoratos G, Cheitlin MD, Conill A, et al. ACC/AHA guidelines for implantation of cardiac pacemakers and antiarrhythmia devices: a report of the American College of Cardiology/American Heart Association Task Force on Practice Guidelines (Committee on Pacemaker Implantation). *J Am Coll Cardiol* 1998;31:1175–1209.

Tang CY, Kerr CR, Connolly SJ. Clinical trials of pacing mode selection. *J Nucl Med* 2000;18:1–23.

Relevant Book Chapters:

Bhargava M, Wilkoff BL. Cardiac pacemakers. In: Topol EJ, ed. *Textbook of cardiovascular medicine*, 3rd ed. Philadelphia: Lippincott Williams and Wilkins Publishers, 2007:1191–1223.

Ellenbogen KA, Kay GN, Wilkoff BL, eds. *Clinical cardiac pacing, defibrillation, and resynchronization therapy*, 3rd ed. Philadelphia: WB Saunders, 2007.

Hayes DL, Zipes DP. Cardiac pacemakers and cardioverter defibrillators. In: Braunwald E, ed. *Heart disease: a textbook of cardiovascular medicine*, 7th ed. Philadelphia: Elsevier Saunders, 2005:767–802.

50 ANTITACHYCARDIA DEVICES

P. Peter Borek and Mandeep Bhargava

I. INTRODUCTION

A. The modern **implantable cardioverter–defibrillator (ICD)** is a multifunctional, multiprogrammable, electronic device designed to abort life-threatening arrhythmias. It is programmed to **automatically detect and manage episodes of ventricular tachycardia (VT), ventricular fibrillation (VF), or bradycardia.** Current ICDs are able to deliver multi-tiered therapies, which may include a combination of **antitachycardia pacing (ATP), cardioversion,** and **defibrillation.** The devices also offer bradycardic support, which may include **rate-responsive single or dual-chamber pacing and**

automatic mode-switch function. The latest addition to the functions noted previously is the capability of these devices to deliver **resynchronization therapy,** which is a significant advancement in the management of heart failure. The devices are also able to **store electrograms (EGMs),** which can be easily retrieved. This function can be of immense use for follow-up management of the patient and programming of the device.

Multiple clinical trials have demonstrated the efficacy of ICDs to accurately detect and manage sudden cardiac death (SCD). The ICDs are superior to conventional therapy with drugs in both **primary and secondary prophylaxis of SCD**. The majority of patients who have indications for an ICD implant are those with left ventricular (LV) dysfunction, both ischemic and nonischemic.

B. Mirowski first introduced the concept of an ICD in the 1960s, but the first human implant was reported in 1980. The early ICD implantations required a **thoracotomy approach** for placement of an epicardial lead system. Subsequent advancements in device and lead technology over the last 20 years have significantly reduced the size of the pulse generator, yet improved the programmability and diagnostic data stored within the device. An improved understanding of VF, defibrillation, and cardiac pacing has resulted in the development of biphasic shock waveforms and transvenous pace/defibrillation lead systems that preclude the need for epicardial patches. As a result, modern ICDs are much smaller devices with expansive programming capability placed by a **transvenous approach.** The newest generation of devices has the added capability of trans-telephonic interrogation.

II. ICD COMPONENTS

A. The current-day ICD is not only an "automatic shock box," but also a sophisticated and intelligent device. It consists of a **generator** and **leads**. The ICD generator consists of a battery, capacitors, DC–DC converter using an oscillator rectifier mechanism, a microprocessor, telemetry communication coils, and their connections. The generator serves as an active electrode within the shocking configuration in most of the modern ICDs and thus is called the **"hot can."** The **battery** used in most of the ICDs is a lithium silver vanadium oxide cell. This can generate approximately 3.2 V at full charge. Because most ICDs use two batteries connected in series, the full initial voltage is approximately 6.4 V. The generator has capacitors that can charge within 7 to 30 seconds to store up to 30 to 40 J of energy. This can be delivered to the heart within 10 to 20 milliseconds when therapy is required.

B. The three essential functions of the ICD—**tachycardia detection, tachycardia therapy, and bradycardia pacing**—are delivered through the active electrodes, which are the noninsulated segments of the leads. Most of the current-day leads have **sensing and pacing electrodes** at the tip and a **distal (right ventricle) and proximal (superior vena cava) shocking coil**. The function of **ventricular sensing and pacing** is achieved by a technology similar to that in pacemakers. This is done through two "dedicated bipolar" electrodes at the distal end of the right ventricular (RV) lead (tip/ring). Sometimes it may be achieved by "integrated bipolar" electrodes, wherein the bipole is formed by the tip of the ventricular lead and the distal shocking coil (tip/coil). Ventricular pacing in **biventricular ICDs** is from the tip of the RV and LV leads, respectively, to either the ring (true bipolar) or the distal shocking coil (integrated bipolar). The sensing could either be from both RV and LV leads but could give rise to false tachycardia detection due to the problem of **"double counting."** It is for this reason that the newer devices restrict the sensing function to the RV lead alone.

C. For the **delivery of shock therapy,** most systems now incorporate a combined RV coil, superior vena cava coil, and active pulse generator can, or sometimes a single RV coil with a hot-can active pulse generator. Modern technology makes it feasible to incorporate all these electrodes and coils in a single lead implantable in a manner similar to a pacemaker,

III. INDICATIONS AND CONTRAINDICATIONS

A. AHA/ACC/ESC Committee for Practice Guidelines 2006 (Guidelines for Management of Patients With Ventricular Arrhythmias and the Prevention of Sudden Cardiac Death). These are the most current guidelines for the implantation of ICDs. The guidelines stratify the various indications as class I, class II (a and b, and class III on the basis of the data from clinical trials and opinion of a panel of experts.

B. Class I indications. These are clinical situations or conditions for which there is evidence and/or general agreement that **ICDs are useful and effective.**

ICD therapy is recommended for secondary prevention of SCD in patients who:

- Survived VF or hemodynamically unstable VT, or
- VT with syncope and have an EF less than 40%

ICD therapy is recommended for primary prevention to reduce total mortality by reducing SCD in patients with New York Heart Association (NYHA) Functional Class II to III who have:

- Ischemic LV dysfunction because of prior myocardial infarction (MI) and are at least more than 40 days post-MI with a left ventricular ejection fraction (LVEF) less than or equal to 30% to 40%.
- Nonischemic dilated cardiomyopathy (DCM) with an LVEF less than or equal to 30% to 35%.

ICD therapy is also indicated in patients with:

- LV dysfunction due to prior MI who present with hemodynamically unstable sustained VT.
- Nonischemic DCM and significant LV dysfunction who have sustained VT.
- Congenital heart disease who are survivors of cardiac arrest when reversible causes have been excluded.
- Hypertrophic cardiomyopathy (HCM) who have sustained VT and/or VF.
- Brugada syndrome with previous cardiac arrest.
- Arrhythmogenic right ventricular dysplasia (ARVD) with documented sustained VT or VF.
- Long QT syndrome with previous cardiac arrest who are also being treated with a β-blocker.

C. Class II indications. These are conditions for which there is **conflicting evidence** about the usefulness of ICD therapy.

Class IIa (Weight of evidence/opinion is in favor of usefulness/efficacy):

Implantation of an ICD is reasonable in the following situations:

- Patients with LV dysfunction due to prior MI who are at least 40 days post-MI, have an LVEF less than or equal to 30% to 35%, and are NYHA Functional Class I.
- Treatment of recurrent sustained VT in patients post-MI with normal or near normal ventricular function.
- Unexplained syncope, significant LV dysfunction, and nonischemic DCM.
- Severe life-threatening ventricular arrhythmias who are not in the acute phase of myocarditis.

Implantation of an ICD for primary prevention is reasonable for patients in the following clinical situations:

- Brugada syndrome with documented VT not resulting in cardiac arrest who have a reasonable expectation of survival with good functional status for more than 1 year.
- Hypertrophic cardiomyopathy with at least one major risk factor for SCD.
- Arrhythmogenic right ventricular cardiomyopathy, including those with LV involvement, history of syncope, or other affected family members.
- Congenital heart disease with unexplained syncope with no definable causes and evidence of LV dysfunction.

Combined ICD therapy and cardiac resynchronization therapy (CRT) can be effective for primary prevention to decrease total mortality by reducing SCD in patients with NYHA Functional Class III or IV HF and who are receiving optimal medical therapy in sinus rhythm with QRS greater than or equal to 120 milliseconds.

Class IIb (Usefulness/efficacy is less well established by evidence/opinion):

ICD therapy may be considered for primary prevention to decrease total mortality by reducing SCD in patients with nonischemic heart disease who have an LVEF less than or equal to 30% to 35% and who are NYHA Functional Class I.

D. Class III indications/contraindications. These are conditions for which there is a general agreement that **ICDs are not useful** and possibly harmful. These include patients with *syncope without any inducible ventricular arrhythmias*, more so in the presence of a normal heart. ICDs should also be avoided in patients with VT and a ***treatable/ablatable** cause* (Wolff-Parkinson-White syndrome, outflow tract VTs, fascicular VTs, and so on) or a ***reversible cause*** (acute MI, myocardial ischemia, electrolyte imbalance, drug toxicity, hypoxia, or sepsis). It is also important to avoid using ICDs in patients with severe ***psychiatric** illnesses* or in patients with ***terminal illnesses***, where the expected life span is less than 12 months. ICDs could do more harm than good in patients with *incessant ventricular arrhythmias* where it is important to control the arrhythmia before ICD implantation to avoid recurrent painful shocks.

IV. IMPLANTATION

A. Device implantation. Currently, available devices are small enough to allow implantation almost exclusively in the **left pectoral region**. Animal studies have shown that the defibrillation efficacy of the hot-can ICDs is superior in the left pectoral or axillary regions followed by the right pectoral and then the abdominal sites. A **right pectoral** system may be necessary in patients who have vascular access problems on the left side or who have undergone pectoral surgery (e.g., mastectomy). For patients with high defibrillation thresholds, additional lead placement, such as a **subcutaneous array/coil** or an epicardial patch, may be necessary. **Epicardial patch** placement is usually reserved for patients who have failed to meet implantation criteria with a transvenous lead system or if there has been previous bilateral pectoral or tricuspid valve replacement surgery.

For pectoral implants, a single 2- to 3-inch incision is made transversely below the clavicle, about 1 cm below and parallel to the deltopectoral groove. Transvenous lead placement is achieved through a subclavian vein puncture or, rarely, by cephalic vein cutdown. An "extrathoracic" subclavian vein puncture or cephalic vein cutdown for access minimizes the risk of pneumothorax and also that for lead failure due to subclavian crush injury.

B. Lead placement. The lead is advanced to the RV apex under fluoroscopic guidance where the tip is secured via an **active fixation screw** or embedded in the trabeculae with **passive fixation tines.** It is important to assess the quality of signals at the time of implant, as it is the best guide to the adequacy of long-term sensing of the lead. The defibrillation threshold is optimized with the lead placed at the RV apex; therefore, this position is often preferred even if there is compromise of the sensing thresholds. If there is already a pacemaker lead in the RV apex, then septal placement of the lead tip is chosen so that the lead tips are at maximal distance from each other to avoid device–device interactions. On certain occasions, placing an additional pacing-sensing lead in the right ventricle may be necessary when the defibrillation efficacy and pace-sense function of the leads are optimized at different locations.

C. Threshold studies. The lead is tested for **pace-sense thresholds** using an external high-voltage system analyzer or pacing system analyzer (PSA). In general, an acute pacing threshold of 2 V or less, R-wave amplitude of 5 mV or more, and lead impedance within the accepted range of the manufacturer (typically 300 to 1,200 O) are necessary to meet implant criteria. The lead is secured within the pocket with a suture sleeve tie-down. If the device uses an atrial and/or an LV lead, then these are implanted at this time. The leads are attached to the pulse generator and the system is placed either in a **submuscular or subcutaneous pocket.** The pulse generator should be placed with the logo "up" toward the skin and excess lead coiled posteriorly to maximize the ability to communicate with an external programming wand. The device is then interrogated to assure appropriate communication. Pace-sense thresholds are again tested by telemetry to demonstrate consistency. Capture of a real-time EGM may identify signal noise in the shock-sensing leads.

D. Defibrillation testing is best assessed by evaluating the defibrillation threshold (DFT), which is defined as the lowest delivered shock strength required for successful defibrillation. Most manufacturers recommend a synchronized sinus test shock to assess the integrity of the device/lead system prior to induction of VF. This is achieved by delivery of a low-energy (less than 2 J) synchronized shock delivered on the QRS complex. This low-energy test allows assessment of sensing as well as shock impedance (typically 35 to 90 Ohm). Following this test, VF is induced with ultrafast burst pacing (30-millisecond intervals), shock on T wave, or application of alternating current (AC). Appropriate ICD detection and effective therapy are verified. Typically, a step-down protocol is incorporated to determine the defibrillation threshold. Two successful therapies that are at least 10 J less than the maximal output of the device are required to meet implant criteria. In general, this approach identifies the level of energy (typically 5 to 15 J) required to achieve a 50% to 75% success rate of defibrillation. Defibrillation therapy is then programmed at a level at least 10 J over the defibrillation threshold. Rarely, a patient may require the addition of a shocking coil in the superior vena cava, subcutaneous patch, or subcutaneous array to achieve an adequate safety margin.

E. Risks and complications. The risks involved with implantation are similar to those of pacemaker insertion. **Operative risks** include bleeding, pneumothorax, hemothorax, infection, myocardial damage, vascular/cardiac perforation, tamponade, thromboemboli, deep venous thrombosis, acceleration of arrhythmias, air embolism, and death. **A rare but dangerous complication** is the occurrence of electromechanical dissociation or refractory VF during defibrillation threshold testing. Due to the nature of the procedure, a separate standby external pacemaker-defibrillator should be immediately available for rescue therapy, should the implanted device fail to appropriately treat an arrhythmia. The overall mortality rate is much less than 1%. **Late complications** include chronic nerve damage, erosion, extrusion, fluid accumulation, infection, formation of hematomas/cysts, keloids, lead migration, lead dislodgment, and venous occlusion.

V. DEVICE REPLACEMENT

A. Battery status is determined by the measured voltage, information retrieved with device interrogation. Generator replacement is generally recommended when the device reaches a battery voltage of around 2.6 V, termed **elective replacement indicator (ERI).** In such situations the generator should be replaced within a few months. With continued depletion of the battery voltage, the generator reaches **end of life (EOL),** a situation that indicates a more urgent need for generator replacement as the battery voltage drops below 2.2 V. This may lead to longer charge times and incomplete or inappropriate function of the device.

B. Pulse generator replacement represents a vulnerable period for the ICD/lead system. A fourfold increased risk of infection has been reported with ICD pulse generator replacement. In the past, manufacturers have had multiple-lead models of variable pin lengths and diameters. Beginning in 1991 they adopted the *3.2-mm international pace-sense standard (IS-1) and 3.2-mm defibrillation standard (DF-1).* Prior to an attempted device replacement, **assessment of the lead model** should be done to verify that the appropriate replacement header or adapters are available at the time of surgery.

C. Leads may be inadvertently damaged during exploration of the pocket or during the exchange of pulse generators. **Intraoperative assessment of lead function** is imperative prior to introducing the replacement generator to the operative field. Replacement of a pace-sense or defibrillation lead may be necessary and require the use of a different device header.

VI. TACHYCARDIA DETECTION AND THERAPY

A. Electrogram and tachycardia sensing. The ICD senses the intracardiac EGM signal via the implanted ventricular sensing electrodes. Recognition of a ventricular arrhythmia mainly depends on the analysis of the R-R intervals (heart rate is determined similarly). Accuracy of the EGMs depends on the **health of the adjacent myocardium and contact with the same.** Accuracy also depends on **far-field signals from the muscles, atrium, or other sources of electromagnetic interference.** The sensed signals are passed through a band pass filter that consists of high- and low-frequency cutoffs to represent true signal events. The accuracy of the signals in the newer devices has been further improved by analysis of the **signal frequency,**

slew rate, amplitude, EGM width, autogain, and autothreshold. These variables are important in helping the device to differentiate VT and VF from other events like atrial fibrillation, sinus tachycardia, and other supraventricular tachycardias, thus reducing the incidence of spurious shocks.

Each EGM event and R-R interval is marked and detected, and there are various algorithms that attempt to identify the events as either normal or various abnormal events. The "abnormal" includes bradycardia that requires pacing, VT requiring antitachycardia pacing or low-energy synchronized shocks, or VF requiring defibrillation. Most of the algorithms depend on the **ventricular rate** criterion. Other variables, such as the **suddenness of onset, variation in cycle length, and change in EGM morphology** help to increase the specificity for diagnosis but at some cost of reduced sensitivity. These need to be adjusted and programmed based on the individual requirement and clinical scenario for every patient.

B. **Event detection** occurs if the device reaches a specified number of intervals programmed by the physician to detect VT or VF, at which point the ICD delivers the prescribed therapy. Most of the devices reconfirm the ongoing episode to avoid therapy for nonsustained events. After delivery of therapy, the device either confirms termination of the episode, or meets criteria for redetection and the next programmed therapy is delivered. The ICD automatically adjusts its sensitivity thresholds following sensed and paced events through an **autogain** mechanism. This allows the device to automatically adjust its sensitivity during a tachycardia episode in response to the changing amplitude of the ventricular signal.

C. **Atrioventricular (AV) sequential devices** incorporate programmable dual-chamber supraventricular criteria to exclude management of supraventricular tachyarrhythmias from inappropriate detection of VT or to identify concurrent VT and supraventricular tachycardia. **Biventricular devices** could pose problems of double counting and unnecessary therapies in patients with the older biventricular devices, where the sensed input is from both the RV and LV leads. Use of newer devices that have sensing inputs from only the RV leads should limit this problem. An additional feature of these devices is the capability to individually program the pacing output and timing of the RV and LV leads through separate ports.

D. **Tachycardia therapy.** Most devices allow for programming of several tachycardia zones. The VT zone is programmed with a lower detection cutoff that would include any clinical VT events. Ideally, the cutoff rate for detection of tachycardia should be above the patient's maximal heart rate to avoid therapy for sinus tachycardia. **Antitachycardia pacing (ATP)** schemes include burst pacing, ramp pacing, and interburst decrement. **Burst pacing** sequences deliver a set of ventricular pulses at a fixed rate faster than that of the VT in an attempt to terminate the re-entry VT by overdriving the circuit. **Ramp pacing** consists of a set of ventricular pulses in which each subsequent paced interval is incrementally shorter than the preceding one. Although this is a more aggressive protocol, there is also a higher chance for the VT degenerating into VF with this therapy. Overall, some studies have shown about 90% success in termination of VT with antitachycardia pacing.

Following a failed ATP attempt, **interburst decrement** allows a more aggressive shortening of the intervals during either a burst or a ramp attempt. The first pulse of a burst or ramp sequence (S_1) is delivered at a calculated percentage of the tachycardia cycle length. The S_1 percentage cycle lengths, number of pulses, interburst decrement, and number of ATP attempts are all programmable features. In addition, **cardioversion therapy (1 to 36 J)** can be programmed in a VT zone. All VT zones have a programmable time limit on episode duration at which point the device defaults to the next zone. Also, if a tachycardia is accelerated to a faster arrhythmia, then the ICD will deliver the therapy appropriate for the rate of the accelerated tachycardia.

E. **Defibrillation therapy.** Successful ICD management of VF can only occur with defibrillation therapy. All devices are programmed with a VF zone due to the risk of acceleration with ATP or cardioversion. Because of the hemodynamic instability seen with fast VT or VF, most devices are typically programmed to manage any sustained episode with rates higher than 180 to 200 beats/minute with defibrillation therapy. The device should be programmed with at least a **10-J safety margin** over the defibrillation threshold observed either at implant or during follow-up testing. Up to six additional shocks may be programmed with maximal outputs programmed at the second or third shock and onward.

VII. BRADYCARDIA DETECTION AND THERAPY

A. All currently available ICDs provide basic VVI pacing with separate programmable post-shock lower rate limit and output. Some dual-chamber devices have been introduced with an atrial lead for diagnostic use only or for AV-synchronized pacing. These devices allow multiple programmable pacing modes including **single- and dual-chamber, fixed-rate, or rate-responsive pacing with automatic mode switch.** These expanded pacing modes have obviated the need for a separate dual-chamber pacemaker that is sometimes necessary in the chronically ill patients who typically receive ICDs. In addition, they may reduce the inappropriate shocks attributed to supraventricular tachycardia. Such devices may also have capabilities to detect and treat atrial arrhythmias in a manner similar to that for the ventricular arrhythmias. However, in patients without any pacing indications, it may actually be detrimental to pace the right ventricle, especially in patients with preexisting LV dysfunction. This has been well demonstrated in the **Dual Chamber and VVI Implantable Defibrillator (DAVID) trial**. Such patients should either be given a single-chamber ICD, or if there are indications for a dual-chamber ICD for tachycardia discrimination or atrial arrhythmias, then they should be programmed for **backup pacing in the VVI mode.**

B. In AV-synchronized devices, the ICD can continue to sense tachyarrhythmias in both chambers regardless of the programmed bradycardic pacing mode. To maintain proper sensing, both atrial and ventricular sensing thresholds are adjusted with auto-gain. The ICD has multiple blanking periods to avoid post-pacing polarization, T-wave oversensing, and cross-talk between chambers. To avoid undersensing of tachyarrhythmias, short cross-chamber blanking periods after paced events and no cross-chamber blanking after sensed events are necessary. The AV synchronous devices have programmable refractory periods available for bradycardia functions, but these refractory periods do not affect tachyarrhythmia detection.

VIII. MAGNET FUNCTION

A. Confusion abounds concerning the function of a magnet with ICDs. The pulse generator contains a reed switch that is closed when a magnet is placed over the device. Closure of the reed switch prevents delivery of tachyarrhythmia therapy. Unlike pacemakers, **bradycardia pacing is not affected by the use of a magnet in ICDs.** Normal device therapy resumes when the magnet is removed and the reed switch opens.

B. One manufacturer, Cardiac Pacemakers, Inc./Guidant (St. Paul, MN), has developed two expanded functions during magnet application. In addition to the inhibition of tachyarrhythmia therapy, magnet application can be used to determine the tachycardia mode of the ICD. If a continuous tone is heard, then the tachycardia mode is programmed "off" (off, storage-only, or monitor-only modes). Alternatively, if a series of intermittent tones (synchronized to the R wave) are heard, then the tachycardia mode is programmed "on" and the device will deliver therapy once the magnet is removed and detection is met. A second additional magnet feature is the change of tachycardia mode with magnet. If this feature is programmed "on," the application of a magnet for more than 30 seconds will change the tachycardia mode. If the device is programmed "off" or "monitor-only" (continuous tone), then the device will be programmed "on" (intermittent tone). If the ICD is programmed "on" (intermittent tone), application of a magnet for more than 30 seconds will program the device "off" (continuous tone). If the device is programmed to storage mode, then application of a magnet has no effect on tachycardia mode and a continuous tone will be heard.

IX. DEVICE–DEVICE INTERACTION

A. Device–device interaction remains a significant issue when multiple-lead systems or devices are used. When a new lead is placed, the lead should be positioned as far from the other leads as possible (at least 2 cm). A dedicated bipolar sensing lead is preferred to minimize the potential of far-field oversensing of the alternate pacing lead.

B. During the implantation procedure, **the devices should be tested for device–device interaction.** To simulate a worst-case scenario, the pacemaker is programmed in a unipolar configuration at high output. The real-time ICD EGM and marker channels are observed for oversensing of the pacemaker output resulting in double counting of the paced QRS complex. This may lead to an inappropriate ICD discharge. Defibrillation testing is performed with the pacemaker programmed to DOO/VOO at high output to verify appropriate VF detection and therapy. Pacing stimuli may lead to ICD undersensing of VT/VF with interpretation of the pacing artifact as "sinus rhythm" and failure to recognize the underlying arrhythmia. In addition, the ICD may affect the pacemaker by resetting the pacemaker pulse generator with a high-voltage shock. The pacemaker is programmed with the sensor "on" during an ICD high-output defibrillation test. The pacemaker is subsequently interrogated to verify appropriate communication and programmed mode. Whenever multiple devices are present and inappropriate ICD discharges are suspected, electrophysiology lab testing for device–device interaction is warranted. Device–device interaction should also be considered when a patient presents with resetting of the programmed mode, output configuration, or failure of communication with the device.

X. MANAGING AND FOLLOWING PATIENTS

A. In the United States, **the government mandates patient registration and tracking.** Once registered, a patient receives a permanent **identification card** to carry at all times. A **Medic Alert** is strongly encouraged. Manufacturer guidelines suggest that patients should **follow up every 1 to 4 months** depending on clinical status. Even if trans-telephonic follow-up is available, it should be supplemented by clinic visits at least on a four-times-monthly basis. Patients should be informed that they are likely to receive therapies. At the follow-up visit, a history of symptoms that might suggest tachyarrhythmias should be obtained. The diagnostic and episode data should be reviewed. Current devices also include stored-episode EGMs to allow review of aborted shocks as well as delivered therapies. Device pacing and sensing thresholds should be obtained. There are no specific guidelines for follow-up testing of ICD defibrillation function. In general, patients experiencing device activation should be evaluated shortly after the event to assess for safe and appropriate device function. When device function or concomitant antiarrhythmic therapy is modified, an evaluation of the sensing, pacing, and defibrillation thresholds is often necessary. Practice patterns vary widely regarding empirical device programming and electrophysiologic testing of modified ICD programming. Some sources recommend that operating a motor vehicle should be avoided for 6 months following a symptomatic arrhythmic event.

B. In general, **ICD pulse generators have 3- to 6-year longevity depending on usage.** The programmer allows evaluation of battery status. As the device approaches the elective replacement interval, follow-up visits should be intensified. In general, **once the device reaches the elective replacement interval, it operates normally for at least 3 months** depending on frequency of therapy. Capacitor deformation occurs during periods when no shocks are delivered and results in longer charge times as well as decreased battery longevity. Current ICDs perform an automatic capacitor reformation that charges the capacitors and delivers the energy to an internal test load. This function improves subsequent charge times and battery longevity. Capacitor reformations should be conducted manually every 3 to 6 months if not conducted automatically.

C. Typically, 40% of patients receive a therapy within the first year after implantation and 10% per year thereafter. **If multiple ICD discharges are experienced, medical attention should be sought emergently.** Failure to discriminate between ventricular and supraventricular rhythms is the most common reason for inappropriate shocks. It is important to evaluate the patients for appropriateness of therapy. The most common cause of **inappropriate shocks** is atrial fibrillation with a fast ventricular rate. Shocks delivered during physical exertion noted to have gradually increasing heart rates and gradually decreasing V-V intervals suggests sinus tachycardia. Therapy is likely to be inappropriate in this setting also. Ideally, the cutoff rate for detection of tachyarrhythmias should be greater than the patient's maximal heart rate. In many cases, the VT rate falls within the patient's achievable sinus rate. Programmable enhancements, such as sudden onset and sustained high rate, can allow sinus tachycardia overlap into the VT zone without delivery of an inappropriate shock. Additional enhancements such as morphology discrimination of the ventricular EGM as well as the introduction of dual-chamber devices with timing intervals, marker channels, and mode-switching capabilities are likely to improve the specificity of device therapy.

D. In the event of multiple ICD discharges, a **magnet can be used to inhibit ICD therapy** so that the underlying rhythm can be appropriately assessed and managed. The device should be interrogated as soon as possible to assess ICD function and facilitate diagnosis. If a supraventricular tachycardia is present, then it should be managed as medically appropriate. For patient comfort, the magnet should be left in place to inhibit ICD therapy until the device can be reprogrammed or the supraventricular tachycardia is terminated. If VF is present, the device is assumed inoperable and cardiopulmonary resuscitation with external defibrillation should be applied.

E. Patients receiving ICDs may suffer from significant psychological and emotional disturbances. **Education and psychological support** are beneficial in improving these patients' quality of life.

XI. ELECTROMAGNETIC INTERFERENCE. Patients should be counseled to **avoid sources of electromagnetic interference** because such interference may cause the pulse generator to become inhibited and either fail to deliver appropriate therapy or deliver inappropriate therapy. Potential sources of electromagnetic interference include **industrial transformers, radiofrequency transmitters such as radar, therapeutic diathermy equipment, arc welding equipment, toy radio transmitters, antitheft devices, and magnetic security wands.** The safe use of medical technologies such as electrosurgery, lithotripsy, external defibrillation, and ionizing irradiation can be accomplished by **deactivating the device before the event.** Shielding of the device is also appropriate when possible. The device should be evaluated for appropriate operation following exposure. **Magnetic resonance imaging (MRI) is contraindicated.** Reports of interference created by cellular phones may be related to either a magnetic field from within the phone or the radiofrequency signal generated by the phone. It is suggested that if an ICD patient wishes to use a cellular phone, it should be held to the ear opposite the device and carried at least 6 to 12 inches from the pulse generator; in addition, the phone should not be carried in a pocket close to the device.

XII. FUTURE. ICD implantation rates have risen tremendously over the last two decades and are expected to rise further with evolving therapies and indications. Multiple clinical studies have demonstrated the role of ICDs in the primary and secondary prevention of SCD. Recent trials have also demonstrated the role of an ICD in combination with cardiac resynchronization therapy (CRT) in reducing mortality and hospital admissions in patients with heart failure. Improvements in electronic technology will continue to expand programming capabilities of these devices while reducing their size. ICD lead technology is also expected to improve, thereby decreasing the number of lead-related complications.

Internal atrial defibrillation therapies for atrial fibrillation as well as other supraventricular arrhythmias are currently available and are undergoing clinical studies. Because atrial defibrillation is painful, programming of the device to a manual, patient-triggered mode may be used. The overall efficacy in terminating atrial fibrillation is about 76% to 90%, with no increased risk of ventricular arrhythmia. Atrial ICDs are also capable of detecting atrial tachyarrhythmias, known precursors of atrial fibrillation, and terminating them via painless rapid atrial pacing.

Due to increasing complexities associated with ICD therapy and recent reports of various device malfunctions, there is ongoing need for surveillance of device performance.

Suggested Readings

ACC/AHA/NASPE 2002 Guideline Update for Implantation of Cardiac Pacemakers and Antiarrhythmia Devices. Summary article. A Report of the American College of Cardiology/American Heart Association Task Force on Practice Guidelines (ACC/AHA/NASPE Committee to Update the 1998 Pacemaker Guidelines). *Circulation* 2002;106:2145–2161.

ACC/AHA/ESC 2006 Guidelines for Management of Patients with Ventricular Arrhythmias and the Prevention of Sudden Cardiac Death. A report of the American College of Cardiology/American Heart Association and the European Society of Cardiology Committee for Practice Guidelines (Writing committee to Develop Guidelines for Management of Patients with Ventricular Arrhythmias and the Prevention of Sudden Cardiac Death). *J Am Coll Cardiol*, 2006;47;

Connolly SJ, Gent M, Roberts RS, et al., for the CIDS Investigators. Canadian Implantable Defibrillator Study: a randomized trial of the implantable cardioverter defibrillator against amiodarone. *Circulation* 2000;101:1297–1302.

Goldberger Z, Lampert R. Implantable cardioverter-defibrillators. Expanding indications and technologies. *JAMA* 2006;295:809–818.

Moss AJ, Zareba W, Hall WJ, et al. Prophylactic implantation of a defibrillator in patients with myocardial infarction and reduced ejection fraction. *N Engl J Med* 2002;346:877–883.

The DAVID Investigators. Dual-chamber pacing or ventricular backup pacing in patients with an implantable defibrillator. *JAMA* 2002;288:3115–3123.

Landmark Articles

Antiarrhythmics Versus Implantable Defibrillators (AVID) Investigators. A comparison of antiarrhythmic drug therapy with implantable defibrillators in patients resuscitated from near-fatal ventricular arrhythmias. *N Engl J Med* 1997;337:1576–1583.

Bigger JT Jr. Prophylactic use of implanted cardiac defibrillators in patients at high risk for ventricular arrhythmias after coronary-artery bypass graft surgery. *N Engl J Med* 1997;337:1569–1575.

Buxton AE, Lee KL, Fisher JD, et al. A randomized study of the prevention of sudden death in patients with coronary artery disease: Multicenter Unsustained Tachycardia Trial Investigators. *N Engl J Med* 1999;341:1882–1890.

Lown B, Axelrod P. Implanted standby defibrillators. *Circulation* 1972;46:637–639.

Mirowski M, Reid PR, Mower MM, et al. Termination of ventricular arrhythmias with an implanted automatic defibrillator in human beings. *N Engl J Med* 1980;303:322–324.

Moss AJ, Hall WJ, Cannom DS, et al. Improved survival with an implanted defibrillator in patients with coronary disease at high risk for ventricular arrhythmias. *N Engl J Med* 1996;335:1933–1940.

Pinski SL, Trohman RG. Implantable cardioverter-defibrillators: implications for the non-electrophysiologist. *Ann Intern Med* 1995;122:770–777.

Key Reviews and Book Chapters

Niebauer MJ, Wilkoff BL. Implantable cardioverter-defibrillators: technical aspects. In: Zipes DP, Jalife J, eds. *Cardiac electrophysiology: from cell to bedside*. Philadelphia: WB Saunders, 2000:949–957.

Pinski SL, Chen PS. Implantable cardioverter-defibrillators. In: Topol EJ, ed. *Textbook of cardiovascular medicine*. Philadelphia: Lippincott–Raven Publishers, 1998:1913–1931.

Pinski SL, Simmons TW, Maloney JD. Troubleshooting antitachycardia pacing in patients with defibrillators. In: Estes NAM, Wang P, Manolis A, eds. *Implantable cardioverter-defibrillators: a comprehensive textbook*. New York: Marcel Dekker, 1994:445–477.

51 CARDIAC RESYNCHRONIZATION THERAPY

P. Peter Borek

I. INTRODUCTION. The prevalence of heart failure (HF) in the United States has increased considerably in the past two decades as a result of the aging population and better medical management of left ventricular dysfunction (LVD). Unfortunately, medical therapy is not completely effective in preventing or reversing progression of HF and, as a result, patients with advanced HF have limited options. A subset of patients with systolic LVD who have associated ventricular conduction delay are at highest risk for HF progression and poor overall outcome. Since the late 1970s, various investigators have shown that left bundle branch block (LBBB), right ventricular (RV) pacing, or intraventricular conduction delay (IVCD) is associated with a less favorable hemodynamic profile in those with LVD and even in normal subjects. The mechanism for this phenomenon is thought to be due to asynchronous and inefficient contraction of opposing areas of the ventricular myocardium. More importantly, *restoring synchronization, either via simultaneous pacing of the RV apex and the left ventricular (LV) free wall or with timed LV free wall activation, can lead to a significant hemodynamic improvement.* In 1994, two investigators in Europe applied cardiac resynchronization therapy (CRT) in the clinical setting for the first time. Subsequent small observational studies suggested benefit from synchronous pacing. Larger randomized clinical trials confirmed those findings. CRT was approved for maximally medically managed patients with persistent New York Heart Association (NYHA) class III or IV HF symptoms due to severe LVD associated with prolonged QRS duration. Further randomized studies, powered for mortality, showed a significant survival benefit with CRT or combination of CRT with a defibrillator (CRT-D). Unfortunately, not all patients who are selected for CRT based on current guidelines respond. Furthermore, some patients who would not be selected for CRT based on the current guidelines may actually benefit from the therapy. One of the major current challenges in this field is the optimal definition of the appropriate and cost-effective use of this expensive technology.

II. MECHANISM OF LV DYSSYNCHRONY. The normal pattern of electrical activation of the ventricular myocardium, once the impulse passes through the atrioventricular (AV) node, starts in the His bundle, followed by simultaneous activation of the right and left bundles of the Purkinje system, and it finally proceeds into the myocardium. The Purkinje system is electrically isolated from the rest of the myocardium until it reaches its exit points at the Purkinje-myocardial junctions. As a result, typical LV myocardial activation occurs from apex to base, simultaneously in the septum and in the LV free wall, and is described as synchronous. Due to tight electromechanical coupling of the myocardium, synchronous ventricular activation is followed by synchronous ventricular contraction.

In the *setting of LBBB, IVCD, or RV pacing, the activation of the LV is not synchronous.* This results from slower conduction of the electrical impulse through the myocardium as compared to the Purkinje system. As a consequence, the activation of the entire LV myocardium takes almost twice as long, with the **posterolateral segments being activated latest.** This dyssynchronous activation pattern leads to increased arrhythmia susceptibility. LV chamber hypertrophy, dilation, and reduced efficiency in the face of reduced coronary reserve lead to increased ischemia susceptibility, creating a vicious cycle that perpetuates this process into more advanced HF. As a result, when comparing patients with similar degrees of LV dysfunction, those with LBBB, IVCD, or RV pacing have a worse overall prognosis. CRT has been shown to reverse this deleterious process. Synchronized pacing has been shown to improve LV function without increasing oxygen demand, suggesting that the improvement is related to better efficiency of the LV chamber.

Interestingly, dyssynchronous activation and contraction have an undesirable effect in patients *without* LV systolic dysfunction as well. When compared to normal controls, patients with LBBB have a lower EF, are more likely to develop HF, and have a tenfold greater cardiovascular morbidity and mortality risk.

III. OTHER TYPES OF DYSSYNCHRONY IN LVD. LV dyssynchrony is often accompanied by AV and interventricular dyssynchrony.

A. AV dyssynchrony. In the setting of PR or QRS prolongation, the atrial contribution to LV filling is abnormal. Atrial systole occurs too early with respect to ventricular diastole, leading to early truncation of passive LV filling. Early atrial systole also causes early rise in diastolic ventricular pressure, leading to diastolic mitral regurgitation (MR). Compromised LV filling and MR cause lower cardiac output. AV synchronization can improve cardiac output in HF by as much as 20%.

B. Interventricular dyssynchrony. Early RV activation present during LBBB, IVCD, or RV pacing leads to early RV contraction, which negatively affects late LV filling. This translates to a decrease in LV preload and a subsequent decrease in cardiac

TABLE 51.1 Commonly used Echocardiographic Measurements of Dyssynchrony

Method	Measurement	Value
M-mode	Septal to posterior wall delay	>130 ms
Pulsed tissue Doppler	Opposing wall delay onset velocity	>60 ms
Color tissue Doppler	Opposing wall delay peak velocity	>65 ms
Color tissue Doppler	12-segment standard deviation	>34 ms
Tissue Doppler radial strain	Septal to posterior wall delay	>130 ms
Tissue speckle tracking radial strain	Septal to posterior wall delay	>130 ms
3D echocardiography	12-segment standard deviation	>36 ms

output. Up to this point, however, interventricular resynchronization has not been shown to be of significant benefit clinically.

IV. ASSESSMENT OF DYSSYNCHRONY (see Table 51.1). **Early clinical trials used prolonged QRS duration (greater than 120 milliseconds) as a surrogate for mechanical dyssynchrony.** This criterion has the advantage of simplicity, but it is not very accurate in defining the presence of dyssynchrony clinically. Studies have revealed that **up to 30% of patients with prolonged QRS do not have mechanical dyssynchrony** as assessed by magnetic resonance imaging (MRI) or echocardiography, which may partly explain why in clinical trials, there is a substantial rate of non-response to CRT. Furthermore, **up to 30% of patients with normal QRS and symptomatic HF have evidence of mechanical dyssynchrony** on echo or MRI and could potentially benefit from resynchronization therapy. Ongoing research is focused on identifying strategies that may best detect mechanical dyssynchrony.

A. Echocardiographic assessment of dyssynchrony. The assessment of cardiac mechanical dyssynchrony was initially assessed with M-Mode and pulsed-wave Doppler. Subsequently, tissue Doppler imaging and tissue synchronization imaging have been used. Three-dimensional echocardiography and speckle tracking technology are currently under investigation.

1. **Pulsed-wave Doppler** has been used to assess interventricular dyssynchrony by measuring the time delay between initiation of RV and LV ejection, known as presystolic ejection period (PSEP). Values greater than 40 milliseconds are considered to be abnormal; however, the clinical utility of this measure remains to be proven.
2. **Septal to posterior wall-motion delay (SPWMD)** as assessed by **M mode** in the parasternal long or short axis view has been used to detect intraventricular dyssynchrony. A value greater than 130 milliseconds has been associated with a greater response to CRT in terms of symptomatic improvement, LV remodeling, and EF increase. Unfortunately, this parameter has significant limitations. It evaluates dyssynchrony in only two segments of the myocardium: the septum and the posterior wall. It is also difficult to obtain in up to 40% of patients due to poor acoustic windows, or is less reliable due to akinesis of the septum or RV pressure overload.
3. **Tissue Doppler imaging (TDI).** This technique uses pulsed-wave Doppler to record myocardial velocities at the basal septum and the basal lateral wall as close as possible to the mitral valve annulus in the four-chamber view. Time from the onset of the QRS to the onset of systolic velocity or to the peak of systolic velocity is measured. So too is the difference in these measurements between the septum and the lateral wall. Values greater than 62 milliseconds for time to systolic velocity initiation and 65 milliseconds for time to peak systolic velocity are abnormal and have predicted a favorable clinical and echocardiographic response to CRT. TDI has excellent temporal resolution and does not require endocardial border identification for determining the degree of delay. The limitations of TDI are: (1) occasional difficulty in identifying the true peak of systolic velocity, and (2) because segments are not assessed simultaneously,

heart rate variability and respiration can lead to false comparisons. To better deal with those two limitations, computer software has been developed that allows post-processing of Doppler data so that all of these measurements are determined from one image. Additional views (apical three-chamber and apical two-chamber) may be used to increase the number of myocardial segments assessed. This technique improves both specificity and sensitivity in the identification of mechanical dyssynchrony, as compared to older, less sophisticated methods.

Another major problem with current methods of TDI is that they assess systolic motion only in the longitudinal plane of the heart and therefore may be prone to artifact from tethering and pulling. The heart contracts in three different planes: longitudinal, radial, and rotational. The latter two are not assessed by conventional TDI but have a greater contribution to ventricular contraction than the longitudinal plane.

4. **Tissue synchronization imaging (TSI)** allows for color guidance that provides the operator with visualization of the mechanical activation pattern of the LV before choosing the sampling regions in the various views during post-processing. Initially, post-processing was done after completion of the study. However, currently, with the aid of improved computer software, the operator can perform the measurements shortly after the frames are obtained at the bedside. These dyssynchrony echo studies take longer than standard echocardiograms and require considerable additional training to perform them well.

B. New echocardiographic indices of dyssynchrony. Some of the newer echocardiographic techniques that are on the horizon focus on eliminating the shortcomings of longitudinal TDI, namely the tethering and pulling artifact and lack of radial and rotational strain assessment.

1. **Strain imaging** performed in the four-chamber and parasternal short axis views incorporates velocity sampling in two nearby points. The sampled velocity difference divided by the separation distance is proportional to strain rate, which when integrated over time can provide the strain value. Strain, unlike velocity, does not depend on tethering or pulling of the myocardium. This is a time-consuming effort that requires extensive off-line post-processing.
2. **Speckle tracking may also be used** to assess for LV strain. Speckles are hyperechoic areas of the myocardium that can be individually identified and tracked through the cardiac cycle on routine echocardiography using specialized software. Both strain and its planar dimensions may be assessed using semi-automated off-line. This is a promising technique, and there are ongoing clinical trials using it to assess for mechanical dyssynchrony.

C. Alternative modalities for dyssynchrony assessment. Tagged MRI imaging is ideal for measuring strain; however, due to its expense, high level of complexity, and contraindication in patients with pacemakers or implantable cardioverter-defibrillators (ICD), it is of limited use with respect to dyssynchrony assessment.

V. ROLE OF CRT. The primary role of CRT is **to improve systolic and diastolic LV performance via an improvement in chamber efficiency,** thereby leading to symptomatic improvements in patients with advance refractory heart failure. The **systolic improvement** is usually noticed **within a week** of device implantation. In clinical trials, the **EF improved by an average of about 5%** with a significant improvement in MR. This was accompanied by symptomatic improvement, as evidenced by increased 6-minute walk time and quality of life index score (QOLS). **The remodeling of the LV takes at least 3 or more months.** On average, the LV systolic and diastolic dimensions decrease significantly following prolonged CRT. In studies in which biventricular (Bi-V) pacing was switched off after prolonged synchronized pacing, the systolic benefits disappeared rapidly; however, the LV dimensions were maintained for a longer period of time, suggesting that actual LV remodeling took place during CRT. There is also evidence that CRT may lead to electrical remodeling of the heart. In patients with LBBB or IVCD, CRT led to shortening of the duration of the native QRS complex. More recently, evidence from randomized clinical trials powered for mortality, in addition to symptomatic improvement, supports the use of CRT alone or in combination with an ICD in patients with ischemic and nonischemic etiologies of severe LV dysfunction.

VI. **SUMMARY OF MAJOR CLINICAL TRIALS IN CRT.** Most clinical trials evaluating CRT have addressed its role in patients in normal sinus rhythm with severe LV dysfunction, class III to IV HF symptoms refractory to medical therapy, and indirect evidence of mechanical dyssynchrony represented by prolonged QRS duration (on average, greater than 120 milliseconds).

A. **PATH-CHF.** A longitudinal study of 41 patients evaluating CRT (Bi-V or LV pacing) versus crossover into no therapy. Primary endpoints of peak VO_2, 6-minute walk, NYHA class, and QOLS significantly improved during CRT.

B. **MUSTIC.** A small prospective randomized trial powered for symptomatic improvement as measured by hospitalization, 6-minute walk, and QOLS in patients in normal sinus rhythm (NSR) or in atrial fibrillation at the time of enrollment. The trial showed significant improvement with CRT, and the benefit was similar in NSR and atrial fibrillation.

C. **MIRACLE.** A moderate-size prospective randomized trial that evaluated morbidity endpoints. Each patient was implanted with a Bi-V device and randomized to Bi-V pacing versus no therapy for 6 months, followed by crossover and subsequent evaluation for symptoms. The trial revealed significant improvement in symptoms with CRT. This trial led to approval of CRT devices by the Food and Drug Administration (FDA).

D. **MIRACLE-ICD.** Moderate-sized prospective randomized trial evaluating the safety and efficacy of combining CRT with ICD therapy for a composite endpoint of mortality, hospitalization, and symptomatic improvement. At 6 months follow-up, the CRT-ICD arm had a significant improvement in the composite endpoint. Combining CRT with ICD was deemed safe.

E. **CARE-HF.** Large, open-label randomized controlled trial powered for mortality benefit with best medical therapy plus CRT versus medical therapy alone in patients with ischemic and nonischemic etiology of LV dysfunction. In addition to the conventional dyssynchrony criteria of QRS duration greater than 150 milliseconds, the trial was first to implement echocardiographic markers of mechanical dyssynchrony in those patients with QRS duration between 120 and 150 milliseconds. At 3 years of follow-up, the primary endpoint of all-cause mortality and hospitalization was significantly different in favor of the CRT group. Furthermore, the secondary endpoint of all-cause mortality reached statistical significance after 3 years of follow-up, and the survival curves continued to separate. Number needed to treat (NNT) with CRT to save one life was estimated at nine patients.

F. **COMPANION.** Large, open-label randomized (1:2:2) prospective trial powered for mortality and hospitalization benefit in patients with ischemic and nonischemic etiology of LV dysfunction comparing medical therapy versus CRT versus CRT-D. In addition to conventional QRS criteria for CRT, patients also had to have had one episode of hospitalization for HF in the year prior to randomization. Primary endpoint of all-cause mortality and hospitalization was significantly different in the device groups as compared to the medically treated group. The secondary endpoint of all-cause mortality was significantly different in the CRT-D group as compared to the medical controls. The CRT group showed a strong trend toward mortality benefit that did not reach statistical significance. The trial was not powered to compare mortality benefits between the two device groups. In the CRT-D group, the mortality benefit was noticed shortly after the beginning of the trial, as compared to 6 to 12 months after study initiation in CARE-HF. The early mortality benefit in this trial was thought to be ICD related. The later benefits were attributed to both ICD and CRT therapies. The results of this trial led to approval of combined CRT-D therapy in the above population of patients.

VII. **NON-RESPONDERS. Up to 30 % of patients who received CRT based on current QRS criteria fail to benefit from the therapy.** Their symptoms do not improve or worsen, and there is no echocardiographic evidence of reverse ventricular remodeling. A clear etiology of the lack of improvement from CRT in those patients has not yet been elucidated. One of the possibilities is that QRS duration alone is not a good indicator of mechanical dyssynchrony, and some patients, despite prolonged QRS duration, do not have mechanical dyssynchrony and worsen when Bi-V pacing is commenced. In subjects with normal baseline LV contraction, Bi-V or LV free-wall pacing has an inferior hemodynamic profile when compared to native conduction. Therefore, it becomes important that CRT be only offered to those that truly have asynchronous contraction. Echocardiography criteria for mechanical dyssynchrony are currently being tested in clinical trials with hopes that they will lead to decreased rates of non-response.

Another potential explanation for the lack of CRT benefit in certain patients is the presence of myocardial scar in the LV free-wall territory. Areas of fibrous myocardium are electrically and mechanically nonviable; therefore, pacing at those sites may be of little value. Studies looking at presence of myocardial scar as it affects response to CRT are currently under way.

Studies are also attempting to evaluate the optimal position for LV lead placement with respect to the segment with the most delayed activation. Typically, in nonischemic DCM with LBBB, the posterobasal segment has the most delayed activation and contraction. This is not always the case in patients with ischemic etiology of LV dysfunction, where occasionally the inferior wall becomes activated the latest. Current echocardiographic techniques that were described earlier are being used to attempt to identify segments of latest contraction on an individual patient basis. However, it is conceivable that, due to limitations in the myocardial venous system, inadvertent placement of the LV lead in an area that is not significantly delayed may lead to adverse hemodynamic effects, also contributing to the high rate of nonresponders.

VIII. CURRENT GUIDELINES AND RECOMMENDATIONS (see Table 51.2). Based on the inclusion criteria in the eight larger randomized trials with CRT, the AHA/ACC 2005 Guideline Update for the Diagnosis and Management of Chronic Heart Failure in the Adult give CRT a class I indication (level of evidence A) in patients with ischemic or nonischemic etiology of depressed LV function, EF less than or equal to 35%, severe HF

TABLE 51.2 Current Recommendations for the use of CRT or CRT-D in Patients with Heart Failure

Recommendation	Class	Level of evidence
Symptomatic HF patients in NYHA classes III–IV despite optimal medical therapy, with LVEF ≤35%, LV dilation with LV end-diastolic diameter >55 mm, normal sinus rhythm, and wide QRS complex (≥120 ms) should be treated with CRT/-D.	I	A for CRT B for CRT-D
Symptomatic HF patients in NYHA classes III–IV despite optimal medical therapy, with LVEF ≤35%, LV dilation, and a concomitant indication for permanent pacing should be treated with CRT/-D.	IIa	C
Symptomatic HF patients in NYHA classes III–IV despite optimal medical therapy, with LVEF ≤35%, LV dilation, permanent atrial fibrillation, and indication for AV junction ablation should be treated with CRT/-D.	IIa	C
Asymptomatic HF patients in NYHA classes I–II, with LVEF ≤35%, and prolonged QRS should not be treated with CRT/-D.	III	None

AV, atrioventricular; CRT, cardiac resynchronization therapy; HF, heart failure; LV, left ventricular; LVEF, left ventricular ejection fraction; NYHA, New York Heart Association.
Adapted from AHA/ACC 2005 Guideline Update for the Diagnosis and Management of Chronic Heart Failure in the Adult and the Task Force for Cardiac Pacing and Cardiac Resynchronization Therapy of the European Society of Cardiology.

symptoms, NYHA class III or IV, on optimal medical therapy, in sinus rhythm with wide QRS complex greater than or equal to 120 milliseconds and LV end-diastolic diameter greater than or equal to 55 to 60 mm. The Task Force for Cardiac Pacing and Cardiac Resynchronization Therapy of the European Society of Cardiology, in collaboration with the European Heart Rhythm Association, provide the following recommendations for CRT:

1. The use of CRT or CRT-D is recommended in HF patients who remain symptomatic in NYHA classes III–IV despite optimal medical therapy, with LVEF less than or equal to 35%, LV dilation with LV end-diastolic diameter greater than 55 mm, normal sinus rhythm and wide QRS complex (greater than or equal to 120 milliseconds). (Class I, Level of evidence A for CRT; Class I, Level of Evidence B for CRT-D.)
2. The use of CRT is also recommended in HF patients with NYHA classes III–IV despite optimal medical therapy, with LVEF ≤35%, LV dilation, and a concomitant indication for permanent pacing (first implant or upgrade of conventional pacemaker). (Class IIa, Level of Evidence C.)
3. The use of CRT is also recommended in HF patients who remain symptomatic in classes III–IV despite optimal medical therapy, with LVEF less than or equal to 35%, LV dilation, permanent atrial fibrillation, and indication for AV junction ablation. (Class IIa, Level of Evidence C.)

IX. IMPLANTATION PROCEDURE. Unlike conventional transvenous pacemaker or ICD implantation that requires lead placement in the right atrium (RA) and/or the right ventricle (RV) only, Bi-V pacing requires LV lead implantation. Initially, this was achieved via a thoracotomy; however, currently up to 98% of Bi-V devices are placed via a transvenous approach. Although now used infrequently, some patients are still referred for a thoracotomy after a failed transvenous approach. Because most patients who qualify for CRT are also candidates for an ICD, current CRT devices have a combined pacemaker/ICD capability. The hybridization of CRT and ICD therapy increases the complexity of programming, follow-up, and troubleshooting of such devices.

The procedure is performed in an electrophysiology (EP) laboratory under sterile conditions. All patients receive preprocedural antibiotics at least 30 minutes before the procedure. A subcutaneous pocket is first prepared, making sure that appropriate hemostasis is achieved. Bi-V device implantation, due to the increased risk imposed by possible coronary sinus (CS) perforation, requires complete reversal of anticoagulation. Typically, a cephalic or axillary vein approach to venous access is used. The RA and RV leads are implanted in a fashion similar to a pacemaker or ICD implantation. The LV lead is placed through the CS in a vein located on the lateral free wall of the LV. Performing an occlusive CS venogram may help identify the appropriate vein. Various sheaths, catheters, and guidewires are used to cannulate the CS and advance the pacing lead into the appropriate vein. Transvenous LV leads can be either unipolar or bipolar. The optimal site for LV lead placement is controversial. Typically, however, the base to mid posterolateral wall is chosen as the optimal site. Before lead insertion, viability in the desired region and phrenic stimulation can be assessed by applying current to a partially insulated guidewire and looking for capture. Once the lead is advanced, its location should be confirmed by fluoroscopy, typically, in the left anterior oblique (LAO) view. The goal is to document base to mid posterolateral LV lead placement and maximal LV-RV lead separation in the left anterior oblique (LAO) view. A steep angulation in the LAO view tends to be most accurate. However, it has been shown that only LV-RV inter-lead distance on the **lateral chest radiograph** is most predictive of CRT response. Pacing thresholds are acceptable if less than 3 V at 0.5 milliseconds. Diaphragmatic capture is excluded by high-voltage pacing. If high pacing threshold or diaphragm capture occurs, the lead should be repositioned. CS trauma is frequent during lead placement, and it may range from dissection to frank perforation. Because the pressure in the venous system is low, serious sequelae are unusual and cardiac tamponade rarely results. After adequate LV lead placement and confirmed appropriate LV lead function, care must be taken during guidewire, CS platform, and stylet removal, so as not to disrupt lead position. Lead dislodgement occurs in as many as 5% to

10% of implantations. The time frame for the majority of dislodgements is the first 24 to 48 hours post implantation, when patients resume activity. For that same reason, patients are encouraged to ambulate while still in-house to prevent any out-of-hospital dislodgement, which may have more serious consequences.

X. PROGRAMMING AND FOLLOW-UP. LV leads may be either unipolar or bipolar; however, it is the unipolar lead with a distal stimulating cathode that is implanted most frequently. The RV lead is typically bipolar with a distal stimulating cathode and a proximal nonstimulating anode. The proximal nonstimulating anode on the RV leads also acts as anode for the LV lead. Most of the contemporary CRT pacing systems employ this shared configuration.

It is possible to convert conventional pacing generators to Bi-V use with special Y-shaped adaptors for separate ventricular leads. Both ventricles are stimulated simultaneously as intended in CRT; however, occasionally, oversensing becomes an issue due to double counting of the LV potentials. In the past, patients with atrial fibrillation who had no need for an atrial lead, had the LV lead connected to the atrial terminal on the generator, and the AV (effective VV) delay was set to the minimum between 0 to 30 milliseconds. This allowed for separate output to the ventricles and lower likelihood of oversensing. Currently, however, special multisite generators with separate ventricular ports are most frequently used. This allows for optimal programming and eliminates the potential complications of biventricular sensing.

Pacing must be **continuous** during CRT in order to obtain maximal benefit. Typically, DDD mode with a short AV delay (80 to 110 milliseconds) to prevent native conduction is employed. If atrial pacing is undesirable due to increased incidence of atrial fibrillation or altered left-sided AV timing, VDD mode may be used. Ventricular pacing is usually simultaneous or with a slight V-V delay. Given the two ventricular inputs (RV and LV), one could foresee that ventricular timing cycles could be quite complex during Bi-V pacing. Therefore, in most of the currently available devices, the RV is the only sensing chamber.

Follow-up of CRT devices includes a 12-lead EKG to assess for Bi-V capture and device interrogation to assess pacing thresholds. In those patients who are deemed nonresponders, echocardiography may be used to optimally time the AV delay based on Doppler mitral valve inflow patterns or Doppler aortic velocity time integral (VTI). Generally speaking, interventricular timing (V-V interval), although programmable, is not taken into consideration during CRT programming. Ongoing research, however, suggests that AV and VV interval programming may lead to a better acute hemodynamic response to CRT in certain patients. Whether this will translate to long-term benefit is uncertain.

XI. LOSS OF CRT. CRT is transiently interrupted in up to 35% of patients and permanently interrupted in 5% at 2 years of follow-up. Fortunately, restoration of CRT can be accomplished via nonsurgical means in the majority of the cases. Pacing parameters, occurrence of atrial arrhythmias, and lead malfunction or dislodgement are common causes of CRT interruption. The goal of continuous pacing during CRT should be reflected in appropriate programming algorithms. Typically, the AV conduction status is what influences continuous delivery of Bi-V pacing. Because the majority of patients who require CRT have an intact AV node, any parameters that allow for preferential native conduction will reduce CRT delivery. Keeping the AV interval as short as possible while maintaining proper ventricular loading is therefore optimal. Atrial arrhythmias are common in advanced HF. Rapid ventricular rate during atrial arrhythmias with rapid AV conduction inactivates Bi-V pacing due to the upper tracking rate limit. Keeping patients in normal sinus rhythm is therefore desirable. Any evidence of lead malfunction or displacement should be dealt with promptly by re-intervention. Loss of CRT results in symptomatic deterioration in HF and hospital admission in many instances.

XII. FUTURE DIRECTIONS. Due to the high rate of nonresponders to CRT, studies focusing on identification of patients with mechanical dyssynchrony via means other than the QRS duration alone are currently under way using the previously described echocardiographic techniques Identification of patients with nonviable myocardium in the LV free wall, who are unlikely to respond to pacing, is important. MRI, nuclear imaging, and CT imaging are currently being evaluated for that purpose. Chronic atrial fibrillation affects up to 15% of patients with severe LV dysfunction. Most of the major CRT trials have excluded patients with chronic atrial fibrillation (all except for MUSTIC-AF). Because Bi-V therapy may not be as effective in patients with lack of AV synchrony, or may not be feasible in patients with rapid ventricular rates, further data is needed to assess whether CRT should be offered to those patients.

The role of CRT in prevention of worsening LV dysfunction must also be addressed, given reports of more rapid progression of HF in NYHA class I and II patients with low ejection fraction and LBBB or IVCD. The MIRACLE-CRT trial is under way and should provide some answers regarding the role of CRT in that setting.

Finally, patients without LV dysfunction who are continuously RV paced are also at increased risk of developing HF. RV pacing creates an acquired LV conduction delay that has been associated with the development of LV dysfunction. The question of whether bradycardia-induced RV-paced patients should be upgraded to Bi-V systems or whether Bi-V systems should be implanted in patients likely to require continuous RV pacing will be answered by the BLOCK-HF trial.

XIII. SUMMARY. CRT has emerged as an effective means for advanced refractory HF therapy in patients with suspected mechanical dyssynchrony. Major clinical trials have proven significant morbidity and mortality benefit from CRT. Combining CRT with ICD therapy provides additional mortality benefits, and as a result, most patients who qualify for CRT receive ICD as well. The rates of nonresponders to CRT are high, considering the complexities related to device implantation and the cost. The current criteria that use QRS duration have been proven to have low specificity for identification of CRT responders. Studies to better assess mechanical LV dyssynchrony, presence of myocardial scar, and feasibility of LV lead implantation in the most delayed area are currently under way. With proven benefits in symptomatic patients in sinus rhythm with LV dysfunction and conduction abnormalities with CRT, the attention is now shifting toward using CRT in similar patients with atrial fibrillation, and toward preventing severe HF development in patients with underlying LV conduction abnormalities.

Key Reviews and Book Chapters

1. Kass DA. Ventricular dyssynchrony and mechanisms of resynchronization therapy. *Eur Heart J* 2004;(Suppl 4): 23–30.
2. Kass DA. Cardiac resynchronization therapy. *J Cardiovasc Electrophysiol* 2005;(Suppl 1):S35–41.
3. Spragg DD, Kass DA. Pathobiology of left ventricular dyssynchrony and resynchronization. *Prog Cardiovasc Dis* 2006;49:26–41.
4. Bax JJ, Abraham T, Barold SS, et al. Cardiac resynchronization therapy: Part 1–issues before device implantation. *J Am Coll Cardiol* 2005;46:2153–2167.
5. Bax JJ, Abraham T, Barold SS, et al. Cardiac resynchronization therapy: Part 2—issues during and after device implantation and unresolved questions. *J Am Coll Cardiol* 2005;46:2168–2182.
6. Hasan A, Abraham WT. Cardiac resynchronization treatment of heart failure. *Annu Rev Med* 2007;58:63–74.
7. Vardas PE, Auricchio A, Blanc JJ, et al. European Society of Cardiology; European Heart Rhythm Association: Guidelines for cardiac pacing and cardiac resynchronization therapy: the task force for cardiac pacing and cardiac resynchronization therapy of the European Society of Cardiology. Developed in collaboration with the European Heart Rhythm Association. *Eur Heart J* 2007;28:2256–2295. Epub Aug 28, 2007.
8. Hunt SA, Abraham WT, Chin MH, et al. American College of Cardiology; American Heart Association Task Force on Practice Guidelines; American College of Chest Physicians; International Society for Heart and Lung Transplantation; Heart Rhythm Society: ACC/AHA 2005 Guideline Update for the Diagnosis and Management of Chronic Heart Failure in the Adult: a report of the American College of Cardiology/American Heart Association Task Force on Practice Guidelines (Writing Committee to Update the 2001 Guidelines for the Evaluation and Management of Heart Failure): developed in collaboration with the American College of Chest Physicians and the International Society for Heart and Lung Transplantation: endorsed by the Heart Rhythm Society. *Circulation* 2005;112:e154–235. Epub Sep 13, 2005.
9. Ellenbogen Kenneth A, Kay Neal G, Lau Chu Pak, et al, eds. *Clinical cardiac pacing, defibrillation and resynchronization therapy*, 3rd ed Philadelphia: Saunders, 2007.

Common Cardiology Procedures XI

RIGHT HEART CATHETERIZATION 52

Kellan E. Ashley and Leslie Cho

I. INTRODUCTION. For many years, right heart catheterization has been an integral part of cardiology. It has led to a new understanding of physiology and has been helpful in diagnosing and treating patients. However, controversy surrounding the use of pulmonary artery (PA) catheterization has led to some confusion, as there have been reports of increased mortality due to PA catheterization in some settings. Nonetheless, it is still the gold standard in hemodynamic monitoring, and its use can be crucial in diagnosing and treating critically ill patients. As evidenced by the ESCAPE (Evaluation Study of Congestive Heart Failure and Pulmonary Artery Catheterization Effectiveness) trial, PA catheters are actually safe when used in the appropriate patient population. In this trial of 433 patients randomized to therapy for class IV heart failure (HF) guided by either clinical assessment or clinical assessment plus PA catheterization, there was no difference in the primary endpoint of days alive out of the hospital during the first 6 months after hospitalization. There was an increase in in-hospital adverse events in the PA catheter group; however, there were no deaths related to PA catheter use and no difference in in-hospital or 30-day mortality between the two groups (see "Suggested Readings" in this chapter).

II. INDICATIONS (see Table 52.1 for ACC recommendations for using PA catheterization).

- **A. Acute myocardial infarction** (MI) complicated by hypotension, congestive heart failure (CHF), sinus tachycardia, right ventricular infarction, or mechanical complications (such as ventricular septal defect [VSD], pericardial tamponade, or acute mitral regurgitation [MR]).
- **B. Assessment of volume status** in patients for whom physical signs may be unreliable.
- **C. Severe left ventricular failure** to guide inotropic, diuretic, and afterload reduction management.
- **D. Differentiation between various shock states** (e.g., cardiogenic, distributive, or hypovolemic) and guidance for therapies.
- **E. Risk stratification for patients during heart transplant evaluation.**
- **F. Cardiac tamponade.** Although echocardiography is the diagnostic test of choice, PA catheterization may be used when echo is not readily available or the echo findings are not diagnostic and the risk or difficulty of pericardiocentesis is high.
- **G. Assessment of the level and magnitude of an intracardiac shunt,** especially if transthoracic echocardiography is nondiagnostic.
- **H. Differentiation between constrictive and restrictive cardiac physiology.**
- **I. Severe pulmonary hypertension.**
- **J. High-risk cardiac patients during pre-, intra-, and postoperative periods** to monitor volume status and cardiac output (CO).

TABLE 52.1	Common Indications for the use of Right Heart Catheterization

Heart Failure

1. To differentiate between cardiogenic and noncardiogenic pulmonary edema.
2. To differentiate between cardiogenic and noncardiogenic shock and to guide its pharmacologic or mechanical support.
3. To guide therapy in patients with biventricular heart failure.
4. To diagnose pericardial tamponade when echocardiography is unavailable or nondiagnostic.
5. Perioperative management of patients with decompensated heart failure (HF) undergoing high-risk surgery.
6. To identify reversible pulmonary hypertension in patients undergoing heart transplant evaluation.

Acute Myocardial Infarction (MI)

1. To differentiate between cardiogenic and hypovolemic shock.
2. To guide pharmacologic and/or mechanical support of cardiogenic shock in patients with or without coronary reperfusion therapy.
3. Short-term guidance of pharmacologic and/or mechanical support in acute mitral regurgitation (MR) before surgery.
4. To establish severity and for short-term guidance of pharmacologic and/or mechanical support of ventricular septal rupture before surgery.
5. To guide management of right ventricular infarction that does not respond to intravascular volume expansion, low doses of inotropic drugs, and/or restoration of heart rate and atrioventricular synchrony.
6. To manage acute pulmonary edema that does not respond to treatment with diuretics, nitroglycerin, other vasodilators, and/or low doses of inotropic drugs.

Perioperative Use in Cardiac Surgery

1. To determine etiology of low cardiac output (hypovolemia vs. ventricular dysfunction) when exam and echocardiography are inconclusive.
2. To differentiate between right and left ventricular dysfunction and pericardial tamponade when exam and echocardiography are inconclusive.
3. To guide management of severe low cardiac output syndrome.
4. To diagnose and guide management of pulmonary hypertension in patients with systemic hypotension and evidence of inadequate organ perfusion.

Primary Pulmonary Hypertension

1. To exclude postcapillary (elevated pulmonary capillary wedge pressure) causes of pulmonary hypertension.
2. To diagnose and establish severity of precapillary (normal pulmonary capillary wedge pressure) pulmonary hypertension.
3. To select and establish the safety and efficacy of long-term vasodilator therapy based on acute hemodynamic response.
4. For hemodynamic assessment before lung transplantation.

Adapted from Mueller, et al. ACC Expert Consensus Document: Present Use of Bedside Right Heart Catheterization in Patients With Cardiac Disease. *JACC* 1998;32:840–864.

K. Severe adult respiratory distress syndrome during positive end-expiratory pressure trials to assess CO.

III. CONTRAINDICATIONS. The absolute contraindications to PA catheter placement are right-sided endocarditis, a mechanical tricuspid or pulmonic valve prosthesis, thrombus or tumor in a right heart chamber, and terminal illness for which aggressive management is considered futile. Relative contraindications are profound coagulopathy (INR greater than 2 or platelet count less than 20,000 to 50,000), bioprosthetic tricuspid or pulmonic valve prosthesis, newly implanted pacemaker or defibrillator (unless fluoroscopic guidance is used), and left bundle-branch block (LBBB). LBBB is a relative contraindication because one of the complications of a PA catheter is right

TABLE 52.2 Complications of Right Heart Catheterization

Related to the introducer	Related to the catheter passage	Related to the catheter
Arterial puncture	Arrhythmia (PVC, NSVT, VF)	Thrombosis
Bleeding from insertion site	Complete heart block or RBBB	Thrombophlebitis
Pneumothorax	Coiling	PA rupture
Nerve injury	Valve trauma	PA infection
Horner's syndrome	PA/RV perforation	Bacteremia +/− endocarditis
Air embolism		Balloon rupture +/− embolization

NSVT, nonsustained ventricular tachycardia; PA, pulmonary artery; PVC, premature ventricular contraction; RBBB, right bundle-branch block; RV, right ventricle; VF, ventricular fibrillation.

bundle-branch block (RBBB), which can lead to complete heart block in patients with existing left bundle-branch block. Temporary pacing should be immediately available when inserting a PA catheter in these patients.

IV. TECHNIQUE

A. Venous introducer insertion. It is important to obtain informed consent from the patient before the procedure. Table 52.2 lists the major complications of PA catheterization. The patient is **prepped and draped** in a sterile fashion. The patient should be draped from head to toe during the catheter insertion, regardless of the insertion site chosen. Multiple sites can be used for introducer placement; however, **a site that can be readily compressed, such as the internal jugular (IJ) vein, is preferred.**

1. The **IJ vein** (see Fig. 52.1) has multiple advantages, such as compressibility and minimal risk of pneumothorax. The disadvantages are the ease of carotid artery puncture and limited neck mobility for patients. The IJ vein can be entered via

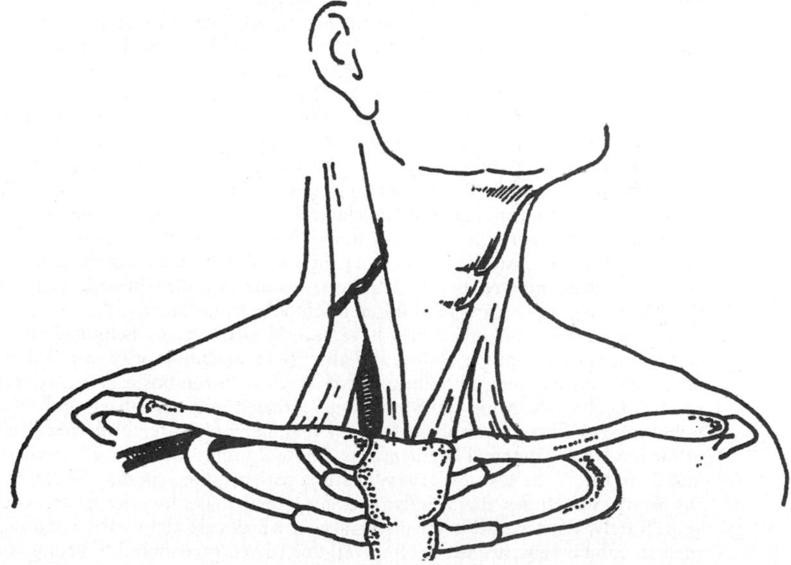

Figure 52.1. Neck anatomy.

an anterior or posterior approach. The right side is generally preferred because the vein runs a direct path to the right atrium. Often, it is easier to access the IJ if the patient is in the Trendelenberg position. The anterior approach uses the triangle created by the two heads of the sternocleidomastoid muscle and the clavicle. A finger should always be placed on the carotid artery to identify its position and to retract it medially. The needle should be inserted at the apex of this triangle and advanced in the direction of the ipsilateral nipple at a 45° angle. The vein can usually be entered 3 to 5 cm from the skin surface. In order to minimize complications, the vein should be found with a finder needle (20-gauge) before using the large-bore catheter (16-gauge) needle. If the vein is not cannulated easily or the patient has poor anatomic landmarks, ultrasound guidance may be used. Lifting the patient's neck allows better visualization of landmarks or the ability to switch sites. Once the IJ vein is cannulated, the catheter-over-guidewire approach should be used to place the introducer. The guidewire minimizes damage to the vessel and should pass smoothly. Never force the guidewire. If difficulty threading the wire is encountered, reattach the syringe and attempt to aspirate venous blood to ensure that the needle tip is still located in the vessel.

An alternative to standard IJ access is the posterior approach. The advantage of this approach is that it minimizes the risk of carotid artery puncture. First, the external jugular vein is located, and the IJ vein is cannulated 1 cm superior to the point where the external jugular vein crosses the lateral edge of the sternocleidomastoid muscle. Another posterior approach is to puncture along the posterior edge of the sternocleidomastoid muscle, two fingerwidths above the clavicle. The needle should be pointing toward the posterior aspect of the upper portion of the manubrium sterni.

2. The **subclavian vein** (see Fig. 52.1) is associated with greater patient comfort and ease of insertion. However, there is an increased risk of pneumothorax and subclavian artery cannulation, especially in patients on mechanical ventilation or with chronic obstructive pulmonary disease (COPD). The vein lies just under the clavicle at the insertion site for the clavicular head of the sternocleidomastoid muscle. This is where the vein should be cannulated. The subclavian artery lies just beneath the anterior scalene muscle, which is just below the subclavian vein, with the lung just underneath the artery. For better landmark definition and separation of the vein from the pleura, a rolled-up towel can be placed between the scapulae. There are two approaches to cannulating the subclavian vein: infraclavicular and supraclavicular. The infraclavicular approach is used more frequently. The needle is inserted under the clavicle at about 1-cm lateral to the sternocleidomastoid muscle insertion point. The needle is then advanced horizontally, nearly parallel to the clavicle, toward the suprasternal notch.

   With the supraclavicular approach, the vein is entered from above. The sternocleidomastoid muscle and the clavicle form an angle, and the needle is inserted at this point at a 45-degree angle. The vein should be cannulated no deeper than 2 cm below the skin surface. If there is uncertainty whether artery or vein has been cannulated, before dilating, transduce pressure through the needle or obtain a blood gas sample to differentiate vein from artery.
3. The **femoral vein** and other sites have several advantages, including ease of cannulation, easy compressibility, and absence of pneumothorax risk. The disadvantages are patient immobility, risk of infection, thrombosis, increased technical difficulty advancing the Swan-Ganz catheter, and risk of femoral artery puncture. For cannulation of the femoral vein, palpate the femoral artery pulse at the level of the inguinal ligament. The femoral vein is located 2 cm medial to and 2 cm below the femoral artery. In some patients, the vein may lie closer to the artery. Sometimes, the Valsalva maneuver may make it easier to access the vein. Rarely, venous cutdown is necessary, in which case right basilic and right median cubital veins are used. However, due to venospasm and difficulty with catheter insertion and advancement, the antecubital route is reserved for those who have failed other routes.

B. Pulmonary artery catheter insertion

1. After the introducer is placed, the PA catheter can be inserted. Always test balloon inflation, flush the ports, and make sure the catheter is properly calibrated before beginning the procedure. After the PA catheter is tested, insert it through the protective sterile covering and then through the introducer. Fluoroscopy and/or pressure waveforms can be used during PA catheter insertion for guidance. The catheter should advance easily; if not, do not force the catheter, but make sure the introducer is properly placed and flushed. Once the catheter has been inserted 15 to 20 cm or after the right atrial tracing is seen, inflate the balloon and advance across the tricuspid valve. The right ventricular tracing should be visualized next, followed by the PA tracing, and, finally, the pulmonary capillary wedge pressure (PCWP) tracing (see Fig. 52.2). Not infrequently, the right ventricular tracing is accompanied by a few premature ventricular ectopic beats. In general, the PA tracing should be reached within 50 to 55 cm if the catheter is inserted from the IJ or subclavian veins or 65 to 70 cm if via a femoral or an arm approach. If the PA tracing has not been visualized by this point, the catheter is likely coiled in the right ventricle. The balloon should be deflated, and the catheter withdrawn. The process is repeated until proper placement is achieved. Once the PCWP tracing is obtained, deflate the balloon and re-obtain the wedge pressure by inflating the balloon with 1.5 cm^3 of air. If the PCWP tracing is obtained even when the balloon is deflated or with less than 1.5 cm^3 of air, the catheter has been advanced too far and needs to be pulled back. The pressure waveform should always be closely monitored when inflating balloon-tipped catheters in order to immediately identify this "overwedging." The likelihood of PA rupture and infarction increases when catheters are overwedged. The PCWP should be obtained at end-expiration. In general, wedging the catheter should be avoided in patients with severe pulmonary hypertension.
2. It is much easier to float the catheter from the right IJ or either subclavian vein. From the femoral veins, it is slightly more difficult. Often, the femoral PA catheter needs to be inserted under fluoroscopic guidance. Alternatively, an S-shaped femoral swan can be used. When using fluoroscopy, the camera should be in the anteroposterior position, and the balloon should be inflated under fluoroscopy. Finally, check the catheter placement and check for pneumothorax after the procedure by obtaining a chest x-ray film. Catheter placement may be difficult in patients with low CO, severe tricuspid regurgitation, pulmonary hypertension, or a dilated right atrium or right ventricle.
3. Catheter advancement may be facilitated by a deep inspiration or, in more difficult cases, by a guidewire with a 0.021 inch diameter. The wire can be placed inside the distal lumen of the catheter, improving the stiffness and making the catheter easier to manipulate. A hemostat can be placed on the end of the guidewire so that it is not lost. Advancing the catheter from the femoral vein can be difficult; therefore, using fluoroscopy and an 0.021-inch guidewire is recommended in order to facilitate the process.

V. COMPLICATIONS (see Table 52.2)

VI. TROUBLESHOOTING (see Table 52.3)

VII. WAVEFORMS (see Fig. 52.2)

A. Right atrial (RA) systole occurs after the *p*-wave on the electrocardiogram (ECG) and produces the *a*-wave on the RA pressure tracing. Atrial relaxation, the *x* descent, occurs with a decline in pressure. Tricuspid valve closure produces a slight upward deflection during the *x* descent, which is known as the *c*-wave. The *c*-wave follows the *a*-wave by the PR interval. The *v*-wave occurs near the end of the *t*-wave on ECG and marks atrial filling during diastole. Finally, the *y* descent marks the opening of the tricuspid valve with emptying of the atrium. In the normal right atrium, the peak *a*-wave is greater than the peak *v*-wave.

B. Right ventricular systole follows the QRS complex of the ECG. With ventricular relaxation, the pressure declines and the tricuspid valve opens. During the continuous filling from the right atrium, a small *a*-wave is produced that marks atrial contraction and occurs after the *p*-wave and just before the QRS on the ECG.

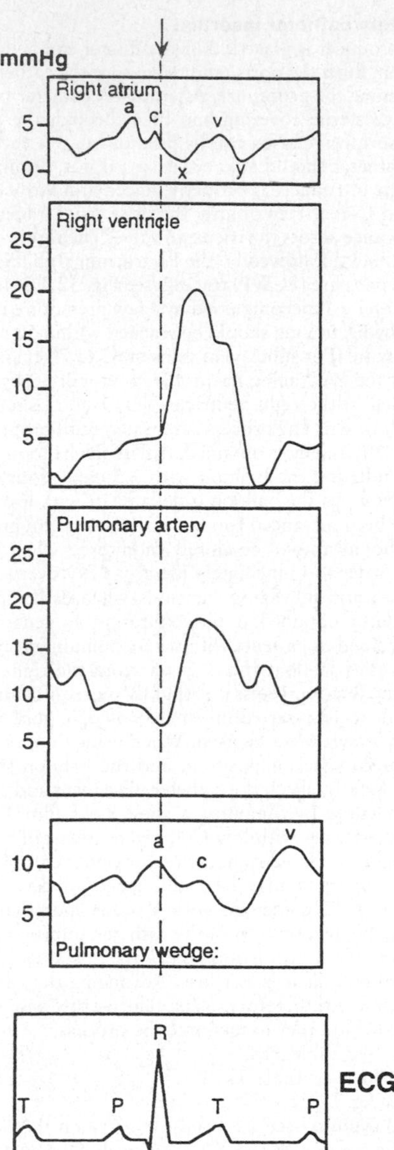

Figure 52.2. Waveforms.

End-diastole is the point just after the *a*-wave and just before ventricular contraction. The peak systolic and end-diastolic measurements are used for right ventricular pressures (RVPs).

C. The normal **pulmonary arterial pressure** tracing contains a *v*-wave, which corresponds to right ventricular systole and follows the QRS complex. During the relaxation period, pulmonic valve closure produces the incisura, a notch during

TABLE 52.3 Troubleshooting in Right Heart Catheterization

Problems	Solutions
Arrhythmia	Catheter may be in the RVOT. Pull the catheter back or advance forward.
No PCWP tracing	Catheter tip is usually not advanced far enough, balloon has ruptured, or the catheter is coiled in the right ventricle. Use fluoroscopy for guidance.
Continuous PCWP tracing	Balloon is inflated or the catheter is too far advanced ("overwedged").
Abnormal tracing	Catheter tip is up against a vessel wall or is too far advanced.
Damped tracing	Tubing is kinked, air or thrombus is in the catheter, or catheter tip is up against the vessel wall. Flush and/or withdraw the catheter.
Change in pressure tracing	Improper calibration, change in patient position, or catheter location.

PCWP, pulmonary capillary wedge pressure; RVOT, right ventricular outflow tract.

pressure decline on the *v*-wave. The trough of the pressure decline marks end-diastole. Pulmonic arterial systolic pressure, end-diastolic pressure, and mean pressure are recorded.

D. The **PCWP tracing** is a transmitted left atrial pressure (LAP). The waveforms are similar to a right atrial pressure (RAP) tracing, with the *a*-wave corresponding to left atrial systole, the *x* descent to relaxation, the *v*-wave to filling, and the *y* descent to emptying. However, in contrast to the RA, the *v*-wave is greater than the *a*-wave in the left atrium and the *c*-wave is not seen due to transmission through the pulmonary vasculature. Mean PCWP, *a*-wave pressure, and *v*-wave pressure are generally recorded.

VIII. PITFALLS OF THE PA CATHETER. The PA catheter remains the gold standard in monitoring hemodynamics; however, proper interpretation of its data is essential. The data are useless unless the catheter is calibrated correctly. The wedge pressure is an accurate measurement of left ventricular filling pressure, except in pulmonary veno-occlusive disease; in mitral stenosis and left atrial myxoma, where PCWP equals LAP but LAP does not correspond to left ventricular end-diastolic pressure (LVEDP); in MR, where LAP is greater than LVEDP; in acute aortic insufficiency and noncompliant ventricle, where LVEDP is greater than LAP; and in severe respiratory failure with high positive end-expiratory pressure. The thermodilution method to assess CO is accurate in most cases, except in patients with severe tricuspid regurgitation, intracardiac shunts, existing catheter thrombosis, and low CO. Serial hemodynamic measurements should be performed with the patient in the same position and only after the catheter has been properly calibrated and aligned at the time of each measurement.

IX. CARDIAC OUTPUT

A. Measurement via thermodilution technique:

1. Prefill syringes with 10 mL of room temperature indicator (usually normal saline), then cap the syringe.
2. Check the position of the catheter. Make sure you can obtain the PCWP tracing with 1.5 cm^3 of air and no less.
3. After properly attaching the tubing to the thermistor, inject the contents of the syringe five separate times. Discard the highest and lowest values, taking the mean measurement of the remaining three values.

B. Calculation of CO using the Fick equation:

1. Obtain patient's weight in kilograms.
2. Draw peripheral arterial blood gas to obtain systemic oxygen saturation ($Ao_2\%$).

TABLE 52.4 Clinical Scenarios in Right Heart Catheterization

Clinical scenarios	Data	Tracing
RV infarct	↑RAP, ↓CO, ↓BP RAP >PCWP, Steep *y* descent, Square root sign (RV diastolic dip and plateau)	Fig. 52.3
Acute mitral regurgitation	↑PCWP, prominent *v* wave	Fig. 52.4
Acute VSD	Oxygen saturation step up from RA to PA	
Noncardiac pulmonary edema	Normal PCWP	
Massive pulmonary embolism	↓BP, ↓CO, ↑PAP, normal PCWP	
Pulmonary hypertension	↑RAP, ↑RVP, ↑PAP, normal PCWP PAP and RV systolic pressure may reach systemic levels	
Tamponade	Diastolic equalization of pressures RAP = RV diastolic pressure = PCWP ↑RAP, ↑RVP, ↑PCWP Paradoxical pulse, blunted *y* descent, prominent *x* descent on RA tracing	Fig. 52.5
Constrictive pericarditis	↑RAP, ↑PCWP Dip and plateau in RV pressure tracing, M- or W-shaped jugular venous pressure tracing	Fig. 52.6
Tricuspid regurgitation	↑RAP, ↑RV EDP Blunted *x* descent, prominent *v* wave, steep *y* descent, and ventricularization of RAP	

BP, blood pressure; CO, cardiac output; EDP, end-diastolic pressure; PA, pulmonary artery; PAP, pulmonary arterial pressure; PCWP, pulmonary capillary wedge pressure; RA, right atrium; RAP, right atrial pressure; RV, right ventricle; RVP, right ventricular pressure; VSD, ventricular septal defect.

3. Draw blood gas from the distal lumen of the PA catheter ($Vo_2\%$).
4. Draw hemoglobin.
5. $CO = [Wt \times 3\ mL\ O_2/kg]/[(Ao_2\% - Vo_2\%) \times 1.36 \times Hgb \times 10]$
6. Oxygen consumption can be measured from a metabolic hood or a Douglas bag. It can also be estimated as 3 mL O_2/kg.

X. CLINICAL SCENARIOS (see Table 52.4)

A. Shock (see Table 52.5). Four classes of shock are characterized: hypovolemic, cardiogenic, distributive, and anaphylactic. Hypovolemic shock is due to a profound decrease in venous return and ventricular preload and can be caused by hemorrhage, dehydration, increased positive intrathoracic pressure, and depressed vasomotor tone. Hemodynamic data consist of decreased blood pressure (BP), CO, and PCWP with increased systemic vascular resistance (SVR). Cardiogenic shock results from failure of the cardiac pump to maintain adequate output and can be caused by a change in loading conditions (decrease in preload due to tamponade or

TABLE 52.5 Interpreting Right Heart Catheterization Data in Shock

	Blood pressure	PCWP	CO	SVR
Distributive	Low	Low	High	Low
Cardiogenic	Low	High	Low	High
Hypovolemic	Low	Low	Low	High

CO, cardiac output; PCWP, pulmonary capillary wedge pressure; SVR, systemic vascular resistance.

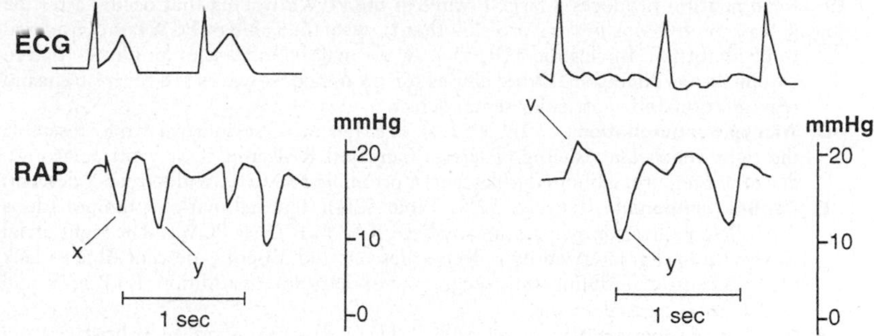

Figure 52.3. Right ventricular infarction without tricuspid regurgitation (*left*); right ventricular infarction with tricuspid regurgitation (*right*).

increase in preload due to ventricular septal defect), contractility (acute ischemia or infarction), or an abrupt increase in afterload. Low BP and CO but high PCWP and SVR characterize cardiogenic shock due to left ventricular dysfunction. In general, predominant elevation of RAP is indicative of right ventricular failure, and isolated elevation of the PCWP is indicative of left ventricular failure. The hemodynamic indices characteristic of distributive shock are low BP, PCWP, and SVR but high CO. A depressed CO as well as low BP, PCWP, and SVR can characterize the late phase of distributive shock. Finally, in terms of hemodynamics, not as much is known about anaphylactic shock. However, there is a hyperkinetic phase, characterized by low SVR and high CO, as well as a later hypokinetic phase, dominated by profound hypovolemia with decreased CO.

B. **Right ventricular failure** (see Fig. 52.3, Table 52.4) may be due to right ventricular infarction, severe pulmonary hypertension, pulmonary embolism, or increased preload due to left-to-right intracardiac shunt. A right ventricle infarct (see Fig. 52.3) produces increased RAP and right ventricular end-diastolic pressure, with low CO and BP. Because the right ventricle dilates and becomes less distensible, a dip-and-plateau pattern on the RVP tracing is seen. On the RAP tracing, there is a steep *y* descent. In the setting of severe tricuspid regurgitation and right ventricle infarction, the dip-and-plateau pattern is lost. A blunted *x* descent, prominent *v*-wave, and steep *y* descent are then seen.

C. **Acute MR** (see Fig. 52.4, Table 52.4) may be due to papillary muscle dysfunction or rupture. In this setting, the left atrium is subjected to increased pressure.

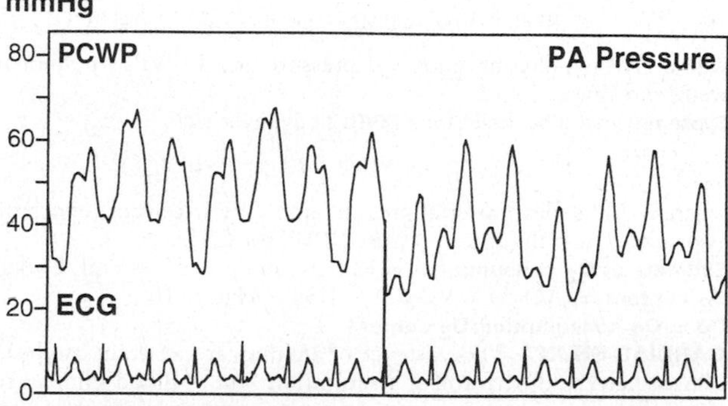

Figure 52.4. Acute mitral regurgitation.

Regurgitation produces a large *v*-wave in the PCWP tracing that occurs after the *T*-wave on ECG. A *v*-wave pressure that is twice the value of PCWP is considered to be abnormal. In chronic MR, the *v*-wave may be modest in amplitude due to chronic atrial dilatation. Other causes for prominent *v*-waves are severe tricuspid regurgitation and ventricular septal defect.

D. Tricuspid regurgitation (see Table 52.4). The right atrial systolic wave may resemble the right ventricular tracing. There is increased RAP and right ventricular end-diastolic pressure, a blunted *x* descent, a prominent *v*-wave, and a steep *y* descent.

E. Cardiac tamponade (see Fig. 52.5, Table 52.4). The hallmark of tamponade is diastolic equalization of pressures, where RAP = RVP = PCWP. The right atrial waveform is characterized by a deep *x* descent and absent *y* descent (due to lack of rapid ventricular filling at the beginning of diastole). In addition, RAP, RVP, and PCWP are increased.

F. Constrictive pericarditis (see Fig. 52.6, Table 52.4) is characterized by brisk ventricular filling during early diastole and limited ventricular filling during late diastole. The constriction results in the elevation and equalization of right and left ventricular end-diastolic pressures. The dip-and-plateau waveform is seen in constrictive pericarditis as well as restrictive cardiomyopathy, right ventricular infarct, and massive pulmonary embolism.

G. Massive pulmonary embolism (see Table 52.4). There is ventricularization of the PA waveform with rapid end-systolic descent and a hardly visible, or absent, dicrotic notch due to obstruction in the pulmonary artery.

H. Restrictive cardiomyopathy (see Table 52.6) includes a heterogeneous group of illnesses, such as hemochromatosis, amyloidosis, and endomyocardial fibrosis. This leads to impaired diastolic filling of the ventricles. There is a prominent *y* descent, but the dip-and-plateau waveform is less pronounced due to a pandiastolic hindrance to ventricular filling.

XI. FORMULAS (see Table 52.7)

1. **Cardiac output (CO)** by Fick equation in L/min:

$$CO = [Wt \times 3\,mLO_2/kg]/[(Ao_2\% - Vo_2\%) \times 1.36 \times Hgb \times 10]$$

where Wt is weight in kilograms, $Ao_2\%$ is systemic arterial oxygen saturation, $Vo_2\%$ is mixed venous oxygen saturation, and Hgb is hemoglobin concentration

2. **Cardiac index (CI)** in L/min per m^2:

$$CI = CO/BSA$$

where BSA is body surface area in m^2.

3. **Stroke volume (SV)** in mL/beat:

$$SV = CO/\text{heart rate (HR)}$$

4. **Pulmonary vascular resistance (PVR)** in dynes $\times$ s/cm^5:

$$PVR = [(\text{mean PAP} - \text{mean PCWP}) \times 80]/[CO]$$

where PAP is pulmonary arterial pressure and PCWP is pulmonary capillary wedge pressure.

5. **Systemic vascular resistance (SVR)** in dynes $\times$ s/cm^5:

$$SVR = [(MAP - CVP) \times 80]/[CO]$$

where MAP is mean arterial pressure and CVP is central venous pressure (can also substitute right atrial pressure [RAP] for CVP).

6. **Estimate of O_2 consumption** = 125 mL/min per m^2 = 3 mL O_2/kg
7. **O_2 content** = $(AO_2\% - VO_2\%) \times 1.36 \times Hgb \times 10$
8. **CO = O_2 consumption/O_2 content**

XII. INTRACARDIAC SHUNT.

The existence of an intracardiac shunt can be evaluated by using a PA catheter and performing a saturation "run." Blood samples for oximetry are obtained from the pulmonary artery as well as regions of the right ventricle, right atrium, superior vena cava, and inferior vena cava. With the catheter positioned in the

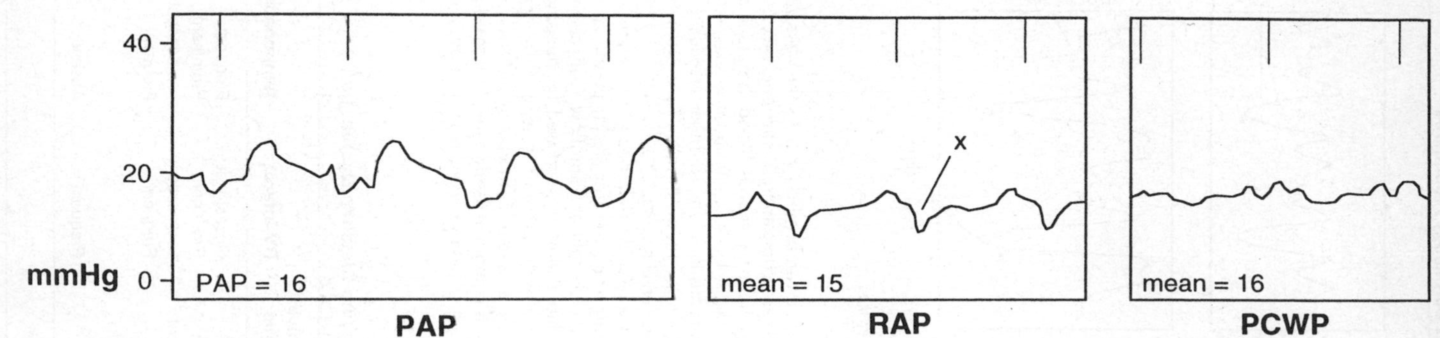

Figure 52.5. Cardiac tamponade.

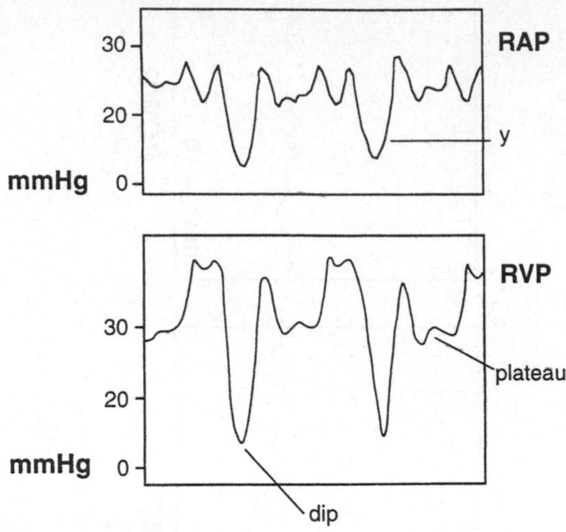

Figure 52.6. Constrictive pericarditis.

PA, CO by the Fick equation can be obtained. As the operator manipulates and pulls the catheter back under fluoroscopic and pressure guidance, a blood sample from each location is aspirated. A pulmonary venous blood sample is collected by inflating the balloon and then aspirating. A left-to-right shunt is suggested when a "step up," or increase, in the oxygen saturation in one chamber exceeds the oxygen saturation of a proximal compartment by more than 7% in the case of an atrial shunt or more than 5% in ventricular or great vessel shunts.

In a normal setting, the effective pulmonary blood flow should equal the systemic blood flow. However, with a left-to-right shunt, pulmonary blood flow is equal to systemic blood flow plus the amount of shunt flow. Conversely, in a right-to-left shunt, the effective pulmonary blood flow is decreased by the amount of shunt flow. The shunt fraction is the ratio of pulmonary to systemic flow, denoted Q_p/Q_s (where Q_p is pulmonary flow and Q_s is systemic flow). For an atrial septal defect, the mixed venous oxygen saturation is computed as the sum of three times the superior vena cava saturation plus the inferior vena cava oxygen saturation, and the total is divided by four.

TABLE 52.6 Differentiating Diastolic Dysfunction

	Constrictive pericarditis	RV Infarct	Tamponade	Restrictive cardiomyopathy
Pulsus paradoxus	Rare	Occasional	Frequent	Rare
RA waveforms	Prominent *y* descent	Prominent *y* descent	Prominent *x* descent	Prominent *y* descent
Equalization of diastolic pressures	Frequent	Frequent	Frequent	Rare
Dip and plateau	Frequent	Frequent	Absent	Frequent

RA, right atrial; RV, right ventricular.

TABLE 52.7 Normal Values and Formulas

	Formula	Normal values
RA		0–8 mm Hg
RV		Systolic 15–30 mm Hg Diastolic 0–8 mm Hg
PA		Systolic 15–30 mm Hg Diastolic 3–12 mm Hg
PCWP		6–12 mm Hg
CO	Fick equation: [Wt x 3 mL/kg]/[(Ao_2% – Vo_2%) × 1.36 × Hgb × 10]	4–8 L/min
CI	CO/BSA	2.8–4.2 L/min/m^2
SV	CO/HR	40–120 cm^3/beat
SVR	[(MAP – CVP) × 80]/CO	770–1,500 dynes s/cm^2
PVR	[(PAP – PCWP) × 80]/CO	20–120 dynes s/cm^2
Shunt fraction (Q_p/Q_s)	[AO_2% – VO_2%]/[PVO_2% – PAO_2%]	>2.0 Large defect 1.5–2.0 Small defect <1.5 Right to left shunt

Ao_2%, peripheral arterial oxygen saturation; BSA, body surface area; CI, cardiac index; CO, cardiac output; CVP, central venous pressure; Hgb, hemoglobin; HR, heart rate; MAP, mean arterial pressure; PA, pulmonary artery; PAO_2%, pulmonary artery oxygen saturation; PAP, pulmonary arterial pressure; PCWP, pulmonary capillary wedge pressure; PVO_2%, pulmonary vein oxygen saturation; PVR, pulmonary vascular resistance; Q_p, pulmonary flow; Q_s, systenic flow; RA, right atrium; RV, right ventricle; SV, stroke volume; SVR, systemic vascular resistance; Vo_2%, mixed venous oxygen saturation, Wt, weight in kilograms.

A. Calculation for left-to-right shunt

1. **Shunt fraction = pulmonary flow in L/min (Q_p)/systemic flow in L/min (Q_s)**
2. **Q_p = O_2 consumption/[10 × (PVO_2% − PAO_2%)]**
   where PVO_2% is pulmonary vein oxygen saturation and PAO_2% is pulmonary artery oxygen saturation.
3. **Q_s = O_2 consumption/[10 × (AO_2% − MVO_2%)]**
   where AO_2% is peripheral arterial oxygen saturation and MVO_2% is mixed venous oxygen saturation.
4. **Simplified calculation** using saturation only:

$$Q_p/Q_s = (AO_2\% - MVO_2\%)/(PVO_2\% - PAO_2\%)$$

Important note: A shunt fraction ratio of greater than 1.5 often necessitates closure.

Landmark Articles

Chatterjee K, Swan HJ, Ganz W, et al. Use of a balloon-tipped flotation electrode catheter for cardiac monitoring. *Am J Cardiol* 1975;36:56–61.

The ESCAPE Investigators. Evaluation Study of Congestive Heart Failure and Pulmonary Artery Catheterization Effectiveness. *JAMA* 2005;294:1625–1633.

Segal J, Pearl RG, Ford AJ Jr, et al. Instantaneous and continuous cardiac output obtained with a Doppler pulmonary artery catheter. *J Am Coll Cardiol* 1989;13:1382–1392.

Swan HJ, Ganz W, Forrester J, et al. Catheterization of the heart in man with use of a flow-directed balloon-tipped catheter. *N Engl J Med* 1970;283:447–451.

Key Reviews

Amin DK, Shah PK, Swan HJ. The Swan-Ganz catheter: choosing and using the equipment. *J Crit Illness* 1986;1:24–32.

Amin DK, Shah PK, Swan HJ. The Swan-Ganz catheter: tips on interpreting results. *J Crit Illness* 1986;1:32–38.

Mueller HS, Chatterjee K, Davis KB, et al. Present use of bedside right heart catheterization in patients with cardiac disease. *J Am Coll Cardiol* 1998;32:840–864.
Swan HJ, Shah PK. The rationale for bedside hemodynamic monitoring. *J Crit Illness* 1986;1:39–45.

Relevant Book Chapters

Kern MJ. *The cardiac catheterization handbook,* 2nd ed. St. Louis: Mosby–Year Book, 1995.
Marini J. *The ICU book*. Baltimore: Williams & Wilkins, 1987.
Perret C, Tagan D, Feihl F, et al. *The pulmonary artery catheter in critical care: a concise handbook*. Cambridge, MA: Blackwell Science, 1996.

53 TEMPORARY TRANSVENOUS PACING

George Thomas

I. INDICATIONS

A. Acute hemodynamically significant bradycardia or asystole. Temporary pacing is indicated for patients with acute hemodynamically significant bradycardia or asystole. Reversible causes such as digitalis, antiarrhythmic agents, and electrolyte disturbances such as hyperkalemia should be determined and reversed.

B. Termination of tachycardias (overdrive pacing). Temporary pacing is indicated for overdrive pacing and termination of atrial flutter (type I with long excitable gap), or supraventricular tachycardia due a reentrant mechanism.

C. Bridge to permanent pacing. Temporary pacing may be used as a bridge to permanent pacing in patients with complete heart block, high-grade second-degree block, severe sinus node dysfunction, and asystole. Generally, temporary pacing in this setting is for patients with an acute illness (endocarditis, systemic infection elsewhere) that delays permanent pacemaker placement.

D. Ventricular tachycardia. Temporary pacing is indicated in patients with bradycardia-dependent ventricular tachycardia and recurrent tachyarrhythmias secondary to long QT syndrome or pause-dependent ventricular tachycardia. Monomorphic ventricular tachycardia can be terminated with antitachycardia pacing (ATP) through a ventricular temporary wire by pacing at a rate faster than the tachycardia.

E. Acute myocardial infarction. Indications for temporary pacing in this setting include **development of a new bifasicular block** (right bundle-branch block with either left-axis [left anterior hemiblock] or right-axis deviation [left posterior hemiblock]), **new left bundle-branch block (LBBB) with first-degree atrioventricular (AV) block, alternating left and right bundle-branch block (RBBB), Mobitz type II block, and complete heart block.** *Patients with* **right ventricular infarction and loss of AV synchrony may benefit from AV sequential pacing.**

F. Condition where there is a chance for recovery. In certain forms of myocarditis with heart block, such as Lyme disease, or post cardiac surgery, temporary pacing can be used because there is a significant chance of recovery of conduction.

G. Acute aortic regurgitation. Pacing to increase heart rate in patients with acute aortic regurgiation who have elevated left ventricular end-diastolic pressure (LVEDP) can reduce diastolic filling time and improve hemodynamics.

H. Prophylactic. Prophylactic temporary pacing is considered in patients with undergoing right heart catheterization and/or myocardial biopsy, complex interverntion to the right coronary artery as it supplies the AV node in 90% of individuals, and cardioversion in patients with the sick sinus syndrome, although generally the use of trancutaneous pacing back up is used instead. Patients who are undergoing alcohol septal ablation receive prophylactic transvenous pacers, given the significant risk of complete heart block during the procedure.

II. RELATIVE CONTRAINDICATIONS

A. Poor vascular access

B. Bleeding disorders or anticoagulant therapy. If the international normalized ratio (INR) is greater than 1.8 and platelets are less than 50,000, these conditions should be corrected prior to placement of a transvenous pacer if possible.

III. PATIENT PREPARATION

A. Informed consent should be obtained for the procedure. However, if the patient is hemodynamically unstable because of a cardiac arrhythmia that could be improved with a pacemaker, this procedure is indicated emergently.

B. If the procedure is elective, peripheral intravenous access should be obtained before the start of the procedure.

C. The procedure should be performed in a monitored setting that is equipped for cardiopulmonary resuscitation and with fluoroscopy available.

IV. TECHNIQUE

A. Sites. The preferred site for pacemaker insertion is the **internal jugular vein.** The subclavian vein, femoral vein, and external jubgular vein can also be used. However, if a permanent pacemaker will eventually be inserted, the subclavian vein sites should be avoided, if possible. The easiest access in the catheterization lab is usually the femoral vein.

B. Position. The patient should be placed supine in bed. The patient may be placed in the Trendelenberg position for internal jugular and subclavian vein cannulation.

C. Placement

1. A 5F venous sheath is inserted into one of the central veins and 5F pacing catheters are used. The pacing catheter is advanced under fluoroscopy near the right ventricular apex for ventricular pacing and to the right atrial appendage for atrial pacing. The catheter is advanced to the tricuspid valve and turned either clockwise or counterclockwise to direct the tip anteriorly. An attempt is made to cross the valve directly. If unsuccessful, gentle pressure is applied and the catheter is torqued, allowing the middle portion to prolapse across the valve into the right ventricle. If the tricuspid valve is difficult to traverse, it may be possible to enter the right ventricle by looping the tip of the catheter against the lateral atrial wall and then rotating the loop medially against the atrial septum with the catheter tip just above the tricuspid valve. Another option is to increase the tip bend before attempting to traverse the right ventricle. Once the catheter has entered the right ventricle, it is rotated so that the tip points inferiorly to the apex with minimal movement in systole. The lead can also be advanced in the right ventricular outflow tract, then slowly pulled back until it drops, and then advanced into the apex as it drops. Some degree of buckling is acceptable; however, excessive buckling increases the risk of perforation. Ideally, the pacemaker tip should be near the apex of the right ventricle. The ideal catheter placement site is on the diaphragmatic surface or "floor" of the right ventricle anywhere between its midpoint and its apex. The floor of the more proximal ventricle is a second choice. The true apex is not a good choice for placement of the catheter tip. The paced electrocardiogram from this location usually shows a LBBB pattern with left-axis deviation. Ventricular pacing can also be done with the tip in the right ventricular outflow tract if the catheter cannot be placed on the floor of the right ventricle in a stable position. The pacer tip is considerably less stable at this site compared to the right ventricle floor and is more likely to be displaced; however, this is a very good position for a screw-in temporary pacing wire Pacing from this location will show a LBBB pattern with an inferior axis. The threshold may be higher with the tip in the right ventricular outflow tract. Use of a balloon-tipped temporary pacing electrode can aid in the advancement of the electrode into the proper position. In addition, echocardiographic guidance can be used to help guide lead placement in situations where fluoroscopy is not available or advisable (e.g., pregnant women).

2. For atrial pacing the right atrium is the easiest chamber to reach and pace, but the most stable position is usually found in the right atrial appendage. For atrial pacing, a 5F J-tipped atrial pacing catheter is used. Alternatively, a temporary screw-in lead can be placed in a stable position with good pacing and sensing thresholds. The atrial appendage is directed anteriorly above the tricuspid annulus, and multiple planes are frequently helpful in verifying location. (The catheter appears as a "J" in the left anterior oblique projection or as an "L" in the right anterior oblique projection.)
3. Both atrial and ventricular pacing may be performed by placing the catheter in the coronary sinus. The coronary sinus in its proximal portion courses along the left atrium. Ventricular pacing may be achieved by positioning the catheter in a great cardiac vein off the coronary sinus. The threshold in the coronary sinus is frequently high, but sometimes it may be a more stable location than the atrial appendage. Post–heart surgery patients often may have had their right atrial appendage resected, and steerable electrophysiologic pacing catheters may be useful in such patients.
4. For patients who need extended temporary pacing (those with pacemaker infections, or Lyme disease), a permanent pacing wire can be placed in the approriate chamber percutaneously and sutured to the skin. This can be connected to a temporary pulse genator. In addition, it can be attached to a resterilized permanent device that can be secured to the skin as well. This leads to a very stable intermediate term pacing system.

D. Testing. Once a catheter is in a stable position, threshold testing should be performed. The distal electrode on the pacing catheter is used as the cathode and connects with the negative terminal, and the ring is used as the anode and connects with the positive terminal of the generator. The pacing catheter is attached via a cable to the pacemaker generator. Pacing is started at a rate 10 to 20 beats faster than the intrinsic rate with 5-mA output. If capture is not seen at this point, the catheter needs to be repositioned. Once capture is seen, the output is slowly decreased until loss of capture is seen. The lowest capturing current is the **pacing threshold**. If the catheter is in good position, the threshold should be less than 1 mA. Pacing output should be three times the threshold, but pacing is usually performed at a minimum of 5 mA (even if three times the threshold is less than 5 mA). This is because minor dislodgment can cause major changes in threshold and adds a safety margin. To determine sensing, the sensing setting is gradually decreased (increased millivolts) until asynchronous pacing is seen. This is the **sensing threshold**. The pacer is set at twice the sensing threshold. For dual-chamber pacing, the AV interval will need to be programmed. A default of 150 milliseconds is frequently used, but the optimal AV delay may be different in individual patients. Patients with diastolic ventricular dysfunction may need longer AV delay for ventricular filling. In patients with marginal cardiac reserve, obtaining cardiac output measurements at various AV intervals and heart rates may help determine the optimal AV interval and heart rate.

E. Tachycardia termination. Reentrant tachyarrhythmias may be pace terminated. This involves pacing the chamber in which the reentrant circuit exists. Overdrive pacing is initiated at 10 to 15 beats faster than the tachycardia. Pacing is done for several captured beats up to 10 to 15 seconds and then abruptly stopped. If tachycardia persists, the pacing rate is sequentially increased by 10 beats and pacing repeated. The major complication of this technique is conversion to a faster or unstable rhythm. The advantage is that posttachycardia pauses can be managed with pacing if necessary, and direct current cardioversion may be avoided.

V. CHEST RADIOGRAPHY

A. Postprocedure chest radiograph must be evaluated for pneumothorax.

B. For right ventricular apex pacing, the electrode tip should be located to the left of the spine, and directed inferiorly and anteriorly.

C. For pacing through the coronary sinus, the tip is to the left of the spine, directed posteriorly and superiorly.

VI. PACER CARE

A. Check the catheter insertion site daily for signs of infection and apply a new sterile dressing at intervals.

B. Obtain a daily 12-lead surface electrocardiogram, ideally with and without pacing, to assess changes in native conduction and appropriate pacemaker sensing and capture.

C. Check pacemaker function daily by determining the sensing and pacing threshold, and check the underlying rhythm daily by decreasing the pacing rate gradually to "off." Abrupt termination in pacing may increase the risk of long pauses.

VII. COMPLICATIONS

A. Related to **central venous access** such as pneumothorax, hemothorax, air embolism, thrombosis, and infection.

B. **Cardiac arrhythmias** such as premature ventricular contractions, premature atrial contractions, ventricular tachycardia, and RBBB.

C. **Myocardial perforation with cardiac tamponade.** The unipolar recording from the tip normally shows pronounced ST elevation in comparison with the proximal electrode. ST depression from the tip is associated with perforation.

D. **Pacemaker dysfunction** with generator failure, over- or undersensing, electrode displacement with failure to capture.

E. **Complete heart block** in patients with preexisting LBBB caused by catheter irritation of the right bundle.

VIII. TRANSCUTANEOUS PACING.

Transcutaneous ventricular pacing involves placement of large-surface-area, high-impedance electrodes (Zoll pads) on the anterior and posterior chest walls. It usually requires long pulse widths (20 to 40 milliseconds) and high outputs of up to 100 to 200 mA. Transcutaneous pacing may be useful when transvenous pacing is contraindicated and in code situations. It avoids the complications associated with transvenous pacers such as pneumothorax, right ventricle perforation, infection, bleeding, and venous thrombosis. The major drawbacks are failure to capture and patient discomfort.

IX. TRANSESOPHAGEAL PACING.

Using a flexible electrode placed in the fundus of the stomach, the ventricular can be paced through the esophagus. This is useful when transvenous pacing cannot be performed, and transcutaneous pacing is unsuccessful or uncomfortable.

Suggested Readings

Bhargava M, Wilkoff BL. Cardiac pacemakers. In: Califf RM, Prystowsky EN, Thomas JD, et al., eds. *Textbook of cardiovascular medicine*, 3rd ed. Lippincott Williams & Wilkins, 2007:1191–1212.

Bitar S, Kern MJ. Angiographic data. In: Kern MJ, ed. *The cardiac catheterization handbook*. St. Louis: Mosby, 2003:320–325.

Hayes DL, Zipes DP. Cardiac pacemakers and antiarrhythmic devices. In: Braunwald E, ed. *Heart disease: a textbook of cardiovascular medicine,* 8th ed. Philadelphia: WB Saunders, 2008:831–862.

54 PERICARDIOCENTESIS

Christian Gring and Brian P. Griffin

I. INTRODUCTION. Pericardiocentesis is an important therapeutic and diagnostic procedure in cardiology. Most often it is used to relieve tamponade and identify causes of pericardial effusions. When performed correctly by experienced operators, pericardiocentesis has proven to be both an effective and safe procedure.

II. INDICATIONS

A. Alleviation of cardiac tamponade. Cardiac tamponade is a clinical diagnosis characterized by hypotension, tachycardia, distended neck veins, and distant heart sounds. Echocardiographic data provide confirmatory evidence for this diagnosis and include effusion (regional or circumferential), inferior vena cava plethora, collapse of the right atrium and right ventricle, and respiratory variation of blood flow through the tricuspid and mitral valves. Up to 30 mL of fluid is normally found in the pericardium. The additional volume of fluid required to cause hemodynamic compromise is variable and is dependent upon several factors, including the patient's volume status, the rapidity of fluid accumulation, and intrathoracic pressure (positive end-expiratory pressure increases intrathoracic pressure, impairing right heart filling and exacerbating tamponade physiology). Therefore, a relatively small but rapidly accumulating effusion can cause tamponade, particularly in the intravascularly depleted patient.

B. Evaluation of and therapy for pericardial effusion

1. After open heart surgery. Effusions after open heart surgery are common; rarely, they may be of hemodynamic significance. The incidence of large effusion/tamponade varies with the type of surgery: data from the Mayo Clinic suggest that the incidence of large effusion/tamponade after coronary artery bypass grafting is 1%, whereas post–heart transplantation patients had the highest incidence of tamponade at 8%. Of note, most episodes of postoperative tamponade were secondary to early, and, frequently, supratherapeutic, anticoagulation (1).

2. Idiopathic. In patients presenting with large, idiopathic effusions, evaluation of pericardial fluid, including cytologic examination, culture, cell counts, and chemistries, frequently assists in diagnosis. In fact, data suggest that the causes of most effusions can be diagnosed with history, physical examination, laboratory evaluation, and pericardial fluid analysis. Fluid analysis has been shown to be more helpful than pericardial tissue biopsy for culture of viral and bacterial pathogens (2), and cytology is positive in 65% to 85% of cases of malignant effusion (3).

3. Malignant. Malignant pericardial effusions are a rare manifestation of metastatic disease. Fluid cytology is usually positive and can be of value if the primary tumor is unknown. Lung, breast, and hematologic cancers are the most common etiologic factors. Controversy exists regarding the most appropriate management of malignant effusions: frequently surgical approaches are used because of concerns about reaccumulation. However, several studies have indicated that when a pericardial drain is left in place for several days, the risk of reaccumulation is low—approximately 12%. Sclerotherapy has a similar failure rate, and the 30-day mortality risk of a pericardial window is approximately 8% (4). Therefore, pericardiocentesis with drain placement is a very reasonable initial procedure for diagnosis and management of malignant effusions.

III. CONTRAINDICATIONS

A. Absolute. In emergent scenarios of cardiac tamponade, when circulatory collapse is imminent, there are no absolute contraindications. In these instances, pericardiocentesis can be a life-saving intervention.

B. Relative

1. **Anticoagulation.** Risk of bleeding is low with pericardiocentesis; however, if time permits, prothrombin time (PT) and partial thromboplastin time (PTT) should be obtained in all patients undergoing pericardiocentesis. A PT international normalized ratio (INR) greater than 1.8 or PTT greater than twice normal should be managed with fresh frozen plasma before intervention.
2. **Thrombocytopenia.** Platelet counts should be greater than 50,000.
3. **Traumatic hemopericardium.** A patient with traumatic hemopericardium should be treated surgically.
4. **Type A aortic dissection.** Typically, hemorrhagic effusions secondary to type A dissections are treated emergently with surgery. However, in situations where tamponade and circulatory collapse are imminent, small volume (10 to 25 cm^3) pericardiocentesis is indicated to stabilize patients before surgery. Data suggest that larger volume taps may be detrimental (5).
5. **Subacute free wall rupture.** As with dissections, free wall ruptures are best addressed surgically, but small volume taps may be necessary to stabilize patients in preparation for operative repair.
6. **Small or posteriorly located effusions** are technically more difficult to tap and have increased risk of complication. Echocardiographic guidance is paramount if pericardiocentesis is attempted.
7. **Purulent effusions.** If anticipated, grossly infected pericardial fluid should be managed surgically. Likewise, if a diagnostic tap reveals pus in the pericardium, surgical intervention is mandatory.
8. **Malignant effusion.** As stated previously, management of malignant effusions is controversial. Although pericardiocentesis is an effective and proven first-line therapy, recurrent effusions should be considered for pericardial window.

IV. PATIENT PREPARATION.

Ideally, pericardiocentesis is performed in a laboratory equipped for fluoroscopy and invasive hemodynamic monitoring.

A. Informed consent. Patients should receive a clear explanation of the risks and benefits of pericardiocentesis, including the rationale for performing the procedure.

B. Monitoring. Patients should have heart rate, blood pressure, and oxygen saturations measured throughout the procedure. In addition, electrocardiographic monitoring is necessary. Worsening hemodynamics or falling oxygenation should alert the operator to the possibility of a procedural complication. Frequent ectopy (premature ventricular contractions, premature atrial contractions (PACs), or nonsustained ventricular tachycardia) may indicate impending perforation of a cardiac chamber. Some authorities recommend pulmonary artery catheter placement prior to performing a tap; however, for routine cases this is not necessary.

V. TECHNIQUES

A. Echo guided. Currently, echocardiographically guided pericardiocentesis is the standard approach at most institutions. Patients are placed supine or in a slight left lateral decubitus position. The head is elevated approximately 30 degrees, and a complete echocardiographic evaluation is performed with standard parasternal, apical, and subcostal views. Attention is focused on the site where the greatest amount of pericardial fluid is closest to the skin surface. In addition, the liver should be identified to avoid accidental laceration during the procedure. Because it is air filled, lung tissue will block ultrasound waves and preclude imaging of the heart; consequently,, the risk of pneumothorax is low if a good echocardiographic window is selected for the tap. While imaging, **it is imperative to take note of the distance to the fluid pocket as well as the probe trajectory.** Obviously the trajectory of the needle during the pericardiocentesis should be identical to the echocardiographic probe's when imaging.

1. **Prepping the patient.** Once the best window is selected, the probe's location is marked with a permanent marker and scrubbed with sterile povidone iodine

solution. The entire torso is draped with sterile towels. The patient should not move between the echocardiographic examination and procedure.

2. **Marking the needle.** Using a sterile hemostat, a mark should be made on the pericardiocentesis needle at the approximate distance between the skin and effusion that was noted on the echocardiogram. In some instances, particularly in obese patients, longer needles will be needed. It is imperative to know in these situations how far the needle should be inserted before pericardial fluid is expected.
3. **Anesthetic.** Local anesthetic (e.g., 1% lidocaine) is applied to the skin over the mark. Then deeper anesthetic is given over the superior aspect of the rib (if a chest wall approach is used).
4. **Entering the pericardium.** Using a three-way stopcock, an 18-gauge Cook needle is attached to a syringe that contains a few more milliliters of local anesthetic. The needle is advanced through the anesthetized tract, over the rib, along the same trajectory as the echocardiographic probe, until fluid is aspirated. Alternatively, a sheathed catheter may be used instead of the Cook needle. Upon aspiration of fluid, the catheter is advanced over the needle, and the needle is withdrawn.
5. **Confirming catheter/needle placement.** While imaging from a remote location, agitated saline may be injected through the stopcock. The appearance of bubbles in the pericardial space confirms an appropriate location. Bubbles appearing within a cardiac chamber suggest that the heart has been perforated and that the needle or catheter should be withdrawn. If agitated saline cannot be visualized, one should consider intrathoracic needle position. If effusions are large, the agitated saline may not be visible from all echocardiographic windows; occasionally it may be necessary to reinject saline and image from an alternative location.
6. **Placing the pericardial catheter.** Once the intrapericardial position is confirmed, a floppy-tipped, 0.035-inch guidewire is inserted through the needle into the pericardial space. A blade scalpel is then used to nick the skin over the needle, the needle in withdrawn, and a 6F dilator is used to broaden the tract into the pericardium. Finally, the dilator is removed and a 6F to 8F pigtail angiocatheter with sideholes is threaded over the wire well into the pericardial space. The wire is removed, and catheter placement can again be confirmed with agitated saline injection. With a three-way stopcock, the catheter is then attached to a 30-cm length of plastic tubing, which in turn may be connected to a vacuum bottle or drainage bag. The catheter should be sutured in place.
7. **Bloody pericardial fluid or frank blood?** Occasionally, very bloody fluid may be aspirated during pericardiocentesis, and confirmation of the needle placement may be difficult. Therefore, differentiating between blood (chamber perforation) and bloody effusion can be challenging. A few milliliters of the aspirate can be placed on a gauze pad; classical teaching suggests that if the fluid coagulates, it is blood from chamber perforation. Conversely, fluid that spreads out on the gauze forming a pinkish halo suggests an intrapericardial origin. In reality, effusions caused by cardiac rupture, dissection, or ongoing bleeding into the pericardial space may clot upon aspiration; this fluid should be sent for hematocrit (to confirm that it is blood), and cardiothoracic surgery consultation should take place emergently.
8. **Real-time echocardiographic imaging.** With the technique described previously, echocardiographic guidance is not performed in real time; that is, imaging is not performed as the pericardium is punctured. A recently developed device may change this. The ColorMark (Echocath, Inc., Princeton, NJ) is a battery-operated generator that produces an electrical current, which is then converted to a mechanical vibration by a piezoelectric clip. This clip attaches directly to the pericardiocentesis needle and induces a high-frequency, low-amplitude vibration through the needle that can be imaged by color Doppler. Therefore, the needle tip can be imaged in real time from a remote location as it enters the

pericardial space. This technology has not yet been widely adopted, but initial studies are promising (6).

B. Electrocardiographic guidance. Electrocardiographically guided pericardiocentesis may be used if echocardiography is unavailable, or it may be used in conjunction with echocardiography. However, most authorities agree that electrocardiographic guidance adds little to the safety of a carefully performed echocardiographically guided procedure. If used instead of echocardiography, a subxiphoid approach is typically preferred:

1. The patient is positioned at a 45-degree incline.
2. Electrocardiographic limb leads are attached to the patient in the usual fashion.
3. The xiphoid process is identified, and a point just inferior and to the left of the process is marked.
4. The region is prepared and draped sterilely, and local anesthetic is given around the mark with a 25-gauge needle.
5. A 21-gauge steel spinal needle is attached to a syringe filled with local anesthetic. The needle should be approximately 10-cm long. With a sterile alligator clip, the V lead of the electrocardiography monitor is attached to the metal hub of the spinal needle.
6. Aiming at the patient's left shoulder and at a 30-degree angle to the patient, the needle is advanced beneath the costal margin. Local anesthetic is injected as needed, and gentle suction should be applied to the syringe when advancing.
7. ST elevation or premature ventricular contractions on the electrocardiography monitor indicates that the needle is encountering the right ventricle. PR-segment elevation or frequent PACs indicate that the needle is penetrating the right atrium. In the average adult, **the distance from skin to pericardium is approximately 6 to 8 cm** (7).
8. Once in the pericardial space, a catheter may be placed as described previously.

C. Fluoroscopic guidance. Fluoroscopy can be used as well to guide pericardiocentesis, although this approach has largely been supplanted by echocardiography. With fluoroscopy, a subxiphoid approach is again used. The needle is directed to the left shoulder and toward the anterior diaphragmatic border of the right ventricle. Upon penetration into the pericardial space, needle position is confirmed with injection of radiopaque contrast media (8). A drainage catheter may then be placed as described earlier.

D. Blind approach. In emergent conditions, blind pericardiocentesis may be necessary. A subcostal approach is used. However, because of the significantly higher rates of complications, blind taps should be avoided unless absolutely necessary.

VI. DIAGNOSTIC STUDIES. If the cause of the pericardial effusion is not clear, fluid should be sent for analysis. The primary causes of idiopathic effusions depend somewhat on the patient population but include tuberculosis, viral infection, uremia, collagen vascular disease, neoplasia, surgery, and myocardial infarction (2,9,10). Therefore, fluid should be sent for bacterial, mycobacterial, and viral cultures; cytologic examination; acid-fast bacillus smear; cell count; protein; and lactate dehydrogenase. Blood samples should be sent for chemistry, acute and convalescent titers of cytomegalovirus and coxsackievirus B (if infection is likely), antinuclear antibody, and rheumatoid factor (if connective tissue disease is suspected). Consideration should also be given to placing a tuberculin purified protein derivative skin test.

VII. COMPLICATIONS. Using echocardiographic guidance, the rate of complications is very low. The largest series of echo-guided pericardiocenteses comes from the Mayo Clinic. Among the 1,127 procedures studied, major complications occurred in 1.2% of cases, and included one death from right ventricular perforation, five nonfatal perforations that required surgery, one intercostal artery laceration, five pneumothoraces, one episode of sustained ventricular tachycardia, and one episode of bacteremia. Minor complications occurred 3.5% of the time and included 11 chamber perforations that sealed spontaneously, eight self-limited pneumothoraces, nine pleuropericardial fistulas, and two episodes of nonsustained ventricular tachycardia (11).

Fluoroscopy appears to have higher rates of complications. In one series of 352 procedures, complications included 2 (0.6%) deaths, 23 (5.6%) chamber perforations

(3 requiring surgery), 5 (1.4%) arterial bleeds (3 diaphragmatic, 1 posterior descending artery, and 1 left internal mammary artery), and 2 pneumothoraces (8).

Blind pericardiocentesis has been associated with morbidity rates as high as 20% and mortality rates as high as 6% (11).

Therefore, complications are relatively rare, although one must be mindful of the following:

A. Pneumothorax. Usually effectively avoided with echocardiographic imaging.

B. Chamber entry/cardiac laceration. Usually asymptomatic and self-sealing, particularly if the left ventricle is entered. Right ventricular perforations have a somewhat higher likelihood of bleeding when perforated, but right atrial lacerations carry the highest risk. If laceration is suspected, the needle or catheter should be withdrawn and the patient should be observed overnight in an intensive care setting. Serial echocardiograms are indicated to assess for changes in effusion size.

C. Arterial laceration. The left mammary runs down the chest wall about 5 cm lateral to the sternum. Left chest wall and subxiphoid approaches must take this anatomy into consideration. The posterior descending artery can be lacerated on subxiphoid approaches if the needle is aimed too medially. On a chest wall approach, the intercostal arteries are avoided by passing the catheter just superior to the rib.

D. Infection. Sterile technique during the procedure and meticulous catheter care afterward if a drain is left in place minimize this risk. As the Mayo series suggests, the risk of catheter-related infection is very low, even among cancer patients.

E. Death. This is exceptionally rare when procedures are performed by experienced operators with echocardiographic guidance. Moreover, the mortality rate is much lower than that associated with surgical drainage techniques (4).

VIII. POSTPROCEDURE CARE

A. Chest radiography. A postprocedure chest film should be obtained in all patients to exclude pneumothorax.

B. Monitoring. Patients should be observed for 1 to 2 hours following the pericardiocentesis. Patients without significant comorbidities who have uncomplicated diagnostic taps do not require inpatient care following the procedure (12).

C. Drain care (13). Care of an indwelling pericardial catheter is similar to that for any central line. After the catheter is sutured in place, the site is treated with an antibacterial ointment and then dressed sterilely. The dressing should be changed every 2 or 3 days.

1. The drain should be aspirated every 6 hours. Continuous drainage can also be used, but the risk of catheter obstruction is higher. Following aspiration, the catheter is flushed with sterile saline.
2. If the fluid becomes purulent or the patient becomes septic, the catheter must be removed.
3. Strict record of the volume of fluid draining from the catheter must be kept. When the drainage is less than 50 cm^3/day, the pigtail can be pulled.

D. Follow-up echocardiography. Before pulling the drain, an echocardiogram should be obtained to ensure resolution of the effusion.

E. Patient care. Patients may be ambulatory with the drain securely in place. Pericardial pain is best managed with nonsteroidal analgesics.

References

1. Tsang TS, Barnes ME, Hayes SN, Freeman WK, Dearani JA, Butler SL, Seward JB. Clinical and echocardiographic characteristics of significant pericardial effusions following cardiothoracic surgery and outcomes of echo-guided pericardiocentesis for management: *Mayo Clinic experience*, 1979–1998. *Chest* 116(2):322–31, 1999.
2. Corey GR, Campbell PT, Van Trigt P, Kenney RT, O'Connor CM, Sheikh KH, Kisslo JA, Wall TC. Etiology of large pericardial effusions. *American Journal of Medicine* 95(2):209–13, 1993.
3. Vaitkus PT, Herrmann HC, LeWinter MM. Treatment of malignant pericardial effusion. *JAMA* 272(1):59–64, 1994.
4. Tsang TS, Seward JB, Barnes ME, Bailey KR, Sinak LJ, Urban LH, Hayes SN. Outcomes of primary and secondary treatment of pericardial effusion in patients with malignancy. *Mayo Clinic Proceedings* 75(3):248–53, 2000.
5. Isselbacher EM, Cigarroa JE, Eagle KA. Cardiac tamponade complicating proximal aortic dissection. Is pericardiocentesis harmful? *Circulation* 90(5):2375–8, 1994.
6. Armstrong G, Cardon L, Vilkomerson D, Lipson D, Wong J, Rodriguez LL, Thomas JD, Griffin BP. Localization of needle tip with color Doppler during pericardiocentesis: In vitro validation and initial clinical application. *Journal of the American Society of Echocardiography* 14:29–37, 2001.

7. Miller JI. Surgical management of pericardial disease. Schlant RC, Alexander RW, eds. *Hurst's the heart,* 8th ed. New York: McGraw-Hill, 1994:1675–1680.
8. Duvernoy O, Borowiec J, Helmius G, Erikson U. Complications of percutaneous pericardiocentesis under fluoroscopic guidance. *Acta Radiologica* 33(4):309–13, 1992.
9. Gibbs CR, Watson RD, Singh SP, Lip GY. Management of pericardial effusion by drainage: a survey of 10 years' experience in a city centre general hospital serving a multiracial population. *Postgraduate Medical Journal* 76(902):809–13, 2000.
10. Soler-Soler J, Sagrista-Sauleda J, Permanyer-Miralda G. Management of pericardial effusion. *Heart* 86(2):235–40, 2001.
11. Tsang TS, Enriquez-Sarano M, Freeman WK, Barnes ME, Sinak LJ, Gersh BJ, Bailey KR, Seward JB. Consecutive 1127 therapeutic echocardiographically guided pericardiocenteses: clinical profile, practice patterns, and outcomes spanning 21 years. *Mayo Clinic Proceedings* 77:429–36, 2002.
12. Drummond JB, Seward JB, Tsang TS, Hayes SN, Miller FA Jr. Outpatient two-dimensional echocardiography-guided pericardiocentesis. *Journal of the American Society of Echocardiography* 11(5):433–5, 1998.
13. Tsang TS, Freeman WK, Sinak LJ, Seward JB. Echocardiographically guided pericardiocentesis: evolution and state-of-the-art technique. *Mayo Clinic Proceedings* 73(7):647–52, 1998.

ELECTRICAL CARDIOVERSION 55

Thomas D. Callahan and Robert A. Schweikert

I. INTRODUCTION. Delivery of electrical countershock to terminate cardiac arrhythmias is a safe and effective technique that is routinely performed in most hospitals. *Cardioversion* is defined by delivery of energy synchronized to the QRS complex, whereas random delivery of shock during the cardiac cycle (usually done for terminating ventricular fibrillation) is termed *defibrillation.*

II. MECHANISM. Although it has long been recognized that application of an electrical shock to the myocardium can restore a normal rhythm, knowledge of the fundamental mechanism underlying defibrillation remains incomplete. A rapidly delivered electric shock depolarizes the myocardial cells and creates a zone of myocardium with an extended refractory period. Activation fronts encountering tissue with a prolonged refractory period will not be able to propagate, thus terminating both macro- and microreentrant circuits. Atrial and ventricular fibrillation are generally agreed to be more electrically stable rhythms, and thus require higher current delivery for termination. The most common waveform shapes used in external defibrillation are the monophasic and biphasic waveforms. In biphasic waveforms, the polarity at each electrode reverses partway through the defibrillation waveform. Use of a biphasic waveform in cardioversion and defibrillation has been shown to be associated with an increased efficacy and may reduce the development of post-shock arrhythmias.

III. INDICATIONS AND CONTRAINDICATIONS. The indications and contraindications of cardioversion are listed in Tables 55.1 and 55.2. **Cardioversion should not be performed in patients in whom the rhythm is sinus or the abnormal rhythm is secondary to increased automaticity (e.g., multifocal atrial tachycardia, junctional tachycardia). If the presenting rhythm is ventricular fibrillation or ventricular tachycardia with hemodynamic compromise, the only clear contraindication to defibrillation is clear expression of the patient's (or patient's surrogate's) informed wish not to be resuscitated.**

IV. PROCEDURE

A. Patient preparation

1. **Informed consent** should be obtained from the patient or surrogate (if patient is unable to comprehend and give meaningful informed consent).

TABLE 55.1 Indications and Contraindications of Cardioversion

INDICATIONS

Cardioversion

1. Atrial fibrillation/atrial flutter
   - **a.** Patient with atrial fibrillation/atrial flutter >48-h (or unknown) duration and anticoagulation for >3–4 wk (INR 2–3)
   - **b.** Acute onset atrial fibrillation/flutter with associated hemodynamic compromise, e.g.,
     1. Angina pectoris
     2. Myocardial infarction
     3. Pulmonary edema
     4. Hypotension
     5. Heart failure
   - **c.** Atrial fibrillation/flutter of unknown duration and absence of thrombus in left atrium or left atrial appendage on biplane transesophageal echocardiogram
   - **d.** Atrial fibrillation/flutter <48-h duration → anticoagulation optional—depending on risk
2. Atrial tachycardia
3. Atrioventricular nodal reentrant tachycardia
4. Reentry tachycardias associated with Wolf-Parkinson-White syndrome
5. Ventricular tachycardia

Defibrillation

1. Ventricular fibrillation
2. Ventricular tachycardia with hemodynamic instability

CONTRAINDICATIONS

Cardioversion

1. Known atrial thrombus and no emergent indication
2. Sinus rhythm/tachycardia
3. Tachycardias associated with increased automaticity
   - **a.** Multifocal atrial tachycardia
   - **b.** Junctional tachycardia
4. Digitalis toxicity
5. Severe electrolyte imbalance and nonemergent indication
6. Unknown duration of atrial fibrillation or atrial flutter in a non-anticoagulated patient in the absence of transesophageal echocardiogram
7. Patient who cannot be safely sedated

Defibrillation

1. Prior expression of patients who wish not to be resuscitated

INR, International normalized ratio.

2. In elective cases, patient should **fast for a minimum of 6 to 8 hours.**
3. A review of the patient's medical **history and a focused physical examination** should be performed. **Special attention should be paid to the airway.** Inability to visualize the uvula, inability to open the mouth with at least 2 cm between the teeth, or difficulty in extending the neck are factors that may make potential intubation difficult and may suggest the need for the presence of an anesthesiologist during the procedure.
4. Patient's **medication and anticoagulation status** (for patients in atrial fibrillation or flutter should be confirmed [Table 55.3]). Because patients may not always have symptoms with arrhythmias such as atrial fibrillation and atrial flutter, convincing historical or electrocardiographic evidence of the tachycardia initiating within 48 hours of cardioversion should be documented before cardioverting a patient with atrial fibrillation or atrial flutter without adequate anticoagulation.
5. A 12-lead electrocardiogram (ECG) should be obtained to **confirm the presenting rhythm,** as well as to discern any suggestion of electrolyte abnormality (hypo- or hyperkalemia) or drug toxicity (digitalis). If any of those are suspected,

TABLE 55.2 Indications for Cardioversion in Patients with Atrial Fibrillation

Class I

1. Immediate electrical cardioversion in patients with paroxysmal AF and a rapid ventricular response who have electrocardiographic evidence of acute MI or symptomatic hypotension, angina, or HF that does not respond promptly to pharmacologic measures.
2. Cardioversion in patients without hemodynamic instability when symptoms of AF are unacceptable

Class IIa

1. Electrical cardioversion to accelerate restoration of sinus rhythm in patients with a first-detected episode of AF.
2. Electrical cardioversion in patients with persistent AF when early recurrence is unlikely.
3. Repeated cardioversion followed by prophylactic drug therapy in patients who relapse to AF without antiarrhythmic medication after successful cardioversion.

Class III

1. Electrical cardioversion in patients who display spontaneous alteration between AF and sinus rhythm over short periods of time.
2. Additional cardioversion in patients with short periods of sinus rhythm who relapse to AF despite multiple cardioversion procedures and prophylactic antiarrhythmic drug treatment.

AF, atrial fibrillation; HF, heart failure; MI, myocardial infarction.
Adapted from ACC/AHA/ESC 2001 Guidelines

appropriate blood levels should be checked. Routine measurement of digoxin levels is not recommended.

6. **Peripheral venous access** should be obtained for elective cases.
7. A good-quality **continuous ECG** should be obtained. Good contact of the skin and electrodes is essential, and proper skin preparation, including shaving of the chest hair (if present), is recommended.

TABLE 55.3 Anticoagulation Status and Cardioversion for Atrial Fibrillation/Flutter[a]

Anticoagulation before cardioversion

1. Administer oral anticoagulation and ensure therapeutic INR (>2) for a minimum of 3–4 weeks prior to cardioversion (target INR 2–3)

or

2. Anticoagulate with heparin to achieve a PTT 1.5–2 times control, and screen for thrombus in left atrium or left atrial appendage by transesophageal echocardiography
   a. If no thrombus, cardiovert and continue heparin while loading Coumadin until INR is therapeutic (>2)

   or

   b. If thrombus is visualized, anticoagulate for 3–4 wk (target INR 2–3) and recheck transesophageal echocardiogram to confirm thrombus is resolved prior to cardioversion
3. If emergent indication
   Administer heparin (unless contraindicated) to achieve PTT 1.5–2 times control prior to or immediately after cardioversion

Anticoagulation after cardioversion

Oral anticoagulation for at least 3–4 wk with target INR 2–3 if no contraindications

[a]Limited data support the use of low–molecular-weight heparin (LMWH) before or after cardioversion (Level of evidence: C). Use of LMWH in such clinical situations must be individualized after careful determination of the risks and benefits involved.
INR, international normalized ratio; PTT, partial thromboplastin time.

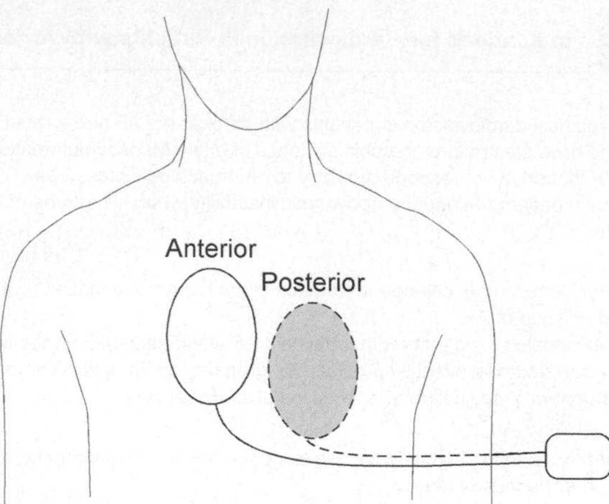

Figure 55.1. Right parasternal–left paravertebral electrode patch position.

8. **Oxygen and airway management** equipment (including suction with suction catheters, bag-valve-mask, laryngoscope, endotracheal tubes, and pulse oximeter) is required and should be checked prior to the procedure.

B. Technique

1. Once the patient is adequately prepared and an appropriately trained physician is present, **cardioversion patches are placed and the patient is sedated.**
2. **Electrode placement.** Patches or paddles may be placed in the anteroapical or the anteroposterior position.
   a. Although the anteroapical position is easy to use in an emergency, it is associated with a lower delivery of current to the myocardium.
   b. The left anteroposterior position is commonly used for cardioversion of atrial arrhythmias because it is associated with a smaller interelectrode distance and a lesser interposition of lung parenchyma. This enhances delivery of current to the atria and improves the success of cardioversion.
   c. The right parasternal–left paravertebral position is associated with better current delivery to both atria and is particularly useful in patients with atrial abnormalities. (e.g., atrial septal defect, rheumatic valve disease). This electrode position is favored in our laboratory for cardioversion of atrial fibrillation (Fig. 55.1).
   d. Although internal cardioversion (using a right atrial catheter and a coronary sinus catheter as electrodes, or using a right atrial and a posteriorly placed external electrode) has been used in the past for cardioverting morbidly obese patients or patients who are resistant to external cardioversion, it is now rarely necessary, given the widespread availability of biphasic cardioversion.
3. **Sedation.** Short-acting sedatives should be administered before all elective cardioversions, since the procedure is uncomfortable. Commonly used agents include methohexital (0.5 to 0.6 mg/kg body weight, repeated in 4 to 7 minutes as needed), etomidate (0.2 to 0.6 mg/kg body weight over 30 to 60 seconds), and midazolam (0.5 to 2 mg over 2 minutes, repeated every 2 to 3 minutes if necessary). Adequate sedation is confirmed by lack of response to verbal and pressure stimuli and loss of eyelash reflex. Airway, breathing, and oxygenation should be monitored until the patient makes a complete recovery and appropriate support is provided as needed.
4. **Energy selection.** Success of cardioversion is dependent on adequate energy delivery to the heart. This in turn is dependent on the energy output, current vector, and the transthoracic impedence.

TABLE 55.4 Initial Energy Selection for Commonly Encountered Arrhythmias

Arrhythmia	Energy Output (J)	
	Monophasic	Biphasic
Ventricular fibrillation (or unstable ventricular tachycardia)	200	120
Atrial fibrillation	200	100
Atrial flutter	50	50
Supraventricular tachycardia	150	100
Ventricular tachycardia (stable)	100	50–100

a. The commonly used energy selection for various arrhythmias is outlined in Table 55.4. The energy selected differs between monophasic and biphasic devices.

b. Impedance is defined as opposition to electrical flow or current. Higher impedance results in a reduction in current delivery to the myocardium. Therefore, initial energy selection should be individually tailored after consideration of important patient factors such as body habitus and the presence of lung disease, which may affect impedance. In addition, all efforts must be made to reduce impedance. A key factor that modulates impedance is electrode size, with optimal size approximating the size of the heart. Although smaller electrodes increase impedance, larger ones are associated with current wastage. The optimal diameter of an electrode for an adult patient is approximately 12 cm. Other measures to reduce impedance include application of pressure on the electrodes (approximately 12 kg) during shock delivery, shock during end-expiration, better skin–electrode interface and use of conducting gels, and repeat administration of shocks. Conversely, increasing interelectrode distance and interposition of soft tissue or pulmonary parenchyma reduces impedance.

5. **Synchronization.** Once the underlying rhythm is confirmed and a good-equality ECG is obtained, the synchronize mode is switched on (except for defibrillation where mode must be asynchronous). Synchronization is essential to prevent delivery of shock during the vulnerable period (from 80 milliseconds before to 30 milliseconds after the apex of T wave) with resultant ventricular fibrillation. Defibrillators are designed to time the shock to the R wave during synchronization mode. The position of the timing artifact on R wave is confirmed on the monitor and on a printout, because rarely the defibrillator may synchronize to the T wave. Conversely, when defibrillating, the mode must be asynchronous because lack of identifiable QRS complex prevents a defibrillator in the synchronous mode from discharging.

6. **Delivery of shock.** Once the patient is adequately prepared, the electrodes are adequately positioned, and the appropriate output and mode are selected, the adequacy of sedation should be reconfirmed. The defibrillator capacitors are charged, the ancillary staff are warned to stay clear of the patient, proper synchronization is reconfirmed, and the appropriate shock is delivered. The patient is immediately assessed for adequacy of airway, breathing, and circulation. The ECG is inspected to confirm rhythm, and if sedation is still adequate, the procedure is repeated if necessary. The patient is monitored until completely recovered (generally 1 hour). Anticoagulation and antiarrhythmic medications (if any) must be addressed before discharge.

V. COMPLICATIONS OF CARDIOVERSION.

Complications after cardioversion are uncommon but include:

A. Embolism. One percent to to 7% of patients in atrial fibrillation not anticoagulated before cardioversion develop arterial embolization after the procedure. In appropriately anticoagulated patients, the incidence of embolism is extremely low. In the Assessment of Cardioversion Using Transesophageal Echocardiography (ACUTE) trial, comparing anticoagulation for 3 weeks before cardioversion to transesophageal echocardiography (TEE)–guided therapy, the incidence of embolism was 0.5% in the conventional arm and 0.8% in the TEE-guided arm. TEE-guided cardioversion is now widely used in patients who require cardioversion urgently, but who have not been adequately anticoagulated for 3 weeks.

B. Arrhythmias. It is not uncommon for patients to have premature atrial contractions or premature ventricular contractions after cardioversion. Although some patients exhibit transient sinus arrest or atrioventricular block, this is usually self-limited. However, ability to provide emergent temporary transthoracic pacing should be available for the rare patient who needs it. Malignant ventricular tachyarrhythmias are rare but may occur if the shock is delivered during the vulnerable period. The risk of malignant tachyarrhythmias is increased in the setting of hypokalemia or digoxin toxicity.

C. Injuries. The incidence and severity of chest wall burns can be reduced by the use of conductive gel, good skin and electrode contact, and use of lowest effective energy output.

D. Airway compromise. Excessive sedation may be associated with respiratory depression. This is more likely in the elderly or in those with hepatic or renal dysfunction. Appropriate adjustment of dose and monitoring of airway and oxygenation until complete recovery will minimize any undue effects of excessive sedation.

E. Myocardial depression. Cardioversion is a safe procedure with a wide margin of safety. Transient ST-segment elevation without apparent myocardial damage and minor elevations in creatine kinase-myocardial band (CK-MB) isoenzyme or in troponin I have been reported in rare instances. Rarely patients have developed pulmonary edema after direct-current cardioversion.

F. Injuries to the operator. Injuries to the operator are rare, with an incidence of less than 1 in 1,700 in one series. Most are minor electrical injuries and manifest as extremity paresthesias. Major electrocution is extremely rare, and the reported cases have all been associated with equipment malfunction. Cardioversion in the presence of wet skin or nitroglycerin ointment can lead to arcing and may present a fire hazard.

VI. TROUBLESHOOTING

A. Monitor does not work. This is usually related to a mechanical problem. The power source, lead connections, and monitor lead electrode patches should be checked.

B. Timing artifact falls on T wave. Monitoring lead should be changed and the correct position of the timing artifact confirmed prior to cardioversion.

C. Capacitor does not discharge. When operating in the synchronized mode, the capacitor will not discharge until it recognizes a synchronized QRS. The switch should be pressed until the capacitor discharges. If this method fails, the monitoring lead should be changed and cardioversion attempted again.

D. Cardioversion unsuccessful

1. The first step should be to repeat the ECG to check the underlying rhythm to confirm diagnosis and to differentiate between failure to cardiovert and successful cardioversion that is followed by recurrence of the presenting arrhythmia.
2. For patients who truly fail to cardiovert, a higher energy level may be considered for a repeat attempt. A biphasic device should be used if available and all possible measures to reduce impedance applied (IV.B.4.b).
3. Unsuccessful cardioversion may be secondary to a deranged metabolic milieu, and reversible causes (such as electrolyte imbalance or thyrotoxicosis) should be corrected.
4. Patients who are on amiodarone long-term may present with atrial fibrillation as the first manifestation of amiodarone-induced hyperthyroidism, which may in turn make cardioversion more difficult.
5. In resistant cases where a biphasic device is unavailable, reversing the polarity of the electrodes with cardioversion at maximal energy, using two defibrillators to increase current, or internal cardioversion may be an option.

6. Use of appropriate antiarrhythmic drugs may facilitate cardioversion and maintenance of sinus rhythm, and the procedure may be repeated after loading with appropriate drugs. Pretreatment with 1 mg ibutilide has been shown to increase the likelihood of successful cardioversion. Ibutilide administration has been associated with the development of torsade de pointes. At our institution, patients pretreated with ibutilide are also given 1 g of IV magnesium sulfate in order to minimize this risk.
7. Predictors of unsuccessful cardioversion in chronic atrial fibrillation include long duration of atrial fibrillation, underlying structural heart disease, left atrial enlargement, and cardiomegaly.

VII. SPECIAL SITUATIONS

A. Preexisting permanent pacemaker or implantable cardioverter–defibrillator. Electric current can conduct along the implanted electrode lead and cause myocardial injury. This may manifest as a temporary or permanent increase in stimulation threshold, and, when pronounced, this may manifest as failure of capture-exit block. This can be avoided by **positioning electrodes away from the device**; therefore, the anteroposterior position is preferred. The device should be interrogated before and after cardioversion.

B. Pregnancy. Successful cardioversion has been carried out in all trimesters of pregnancy without ill effects to the mother or the fetus.

VIII. AUTOMATIC EXTERNAL DEFIBRILLATORS. The automatic external defibrillator (AED) is a battery-operated microprocessor-based defibrillator that identifies tachyarrhythmias and, upon activation, delivers a shock to terminate them. This device is designed for use on an unresponsive patient with cardiac arrest. The system includes external self-adhesive pads that are applied on the victim, after which the device is switched on and cardiopulmonary resuscitation temporarily discontinued. The device analyzes the rhythm and advises the operator to press a switch to deliver a nonsynchronized shock, reanalyzes the resulting rhythm, and advises further delivery of shock if indicated. These devices are easy to use and designed to be used in the field by lay people. In various studies the sensitivity and specificity of detection and success of termination of ventricular fibrillation and ventricular tachycardia has been greater than 90%, with a significant reduction in the response time for the first shock.

ACKNOWLEDGMENTS

The authors thank Drs. Hitinder S. Gurm and Robert A. Schweikert for their contributions to earlier editions of this chapter.

Landmark Articles

Bjerkelund CJ, Orning OM. The efficacy of anticoagulant therapy in preventing embolism related to D.C. electrical conversion of atrial fibrillation. *Am J Cardiol* 1969;23: 208–216.

Gall NP, Murgatroyd FD. Electrical cardioversion for AF-the state of the art. *Pacing Clin Electrophysiol* 2007;30:554–567.

Klein AL, Grimm RA, Murray RD, et al. Use of transesophageal echocardiography to guide cardioversion in patients with atrial fibrillation. *N Engl J Med* 2001;344:1411–1420.

Lown B, Amarasingham R, Neuman J. New method for terminating cardiac arrhythmias: use of synchronised capacitor discharge. *JAMA* 1962;182:548–555.

Mittal S, Ayati S, Stein KM, et al. Transthoracic cardioversion of atrial fibrillation: comparison of rectilinear biphasic versus damped sine wave monophasic shocks. *Circulation* 2000;101:1282–1287.

Mittal S, Stein KM, Markowitz SM, et al. An update on electrical cardioversion of atrial fibrillation. *Card Electrophysiol Rev* 2003;7:285–289.

Oral H, Souza J, Michaud G, et al. Facilitation transthoracic cardioversion of atrial fibrillation with ibutilide pretreatment. *N Engl J Med* 1999; 340:1849–1854.

Book Chapters

Miller JM, Zipes DP. Therapy for cardiac arrhythmias. In: Zipes DP, Libby P, Bonow RO, et al., eds. *Braunwald's heart disease: a textbook of cardiovascular medicine,* 8th ed. Saunders-Elsevier: Philadelphia, 2008:801–803.

Walcott G, Ideker R. Principles of defibrillation: from cellular physiology to fields and waveforms. In: Ellenbogen KA, Kay, GN, Lau C, eds. *Clinical cardiac pacing, defibrillation, and reshynchronization therapy*, 3rd ed. Philadelphia, PA: Saunders-Elsevier, 2007:59–74.

56 ENDOMYOCARDIAL BIOPSY

Wilfried Mullens and Zuheir Abrahams

I. INDICATIONS AND CONTRAINDICATIONS. Use of endomyocardial biopsy (EMB) as a diagnostic tool for patients with systolic or diastolic dysfunction has decreased during the last 5 years with the introduction of more advanced noninvasive imaging techniques such as magnetic resonance imaging (MRI). The major indication for EMB nowadays is monitoring for allograft rejection after cardiac transplantation, as well as ruling out some potentially treatable forms of myocarditis. The role for this procedure in other disorders, such as arrhythmogenic right ventricular dysplasia, remains controversial because the diagnostic accuracy must be considered in relation to the lack of proven effective therapy. Potential indications and contraindications for EMB are listed in Tables 56.1, 56.2, and 56.3.

II. PATIENT PREPARATION. As with any other procedure, extensive patient education and informed consent are necessary before starting the procedure. Patients undergoing EMB have to be aware that there is a very small chance (less than 1% in experienced hands) of cardiac perforation, with potential urgent cardiovascular surgery and even death as a consequence.

Sedation is seldom needed but might help more anxious patients better tolerate the procedure. Monitoring of heart rate by continuous electrocardiographic registration, blood pressure (noninvasively), and pulse oximetry are needed throughout the procedure. Monitoring the patient for a couple of hours after the procedure is essential, as evidence for myocardial perforation with subsequent pericardial effusion might only become apparent some time after the EMB. The patient is always positioned flat regardless of the venous approach. Venous access may be obtained through the internal jugular (most common), subclavian, or femoral veins. Use of an ultrasound or different maneuvers to increase central venous pressure such as Valsalva, leg elevation with a wedge, and Trendelenburg position can be helpful in obtaining venous access. Most centers use fluoroscopy as the imaging method of choice to guide the EMB. However, echocardiography can also be used, particularly when radiation exposure needs to be minimized, such as in pregnant women.

III. DEVICES

A. Sheath. Venous access is obtained using the Seldinger technique, and the sheath is always placed with the help of a guidewire so as not to damage any cardiovascular structures. A standard short sheath (11-cm, 7F or 8F) is generally sufficient for the right internal jugular or any subclavian approach. The intermediate length sheath (24 or 35 cm) may be helpfull to straighten venous angulations or to avoid damaging the vessel wall or a suture line in case of a heart transplantation when inserting the bioptome. For the left internal jugular approach, a longer sheath (40 cm, 7F) is used with a single- or double-curved tip according to the operators preference and the venous and cardiac anatomy. For a femoral approach, a curved 7F, 85-cm-long transseptal sheath is used, as it can be easily positioned into the right ventricle.

B. Bioptome. There are two basic types of bioptomes: (1) independent and stiff, which does not require a long sheath but does rely on the operator's skills to be maneuvered safely into the right ventricle; and (2) flexible, which requires a longer sheath advanced into the right ventricle for positioning. Resterilizable and reusable bioptomes are widely used, but disposable bioptomes are also available. For internal jugular and subclavian approaches, 50-cm-long bioptomes are used, whereas for femoral access, the bioptomes used are longer (up to 105 cm).

TABLE 56.1 Common Indications for Endomyocardial Biopsy

Clinical scenarios	Class of recommendation
New-onset heart failure of <2 weeks duration associated with a normal-sized or dilated left ventricle and hemodynamic compromise	I
New-onset heart failure of 2 weeks to 3 months duration associated with a dilated left ventricle and new ventricular arrhythmias, 2nd or 3rd heart block, or failure to respond to usual care within 1 to 2 weeks	I
Heart failure of >3 months duration associated with a dilated left ventricle and new ventricular arrhythmias, 2nd or 3rd degree heart block, or failure to respond to usual care within 1 to 2 weeks	IIa
Heart failure associated with a DCM of any duration associated with suspected allergic reaction and/or eosinophilia	IIa
Heart failure associated with suspected anthracycline cardiomyopathy	IIa
Heart failure associated with unexplained restrictive cardiomyopathy	IIa
Suspected cardiac tumors	IIa
Unexplained cardiomyopathy in children	IIa

DCM, dilated cardiomyopathy.
Adapted from AHA/ACC/ESC 2007 Consensus Statement.

TABLE 56.2 Conditions Involving the Heart in which Endomyocardial Biopsy Can Establish the Diagnosis, Listed According to the Presence or Absence of Proven Effective Therapy

Treatable conditions	Less treatable conditions
Cardiac allograft rejection	Myocarditis (non–giant cell)
Cardiac amyloidosis	Arrhythmogenic right ventricular dysplasia
Giant cell myocarditis	Glycogen storage disease
Hypereosinophilic syndrome	Rheumatic carditis
Staging of anthracycline toxicity	Chagas disease
Cardiac sarcoidosis	
Cardiac hemochromatosis	
Lyme carditis	
Fabry's disease	

TABLE 56.3 Relative Contraindications for Endomyocardial Biopsy

- Informed consent not obtained
- Patient not cooperative (confused, agitated, etc.)
- Profound hemodynamic compromise
- No cardiac surgery back-up available
- Coagulopathy (INR >1.5)
- Mechanical tricuspid prosthesis
- Significant right-to-left shunt (risk of air embolus)
- Thinning of myocardium after MI or in case of ARVD
- RA or RV thrombus

ARVD, arrhythmogenic right ventricular dysplasia; INR, international normalized ratio; MI, myocardial infarction; RA, right atrial; RV, right ventricular.

IV. TECHNIQUE. Right ventricular endomyocardial biopsies can be performed from either right or left internal jugular, subclavian, or femoral veins. If necessary, a left ventricular endomyocardial biopsy can be obtained via the femoral artery approach, although this is rarely necessary.

A. Right ventricular biopsy

1. **Internal jugular vein approach.** After standard preparation and local anesthesia, the required anatomic landmarks (see Chapter 53) are identified. A vein-localizing pilot puncture is sometimes made with a 22-gauge needle. Following the same directions, the internal jugular vein is punctured with the larger-bore 18-gauge (Cook) needle, and the sheath is introduced using standard technique. The bioptome, with jaws closed and tip straightened, is advanced under fluoroscopic or echocardiographic guidance across the atrial suture line (in allografts) until its tip lies against the lower third of the lateral right atrial wall. It is then rotated gently counterclockwise and simultaneously advanced into the right ventricular cavity. During this procedure, the tip is gently unstraightened. Rotation is continued until the catheter reaches the apical half of the right ventricle and the handle clamp points in the posterior direction. At this point, the tip of the bioptome rests on the interventricular septum. The position is confirmed by lack of further advancement, generation of premature ventricular contractions, and fluoroscopic findings. Generation of premature atrial contractions or absence of ventricular ectopy may indicate that the bioptome was advanced in the right atrium or in the coronary sinus. If there is any doubt about the position, the bioptome is withdrawn and the process repeated. Once in the desired position, the bioptome is withdrawn about 0.5 to 1 cm and advanced again after the jaws have been opened. When it touches the endocardium, the jaws are closed and the bioptome is gently withdrawn with its jaws closed under continous fluoroscopic guidance. A small tug is often felt while withdrawing, but excessive tugging and multiple premature ventricular contractions should prompt consideration of repositioning. Usually four to six biopsy specimens are obtained in different areas of the septum to reduce sampling error. Once the procedure is completed, the venous sheath is removed and hemostasis achieved. Patients are observed for about 2 to 4 hours before discharge to home.
2. **Femoral vein approach.** After standard preparation and local anesthesia, the required anatomic landmarks (see Chapter 52) are identified. The right (more common) or the left femoral vein is punctured with a 18-gauge (Cook) needle and a 0.038-inch guidewire is advanced up to the right atrium. A long (85-cm) 7F sheath with dilator is advanced over the wire, and on entering right atrium the dilator is withdrawn. The tricuspid valve is crossed with the help of the guidewire (a balloon-tipped catheter can also be used), and the sheath is advanced into the right ventricle. The pressure tracing, occurrence of ventricular ectopy, as well as fluoroscopy are used to confirm position pointing to the interventricular septum. The side port of the sheath may be connected to a slow continuous intravenous infusion to prevent clot formation inside the sheath, especially if a long procedure is anticipated. A long nonsteerable bioptome is advanced through the sheath and is used to acquire samples. Biopsies are taken in a manner similar to that of the internal jugular vein approach.
3. **Subclavian vein approach.** After standard preparation and local anesthesia, the required anatomic landmarks (see Chapter 52) are identified. The subclavian vein is punctured using an 18-gauge (Cook) needle followed by insertion of the sheath. The occurrence of ventricular ectopy and fluoroscopic images are used to confirm a position pointing toward the interventricular septum. Biopsies are taken as with the internal jugular vein approach.

B. Left ventricular biopsy

1. **Femoral arterial approach.** After standard preparation and local anesthesia, the required anatomic landmarks are identified. The right (more common) or left femoral artery is punctured with an 18-gauge (Cook) needle, and a short

8F sheath is inserted while a 0.035-inch exchange long guidewire is advanced up to the ascending aorta. A regular-length 7F pigtail catheter is advanced over the wire, and the aortic valve is crossed in the conventional manner. Afterward, the pigtail catheter is removed, while leaving the guidewire in the left ventricle, and exchanged with an 8F long, curved guiding sheath. The tip of this sheath is directed toward the interventricular septum, distal to the mitral apparatus, away from the thinner posterobasal wall. The position of the sheath is carefully reconfirmed (fluoroscopic images in two angulations and pressure tracings), and 5000 U heparin is given intravenously before insertion of the bioptome. A long, nonsteerable bioptome is then advanced through the guiding sheath, and biopsy samples are collected as with right ventricular biopsy. It is important to note that catheters must be aspirated and flushed after each biopsy, since air can enter the sheath and clots can form in the sheath after removing the bioptome. Heparin is not reversed with protamine at the end of the procedure as it is thought to minimize thrombus formation at the biopsy sites.

V. COMPLICATIONS. In general, EMB can be performed more safely in heart transplant recipients than in patients with native hearts, because of the scarred and thickened pericardium in transplanted patients.

A. Mortality. Procedure-related deaths have been reported to be less than 0.05% in contemporary series.

B. Cardiac perforation and tamponade. The reported incidence of cardiac perforation is 0.3% to 0.5%, which can rapidly result in tamponade. The risk can be minimized by careful monitoring of catheter position to ensure that biopsies are obtained from the thicker interventricular septum and by gentle catheter advancement and EMB procurement. Symptoms of chest pain during or after the procedure, shortness of breath, a pericardial rub, or altered hemodynamics should suggest potential perforation and should prompt urgent echocardiography to rule out a new pericardial effusion or tamponade. Patients in whom a new pericardial effusion is suspected or detected should be monitored in the hospital for evidence of increasing pericardial effusion or tamponade, and an echocardiogram should be repeated at intervals as necessary and before discharge.

In patients early after heart transplantation, the atrial suture line also poses a higher risk for perforation. Very gentle advancement of the bioptome (and pulling back if any resistance is felt) and use of a longer sheath to pass the suture line if needed will reduce this risk. Patients with suspected perforation should be closely monitored and echocardiography, fluoroscopy, and cardiac tomography scanning can be used to confirm the diagnosis.

For both complications, careful monitoring is usually sufficient, although pericardiocentesis or even urgent cardiac surgery may be necessary if hemodynamic compromise develops.

C. Thromboembolism. Right-sided thromboembolism during EMB is possible in theory, but does not cause any clinically significant sequelae if it occurs. The risk of arterial embolization during left ventricular EMB is higher, owing to the longer sheath, and may have catastrophic consequences. Using heparin during a left-sided approach, and aspirating air and flushing the sheath before inserting the bioptome minimize the risk of embolism.

D. Arrhythmia. Occasionally a sustained atrial or, less commonly, a ventricular tachycardia is induced by EMB. These arrhythmias are almost always stopped by touching the wall of the right atrium or ventricle with the bioptome. Bradyarrhythmic episodes or bundle-branch block induced by EMB are very rare and respond only to β_1 stimulants and not to atropine in heart transplantation patients.

E. Tricuspid valve (or mitral valve for left ventricular biopsy) dysfunction. The bioptome can damage the chordae or papillary muscle and produce significant valvular regurgitation. The risk of this complication is minimized by careful confirmation of bioptome position before sampling. The cumulative risk of this complication is greater in heart transplantation patients because they undergo many EMB procedures.

F. Damage to vena cava, coronary sinus, hepatic vein, and coronary arteries. Gentle advancement of the bioptome, use of a longer sheath, retraction of bioptome whenever resistance is felt, and position confirmation with multiple fluoroscopic views can minimize these complications. Fistula formation from a coronary artery branch to the right ventricle has occurred following EMB but is of no clinical significance.

G. Local complications. Hematoma, local infection, injury to lung (pneumothorax, incidence 0.9%) and nerve (recurrent laryngeal palsy and Horner's syndrome) are possible but rare while achieving vascular access. Careful identification of anatomic landmarks reduce the risk.

H. Pain. The EMB itself is usually painless, but some patients experience some mild degree of pain when the bioptome touches the heart or when a biospy is taken.

ACKNOWLEDGMENT

The authors would like to thank Dr. Milind Shah for his contributions to earlier editions of this chapter.

Suggested Readings

Baim D, Grossman W. *Grossman's cardiac catheterization, angiography, and intervention,* 7th ed. Baltimore: Williams & Wilkins, 1996:395–412.

Cooper LT, Baughman KL, Feldman AM, et al. The role of endomyocardial biopsy in the management of cardiovascular disease: a scientific statement from the American Heart Association, the American College of Cardiology, and the European Society of Cardiology. *Circulation* 2007;116:2216–2233.

Kern M. *The cardiac catheterization handbook,* 4th ed. St. Louis: Mosby, 2003:421–428.

57 INTRAAORTIC BALLOON COUNTERPULSATION

Apur R. Kamdar

I. INTRODUCTION. Intraaortic balloon counterpulsation (IABC) is usually used to **support hemodynamics** in cardiogenic shock and to **relieve medically refractory ischemia** in patients with severe coronary disease. The duration of support with an intraaortic balloon pump (IABP) is typically short (2–3 days), because multiple complications can develop in patients treated with IABC. Therefore, patients considered for IABC should be carefully selected and should be closely monitored in a critical care setting while the IABP is in place.

II. INDICATIONS

A. Cardiogenic shock

1. Bridge to revascularization. IABC provides temporary hemodynamic stabilization for patients with cardiogenic shock caused by acute myocardial infarction (MI). Hospital survival rates for cardiogenic shock with balloon pump support alone without revascularization are poor (5% to 20%). Early revascularization with percutaneous transluminal coronary angioplasty (PTCA) improves survival rates in cardiogenic shock caused by acute MI.

a. In the **Global Utilization of Streptokinase and Tissue Plasminogen Activator for Occluded Coronary Arteries (GUSTO I)** trial comparing fibrinolytic regimens for acute ST elevation MI, PTCA was the only factor associated with a lower 30-day mortality rate in 2972 patients with cardiogenic shock.

b. In addition, early placement of an IABP in this cohort of patients was associated with lower 30-day and 1-year mortality rates.

c. Cardiogenic shock and hemodynamic support during or after PCI are the primary reasons for IABP placement in more than half of all patients treated with IABC. IABP placement is a **ACC/AHA class I** recommendation in patients with STEMI presenting with cardiogenic shock when shock is not quickly reversed with pharmacologic therapy. The IABP in this setting is a stabilizing measure for angiography and prompt revascularization.

2. Bridge to a tertiary center. Thrombolytic therapy alone in patients with cardiogenic shock is less successful than mechanical reperfusion. However, the addition of IABC to thrombolysis can improve outcomes in patients with cardiogenic shock. In 46 patients with acute MI and cardiogenic shock treated at community hospitals without angioplasty capabilities, simultaneous treatment with thrombolysis and IABC was associated with an improved 1-year survival rate (67% vs. 32%) and successful transfer to a tertiary facility for revascularization when thrombolysis failed.

B. Acute MI catheter-based reperfusion. The **benefits** of IABC for patients with acute MI without cardiogenic shock treated with catheter-based reperfusion are **uncertain.**

1. In a randomized trial of 182 hemodynamically stable patients who underwent direct PTCA for acute MI, prophylactic IABC for 2 days after the procedure reduced recurrent ischemia and reocclusion of the infarct-related artery but had no effect on survival or reinfarction.

2. In the **Primary Angioplasty in Myocardial Infarction II (PAMI II)** trial, 437 high-risk patients (age greater than 70 years, multivessel coronary disease, reduced ejection fraction, vein graft disease, or persistent ventricular arrhythmias) treated with direct PTCA for acute MI were randomized to ±1 to 2 days of IABC after PTCA. Patients treated with IABC had a slight reduction in recurrent ischemia but had no reduction in mortality, reinfarction, or infarct-related artery reocclusion. Thus, hemodynamically stable patients with acute MI treated with catheter-based reperfusion are not likely to benefit from IABP support after the intervention.

C. High-risk percutaneous revascularization. Patients at high risk for complications during percutaneous revascularization include those with unprotected left main coronary disease, left ventricular dysfunction (ejection fraction less than 40%), the target vessel supplying more than 40% of the myocardial territory, or severe congestive heart failure (CHF). Placement of an IABP in these high-risk patients affords the operator a longer duration of ischemia during balloon inflation before CHF and hypotension may develop.

1. In a study of 219 patients undergoing unprotected left main trunk stenting, elective IABP placement was associated with fewer intraprocedural major adverse cardiac events, including combined endpoints of severe hypotension, MI, need for urgent bypass surgery, and death.

2. Although there are no specific recommendations for when to use IABC during high-risk coronary interventions, improved percutaneous revascularization techniques with coronary stents and adjunctive glycoprotein IIb/IIIa receptor antagonists have reduced the need for prophylactic IABP placement in high-risk patients.

D. Mechanical complications of acute MI. Acute mitral regurgitation (MR) and **ventricular septal defect** are devastating complications of acute MI and frequently cause rapid deterioration progressing to cardiogenic shock. An IABP should be placed before surgical repair in patients with hemodynamically significant MR or ventricular septal defect after an MI. Placement of an IABP in the setting of STEMI and secondary acute mitral valve regurgitation is an **ACC/AHA class I** indication. Similarly, insertion of an IABP and prompt surgical referral are **class I** recommendations.

E. Refractory unstable angina. Patients with severe coronary disease who have refractory ischemia or hemodynamic instability show **dramatic improvement** when IABC is used before revascularization. The ACC/AHA clinical guidelines assign a **class I** recommendation in STEMI patients and a **class IIa** recommendation in UA/NSTEMI patients for IABP placement in patients with severe ischemia that is continuingor recurs frequentlydespite intensive medical therapy. In the setting of STEMI, refractory pulmonary congestion carries a **class IIb** recommendation for IABP placement.

F. Weaning from cardiopulmonary bypass/postoperative pump failure. Patients with severe left ventricular dysfunction or those with prolonged runs on cardiopulmonary bypass can be difficult to wean from bypass after open heart surgery because of stunned myocardium from prolonged cardioplegic arrest. For these patients, IABP support improves hemodynamics and facilitates weaning from cardiopulmonary bypass.

G. End-stage cardiomyopathy/bridge to cardiac transplantation. An IABP improves cardiac output and lowers filling pressures in patients with dilated and ischemic cardiomyopathy. It can be used for hemodynamic support before cardiac transplantation.

1. **Disadvantages** of prolonged IABP support in patients awaiting cardiac transplantation include a high risk of infection and the need for continuous bed rest.
2. However, with improved inotropic therapy and implantable left ventricular assist devices for patients awaiting cardiac transplantation, IABC is now used infrequently for prolonged mechanical support in patients with end-stage cardiomyopathy.

H. Refractory ventricular arrhythmias. Incessant ventricular tachycardia compromises left ventricular filling, reduces stroke volume, and causes or exacerbates ischemia. IABC improved hemodynamics, lessened ischemia, and controlled refractory ventricular arrhythmias in 86% of patients in a large case series. Placement of IABP support in patients with STEMI and refractory polymorphic VT carries an **ACC/AHA class IIa** recommendation.

I. Support during noncardiac surgery. Patients with severe coronary disease, recent MI, and severe left ventricular dysfunction are at high risk for cardiac complications when they undergo noncardiac surgery. Case reports have demonstrated that high-risk patients are stabilized hemodynamically and have acceptable postoperative outcomes when prophylactic IABP support is used during and after noncardiac surgical procedures.

J. Decompensated aortic stenosis can be managed with temporary IABP support to improve the stroke volume and reduce the transvalvular gradient before aortic valve replacement. However, because aortic insufficiency often accompanies severe aortic stenosis, careful monitoring early after initiation of IABC is recommended to ensure that aortic insufficiency is not worsened by the balloon pump.

III. CONTRAINDICATIONS

A. Aortic dissection. Any type of aortic dissection precludes IABP use because of the potential of the balloon catheter to extend the dissection and to worsen ischemia of a peripheral vascular bed that may be involved by the dissection.

B. Abdominal or thoracic aneurysm. Using IABP with an abdominal or thoracic aneurysm can precipitate an acute aortic dissection, dislodgement of atheroemboli, or aortic rupture, so the presence of an aneurysm is a contraindication to IABP use.

C. Severe peripheral vascular disease

1. The majority of the complications of IABC are caused by vascular insufficiency in the accessed leg because of the **large size of the balloon sheath and catheter and the concomitant presence of peripheral vascular disease** in patients who typically need IABC. The IABP catheters are commonly available in two sizes, 8F and 9.5F, and the corresponding sheaths are 8F and 9.5F. Recently, 7F and 7.5F catheters have been introduced and may be associated with less obstruction of arterial flow in patients with peripheral vascular disease or small arteries.

2. **Limb ischemia and threatened limb viability** can occur when peripheral perfusion is compromised by the balloon catheter and sheath. The IABP catheter can be inserted without a sheath to reduce the diameter of obstruction in the iliac vessels, but in patients with tortuous aortoiliac vessels, sheathless IABP insertion can be difficult (see V.C).
3. Thus, severe peripheral vascular disease is a contraindication to IABP insertion, depending on the necessity of IABP support and the degree of vascular compromise.

D. Descending aortic and peripheral vascular grafts

1. **Prosthetic descending aortic grafts and iliofemoral vascular grafts** are relative contraindications to IABC. Consultation with a vascular surgeon is recommended before attempting balloon pump insertion in these patients.
2. **Iliac artery stents** are not an absolute contraindication to IABP placement. However, passage of the guidewire and balloon catheter through the stent must be performed under direct fluoroscopic guidance.

E. Coagulopathy or contraindication to heparin

1. The balloon catheter is thrombogenic, and intravenous heparin is commonly given while the IABP is in place to prevent the development of thrombi on the balloon surface. Patients with a contraindication to heparin, such as those with prior heparin-induced thrombocytopenia, can be **anticoagulated with alternative agents** such as direct thrombin inhibitors like bivalirudin.
2. After cardiac surgery, heparin can be avoided because of the increased risk of intrathoracic bleeding, but IABP support in such patients is usually of short duration. In nonsurgical patients, if an anticoagulant cannot be given or if a severe coagulopathy exists that could precipitate bleeding at the access site, IABC is discouraged but could safely be undertaken for a short period.

F. Moderate to severe aortic insufficiency. By inflating during diastole, the IABP can worsen aortic insufficiency when blood is displaced to the proximal aorta. No consensus exists as to what degree of aortic insufficiency absolutely contraindicates IABP use. Therefore, **careful monitoring** of patients with aortic insufficiency who absolutely need IABP support is recommended.

IV. HEMODYNAMICS OF BALLOON PUMP FUNCTION

A. Decreased afterload

1. As systole begins, the intraaortic balloon rapidly deflates and creates negative pressure in the aorta, which reduces afterload and improves forward flow from the left ventricle. Afterload reduction occurs because the aortic end-diastolic pressure is reduced, resulting in an increase in cardiac output of approximately 20% and a decrease in the mean pulmonary capillary wedge pressure of approximately 20%.
2. The **overall hemodynamic benefit** of IABP appears to be a reduction in left ventricular wall stress from decreased filling pressures and decreased afterload, which in turn improves stroke volume and cardiac output (see Figs. 57.1 and 57.2).

B. Augmented coronary perfusion

1. When the balloon inflates during diastole, it displaces blood to the proximal aorta and augments aortic diastolic pressure and, thus, coronary perfusion pressure. The augmentation of coronary perfusion pressure is more dramatic when systemic hypotension is present (see Figs. 57.1 and 57.2).
2. Doppler flow studies have demonstrated that peak coronary flow velocity is increased with IABP support, but there is no improvement in coronary flow past critical coronary stenoses (unless the obstructions are first relieved with percutaneous revascularization). Also, collateral coronary flow does not increase with IABP support. Thus, with severe, nonrevascularized coronary disease, IABP relieves ischemia more through decreased left ventricular wall stress and decreased myocardial oxygen demand than through increased coronary perfusion.

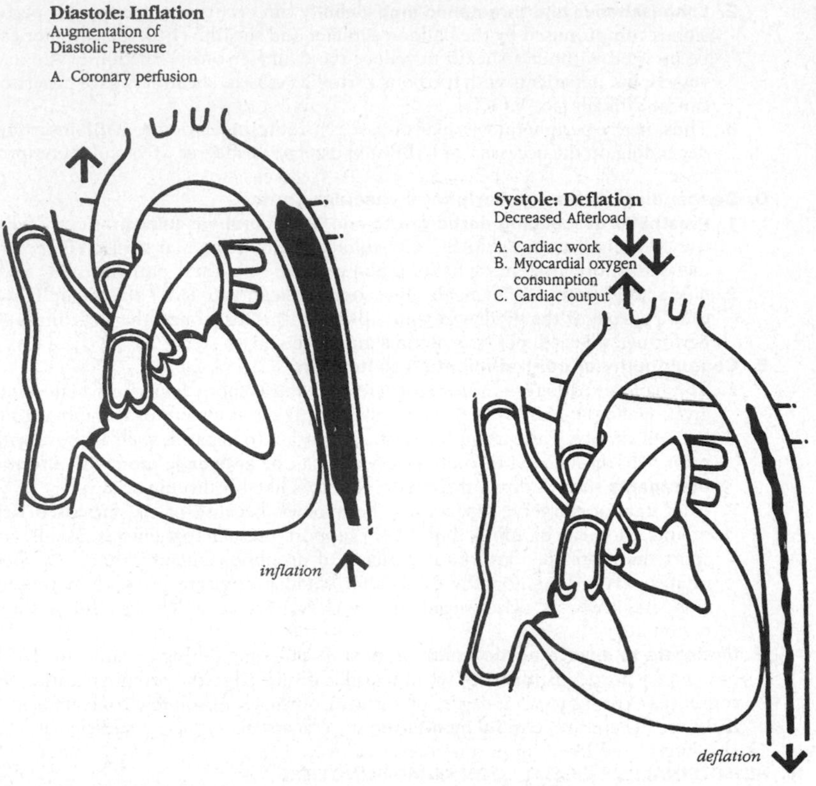

Diastole: Inflation
Augmentation of Diastolic Pressure
A. Coronary perfusion

inflation

Systole: Deflation
Decreased Afterload
A. Cardiac work
B. Myocardial oxygen consumption
C. Cardiac output

deflation

Figure 57.1. By inflating during diastole, the intraaortic balloon pump increases coronary perfusion. Deflation of the balloon at the onset of systole decreases myocardial wall stress and oxygen demand and increases cardiac output. (Courtesy of Datascope Corp.)

V. INSERTION TECHNIQUE/PATIENT EVALUATION AND MONITORING

A. Balloon sizing is based on the patient's height. Four common balloon sizes are available: 50 cm^3 for patients taller than 6 ft; 40 cm^3 for patients between 5 ft 4 inch and 6 ft; 34 cm^3 for patients between 5 ft and 5 ft 4 inch; and 25 cm^3 for patients shorter than 5 ft. Balloon length and diameter increases with each larger size. The 40-cm^3 balloon is most commonly used, whereas the 50-cm^3 balloon is rarely used because the balloon is too long for most patients.

B. Evaluating peripheral vasculature. Proximal and distal pulses are assessed in both legs, and ankle/brachial indices can also be determined. The leg with the strongest pulses and/or the best ankle/brachial index score should be chosen for access.

C. Insertion technique

1. Gaining access/sheath insertion. After careful evaluation of clotting parameters and peripheral vasculature, the leg chosen for access should be shaved and prepped with antiseptic solution from the umbilicus to the knee. After infiltration with a local anesthetic, the femoral artery is accessed with an 18-gauge introducer needle, and a 0.030-inch × 145-cm J-tipped guidewire is advanced through the needle to the aortic arch under **fluoroscopic guidance.** A smaller 5F dilator is first inserted over the wire to dilate the subcutaneous tissues. Then the sheath, loaded with a larger dilator that is 1F smaller than the sheath, is

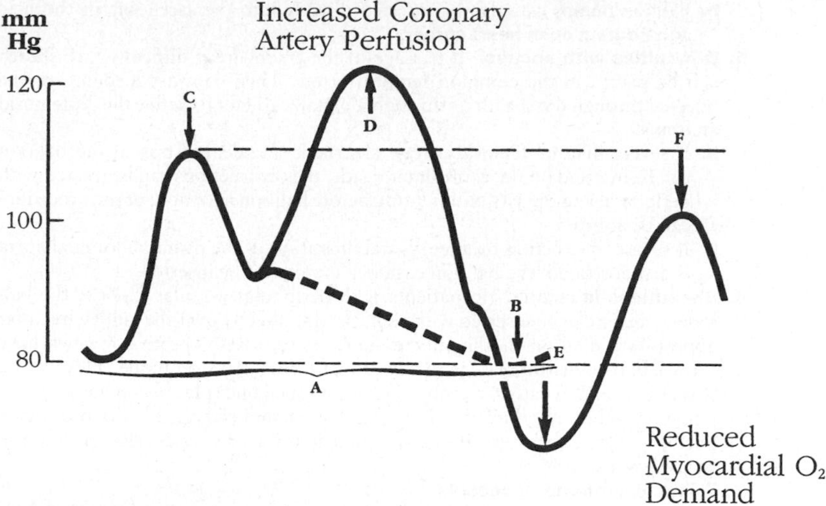

A. One Complete Cardiac Cycle
B. Unassisted Aortic End Diastolic Pressure
C. Unassisted Systolic Pressure
D. Diastolic Augmentation
E. Assisted Aortic End Diastolic Pressure
F. Reduced Systolic Pressure

Figure 57.2. Proper timing of balloon function occurs when the balloon inflates on the downslope of the systolic pressure waveform and deflates before the onset of the next systolic waveform. The intraaortic balloon pump inflation in diastole increases diastolic pressure to improve coronary artery perfusion and to increase mean arterial pressure. In addition, aortic end-diastolic pressure is reduced when the balloon deflates in end-diastole to lower afterload and myocardial oxygen demand. (Courtesy of Datascope Corp.)

inserted over the guidewire. The guidewire should be left in place in the aortic arch.

2. **Balloon insertion.** The two balloon catheter sizes commonly available are 8F and 9.5F. A 7F and 7.5F size catheter and sheath have become available recently, but use has been limited. The most common sheath used is 8F, with an 8F balloon. The prewrapped balloon is inserted over the guidewire and is advanced until the proximal tip is positioned 1 cm below the left subclavian artery and 2 cm above the carina. The guidewire is then removed, and the distal tip of the balloon is visualized under fluoroscopic guidance to ensure that it is out of the sheath.
3. **Insertion without fluoroscopy.** Fluoroscopic guidance is recommended for placement of the IABP. However, if fluoroscopy is unavailable, the distance from the angle of Louis to the umbilicus and then to the common femoral artery insertion site is measured to determine the approximate distance the balloon must be advanced.
4. **Surgical insertion**
   a. Occasionally, balloon pumps can be inserted surgically **by directly exposing the common femoral artery** or by suturing a 6- to 12-mm prosthetic graft end-to-side to the femoral artery to provide a conduit for the catheter. Distal limb ischemia is reduced with these methods, but grafts must be removed surgically, and the femoral artery has to be directly repaired after IABP removal when surgical access is used.

b. Balloon pumps can also be inserted directly into the ascending or thoracic aorta **during open heart surgery.**

5. **Difficulties with access.** If passage of the guidewire is difficult, a 5F sheath can be placed in the common femoral artery. Then contrast medium can be injected through the sheath or through a pigtail catheter to define the iliofemoral anatomy.
   a. If severe iliac or femoral artery obstruction is demonstrated, the balloon can be inserted on the contralateral side, the obstructions can be treated with peripheral angioplasty and stenting before balloon insertion, or the procedure can be aborted.
   b. If severe obstruction or aneurysmal dilatation of the distal abdominal aorta is demonstrated, the balloon catheter should not be inserted.
6. **Sheathless insertion.** In patients with peripheral vascular disease, the balloon catheter can be inserted without a sheath, directly over the guidewire, after appropriate dilation of the subcutaneous tissue. Retrospective reviews have shown that lower-limb ischemia is reduced with this technique. However, a sheathless balloon catheter cannot be repositioned once placed and has a greater potential to become infected from skin flora than a sheathed balloon catheter. Smaller balloon catheters and stiffer guidewires are being developed to aid in sheathless insertion.
7. **Tortuous iliofemoral vessels**
   a. When the tortuosity of the iliofemoral vessels prevents passage of the 0.030-inch guidewire supplied in the IABP kit, a 0.035-inch Wholey wire can be used to traverse the tortuous vessels. A long (45 or 60 cm) flexible sheath is then placed in the descending aorta past the tortuous iliac vessels.
   b. A superstiff 0.038-inch wire is then exchanged through the sheath. The 11-inch IABP sheath is inserted over the superstiff wire, which provides more support for placement of the less flexible IABP sheath. The superstiff wire is then exchanged for the 0.030-inch standard IABP wire through the sheath, and the balloon catheter is inserted over this wire into the proper position.

D. **Initial setup**
1. After insertion, the helium gas line of the balloon catheter is connected to the IABP console, and the central lumen of the catheter is attached to an arterial pressure monitor device on the console with pressure tubing, after allowing the line to back-bleed.
2. Balloon autoinflation is initiated from the console, the arterial line attached to the central lumen of the catheter is flushed, and the initial IABP inflation is at 1:2 (per cardiac cycle) while the timing is adjusted (VI).
3. Balloon inflation is then observed under fluoroscopic guidance to ensure that the balloon is completely out of the sheath. If the balloon is kinked or is not inflating fully, it should be repositioned by pulling the sheath back a few inches, or it should be manually inflated.
4. Finally, the sheath and balloon catheter are sutured in place, dressed using sterile technique, and the inflation is changed to 1:1.

E. **Monitoring**
1. **A chest x-ray film is immediately obtained after IABP** placement to verify the catheter position, even if fluoroscopic guidance has been used.
2. **Intravenous heparin** is started once the balloon and sheath are secure to maintain the activated partial thromboplastin time (aPTT) at 50 to 70 seconds.
3. **Daily chest x-ray films** are recommended while the IABP is in place so that the physician can check the position of the catheter. If the catheter needs to be repositioned, it can be manipulated through a sterile plastic sleeve placed over the part of the catheter that extrudes from the sheath.
4. Daily hemoglobin and platelet counts are followed to monitor for hemolysis and thrombocytopenia.

F. **Care of the patient with an IABP**
1. All patients with an IABP in place should be observed closely in a **critical care setting. The patient should be kept supine in bed,** and peripheral pulses should

be regularly evaluated for **possible limb ishemia** (dorsalis pedis/posterior tibial pulses should be checked every 6–8 hours and/or with use of Doppler).

2. **The accessed leg should be secured** to prevent inadvertent or involuntary movement by the patient.
3. **Use of prophylactic antibiotics is not recommended** while the IABP is in place.
4. **Blood samples generally should not be obtained from the central lumen of the IABP** because the risk of clotting the lumen is increased, and air or small thrombi can be injected through the central lumen during flushing of the tubing after blood withdrawal.

VI. BALLOON PUMP TRIGGERING AND TIMING

A. Triggering. Balloon pump inflation can be triggered by the surface electrocardiogram (ECG), the arterial pressure waveform, a paced rhythm, or an internal asynchronous mode.

1. Preferably, the surface ECG is used to trigger IABP inflation, which is appropriately delayed after the R wave to begin at the time in the cardiac cycle when the aortic valve closes (dicrotic notch).
2. If the IABP fails to trigger properly from the surface ECG, change the lead being evaluated, check surface electrode placement, or increase the QRS gain on the console monitor.
3. For patients with poor surface electrocardiographic tracings, the balloon can be triggered from the central arterial pressure waveform. Pacing spikes should be used to trigger the balloon in patients who are 100% paced.
4. When the patient is arresting or when the other triggering mechanisms are not working correctly, an internal asynchronous mode can be used to trigger the balloon to inflate at a regular interval.

B. Timing. Ideal balloon pump timing occurs when the balloon inflates on the downslope of the systolic pressure waveform before the dicrotic notch and deflates before the onset of the next systolic pressure waveform (see Fig. 57.2). Timing is usually adjusted manually but can be automatically adjusted by internal algorithms programmed in the console.

1. **Early inflation** (see Fig. 57.3) is inflation of the IABP before aortic valve closure (dicrotic notch).
   - **a.** There is premature closure of the aortic valve with increased afterload, left ventricular wall stress, and myocardial oxygen demand. Stroke volume is decreased.
   - **b.** It is corrected by delaying inflation until after aortic valve closure.

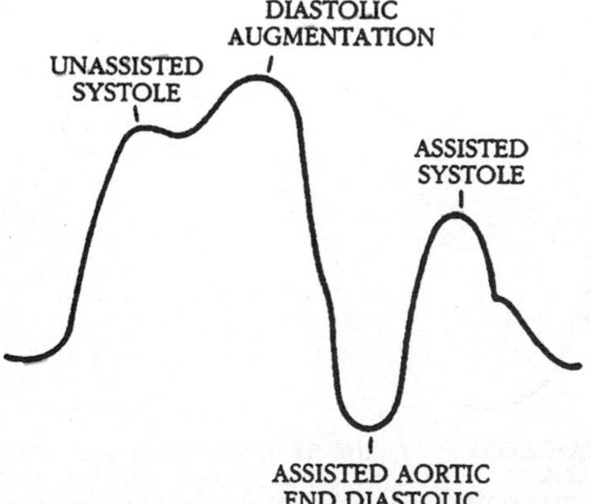

Figure 57.3. With early balloon inflation, the aortic valve closes prematurely, and left ventricular wall stress and myocardial oxygen demand are increased. (Courtesy of Datascope Corp.)

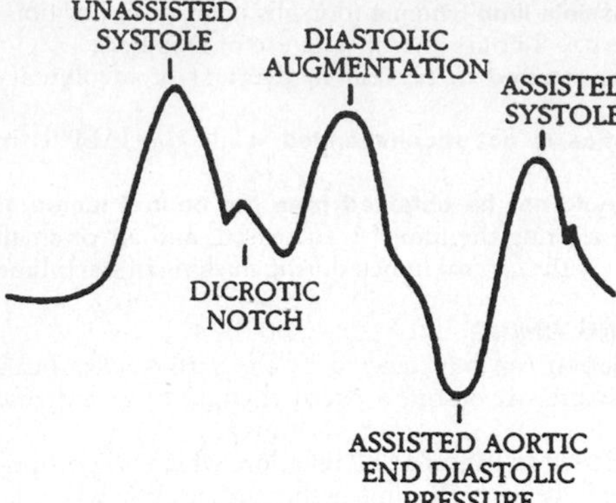

Figure 57.4. With late balloon inflation, there is suboptimal augmentation of diastolic aortic pressure and coronary perfusion. (Courtesy of Datascope Corp.)

2. **Late inflation** (see Fig. 57.4) is inflation of the IABP well after closure of the aortic valve.
   a. There is diminished diastolic pressure augmentation and suboptimal coronary perfusion.
   b. It is corrected by adjusting inflation to occur just before the dicrotic notch.
3. **Early deflation** (see Fig. 57.5) is deflation of the IABP before isovolumic left ventricular contraction.
   a. There is suboptimal diastolic augmentation, coronary perfusion, and afterload reduction, which then causes increased myocardial oxygen demand.
   b. It is corrected by delaying deflation until just before the onset of systole.
4. **Late deflation** (see Fig. 57.6) is deflation of the IABP after the onset of systole.
   a. There is impaired left ventricular emptying, increased afterload and preload, increased myocardial oxygen consumption, and reduced stroke volume.
   b. It is corrected by adjusting deflation to occur just before the onset of systole.
5. **During arrhythmias.** Adequate augmentation with the balloon pump is difficult to achieve with tachyarrhythmias. When heart rates approach 150 beats/min, there is insufficient time for the helium gas to shuttle in and out of the balloon with each inflation. With rapid atrial fibrillation, variable systolic pressure waveforms caused by inadequate left ventricular filling and rapid pulse rates make augmentation especially difficult. Adjusting balloon inflation to 1:2 can sometimes improve augmentation with tachyarrhythmias.

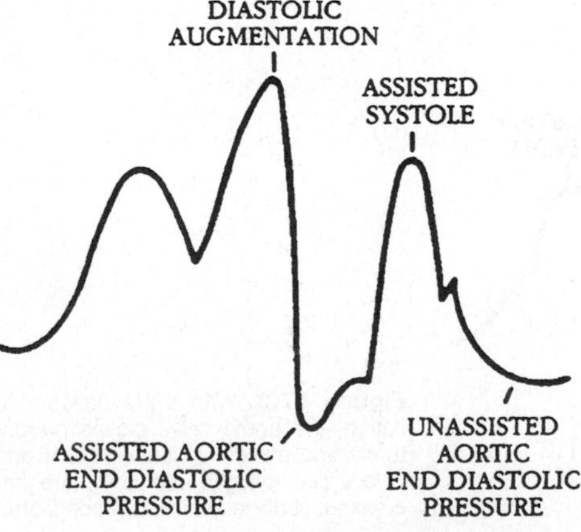

Figure 57.5. With early balloon deflation, there is suboptimal augmentation of coronary perfusion and afterload reduction. (Courtesy of Datascope Corp.)

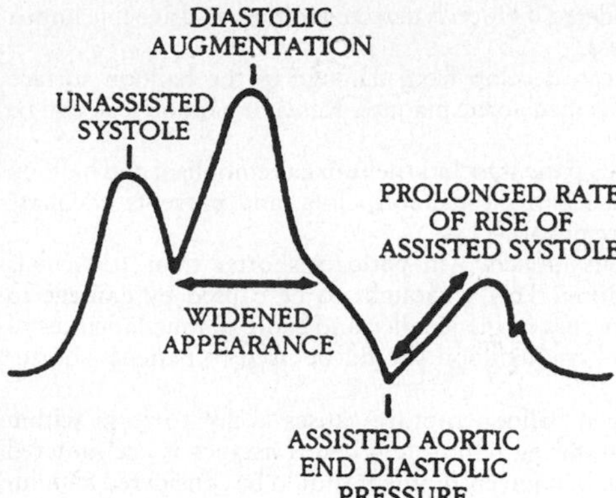

Figure 57.6. With late balloon deflation, there is no afterload reduction, and myocardial oxygen consumption is increased. (Courtesy of Datascope Corp.)

C. Troubleshooting. In the situation of **console alarms,** there may be:

1. **Loose connections** in the gas drive line or arterial pressure tubing.
2. **Blood in the tubing.** If blood is detected in the gas drive lumen, put the balloon catheter on standby and evaluate for balloon rupture or entrapment (VII).
3. **Poor augmentation**
   a. Adjust the timing.
   b. Change the triggering mechanism (VI.A).
   c. Evaluate inflation/deflation of the balloon and the catheter position under fluoroscopic guidance to detect balloon kinking.
   d. If the IABP is thought to be positioned in a false lumen of the aorta because of poor augmentation, 10 to 20 mL of contrast media can be injected through the central lumen of the catheter to evaluate the position under fluoroscopy.

VII. COMPLICATIONS

A. Vascular. Common vascular complications of IABP include limb ischemia, hematoma around the access site, and bleeding from the access site. Rates of vascular complications have varied in the literature from 5% to 20%, depending on the patient populations studied. However, a contemporary series showed the incidence of limb ischemia to be 2.3% and incidence of major limb ischemia to be 0.5% in 5,495 consecutive patients with IABP. Diabetes, female sex, preexisting peripheral vascular disease, history of smoking, and catheter size are all independent risk factors that are strongly associated with the development of ischemic vascular complications from IABP use.

1. **Ischemia**
   a. If ischemia develops in the accessed leg, the balloon catheter and sheath should be removed and hemostasis obtained at the access site.
   b. If ischemia is still present, consultation with a vascular surgeon is indicated. Surgical intervention for ischemic limbs caused by IABP catheters includes thrombectomy, surgical bypass grafting, and, rarely, amputation.
2. **Bleeding**
   a. Bleeding around the access site develops in 1% to 5% of patients treated with IABP. It is usually controlled with prolonged manual pressure at the access site.
   b. Hematomas that develop at the access site may require transfusion of blood products and, occasionally, direct arterial repair.
   c. Pseudoaneurysms after IABP removal are rare but often require surgical correction.

B. Infection. Infectious complications are rare and include access site infections, catheter infections, and bacteremia. No studies have addressed how frequently balloon catheters become infected and how frequently they need to be changed to limit infectious complications.

C. Balloon rupture should be considered if blood is detected in the gas drive line lumen or if balloon augmentation ceases.

1. Small leaks in the balloon can develop from damage to the balloon surface caused by inflation against calcified aortic plaques. Rates of balloon leak can be as high as 4.2%.
2. Potential complications for the patient include helium gas embolism and balloon entrapment when blood leaks into the balloon, clots, and prevents adequate deflation of the balloon for removal.
3. Use of standard-size balloons (40 cm^3) in patients shorter than 170 cm is associated with balloon rupture. This is thought to be caused by damage to the balloon when inflation occurs in the smaller and more plaque-laden distal abdominal aorta. Thus, a 34-cm^3 balloon should be used in patients shorter than 170 cm.

D. Balloon entrapment occurs when balloon rupture causes a clot to form within the balloon to prevent deflation during removal. When resistance is encountered during balloon catheter removal, balloon entrapment should be considered and fluoroscopy immediately carried out to assess the position of the retained catheter.

1. Management of balloon entrapment usually involves surgical extraction because forceful removal of a partially deflated balloon catheter could cause serious vascular injury.
2. Case reports have documented successful lysis of clots within the balloon by instilling thrombolytic agents through the gas drive lumen of the IABP catheter. The balloons were deflated after clot lysis and the catheters successfully removed.

E. Red blood cell and platelet destruction. Due to the shear forces of the balloon catheter, hemolytic anemia and mild thrombocytopenia can occur during IABP support. Daily hemoglobin and platelet values should be checked. Platelet counts less than 50,000 are unlikely to be caused by the IABP, and alternative causes should be sought.

F. Other complications. Rare complications of IABP use include acute renal failure, mesenteric ischemia, and paraplegia from plaque embolization to or thrombosis of the renal, mesenteric, or spinal arteries, respectively. Aortic dissections and aortic perforations, though rare, usually occur during insertion.

VIII. REMOVING THE IABP CATHETER

A. Weaning. Whether IABC needs to be weaned before the balloon catheter is removed depends on multiple factors, including the duration of support, the hemodynamic status of the patient, and left ventricular function.

1. The usual practice is to change IABP inflation to 1:2 for a few hours and then to 1:3 with close hemodynamic monitoring.
2. At the same time, intravenous inotropic drugs are used to simulate the IABP's hemodynamic effects. Dobutamine or milrinone is used to maintain an adequate cardiac output, and nitroprusside is used to replace the afterload reduction provided by the IABP.
3. If weaning is tolerated hemodynamically, the balloon can then be removed.

B. Withdrawal of the balloon catheter and sheath

1. Intravenous heparin should be discontinued for at least 4 hours before removal of the catheter. The activated coagulation time is checked until it falls below 150 seconds.
2. Percutaneously placed catheters can then be removed manually, but surgically placed catheters must be removed with direct arterial repair.
3. To begin removal of the balloon catheter, the balloon is changed to standby and the gas drive line is disconnected. Then, the balloon catheter is pulled back until resistance is met, indicating that the catheter is in the sheath. The sheath and the balloon catheter are then withdrawn together as a unit, but excessive force should never be applied.

C. Hemostasis

1. After the balloon is withdrawn, the puncture site is allowed to bleed back for 1 to 2 seconds while pressure is held distal to the puncture site to evacuate proximal thrombi.

2. Then manual pressure is applied proximal to the puncture site, and back-bleeding is repeated to evacuate distal thrombi.
3. Manual pressure is then applied for 30 to 45 minutes over the puncture site until adequate hemostasis is achieved.
4. A compressive dressing is applied thereafter.

D. Monitoring during IABP removal

1. During the application of manual pressure to the puncture site, the distal pulses in the leg should be continually assessed, and pressure should be adjusted to maintain adequate distal perfusion.
2. The patient should be confined to strict bed rest for 6 to 12 hours after the catheter and sheath have been removed, and the leg should be periodically assessed for signs of ischemia.

IX. CHANGING THE IABP CATHETER

A. Reasons for changing the IABP

1. When patients require prolonged IABP support, some clinicians change the catheter and sheath every 4 to 5 days to prevent infectious complications. However, there is no consensus regarding this dilemma.
2. Other reasons for changing the IABP include balloon entrapment and rupture, kinking of the catheter or sheath (which prevents adequate balloon inflation), or fever (which may indicate bacteremia from a line infection).

B. Simultaneous change. In patients who are critically dependent on IABP support and who need the IABP changed for one of the above reasons, the catheter and sheath must be changed simultaneously with placement of a new IABP.

1. Contralateral femoral artery

a. When the contralateral femoral artery can be used, it is accessed and the sheath is placed. A guidewire is then positioned in the aortic arch while the old balloon is on standby.
b. Counterpulsation is reinitiated, and the new balloon catheter is prepared and readied for use.
c. The old balloon is then deflated and quickly withdrawn, while the new balloon catheter is placed over the guidewire from the contralateral femoral artery. This technique limits the period without IABP support during the change to less than 30 seconds.
d. Anticoagulation can safely be discontinued before and after a simultaneous change to aid in achieving hemostasis at the old access site.

2. Same femoral artery

a. When the contralateral femoral artery cannot be used, the old catheter and sheath must be removed and changed under direct vision.
b. The accessed femoral artery is exposed surgically, and a purse-string suture is placed around the preexisting sheath.
c. The old sheath is then removed, and tension is applied to the suture for hemostasis.
   (1) The small dilator in the catheter package is directly inserted into the previous puncture site, and the guidewire is advanced to the aortic arch through it.
   (2) The sheath is advanced over the guidewire into the proper position, and the purse-string suture is tied down.
   (3) The balloon catheter is then inserted via the sheath, and the soft tissue and skin incision are closed with sutures.
d. In emergency situations, the preexisting sheath can be rewired and a new balloon catheter inserted through the old sheath. However, infectious complications are high with this approach.

ACKNOWLEDGMENT

The author thanks Dr. Matthew T. Roe for his contributions to earlier editions of this chapter.

Landmark Articles

Holmes DR Jr, Bates ER, Kleinman NS, et al. Contemporary reperfusion therapy for cardiogenic shock: the GUSTO-I trial experience. *J Am Coll Cardiol* 1995;26:668–674.

Anderson RD, Ohman EM, Holmes DR Jr, et al. Use of intraaortic balloon counterpulsation in patients presenting with cardiogenic shock: observations from the GUSTO-I study. *J Am Coll Cardiol* 1997;30:708–715.

Stone GW, Ohman EM, Miller MF, et al. Contemporary utilization and outcomes of intra-aortic balloon counterpulsation in acute myocardial infarction: The benchmark registry. *J Am Coll Cardiol* 2003;41:1940–1945.

Kovack PJ, Rasak MA, Bates ER, et al. Thrombolysis plus aortic counterpulsation: improved survival in patients who present to community hospitals with cardiogenic shock. *J Am Coll Cardiol* 1997;29:1454–1458.

Braunwald EG, Mark DB, Jones RH, et al. Unstable angina: diagnosis and management. Clinical Practice Guideline No. 10. AHCPR Publication No. 94-0602. Rockville, MD: Agency for Health Care Policy Research and the National Heart, Lung, and Blood Institute, Public Health Service, US Department of Health and Human Services, May 1994.

Ohman EM, George BS, White CJ, et al. Use of aortic counterpulsation to improve sustained coronary artery patency during acute myocardial infarction: results of a randomized trial. *Circulation* 1994;90:792–799.

Stone GW, Marsalese D, Brodie BR, et al. A prospective, randomized evaluation of prophylactic intraaortic balloon counterpulsation in high-risk patients with acute myocardial infarction treated with primary angioplasty. *J Am Coll Cardiol* 1997;29:1459–1467.

Briguori C, Airoldi F, Chieffo A, et al. Elective versus provisional intraaortic balloon pumping in unprotected left main stenting. *Am Heart J* 2006;152:565–572.

Antman EM, Hand M, Armstrong PW, et al. 2007 Focused Update of the ACC/AHA 2004 Guidelines for the Management of Patients With ST-Elevation Myocardial Infarction: a report of the American College of Cardiology/American Heart Association Task Force on Practice Guidelines: developed in collaboration With the Canadian Cardiovascular Society endorsed by the American Academy of Family Physicians: 2007 Writing Group to Review New Evidence and Update the ACC/AHA 2004 Guidelines for the Management of Patients With ST-Elevation Myocardial Infarction, Writing on Behalf of the 2004 Writing Committee. *Circulation* 2008;117:296–329.

Anderson JL, Adams CD, Antman EM, et al. ACC/AHA 2007 guidelines for the management of patients with unstable angina/non-ST-elevation myocardial infarction. A report of the American College of Cardiology/American Heart Association Task Force on Practice Guidelines. *J Am Coll Cardiol* 2007;50:e1–e157.

Ohman EM, George BS, White CJ, et al. Use of aortic counterpulsation to improve sustained coronary artery patency during acute myocardial infarction. *Circulation* 1994;90:792–799.

Patel JJ, Kopisyansky C, Boston B, et al. Prospective evaluation of complications associated with percutaneous intraaortic balloon counterpulsation. *Am J Cardiol* 1995;76:1205–1207.

Stone GW, Marsalese D, Brodie BR, et al. A prospective, randomized evaluation of prophylactic intraaortic balloon counterpulsation in high risk patients with acute myocardial infarction treated with primary angioplasty. *J Am Coll Cardiol* 1997;29:1459–1467.

Key Reviews

Aguirre FV, Kern MJ, Bach R, et al. Intraaortic balloon pump support during high-risk coronary angioplasty. *Cardiology* 1994;84:175–186.

Kantrowitz A, Cardona RR, Freed PS. Percutaneous intra-aortic balloon counterpulsation. *Crit Care Clin* 1992;8:819–837.

Kern MJ. Intra-aortic balloon counterpulsation. *Coronary Artery Dis* 1991;2:649–660.

Mueller HS. Role of intra-aortic counterpulsation in cardiogenic shock and acute myocardial infarction. *Cardiology* 1994;84:168–174.

Relevant Book Chapters

Burkhoff D. Intra-aortic balloon counterpulsation and other circulatory assist devices. In: Baim D. *Grossman's cardiac catheterization, angiography, and intervention,* 7th ed. Baltimore: Williams & Wilkins, 2006:412–429.

Maccioli GA, ed. *Intra-aortic balloon pump therapy.* Baltimore: Williams & Wilkins, 1997.

LEFT HEART CATHETERIZATION

Saif Anwaruddin

58

I. INTRODUCTION. In 1958, Dr. Mason Sones and his colleagues at the Cleveland Clinic performed the first selective coronary arteriographic procedure. Since then, left heart catheterization (LHC) has become a crucial part of diagnostic cardiology. More than 1.5 million cardiac catheterizations are performed yearly in the United States. Despite the advent of other imaging modalities, coronary arteriography remains the clinical gold standard for determining the presence of significant coronary artery disease (CAD).

LHC is an invasive procedure with serious risks. To be competent in LHC, at a minimum, a cardiologist-in-training must perform 300 catheterizations, serving as primary operator on 200. If in a training phase, the operator must be supervised by a cardiologist who is already competent in the procedure. Of note, there is often a tendency, once a lesion is noted on coronary arteriography, to proceed with percutaneous intervention. Therefore, before LHC is performed there should be a plan regarding how to use the information obtained.

II. INDICATIONS. The American College of Cardiology along with the American Heart Association (ACC/AHA) have categorized reasonable indications for LHC as class I, when there is consensus that LHC is indicated, or class II, when there is no consensus that LHC is indicated but nonetheless the procedure is frequently performed.

A. Acute myocardial infarction (MI). LHC is given a class I indication for routine use in acute MI, particularly in those who will likely undergo primary PCI, in those in cardiogenic shock or other evidence of hemodynamic instability, or those with mechanical complications who are likely to go on to surgical repair. It can be used with the goal of performing primary angioplasty for patients with acute ST elevation MI. There is evidence of the benefit of an early invasive strategy in stable patients with non–ST-segment elevation MI. In patients with non–ST-segment elevation MI, an early invasive strategy has received a class I indication in the presence of the following risk features: elevated cardiac troponins, new or presumed new ST-segment depression, heart failure (HF), depressed ventricular function, hemodynamic instability, sustained ventricular tachycardia, previous bypass surgery, and previous coronary intervention in the last 6 months. Patients with persistent pain or unresolved electrocardiographic changes after thrombolytic therapy are also class I candidates for LHC. Routine LHC soon after thrombolytic therapy in a patient who appears to have clinically reperfused is a class IIb indication.

B. Unstable angina. LHC is given a class I indication in the patient with refractory unstable angina that cannot be controlled by medical therapy. Its role in unstable angina that can be medically controlled is controversial.

C. Chronic stable angina. LHC is given a class I indication for purposes of revascularization in chronic stable angina for patients whose angina is poorly controlled by medicines or who are intolerant of antianginal medications.

D. Abnormal stress test. A stress test that is positive at a low work load (6.5 metabolic equivalents of oxygen consumption) or that is classified as high risk is a class I indication for LHC. An ST depression of 2 mm, especially in multiple leads or persisting into recovery 6 minutes, an ST elevation of 2 mm in leads without Q waves, a drop in blood pressure of more than 10 mm Hg with exercise, or development of ventricular tachycardia with exercise constitutes a high-risk stress test. A high-risk stress test on a concomitant imaging modality showing left ventricle dilatation, a drop in ejection fraction of 10%, or multiple areas of ischemia is a class I indication for catheterization. These indications hold true even if the patient is asymptomatic. Positive stress tests without high-risk criteria are class II indications for LHC.

E. Ventricular arrhythmia. A history of sustained polymorphic ventricular tachycardia, without obvious metabolic cause, is considered a class I indication for LHC.

F. Left ventricular dysfunction. LHC can provide an estimate of left ventricular function and regional wall motion. Left ventricular dysfunction of unknown cause, with an ejection fraction of less than 40%, is a class I indication for LHC to rule out CAD.

G. Valvular heart disease. LHC can be performed to assess the severity of outflow tract obstruction (aortic stenosis, hypertrophic obstructive cardiomyopathy). It can also help quantify aortic and mitral regurgitation (MR). With the advancements in Doppler and color echocardiography, the major role of cardiac catheterization is to provide confirmatory data and to rule out CAD as part of the operative workup. LHC has a class I indication in patients requiring valve surgery who are at risk for CAD. Most centers perform LHC before valve surgery for men older than 40 and women older than 50 to rule out clinically silent CAD. Younger patients may require LHC if cardiac risk factors are present.

H. Preoperative. LHC is performed before ascending aortic aneurysm surgery or some cases of ascending aortic dissection surgery. It is also performed on patients with congenital heart disease to evaluate lesions such as ventricular septal defects and to rule out concomitant coronary anomalies or atherosclerotic disease, if symptomatic. In patients with angina or a positive stress test who are to undergo high-risk surgery, LHC is given a class I indication.

III. CONTRAINDICATIONS. The following are relative contraindications to LHC.

A. Coagulopathy. Coagulopathy must be corrected before elective catheterization. The usual recommendation for patients on warfarin (Coumadin) is to discontinue it 72 hours before the procedure. In elective cases, an international normalized ratio (INR) of less than 1.8 is a cutoff that is often used. If the patient is heparinized, this is usually stopped 2 hours before the procedure. A platelet count less than 50,000 substantially increases the risk of bleeding. After thrombolytic therapy, bleeding is more likely and elective catheterization is best deferred. However, if the indication for the procedure is urgent, it is possible to proceed with caution, with blood products ready for support as needed. Antecedent glycoprotein IIb/IIIa inhibitor therapy poses much less of a risk. Body habitus is also a factor in deciding what level of anticoagulation is acceptable before a catheterization. Obesity increases the chances of bleeding (if multiple attempts at access are needed) and makes bleeding more difficult to detect. Finally, the availability of closure devices makes it possible to seal the artery after the procedure.

B. Renal failure. A rising creatinine is generally a reason to defer elective cardiac catheterization. In a patient on dialysis, catheterization is generally timed immediately after the dialysis. In a patient with stable but moderately severe renal failure, catheterization may be performed with an awareness of the increased risk of needing dialysis.

C. Dye allergy. A history of allergy to previous contrast administration should be sought. Although an allergy to shellfish and seafood has been linked to contrast reactions in some studies, other studies dispute such a relationship. Individuals with a history of asthma or atopy are at increased risk of developing contrast allergies. Treatment of patients with a history of dye allergy is described below.

D. Infection. Active infection is a reason to defer elective cardiac catheterization. Local skin infection at the site of the potential puncture is also undesirable. Fungal infection in groin creases should be controlled before elective cardiac catheterization by the femoral approach; this is a particular concern in obese patients. Alternatively, LHC may be performed through a brachial approach in patients with fungal infection in groin creases.

E. Laboratory abnormalities. Severe anemia, hypokalemia, or hyperkalemia should be corrected before the elective procedure. In the presence of digitalis toxicity, elective catheterization is best deferred.

F. Decompensated HF. Severe HF raises the risks of cardiac catheterization. It is best to optimize medical therapy before elective catheterization. At a minimum, the patient should be able to lie supine without respiratory insufficiency.

G. Severe peripheral vascular disease. Symptoms of claudication warrant careful assessment of pulses. An inadequate lower-extremity pulse favors an upper-extremity approach. A synthetic vascular graft that is older than 6 months is not a strict contraindication to catheterization, but special care should be taken in gaining access as well as in obtaining hemostasis. However, the risk of embolization of friable atheroma or thrombus is heightened, and this risk increases with the age of the graft.

H. Abdominal aortic aneurysm (AAA). Presence of an AAA requires special care during a cardiac catheterization (see subsequent text). An arm approach obviates the need to cross the AAA altogether.

I. Uncontrolled severe hypertension. Blood pressure should be controlled before elective cardiac catheterization to maximize the safety of the procedure. In particular, severe bleeding can occur at the access site after sheath removal if the patient is very hypertensive, especially if above 180 per 100 mm Hg.

IV. PATIENT PREPARATION

A. Informed consent. A detailed discussion with the patient (and family) should outline the indication for the procedure, as well as the alternative treatment and diagnostic options. Specific mention of the serious risks of complications, such as death, MI, stroke, and kidney failure, must be made (see complications in subsequent text). The possible need for emergency coronary artery bypass grafting (CABG) should be noted. The risk of serious complications should be individualized. Informed consent should be documented in the medical record.

B. Precatheterization assessment. Before proceeding with an LHC, a detailed clinical assessment is necessary, including a comprehensive history and physical examination. All peripheral pulses should be palpated, and arterial bruits, if any, should be documented before the catheterization as a baseline for future reference. In addition, laboratory data, including a comprehensive metabolic panel, complete blood count, and coagulation studies should be obtained on all patients. Abnormalities on the laboratory parameters, if any, should be addressed before proceeding with the LHC.

C. Medications. If percutaneous coronary intervention is likely, pretreatment with aspirin 325 mg by mouth (PO) should be given before the catheterization, as it has been shown to improve outcomes with angioplasty. If stenting is a strong possibility, clopidogrel 300 mg PO should be given as a loading dose before the procedure. Metformin should be stopped at the time of the procedure, although the risk of lactic acidosis is extremely low in a patient with normal creatinine.

D. Education. Patients should be warned that they might feel a hot sensation lasting about 30 seconds due to the injection of ionic contrast dye. Some patients may also feel nauseated. Patients should be specifically instructed to cough when they hear anyone in the room say "cough." This maneuver accelerates resolution of dye-induced bradycardia.

E. Equipment. Before performing a cardiac catheterization, it is essential to ensure that the monitoring equipment is fully functional. Continuous electrocardiographic monitoring of heart rate (HR), rhythm, and ST segments, an automated blood pressure cuff, and continuous pulse oximetry are mandatory. Resuscitation equipment should be tested and ready. In particular, defibrillators and intubation trays must be next to the patient. If a long procedure is anticipated, many operators prefer placement of a Foley or Texas urinary catheter. Before actually beginning the procedure, the fluoroscopy and cine equipment should be tested by taking a picture of the patient's nameplate. The usual frame rate of cine film is set at 30 frames per second; 60 frames per second can be useful for tachycardic patients. In thin individuals who are bradycardic (less than 60 beats/min), the frame rate can be lowered to 15 frames per second. In addition, the table should move freely to the level of the patient's groin.

F. Contrast dye

1. Choice of contrast. Ionic contrast dye was historically used during most cardiac catheterizations. In most circumstances, low osmolar nonionic dye, which is now only slightly more expensive, can be used (2). The literature supports that nonionic dye produces less left ventricular dysfunction, bradycardia, and hypotension, as well as less nausea and emesis. Thus, it is useful in cases of suspected left main stenosis, severe left ventricular dysfunction, and severe aortic stenosis. Other indications for nonionic dye are severe renal dysfunction and a reported allergy to contrast dye. However, no reduction in acute renal failure or anaphylactoid reaction has been conclusively demonstrated with the use of nonionic dye. There is evidence that nonionic contrast is more thrombogenic than ionic contrast. Therefore, it should be used carefully in patients with acute coronary syndromes. Whenever nonionic contrast is used, 5 IU of heparin per cubic centimeter of contrast should be added.

2. Dye allergy

a. Premedication. If a patient reports an allergy to contrast dye or a history of prior anaphylactoid reaction, it is customary to premedicate with prednisone 40 mg PO q6h ×4 doses or with hydrocortisone 100 mg intravenously (IV) ×1 at least 6 hours before the procedure, and with cimetidine (Tagamet) 400 mg IV × 1 and diphenhydramine (Benadryl) 50 mg IV ×1. With a history of possible life-threatening dye allergies, it is also prudent to administer small quantities of dye (1 mL) and observe for a few minutes before proceeding.

b. Treatment. If a patient develops signs of an allergic reaction, treatment should be prompt. If signs such as hives or rash develop, treatment with diphenhydramine is usually sufficient. Hydrocortisone is also often given, though its effects would not be manifest for several hours. In cases of oropharyngeal edema, bronchospasm, or hypotension, 0.3 mL of 1:1,000 epinephrine should be administered subcutaneously. With refractory symptoms, 10 μg/min of intravenous epinephrine can be administered until symptoms abate.

c. Latex allergy has become increasingly recognized as a clinical entity, especially in patients who are health care workers. True latex allergy can include urticaria, angioedema, laryngospasm, bronchospasm, and anaphylaxis. If a patient describes a possible latex allergy, allergy testing, including skin testing and rapid antigen serum testing, should be considered. Patients with latex allergy should be scheduled as the first case of the day in order to avoid latex dust from previous procedures. Written protocols outlining materials to be avoided should be strictly followed. A cart with latex-free items should be made available. The sheath is a source of latex exposure. Therefore, a sheathless approach involving catheter exchanges over a wire is preferred.

d. Sedation. Commonly used sedatives include the benzodiazepines midazolam 1 to 2 mg IV or lorazepam 1 to 2 mg IV. Some operators use fentanyl 25 mg IV or morphine 1 to 2 mg IV for pain relief. Diphenhydramine 25 or 50 mg IV can also be used for sedation. Continuous pulse oximetry should be followed to ensure that sedation has not been excessive.

e. Radiation safety. Radiation poses a threat to laboratory personnel; therefore, every effort should be made to reduce exposure. The source is scatter from the x-ray beam originating under the table. Lead aprons (with at least 0.5-mm-thickness lead lining) and thyroid collars are mandatory to minimize radiation exposure. Leaded eyeglasses should also be considered. In addition, radiation badges are worn inside the lead apron and outside the thyroid collar to monitor cumulative radiation exposure. A leaded acrylic shield should be used between the patient and the operator closest to the patient. Standing further from the table also reduces radiation exposure by the inverse square of the distance. A number of additional steps can be taken to minimize radiation to both the operator and the patient. Fluoroscopy and, in particular, cine time should be minimized. The image intensifier should be positioned as close as possible to the patient to reduce radiation scatter. To decrease radiation, higher magnification should be used judiciously. "Coning down" on a region of interest with the use of collimators can also reduce the amount of radiation, as can the use of lung field collimators. Right anterior oblique (RAO) views produce less radiation scatter for the operator than left anterior oblique (LAO) views. Higher cine frame rates increase radiation exposure; use of 15 or 30 frames per second produces less radiation exposure than use of 60 frames per second. In the rare situation that a pregnant patient needs catheterization, a lead apron should be used. This precaution should also be taken for premenopausal women.

V. ACCESS SITE

A. Femoral artery. Femoral artery cannulation is the most common form of arterial access for cardiac catheterization (see Fig. 58.1). The patient is first positioned appropriately, with the knees about 12 inches apart. The table should allow enough movement to perform fluoroscopy of the groin. Anatomic landmarks are then identified. The inguinal ligament is located. Then the femoral pulse is palpated approximately 2 cm (finger breadths) below the inguinal ligament; this marks the site of arterial access. Alternatively, fluoroscopy can be used to locate the femoral head.

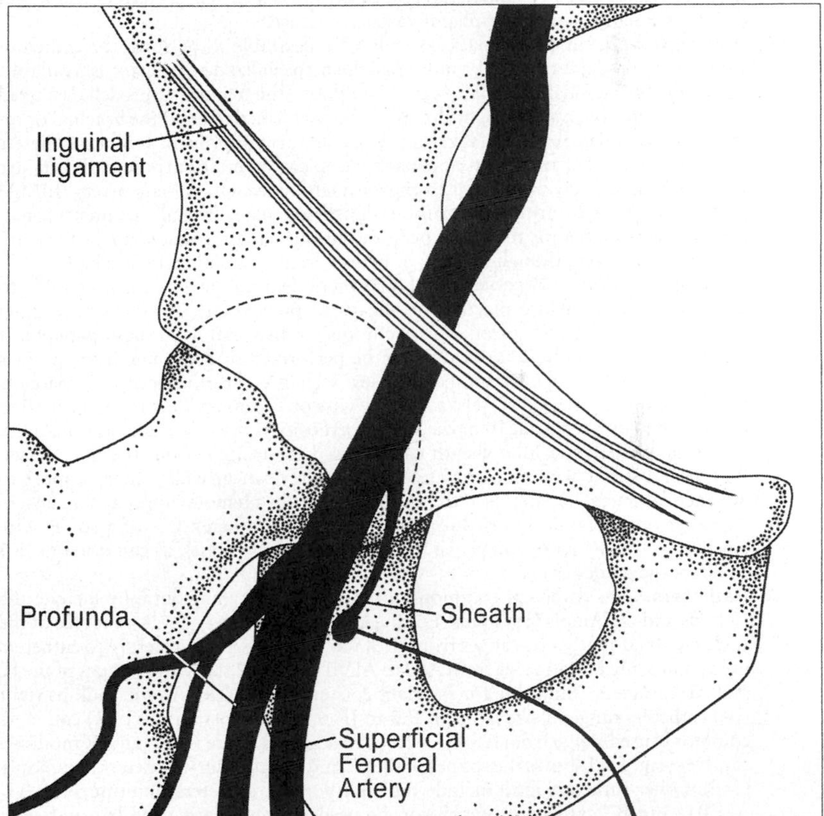

Figure 58.1. Landmarks for right femoral artery puncture.

The entry point on the skin is located over the inferior border of the femoral head. Care must be taken not to enter the artery above the inguinal ligament, as this increases the chance of retroperitoneal bleeding. Arterial entry that is too low must also be avoided, as this can lead to pseudoaneurysm or arteriovenous fistula formation. Once the site of entry has been identified (and marked, if so desired), the area is cleaned with povidone iodine (Betadine) and surgically draped. Local anesthesia is given slowly (it hurts less when delivered slowly) while the clinician observes the heart rate monitor and watches for signs of a vagal reaction (nausea, lightheadedness, yawning). The usual choice is procaine 1%. A subcutaneous wheal is raised with about 3 mL using a 25-gauge needle. Next, an additional 6 to 10 mL is delivered to the deeper tissues with a 22-gauge needle. In patients who are allergic to ester-type anesthetics, lidocaine 2% can be used. Once the site is anesthetized, an 18-gauge Cook needle is inserted into the artery. Upon nearing the artery, a side-to-side motion of the needle indicates a position either medial or lateral to the artery. Up-and-down motion indicates correct positioning. In addition, when the needle is above the artery, it transmits the arterial pulsation to the fingertips. Once brisk arterial blood return is established, a 0.035-inch J-tipped 45-cm guidewire is inserted, the needle is withdrawn, and an arterial sheath with a dilator is placed over the wire. Then the wire and dilator are removed. The sheath is then flushed with saline. A 5F or 6F sheath is generally used for diagnostic catheterizations in the United States, though 4F sheaths are often used in Europe. An 8F sheath is used for acute cases or planned interventions. A 5F sheath is preferred over larger sheaths for patients with peripheral vascular disease.

B. Arm approach. In certain patients it may be desirable to perform the catheterization by a brachial or radial route, for which specialized equipment is available. Percutaneous brachial or radial access is similar to the femoral approach described above. In addition, a surgical cut-down can be performed to enter the brachial or radial arteries under direct visualization. For a left arm approach, Judkins catheters are adequate. For a right arm approach, Amplatz or multipurpose catheters are used, although it may be difficult to engage a left internal mammary artery (LIMA) graft from the right arm; a specially designed brachial internal mammary artery catheter is available for the latter purpose. In rare circumstances, an axillary approach can be used, though the rate of neurovascular complications is higher.

C. Special situations. In patients with prosthetic femoral grafts, it is preferable to use a dilator first before placing the sheath to prevent the sheath from kinking as it passes through the graft. This technique is also useful in obese patients. If a synthetic graft is old, fluoroscopy can be performed to determine if the graft is heavily calcified—a sign that it may not seal well after sheath removal. In patients with tortuous or diseased vessels, a Wholey wire or Terumo glidewire can be used to get catheters up the aorta. If marked iliac tortuosity is present and causes inability to torque catheters, a long sheath can be used to straighten out the iliac vessel. At times, a stiffer wire (such as an Amplatz wire) can provide better support to advance catheters. In patients with an AAA for whom a femoral approach is chosen, exchange wires should be used for every change of catheter. Use of a softer wire (such as a Wholey wire) can prove less traumatic to the vessel, as can use of a JR4 to direct the guidewire.

D. Catheters. The catheters commonly used for coronary angiography include the Judkins and the Amplatz systems. For the left coronary artery (LCA), the size of the Judkins left (JL) catheters ranges from JL 3.5 to JL 6. The Amplatz left (AL) catheters used commonly range in size from AL I to AL III (Fig. 58.2 shows the shapes of the JL and AL catheters). Similarly for the right coronary artery (RCA), the Judkins right (JR) catheters range in size from JR 3.5 to JR 6. The Amplatz right (AR) catheters commonly used range from AR I to AR III. In addition, there is also an AR modified catheter (Fig. 58.3 shows the shapes of the JR and AR coronary catheters commonly used). Other catheters used include the multipurpose catheters (multipurpose A1, A2, B1, and B2 catheters), which can be used for cannulating the left and right coronary arteries and bypass grafts. For coronary bypass grafts, the right or the left coronary bypass catheters may be used. The internal mammary artery may be

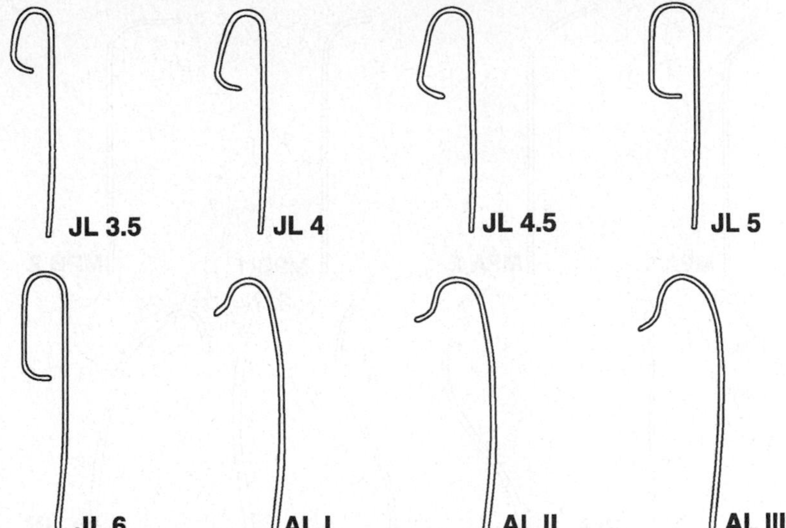

Figure 58.2. Catheters used for cannulating the left coronary artery. JL, Judkins left; AL, Amplatz left.

cannulated using either the internal mammary or the internal mammary special catheters (see Fig. 58.4).

VI. TECHNIQUE

A. Engaging the vessel

1. **LCA.** Catheters are flushed with heparinized saline and passed through the sheath over a J-tipped guidewire. Using fluoroscopic guidance in the LAO

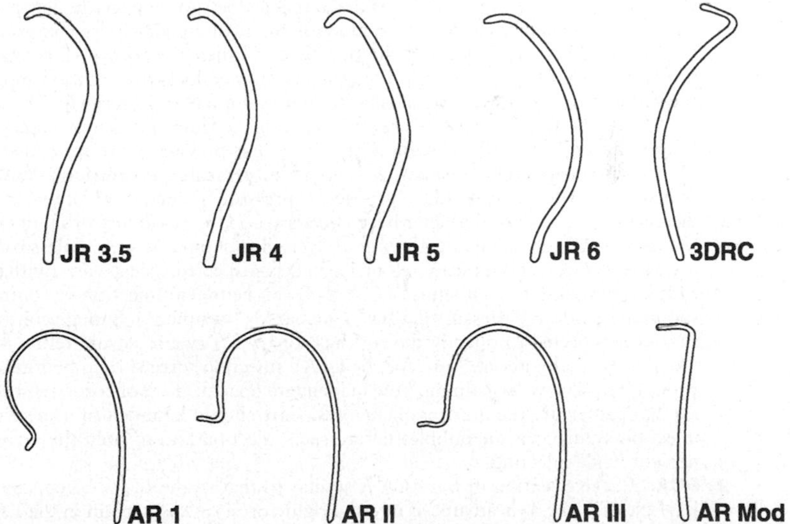

Figure 58.3. Catheters used for cannulating the right coronary artery. JR, Judkins right; AR, Amplatz right; 3DRC, no torque right coronary catheter.

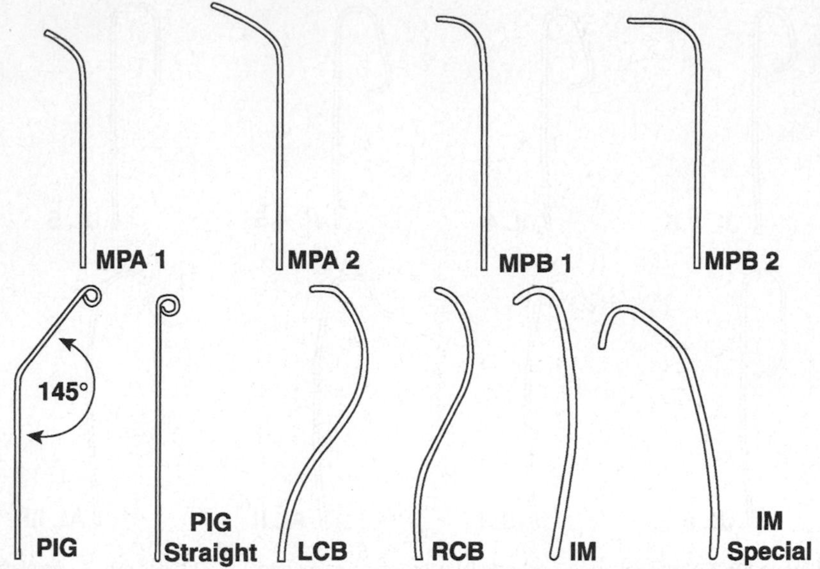

Figure 58.4. Other catheters used for cardiac catheterization. MP, multipurpose; PIG, pigtail; LCB, left coronary bypass catheter; RCB, right coronary bypass catheter; IM, internal mammary.

projection, the left main coronary artery is cannulated, typically with a JL 4 (see Fig. 58.2). The catheter tip should be coaxial to the left main coronary artery, meaning that its tip should not be touching the upper wall of the left main coronary artery. In a small person, a JL 3.5 (see Fig. 58.2) catheter can be used. In a larger person or a person with a dilated aorta, a JL 5 or even a JL 6 (see Fig. 58.2) can be used. If the catheter does not engage the left main ostium easily, a slight clockwise or, more often, a counterclockwise rotation of the catheter hub may help. With the JL catheters, unless the aorta is dilated and provides no hinge point for the JL catheter, counterclockwise rotation moves the catheter tip anteriorly and clockwise rotation moves it posteriorly.

Care should be taken to prevent the catheter from too deeply engaging ("deep-seating") the left main coronary artery. The pressure waveform must be observed for **damping** (a decrease in the systolic pressure) or **ventricularization** (when the waveform looks like a ventricular pressure tracing), both of which indicate a need to pull the catheter back and also raise the possibility of significant left main CAD. An adequate amount of dye reflux should be seen, unless ostial disease is present. If significant left main CAD is suspected, a cusp view (with the catheter placed in the left sinus of Valsalva) can be taken. Injection of contrast should be gentle and pressure gradually increased ("ramping"). Enough contrast should be injected to opacify the entire coronary artery and ensure reflux into the aorta (usually about 8 mL for the LCA). Injection force should be forceful enough to prevent "streaming," the inadequate opacification of coronary arteries that can create the illusion of stenoses. Care should be taken to inspect the injection syringe for air bubbles before each injection and to hold the syringe upright while injecting.

2. **RCA.** Catheterization of the RCA is similar to that of the LCA, except that a JR 4 (see Fig. 58.3) is advanced into the right coronary cusp, again in the LAO projection. The RCA is usually located anteriorly in the right sinus, in a position that is lower than the LCA ostium. As the catheter is slowly pulled back 2 cm above the aortic valve, it is rotated clockwise, causing it to engage. With the JR

catheter, clockwise rotation moves the catheter anteriorly. In addition, clockwise rotation can cause the catheter to dip downward. Thus, it may be necessary to apply backward traction on the catheter as it is being rotated clockwise. Sometimes it is necessary to repeat the clockwise rotation at different levels in order to engage the right coronary ostium. If the JR 4 does not easily engage the RCA or if the pressure dampens, ostial disease, spasm, selective intubation of the conus (which arises separately 50% of the time), or anatomic variation in the direction of the proximal RCA should be suspected. A cusp view can be taken to clarify these situations. Care should be taken to avoid subselectively intubating the conus branch.

If difficulty is encountered in engaging the RCA because of the orientation of the ostium, a 3DR or a no-torque right catheter can be useful (see Fig. 58.3). Both catheters are designed to be placed above the aortic valve and pulled back without torquing maneuvers. An Amplatz or multipurpose catheter (see Figs. 58.3 and 58.4) can be useful for an upwardly angled ostium. An anterior or posterior origin can often be engaged with an Amplatz catheter. The most common cause of an incomplete LHC is a high and anterior RCA. In order to locate its ostium, less clockwise torque should be applied to the catheter so that it faces more anteriorly. Then the catheter can search for the ostium superior to the usual location. Less dye is needed to opacify the RCA than the LCA; over-injection can cause ventricular fibrillation. Sometimes, if a catheter is tenuously engaged, particularly in the right coronary ostium, a deep breath can dislodge it and should be avoided.

3. **LIMA.** Catheterization of the LIMA is done either in the posteroanterior or shallow LAO projection. First, the catheter (usually a JR 4 catheter or a LIMA catheter; see Figs. 58.3 and 58.4) is positioned by pulling it back in the aorta while applying counterclockwise torque until it enters the left subclavian artery. At this point many operators will obtain an angiogram of the left subclavian artery to rule out a stenosis proximal to the LIMA and to give a hint of the angle of takeoff of the LIMA. Next, the wire (J-tipped guidewire or Wholey wire) is advanced into the subclavian artery. Next, the catheter is advanced over the wire into the subclavian artery, the wire is removed, and the catheter is slowly pulled back with a slight counterclockwise rotation until it engages the ostium of the LIMA. Movements around the ostium must be gentle to reduce the risk of dissection of the vessel; frequent test injections are helpful. In addition, if a 6F sheath is in place, switching to a 5F catheter will likely result in less trauma to the ostium of the LIMA. Turning the head to the left or right and pulling the arm caudally are maneuvers that can help engage the LIMA. If the ostium points downward at a sharp angle, the LIMA catheter is more likely to engage it selectively. The special LIMA catheter provides a slightly different angulation. It is best to use nonionic contrast to minimize the pain caused by ionic dye running through the arteries of the chest wall. If the ostium cannot be engaged successfully, a nonselective angiogram can be taken with the tip of the catheter as close to the ostium as possible. A blood pressure cuff should be inflated above systolic pressure in the left arm to facilitate dye movement down the LIMA.
4. **Right internal mammary artery (RIMA).** Catheterization of the RIMA is similar to that of the LIMA. The catheter (either JR 4 or LIMA; see Figs. 58.3 and 58.4) is placed in the brachiocephalic trunk by pulling back in the aorta while applying counterclockwise rotation. The wire is advanced into the right subclavian artery. Care must be taken to avoid the right carotid artery. The wire is removed and the catheter is pulled back until it engages the ostium of the RIMA.
5. **Saphenous vein grafts (SVGs).** Catheterization of SVGs depends on the specific type of graft. The grafts are by necessity anastomosed to the anterior surface of the aorta. The orientation of SVGs from caudal to cranial is usually as follows: RCA, left anterior descending artery (LAD), diagonal branches of LAD, and marginal branches of left circumflex artery (LCX). In the LAO view, grafts to the RCA usually point to the patient's right, whereas grafts to the left system are usually oriented more to the patient's left. It is the practice of some

surgeons to place circular graft markers around the ostia of the vein grafts on the outer surface of the aorta. In the steep LAO projection, the catheter tip should extend beyond the plane of these markers, if the catheter is truly engaged in a vein graft. Injections into presumed vein graft stumps should be forceful to ensure that the graft is truly occluded, as opposed to poor opacification from a tenuously engaged catheter. Review of the operative note is mandatory before catheterization in order to know where grafts were placed. In particular, it should be noted whether any LIMA or RIMA grafts are *in situ* or free (attached to the aorta). A previous catheterization, if done, should be reviewed. Particular attention should be paid to the location of the grafts. The relative relationship to surgical clips should be noted, as this will save time and effort in finding grafts during the catheterization. If a graft cannot be found or a stump identified during a catheterization, an aortogram should be performed (VI.E).

a. **SVG to RCA.** Engaging this graft can be as simple as pulling back on the JR 4 as it sits in the ostium to the RCA while in the LAO projection. Often this graft has a steep downward orientation from the aorta. In this situation, a multipurpose catheter can be useful in engaging the graft. The multipurpose catheter can enter deeply into the graft if not handled carefully. Alternatively, a right bypass catheter or a right modified Amplatz catheter can be useful in engaging the RCA graft.

b. **SVG to LAD.** The graft to the LAD is most easily engaged in the RAO view. To engage this graft, it is necessary to withdraw the catheter from the SVG to the RCA by pulling back. If the catheter does not fall into place, clockwise rotation of the JR 4 at an area cranial to the SVG to RCA graft ostium will locate the LAD graft. It may be necessary to move the catheter up and down along the anterior surface of the aorta several times. Left bypass, left Amplatz, and multipurpose catheters are all alternative catheters that can be used. A similar clockwise rotation to move the catheter tip along the anterior aortic surface is necessary.

c. **SVG to LCX.** To engage this graft, it is necessary to withdraw the catheter from the SVG to the LAD by pulling back, while remaining in the RAO projection. If the catheter does not fall into place, clockwise rotation of the JR 4 at an area cranial to the SVG to LAD graft ostium will locate the LCX graft. The technique is otherwise similar to that for engaging the graft to the LAD.

B. Imaging the vessels

1. **Normal coronary anatomy.** The left main coronary artery originates from the left coronary cusp. It usually bifurcates into a LAD and a LCX, though it sometimes trifurcates to include a ramus intermedius. The LAD courses along the anterior interventricular groove, supplying numerous septal perforators to the septum, and a variable number of diagonal branches to the anterolateral wall of the left ventricle, and usually continues to the apex. The LCX courses along the left atrioventricular (AV) groove, providing a variable number of marginal branches to supply the lateral wall. In some institutions the first marginal branch is called the high lateral branch of the circumflex, with subsequent branches called lateral or posterolateral branches, depending on their destination. The LCX continues in the AV groove for a variable distance. In patients in whom the LCX is dominant (see subsequent text), the LCX reaches the posterior interventricular groove and gives rise to a posterior descending artery (PDA) branch.

   The RCA originates from the right coronary cusp and courses along the right AV groove, providing atrial branches (to the right atrium) and marginal branches (to the right ventricle). A conus branch originates as the first branch from the proximal RCA to supply the right ventricular outflow tract; about half of the time, this branch has an ostium that is separate from the RCA ostium. It is usually unnecessary to visualize a separate conus branch, unless collaterals to the LAD are suspected. The RCA gives off a branch to the sinus node about 60% of the time (otherwise a left atrial branch of the LCX serves this function). The first major branch the distal RCA gives off is the PDA, in a right dominant system. **Dominance** refers to which artery gives off a PDA and supplies the posterior part of the heart. In about 85% of patients, this will be the RCA; in 7% the RCA and LCX will be codominant; and in another 8% the LCX will be dominant. The PDA courses along the inferior interventricular groove, providing septal perforators to supply the inferior septum. After giving off a PDA, the RCA continues as a posterolateral segment supplying a variable number of posterior ventricular branches. From this posterolateral segment, the RCA usually (90% of the time) provides a branch to supply the AV node.

2. **Basic principles.** Several views of the coronary arteries are required to prevent excessive overlap of vessel segments and to delineate the severity of stenoses. A general principle that is useful is that in an RAO view the spine is on the left of the screen, whereas in an LAO view the spine is on the right of the screen. Cranial views bring the silhouette of the diaphragm into the field of view. The diagonal and obtuse marginal branches tend to move in synchrony, because they supply the lateral aspect of the heart, whereas the LAD is located on the anterior portion of the heart. The AV continuation of the LCX lies in the AV groove, and (in patients in sinus rhythm) it has an "atrial kick" to it. This sort of atrial kick can also be seen in atrial branches from either the LCX or the RCA. In the RAO view, a diagonal branch, and not the LAD itself, usually lies on the heart border. In the LAO view, the LAD runs along the border of the heart silhouette, not the diagonal branches. Caudal angulation tends to move posterior vessels (such as the posterolateral branches of the RCA or the obtuse marginal branches of the LCX) inferiorly. Cranial angulation tends to move posterior vessels superiorly.

   Patients should be instructed to take in a deep breath and hold it before most views for the purpose of moving the diaphragm out of the way. The RAO cranial view can be done at end-expiration, in order to facilitate the splaying out of the diagonals from the LAD, or at end-inspiration to view the proximal LCX. The LAO caudal can be done at end expiration to visualize the left main and ostial LAD, or at end-inspiration to view the LCX. Panning motion should be smooth and slow. It is best to wait for two to three systolic cycles and focus on proximal vessels before panning down the length of the artery of interest. It is important to pan to look for collaterals.

3. **Different views** (see Figs. 58.5 to 58.11)

   a. **LCA.** There is wide variation in the sequence of views obtained. Many operators start with a posteroanterior view and focus on the left main coronary artery, sometimes with a coned-down view to improve resolution. The problem with a pure posteroanterior view is that there is significant overlap with the spine. Therefore, a little bit of RAO angulation ("shallow RAO") can be used to get the coronaries off the spine. A steeper amount of RAO provides greater separation of the LAD from the LCX. A slight amount of caudal angulation can be used to decrease the foreshortening of the proximal circumflex in the straight RAO view and to place the diagonals below the LAD. Therefore, a **20° RAO, 20° caudal** is often the first view, displaying the entire left coronary system. This view also provides a good view of the proximal LCX and of the origin of a ramus intermedius branch, if present. The contour collimator (called the wedge or shield) should be moved to the upper right of the screen. A **30° RAO, 25° cranial** view can be used to separate the diagonals from the LAD, placing them above the LAD. The wedge should be placed in the upper right of the screen. A **posterior-anterior view (PA) with 40° cranial** angulation can be useful in viewing the mid and distal portions of the LAD. The **45° LAO, 30° cranial** view is good for separating the LAD from its diagonal branches, especially for vertically oriented hearts. There should be enough LAO angulation to get the LAD off the spine. This view can also be good for a left-sided PDA branch. Steeper degrees of LAO further separate the LAD from the LCX and can get the LCX off the spine, but they can also cause the origins of the diagonals to overlap the LAD and cause the distal LAD to overlap the diaphragm. The **45° LAO, 30° caudal** ("spider"

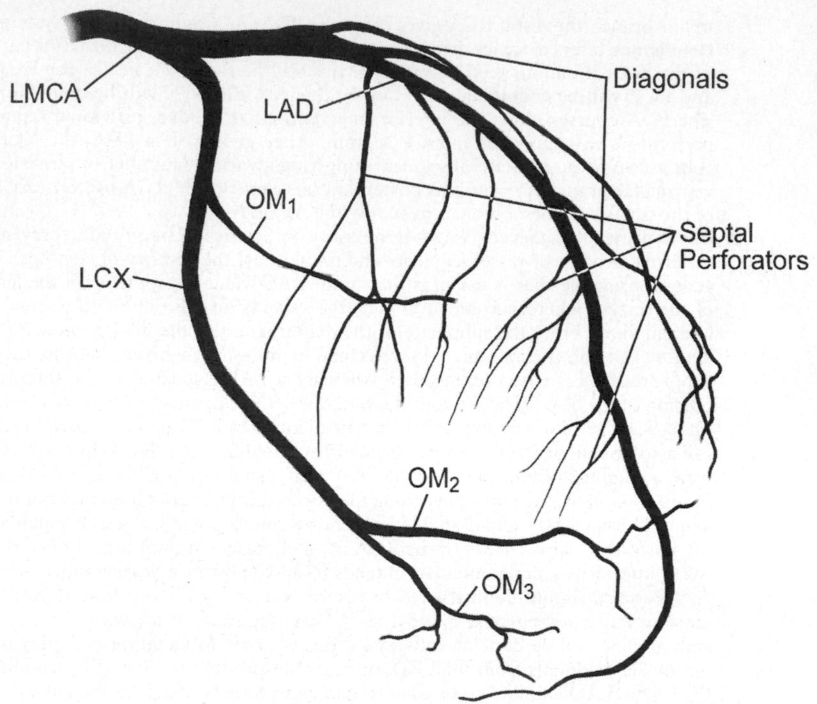

Figure 58.5. Posteroanterior view of left coronary artery. LMCA, left main coronary artery; LCX, left circumflex coronary artery; LAD, left anterior descending artery; OM_1, obtuse marginal branch 1; OM_2, obtuse marginal branch 2; OM_3, obtuse marginal branch 3.

view) is useful for looking at the left main coronary artery and the proximal origin of the LCX. The proximal LAD is also seen but is foreshortened, unless the heart is horizontal in orientation. There must be enough LAO to get the cardiac silhouette off the spine. There is usually no need for a wedge, as it increases the haziness of this view further. Minimal to no panning is required. The **lateral** view provides delineation of the mid-LAD. In addition, the distal LAD does not overlap the diaphragm, and the LCX is off the spine. The patient's hands should be placed behind the head for the lateral view. The shield should be placed above the course of the LAD. Panning involves dropping the table height and moving the table cranially. The **PA with 30° caudal** angulation provides a good view of the LCX.

b. **RCA.** The RCA is usually viewed in LAO and RAO views. The **30° RAO** provides a good view of the proximal and mid-RCA and also of the PDA, which is laid out lengthwise. Cranial angulation can help separate the PDA from the distal vessel. The **40° LAO** view provides a good view of the proximal and mid-RCA, and if cranial angulation is added, a good view of the posterolateral arteries. The **PA with 30° cranial** can provide a useful view of the origins of the PDA and posterolateral branches. The lateral view of the RCA can provide a good view of the mid-RCA. In the RAO view, the right atrium and ventricle are separated by the RCA in the AV groove. Thus, atrial branches will be directed toward the atrium and marginal branches will be directed to the ventricle.

c. **Bypass grafts.** An LAO and an RAO view are required to visualize the body of the graft. Additional views are dictated by the grafted vessel. A particularly

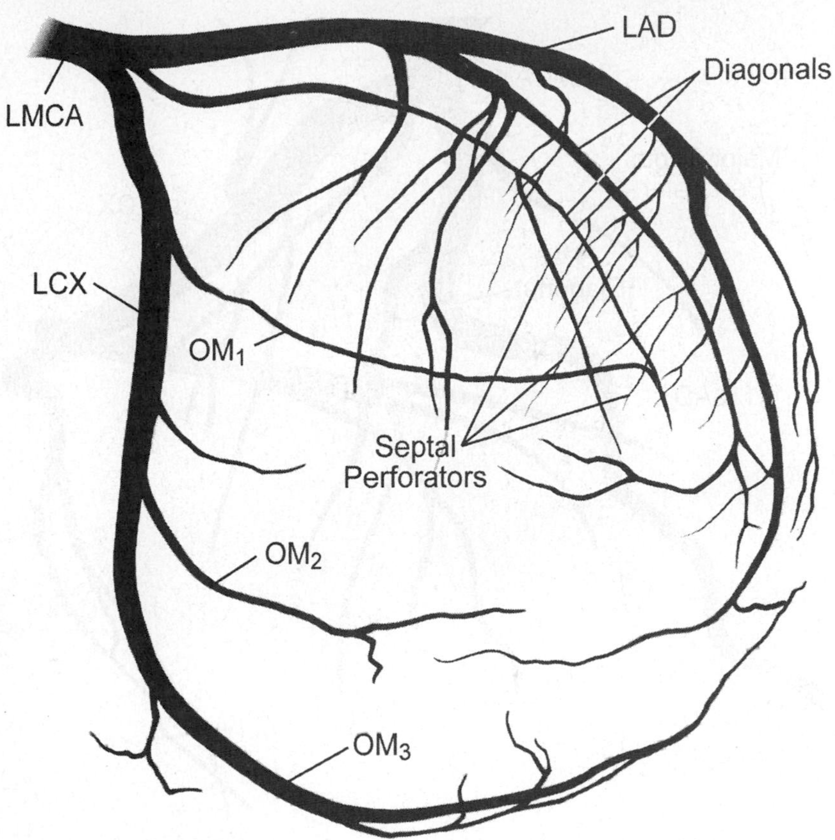

Figure 58.6. Right anterior oblique caudal view of left coronary artery. LMCA, left main coronary artery; LCX, left circumflex coronary artery; LAD, left anterior descending artery; OM_1, obtuse marginal branch 1; OM_2, obtuse marginal branch 2; OM_3, obtuse marginal branch 3.

useful view for the LIMA-LAD anastomosis is the lateral view; cranial LAO and cranial RAO views can also be useful. The graft to the diagonal can be visualized in the cranial LAO and cranial RAO views. The graft to the marginal branch can be seen in the RAO and lateral views. The graft to the distal RCA can be visualized in the cranial LAO and lateral views.

4. **Congenital coronary anomalies.** Coronary artery anomalies should be suspected if there is an absent coronary artery and a large area of myocardium that appears nonperfused (3). The most common anomaly is an absent left main coronary artery trunk, in which the LAD and LCX have separate ostia (incidence 0.47%). If the LAD is first cannulated, the LCX can be engaged with a clockwise rotation; sometimes one size larger catheter (JL 5) is needed. Likewise, if the LCX is first cannulated, counterclockwise rotation, perhaps with a size smaller catheter (JL 3.5), is needed to engage the LAD. The next most common anomaly is the LCX originating from the right sinus of Valsalva (0.45%). The next most common anomaly is the RCA originating from the ascending aorta above the sinus of Valsalva (0.18%). The RCA originating from the left sinus of Valsalva is the next most common anomaly, originating superior and anterior to the left main (0.13%).

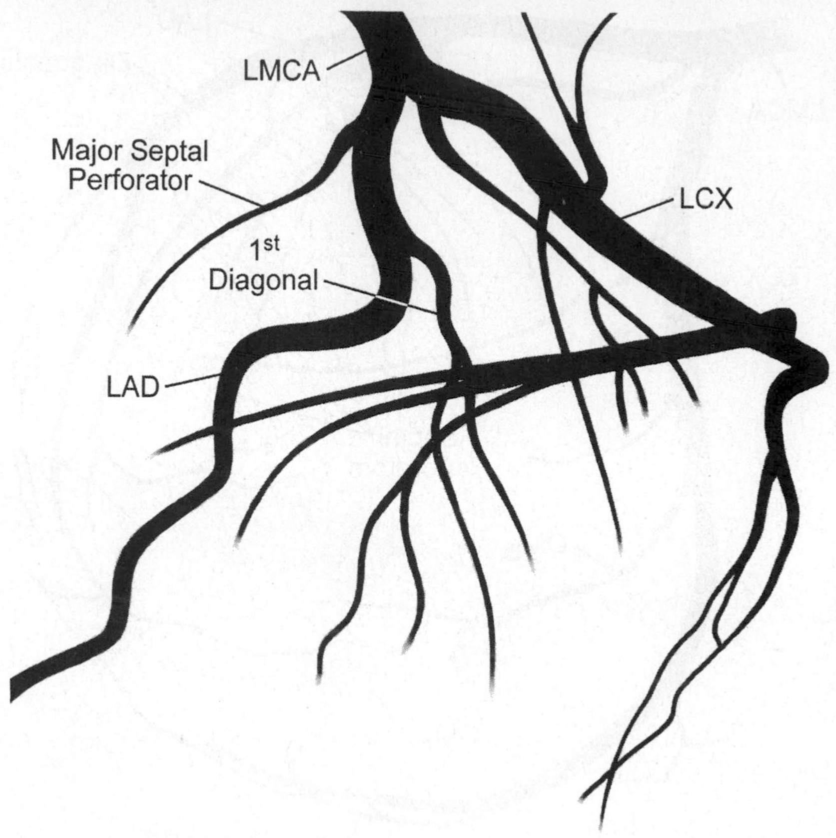

Figure 58.7. Left anterior oblique cranial view of left coronary artery. LMCA, left main coronary artery; LCX, left circumflex coronary artery; LAD, left anterior descending artery.

The origin of the left main artery from the right sinus is even less common (0.02%), but it can result in sudden death if the left main artery passes between the aorta and the pulmonary artery (extremely rare). The left main artery can also pass into the ventricular septum (most common), anterior to the pulmonary artery or posterior to the aorta. The 30° RAO view can help define the relationship between the coronary artery and the great vessels. If the course is septal, septal perforators can be seen originating from the left main.

The other coronary anomalies occur much less frequently. The Amplatz (left or right, depending on the cusp of origin) and multipurpose catheters are especially useful in cannulating anomalous coronary arteries.

Though not truly a congenital anomaly, every angiographer should be aware of **myocardial bridging.** This is an apparent narrowing of a coronary artery (usually the mid-LAD) that is present only during systole. There have been reports of bridging involving the diagonal branches of the LAD, the marginal branches of the LCX, and the distal RCA. Because the majority of coronary blood flow occurs during diastole, myocardial bridges are rarely pathologic, but there have been patients treated with CABG and, more recently, stenting. Nitroglycerin, by dilating epicardial vessels, can make bridging seem even more pronounced. A phenomenon similar to bridging can occur in hypertrophic

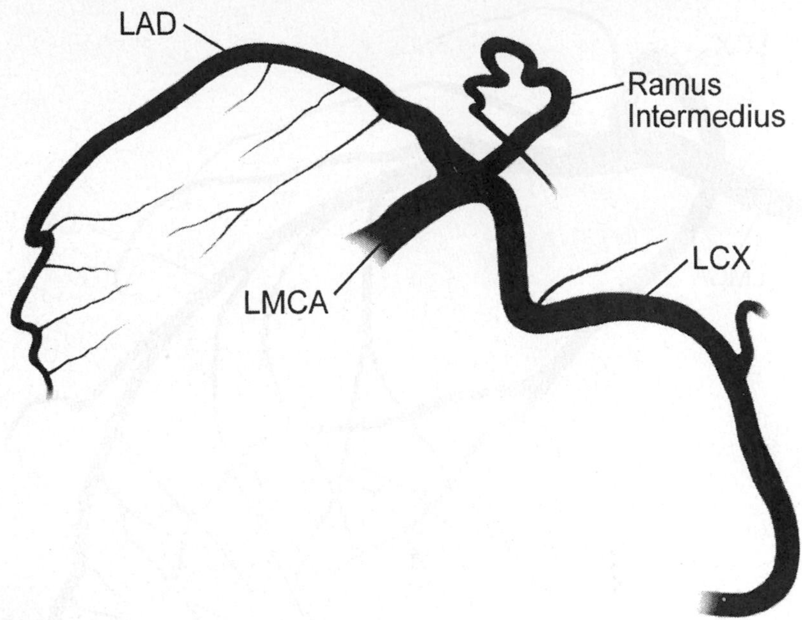

Figure 58.8. Left anterior oblique caudal view of left coronary artery. LMCA, left main coronary artery; LCX, left circumflex coronary artery; LAD, left anterior descending artery.

obstructive cardiomyopathy, in which septal perforators from the LAD can become obliterated during systole.

5. **Quantification of coronary stenosis.** It is important to always obtain at least two perpendicular views of each coronary artery lesion. A single view, or even multiple views, can miss an eccentric lesion. Severity of a lesion is based on percent diameter stenosis compared to a "normal" reference segment. Lesions are generally classified as severe if 70% or more are in the LAD, LCX, and RCA or 50% are in the left main artery. In measuring the size of vessels and stenoses, it is useful to note that a 6F catheter has an external diameter of 2 mm. Formal quantitative coronary angiography or use of calipers can improve the measurement of coronary artery stenoses. Quantitative coronary angiography decreases the inter- and intraobserver variability of grading stenosis severity. The minimal luminal diameter in the most severe view correlates best with perfusion imaging; minimal luminal diameters less than 1.2 to 1.5 mm in proximal vessels typically reduce hyperemic flow.
6. **Limitations of coronary angiography.** Sometimes the severity of a lesion is difficult to gauge based on visual angiographic estimates alone, particularly in the presence of diffuse disease. Angiography only provides an outline of the lumen, the so-called luminogram. In addition, the angiogram can underestimate the presence of atheroma because of outward remodeling of the arterial wall (the Glagov phenomenon). Furthermore, angiography can only visualize arteries greater than 200 μm in diameter. The physiologic importance of 40% to 70% stenoses cannot be determined by angiography alone, and flow limitation should be demonstrated before percutaneous intervention. Techniques such as intravascular ultrasound and the Doppler pressure wire can aid in determining whether ambiguous lesions on angiography are significant. Intravascular ultrasound provides a 360° tomographic view of the vessel lumen rather than a two-dimensional luminogram. Diagnostic applications of intravascular

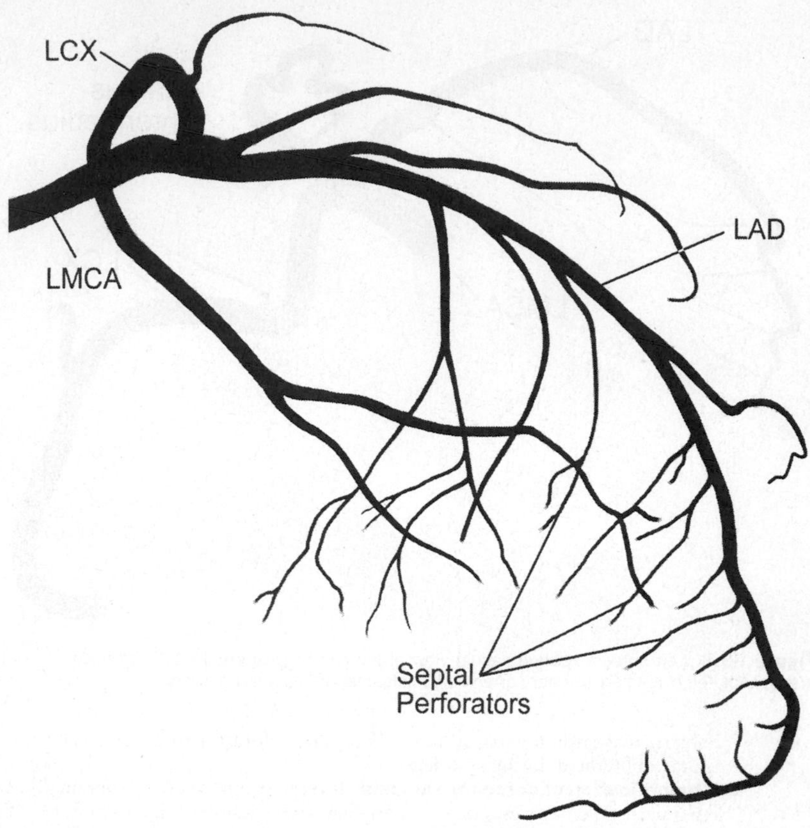

Figure 58.9. Right anterior oblique cranial view of left coronary artery. LMCA, left main coronary artery; LCX, left circumflex coronary artery; LAD, left anterior descending artery.

ultrasound include imaging of angiographically indeterminate lesions, assessment of left main CAD, detection of transplant coronary vasculopathy, and identification of vulnerable plaques. Intravascular ultrasound can also be used during coronary interventions to help guide angioplasty, atherectomy, and stent placement.

C. Crossing the aortic valve

1. Normal aortic valve. The pigtail catheter is most commonly used to cross native aortic valves. Tissue valves can also be crossed, but crossing mechanical valves (e.g., St. Jude, Björk-Shiley, Medtronic-Hall) risks catheter entrapment and is best avoided. The catheter should be made to loop above the aortic valve. Pulling back very slowly, the catheter should give, and it can then be rapidly advanced into the left ventricle during systole. Having the patient take a deep breath and hold it while the pigtail catheter is being unlooped can facilitate the passage of the catheter into the left ventricle. Sometimes the guidewire itself may be useful in crossing the valve, in which case the catheter is simply advanced over the guidewire into the left ventricle. A single operator can cross the aortic valve without assistance, but if two operators are present, one can move the catheter and change its orientation while the other moves the wire back and forth. The pressure in the left ventricle is recorded

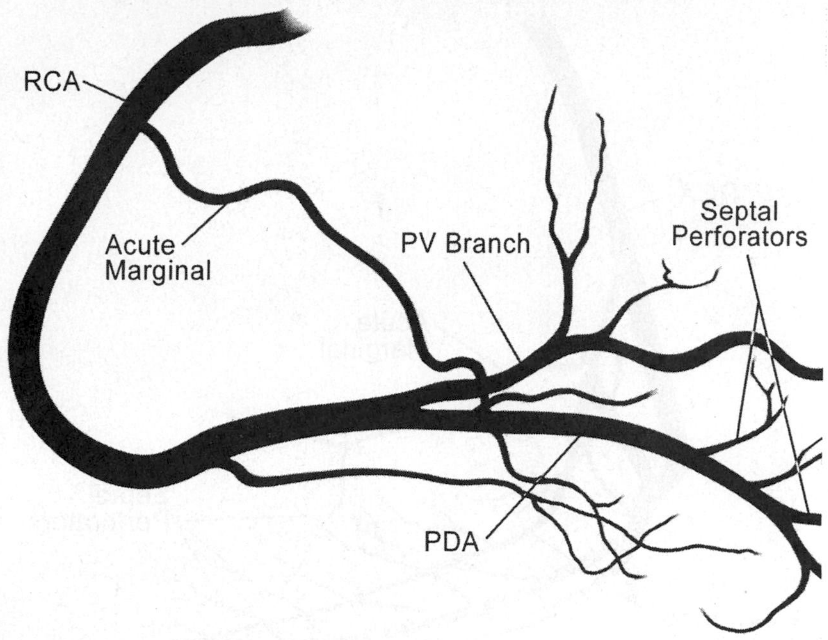

Figure 58.10. Left anterior oblique view of right coronary artery. RCA, right coronary artery; PV branch, posteroventricular branch; PDA, posterior descending artery.

continuously; the catheter is pulled back into the aorta in a single motion to determine the aortic pressure, and the pullback pressure gradient can be calculated.

2. **Aortic stenosis.** In more severe cases of aortic stenosis, difficulty may be encountered in passing any catheter across the aortic valve. In this circumstance a 0.038-inch straight-tipped wire can be used to cross the valve. If this method is elected, some operators recommend a 5,000-U bolus of heparin. The timer should be started, and no more than 3 to 4 minutes should be allowed per attempt at crossing. Between each attempt the wire should be withdrawn and wiped, blood aspirated and discarded, and the catheter flushed. Special care must be used during this maneuver to avoid perforating the aortic cusps or potentially dissecting the coronary ostia. If a 6F sheath is used, a 5F pigtail catheter often provides the correct angle for wire passage; in addition, simultaneous aortic and femoral pressures can be recorded and compared to the left ventricular pressure simultaneously using two transducers. A JR 4 or AL I catheter can also provide the correct orientation for wire passage across the aortic valve. The combination of a Feldman catheter and Rosen wire is an alternative approach to cross stenotic aortic valves. Another way to determine the pressure gradient is to use a double-lumen pigtail catheter and measure the left ventricular and aortic pressures simultaneously. Chapter 50 on right heart catheterization and hemodynamic measurements discusses the method to calculate the aortic gradient.

D. Left ventriculography

1. **Setting up the view.** The pigtail catheter (commonly the angled version) is positioned in the midcavity of the left ventricle. The pigtail should look like a "6" in the RAO projection. If the pigtail twists with each beat, this indicates it is caught in the mitral valve apparatus and needs to be repositioned. The monitor

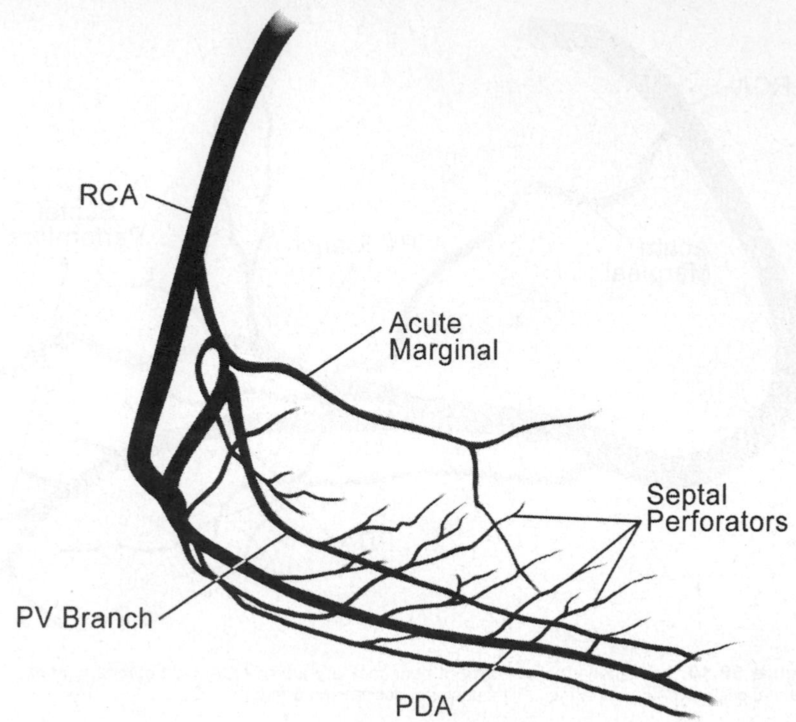

Figure 58.11. Right anterior oblique view of right coronary artery. RCA, right coronary artery; PV branch, posteroventricular branch; PDA, posterior descending artery.

should be observed for ectopy. Once a stable rhythm is present, ventriculography can proceed. First, the left ventricular end-diastolic pressure (LVEDP) should be measured on a 40 scale. In patients with an elevated LVEDP (greater than 25 mm Hg), a left ventriculogram is generally contraindicated. If the decision to proceed with the left ventriculogram is made, sublingual nitroglycerin should first be given to lower the LVEDP. With more moderate degrees of left ventricular dysfunction, nonionic dye, which is less of a myocardial depressant, can be used. Digital subtraction can be used instead of cinefluoroscopy to obtain the left ventriculogram. This allows a smaller amount of contrast to be used. With digital subtraction, the view must be carefully centered because panning is not possible. **The left ventriculogram is best avoided in patients with critical aortic stenosis, significant left main artery disease, or severe left ventricular dysfunction.**

2. **Views.** The **30° RAO** view is used to look at overall left ventricular function. In particular, the anterior, apical, and inferior walls can be assessed (see Fig. 58.12). Some operators routinely pan to the LIMA to assess its patency in a patient who might require CABG. The RAO view is also useful to assess mitral leaflet prolapse and MR. The LAO cranial view can also be used to assess MR, and it avoids the overlap of the aorta with the left atrium that occurs in the RAO view. **MR** can be graded on a scale of 1 to 4; 1 represents trace MR, with mild left atrial opacification that clears with one beat; 2 represents a mild to moderate degree of opacification, though less than the left ventricle; 3 represents moderate to severe opacification of the left atrium equal to the left

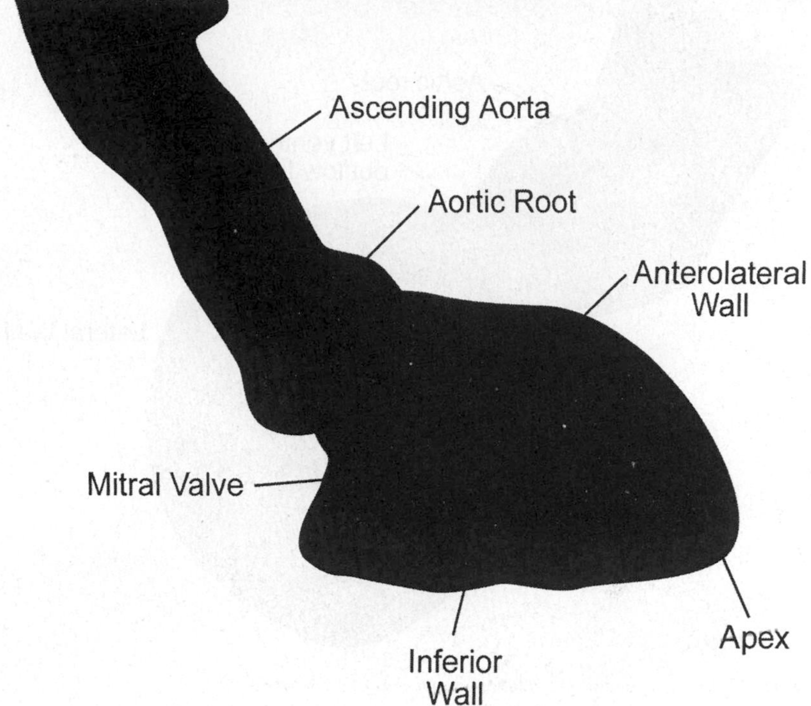

Figure 58.12. Thirty-degree right anterior oblique view of the left ventricle.

ventricle; and 4 represents complete opacification of the left atrium greater than the left ventricle. Panning toward the left atrium may be needed if MR is present. The catheter itself can cause MR if it is caught in the mitral valve apparatus or if it induces premature ventricular contractions. The correlation between angiographic and echocardiographic MR is excellent. The **60° LAO** projection allows evaluation of the septum and the posterior and lateral walls (see Fig. 58.13). Ventricular septal defects are best identified in the LAO projection with slight cranial angulation. If biplane imaging capability exists, RAO and LAO views of the left ventricle can be obtained simultaneously.

3. **Settings.** For a ventriculogram, the flow injector can be set at a rate of 10 to 15 mL/second for a total volume of about 35 to 50 mL, with a rate rise of 0.4 second (to minimize ectopy and to keep the catheter from moving abruptly) and a pressure of 600 PSI. The exact settings will vary depending on the size of the heart and the need to limit contrast.

E. **Aortography.** Aortography is usually performed in the LAO position, with the catheter about 2 cm above the aortic leaflets. Compared to a ventriculogram, a larger volume of contrast is needed to opacify the aorta. The flow injector is set to a higher total volume than for the left ventriculogram, usually about 60 mL at 20 to 25 mL/second. No rate rise is necessary (other than to keep smaller catheters from moving), and a pressure limit of 600 is used. **Aortic insufficiency** can be identified with a grading system similar to that for MR; 1 represents trace aortic insufficiency that clears from the left ventricle with each beat; 2 represents mild left ventricular opacification that takes more than one beat to clear; 3 represents

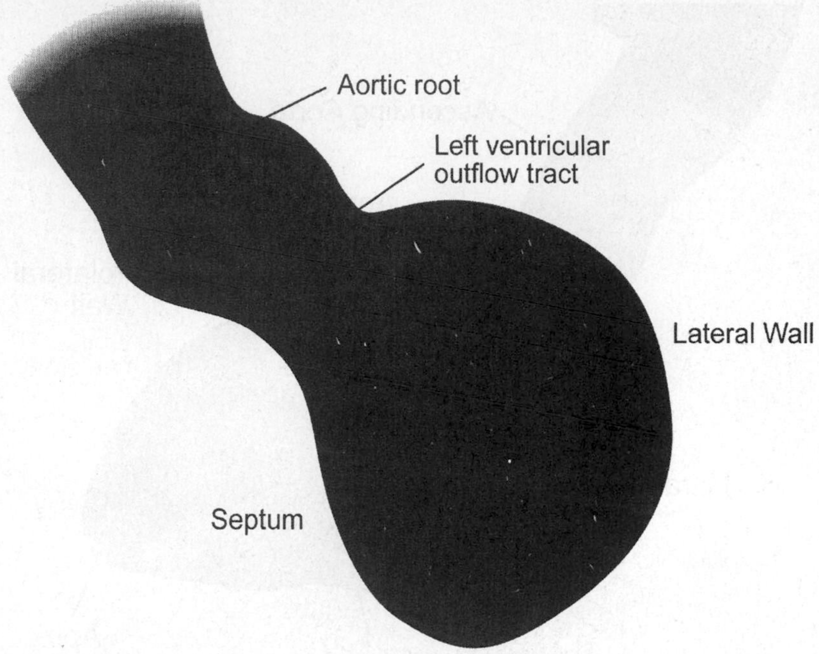

Figure 58.13. Sixty-degree left anterior oblique view of the left ventricle.

moderate left ventricular opacification equal to the aortic root; and 4 represents complete opacification of the left ventricle greater than the aortic root. Diseases of the aorta such as aneurysms or dissection can also be identified. An aortogram can also aid in nonselective visualization of anomalous coronary arteries or grafts that are difficult to engage. However, the absence of filling of a bypass graft on an aortogram does not exclude its presence. The aorta must be well and heavily opacified to ensure that grafts are seen.

An aortogram can be performed with the pigtail catheter placed in the descending aorta slightly above the level of the origins of the renal arteries (the L_1 vertebral body) to rule out **renal artery stenosis.** A JR 4 can be used to obtain selective renal arteriograms by turning the tip of the catheter so that it points to either the left or right in the posteroanterior view. The catheter is then pulled gradually back when it is in the vicinity of the renal artery ostia until it engages. Digital acquisition should be used.

Carotid angiography is sometimes necessary to confirm the degree of carotid artery stenosis seen on a noninvasive study. A variety of catheters (the Headhunter and Newton series) can be used to selectively cannulate the common carotid artery. These catheters are advanced to the aortic arch over a guidewire and pulled back to engage the artery of interest. A Newton 5 can be used to engage the right common carotid artery and a Newton 2, with its smaller curve, can be used to engage the left common carotid artery. There is a 0.5% to 1% risk of stroke with this procedure. Digital acquisition and use of nonionic contrast are mandatory.

F. Provocative testing. In patients in whom coronary artery spasm is suspected, intravenous methylergonovine can be given to provoke spasm (4). Once significant angiographic stenosis has been ruled out, 0.05 mg of intravenous methylergonovine is administered. If the patient develops his or her typical chest pain or ST elevation on electrocardiographic monitoring, the coronary arteries are catheterized immediately. The electrocardiographic changes can help determine which coronary artery to cannulate first. If there are no electrocardiographic changes or chest pain, the right coronary (which is statistically more likely to have spasm) and then the left coronary should be recatheterized 5 minutes after the methylergonovine has been administered. A positive response consists of a focal area of spasm that is relieved by intracoronary nitroglycerin (a usual dose of 100 to 200 μg). Diffuse spasm can be physiologic, and it is also managed with nitroglycerin and verapamil (also 100 to 200 μg). Because the half-life of methylergonovine is longer than that of sublingual nitroglycerin, it is important to realize that spasm can recur after a dose of nitroglycerin. If the initial dose of methylergonovine does not provoke a response, an additional dose of 0.2 mg can be given a few minutes after the first. Alternatively, some operators prefer giving a single dose of 0.2 mg.

VII. POSTCATHETERIZATION CARE

A. Sheath removal. The sheath is removed once the procedure is complete. Adequate local anesthesia should be reinjected if the previously given dose has lost its efficacy. After the sheath is removed, hemostasis is generally obtained with direct manual pressure of the fingertips over the pulse, without sterile gauze to obscure the view. Pressure is held for approximately 20 minutes (about 3 minutes for each French size) until there is no bleeding. To shorten the time of manual pressure, a new device called the Syvek patch (Marine Polymer Technologies) is available. This is paper-based and is made up of algae. It is supposed to accelerate the process of hemostasis when used on the skin over the arteriotomy site while holding manual pressure. Another similar device is the Chito Seal (Abbott), which is a patch that can be applied to stop bleeding from femoral arteriotomy sites. Manual pressure is held for about 10 minutes when using this patch. In patients who have coagulopathy, poorly controlled hypertension, or aortic regurgitation with a wide pulse pressure, a longer duration of pressure is necessary. Care must be taken to intermittently allow adequate blood flow to the distal extremity. It is therefore best if one can directly visualize the extremity to assess its color. If both arterial and venous sheaths are present, it is best to remove the venous sheath first and obtain hemostasis before removing the arterial sheath. In patients with severe aortic stenosis or significant left main CAD, laboratory personnel should be prepared to rapidly manage a vagal episode, which can be life threatening in these situations. Adequate administration of anesthesia before removal of the sheath decreases the chance of a vagal reaction.

Bed rest is generally required for 6 hours after a femoral sheath is removed, although some operators require 1 hour for each French size. In fact, 2 hours is a sufficient period of bed rest for 5F sheaths. Two hours of keeping the arm straight are necessary after a brachial or radial procedure. During the postprocedure observation period it is necessary to monitor heart rate, temperature, blood pressure, urine output, distal pulses, and the access site (for pain, bleeding, or hematoma). Using sandbags over the groin site is discouraged. Before discharge it is best to have the patient ambulate under observation. Specific discharge instructions should include the possibility of late access-site bleeding and the need to hold pressure and call for emergency help.

Intravenous fluids are often given after a cardiac catheterization. The osmotic load of the contrast dye can cause a large diuresis. Intravenous fluids (e.g., normal saline at 100 mL/hour for several hours) can prevent volume depletion. Care should be used in patients with a history of congestive heart failure (CHF), in whom liberal intravenous fluids could contribute to pulmonary edema.

B. Compression/closure devices. The use of femoral artery closure devices offers the advantages of improved patient comfort, potentially lower complication rates, early sheath removal, early hospital discharge, and in some patients anticoagulation may be continued without interruption. The currently available products include compression devices such as the FemoStop (RADI Medical

Systems) and the C clamp, biosealants (Duett, vascular solutions), collagen plugs (Vasoseal; Datascope), vascular sandwiches (Angioseal; Daig), and percutaneous sutures (Perclose, Prostar, Techstar; Abbott).

1. The **FemoStop** is a pneumatic compression device that can be used for holding pressure in cases of prolonged bleeding. The **C clamp** is a mechanical clamp that can also be used for holding prolonged pressure. If either of these devices is employed, direct supervision of the patient is required.
2. **Biosealant** (Duett) devices consist of a procoagulant mixture of collagen and thrombin that is deployed in the tissues surrounding the arterial puncture site through a balloon catheter. This device allows early ambulation. The disadvantages of this device include delayed reuse of the arteriotomy site (repeat arterial puncture cannot be performed for about 3 months) and possibility of infection due to the foreign material introduced; it can also be cumbersome to deploy, and in rare cases, inadvertent deployment of the procoagulant mixture into the femoral artery may result in arterial occlusion requiring surgical intervention.
3. The **Angioseal** (St. Jude/Kensey Nash) hemostatic puncture closure device can be used to obtain hemostasis in an uncomplicated femoral procedure if an 8F or smaller sheath was used. Before deploying the Angioseal, it is advisable to obtain an angiogram of the femoral artery to ensure that the entry site of sheath is above the bifurcation of the common femoral artery. It is available in 6F and 8F sizes. A biodegradable collagen plug is deployed to the femoral artery puncture site using a guidewire and special sheath. No manual pressure is required, and ambulation can begin after 1 hour. The Angioseal device is user friendly due to its ease of deployment and general reliability. The disadvantage of this device is the introduction of foreign material that could be a potential source of infection, and repeat arterial puncture cannot be performed at the same site for about 45 to 60 days.
4. The **Vasoseal** (Datascope) is a collagen plug that is placed over the femoral artery puncture site. It comes in several sizes; to determine the appropriate size, it is necessary to place a depth marker on the needle during the initial arterial puncture. Ambulation can begin 1 hour after placement.
5. The **Perclose** (Abbott) is a percutaneous vascular suture device that allows immediate ambulation (of course, after the effects of any sedation given during the procedure have worn off). Before its use, a 35-degree RAO view of the right femoral artery should be taken to ensure that the sheath has been placed above the femoral artery bifurcation. The device is currently available in 6F, 8F, and 10F sizes. Other improved devices are likely to be available in the near future.
6. The **StarClose Vascular Closure System** (Abbott) is a percutaneous vascular closure device that employs a nitinol clip. Before its use, a view of the right femoral artery should be taken to ensure that the sheath has been placed above the femoral artery bifurcation. The device is delivered through a sheath onto the arteriotomy site, and the clip takes hold of the tissue in a circular manner and closes off the arteriotomy site.

VIII. COMPLICATIONS

A. **Death.** There is a 0.1% risk of death from LHC. This risk is substantially higher in patients undergoing urgent catheterization for acute coronary syndromes. In addition, patients with left main CAD, severe aortic stenosis, or severe left ventricular dysfunction are known to be patient subgroups with a particularly increased risk. Advanced age increases the risk of death.

B. **MI.** There is a 0.05% risk of MI from LHC. MI can result from coronary dissection, disruption of a preexisting atheromatous plaque, a large air embolus, or a thrombus. Patients with acute coronary syndromes have a higher risk of MI.

C. **Stroke.** Stroke occurs in 0.05% of catheterizations. There is a risk of stroke from an inadvertent air embolus or thrombus. Presence of aortic atheroma is a risk factor for embolic complications. Dislodgement of atheromatous debris in the aorta can lead to a stroke. This risk can be minimized by use of 260-cm exchange wires for catheter changes in patients with known severe aortic disease.

D. Coronary artery dissection. Engagement of the coronary arteries can rarely cause dissection. It is most often due to injection of contrast through a catheter that is not coaxial to the coronary artery, causing rupture of a preexisting plaque, or placement of the catheter too deeply into the coronary artery (so-called deep throating). Particular caution should be used with Amplatz catheters. In cases of left main coronary artery dissection, a stent can be placed emergently and the patient can be placed on peripheral cardiopulmonary support until the surgical team can be mobilized.

E. Coronary artery spasm. Engagement of the coronary arteries, in particular the RCA, can cause spasm. This is best treated with withdrawal of the catheter. Subsequent reengagement and administration of intracoronary nitroglycerin (100 to 200 μg) may also be necessary for more rapid resolution of spasm.

F. Renal failure. Contrast dye can precipitate renal failure in any patient, although certain patients (those with elevated creatinine, diabetes, proteinuria, or dehydration) are at higher risk. Adequate prehydration with normal saline can reduce this risk. In some cases (especially in diabetics with renal insufficiency and those with renal artery stenoses), patients may need to be admitted to the hospital for hydration with 0.45% saline for several hours before the LHC to minimize risk of contrast-induced nephrotoxicity. The use of the antioxidant *N*-acetylcysteine (600 mg orally twice daily) before and after exposure to radiocontrast along with 0.45% saline prevented the decrease in renal function in patients with chronic renal insufficiency exposed to nonionic low-osmolality contrast agent. This study, however, enrolled only 83 patients. Other studies have examined the role of sodium bicarbonate infusions in preventing contrast-induced nephropathy. Several small studies have shown benefit with the use of sodium bicarbonate infusions (3 ampules sodium bicarbonate in 1L NS, infused at 3 mL/kg per hour for 1 hour before procedure and 1 mL/kg per hour during the procedure and for 6 hours following) or sodium bicarbonate plus *N*-acetylcysteine in preventing contrast-induced renal function. In a study of 129 patients with serum creatinine concentrations of 1.5 to 3.5 mg/dL who underwent coronary or aortofemoral angiography, use of the isoosmolar, dimeric, nonionic contrast medium iodixanol was associated with decreased risk of nephropathy, compared with the low-osmolar, nonionic, monomeric contrast medium iohexol. The best way to minimize contrast-induced renal failure is to limit the amount of dye used. Using less than 30 mL of contrast dye dramatically reduces the incidence of renal failure in even the highest-risk patients (7). Biplane cineangiography can maximize the amount of information obtained with each view.

G. Emergency CABG. There is a risk of needing emergency CABG as a complication of the catheterization (e.g., dissection of the left main coronary artery). There is also the possibility of identification of critical disease, such as severe left main CAD, that may prompt emergency CABG as the most expedient treatment.

H. Arrhythmias. A risk of ventricular fibrillation (0.5%) exists with catheterization. This rhythm is treated with electrical defibrillation. In particular, overinjection of contrast into the RCA can cause ventricular fibrillation. Contrast dye (less so nonionic dye) can cause transient bradycardia, best dealt with by having the patient cough and by minimizing the amount of dye injected with each angiographic procedure.

I. HF. The osmotic load of contrast dye can put a patient with diminished cardiac or renal function into overt pulmonary edema. In patients with severe cardiac or renal disease, injection of contrast should be limited, and use of nonionic, low-osmolar dye should be considered.

J. Vagal reaction. If a patient develops hypotension and/or bradycardia, a vagal reaction should be considered. It is common to see this when local anesthetic is being administered or when the sheath is being removed. Atropine 1 mg IV should be available and given in these situations. Adequate anesthesia can help prevent such reactions. In a patient with severe aortic stenosis or left main CAD, a vagal reaction can start a downward spiral that leads to death. Levophed (about 10 μg) should always be available and used immediately in such cases of hypotension.

K. Vascular

1. **Femoral.** Pseudoaneurysms, arteriovenous fistulas, arterial thrombosis, and peripheral emboli are possible vascular complications. Careful technique can minimize these events. In particular, paying attention to puncture location and obtaining adequate hemostasis after sheath removal are the best ways to decrease vascular complications. For example, the smaller sheaths (5F) are preferred in patients with significant peripheral vascular disease. Frequent aspiration and discarding of blood from the arterial sheath, followed by gentle flushing, is useful. If an attempted cannulation is unsuccessful but an arterial puncture has been made, the needle should be withdrawn and adequate manual pressure held (about 5 minutes). If a venous puncture has been made inadvertently, the needle should be removed and pressure held (for about 3 minutes). Proceeding directly to arterial puncture without removing the needle and holding pressure increases the chance of arteriovenous fistula formation. If a venous puncture is planned, it should be made lower than the arterial puncture site. Bruits should be auscultated both before and after the procedure. A new bruit may indicate a vascular complication. **Ultrasound** is an essential part of managing groin complications. If there is a large pseudoaneurysm present, surgery may be required after a trial of ultrasound-guided compression. Percutaneous injection of thrombin into the pseudoaneurysm has proven to be a more effective alternative to compression. Small pseudoaneurysms (less than 2 cm) tend to close spontaneously but should be followed by serial ultrasound examinations. An arteriovenous fistula that does not close spontaneously in 2 to 4 weeks may require surgical repair.
2. **Brachial/radial.** When using an upper-extremity approach, blood pressure should first be checked in both arms. If there is a difference between arms, peripheral vascular disease should be suspected and the side with the higher blood pressure should be used. For a radial approach, an Allen test must be performed to assess the patency of collateral ulnar circulation. The rate of vascular complications such as thrombosis is higher with the upper-extremity approach than with the femoral approach.

L. Bleeding. Access site bleeding can be significant. If there is a great deal of oozing around the sheath, it can be exchanged for a sheath one French size larger. Adequate manual pressure is usually sufficient to stop bleeding after sheath removal. It is typical practice to check the activated clotting time on patients who had been on heparin before the procedure and only proceed with sheath removal if the clotting time is below 160. Some institutions use protamine (1 mg per 100 U heparin) to reverse heparinization, but this exposes the patient to the potential for allergic reactions to protamine (namely, hypotension). Even more concerning is **retroperitoneal bleeding.** If a patient complains of severe back pain after a catheterization, this should be considered. An unexpected drop in hemoglobin after a catheterization should also raise this possibility. Obese patients, in particular, can have a major bleed without obvious external signs. Noncontrast computed tomography (CT) scan of the abdomen and pelvis can diagnose a retroperitoneal bleed, but it is important to assess the patient's clinical stability before sending them to such a study.

M. Infection. There is a risk of infection, as with any invasive procedure. This risk can be minimized with proper attention to sterile technique. There is usually no need for prophylactic antibiotics. However, some operators do give antibiotics after use of a percutaneous vascular suture device in patients who are at elevated risk for infection, such as obese or diabetic patients. Endocarditis prophylaxis for patients with valvular heart disease or prosthetic valves is unnecessary.

N. Neuropathy. There is a slight risk of damage to the femoral nerve from inadvertent puncture. Femoral hematoma (or retroperitoneal bleeding) can also cause compromise of the femoral nerve. Function usually improves with time, but complete recovery can take several months.

O. Allergy. As discussed above, contrast dye can cause adverse reactions, ranging from hives to anaphylaxis. Severe anaphylactoid reactions to contrast dye occur in about 0.1% of cases. Local anesthetic can also cause problems due to specific allergies to the amide or ester component, or to the preservative. A variety of agents are available. Procaine (an ester agent), lidocaine (an amide agent), and bupivacaine (a preservative-free amide agent) are alternative agents.

ACKNOWLEDGMENTS

The authors thank Drs. Niranjan Seshadri and Deepak L. Bhatt for their contributions to this chapter.

Suggested Readings

Aspelin P, Aubry P, Fransson SG, et al. Nephrotoxicity in High-Risk Patients Study of Iso-osmolar and Low-Osmolar Non-ionic Contrast Media Study Investigators. *N Engl J Med* 2003;348:551–553.

Bashore TM, et al. American College of Cardiology/Society for Cardiac Angiography and Interventions clinical expert consensus document on cardiac catheterization laboratory standards. *J Am Coll Cardiol* 2001;37:2170–2214.

Tepel M, van der Giet M, Schwarzfeld C, et al. Prevention of radiographic-contrast-agent-induced reductions in renal function by acetylcysteine. *N Engl J Med* 2000;343:180–184.

Landmark Articles

Heupler FA, Proudfit WL, Razavi M, et al. Ergonovine maleate provocative test for coronary arterial spasm. *Am J Cardiol* 1978;41:631–640.

Manske CL, Sprafka JM, Strony JT, et al. Contrast nephropathy in azotemic diabetic patients undergoing coronary angiography. *Am J Med* 1990;89:615–620.

Matthai WH, Kussmal WG, Krol J, et al. A comparison of low- with high-osmolar contrast agents in cardiac angiography: identification of criteria for selective use. *Circulation* 1994;89:291–301.

Yamanaka O, Hobbs RE. Coronary artery anomalies in 126,595 patients undergoing coronary arteriography. *Catheter Cardiovasc Diagn* 1990;21:28–40.

Key Reviews

Boucher RA, Myler RK, Clark DA, et al. Coronary angiography and angioplasty. *Catheter Cardiovasc Diagn* 1988;14:269–285.

Ziada KM, Kapadia SR, Tuzcu EM, et al. The current status of intravascular ultrasound imaging. *Curr Prob Cardiol* 1999;24:541–616.

Relevant Book Chapters

Baim DS, Grossman W. *Cardiac catheterization, angiography, and intervention,* 7th ed. Philadelphia: Lippincott Williams & Wilkins, 2006: 187–221

Baum S. *Abram's angiography,* 4th ed. Boston: Little, Brown and Company, 1997:241–252.

Bhatt DL, Heupler FA Jr. Coronary angiography. In: Topol EJ, ed. *Textbook of Cardiovascular Medicine,* 3rd ed. Philadelphia: Lippincott Williams & Wilkins, 2007:1226–1242.

Ellis SG. Coronary angiography. In: Fuster V, Ross R, Topol E, eds. *Atherosclerosis and coronary artery disease,* vol. 2. Philadelphia: Lippincott–Raven Publishers, 1996:1433–1450.

Green CE. *Coronary cinematography.* Philadelphia: Lippincott–Raven Publishers, 1996:39–68.

Kern MJ. *The cardiac catheterization handbook,* 3rd ed. St. Louis: Mosby–Year Book, 1999:278–390.

Tilkian AG, Daily EK. *Cardiovascular procedures: diagnostic techniques and therapeutic procedures.* St. Louis: Mosby, 1986:117–151.

59 PERCUTANEOUS CORONARY INTERVENTION

Matthew C. Becker

I. INTRODUCTION

A. Coronary atherosclerosis may result in a flow-limiting stenosis that leads to myocardial ischemia and/or myocardial infarction (MI). Andreas Gruntzig first managed these lesions percutaneously on September 16, 1977, when he advanced a fixed-wire, distensible balloon across a coronary stenosis and briefly inflated it to 6 atm (90 psi). This procedure was termed percutaneous transluminal coronary angioplasty (PTCA). With the advent of stents and other therapeutic coronary devices, these procedures are now more broadly termed percutaneous coronary intervention (PCI). It is estimated that more than 1 million PCI procedures are completed in the United States and approximately 2 million worldwide annually.

B. The field of interventional cardiology continues to rapidly evolve as a result of many important advances in equipment, strategies, and adjunctive medication. These advances have been paralleled by a concomitant improvement in the safety and efficacy profile of PCI. The assimilation of a large body of basic and clinical research encompassing all areas of interventional cardiology continue to redefine the standard of care paradigm. As a result, the American Heart Association (AHA), the American College of Cardiology (ACC), and the American Board of Internal Medicine have established PCI guidelines and board certification for interventional cardiology.

II. PCI INDICATIONS

A. Central tenet. Although there is no substitute for sound clinical judgment, PCI is generally reserved for patients in whom there is an objective demonstration of myocardial ischemia or symptoms as well as angiographic demonstration of obstructive coronary disease. PCI may not be indicated for asymptomatic or mildly symptomatic patients who have only a small area of viable or jeopardized myocardium, have no objective evidence of myocardial ischemia, have other life-limiting disease processes, or have lesions that have a low likelihood of success (Tables 59.1 and 59.2).

B. ST-Segment-Elevation MI (STEMI). Primary **PCI should be the preferred treatment strategy for patients presenting with STEMI to a facility experienced with and capable of performing PCI.** Randomized trials have demonstrated that clinical outcomes are improved when such patients are emergently transferred to centers able to perform primary PCI as opposed to therapy with thrombolytics—despite a significant delay (mean time of 44 minutes) in time to therapy due to transport. This seems especially true of patients presenting 3 to 12 hours after symptom onset, where the superiority of primary PCI clearly becomes evident. In those presenting within 3 hours of symptom onset, the mortality data would suggest that either therapy is equally efficacious in appropriate candidates.

1. Primary PCI is indicated in patients presenting with STEMI less than 12 hours from symptom onset (or more than 12 hours with persistent symptoms), provided that the door-to-balloon time is anticipated to be less than 90 minutes and is performed by an experienced operator at a high-volume center (i.e., greater than 200 PCI procedures per year, of which at least 36 are for the indication of STEMI).
2. Primary PCI is also indicated in patients presenting with an appropriate clinical history and a presumed new left bundle-branch block (LBBB).

TABLE 59.1	Standard Pre-percutaneous Coronary Intervention Evaluation
History ■ Symptoms (angina, dyspnea, paroxysmal nocturnal dyspnea, syncope) ■ Previous MI ■ Previous cardiac interventions (PCI, CABG) ■ Comorbidities (diabetes mellitus, hyperlipidemia, hypertension, etc.) Medications (glucophage, statins, aspirin, thienopyridines, etc.) Allergies (contrast dye, latex, etc.) Physical exam (murmurs, jugular venous pressure, pulses, bruits, edema) Laboratory data (creatinine, potassium, hemoglobin, platelets, INR) Other tests (ECG, echocardiogram, stress tests) Informed consent including risks, benefits, alternatives	

CABG, coronary artery bypass grafting; ECG, electrocardiogram; INR, international normalized ratio; MI, myocardial infarction; PCI, percutaneous coronary intervention.

3. Patients younger than 75 years old presenting with STEMI complicated by cardiogenic shock within 36 hours of symptom onset who are otherwise candidates for revascularization within 18 hours of onset of shock should be considered for primary PCI unless otherwise contraindicated. Primary PCI is reasonable in *selected* patients younger than 75 years old presenting with shock complicating STEMI within 36 hours if the patients are known to have good prior functional status, agree to invasive management strategy, and are otherwise suitable for revascularization.
4. Primary PCI is indicated for patients with STEMI complicated by severe congestive heart failure (CHF) (i.e., Killip class III) presenting within 12 hours of symptom onset.
5. In addition, primary PCI should be considered for patients that are ineligible for thrombolytic therapy or for those who require rescue angioplasty after failed thrombolytic therapy. At the Cleveland Clinic (CC), successful thrombolysis is defined as the patient being pain free, hemodynamically stable, and having more than 70% ST-segment resolution at 90 minutes. For cardiogenic shock patients, keep in mind that 14% of patients in the SHould we emergently revascularize Occluded coronaries for Cardiogenic shocK (SHOCK) trial presented with mechanical complications [i.e., ventricular septal defect (VSD), mitral regurgitation (MR), and free wall rupture].

TABLE 59.2	Considerations for Every Percutaneous Coronary Intervention

Review clinical and angiographic risk factors
Develop strategy and anticipate problems
  Surgical backup
  Access
  Anticoagulation and antiplatelet therapy
  Consider diagnostic adjuncts (e.g., PA line)
  Consider therapeutic mechanical adjuncts (e.g., IABP)
  Guide wire
  Device (e.g., angioplasty, stent)
  Closure of vascular access site
  Post-PCI destination (telemetry ward, CICU)	

CICU, cardiac intensive care unit; IABP, intraaortic balloon pump; PA, pulmonary artery; PCI, percutaneous coronary intervention.

6. Facilitated PCI (i.e., fibrinolytics immediately before planned PCI) may be considered in selected higher-risk patients when primary PCI is not immediately available and bleeding risk is low. However, clinical data thus far have failed to clearly document a significant advantage to this strategy, and ongoing trials are poised to provide more information on this topic.
7. Rescue PCI (i.e., PCI within 12 hours of thrombolytic therapy with persistent ischemia) is reasonable in patients developing electrical or hemodynamic instability, CHF, or shock within 36 hours of MI or if there is evidence of residual ischemia. The Randomized Evaluation of Salvage Angioplasty with Combined Utilization of Endpoints (RESCUE) trial demonstrated a significant in-hospital and combined mortality benefit associated with rescue PCI that persisted beyond 1 year of follow-up in patients that were judged to have failed thrombolysis in the setting of anterior wall STEMI.
8. Immediate PCI is not recommended in STEMI patients who underwent successful thrombolysis except in cases of recurrent MI, shock, or objective demonstration of ischemia during recovery. In addition, it is reasonable to perform routine left heart catheterization (LHC) with PCI in patients that were treated with fibrinolytics that have a post-MI (ejection fraction) EF of less than 40%, malignant ventricular arrhythmia, or heart failure (HF) during the acute event.

C. **Acute coronary syndrome (ACS).** Unstable angina (UA) and non–ST-segment elevation myocardial infarction (NSTEMI) are considered part of the spectrum of the ACS. Because the primary difference in the two entities is the presence of ischemia severe enough to result in myocardial necrosis as evidenced by positive serum biomarkers, differentiation at presentation is impossible. As a result, UA/NSTEMI are treated as a single entity in the ACC/AHA Guidelines. Given that individual patients presenting with UA/NSTEMI are at widely varying risk for subsequent morbidity and mortality, early and aggressive risk stratification including cardiac catheterization with subsequent percutaneous or surgical revascularization (rather than noninvasive stress testing) is recommended. This recommendation is supported by a number of clinical trials comparing an early invasive to delayed conservative strategy. Both the FRagmin and Fast Revascularization during InStability in Coronary artery disease Investigators (FRISC II) and TACTICS-TIMI 18 trials demonstrated a reduction in the rate of death or MI in the early invasive group. However, this benefit was primarily driven by a reduction in MI and observed in the troponin positive patients. More recently, two large meta-analyses that included results from the recently published Invasive Versus Conservative Treatment in Unstable Coronary Syndromes (ICTUS) and Randomized Intervention Treatment of Angina (RITA-3) trials concluded that an early invasive strategy was superior to the delayed conservative approach because of a significant reduction in both mortality and nonfatal MI from hospital discharge to the end of follow-up. Recently, the 5-year follow-up data from both RITA-3 and FRISC II trials have been published and indicate a significant and persistent reduction in the endpoint of death or MI. Not surprisingly, there was also a sigificant reduction in severe angina and rehospitalization associated with an early aggressive strategy. There are, however, several studies that would suggest improved outcomes using a delayed conservative strategy, such as the ICTUS and Veterans Affairs Non-Q Wave Infarction Strategies In Hospital (VANQWISH) trials. Consisting of a moderate-high risk NSTEMI population, the ICTUS trial randomized patients to either an early invasive or selectively invasive strategy (i.e., angiography only for refractory angina, hemodynamic instability, or significant ischemia). Although there was a significant increase in periprocedural MI in the early invasive group, there was no difference between the groups in regard to the primary endpoint (death, nonfatal MI, or rehospitalization for angina within 1 year) at trial end. There was, however, a significant reduction in the rate of rehospitalization in the early invasive group. The applicability of the VANQWISH trial, which showed inferiority of an early invasive approach, is questionable given the high surgical mortality rate (approximately 11%), the lack of stents and antiplatelet adjuncts during PCI, and the inclusion of MI patients who received fibrinolytic therapy.

1. The most recent AHA/ACC guidelines (Table 59.3) recommend that an early invasive revascularization strategy is indicated in patients without serious or life-limiting illnesses presenting with UA/NSTEMI with the following **high-risk features**:
   a. Positive serum cardiac biomarkers (i.e., troponin I or T)
   b. Dynamic electrocardiographic changes (i.e., new ST-segment depression or transient ST elevation)
   c. HF or objective evidence of new left ventricular (LV) dysfunction
   d. Shock or evidence of hemodynamic instability
   e. Recurrent ischemia despite adequate medical therapy
   f. Malignant ventricular arrhythmia

TABLE 59.3 2007 American College of Cardiology/American Heart Association (ACC/AHA) Percutaneous Coronary Intervention Guidelines

ST elevation MI	Class	Level of evidence
Primary PCI STEMI patients presenting to a hospital with PCI capability should be treated with primary PCI within 90 minutes of first medical contact.	I	A
Fibrinolytic therapy. STEMI patients presenting to a hospital without PCI capability and who cannot be transferred to a PCI center and undergo PCI within 90 minutes of first medical contact should be treated with fibrinolytic therapy within 30 minutes of hospital presentation as a systems goal unless fibrinolytic therapy is contraindicated.	I	B
Rescue PCI. Coronary angiography with intent to perform PCI (or emergency CABG) is recommended for patients who have received fibrinolytic therapy and have shock (<75 years of age – [*LOE* B]), CHF (B), or hemodynamically compromising arrythmias (C)	I	B,B,C
Facilitated PCI. Regimens *other than* full-dose fibrinolytic therapy might be considered as a reperfusion strategy when patients are at high risk, PCI is not immediately available within 90 minutes, and bleeding risk is low (younger age, absence of poorly controlled hypertension, normal body weight).	IIb	C
Unstable angina/Non ST elevation MI		
Early Invasive strategy. Patients presenting with: ■ Recurrent angina/ischemia at rest or with low-level activities despite intensive anti-ischemic therapy ■ Recurrent angina/ischemia with CHF symptoms ■ New or worsening MR ■ High-risk findings on noninvasive stress testing ■ Depressed LV systolic function (e.g., EF <0.40) ■ Hemodynamic instability or rest angina accompanied by hypotension ■ Sustained ventricular tachycardia ■ PCI within 6 months or prior CABG	I	B
Early Conservative Strategy Decisions regarding coronary angiography in patients who lack high risk features according to findings on clinical examination/noninvasive testing can be individualized based on patient preferences.	I	B

CABG, coronary artery bypass grafting; CHF, congestive heart failure; LV, left ventricular; MI, myocardial infarction; MR, mitral regurgitation; PCI, percutaneous coronary intervention; STEMI, ST-Segment-Elevation MI.

g. History of PCI in the preceeding 6 months or coronary artery bypass grafting (CABG) at any time in the past

2. In **stable** patients presenting with UA/NSTEMI who lack these high-risk features, either an early invasive or conservative strategy may be considered.

3. Patients presenting with UA/NSTEMI because of significant (i.e., >50% stenosis) left main trunk (LMT) disease who are **not candidates** for revascularization via CABG may be considered for high-risk PCI.

4. Patients **lacking** the above-noted high-risk features associated with UA/NSTEMI found to have a saphenous vein graft (SVG) lesion or multiple lesions of the native coronary circulation may be considered for PCI if they are not candidates for reoperative surgery.

D. Chronic stable angina. It is estimated that more than 85% of all PCI procedures are performed in the elective setting for chronic stable angina.

1. **PCI versus Medical Therapy.** Although PCI has been shown to be more effective than medical therapy alone in decreasing the frequency of anginal symptoms and improving exercise capacity, it has never been demonstrated to reduce the rate of MI or mortality. Data from the Clinical Outcomes Utilizing Revascularization and Aggressive Drug Evaluation (COURAGE) trial—which prospectively randomized 2287 patients with objective evidence of ischemia to either aggressive medical therapy or elective PCI—suggests that PCI in addition to optimal medical therapy **does not** reduce the incidence of death, MI, or other major cardiovascular morbidity. This is in contrast to data from the much smaller Asymptomatic Cardiac Ischemia Pilot (ACIP) study that demonstrated a mortality benefit associated with revascularization (i.e., PCI or CABG) in patients with asymptomatic ischemia, especially those with diabetes mellitus. These data, therefore, suggest that in the setting of chronic stable angina, a physician has the option of controlling anginal symptoms with either medication or PCI as dictated by individual patient characteristics or preferences.

2. **PCI versus CABG surgery.** In the Bypass Angioplasty Revascularization Investigators (BARI) trial, balloon angioplasty, as compared to CABG, provided shorter convalescent time and similar survival rates, except in the diabetic subpopulation. In addition, patients undergoing CABG had a greater improvement in functional status and fewer repeat procedures. The Arterial Revascularization Therapies Study (ARTS) trial had similar findings except that the use of bare metal stents (BMS) reduced the rate of restenosis. The ARTS II trial compared PCI with drug-eluting stents (DES) to the CABG group from the ARTS I trial using Bayesian analysis and found similar rates of freedom from death, cerebrovascular events, MI, or repeat percutaneous or surgical revascularization procedure at 1 year. In general, the benefits of CABG are greater durability and more complete revascularization. The advantages of PCI are the avoidance of general anesthesia, sternotomy, extracorporeal bypass, central nervous system complications, and prolonged convalescence. PCI disadvantages include restenosis, chronic antiplatelet therapy requirement, late thrombosis (risk appears to be greater with DES), and incomplete revascularization due to diffuse disease. Therefore, although the available data suggest that CABG is favored for patients with diabetes with multivessel disease including the proximal left anterior descending (LAD), reduced LV systolic function, unprotected left main or diffuse coronary disease, the advances associated with modern PCI appear to be eroding this advantage.

III. CONTRAINDICATIONS. The only absolute contraindication to PCI is significant active bleeding, given the absolute need to anticoagulate and given antiplatelet therapy. Relative contraindications include a bleeding diathesis, unsuitable or high-risk coronary anatomy (e.g., chronic total occlusion in the absence of ischemia, diffuse distal disease, and most cases of unprotected left main trunk stenosis), recurrent restenosis despite brachytherapy, and a short life expectancy because of a comorbid condition.

IV. PROGNOSIS. A patient's clinical status and coronary angiogram are powerful predictors of outcome. Certain clinical and angiographic variables have repeatedly been associated with adverse events (Table 59.4).

TABLE 59.4 Clinical and Angiographic Predictors of Adverse Outcomes

Clinical predictors	Angiographic predictors
■ Older age	■ Thrombus
■ Unstable angina	■ Bypass graft
■ Acute MI	■ Left main trunk
■ Cardiogenic shock	■ Lesion >20 mm in length
■ CHF	■ Excessive tortuosity of proximal segment
■ Left ventricular function	■ Extremely angulated lesions >90°
■ Multivessel coronary disease	■ Total occlusion >3 months old and/or bridging collaterals
■ Diabetes mellitus	■ Inability to protect major side branches
■ Renal impairment	■ Degenerated vein grafts with friable lesions
■ Peripheral vascular disease	■ Unprotected left main trunk
■ Small body size	

CHF, congestive heart failure; MI, myocardial infarction.

V. ANGIOGRAPHIC/PROCEDURAL/CLINICAL SUCCESS. Angiographic success is defined as a residual stenosis less than 50% with PTCA or less than 20% with stenting, and is achieved in 96% to 99% of patients. The definition of procedural success is angiographic success without major in-hospital complications (i.e., death, CABG, or MI). Clinical success is defined as procedural success with relief of the symptoms and signs of myocardial ischemia.

VI. COMPLICATIONS

A. The incidence of complications (death 0.5% to 1.4%, periprocedural MI [as defined by creatinine kinase-myocardial band (CK-MB) elevation greater than three times the upper limit of normal] up to 8%, and emergency CABG surgery 0.2% to 0.3%) has consistently decreased over the past 20 years because of the advent of stents, new and more effective antiplatelet therapies, improved equipment, and inceasing reliance upon evidence-based strategies.

B. Abrupt closure is the most common cause of a major adverse cardiac event (MACE) and typically occurs within 6 hours of intervention. The most common cause of abrupt closure is suboptimal stent expansion or dissection followed by thrombus, spasm, and sidebranch occlusion. In the mid-1980s, the risk of abrupt closure approached 5%. The common use of periprocedural glycoprotein IIb/IIIa and/or direct thrombin-inhibiting anticoagulants and stent deployment has reduced this risk to less than 1% in modern practice. Risk factors for abrupt closure include presentation with acute MI, poor coronary flow post-intervention (i.e., less thanTIMI II), complex lesion morphology (i.e., class C lesions), and suboptimal result as judged by angiography or intravascular ultrasonography (IVUS) imaging.

C. Athero- and thromboembolism probably occur to varying degrees in all interventions, but they are most frequently encountered in cases involving degenerated vein grafts, patients presenting with acute coronary syndromes, and in cases using directional/rotational atherectomy. Distal embolization can result in no reflow (decreased coronary flow), abrupt closure, and periprocedural MI. Preventing thromboembolization to the distal vascular bed can best be accomplished with medications (anticoagulant and antiplatelet therapy) and devices (Possis AngioJet, PercuSurge GuardWire, and Export catheter and filter devices). Preventing atheroembolization (i.e., atherosclerotic plaque contents) is best accomplished by using devices (i.e., PercuSurge GuardWire, filter devices) that trap and remove the debris before it reaches the distal vascular bed. Vasodilators such as adenosine (36 to 72 μg repeatedly), nitroprusside (50 to 200 μg), and verapamil (200 μg) have been shown to prevent and manage no reflow but have no effect in preventing CK-MB elevation.

D. Coronary perforation is estimated to occur in 0.1% to 1.14% of PTCA cases, 0.25% to 0.70% of cases using directional atherectomy, up to 1.3% in cases of rotational atherectomy, 1.3% to 2.1% of cases using extractional atherectomy, and 1.9% to 2.0% following excimer laser angioplasty. Contrast extravasation is typically evident in 80% to 90% of perforation at the time of intervention. However, up to 20% of cases can present several hours after the procedure and are frequently because of hydrophilic wire perforation of a small vessel. Treatment usually requires prolonged balloon inflation (consider a perfusion balloon) and reversal of anticoagulation. Transthoracic echocardiography should be immediately performed in the setting of clinical instability in order to evaluate for the presence of a pericardial effusion and/or tamponade, in which case urgent pericardiocentesis is required. Covered stents, coils, or surgical repair may be required for definitive management.

E. Vascular access site complications remain the most common PTCA complication and occur in up to 5% of patients. The most common are blood transfusion (3%), arteriovenous fistula (less than 2%), pseudoaneurysm (up to 5%), acute arterial occlusion (less than 1%), and infections (less than 0.1%). Shorter anticoagulation regimens, weight-adjusted heparin, earlier sheath removal, vigilant monitoring of activated clotting times (ACTs), smaller sheaths, and avoidance of routine venous sheath insertion have all contributed to a reduction in complications. Stopping heparin after PCI and substituting clopidogrel for warfarin has also resulted in a reduction of bleeding and coronary complications.

F. Contrast-induced nephropathy (CIN) occurs in 3% to 7% of patients, and the risk increases tenfold for serum creatinine greater than 2.0 mg/dL, especially in the presence of diabetes mellitus. Renal failure prevention is best accomplished by infusing saline before catheterization, giving *N*-acetylcysteine 600 mg PO bid for 1 day before and after the day of catheterization, using nonionic contrast dye, and conservative use of contrast. In addition, the use of a laboratory equipped with biplane imaging can significantly reduce the volume of contrast required. Recent data from several small studies suggest that intravenous infusion of 3 ampules of sodium bicarbonate added to 1 liter of D5W solution infused 6 to 12 hours before contrast exposure may significantly reduce the risk of CIN as compared to hydration alone in patients with diabetes or moderately reduced glomerular filtration rate (GFR).

G. Contrast-mediated reactions can be serious. Anaphylactoid reactions occur in 1% to 2% of patients receiving iodinated contrast. These reactions can be severe in 0.10% to 0.23% of patients. The risk of a severe reaction can be effectively decreased by using nonionic contrast, preprocedural corticosteroids (i.e., prednisone 40 to 60 mg) given the evening before and the morning of the procedure, and the use of H_1 or H_2 blockers. In the circumstance that a patient presents for PCI without having undergone preprocedural steroid preparation, administration of hydrocortisone 100 mg IV and diphenhydramine 25 to 50 mg IV 60 to 120 minutes before the injection of contrast is a safe and feasible alternative.

H. In-stent thrombosis typically occurs during the first 2 to 4 weeks after stent implantation and typically results in MI. If both aspirin and clopidogrel are taken on a daily basis, the risk is less than 1%. Following BMS implantation, the vascular endothelium typically grows over the stent struts in 2 to 4 weeks, thereby eliminating contact between the stent and circulating platelets with a concomitant reduction in thrombotic risk. It is for this reason that BMS is a favored option in patients requiring PCI before major surgery or that possess a significant contraindication to long-term antiplatelet therapy. **In contrast to the re-endothelialization process of the BMS, re-endothelialization following DES implantation is significantly retarded because of the anti-proliferative effect of the coating agent**, thereby allowing for strut/platelet contact up to several years post-PCI. It is hypothesized that this pathophysiology accounts for the increasing reports of very late stent thrombosis (greater than 1 year post-PCI) in patients that have received DES and discontinued their antiplatelet therapy at 1 year, as has been the recommendation in the early years of the DES era. This situation is somewhat similar to that of brachytherapy.

Brachytherapy inhibits vascular endothelial proliferation, thereby potentially leaving bare stent exposed to the blood and necessitating prolonged antiplatelet therapy with aspirin and clopidogrel.

VII. EXPERIENCED OPERATORS/CENTERS

A. Procedural volume is an important predictor for PCI complications. **Elective PCI** should be performed in high-volume centers (more than 200 interventions per year, with an ideal minimum of more than 400 cases per year) by operators with an acceptable annual volume (more than 75 cases per year) at institutions with fully equipped interventional laboratories, experienced support staff, and an on-site cardiovascular surgical program. **Primary PCI for STEMI** should be performed in similarly experienced/skilled centers by operators who perform more than 75 elective cases per year and intervene on at least 11 cases of STEMI per year. **Elective PCI should not be** performed by low-volume operators (less than 75 cases per year) in low-volume centers (less than 200 cases per year), regardless of the availability of on-site cardiothoracic surgery, because of the increased risk of suboptimal outcomes. Referral to a larger regional center is recommended in this situation.

B. In cases of STEMI, there is an inverse relationship between the number of primary angioplasty procedures performed by an operator and in-hospital mortality. The data suggest that both door-to-balloon time and in-hospital mortality are significantly lower in institutions that perform a minimum of 36 primary angioplasty procedures per year.

VIII. SURGICAL BACKUP.

Emergency surgical intervention is a rare event and is required in 0.3% to 1.0% of cases of PCI, usually because of complications that cannot be addressed percutaneously or to provide urgent hemodynamic support. The most common reasons for emergency CABG surgery are dissection resulting in acute vessel closure, perforation, inability to retrieve a stent or other device, or aortic dissection. Emergency CABG after PCI has a mortality rate of 15% and periprocedural MI rate of 12%. The internal mammary artery may not be harvested, and surgery should not be delayed due to abciximab. Perfusion balloons may temporize a life-threatening perforation or dissection, and an intraaortic balloon pump can minimize ischemic injury and stabilize hemodynamics. Data from the Atlantic Cardiovascular Patient Outcomes Research Team (C-PORT) and PAMI with No Surgery On-Site (PAMI-No SOS) trials suggest that **primary PCI for STEMI** can be safely and effectively performed in centers that **do not** perform elective PCI and do not have on-site cardiac surgery capabilities if they implement a carefully developed and proven strategy capable of rapid and effective PCI (including an experienced operator with more than 75 total PCIs and at least 11 primary PCIs for STEMI per year) with a predetermined transfer plan to a nearby center with on-site surgical backup.

IX. SHEATHS, GUIDES, AND WIRES

A. Typical arterial access involves placing a 6F to 8F short sheath in the common femoral artery using the modified Seldinger technique. Using fluoroscopic guidance when entering the femoral artery above the inferior femoral head but below the pelvic rim increases the likelihood of entering the common femoral artery at a compressible site. The superficial/profunda femoral artery bifurcation is best seen in the ipsilateral 30-degree to 40-degree projection. The brachial and radial arteries can accommodate up to 7F and 6F sheaths, respectively. Ulnar artery and digital arch patency should be confirmed via the Allen test in case the radial artery becomes occluded (approximately 5%). Radial access improves hemostasis and earlier ambulation but increases radiation exposure, lengthens the procedure, and limits the choice of coronary equipment (6F compatible).

B. Large guide size (8F) provides extra support and permits use of rotational atherectomy, along with such devices as the PercuSurge GuardWire and kissing balloons. For straightforward lesions, a 6F system is typically adequate. The XB (extra backup) and Amplatz guiding catheters provide good support; the Amplatz guide is especially effective in the case of an acutely angled left circumflex artery. The Amplatz guide catheter is the most likely catheter to traumatize the LMT in inexperienced hands due to its tendency to deeply engage the vessel. Many experienced interventionalists choose to remove this catheter over the J-tipped guidewire to provide support to the distal tip. Great care should be taken to avoid atheroembolism and air embolism after advancing a guiding catheter through the aorta. This is accomplished by allowing blood to bleed backwards after engaging the coronary ostium and aspirating blood through the extension tubing into the manifold to remove any air before injecting contrast.

C. A coronary lesion is initially crossed with an 0.014-inch-diameter coronary wire, which serves as a "rail" for coronary devices such as balloons and stents. A key principle of endovascular intervention is not to lose wire position once a lesion is crossed. The choice of a wire depends on the wire tip's stiffness, slipperiness, and support characteristics. Stiff tips are helpful for tough chronic total occlusion but increase the risk of vessel dissection or perforation. Hydrophilic wires are quite slippery and can cross tortuous high-grade lesions quite easily but can also cause dissection or end-vessel perforation. Support wires typically have stiff tips but are primarily used as a supportive rail to deliver coronary equipment to the lesion. Both short (approximately 190-cm) and long (approximately 300-cm) wires are available. Classic over-the-wire equipment typically requires two people and a long wire for equipment exchange. Rapid-exchange technology uses a short monorail that allows use of a short, less cumbersome wire that requires only one operator and no fluoroscopy during equipment exchanges.

X. DIAGNOSTIC ADJUNCTS

A. Intravascular ultrasound (anatomic)

1. An intravascular ultrasonography (IVUS) catheter generates a cross-sectional tomographic image of both the lumen and the vessel wall. This complementary imaging modality can be invaluable when repeated angiographic views fail to determine the mechanism and/or significance of a coronary lesion. IVUS has proven helpful in assessing adequacy of coronary stent deployment, mechanism of in-stent restenosis (neointimal hyperplasia versus inadequate stent expansion), a coronary lesion at a location difficult to image by angiography, a suboptimal angiographic result after PCI, coronary allograft vasculopathy after cardiac transplantation, coronary calcium when considering rotational atherectomy, and plaque location/circumferential distribution to guide directional coronary atherectomy (DCA). IVUS may also be used to gauge lesion characteristics in order to assist in the optimal selection of a revascularization device or technique. However, the routine use of IVUS to optimally size stents and ensure adequate expansion has not been found to reduce restenosis rates.
2. IVUS provides anatomic, not physiologic, information. However, a lumen area less than 4.0 mm^2 in the left anterior descending (LAD), left circumflex, or right coronary artery or less than 6.0 to 7.0 mm^2 in the left main suggests the presence of a hemodynamically significant lesion.

B. Angioscopy (anatomic). Angioscopy uses a balloon-tipped catheter with a fiberoptic viewport at the distal tip that allows direct visualization of the lumen. Angioscopically evident thrombus has been shown to be angiographically silent in up to 50% of patients. This imaging modality is only used for research purposes.

C. Coronary flow reserve (physiologic)

1. A 0.014-inch wire capable of measuring coronary flow velocity permits assessment of epicardial and microvascular resistance. This information is helpful in determining whether a moderate-grade coronary stenosis (i.e., 30% to 70% stenosis) is hemodynamically significant. The ratio of hyperemic to basal flow is known as the coronary flow reserve (CFR) and is determined by giving an intracoronary vasodilator such as adenosine (36 to 64 μg). A normal coronary flow reserve is 3 to 5. A CFR less than 2.0 is abnormal and is consistent with a flow-limiting epicardial stenosis or increased microvascular tone.
2. The effect of the microvasculature can be eliminated by measuring the CFR in two vessels: the lesion-containing vessel and a normal-appearing vessel. This allows calculation of the relative coronary flow reserve velocity ($rCFR = CFR_{target}/CFR_{reference}$). A nonhemodynamically significant stenosis has an rCFR value of less than 0.8 and is similar in prognostic value to negative stress testing.

Unlike fraction flow reserve (FFR), CFR depends on hemodynamic and microcirculatory changes. In general, FFR is the preferred diagnostic modality for assessing the hemodynamic significance of a coronary lesion.

D. FFR (physiologic). A 0.014-inch wire with a pressure transducer is placed distal to a coronary stenosis and the translesional gradient measured. This allows calculation of the FFR, which is the ratio of this distal coronary pressure to aortic pressure during maximal hyperemia. A vasodilator such as adenosine [intravenous (IV) infusion 140 μg/kg per minute or intracoronary 36 to 64 μg] is used. A coronary artery without flow-limiting coronary obstruction would have an FFR of 1.0. An FFR value of less than 0.75 is consistent with a hemodynamically significant obstruction and positively correlates with myocardial ischemia on stress testing. Unlike the CFR, the FFR reflects only the epicardial artery lesion. Prospective studies have also demonstrated that FFR is able to risk stratify post-PCI patients for the development of future complications such as in-stent restenosis (ISR).

E. Pulmonary artery catheter (physiologic). A balloon-tipped Swan-Ganz catheter advanced to the pulmonary arteries allows measurement of right and left heart filling pressures as well as the cardiac output. This information can be helpful in patients presenting in cardiogenic shock, during high-risk PCI in the setting of severe LV dysfunction, when there is a question of pericardial tamponade, or when the cause of hemodynamic deterioration is unclear.

XI. THERAPEUTIC DEVICES

A. PTCA. The coronary balloon remains the backbone of endovascular intervention although its sole use is in decline. The initial gain in the coronary lumen achieved by balloon inflation results in localized dissection of the intima (and often the media) plus distension of the adventitia. The dissection is covered by platelet-rich thrombus and later by new intimal layers. As a result of these inevitable dissections, the abrupt closure rate is 4% to 7%, although the use of glycoprotein IIb/IIIa inhibitors has reduced this rate. The 6-month angiographic restenosis rate of 30% to 40% is another downside to PTCA. Furthermore, the risk of cardiac morbidity, including anginal symptoms, progressively increases with subsequent episodes of ISR following balloon angioplasty. It is recommended that patients determined to have significant ISR following PTCA should be strongly considered for coronary stent implantation.

There are two specific situations where PTCA still has great utility: 1) patients presenting with ACS found to have multivessel disease suitable for urgent/emergent CABG (e.g., PTCA alone rapidly restores patency to the infarct-related artery yet avoids the need for antiplatelet therapy, thereby allowing the patient to proceed to surgery without delay); and 2) patients found to have significant coronary disease in the preoperative setting (PTCA alone may allow revascularization while avoiding the requirement of antiplatelet therapy that would delay surgery). However, in most settings, BMS can provide superior long-term results with only a 6-week minimum requirement for antiplatelet therapy (see subsequent text).

B. Bare metal stents

1. Present-day coronary stents are flexible, laser-cut and polished, balloon-mounted and expandable, stainless steel, slotted tubes. These have proven effective in treating dissections and reducing the incidence of abrupt closure, emergency CABG (less than 1%), and restenosis. The procedural success rate for a coronary intervention approaches 98%. First implemented in the late 1980s for emergency treatment of coronary dissection after angioplasty, the early era of the intracoronary stent was plagued by high rates of subacute closure despite intensive anticoagulation regimens that often led to bleeding complications and prolonged hospitalization. Evolution of stent design and interventional technique led to a rapid reduction in procedural complication rates, such that in 1993 the Belgium Netherlands Stent (BENESTENT) and the North American Stent Restenosis (STRESS) studies both demonstrated a significant reduction in the rate of ISR and repeat revascularization, as compared to PTCA. Although subacute vessel closure may occur in up to 3% of cases following stent implantation, elastic recoil and negative remodeling are drastically reduced.

Compared to PTCA alone, stents reduce restenosis by approximately 30% in patients with chronic total occlusions, ACS, balloon restenosis, and focal de novo lesions in native coronary arteries with reference vessel diameter (RVD) greater than 2.75 mm. In SVG intervention, stents provide a higher procedural success rate and lower adverse cardiac event rate than PTCA alone. However, although stents reduce the rate of restenosis and repeat revascularization as compared to PTCA alone, they have not been shown to reduce the incidence of death or MI.

2. Bare metal stents are by no means immune to restenosis, however, as neointimal hyperplasia results in significant ISR in 17% to 30% of patients. This risk is increased in patients with small reference vessel size, smaller postprocedural luminal diameter, or high degree of residual stenosis, long lesion length, diabetes, lesion location in the LAD, and presence of untreated edge dissection during the procedure.
3. Bare metal stents have been shown to reduce rates of ISR by approximately 5% and MACE by 7% in small vessels (i.e., RVD less than 3mm) as compared to PTCA (especially when there is a suboptimal result); however, the difference is much smaller than that observed in larger vessels.

C. DES. The Achilles heel of bare-metal stents has been in-stent restenosis. Antiproliferative agents such as sirolimus and paclitaxel arrest cell division during the mitotic growth phase. The use of polymers to coat these agents onto a stent's surface has dramatically reduced neointimal hyperplasia to almost negligible levels.

1. **Clinical data.** The Randomized Study with the Sirolimus-Coated Bx Velocity (RAVEL) trial randomized 238 patients with significant lesions in 2.5- to 3.5-mm diameter vessels to an 18-mm rapamycin-eluting stent versus a standard bare metal stent. The rapamycin group had a 6-month angiographic restenosis rate (i.e., more than 50% lumen diameter) of 0% and a MACE (death/MI/target lesion revascularization) rate of 3.3% compared to 26% and 27.1%, respectively, for the bare metal stent group. The SIRIUS trial randomly compared 1058 patients with complex coronary disease encompassing lesion lengths between 15 and 30 mm with vessel diameters 2.5 to 3.5 mm to either BMS or sirolimus eluting stents (SES). SES implantation resulted in a 12% reduction in both the combined endpoint of death, MI, or target vessel revascularization (TVR) and in target lesion revascularization (TLR). This benefit was especially significant in the diabetic subset included in this trial (279 patients), which were noted to have a 14% reduction in the rate of TLR. The TAXUS-IV trial randomly compared 1314 patients with complex native vessel coronary disease (lesion length 10 to 28 mm and diameter 2.5 to 3.75 mm) to either BMS or paclitaxel-eluting stents (PES) and demonstrated 7% reduction in 9-month rates of TVR and 8% reduction in TLR in those assigned to the PES. The SIRTAX trial randomly assigned 1012 patients presenting to the catheterization laboratory to either SES or PES and demonstrated a significant reduction (10.8% vs. 6.2%) in the rate of MACE, primarily due to reduction in the rate of TLR observed in the SES group.
2. **Late thrombosis.** Although DES have dramatically reduced the incidence of ISR and MACE, especially in diabetics and complex coronary lesions, a mounting body of evidence suggests an increased risk of **late thrombosis** (i.e., 30 to 180 days postintervention). Following the discontinuation of antiplatelet therapies (such as clopidogrel and aspirin), several studies have demonstrated a small but significant increase in late thrombosis. This risk appears to be related to delayed endothelialization of the stent because of the presence of the antiproliferative coating agents.

D. Covered stents. Covered stents use a material such as polytetrafluoroethylene (PTFE), which covers the stent struts and seals off the vessel wall from the stent lumen. The JOMED covered stent has PTFE sandwiched between two Jostents. This covered stent is approved for coronary perforation by the Food and Drug Administration (FDA). FDA approval can be obtained on a case-by-case basis for coronary aneurysms.

E. Cutting balloon atherectomy

1. These balloons were initially developed in the present era in order to create a "controlled dissection." A cutting balloon has three to four, longitudinally mounted, razor-sharp atherotomes. These atherotomes cut into both plaque and vessel wall and allow vessel dilatation at a lower balloon pressure. Success in the treatment of balloon-resistant lesions led to FDA approval in 1995. Although randomized data have shown no difference between cutting balloon (CB) angioplasty and PTCA, many operators will use this device in lesions with high elastic recoil (i.e., ostial or bifurcation lesions) before DES.
2. Cutting balloons have also found a niche in the treatment of in-stent restenosis. Regular balloons often slip when inflated across these rubbery lesions. The Restenosis Reduction by Cutting Balloon Evaluation III (REDUCE III) trial randomized 521 patients to CB or PTCA before stenting (with angiographic or IVUS guidance) and demonstrated a significantly lower rate of angiographic restenosis in the CB before stenting group, primarily with IVUS guidance.
3. Care must be taken not to oversize cutting balloons, because perforation can occur. Placing these balloons through stent struts or down tortuous vessels can result in atherotome entrapment, as can a perforated balloon. These balloons should only be inflated to 6 to 10 atm in order to decrease the likelihood of balloon rupture.

F. Rotational atherectomy (RA)

1. RA uses a 160,000 rpm, diamond-coated burr (i.e., drill bit) that is advanced over a 0.009-inch wire to the coronary lesion. Slow advancement and intermittent light forward pressure in a sanding fashion results in particles smaller than the diamond bits (5 to 7 μm). The process generates microparticular debris that embolize and may attenuate the coronary microcirculation, inducing transient myocardial stunning, periprocedural MI, and LV dysfunction in the region of the target vessel. Therefore, although limited clinical data suggest that RA can be safely performed in patients with depressed LV function in the hands of an experienced operator, it is not recommended. The majority of these particles travel through the coronary microcirculation and are cleared by the liver, lung, and spleen.
2. Compared to plain balloon angioplasty, rotational atherectomy increases the chance of procedural success but has not been shown to reduce the risk of restenosis or major adverse cardiac events in de novo or restenotic lesions. Although the use of rotational atherectomy has declined, it is recommended before stenting in patients with severely calcifed lesions, undilatable lesions, chronic total occlusions, and bifurcation lesions to help ensure proper stent expansion and apposition in balloon-resistant lesions.
3. Familiarity with the device is essential. Sluggish coronary flow can occur, requiring a vasodilator such as verapamil, nitroprusside, or adenosine. Perforation occurs in approximately 1% of patients, typically when significant tortuosity forces the burr to the outside edge of a curve. Prophylactic pacing or aminophylline is frequently required if rotational atherectomy is performed in the vessel supplying the atrioventricular (AV) node. Rotational atherectomy is typically contraindicated in patients with thrombus, dissection, or severely reduced LV systolic dysfunction. Glycoprotein IIb/IIIa inhibitors decrease the risk of CK-MB elevation.

G. DCA

1. John Simpson developed DCA in the 1980s in response to the high rate of balloon angioplasty complications. DCA uses a sharp blade that repeatedly shaves off eccentric plaque and requires intravascular ultrasound to ensure adequate debulking. This revascularization technique is effective in treating fibrotic, noncalcified, ostial, bifurcation, branch ostial, or bulky eccentric lesions in large proximal vessels (greater than 3 mm) and requires an experienced operator for safe and effective use. The FDA approved this device in 1990. The device initially required a 10F guiding catheter, but the present-day version requires only an 8F guiding catheter.

2. Despite multiple randomized prospective trials, optimal DCA has never been shown to have lower rates of TVR when compared to plain balloon angioplasty or stenting. The Atherectomy Before MULTI-LINK Improves Lumen Gain and Clinical Outcomes (AMIGO) and the Debulking and Stenting in Restenosis Elimination (DESIRE) trials compared DCA before stenting to stenting alone and failed to show any improvement in angiographic or clinical restenosis. As a result, DCA has little role in present-day interventional cardiology, although some cardiologists continue to use it for debulking bifurcation lesions and other eccentric, noncalcified, nonthrombotic lesions.

H. Excimer laser

1. The excimer (*exci*ted and di*mer*) laser catheter (ELCA) tip is brought into contact with the target lesion. It creates ultraviolet light (308 nm) at a rate of 25 to 40 pulses per second from a high-energy, metastable, dimeric molecule of xenon and chloride. This provides 45 mJ/mm^2, which can ablate 0.5 mm of tissue per second and reduces the target tissue to gas and subcellular debris. The size of the lumen created is equivalent to that of the catheter.
2. The ELCA was approved by the FDA in 1992 for total occlusions, moderately calcified stenoses, balloon crossing/dilatation failures, ostial lesions, bypass grafts, and long diffuse disease. It is contraindicated in angulated lesions, coronary dissection, thrombotic lesions, and severely calcified lesions. However, long-term clinical data has failed to demonstrate a significant restenosis benefit, and routine use increases the complication rate in comparison with plain balloon angioplasty. Therefore, the ACC/AHA PCI Guidelines do not suggest use of ELCA as a primary strategy for revascularization. ELCA has little role in present-day interventional cardiology.

I. Mechanical thrombectomy: Possis AngioJet. The Possis AngioJet is the dominant mechanical thrombectomy device. The device is a 5F double lumen, flexible catheter that contains a hypotube through which six high-speed saline jets create a low-pressure area at the tip (approximately −760 mmHg), which serve to macerate and aspirate the thrombus back into the catheter lumen in accordance with the Venturi-Bernoulli principle. This catheter has proven to be successful in thrombotic vein grafts, for which it received FDA approval in 1998. It is currently being studied in acute myocardial infarction (AMI). Temporary prophylactic pacing is recommended when treating vessels supplying the inferior wall, because of temporary AV block. Temporary ST-segment elevation is frequent. Perforation can occur in vessels less than 2.0 mm in diameter due to the high-pressure saline injection. Although small studies using the AngioJet in the setting of ACS have been encouraging, prospective randomized data demonstrating a clinical benefit have been lacking. The AngioJet Rheolytic Thrombectomy In Patients Undergoing Primary Angioplasty for Acute Myocardial Infarction (AiMI) trial randomized patients with acute MI to AngioJet thrombectomy followed by PCI or PCI alone and concluded that mortality rates (4.6% vs. 0.8%, $p < 0.02$), infarct size (12.5 ± 12.1% vs. 9.8 ± 10.9%, $p = 0.02$), and MACE rates (6.7% vs. 1.7%, $p < 0.01$) were considerably **higher** in those undergoing thrombectomy.

J. PercuSurge GuardWire

1. Atheromatous embolization is a frequent and dreaded complication of degenerated SVG intervention. The first distal emboli protection device approved by the FDA was the PercuSurge GuardWire and Export catheter. The PercuSurge GuardWire is a 0.014-inch hypotube (i.e., hollow tube) with a balloon mounted on the distal end near the fixed floppy wire. The deflated balloon is steered across the SVG lesion and inflated in a distal portion of the graft. This results in cessation of blood flow in the SVG. Angioplasty and stenting are then performed, followed by removal of the column of blood with the Export catheter. The PercuSurge GuardWire balloon is then deflated and flow is restored. In experienced hands, this procedure can be performed in 4 to 6 minutes.
2. In the Saphenous Vein Graft Angioplasty Free of Emboli Randomized (SAFER) trial, the use of the PercuSurge GuardWire resulted in the recovery of atheromatous debris (83 to 204 μm) in 93% of cases and a 42% reduction in MACE

(i.e., death or MI). There was also a lower incidence of periprocedural slow flow.

3. Randomized data have failed to demonstrate the benefit of using the PercuSurge GuardWire in the setting of STEMI. The Enhanced Myocardial Efficacy and Removal by Aspiration of Liberated Debris (EMERALD) trial found no benefit to using the PercuSurge Guard Wire in regards to angiographically assessed myocardial reperfusion, ST segment elevation resolution, or infarct size at 30 days.

K. Filters. Collapsible microporous polyurethane net attached to a nitinol ring anchored distally to a 0.014-inch guidewire that can be advanced across high-risk SVG or carotid stenoses and then deployed downstream of the lesion. When deployed, these porous devices appear as a windsock or umbrella and allow blood to flow through while filtering any debris larger than 80 to 100 μm. Advantages are ease of use and avoidance of prolonged ischemia. Potential disadvantages are incomplete sealing, passage of smaller particles through the filter pores, overloading of the device, and spillage during device retrieval. The FilterWire EX Randomized Evaluation (FIRE) trial prospectively randomized 650 patients undergoing PCI to diseased SVGs to either the EPI FilterWire EX or the PercuSurge GuardWire embolic protection device and revealed equal efficacy of both types of devices in regards to the primary endpoint of death, periprocedural MI, or TLR at 30 days. This trial led to FDA approval of the FilterWire EX for use in degenerated SVGs.

XII. POST-CABG SURGERY PATIENTS (i.e., SVG INTERVENTIONS)

A. Saphenous vein bypass grafts are frequently used in CABG surgery. However, 7% occlude the first week, 15% to 20% occlude the first year, and by the tenth year 50% of SVGs are occluded and 25% are severely degenerated. Redo CABG is high-risk surgery with high rates of morbidity and mortality that approach 7% to 10% nationally. At the Cleveland Clinic, the rate is 1.8%. A patient with a patent internal mammary artery graft to the LAD artery makes surgery less appealing. Patients with no arterial conduit, multiple failed SVGs, multivessel disease, and depressed LV systolic function are ideal candidates for redo surgery.

B. Early postoperative ischemia within the first 30 days usually reflects graft failure (often secondary to thrombosis) or incomplete revascularization, and urgent coronary angiography is indicated. Emergency PCI of the graft, even across suture lines, has been safely performed within days of surgery. Intracoronary thrombolytics should be used with caution. Mechanical thrombectomy is a safer choice. Given that SVG flow is pressure dependent, intraaortic balloon pump (IABP) use should be strongly considered in patients that present with hypotension or depressed LV function.

C. Recurrent ischemia 1 to 12 months after CABG surgery usually reflects perianastomotic graft stenosis. Distal anastomotic stenoses respond well to balloon inflation only. Midshaft vein graft stenoses are usually due to intimal hyperplasia.

D. Recurrent ischemia more than 1 year after CABG surgery usually reflects the development of atherosclerosis. SVGs have greater plaque burden than native coronary arteries, and aspirates are composed of atherosclerotic rather than thrombotic elements. This may explain the lack of benefit seen with glycoprotein IIb/IIIa inhibitors. Unprotected PCI (i.e., no PercuSurge GuardWire or filter device) results in varying degrees of atheroembolization with 15% of patients having a CK-MB more than five times normal. Therefore, use of distal protection devices during SVG interventions is strongly encouraged when technically feasible.

XIII. RESTENOSIS

A. Restenosis is the most commonly occurring late PTCA complication and typically occurs within 6 months. Post-PTCA restenosis is primarily due to vessel contracture, elastic recoil, negative vessel remodeling, and neointimal hyperplasia. In-stent restenosis is almost entirely due to neointimal hyperplasia. Not surprisingly, focal restenosis has a better outcome and response to treatment than does diffuse restenosis. The predictors of restenosis are diabetes, unstable angina, acute MI, prior restenosis, small vessel diameter, total occlusion, long lesion length, SVG, proximal LAD, higher percent stenosis after the procedure, and smaller minimal luminal diameter after the procedure. Strategies to decrease restenosis include maximizing stent expansion (i.e., bigger is better) and minimizing the distance of arterial injury.

B. Post-PTCA. Balloon angioplasty alone has a 6-month restenosis rate of 32% to 40%. For restenotic lesions managed with PTCA, the restenosis rate is comparable to de novo lesions. For a third episode of restenosis, PTCA has a restenosis rate approaching 50% (not 100%). With PTCA alone, late patency is 93% after three procedures. Only 1.6% of lesions require four or more procedures. Atheroablative approaches, such as excimer laser and rotational atherectomy, have not proven superior for managing restenosis. However, stents are superior to PTCA, with a 6-month TVR rate of 10% versus 32%.

C. In-stent restenosis. The risk of recurrent ISR after balloon angioplasty is 10% for focal ISR, 50% for diffuse restenosis, and 80% for total stent occlusion. Atheroablative approaches, such as use of the cutting balloon and rotational atherectomy, have not proven clinically superior to PTCA. ISR occurs in 17% to 32% of patients treated with BMS depending upon such variables as vessel size, lesion length, diabetes mellitus, smaller postprocedure minimal luminal diameter, higher residual percent stenosis, and vessel location. The observed rate is significantly lower with DES. The introduction of DES in 2003 has dramatically reduced the incidence of ISR and the rate of TVR as compared to the BMS. In the RAVEL trial, patients randomized to SES had a 5.8% rate of restenosis at 1 year follow-up as compared to 29% in the BMS group. Three-year follow-up from this trial revealed an 11.4% rate of TVR in the SES group, thus documenting the long-term efficacy of the DES platform. Results from the Sirolimus Balloon Expandable Stent in the Treatment of Patients with De Novo Native Coronary Artery Lesions (SIRIUS) trial reported a 4.1% rate of TVR because of reduction in the incidence of neointimal hyperplasia as assessed by IVUS. The paclitaxel-coated stents have similar rates of efficacy as demonstrated by the TAXUS-IV trial, wherein patients treated with PES were noted to have an 8% rate of ISR (vs. 27% in the BMS group) at 9 months and 3% TVR. The REALITY trial is the largest trial to date comparing the paclitaxel to the sirolimus-eluting stent, and it concluded that although the sirolimus stent was associated with a significantly lower rate of late lumen loss (0.09 versus 0.31 mm) at 8 months, this did not translate into a meaningful difference in the rate of TVR (6.0% vs. 6.1%). Similar findings were reported by the SIRTAX trial, where use of SES was associated with a significantly lower rate of agiographic restenosis (6.6% vs. 11.7%) as compared to PES—although in this case, TVR was significantly reduced in the SES group (4.8% vs. 8.3%). The Intracoronary Stenting or Angioplasty for Restonosis Reduction—Drug-Eluting Stents for In-Stent Restonosis (ISAR-DESIRE) trial compared SES and PES to balloon angioplasty in 300 patients with ISR following BMS and demonstrated a significant reduction in restenosis at 6-month follow-up in the DES groups as compared to angioplasty alone (8% vs. 33%). Therefore, repeat PCI with either of the approved DES is reasonable for treatment of ISR. Overall, rate of death and MI are very low regardless of which stent is chosen. At present, both the sirolimus- and paclitaxel-coated stents appear to have nearly equal safety and efficacy data, and no compelling data exist for which to recommend one over the other. Predictors of restenosis are vessel size, lesion length, diabetes mellitus, smaller postprocedure minimal luminal diameter, higher residual percent stenosis, and LAD lesions leading to the concept "bigger is better." The risk of recurrent ISR after balloon angioplasty is 10% for focal in-stent restenosis, 50% for diffuse restenosis, and 80% for total stent occlusion. Atheroablative approaches, such as use of the cutting balloon and rotational atherectomy, have not proven clinically superior to PTCA. The routine use of stents-within-a-stent (i.e., stent sandwich) is generally not advised. IVUS is appropriate to ensure good stent expansion.

D. Brachytherapy. Brachytherapy damages chromosomes and prevents cell division, thereby inhibiting neointimal hyperplasia. Both beta and gamma brachytherapy catheter-based systems use closed-end lumen catheters that deliver the source and keep it out of contact with the blood, allowing reuse. Both gamma (iridium 192) and beta (phosphorus 32, strontium 90) brachytherapy result in approximately a 50% reduction in in-stent restenosis compared to balloon angioplasty alone. It is important to ensure brachytherapy delivery to all balloon-injured segments in the target vessel, or else inadequate radiation to an injured segment can cause neointimal proliferation. Brachytherapy can only be used once in each vessel, and long-term dual-antiplatelet therapy with aspirin and clopidogrel is essential given the risk of late in-stent thrombosis.

XIV. PHARMACOLOGIC ADJUNCTIVE THERAPY

A. Antithrombins. Antithrombins prevent the generation of thrombin and/or inhibit the activity of thrombin. An antithrombin such as unfractionated heparin, bivalirudin (direct thrombin inhibitor), or enoxaparin (low molecular weight heparin) should be used during all coronary interventions to prevent thrombus formation on the equipment. This principle applies even to patients with a high international normalized ratio (INR).

B. Unfractionated heparin

1. Heparin is a cofactor that dramatically accelerates the action of antithrombin several thousand-fold. Antithrombin inactivates both thrombin and activated factor X. Heparin binds to a variety of sites throughout the body because of its highly negative charge (e.g., endothelial cells, macrophages, plasma proteins) resulting in nonlinear anticoagulant effects at low to moderate doses. Circulating plasma levels are achieved only when the receptors are saturated. Subsequent clearance is largely renal, with a half-life of 60 to 90 minutes. The typical dose is a 100 Units/kg bolus if no glycoprotein IIb/IIIa inhibitor is given. If a glycoprotein IIb/IIIa inhibitor is given, then 50 to 70 Units/kg of heparin are infused as a bolus. No maintenance infusion is given.
2. ACT is used to indicate the level of anticoagulation, because the partial thromboplastin time cannot be applied to higher levels of anticoagulation. An ACT greater than 400 seconds is associated with an increased risk of bleeding complications, although the ACT is inversely correlated to the likelihood of abrupt vessel closure. A minimal ACT has not been identified. Without a glycoprotein IIb/IIIa inhibitor, the goal ACT is 300 to 350 seconds (Hemochron) or 250 to 300 seconds (HemoTec). With a glycoprotein IIb/IIIa inhibitor, the goal ACT should be more than 200 seconds for either Hemochron or HemoTec devices. The ACT should be checked every 30 minutes. Every cardiac catheterization laboratory should have the ability to rapidly measure the ACT.
3. In uncomplicated PCI cases, prolonged postprocedural heparin infusions increase bleeding complications and do not lower the likelihood of abrupt vessel closure or the rate of restenosis. The sheath should be removed when the ACT is less than 180 seconds.
4. Prolonged or repeated exposure to unfractionated heparin can result in thrombocytopenia. Nonimmunologic, heparin-induced thrombocytopenia (HIT-1) is due to heparin-induced platelet aggregation resulting in a mild lowering of the platelet count. Immunologic, heparin-induced thrombocytopenia (HIT-2) is a serious event in which IgG production directed at the platelet can lead to intravascular thrombosis. Heparin-related antibodies have a 70% sensitivity for detecting this disorder.

C. Low molecular weight heparin (LMWH)

1. Factor Xa is necessary for the production of thrombin. LMWH is made via heparin saccharide depolymerization and results in more predictable factor Xa inhibition. LMWHs are increasingly being used in the setting of ACS as a result of data suggesting a possible reduction in the combination of recurrent angina, MI, and death associated with the use of enoxaparin as compared to unfractionated heparin (ESSENCE and TIMI IIb trials). This may, however, come at the expense of increased major hemorrhage. As a result, many patients are receiving enoxaparin at the time of presentation to the cardiac catheterization laboratory. Results of the Superior Yield of the New Strategy of Enoxaparin, Revascularization, and Glycoprotein IIb/IIIa inhibitors (SYNERGY) trial demonstrated that rates of major ischemic complications in patients treated with either UFH or

enoxaparin undergoing early PCI due to NSTEMI were similar. It should be noted, however, that "cross-over" from one agent to another did result in a significantly increased risk of bleeding and should be avoided if possible. Thus, use of LMWH is a reasonable alternative to UFH in patients undergoing PCI due to ACS.

2. If a hospitalized patient has been given subcutaneous enoxaparin, a reasonable strategy is as follows. If PCI is performed within 8 hours of subcutaneous enoxaparin administration, then no additional heparin is required. If PCI is performed within 8 to 12 hours, an additional intravenous dose of 0.3 mg/kg of enoxaparin should be administered. If PCI is performed more than 12 hours after enoxaparin injection, standard doses of unfractionated heparin can be used.
3. When using LMWH, ACT measurement does not reflect the degree of anticoagulation. Currently, there is no rapid method for determining factor Xa activity, and it is unclear if monitoring is even necessary. This inability to confirm adequate antithrombin activity with a bedside test makes some interventional cardiologists uncomfortable. Significant anti-factor Xa activity persists for about 12 hours.
4. LMWH is only partially reversed with protamine. Dosing LMWH in obese patients provides a much less reliable level of anticoagulation. Extreme caution should be exercised in patients with moderate-to-severe renal insufficiency (i.e., creatinine clearance less than 30 mL/min), as the renal elimination of LMWH may result in unexpectedly high degrees of anticoagulation for a prolonged period. In these cases, most interventionalists will use an alternative antithrombotic agent.
5. Fondaparinux is a synthetic pentasaccharide that binds to antithrombin and induces a conformational change that increases its affinity for factor Xa. Fondaparinux has compared favorably to LMWH in both the NSTEMI and STEMI settings. The OASIS-5 trial randomized 20,078 patients presenting with NSTEMI to fondaparinux (2.5 mg/day) or enoxaparin (1 mg/kg twice daily). Although there was no significant difference between the groups with regard to the primary endpoint (death, MI, or refractory ischemia at 9 days), there was a significant reduction in the rate of major bleeding associated with fondaparinux (2.2% vs. 4.1%, HR 0.52, 95% CI 0.44 to 0.61). The benefit of fondaparinux in STEMI was demonstrated by the OASIS-6 trial, in which patients were randomized to fondaparinux (2.5 mg/day) or placebo. Overall, use of fondaparinux was associated with a significant reduction in the primary endpoint of death or reinfarction at 30 days (9.7% vs. 11.2%, HR 0.86, 95% CI 0.77 to 0.96). However, this benefit was not realized in the patients that had an indication for concomitant heparin therapy.

D. Direct thrombin inhibitors (bivalirudin)

1. The initial direct thrombin inhibitor was isolated from leech saliva, although now these materials are synthesized by recombinant technology. These agents directly inhibit clot-bound thrombin without requiring an antithrombin cofactor. Direct thrombin inhibitors are better able to block both fluid-phase and clot-bound thrombin, which may be particularly important in a thrombus's platelet-rich environment.
2. A hirudin analog, bivalirudin is becoming increasingly more common in catheterization laboratories and is an important anticoagulant for patients undergoing PCI. Initially approved for use in PCI in patients with heparin-induced thrombocytopenia, bivalirudin is now considered a safe alternative to the combination of UFH and GP IIb/IIIa inhibitors in low-risk patients undergoing elective PCI. The REPLACE-2 trial compared bivalirudin to abciximab/unfractionated heparin in a prospective, randomized, double-blind fashion and found it to be associated with fewer bleeding-associated complications and a statistically noninferior rate of MACEs.
3. Bivalirudin is given as a 1 mg/kg bolus followed by a 4-hour maintenance infusion of 2.5 mg/kg per hour followed by 0.2 mg/kg per hour. A given

bivalirudin dose provides a more predictable ACT than does unfractionated heparin. The half-life is 25 minutes in patients with normal renal function, although in dialysis-dependent patients the half-life may be as long as 3.5 hours. The maintenance infusion can be discontinued after completion of the coronary intervention. If a vascular closure device is not used, the sheath can typically be removed in 1 to 2 hours given the drug's short half-life. Unfortunately, the effects of bivalirudin cannot be reversed.

E. Warfarin. Routine warfarin is no longer recommended unless a patient has a mechanical prosthetic valve, atrial fibrillation, or intracardiac thrombus. Dual antiplatelet therapy has proven superior. An INR greater than 1.6 is a strong relative contraindication to cardiac catheterization. If emergent cardiac catheterization is required due to acute coronary syndrome or MI, consider accessing the radial artery because hemostasis is rarely an issue with this approach.

F. Antiplatelet therapy

1. Platelets are essential in thrombus formation, and some form of antiplatelet therapy is typically given at the time of PCI.
2. **Thromboxane A_2 inhibitor (aspirin).** Aspirin impairs platelet aggregation by irreversibly inhibiting platelet cyclooxygenase and thromboxane A_2 production. A loading dose of 325 mg of aspirin should ideally be given at least 2 hours before PCI and be continued at 325 mg daily for at least 1 month following the procedure. In the case of DES, higher-dose aspirin may be continued for longer periods. Secondary prevention trials have shown aspirin to reduce death, MI, and stroke by 27%. In PCI patients, aspirin reduces abrupt vessel closure.
3. **ADP receptor antagonists (clopidogrel, ticlopidine, prasugrel)**
   - **a.** Thienopyridines such as clopidogrel and ticlopidine inhibit adenosine diphosphate (ADP)–induced platelet aggregation by the P2Y12 receptor. Clopidogrel is preferred to ticlopidine because of its better safety profile, although both require hepatic metabolism for activation.
   - **b.** Ticlopidine was the first thienopyridine in clinical practice, and its use was based on several trials showing dual antiplatelet therapy with aspirin and ticlopidine (250 mg bid) to be superior to aspirin alone or dual aspirin/warfarin therapy. However, maximal platelet inhibition requires 5 to 7 days, and inadequate pretreatment (i.e., starting ticlopidine on the day of stent implantation) resulted in an increase in stent thrombosis in the first 24 hours.
   - **c.** Ticlopidine is also poorly tolerated with prolonged use, resulting in 20% of patients discontinuing the drug due to nausea, diarrhea, and rash. Neutropenia and thrombotic thrombocytopenic purpura (TTP) occur in 1% to 3% and 0.03% of patients, respectively. The complete blood count (CBC) should be serially examined in the first several months of use (q 2 weeks × 3 months).
   - **d.** Clopidogrel is better tolerated than ticlopidine and has largely replaced it in clinical practice in the United States. In two randomized, prospective, double-blind trials comparing aspirin therapy with clopidogrel or ticlopidine, clopidogrel was at least equivalent and had significantly fewer side effects. The risk of TTP is the same as the general population (11 in 3 million) and neutropenia is not an issue, making blood count monitoring unnecessary. In patients presenting with ACS, pretreatment and long-term therapy with clopidogrel improves patient outcomes. In the PCI-CURE trial, pretreatment with aspirin and 300 mg of clopidogrel followed by 8 months of 75 mg of clopidogrel daily resulted in a significant reduction in the combined endpoint of cardiovascular death, MI, or urgent TVR without a significant increase in bleeding. The CREDO trial examined the use of a loading dose of 300 mg of clopidogrel within 24 hours of PCI followed by either 28 days or 1 year of clopidogrel following PCI. It was reported that clopidogrel therapy was associated with a significant reduction in the combined endpoint of death, MI, or urgent TVR at 1 year. Additionally, the maximal benefit of pretreatment was noted at 24 hours before PCI. The ISAR-REACT

trial demonstrated that a higher 600 mg loading dose of clopidogrel before low-risk, elective PCI compares favorably to abciximab. In the ARMYDA-2 trial, patients presenting with UA/NSTEMI given the 600 mg loading dose of clopidogrel experienced a lower rate of death, MI, or TVR as compared to those receiving the traditional 300 mg loading dose. Thus, although it is recommended that a 300 mg loading dose of clopidogrel be given at least 6 hours before PCI, many interventionalists use the higher 600 mg loading dose as a result of the above data. Clopidogrel loading has also been shown to be beneficial in the setting of STEMI, in conjunction with fibrinolytic therapy in both the TIMI 28-CLARITY and COMMIT/CCS-2 trials. It should be noted that routine clopidogrel pretreatment is **somewhat controversial**, given clopidogrel's increased risk of bleeding in the event that a patient requires emergent CABG surgery.

e. Prasugrel is a novel thienopyridine prodrug that requires conversion to an active metabolite with high affinity for the platelet P2Y12 receptor site, resulting in a potent antiplatelet effect. The TRITON-TIMI 38 trial randomized 13,608 patients with moderate-to-high risk ACS with scheduled PCI to either prasugrel or clopidogrel therapy and found a significant reduction in the primary efficacy endpoint of death from cardiovascular causes, nonfatal MI, or nonfatal stroke associated with prasugrel therapy. Prasugrel was also associated with a reduction in rates of MI, TVR, and stent thrombosis. However, of some concern was a significant increase in major (HR 1.32; 95% CI, 1.03 to 1.68; p = 0.03) and life-threatening (1.4% vs. 0.9%, p = 0.01) bleeding observed in the prasugrel group.

G. Glycoprotein IIb/IIIa inhibitors (abciximab, eptifibatide, tirofiban)

1. Glycoprotein IIb/IIIa receptor inhibition prevents these receptors from binding to fibrin and forming the platelet–fibrin crosslinking that is required for thrombus formation. Glycoprotein IIb/IIIa receptor occupancy greater than 80% prevents the development of thrombus.
2. **Abciximab** is a human-murine chimeric antibody fragment that binds the glycoprotein IIb/IIIa receptor with high affinity resulting in a slow dissociation rate (i.e., noncompetitive inhibition). Although abciximab remains detectable on platelets for the lifetime of the platelet, it is rapidly cleared from plasma, allowing platelet aggregation to return to normal in 12 to 36 hours. Rapid reversal of platelet inhibition in the event of bleeding requires discontinuation of the abciximab infusion, waiting 30 minutes for plasma clearance, and platelet infusion (12 units) so as to provide functional platelets. Profound thrombocytopenia occurs in 0.4% to 1.1% of patients. Platelet counts should be measured within the first 2 to 4 hours and the following day. Abciximab readministration has not been associated with hypersensitivity or anaphylaxis, although the risk of profound thrombocytopenia is somewhat higher (2.2%).
3. **Eptifibatide** is a cyclic heptapeptide and **tirofiban** is a tyrosine derivative nonpeptide mimetic. Both act as competitive inhibitors requiring high levels for adequate inhibition. Both have a short plasma half-life (2.0 to 2.5 hours) with platelet aggregation normalizing in 30 minutes to 4 hours. In the event of bleeding, the infusion should be stopped. Unlike abciximab, the effect cannot be reversed and platelets remain inhibited until plasma drug levels fall. Profound thrombocytopenia is rare (0.0% to 0.3%).
4. The use of glycoprotein IIb/IIIa inhibitors during PCI prevents 65 adverse events per 1000 treated patients and is arguably beneficial for all types of intervention. These benefits are particularly enhanced for unstable angina, diabetes mellitus, and bailout stenting. Abciximab showed an absolute 4.5% to 6.5% reduction in the 30-day composite endpoint of death, MI, and target vessel revascularization. Eptifibatide showed a 3.7% absolute risk reduction in this composite endpoint. In a direct head-to-head comparison, abciximab was superior to tirofiban at 30 days but was statistically similar at 6 months.

H. Intracoronary vasodilators. PCI can result in no reflow, which is defined as a reduction in coronary flow without an obstructive lesion. The most probable causes of no-reflow are microvascular spasm and distal embolization. Potent microvascular vasodilators, such as adenosine (36 to 72 μg), nicardipine (100 to 200 μg), nitroprusside (50 to 200 μg), or verapamil (200 μg), often restore normal flow. Nitroglycerin is a logical choice for relieving epicardial spasm but has no effect on the microvasculature. Immediately before SVG intervention, verapamil pretreatment has been shown to prevent no reflow but has never been shown to reduce the risk of CK-MB elevation.

XV. SUPPORTIVE ADJUNCTIVE THERAPY

A. Pacemaker. A temporary pacing wire placed by fluoroscopy into the right ventricle should be considered for patients undergoing rotational atherectomy or rheolytic thrombectomy (i.e., Possis AngioJet) in the artery supplying the AV node. For rotational atherectomy patients, pretreatment with aminophylline is a reasonable alternative. If ionic contrast injection causes bradycardia, simply change to nonionic contrast.

B. IABP. An IABP should be inserted for hemodynamic support when a patient develops cardiogenic shock. There is a low threshold for IABP insertion in high-risk PCI patients (e.g., poor ventricular function, large area of myocardial ischemia, critical LMT disease, cardiogenic shock). Because of the inherent risk of complications, such as atheroembolism, distal limb ischemia, infection, and thrombocytopenia, IABP should be reserved for selected patients in whom there is an appropriate risk/benefit ratio.

C. Percutaneous cardiopulmonary support is a rarely performed but occasionally life-saving procedure that requires the placement of very large caliber catheters (24F) in the aorta and inferior vena cava via the femoral artery and vein, respectively. A perfusionist is required to provide extracorporeal membrane oxygen support. Systemic perfusion to vital organs can be preserved regardless of cardiac status, even in instances of asystole and incessant ventricular tachycardia. Unfortunately, the vascular complication rate approaches 40%. The Tandem Heart™ is a new form of percutaneous cardiopulmonary support. Functioning as a percutaneous left atrial-to-femoral arterial ventricular assist device, a venous catheter is inserted into the left atrium via transseptal puncture (Brockenbrough catheter), and an arterial cannula is inserted into the iliac artery for the return of blood. The Tandem Heart device can be quickly positioned, generally in less than 30 minutes. It is primarily used for emergent, short-term hemodynamic stabilization until definitive revascularization can be achieved.

XVI. POST-PCI MANAGEMENT

A. Antiplatelet therapy. Following implantation of BMS, patients should be treated with aspirin 325 mg daily for 1 month, 3 months in the setting of SES, and 6 months for PES. Thereafter, 75 to 162 mg of aspirin daily should be maintained indefinitely. In addition, clopidogrel 75 mg daily should be instituted for at least 4 to 6 weeks following BMS implantation (unless the patient has a clear bleeding diathesis, in which case the ACC/AHA Guidelines suggest that 2 to 4 weeks may suffice). Following sirolimus coated stents, 3 months of clopidogrel therapy is recommended, with 6 months recommended for patients following paclitaxel coated stents. Given the recent evidence that there is a small but definite risk of abrupt late thrombosis in DES (regardless of drug coating used), many interventionalists are opting to continue dual antiplatelet therapy *indefinitely* in patients in whom there is not an increased bleeding risk. In patients with a history of aspirin or clopidogrel resistance or prior stent thrombosis, a platelet aggregation assay may be considered. Less than 50% inhibition may indicate patients in whom treatment with clopidogrel 75 mg twice daily (or 150 mg daily) is beneficial.

B. Access site care

1. The groin or arm access site should be examined for hematoma, pseudoaneurysm (systolic bruit), and arteriovenous fistulas (continuous murmur). A pulsatile mass also suggests a pseudoaneurysm. Ultrasound studies can confirm the diagnosis of pseudoaneurysm or arteriovenous fistula. Suprainguinal tenderness, back pain, lower quadrant abdominal pain, or hypotension should make one suspicious for retroperitoneal hemorrhage and can be confirmed by computed

tomography (CT). A hemoglobin level 1 day after PCI should be routine, and a decrease greater than 2 g/dL is concerning. Distal pulses should be examined as well. Pulselessness, pain, pallor, paresthesias, and a cool extremity suggest an acute arterial occlusion.

2. **Pseudoaneurysms** smaller than 2 cm often close spontaneously; those 2 to 3 cm can often be closed by external, ultrasound-guided compression (90% success rate); and those larger than 3 cm generally require surgical correction. Another frequently successful option is thrombin injection if the pseudoaneurysm has a thin neck.
3. **Arteriovenous fistulas** are typically small and inconsequential, rarely causing high-output failure. Indications for ultrasound-guided compression (success rate greater than 80%) or surgical closure include significant shunting, extremity swelling/tenderness, CHF, and deep venous thrombosis (DVT).
4. A **retroperitoneal hemorrhage** can be treated by supportive care (i.e., transfusions, close observation, bedrest) in more than 80% of cases. Anticoagulation must be reversed, and frequent hemodynamic monitoring in an experienced ICU is required. If required, transportation to CT scan should be deferred until the patient is hemodynamically stable. If the bleeding does not spontaneously stop, the patient may require vascular surgery consultation. Other options include balloon tamponade or coil embolization if a small sidebranch is the culprit.
5. **Acute arterial occlusion** may be due to dissection or thromboembolism. Both typically require angiography of the affected extremity with access from another extremity (e.g., with a cold right leg after right femoral artery access, left femoral access should be obtained and an angiogram can be performed of the right lower extremity by crossing over to the right common iliac artery). Dissection typically requires prolonged balloon inflation and possible stenting or surgery. Stenting at the common femoral artery is discouraged, because it is a flexion point and a frequent site of attaching bypass grafts. Thromboembolism can be treated with surgical (Fogarty catheter) or percutaneous mechanical thrombectomy (Possis AngioJet).

C. **Monitoring for myocardial ischemia.** A 12-lead ECG should be obtained before and after PCI in order to have a baseline. The patient should be monitored on a cardiac ward that has continuous electrocardiographic monitoring and nurses familiar with routine post-PCI care. The CK and CK-MB levels should be measured 12 hours after the intervention. A procedural MI is presently defined as a CK-MB more than 3 times the normal (assuming a normal baseline CK-MB). Elevated CK, CK-MB, or electrocardiographic abnormalities occur in 5% to 30% of patients. Mechanisms include distal embolization, sidebranch occlusion, dissection, and spasm. Troponin levels are not routinely measured after PCI.

D. **Monitoring for contrast-induced nephropathy.** Nonsteroidal anti-inflammatory drugs, cyclosporine, and metformin should be withheld for 24 to 48 hours beforehand and for 48 hours afterward. Postprocedure saline hydration is continued at 75 to 150 mL/hour for 1 to 2 liters. Renal function (serum creatinine) should be monitored in patients with diabetes and renal dysfunction.

E. **Secondary prevention.** After PCI, patients are typically motivated and receptive to counseling regarding smoking cessation, exercise, diet, and weight loss. Blood pressure should be less than 140/90 mm Hg in all patients and less than 130/85 mm Hg in diabetics. Each person should be taking an aspirin, statin, angiotensin-converting enzyme inhibitor, and beta blocker unless contraindicated. In addition to obtaining a complete lipid profile, check lipoprotein (a), serum homocysteine, and ultra-sensitive C-reactive protein levels.

F. **Stress testing.** The goal is to recognize restenosis. Routine exercise testing in all PCI patients 4 to 6 months later is not necessary. The problem is that 25% of asymptomatic patients have myocardial ischemia by exercise testing, and we know that myocardial ischemia, whether symptomatic or silent, worsens prognosis. The ACC recommends selective testing in patients with decreased LV function, multivessel or proximal LAD intervention, previous sudden death, diabetes, hazardous occupations, and suboptimal PCI result. Exercise treadmill testing (ETT) alone is less sensitive than ETT with single photon emission CT or echocardiography.

ACKNOWLEDGMENT

The author thanks Dr. Kent W. Dauterman for his contributions to earlier editions of this chapter.

References

1. Anderson JL, et al. ACC/AHA 2007 Guidelines for the Management of Patients With Unstable Angina/Non–ST-Elevation Myocardial Infarction. J Am Coll Cardiol 2007;50:652–726.
2. Hochman JS, et al. One-year survival following early revascularization for cardiogenic shock. JAMA 2001;285:190–192.
3. Sabatine MS, et al. Addition of clopidogrel to aspirin and fibrinolytic therapy for myocardial infarction with ST-segment elevation (CLARITY TIMI 28 study). *N Engl J Med* 2005;352:1179–1189.
4. Keeley EC, et al. Comparison of primary and facilitated percutaneous coronary interventions for ST-elevation myocardial infarction: quantitative review of randomized trials. *Lancet* 2006;367:579–588.
5. Ellis SG, et al. Review of immediate angioplasty after fibrinolytic therapy for acute myocardial Infarction: insights from the RESCUE I, RESCUE II, and other contemporary clinical experiences. *Am Heart J* 2000;139:1046–1053.
6. de Lemos JA, Braunwald E. ST segment resolution as a tool for assessing the efficacy of reperfusion therapy. *J Am Coll Cardiol* 2001;38:1283–1294.
7. Hochman JS, et al. Cardiogenic shock complicating acute myocardial infarction—etiologies, management and outcome: a report from the SHOCK Trial Registry. Should we emergently revascularize occluded coronaries for cardiogenic shock? *J Am Coll Cardiol* 2000;36[3 Suppl A]:1063–1070.
8. Fox KA, et al. Interventional versus conservative treatment for patients with unstable angina or non-ST-elevation myocardial infarction: the British Heart Foundation RITA 3 randomised trial. Randomized Intervention Trial of unstable Angina. *Lancet* 2002;360:743–751.
9. Cannon CP, et al. Comparison of early invasive and conservative strategies in patients with unstable coronary syndromes treated with the glycoprotein IIb/IIIa inhibitor tirofiban. *N Engl J Med* 2001;344:1879–1887.
10. Wallentin L, et al. Outcome at 1 year after an invasive compared with a non-invasive strategy in unstable coronary-artery disease: the FRISC II invasive randomised trial. FRISC II Investigators. Fast revascularisation during instability in coronary artery disease. *Lancet* 2000;356:9–16.
11. Mahaffey KW, et al. Enoxaparin vs unfractionated heparin in high-risk patients with non–ST-segment elevation acute coronary syndromes managed with an intended early invasive strategy (SYNERGY trial). *JAMA* 2004;292:45–54.
12. Boden WE, et al. Outcomes in patients with acute non-Q-wave myocardial infarction randomly assigned to an invasive as compared with a conservative management strategy. Veterans Affairs Non-Q-Wave Infarction Strategies in Hospital (VANQWISH) Trial Investigators. *N Engl J Med* 1998;338:1785–1792.
13. de Winter, et al. Early invasive versus selectively invasive management for acute coronary syndromes. *N Engl J Med* 2005;353:1095–1104.
14. Davies RF, et al. Asymptomatic Cardiac Ischemia Pilot (ACIP) study two-year follow-up: outcomes of patients randomized to initial strategies of medical therapy versus revascularization. *Circulation* 1997;95:2037–2043.
15. Chen Z, et al. Addition of clopidogrel to aspirin in 45,852 patients with acute myocardial infarction: randomised placebo-controlled trial. *Lancet* 2005;366:1607–1621 (COMMIT/CCS-2 Study).
16. Boden WE, et al. Optimal medical therapy with or without PCI for stable coronary disease. *N Engl J Med* 2007;356:1503–1516.
17. Stone PH, et al. Asymptomatic Cardiac Ischemia Pilot (ACIP) Study. *Circulation* 1996;94:1537–1544.
18. The Bypass Angioplasty Revascularization Investigation (BARI) Investigators. Comparison of coronary bypass surgery with angioplasty in patients with multivessel disease. *N Engl J Med* 1996;335:217–225.
19. Serruys PW, et al. Comparison of coronary-artery bypass surgery and stenting for the treatment of multivessel disease. *N Engl J Med* 2001;344:1117–1124.
20. Aversano T, et al. Thrombolytic therapy vs primary percutaneous coronary intervention for myocardial infarction in patients presenting to hospitals without on-site cardiac surgery: a randomized controlled trial. *JAMA* 2002;287:1943–1951.
21. Seshadri N, et al. Emergency coronary artery bypass surgery in the contemporary percutaneous coronary intervention era. *Circulation* 2002;106:2346–2350.
22. Kastrati A, et al. A randomized trial comparing stenting with balloon angioplasty in small vessels in patients with symptomatic coronary artery disease. ISAR-SMART Study Investigators. Intracoronary Stenting or Angioplasty for Restenosis Reduction in Small Arteries. *Circulation* 2000;102:2593–2598.
23. Kastrati A, et al. Abciximab in patients with acute coronary syndromes undergoing percutaneous coronary intervention after clopidogrel pretreatment: The ISAR-REACT 2 randomized trial. *JAMA* 2006;295:1531–1538.
24. Rubartelli P, et al. Stent implantation versus balloon angioplasty in chronic coronary occlusions: results from the GISSOC trial. Gruppo Italiano di Studio sullo Stent nelle Occlusioni Coronariche. *J Am Coll Cardiol* 1998;32:90–96.
25. Buller CE, et al. Primary stenting versus balloon angioplasty in occluded coronary arteries: the Total Occlusion Study of Canada (TOSCA). *Circulation* 1999;100:236–242.
26. Stone GW, et al. Comparison of angioplasty with stenting, with or without abciximab, in acute myocardial infarction. *N Engl J Med* 2002;346:957–966.
27. Hochman JS, et al. The Occluded Artery Trial (OAT). *N Engl J Med* 2006;355:2395–2407.
28. Fischman DL, et al. A randomized comparison of coronary-stent placement and balloon angioplasty in the treatment of coronary artery disease. Stent Restenosis Study Investigators. *N Engl J Med* 1994;331:496–501.
29. Serruys PW, et al. A comparison of balloon-expandable-stent implantation with balloon angioplasty in patients with coronary artery disease. Benestent Study Group. *N Engl J Med* 1994;331:489–495.

30. Betriu A, et al. Randomized comparison of coronary stent implantation and balloon angioplasty in the treatment of de novo coronary artery lesions (START): a four-year follow-up. *J Am Coll Cardiol* 1999;34:1498–1506.
31. Weaver WD, et al. Optimum percutaneous transluminal coronary angioplasty compared with routine stent strategy trial (OPUS-1): a randomised trial. *Lancet* 2000;355:2199–2203.
32. Savage MP, et al. Stent placement compared with balloon angioplasty for obstructed coronary bypass grafts. Saphenous Vein De Novo Trial Investigators. *N Engl J Med* 1997;337:740–747.
33. Cutlip DE, et al. Stent thrombosis in the modern era: a pooled analysis of multicenter coronary stent clinical trials. *Circulation* 2001;103:1967–1971.
34. Morice MC, et al. A randomized comparison of a sirolimus-eluting stent with a standard stent for coronary revascularization. *N Engl J Med* 2002;346:1773–1780.
35. Reifart N, et al. Randomized comparison of angioplasty of complex coronary lesions at a single center. Excimer Laser, Rotational Atherectomy, and Balloon Angioplasty Comparison (ERBAC) Study. *Circulation* 1997;96:91–98.
36. von Dahl J, et al. Rotational atherectomy does not reduce recurrent in-stent restenosis: results of the angioplasty versus rotational atherectomy for treatment of diffuse in-stent restenosis trial (ARTIST). *Circulation* 2002;105:583–588.
37. Topol EJ, et al. A comparison of directional atherectomy with coronary angioplasty in patients with coronary artery disease. The CAVEAT Study Group. *N Engl J Med* 1993;329:221–227.
38. Holmes DR Jr, et al. A multicenter, randomized trial of coronary angioplasty versus directional atherectomy for patients with saphenous vein bypass graft lesions. CAVEAT-II Investigators. *Circulation* 1995;91:1966–1974.
39. Baim DS, et al. Final results of the Balloon vs Optimal Atherectomy Trial (BOAT). *Circulation* 1998;97:322–331.
40. Kuntz RE, et al. A trial comparing rheolytic thrombectomy with intracoronary urokinase for coronary and vein graft thrombus (the Vein Graft AngioJet Study) [VeGAS 2]. *Am J Cardiol* 2002;89:326–330.
41. Baim DS, et al. Randomized trial of a distal embolic protection device during percutaneous intervention of saphenous vein aorto-coronary bypass grafts. *Circulation* 2002;105:1285–1290.
42. Leon MB, et al. Localized intracoronary gamma-radiation therapy to inhibit the recurrence of restenosis after stenting. *N Engl J Med* 2001;344:250–256.
43. King SP, et al. Arterial Revascularization Therapies (ARTS I) trial. *JACC* 2001;37:1016.
44. Waksman R, et al. Intravascular gamma radiation for in-stent restenosis in saphenous-vein bypass grafts. *N Engl J Med* 2002;346:1194–1199.
45. Waksman R, et al. Intracoronary gamma-radiation therapy after angioplasty inhibits recurrence in patients with in-stent restenosis. *Circulation* 2000;101:2165–2171.
46. Leon MB, et al. A clinical trial comparing three antithrombotic-drug regimens after coronary-artery stenting. Stent Anticoagulation Restenosis Study Investigators. *N Engl J Med* 1998;339:1665–1671.
47. Stone GW, et al. Acute Catheterization and Urgent Intervention Triage strategY (ACUITY) trial. *N Engl J Med* 2006;355:2249–2250.
48. Schomig A, et al. A randomized comparison of antiplatelet and anticoagulant therapy after the placement of coronary-artery stents. *N Engl J Med* 1996;334:1084–1089.
49. Wiviot SD, et al. Prasugrel versus clopidogrel in patients with acute coronary syndromes. The TRITON TIMI 38 Study. *N Engl J Med* 2007;357:2001–2015.
50. Taniuchi M, Kurz HI, Lasala JM. Randomized comparison of ticlopidine and clopidogrel after intracoronary stent implantation in a broad patient population. *Circulation* 2001;104:539–543.
51. Mehta SR, et al. Effects of pretreatment with clopidogrel and aspirin followed by long-term therapy in patients undergoing percutaneous coronary intervention: the PCI-CURE study. *Lancet* 2001;358:527–533.
52. Steinhubl SR, et al. Early and sustained dual oral antiplatelet therapy following percutaneous coronary intervention: a randomized controlled trial. *JAMA* 2002;288:2411–2420.
53. The EPIC Investigators. Use of a monoclonal antibody directed against the platelet glycoprotein IIb/IIIa receptor in high-risk coronary angioplasty. *N Engl J Med* 1994;330:956–961.
54. The EPILOG Investigators. Platelet glycoprotein IIb/IIIa receptor blockade and low-dose heparin during percutaneous coronary revascularization. *N Engl J Med* 1997;336:1689–1696.
55. The EPISTENT Investigators. Randomised placebo-controlled and balloon-angioplasty-controlled trial to assess safety of coronary stenting with use of platelet glycoprotein-IIb/IIIa blockade. Evaluation of Platelet IIb/IIIa Inhibitor for Stenting. *Lancet* 1998;352:87–92.
56. Randomised placebo-controlled trial of abciximab before and during coronary intervention in refractory unstable angina: the CAPTURE Study. *Lancet* 1997;349:1429–1435.
57. O'Shea JC, et al. Platelet glycoprotein IIb/IIIa integrin blockade with eptifibatide in coronary stent intervention: the ESPRIT trial: a randomized controlled trial. *JAMA* 2001;285:2468–2473.
58. Moliterno DJ, et al. Outcomes at 6 months for the direct comparison of tirofiban and abciximab during percutaneous coronary revascularisation with stent placement: the TARGET follow-up study. *Lancet* 2002;360:355–360.
59. Ohman EM, et al. Use of aortic counterpulsation to improve sustained coronary artery patency during acute myocardial infarction. Results of a randomized trial. The Randomized IABP Study Group. *Circulation* 1994;90:792–799.
60. Stone GW, et al. A prospective, randomized evaluation of prophylactic intraaortic balloon counterpulsation in high risk patients with acute myocardial infarction treated with primary angioplasty. Second Primary Angioplasty in Myocardial Infarction (PAMI-II) Trial Investigators. *J Am Coll Cardiol* 1997;29:1459–1467.

TRANSTHORACIC ECHOCARDIOGRAPHY

60

Ron Jacob

I. INTRODUCTION. Transthoracic echocardiography is a reliable and versatile tool for the assessment of cardiac structure, function, and pathophysiology.

II. INDICATIONS. Common indications and corresponding aims of the echocardiographic evaluation are listed in Table 60.1.

III. TWO-DIMENSIONAL IMAGE ACQUISITION

A. Patient and probe positioning. The probe can be held with the right or left hand depending on the patient side that one chooses to scan from. Standard imaging planes are illustrated in Figures 60.1 to 60.6. The patient should be in the left lateral decubitus position, with the left arm extended behind the head, as this brings the heart into contact with the chest wall. See Table 60.2 for standard examination protocol and Table 60.3 for useful examination tips.

B. Electrocardiographic lead placement. The electrocardiogram allows identification of arrhythmias and timing of cardiac events during the echocardiographic examination, and it is used as a timing marker for digital recording of images. Typically digital "clips" are set to record a predefined number of cardiac cycles (usually one), with timing based on the electrocardiogram. It is important that irregular beats be identified and excluded from the analysis. For example, a postectopic beat will falsely increase the two-dimensional assessment of ejection fraction and the Doppler assessment of transaortic gradient. In general, any Doppler index requires the average of at least three measurements. For patients in atrial fibrillation, 7 to 10 beats should be averaged. For patients with very high heart rates, or with a noisy electrocardiographic signal, the digital clips can be set to record for a predefined period of time (usually 2 seconds).

C. Transducer selection. The adult echocardiographic examination typically begins with a 2.5- to 3.5-MHz phased array transducer. Transducer frequency is important, as at higher frequencies spatial resolution improves but at the expense of reduced depth penetration. Higher-frequency (3.0 to 5.0 MHz) transducers may be used in thin or pediatric patients, or intraoperatively for epiaortic scanning. Therefore, for optimal two-dimensional resolution, select the highest-frequency transducer that will provide adequate far-field penetration.

With regard to transducer frequency for the Doppler examination, lower-frequency transducers can record higher velocities (see Doppler equation later in chapter). The Pedoff probe is a continuous wave, nonimaging probe (typical frequency 1.8 MHz) used mainly to detect higher velocity profiles and confirm velocities obtained by other imaging methods.

D. Tissue harmonic imaging has become the standard imaging modality in many laboratories. It utilizes the fact that as ultrasound waves propagate through tissue, the waveform becomes altered by the tissue, with the generation of new waveforms of higher frequency—multiples of baseline frequency ("harmonics"). Setting the transducer to receive only sound waves of a multiple harmonic frequency, typically twice ("second harmonics"), improves image quality significantly compared with fundamental (standard) imaging, with fewer near-field artifacts and better endocardial definition.One limitation of harmonic imaging is that valve leaflets appear thicker; an artifact generated during image processing that appears to be related to the rapid motion of the leaflets.

E. Contrast echocardiography. Contrast echocardiography is performed by injecting either **agitated saline** or one of the **commercially available contrast agents**

TABLE 60.1 Common Indications and Corresponding AIMS of Echocardiographic Evaluation

Indications	Echocardiographic evaluation
Valvular heart disease	Valve morphology; regurgitation and/or stenosis severity and etiology; ventricular size and function
Infective endocarditis	Vegetation; abscess; fistula; valvular function; ventricular size and function
Coronary artery disease	Wall-motion abnormalities; ventricular function; mitral regurgitation/ ventricular septal defect and other ischemic complications
Congestive heart failure	Systolic function; wall-motion abnormalities; chamber size; valvular pathology; diastolic function
Pericardial disease	Pericardial effusion; pericardial thickening ± calcification; RV size and function; respiratory variations in mitral, tricuspid pulmonary venous and hepatic venous flow; IVC size and respiratory variation; RV/RA collapse
Cardiac tamponade	
Ascending aortic pathology	Aneurysm; atheroma; dissection or intramural hematoma; aortic valve pathology
Pulmonary hypertension	RV systolic pressure; RV and LV function; tricuspid, pulmonary, and mitral valve pathology
	Interatrial shunt; respiratory effects on IVC diameter
Systemic hypertension	LV function; LV wall thickness; evidence of aortic coarctation
Embolic disease	LA and LV thrombus; mitral valve pathology; aortic atheroma; LV function; interatrial shunt
Arrhythmias	LA and LV thrombus; ventricular size and function; atrial dimensions; mitral valve pathology
Syncope	LV outflow tract obstruction; aortic and mitral valve pathology; LV function; congenital abnormalities
Cardiac trauma	Ascending aortic dissection; ascending aortic aneurysm; cardiac tamponade
Congenital heart disease	Congenital anomaly; shunt calculation
Critical illness	LV function; valvular pathology; pericardial effusion/tamponade; right-to-left shunt; volume status

IVC, inferior vena cava; LA, left atrial; LV, left ventricular; RA, right atrial; RV, right ventricular.

into an arm vein. Both are microbubbles that reflect ultrasound waves and opacify intracardiac chambers. Ultrasound waves, especially those of higher power, destroy microbubbles. Therefore, for optimal contrast imaging, it is important to reduce the mechanical index (the output of the machine), typically to 0.4 to 0.6. Agitated saline is saline (preferably mixed with some blood), combined with a small quantity of air, which has been exchanged rapidly using a three-way stopcock between two syringes to create small bubbles. These relatively large (and unstable) bubbles are destroyed in the lung and do not routinely appear in the left side of the heart. The appearance of bubbles within the left atrium (either spontaneously or after a cough or Valsalva maneuver) within three beats after contrast appears within the left atrium, suggests a right-to-left intracardiac shunt—typically a small patent foramen ovale (which is typically not seen with two-dimensional examination alone). Delayed contrast appearance in the left atrium may be caused by intrapulmonary shunting and does not necessarily imply an intracardiac shunt.

Modern commercial contrast agents consist either of an albumin-based shell containing perfluorocarbon gas (Optison) or a synthetic phospholipid shell containing perfluoropropane gas (Definity). These microbubbles are smaller (size of a red blood cell) and more stable, and they cross the pulmonary vasculature, appearing in

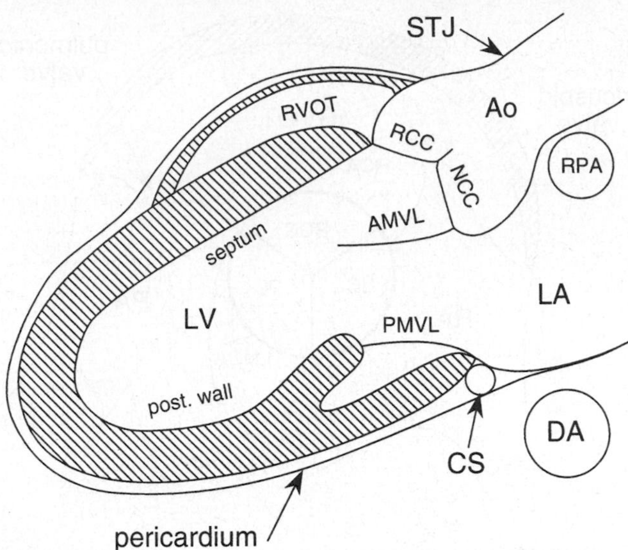

Figure 60.1. Schematic diagram of the parasternal long-axis view in diastole. AML, anterior mitral leaflet; Ao, aorta; CS, coronary sinus; DA, descending aorta; LA, left atrium; LV, left ventricle; NCC, noncoronary cusp; PMVL, posterior mitral valve leaflet; PW, posterior wall; RCC, right coronary cusp; RPA, right pulmonary artery; RVOT, right ventricular outflow tract; STJ, sinotubular junction. (From Otto CM, Pearlman AS. *Otto and Pearlman's textbook of clinical echocardiography.* Philadelphia: WB Saunders, 1995:21–64, with permission.)

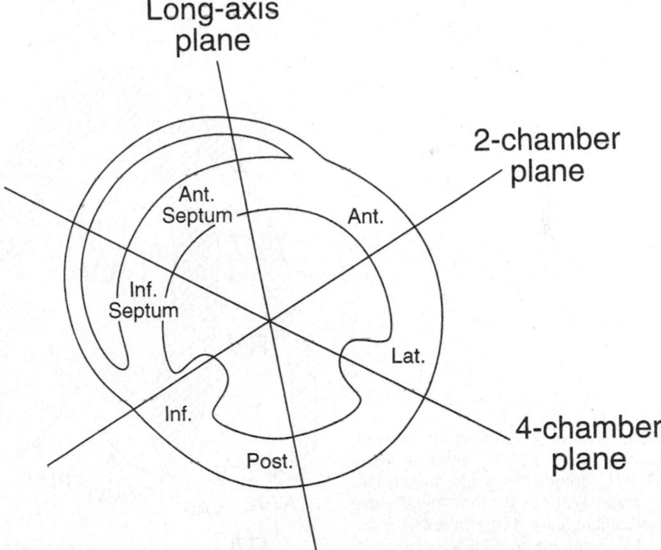

Figure 60.2. Schematic diagram of the parasternal short-axis view at the level of papillary muscles. Ant. Septum, anterior septum; Ant., anterior wall; Inf. Septum, inferior septum; Inf., inferior wall; Lat., lateral wall; Post., posterior wall. (From Otto CM, Pearlman AS. *Otto and Pearlman's textbook of clinical echocardiography.* Philadelphia: WB Saunders, 1995:21–64, with permission.)

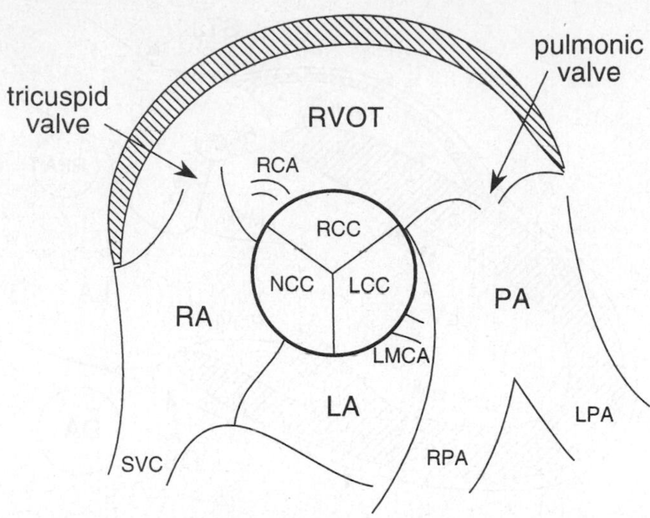

Figure 60.3. Schematic diagram of the parasternal short-axis view at the aortic valve level. LA, left atrium; LCC, left coronary cusp; LMT, left main trunk; LPA, left pulmonary artery; NCC, noncoronary cusp; PA, pulmonary artery; PV, pulmonary valve; RA, right atrium; RCA, right coronary artery; RCC, right coronary cusp; RPA, right pulmonary artery; RVOT, right ventricular outflow tract; SVC, superior vena cava; TV, tricuspid valve. (From Otto CM, Pearlman AS. *Otto and Pearlman's textbook of clinical echocardiography.* Philadelphia: WB Saunders, 1995:21–64, with permission.)

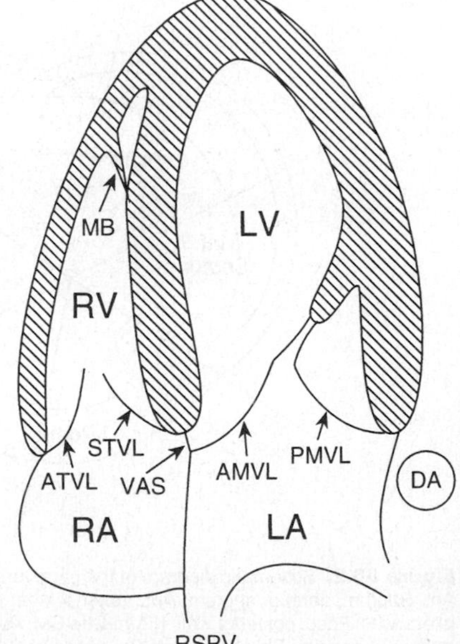

Figure 60.4. Schematic diagram of the apical four-chamber view. AMVL, anterior mitral valve leaflet; ATL, anterior tricuspid leaflet; DA, descending aorta; PMVL, posterior mitral valve leaflet; LA, left atrium; LV, left ventricle; MB, moderator band; RA, right atrium; RUPV, right upper pulmonary vein; RV, right ventricle; STL, septal tricuspid leaflet. (From Otto CM, Pearlman AS. *Otto and Pearlman's textbook of clinical echocardiography.* Philadelphia: WB Saunders, 1995: 21–64, with permission.)

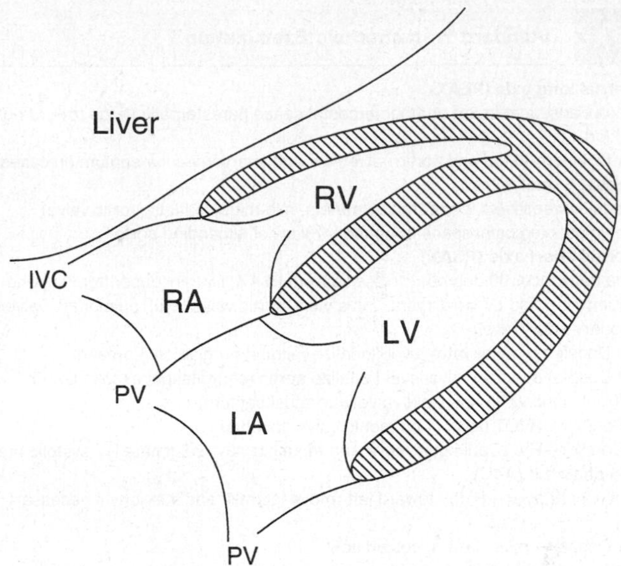

Figure 60.5. Schematic diagram of the four-chamber view from the subcostal approach. IVC, inferior vena cava; LA, left atrium; LV, left ventricle; RA, right atrium; RV, right ventricle. (From Otto CM, Pearlman AS. *Otto and Pearlman's textbook of clinical echocardiography.* Philadelphia: WB Saunders, 1995:21–64, with permission.)

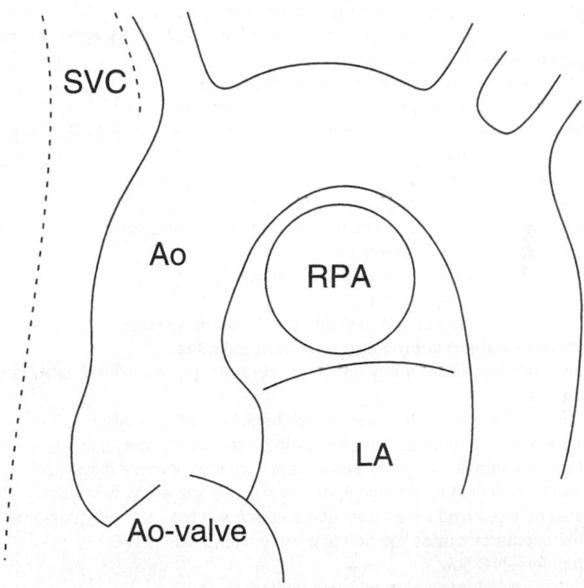

Figure 60.6. Schematic diagram of the aorta and right pulmonary artery from the suprasternal notch window. Ao, aorta; AV, aortic valve; LA, left atrium; RPA, right pulmonary artery; SVC, superior vena cava. (From Otto CM, Pearlman AS. *Otto and Pearlman's textbook of clinical echocardiography.* Philadelphia: WB Saunders, 1995:21–64, with permission.)

TABLE 60.2 Standard Transthoracic Examination

1. **Parasternal long axis (PLAX)**
   - Position transducer in 3rd or 4th intercostal space parasternally (ridge toward right shoulder)
   - Color Doppler—Mitral and aortic valve flow and interventricular septum (in cases of ventricular septal defect)
   - M-mode—three levels (below mitral leaflets, mid-mitral leaflets, aortic valve)
   - Move up an intercostal space to get better view of ascending aorta
2. **Parasternal short axis (PSAX)**
   - Rotate transducer 90 degrees clockwise from PLAX; tilt transducer from superior to inferior (LV apex view, mid-LV view, mitral valve view, aortic valve level, pulmonary valve/main pulmonary artery level)
   - Color Doppler at mitral valve level (localize mitral regurgitation if present)
   - Color Doppler at aortic valve level (localize aortic regurgitation; assess flow in RVOT/pulmonic valve; tricuspid valve; interatrial septum)
   - PW Doppler—RVOT (level of pulmonic valve annulus)
   - CW Doppler—RVOT/pulmonic valve and tricuspid valve (estimate RV systolic pressure)
3. **Apical 4-chamber (A4C)**
   - Transducer at apex—Ridge toward left (move laterally and inferiorly if necessary to get true apex)
   - Color Doppler—mitral flow; tricuspid flow
   - Measure proximal isovelocity surface area if mitral regurgitation (zoom, decrease Nyquist, measure radius)
   - PW Doppler—Mitral inflow—position at level of mitral leaflet tips (gate 1–2 mm)
   - PW Doppler—Pulm. vein (usually right upper PV)—1–2 cm into vein (gate 3–4 mm)
   - CW Doppler—Across mitral valve (stenosis and/or regurgitation, and to calculate proximal isovelocity surface area)
   - CW Doppler—Tricuspid flow (estimate RV systolic pressure)
   - Tilt transducer anteriorly to obtain "5-chamber view," i.e., open up aortic valve/LVOT
   - Color Doppler—LVOT/aortic valve
   - PW Doppler—LVOT—at the level of the aortic annulus
   - CW Doppler—LVOT/aortic valve
   - Tilting transducer posteriorly will bring the coronary sinus in view (along AV junction, emptying into right atrium)
4. **Apical 2-chamber (A2C)**
   - Rotate transducer ~60–90 degrees anticlockwise
   - Tilt posteriorly and rotate clockwise to open out descending aorta
5. **Apical long axis (apical 3-chamber)**
   - Rotate transducer further 30–45 degrees anticlockwise
   - Color Doppler—LVOT/aortic valve
   - Recheck CW Doppler across AV if evaluating for aortic stenosis
6. **Subcostal view—Patient supine and legs bent at knees**
   - Subxiphoid, midline, tilt anteriorly under sternum with groove toward patients left for 4-chamber view
   - Color Doppler across interatrial septum to check for a PFO or ASD
   - Rotate transducer 90 degrees from 4-chamber view until groove is pointing anterosuperiorly
   - Same views as parasternal short axis except rotated 90-degree clockwise
   - Sweep from left to right to get apical, midventricular, and aortic valve level
   - IVC should be visualized when scan plane is directed toward the right mid-clavicular region with some counterclockwise rotation to open out long axis of IVC
   - Color Doppler—IVC flow
   - PW of hepatic veins (may need to angle posteriorly)

(*continued*)

TABLE 60.2 Standard Transthoracic Examination (*Continued*)

7. Suprasternal view—Patient supine, head tilted backward

- Transducer in suprasternal notch, with groove toward left (rotate to about 1 o'clock), parallel to trachea
- Color Doppler in arch and upper descending aorta (especially if suspected coarctation
- PW Doppler in upper descending (if assessing aortic regurgitation severity)

8. Pedoff probe

- Especially for checking maximal aortic valve gradient in aortic stenosis
- Apical position
- Right upper sternal border (aortic stenosis)

AV, atrioventricular; AV, aortic valve; ASD, atrial septal defect; CW, continuous wave; IVC, inferior vena cava; LV, left ventricular; LVOT, left ventricular outflow tract; PFO, patent foramen ovale; PW, pulsed wave; PV, pulmonary vein; RVOT, right ventricular outflow tract.

TABLE 60.3 Tips for Transthoracic Two-Dimensional Examination

1. **Optimize patient position** (left lateral with left hand above head) and **environment** (darken room).
2. Ensure imaging in **harmonics** mode.
3. Consider **contrast** to improve endocardial delineation for technically difficult studies.
4. When parasternal and apical images are limited (body habitus, surgical drains, dressings, etc.), the **subcostal window** may provide the only accessible window.
5. Consider **off-axis views** to enhance visualization of specific structures.
6. Obtain images at **end-expiration,** as the heart is closer to the transducer.
7. **Avoid foreshortening LV apex** (especially in A2C)—true apex may be more inferior and lateral than expected.
8. If **concern of LV thrombus,** zoom and check with low velocity color Doppler to ensure flow throughout. Consider contrast if unclear.
9. If an object is suspicious for an artifact, reassess in other imaging planes.
10. **M-mode** can be useful especially for the accurate timing of cardiac events (especially RV or RA collapse in the setting of possible tamponade, or assessment of possible systolic anterior motion of the mitral valve).
11. Adjust transducer **frequency** to maximum that permits adequate far-field penetration/depth.
12. Set **time gain compensation** in the mid range with lower gain in the near field and higher settings in the far field to compensate for attenuation of the beam with increasing distance from transducer.
13. Use the least amount of **depth** that adequately shows the entire area of interest.
14. Adjust the **transmit gain/output** to optimize image brightness/quality—too low, everything appears black, too high results in a "white-out." Initially set it to high and then adjust downward.
15. Adjust the **"compress"/dynamic range.** Decrease if image quality is poor to produce high-quality contrast images. Increasing it will "soften" images. Typically as compress is increased, the transmit gain should be decreased to maximize the spectrum of the gray scale.
16. Adjust the **focus** (focal zone) to include the area of interest as the beam is narrowest (improves image resolution) within this area, especially when imaging near-field structures (e.g., looking for an apical left ventricular thrombus from the apical windows).
17. Set the **persistence** to low.

LA, left atrial; LV, left ventricular; RA, right atrial; RV, right ventricular.

the left side of the heart where they opacify the left ventricular (LV) cavity. Their primary uses are to improve endocardial definition and to clarify the presence/absence of a suspected LV thrombus/mass. Contrast-enhanced echocardiography for detection of regional wall-motion abnormalities has robust interobserver variability. More recently, contrast has been used to detect myocardial perfusion with results comparable to single positron emission computed tomography (SPECT) imaging. Contrast may be given in a diluted form (1.5 mL mixed with saline up to 10 mL) or in small boluses (typically 0.3 to 0.5 mL) followed by a small amount of saline flush, but should be injected slowly to prevent attenuation artifacts. Contrast also enhances Doppler signals, and agitated saline can be useful to augment the signal from tricuspid regurgitation to better estimate peak right ventricular systolic function (RVSP). Commercial microbubble products (Optison, Definity) can be used to enhance the Doppler envelope in patients with aortic stenosis where the image quality is suboptimal. Newer U.S. Food and Drug Administration (FDA) guidelines recommend careful monitoring of patients after the use of commercial contrast agents, owing to reported rare side-effects after their use.

F. **Machine settings.** To obtain the best images and accurate Doppler information, it is important to optimize the machine settings during different parts of the examination (Tables 60.2 and 60.3).

1. **Time gain compensation.** These controls differentially amplify the echo signals returning from different depths to compensate for attenuation of the ultrasound beam with increasing distance from the transducer. This function is useful with higher frequency transducers, as they are associated with more attenuation at greater depths.
2. **Depth.** Start with the greatest depth to get an overview and then decrease the depth to include all of the target structure. A depth of 16 cm is usually adequate for the apical window and 12 cm for parasternal imaging. Increasing the depth decreases the frame rate, reducing temporal resolution.
3. **Transmit gain.** This adjusts the displayed amplitude (power) of all received signals and, therefore, affects the brightness of echoes displayed. Setting the power too low results in inadequate returning signals and poor image quality, whereas setting it too high results in image white-out.
4. **Compress.** The compress setting is also known as **dynamic range.** It converts the range of returning echo intensities, which may vary a billion-fold in intensity, into 100 to 200 visual shades of brightness or the "gray scale." Increasing the compress will "soften" the image and allow identification of lower-level signals. Decreasing the compress results in the production of high-quality contrast images such that weaker signals are eliminated, noise is reduced, and the strongest echo signals are enhanced. Therefore, the compress/dynamic range is decreased when image quality is poor.
5. **Focus (or position).** The focal zone of the transducer indicates the region of the image at which the ultrasound beam is narrowest and hence where spatial resolution is maximal. Therefore, it is important to reposition the focus to the area of greatest attention/importance, especially those in the near field. When adjusted proximally, however, distal structures may appear blurred as the ultrasound beams scatter.
6. **Persistence.** Temporal averaging of the latest frame with the previous frames to produce a smooth or less noisy display. Fast-moving cardiac structures (e.g., valve leaflets) may appear blurred if the persistence is set above low.

G. **Imaging artifacts**

1. **Acoustic shadowing.** Highly reflective structures block transmission of ultrasound to distal structures, causing poor imaging of these far-field structures. For instance, a mechanical mitral prosthesis prevents good visualization of the left atrium from the apical window.
2. **Reverberation.** This occurs when multiple linear echo signals are generated from a back and forth reflection between two strong reflectors of the ultrasound signal, before the signal returns to the transducer. These appear as multiple parallel irregular dense lines extending from the structure into the far field

(e.g., linear echodensity in the ascending aorta in the parasternal long-axis view simulating a dissection flap, which is a reverberation from a more anteriorly lying structure, such as a rib). Reverberation artifacts will be present at a multiple of the distance between the two strong reflectors—usually at twice the distance between the strong reflectors. Careful analysis of the artifact in multiple views and with color Doppler should be performed. Color flow signals will be seen to pass through the artifact.

3. **Refraction.** Refraction of the ultrasound beam as it passes through a tissue layer can result in a side-by-side double image. This artifact often is seen in parasternal short-axis views of the aortic valve where the image appears to show two aortic valves overlapping.
4. **Beam width artifact.** Ultrasound beams are three-dimensional and are reflected from three-dimensional structures, but they are displayed in a two-dimensional tomographic plane. Strong reflectors at the edge of central beam, especially outside the narrow proximal focal zone, can be superimposed on a structure in the central zone with the resulting appearance of a structure within in the image, that is, outside the two-dimensional tomographic plane (e.g., an aortic valve in the left atrium in the A4C view).
5. **Range ambiguity.** Echo signals from earlier pulse cycles reach the transducer on the next receiving cycle because of re-reflection, resulting in deep structures appearing closer to the transducer than their actual location, and are manifested as the appearance of an anatomically unexpected echo. This can be confirmed by the disappearance of the artifact when the depth setting is changed.
6. **Side lobe artifacts.** In addition to the central beam, transducers produce side lobes 10 to 30-degree off axis. Any echoes returning from structures in these peripheral beams are displayed as if they arose from targets within the main beam. Therefore, strong reflectors may be imaged by these low-intensity side lobes and displayed in an erroneous position on the screen. This is a major source of "clutter" in cardiac cavities. Harmonic echoes have much lower-intensity side lobes, with a resulting reduction in side-lobe artifacts in the image.

IV. M-MODE ECHOCARDIOGRAPHY.

Despite the increasing emphasis on two-dimensional imaging, the M-mode display remains a complementary element of the transthoracic examination. The M-mode cursor should always be guided by two-dimensional imaging to position the scan line along the structure of interest. The image is displayed like a graph, with time on the *x* axis and distance from the transducer on the *y* axis. Its high sampling rate of approximately 1800/second compared with 30/second for two-dimensional echocardiography allows for accurate evaluation of rapidly moving valvular structures and endocardium, and its excellent temporal resolution is useful in the accurate timing of cardiac events. Measurements acquired during the M-mode examination are obtained from the leading echo of the proximal structure to the leading echo of the distal structure. M-Mode echocardiography is especially useful for identifying systolic anterior motion of anterior mitral leaflet, diastolic collapse of the right ventricle, and artifacts.

V. DOPPLER ECHOCARDIOGRAPHY

$$\text{Velocity} = \frac{\text{Doppler frequency shift}}{2\,(\text{transducer frequency}) \times (\text{angle between beam and velocity direction})}$$

A. Doppler principles. Doppler interrogation traditionally was used to measure velocity of red blood cells, but more recently its use has been expanded to evaluate myocardial motion (tissue Doppler and strain rate imaging). Strain rate imaging allows for the estimation of regional myocardial deformation, and, therefore, function. The Doppler principle states that sound frequency increases as the sound source moves toward the observer and decreases as the source moves away. The change in frequency between the transmitted sound and the reflected sound is termed the **Doppler shift.** This Doppler frequency shift relates directly to the velocity component parallel to the ultrasound beam by the **Doppler equation.**

Therefore, the maximal velocity detected is inversely proportional to the transducer frequency; that is, lower transducer frequencies permit higher velocity detection. The Doppler phenomenon is highly angle dependent. The angle between the ultrasound beam and the blood flow jet of interest should be less than 20 degrees, so that the true flow velocity is underestimated by less than 6%. Adhering to this requirement frequently results in off-axis or unusual two-dimensional images. Reference Doppler velocities in the adult examination are shown in Table 60.4.

B. Pulsed-wave Doppler. In the pulsed-wave Doppler mode, a single crystal sends and receives short bursts of ultrasound at a specific pulse repetition frequency (PRF) to a specific location, which are reflected from moving blood cells at this location and received by the same crystal. The maximal velocity that can be measured is limited by the time required to transmit and receive the ultrasound wave. This is called the Nyquist limit (one-half of the PRF). The pulsed-wave signal appears as a wrap around the baseline for velocities greater than the Nyquist velocity. Hence the peak velocity is limited by the depth of the area of interest and also by the transducer frequency (inverse relationship according to the Doppler equation; see previous text). Pulsed-wave Doppler has excellent spatial/depth resolution but has limited capacity to measure high velocities due to the Nyquist limit. It is, therefore, used primarily to measure low velocity flow (less than 2 m/second), at specific sites in the heart.

C. Continuous wave Doppler employs two crystals, one sending and the other receiving continuously. The maximal velocity that can be recorded by continuous wave Doppler is not limited by the PRF or the Nyquist phenomenon. Unlike pulsed-wave Doppler, continuous wave Doppler measures the maximal velocity along the entire ultrasound beam but does not localize to the precise position where the peak velocity is. However, this is often apparent anatomically or can be deduced using pulsed-wave Doppler or color-flow Doppler. **In general, continuous wave Doppler is used to assess high-velocity flow and pulsed-wave Doppler to measure low-velocity flow in specific areas.** Clinical applications of pulsed-wave versus continuous wave Doppler are listed in Table 60.5.

TABLE 60.4 Normal Echo Dimensions in Adults

Factor	Ref. range (cm)		Ref. range (cm)
(i) PARASTERNAL LONG AXIS (M-MODE OR 2D)			
LV end-diastolic Diameter	3.5–5.7	LV end-systolic Diameter	2.3–4.0
Septal thickness (ED)	0.6–1.1	Posterior wall thickness (ED)	0.6–1.1
Aortic root (ED—M-mode)	2.0–3.7	Left atrium (ES)	1.9–4.0
RV end-diastolic Diameter	1.9–3.8		
Aortic annulus (systole—2D)	1.4–2.6	Mid-ascending (2D)	2.1–3.4
(ii) FOUR-CHAMBER VIEW			
LV volume (ED) (cm^3)	96–157	LV volume (ES) (cm^3)	33–68
Ejection fraction (%)	59 ± 6		
Left atrial area (cm^2)			
(iii) DOPPLER VELOCITIES			
Mitral E wave (<50 yr) (cm/s)	72 ± 14	Mitral E wave (>50 yr) (cm/s)	62 ± 14
Mitral A wave (<50 yr) (cm/s)	40 ± 10	Mitral A wave (>50 yr) (cm/s)	59 ± 14
Deceleration time (ms)	140–210		
Ascending aorta (m/s)	1.0–1.7	LV outflow tract (m/s)	0.7–1.1
Pulmonary artery (m/s)	0.5–1.3		
Pulmonary vein S wave (cm/s)	56 ± 13	Pulmonary vein D wave (cm/s)	44 ± 16
Pulmonary vein A reversal (cm/s)	32 ± 7		

ED, end-diastole; ES, end-systole; LV, left ventricular; RV, right ventricular.

TABLE 60.5 Differences and Uses of Pulsed Wave Doppler and Continuous Wave Doppler

Factor	Pulsed wave	Continuous wave
Transducer crystal	Same transmitting and receiving	Different transmitting and receiving
Spatial resolution	Excellent—localizes to precise point	Poor—may be anywhere along the entire beam
Ability to measure high velocity (>2 m/s)	No (limited by Nyquist)	Excellent
Uses	Mitral inflow Pulmonary venous flow LVOT flow Hepatic vein flow Tricuspid Inflow	Gradients in aortic stenosis Gradient and pressure half-time in mitral stenosis Peak velocity in mitral regurgitation and measurement of dP/dt TR velocity—estimate RV systolic pressure

LVOT, left ventricular outflow tract; RV, right ventricular; TR, tricuspid regurgitation.

D. Color-flow imaging. Although spectral (pulsed-wave and continuous wave) Doppler imaging is superior for accurate measurement of specific intracardiac blood flow velocities, the overall pattern of intracardiac flow is best evaluated with color-flow imaging. This codes blood velocity as color shades; with red representing flow toward the transducer and blue flow away. Color-flow Doppler is based on the principle of pulsed-wave Doppler, with multiple sampling volumes at varying depths along a single scan line. A full-color flow map is generated from combining multiple scan lines along the areas of interest. To accurately estimate velocity along a given scan line, the instrument compares the Doppler-shift changes from several successive pulses (typically eight), and this is known as the **burst length.** Where Doppler shifts are detected, pixels representing those areas are designated a color. The color of the pixel is determined by the mean Doppler shift detected at that site. The maximal number of pulses that can be emitted in 1 second is the PRF, which like pulsed-wave Doppler is limited by the depth of the color sector. The number of times per second this entire process can be repeated to provide color information to a specific area equals the frame rate. Frame rate and hence color resolution are, therefore, dependent on the depth of the color sector (dependent on the PRF), the sector width (number of scan lines), the burst length, and the density of the scan lines (determined by the machine).

Color-flow Doppler has limitations similar to that of pulsed-wave Doppler for velocity determination. When the flow velocity is higher than the Nyquist limit (indicated on the color map), color aliasing occurs (depicted as color reversal).

E. Factors affecting color Doppler image. Many factors affect spectral Doppler and color flow Doppler, and it is important to consider these. They can broadly be divided into three groups: machine settings, imaging factors, and hemodynamic factors. See Table 60.6 for tips to optimize Doppler settings.

1. Machine settings

a. Nyquist limit. At any given depth, for color Doppler imaging the Nyquist or aliasing velocity (which is related to the PRF) can be adjusted. Typically it is set to 50 to 60 cm/second. The lowest velocity that is displayed on the color map is related to the Nyquist (minimal displayed velocity = Nyquist × 2/32). Therefore, decreasing the Nyquist increases the lowest velocity displayed, which has the effect of increasing the size of the jet area.

TABLE 60.6 Tips for the Transthoracic Doppler Examination

1. Doppler (all modalities) is very **angle dependent**—angle between the ultrasound beam and the blood flow jet of interest should be less than 20 degrees. In order to achieve this off-axis views are often required.
Pw and Cw doppler
2. Shifting the **Doppler baseline** up or down can double the maximal velocity detected (still <2 m/s) for PW. **3.** Increasing **depth,** decreases the Nyquist limit, and reduces the maximal velocity that can be measured with PW. **4.** Recheck high velocity jets with the **Pedoff (CW)** probe to confirm peak velocity (include right upper sternal border positions when trying to obtain peak aortic stenosis velocity). **5.** Start with high **gain setting** and reduce until noise and clutter are adequately suppressed. **6.** Set **wall filter** to low to avoid overestimation of low velocities. **7.** Decreasing the **compress** enhances the edges of the spectral envelope, increasing it enhances the various velocities displayed within the Doppler envelope. **8.** Initially set **"reject"** at low (20% to 40%) to allow the display of a wide range of signals, then increase to remove signals that obscure the image (i.e., to reduce noise). **9.** Adjust **gate width**—(1–2 mm for mitral inflow and LVOT, 3–4 mm for pulmonary venous flow, 5–10 for Doppler tissue imaging).
Color flow doppler
10. **Narrow** the sector and minimize the **depth** to maximize color resolution (increase frame rate). **11.** Spatial resolution is higher **axial** to the beam than lateral. **12.** Higher **transducer frequencies** result in an increased area of flow disturbance (reduces the Nyquist and increases ability to visualize lower velocities) **13.** Adjust **color gain** until just before noise appears in the color. **14.** Minimize **wall filters** during analysis of PISA/flow convergence, to avoid overestimating low velocities. **15.** Decreasing the **Nyquist limit** increases the size of any regurgitant jet as lower velocities are detected (normally not color coded at higher Nyquist velocities); therefore, set at 50–60 cm/s initially. **16.** Be careful not to miss or underestimate very **eccentric jets** of mitral regurgitation or aortic regurgitation. **17.** Remember that **chamber constraint** reduces the size of a jet.
CW, continuous wave; LVOT, left ventricular outflow tract; PISA, proximal isovelocity surface area; PW, pulsed wave.

b. Transducer frequency. For color flow imaging, higher transducer frequency reduces the peak velocity (Nyquist limit) that can be measured (see Doppler equation above). Lower Nyquist results in an increased color-flow jet area. Therefore, higher frequency transesophageal echocardiography generally produces larger areas of flow disturbance than transthoracic echocardiography. For spectral Doppler imaging, lower-frequency transducers can measure higher velocities.

c. Depth setting. Minimizing the depth setting to encompass only the region of interest maximizes the PRF and frame rate.

d. Gain. Adjust the color gain until just before random noise appears in the color. Increased color gain increases the size of color-flow disturbance. Two-dimensional gain should be decreased during the color Doppler examination to maximize color-flow disturbance because each pixel is assigned to either two-dimensional or color. For pulsed-wave and continuous wave Doppler, start with a high-gain setting until the desired signal is appreciated. The gain is decreased until noise and clutter are adequately suppressed.

e. **Baseline.** Used primarily for unwrapping aliased signals. Generally leave it in the middle of the color bar, but it can be adjusted to maximize the velocity that can be displayed with pulsed-wave or color Doppler. This is also useful for highlighting a specific velocity as in proximal convergence analysis.

f. **Wall filter.** Excludes low-velocity, high-amplitude signals from myocardial motion. If set too high it tends to decrease the color-flow disturbance. A typical initial setting is 400 Hz. The wall filter should be minimized during analysis of the proximal flow convergence region to avoid overestimation of low velocities (i.e., set low for pulsed-wave Doppler and high for continuous wave Doppler).

g. **Beam width.** Especially important with pulsed-wave and continuous wave Doppler. As the ultrasound beam propagates, it spreads out. For example, when sampling pulmonary venous flow with pulse Doppler from the apical view, the sample volume may be at 16-cm depth and the ultrasound beam may be more than 1 cm in width. This can lead to the detection of aortic flow, which is displayed as if it arose along the beam axis (from the pulmonary vein) leading to beam width artifact.

h. **Gate length or sample size.** This is the size of the pulsed-wave Doppler sampling region. It is usually set at 3 to 5 mm. Narrowing the gate focuses the velocity data to a smaller spatial area and can help to improve image quality, but requires very accurate positioning to prevent missing of the appropriate sample area during cardiac motion.

i. **Scale.** Controls the range of Doppler velocities displayed. As the velocity scale increases, the velocity limits increase and the displayed waveform size decreases.

j. **Compress.** For spectral (pulsed-wave and continuous wave) Doppler, the compress setting adjusts the gray scale, which controls image softness. Decrease the compress to enhance the edges of the spectral envelope. Increase the compress to enhance the various velocities displayed within the Doppler spectrum. Set at 30 dB or higher initially.

k. **Reject.** For spectral Doppler, the reject control removes low-amplitude signals ("noise") from the spectral display. The reject control is initially set at a low level (20% to 40% maximum) to allow the display of a wide range of signals. The reject is then increased to remove signals that obscure the image.

2. **Imaging factors**

a. **Interrogation angle.** Color-flow imaging measures only the component of flow that is parallel to the ultrasound beam. This is related to the true flow velocity by the cosine of the angle between the blood flow and the interrogating ultrasound beam. Satisfactory alignment (as parallel to the flow as possible) is vital to record the full and maximal velocity jet with spectral (both pulsed wave and continuous wave) Doppler.

b. **Attenuation.** Loss of signal strength caused by too high a transducer frequency for the required depth results in a reduced area of color-flow disturbance.

c. **Acoustic shadowing.** Loss of signal strength caused by a proximal reflector of ultrasound (e.g., a mechanical prosthetic valve preventing apical imaging of mitral regurgitant jet in the left atrium).

3. **Hemodynamic factors**

a. **Flow volume.** Increasing regurgitant volume results in an increased area of color-flow disturbance, and this is the basis for the common practice of judging the severity of valvular regurgitation by the size of the color jet. However, as outlined in this chapter, many factors affect the size of the color-flow jet area. Therefore, it is important to include other factors in the assessment of regurgitation, such as ventricular and atrial size, the morphologic appearance of the valve, the width of the color jet at its narrowest point (vena contracta), and, in particular, more quantitative analysis using the proximal flow convergence region (proximal isovelocity surface area, PISA). Several cardiac cycles should be inspected with minor adjustments in the angle of interrogation to ensure that the largest jet is visualized.

b. **Driving pressure.** Increased pressure gradient across a regurgitant orifice results in increased color-flow disturbance in the receiving chamber. Color jet size is closely related to jet momentum, given by flow rate multiplied by jet velocity.

c. **Chamber constraint in eccentric jets.** Impingement of a regurgitant jet against walls of the receiving chamber will decrease the size of the color disturbance. For example, severe but eccentric mitral regurgitation may have a very small area of color-flow disturbance because the jet looses momentum to the constraining left atrial wall and appears narrower in a two-dimensional view as it is splayed out over a larger surface area of the wall.

4. **Doppler artifact.** Mirror image artifact can be seen occasionally when the Doppler signal is duplicated on the other side of the baseline.

VI. **COLOR M-MODE (CMM).** This technique, whereby color-flow Doppler is imposed on an M-mode image, permits excellent spatiotemporal distribution of velocity (color) data, although it is limited to the defined scan line. It is a valuable adjunct in the timing of cardiac events, which may not be readily appreciated by two-dimensional and color-flow imaging alone. Its primary use has been in evaluating diastolic filling pattern where the LV inflow CMM pattern typically has two appreciable waves, the first demonstrating the early passive filling wave and the second later wave resulting from atrial contraction (Fig. 60.7). The slope of the early filling wave (velocity of propagation, V_p) is dependent primarily on the rate of relaxation and is reduced with delayed relaxation. It is useful for differentiating a normal mitral inflow pattern (normal V_p), from a pseudonormal filling pattern (where impaired relaxation results in delayed flow propagation into the left ventricle, slower V_p) (Fig. 60.7 and Table 60.7).

Other uses for CMM are in the accurate measurement of aortic regurgitation (AR) jet diameter in the LV outflow tract (LVOT) in the parasternal views for optimal assessment of regurgitant severity and in the detection (with its superior temporal resolution) of diastolic mitral regurgitation, which may be seen in certain conditions (severe acute AR, advanced diastolic dysfunction, complete heart block).

VII. **TISSUE DOPPLER IMAGING (TDI)** is based on adjusting standard Doppler to focus primarily on the low-velocity, high-amplitude motion of the myocardium (usually less

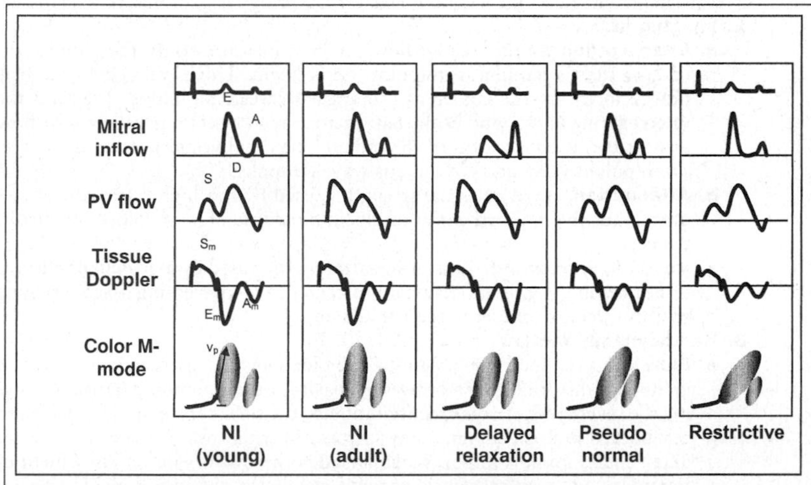

Figure 60.7. Diastolic function/dysfunction staging.

TABLE 60.7 Diastolic Function/Dysfunction Staging

	Normal young	Normal adult	Normal elderly	Delayed relaxation	Pseudo-normal filling	Restrictive filling
Stage	Normal	Normal	Normal	I	II	III
***E/A* ratio**	>1 (often >2)	>1	<1	<1	1–2	>2
DT (ms)	<220	<220	>220	>220	150–200	<150
***S/D* ratio**	<1	≥1	>1	>1	<1	<1
A_r (cm/s)	<35	<35	<35	<35	>35	>25
V_p (cm/s)	>55	>55	<55	<55	<45	<45
E_a (cm/s)	>10	>8	<8	<8	<8	<8

than 20 cm/seconds) instead of the high-velocity, low-amplitude motion of blood. Decreasing the filters (which normally eliminate low-velocity signals) and decreasing the Doppler transmit gain (exclude the low-amplitude blood signals) results in the Doppler focusing primarily on myocardial motion. TDI can be displayed as either pulsed-wave Doppler, typically at one aspect of the mitral annulus (usually septal or lateral) or by color-flow TDI mapping of the entire myocardial area of interest. TDI has been used primarily as an adjunct for the evaluation of LV diastolic function, where the mitral annular TDI pattern shows a systolic (S_a) wave toward the transducer and two diastolic waves away from the transducer (corresponding to early relaxation and late atrial diastolic myocardial motion, labeled E_a and A_a) (Fig. 60.7 and Table 60.7). With worsening diastolic function, E_a velocity decreases and is directly proportional to the rate of relaxation. TDI Annular velocities decrease with age and may be affected by a myocardial infarction in the region adjacent to the annulus or surgery for the mitral valve. Therefore, TDI can be used to help differentiate a normal mitral inflow pattern (normal E_a) from a pseudonormal filling pattern (reduced E_a) (Fig. 60.7 and Table 60.7). TDI can also be used to assess LV filling pressures, myocardial deformation, and ventricular dyssynchrony.

TDI imaging in dyssynchrony assessment

Intraventricular dyssynchrony is said to be present when either of the following parameters are present:

1. A difference in the time to peak velocity of more than 65 milliseconds between opposing walls (basal segments in four-chamber, two-chamber, and three-chamber views yielding a total of six segments).
2. A standard deviation of more than 34 milliseconds in the time to peak velocity (basal and midsegments in four-chamber, two-chamber, and three-chamber views yielding a total of 12 segments). Interventricular dyssynchrony is said to exist when the difference between aortic and pulmonic ejection is greater than 40 milliseconds.

VIII. STRAIN AND STRAIN RATE IMAGING. Tissue strain, a dimensionless entity, is a measure of the relative deformation of tissue. Myocardial deformation in a segment of interest is assessed in reference to the adjacent segment, avoiding errors introduced by translational motion and tethering. Strain rate is the rate of the deformation between two adjacent points of interest along a scan line and is expressed in seconds. A strain rate curve can be derived by analyzing many adjacent segments along a scan line. Doppler techniques for assessing strain are not always ideal due to angle dependence, signal noise, and the need for a high frame rate. Doppler independent techniques such as speckle tracking use ultrasonic reflectors (speckles) within tissues that can be followed from frame to frame through the cardiac cycle. This method can be used to assess radial deformation and torsion of the ventricle. Strain rate is a relatively preload-independent measure of regional myocardial function. Clinical applications include assessment of myocardial ischemia, viability, diastolic function, subclinical LV dysfunction in valve disease, and cardiac involvement in systemic diseases such as diabetes or amyloidosis.

IX. DIASTOLIC FUNCTION. Doppler echocardiography remains the primary modality for assessing LV diastolic function, primarily by integrating information obtained from pulsed-wave Doppler of mitral inflow and pulmonary venous flow combined with two-dimensional assessment of left atrial size. Addition of CMM and TDI modalities can help optimize assessment of degree of diastolic dysfunction and combined mitral inflow/CMM (E/V_p) and mitral inflow/TDI (E/E_a) indices can be used to estimate LV filling pressures.

Traditionally diastolic function was determined solely based on assessment of mitral inflow pattern; however, with worsening diastolic function, a "pseudonormal" pattern appears (due to the opposing effects of delayed LV relaxation and elevated LV filling pressures), and this is indistinguishable from a normal diastolic filling pattern. Pulmonary venous flow can help differentiate these. Conventionally the normal anterograde S/D pattern (S is greater than D) should be reversed (S is less than D) in patients with pseudonormal LV diastolic filling, with an increased retrograde atrial reversal velocity. However, optimal pulmonary venous flow images can be difficult to obtain, and flow patterns can be affected by other factors, including rhythm (atrial fibrillation) and valvular dysfunction (mitral regurgitation). Both CMM (delayed V_p) and TDI (reduced E_a) are useful to help confirm a pseudonormal filling pattern. An additional important key factor in assessing LV diastolic function is left atrial volume indexed to body surface area, which is invariably increased with worsening diastolic function. Significant diastolic dysfunction is unlikely to exist with a normal left atrial volume index. Accurate assessment of diastolic function is important for investigation/diagnosis of patients with primarily LV diastolic heart failure, but is also of major prognostic importance for patients with systolic heart failure.

X. THREE-DIMENSIONAL ECHOCARDIOGRAPHY is now emerging as a realistic imaging modality with improving image quality on newer generation three-dimensional machines. Images are obtained using a transducer that transmits and receives data simultaneously in a three-dimensional volume (voxel). Either real-time three-dimensional images or biplane (orthogonal) simultaneous two-dimensional images can be obtained. The three-dimensional data set can then be manipulated using different software packages to assess function and anatomy. It is of particular benefit for the localization of valvular abnormalities (especially for the complex three-dimensional mitral valve structure), accurate LV volume calculation, guiding surgical interventions (e.g., surgical myectomy for hypertrophic cardiomyopathy), congenital heart disease, and so on. Three-dimensional echocardiography allows for a better assessment of the right ventricle, which has a complicated geometry that is sometimes difficult to assess by two-dimensional echocardiography. Three-dimensional color-flow imaging allows a comprehensive assessment of vena contracta and areas of flow convergence (PISA), which will improve the accuracy in the quantification of valvular regurgitation in the future. With the present technology, image resolution remains inferior to two-dimensional imaging.

XI. DIGITAL ECHOCARDIOGRAPHY. Digital storage of images has many obvious advantages compared with the traditional videotape system, and is becoming the standard in many laboratories. Images can be stored for rapid retrieval, with no degradation of image quality over time. It permits further off-line digital measurement/analysis of images. All modern echocardiography machines have capabilities for digital image acquisition, after which images are transferred over a network to a server, and can be reviewed and further analyzed with one of several commercially available software packages. Optimal image acquisition for digital recording requires additional attention during imaging, as typically only one to two cardiac cycles (timing guided from the electrocardiograph) are recorded to limit the digital size of a study. Therefore, it is vital to ensure that the digital images ("clips") recorded are representative images of a typical cardiac cycle (full cardiac cycle, not a postectopic beat). For atrial fibrillation (with the significant beat-to-beat variability), longer clips are often necessary.

XII. HEMODYNAMIC MEASUREMENT

A. LV volume is best measured using the modified Simpson method (disk summation method). This involves tracing the LV area from two orthogonal views (typically A4C and A2C) and dividing the LV into a number of cylinders of equal height.

Volume is calculated by adding up the totals of all combined cylinders. All modern machines and digital echo reading systems have integrated software to create and combine the volume data after simply tracing the LV areas in both apical views. Three-dimensional echocardiography is superior to two-dimensional echocardiography in the measurement of LV volumes, with greater accuracy and reproduciblity when compared with MRI.

B. Ejection fraction (EF) is the standard measure of LV systolic function. It can be measured using two primary methods:

1. EF from volume data obtained by **Simpson's method:**

$$\text{Stroke volume (SV)} = \text{end-diastolic volume (EDV)} - \text{end-systolic volume (ESV)}$$

$$\text{EF} = \text{SV/EDV} \times 100\%$$

$$\mathbf{EF = EDV - ESV/EDV \times 100\%}$$

2. Quinones method is based on measurement of internal dimensions of the LV:

$$\begin{aligned} \text{EF} &= [(\%\Delta D^2) + (1 - \%\Delta D^2)][\%\Delta L] \\ \%\Delta D^2 &= \text{fractional shortening of the square of the minor axis} \\ &= (\text{LVE}\Delta\text{d}^2 - \text{LVEDs}^2)/\text{LVED}^2 \end{aligned}$$

$\%\Delta L =$ fractional shortening of the long axis, mainly related to apical contraction (15% for normal; 5% for hypokinetic; 0% for akinetic; –5% for dyskinetic; –10% for apical aneurysm)

$$\begin{aligned} \text{LVEDd} &= \text{LV end} - \text{diastolic diameter;} \\ \text{LVEDs} &= \text{LV end} - \text{systolic diameter (PLAX view)} \end{aligned}$$

Newer semiautomated methods in three-dimensional echocardiography using full matrix-array transducers give accurate, reproducible assessments of LV function that are superior to two-dimensional methods when MRI is used as the gold standard.

LV torsion is a newer index by which to assesss LV systolic function using speckle tracking. The difference between clockwise rotation of the base of the heart and the counterclockwise rotation of the apex of the heart (approximately 12 degrees) can be evaluated using speckle tracking.

C. Transvalvular pressure gradient. The **Bernoulli equation** allows measurement of relative pressure differences across valves, shunts, or the LVOT. In its complete form, the Bernoulli equation is too complex for routine clinical use, as it incorporates three main components: convective acceleration; inertial term (flow acceleration); and viscous friction. In many clinical situations, the latter two components can be ignored, leaving the flow gradient across an orifice to be derived from the convective acceleration term alone:

$$\Delta P = 4 \times (V_2^2 - V_1^2)$$

where V_2 is velocity distal to an obstruction and V_1 is velocity proximal to an obstruction.

Flow proximal to a narrowed orifice (V_1) is much lower than the peak flow velocity (V_2) and can frequently be ignored leaving a **simplified Bernoulli equation:**

$$\mathbf{\Delta P = 4V^2}$$

The simplified Bernoulli equation is unreliable when:

1. V_1 is greater than 1.0 m/second, which occurs in serial lesions (subvalvular and valvular stenosis) and mixed stenosis with regurgitation.

2. Viscous resistance becomes significant in the evaluation of long stenoses (e.g., coarctation or a tunnel-like ventricular septal defect)

3. When the inertial term (flow acceleration) is not negligible (flow through normal valves)

It is important to realize that the Bernoulli equation represents the **maximal instantaneous gradient** across a stenosis, which is always higher than the customary peak-to-peak gradient measured in the catheterization laboratory.

Flow within the heart is pulsatile; hence, mean gradients are an important measure and are obtained by integrating the velocity profile over the ejection time. This can be obtained readily with software available on all modern echocardiography machines by simply tracing the area of the velocity profile. The mean pressure gradient is then derived from the mean velocity data using the Bernoulli equation.

D. Intracardiac pressure measurement

1. **Estimated right atrial (RA) pressure** can be derived from the size of the inferior vena cava (IVC) and its response to changes in respiration or a sniff (Table 60.8). Using a dilated IVC to assess elevated RA pressures is not accurate in mechanically ventilated patients; however, a small IVC of less than 1.2 cm in a mechanically ventilated patient is 100% specific for an RA pressure less than 10 mm Hg.
2. **Pulmonary artery systolic pressure (PASP)** is estimated from the tricuspid regurgitation (TR) peak velocity. Providing there is no tricuspid valve obstruction, peak TR velocity will depend on the pressure gradient between the right ventricle and the right atrium [difference between peak right ventricular systolic pressure (RVSP) and RA pressure]. Therefore, estimated RVSP is equal to this pressure difference (determined from the peak TR velocity using the Bernoulli equation) and the estimated RA pressure (Table 60.8). Providing there is no obstruction across the pulmonic valve, the right ventricular systolic pressure will be similar to the **PASP:**

$$\textbf{PASP} = 4 \times (\textbf{peak TR velocity})^2 + \textbf{estimated RA pressure}$$

3. **Pulmonary artery diastolic pressure (PADP)**
Pulmonary regurgitation represents the pressure difference between the pulmonary artery (PA) and the right ventricle. Hence, the end pulmonary regurgitation velocity can be utilized to measure the end-diastolic pressure difference between the PA and right ventricle. The right ventricular end-diastolic pressure should be similar to the RA pressure; therefore, addition of estimated RA pressure to the end-diastolic pressure difference between the PA and the right ventricle will estimate the PADP:

$$\textbf{PADP} = 4 \times (\textbf{end pulmonary regurgitant velocity})^2 + \textbf{estimated RA pressure}$$

4. **Estimated left atrial pressure (LAP)/LV diastolic pressure (LVEDP).** Providing there is no mitral stenosis, LVEDP and LAP should be the same. This important measure of LV diastolic function can be estimated by several methods.
   a. **Deceleration time of mitral inflow (DT).** A DT less than 150 milliseconds is strongly suggestive of an elevated LVEDP/LAP. In very young patients a DT less than 150 milliseconds may be normal. This results from a rapid

TABLE 60.8 Estimation of RA Pressure

IVC	Change with respiration/sniff	Est. RA pressure
Normal (<1.7 cm)	Decrease >50%	0–5 mm Hg
Dilated (>1.7 cm)	Decrease >50%	6–10 mm Hg
Dilated (>1.7 cm)	Decrease <50%	10–15 mm Hg
Dilated (>1.7 cm)	No Change	>15 mm Hg

equalization of pressures secondary to vigorous early diastolic relaxation and is not caused by elevated LAP.

b. Difference between pulmonary venous atrial duration and mitral atrial duration. Normally mitral A wave duration is greater than pulmonary venous atrial reversal (Ar) duration. When LVEDP is increased, the velocity and duration of the mitral A wave decreases, whereas pulmonary vein Ar velocity and duration increase. The difference between the duration of the Ar wave and the mitral A wave correlates with LVEDP. An Ar-A duration of more than 50 milliseconds is specific for an elevated LVEDP greater than 20 mm Hg. This is reliable in patients with reduced ejection fraction but not in patients with normal ejection fraction. The primary limitation with this method is the difficult in accurately measuring the duration of Ar.

c. Combined mitral inflow/CMM index (E/V_p ratio) This index has been demonstrated to correlate with LAP/LVEDP, especially when these filling pressures are elevated. A ratio greater than 2.0 is suggestive of elevated filling pressures. In patients with normal ejection fractions, especially with small ventricles and hyperdynamic function, the flow propagation velocities are not accurate.

d. Combined mitral inflow/DTI index (E/E_a ratio). This index has been shown as a semiquantitative measure of LVEDP. A ratio of more than 10 (using the lateral annulus) or more than 15 (using the septal annulus) correlates with a wedge pressure of greater than 20 mm Hg. A ratio of less than 8 (using the lateral annulus) correlates well with normal filling pressures. For values that fall in between these two limits, the clinician should look at all the other information provided by echocardiography such as left atrial size and pulmonary venous Doppler to assess whether filling pressures are elevated.

E. dP/dt. This index of LV contractility is the rate of pressure increase during isovolumic contraction and is traditionally obtained using invasive pressure transducers. It can be estimated from the continuous wave Doppler mitral regurgitant jet. During isovolumic contraction, there is no change in LAP; therefore, mitral regurgitant velocity changes reflect *dP/dt*, with more rapid increases in mitral regurgitant velocity being associated with increased contractility. The pressure change between 1 m/second and 3 m/second = $4\,(V_2^2 - V_1^2) = 32$ mm Hg. The time difference between 1 m/second and 3 m/second is measured from the mitral regurgitation jet, and *dP/dt* is calculated as follows:

$$dP/dt = 32\ \text{mm Hg/time (s)}$$

This has been demonstrated to correlate well with invasively measured *dP/dt* (normal is greater than 1 200 mm Hg/second).

F. Continuity equation is an application of the principle of conservation of mass, which states that flow across a conduit of varying diameter is equal at all points. This equation is especially useful in the quantifying a stenotic aortic valve area that cannot be accurately planimetered from the transthoracic window. Flow at any point in the heart is the product of the cross-sectional area (CSA) by the flow velocity. As flow velocity varies during ejection in a pulsatile system, individual velocities must be integrated to measure total volume of flow (velocity time integral, VTI). This is determined by tracing the spectral Doppler profile, using standard measurement software built into all echocardiography machines.

Flow at any point = CSA x VTI

For calculation of aortic valve area (AVA) based on the continuity equation:

$$\text{Flow across the LVOT} = \text{flow across the aortic valve}$$

$$\text{Area}_{\text{LVOT}} \times \text{VTI}_{\text{LVOT}} = \text{Area}_{\text{aortic valve}} \times \text{VTI}_{\text{aortic valve}}$$

$$\text{Area}_{\text{aortic valve}} = \text{Area}_{\text{LVOT}} \times \text{VTI}_{\text{LVOT}}/\text{VTI}_{\text{aortic valve}}$$

$$\text{Area}_{\text{aortic valve}} = (\text{diameter}_{\text{LVOT}}/2)^2 \times \pi \times \text{VTI}_{\text{LVOT}}/\text{VTI}_{\text{aortic valve}}$$

$$\mathbf{Area_{aortic\ valve} = (diameter_{LVOT})^2 \times 0.785 \times VTI_{LVOT}/VTI_{aortic\ valve}}$$

The greatest source of error in this equation is in the measurement of the LVOT diameter, which as it is squared will magnify any initial measurement error. It can be difficult to define accurately in some calcified valves. The **dimensionless index** (DI) is the ratio of the LVOT and aortic valve VTIs, and it is preferable to use this to assess aortic stenosis when accurate measurement of the LVOT diameter is not possible. A DI less than 0.25 suggests severe aortic stenosis.

$$\mathbf{Dimensionless\ index = VTI_{LVOT}/VTI_{aortic\ valve}}$$

Of note the flow across the LVOT per beat is the stroke volume, which can thus be calculated from the produce of the LVOT diameter and flow velocity (VTI_{LVOT})

$$\mathbf{Stroke\ volume = (diameter_{LVOT})^2 \times 0.785 \times VTI_{LVOT}}$$

G. Volumetric method to assess regurgitant volume/regurgitant fraction. This is based on the conservation of flow, with total flow across a regurgitant valve being equal to the sum of the forward flow and the regurgitant flow. For example, for mitral regurgitation:

$$\text{Total transmitral flow volume} = \text{forward flow volume (LVOT flow)} + \text{regurgitant volume}$$

(LVOT flow can be assumed to be the same as the forward flow providing there is no AR.)

$$\text{Regurgitant volume} = \text{mitral forward flow} - \text{LVOT flow}$$

$$\mathbf{Regurgitant\ volume = (diameter_{mitral}{}^2 \times 0.785\ VTI_{MV}) - (diameter_{LVOT}{}^2 \times 0.785 \times VTI_{LVOT})}$$

$$\mathbf{Regurgitant\ fraction = regurgitant\ volume/total\ mitral\ flow}$$

H. The PISA method is another application of the principle of conservation of mass. It is based on the phenomenon that flow accelerates proximal to a narrowed orifice. This is illustrated by the acceleration of water in a bathtub before it enters the drain pipe. As flow accelerates, it exceeds the Nyquist limit and the color reverses. This is seen as a colored ("isovelocity") hemisphere with color flow imaging, with the velocity of flow at the surface of this hemisphere being the aliasing velocity (Nyquist limit) of color flow in that direction. Decreasing the aliasing velocity will increase the size of the hemisphere as the velocity at which color changes is reduced. In keeping with conservation of mass, blood flow at the surface of this hemisphere is the same as flow through the regurgitant orifice, and this is the basis of using the PISA method to estimate the regurgitant orifice area (ROA) of a valve. PISA has been most extensively used to estimate the mitral ROA to quantify mitral regurgitation.

$$\text{Flow at surface of hemisphere} = \text{flow through regurgitant orifice}$$

$$\text{Surface area of hemisphere} \times \text{velocity at hemisphere} = \text{ROA} \times \text{peak velocity of regurgitation}$$

$$2 \times \pi(\text{radius})^2 \times \text{aliasing velocity} = \text{ROA} \times \text{peak MR velocity}$$

$$\mathbf{ROA = 2 \times \pi(radius)^2 \times aliasing\ velocity/MR_{CW}\ peak\ velocity}$$

Therefore, the radius of the PISA hemisphere, the aliasing velocity, and the peak MR velocity are the measurements needed to calculate ROA. The greatest source of error is in defining where the ROA is, so as to accurately calculate the radius.

This method can also be used to measure mitral valve area in mitral stenosis (where forward flow convergence is seen and measured) and the aortic ROA in AR, although it may be difficult to obtain satisfactory visualization of the aortic PISA for quantification from the apical long axis (best view to appropriately line up AR jet with the Doppler). When the jet is eccentric, and a full hemisphere is not visible, an angle correction should be considered. The PISA equation for MR can be simplified if the aliasing velocity is set to 40 cm/seconds and it is assumed that peak MR velocity will be 5 m/seconds (equates to a normal LV-to-LA pressure gradient of 100 mm Hg). Using these two constants, the PISA equation is simplified to:

$$\mathbf{ROA = (radius)^2/2}$$

Peak MR velocity will increase or decrease depending on changes in LV systolic pressure and LAP and cannot always be assumed to be 5 m/second. However, this method is useful for semiquantification and rapid assessment. Regurgitant volume can be calculated as follows:

$$\mathbf{Regurgitant\ volume = ROA \times VTI_{MRjet}}$$

I. Pressure half-time ($P\frac{1}{2}$) is used to estimate mitral valve area, as the time for the pressure to fall by half across a stenotic valve is proportional to the degree of stenosis. It is the time interval for the peak pressure gradient to fall by half. Using the Bernoulli equation to convert pressure to velocity, there is a constant relationship between peak velocity and the velocity at $P\frac{1}{2}$.

$$\text{Pressure at half the peak pressure} = \tfrac{1}{2}\ \text{peak pressure}$$

$$4 \times (V\tfrac{1}{2})^2 = \tfrac{1}{2}(4 \times V_{max}^2) \rightarrow V\tfrac{1}{2} = V_{max} \div \sqrt{2}$$

In addition, the $P\frac{1}{2}$ has a constant relationship to the deceleration time (DT) of the early mitral filling wave and is usually estimated from the following:

$$P\tfrac{1}{2} = 0.29 \times \text{DT}$$

Hence, $P\frac{1}{2}$ can easily be measured using the DT or simply measuring the time interval from peak to $\frac{1}{2}$ (which is determined from the V_{max}). All or most echocardiographic measurement software packages automatically calculate $P\frac{1}{2}$ when the slope of the continuous wave Doppler of the mitral inflow jet is measured. For mitral stenosis, an empirical constant has been validated to correlate $P\frac{1}{2}$ and mitral valve area (MVA).

$$\mathbf{MVA = 220/P\tfrac{1}{2}}$$

This has only been validated for native valves and will overestimate valve areas for prosthetic valves. The other primary use of $P\frac{1}{2}$ is to help quantify AR. The $P\frac{1}{2}$ of the AR Doppler velocity jet becomes shorter with worsening AR, as the more severe the AR, the more rapidly the pressure in the aorta and the left ventricle equilibrate. A $P\frac{1}{2}$ less than 250 milliseconds suggests severe AR. There are many limitations with this, including the fact that $P\frac{1}{2}$ is affected by aortic and LV compliance and by change in systemic vascular resistance.

ACKNOWLEDGMENTS

The author thanks Drs. Patrick J. Nash, Steven Lin, and Guy Armstrong for their contributions to earlier editions of this chapter.

Landmark Articles

Edwards WD, Tajik AJ, Seward JB. Standard nomenclature and anatomic basis for regional tomographic analysis of the heart. *Mayo Clin Proc* 1981;56:479–497.

Lester SJ, Tajik AJ, Nishimura RA, et al. Unlocking the mysteries of diastolic function: deciphering the Rosetta Stone 10 years later. *J Am Coll Cardiol* 2008;51:679–689.

Nishimura RA, Tajik AJ. Quantitative hemodynamics by Doppler echocardiography: a noninvasive alternative to cardiac catheterization. *Prog Cardiovasc Dis* 1994;36:309–342.

Thomas JD, Popovic ZB. Assessment of left ventricular function by cardiac ultrasound. *J Am Coll Cardiol* 2006;48:2012–2025.

Thomas JD, Rubin DN. Tissue harmonic imaging: why does it work? *J Am Soc Echocardiogr* 1998;11:803–808.

Relevant Guidelines

Douglas PS, et al. ACCF/ASE/ACEP/ASNC/SCAI/SCCT/SCMR 2007 appropriateness criteria for transthoracic and transesophageal echocardiography: a report of the American College of Cardiology Foundation Quality Strategic Directions Committee Appropriateness Criteria Working Group, American Society of Echocardiography, American College of Emergency Physicians, American Society of Nuclear Cardiology, Society for Cardiovascular Angiography and Interventions, Society of Cardiovascular Computed Tomography, and the Society for Cardiovascular Magnetic Resonance endorsed by the American College of Chest Physicians and the Society of Critical Care Medicine. *J Am Coll Cardiol* 2007;50:187–204.

Relevant Books Chapters

Feigenbaum H. *Echocardiography,* 6th ed. Philadelphia: Lea & Febiger, 2005:1–75.

Oh JK, Seward JB, Tajik AJ. *The echo manual.* Philadelphia: Lippincott Wiliams & Wilkins, 2006:1–28.

Otto CM, Pearlman AS. *Otto and Pearlman's textbook of clinical echocardiography.* Philadelphia: WB Saunders, 1995:21–64.

Topol EJ. *Textbook of cardiovascular medicine.* Philadelphia: Lippincott Williams & Wilkins, 2007:806–819.

Weyman A. *Principles and practice of echocardiography,* 2nd ed. Philadelphia: Lea & Febiger, 1994:3–28.

61 TRANSESOPHAGEAL ECHOCARDIOGRAPHY

Deepu Nair and Maran Thamilarasan

I. INDICATIONS. In general, transesophageal echocardiography (TEE) is performed when there is a clinical question for which the information obtained by transthoracic echocardiography (TTE) is insufficient. This may be to better define pathology that has been identified by TTE or to obtain better images when transthoracic images are inadequate. The close position of the esophagus to the heart allows for improved visualization of many cardiac structures, particularly those that are posteriorly located. In addition, higher-frequency probes can be used, given the shorter distance between the probe and the heart, further enhancing resolution. However, imaging planes are somewhat constrained by the relative position of the esophagus and heart, and some structures (e.g., prosthetic aortic valve) and certain Doppler measurements may be better assessed by TTE.

Indications for TEE in various conditions and clinical situations are listed in Table 61.1. Very common indications include examination to rule out a cardiac source of embolus and assessment of valves for endocarditis and accompanying complications, such as abscess. The assessment of native and prosthetic valvular function, in terms of degree and mechanism of regurgitation or stenosis, is a frequent indication for TEE. Acoustic shadowing by prosthetic valves, particularly in the mitral position, poses less of a problem for TEE than it does for TTE. Given the rising prevalence of atrial fibrillation, another frequent indication for TEE is to assess left atrial and atrial appendage pathology and function, particularly prior to cardioversion. Congenital cardiovascular abnormalities, as well as tumors and masses, can also be well delineated by TEE. Because of its ability to assess the ascending aorta, arch, and descending aorta, TEE also has an important role in the diagnosis of aortic dissection, aneurysms, and atheroma.

TABLE 61.1 Class I Indications for TEE if TTE is Equivocal

Condition	Indication
Native valve endocarditis	Evaluation of native valves, especially with *Staphylococcus* bacteremia and fungemia without known source Detection of abscesses/shunts Evaluation of patients with high-suspicion and negative cultures
Valvular heart disease	Guiding performance of interventional techniques and surgery (e.g., balloon valvotomy, valve repair) Assessment of suspected papillary muscle rupture
Prosthetic valves	Evaluation of suspected prosthetic dysfunction (stenosis, thrombosis, or regurgitation) Evaluation of suspected endocarditis with negative cultures Evaluation of bacteremia without known source Re-evaluation in complex endocarditis
Acute myocardial ischemic syndromes	Assessment of mechanical complications or mural thrombus
Cardiomyopathy	Assessment of LV size and function
Hypotension	Evaluation of unexplained hypotension, especially in the ICU
Right heart failure	Identification of cardiac etiology of edema with elevated central venous pressure
Aortic aneurysm	Characterize aneurysm Characterize aortic root in patient (or first-degree relative of patient) with Marfan's syndrome or other connective tissue disorders Follow-up surgically repaired aortic dissection
Aortic dissection	Evaluate entire aorta for suspected dissection[a]
Intraoperative	Assessment of valve repair/replacement and evaluation of systolic function
Pericardial disease	Assessment of early postoperative bleeding, which may result in localized accumulation of blood clots (especially posteriorly)
Dyspnea	Differentiate cardiac vs. noncardiac cause in patients in whom clinical/laboratory clues are ambiguous
Cardioembolic source	Identification of atrial thrombus or spontaneous echo contrast[a] Identification of patent foramen ovale, atrial septal defect or atrial septal aneurysm[a] Identification of aortic atheroma[a]
Atrial fibrillation, pre-cardioversion	Atrial fibrillation >48 hours without prior prolonged anticoagulation[a] Urgent cardioversion when precardioversion anticoagulation is undesirable[a] Prior cardioembolic events thought due to intra-atrial thrombus[a] Prior intra-atrial thrombus[a]
Trauma	Evaluation of patient with blunt trauma to chest and suspected effusion or tamponade Evaluation of widened mediastinum in patient with suspected aortic injury
Congenital heart disease	Identification of site of origin and initial course of coronary arteries

[a]TEE is indicated as a primary study for these indications.
Adapted from 2003 ACC/AHA/ASE Guideline Update (see references).

TEE is a useful imaging modality in both the operating room and cardiac catheterization laboratory. In cardiothoracic surgery, TEE is used to assess the mechanism of valvular abnormalities and subsequently evaluate the efficacy of valve repair or replacement. TEE can be used to guide the location of the aortic cross-clamp so that segments with severe atheromatous involvement can be avoided, thereby reducing the risk of embolization. In addition, TEE can provide an assessment of left ventricular function and regional wall motion. As newer transcatheter approaches have become common, including atrial septal defect closure and percutaneous valve procedures, TEE has been increasingly utilized to help guide catheter position and evaluate the success and complications of the procedure.

II. CONTRAINDICATIONS

A. There are few **absolute** contraindications to the performance of TEE (Table 61.2). These include the **presence of pharyngeal or esophageal obstruction, active upper gastrointestinal bleeding, recent esophageal or gastric surgery,** and **suspected or known perforated viscus.** If there is instability of the cervical vertebrae, then the examination cannot be performed.

B. Relative contraindications include the **presence of esophageal varices** and **suspected esophageal diverticulum.** In these cases it is prudent to obtain gastrointestinal evaluation before proceeding, if the study must be performed. Severe cervical arthritis, in which patients may have difficulty with neck flexion, may make it difficult to pass the probe. Oropharyngeal pathology, anatomic distortion, or extreme muscle weakness can likewise make it difficult to proceed with the examination.

C. Severe cardiopulmonary disease is not a contraindication to evaluation by TEE (on the contrary, TEE can often provide critical information when used in these patients), but the operator must be particularly careful to minimize any stress on the patient. This is particularly true in **suspected aortic dissection,** where any sudden increase in blood pressure caused by patient discomfort could result in extension of the dissection. In cases where there is **respiratory instability,** endotracheal intubation with assisted ventilation should be considered prior to the procedure. Patients who are **hypotensive** may not be able to receive sedative agents, as these agents could lead to further hemodynamic compromise. In such patients the examination may have to be performed with topical anesthesia alone. This is obviously much more difficult for the patient, and TEE should be done only if critical information is not obtainable by other methods.

D. Given the invasive nature of the procedure, prudence must be observed in patients who are prone to **bleeding.** The procedure is commonly performed on patients who are anticoagulated, such as in those with atrial arrhythmias prior to cardioversion. However, there is increased risk in those who are over-anticoagulated. Although no set guidelines exist, it would seem advisable to **delay the examination if possible in patients with an international normalized ratio (INR) greater than 5 or a partial thromboplastin time greater than 100 seconds. Thrombocytopenia** may also

TABLE 61.2 Transesophageal Echocardiography Contraindications

Absolute
Esophageal or pharyngeal obstruction
Suspected or known perforated viscus
Gastrointestinal bleeding that has not been evaluated
Instability of cervical vertebrae
Uncooperative patient
Relative
Esophageal varices or diverticula
Cervical arthritis
Oropharyngeal distortion
Bleeding diathesis or overanticoagulation

increase the risk, particularly with platelet counts **less than 50,000/mm^3**. The TEE can still be performed if needed, as the absolute risk remains low, but meticulous attention must be given to nontraumatic esophageal intubation.

E. Esophageal infections, such as those that occur in the context of human immunodeficiency virus (HIV), do not necessarily represent contraindications to the procedure. **Patient discomfort** caused by the presence of the probe in the esophagus may preclude the examination. Universal precautions should be followed (as they should for any patient). The standard disinfectants used to clean the probe will inactivate HIV.

F. A patient who is very uncooperative is at significant risk for complications from the procedure. In such a case, consideration should be given to aborting the TEE.

III. PERSONNEL. The American Society of Echocardiography has proposed the following guidelines for operators who wish to perform TEE: as background, interpretation of a minimum of 300 transthoracic echocardiograms; a minimum of 25 esophageal intubations under the guidance of a gastroenterologist or a skilled transesophageal echocardiographer; and a minimum of 50 TEE examinations during training. Furthermore, operators should perform a minimum of 50 to 75 TEE examinations yearly to maintain competency.

The presence of a skilled assistant is invaluable during the procedure. The assistant should be either a sonographer or a registered nurse. The role of the assistant is to monitor vital signs during the procedure, ensure proper suctioning of oropharyngeal secretions, and administer medications.

IV. EQUIPMENT. Necessary equipment is listed in Table 61.3.

V. THE TRANSESOPHAGEAL PROBE. The probe is a modification of the standard gastroscope, with transducers in place of fiberoptics. The conventional rotary controls with inner and outer dials are present. The inner dial typically guides anteflexion and retroflexion, whereas the outer dial controls medial and lateral movement of the tip. A locking mechanism is present, which must not be in effect when the probe is advanced or withdrawn, as esophageal trauma may result. The multiplane probe also has a lever control to guide rotation. Biplane probes are no longer in common use as they require switching between the transverse and longitudinal planes by a control switch on the echo machine. Advancement and withdrawal of the probe, rotation of the probe about its long axis, and the manipulations available using the above rotary controls constitute the means by which specific images can be obtained (diagrammed in Fig. 61.1).

VI. PATIENT PREPARATION (Table 61.4). The patient should have had nothing by mouth (NPO) for at least 4 hours before the procedure. The clinician can rule out possible contraindications by asking for a history of odynophagia or dysphagia. It is important

TABLE 61.3 Equipment for Transesophageal Echocardiography

1. Echo machine and probe (calibrate prior to intubation)
2. Sphygmomanometer
3. ECG rhythm monitor
4. Pulse oximeter
5. Supplemental oxygen
6. Wall suction with Yankauer
7. Intravenous lines and tubing
8. Topical anesthetic agents
9. Sedative medications
10. Bite block
11. Gloves and goggles
12. Emergency equipment
    - a. Drugs (e.g., atropine, epinephrine, narcan, flumazenil, lidocaine)
    - b. Defibrillator
    - c. Intubation supplies

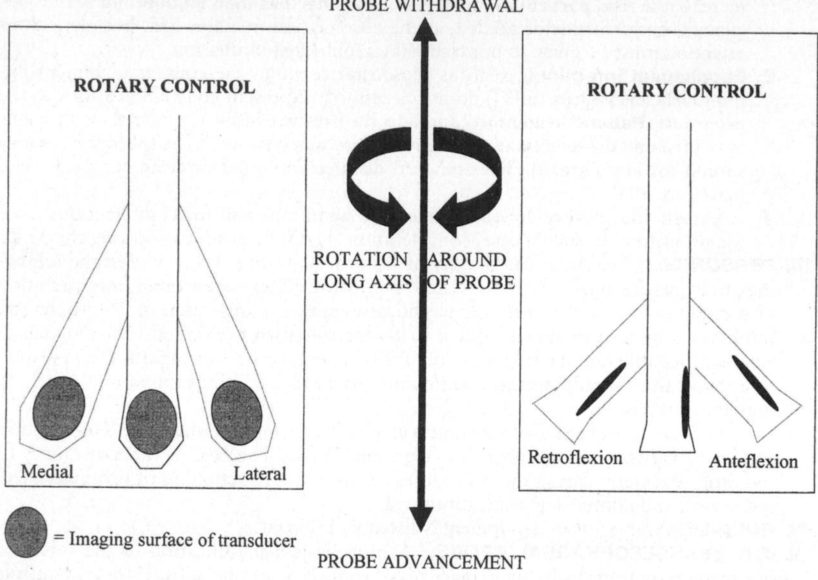

Figure 61.1. Specific images can be obtained by advancement and withdrawal of the probe, by rotation of the probe about its long axis, and by the manipulations that are possible using rotary controls.

to be aware of any history of radiation therapy to the mediastinum or cervical region that may have resulted in stricture formation.

The extent of previous workup for any history of gastrointestinal bleeding must be reviewed. The clinician should review recent lab studies, paying particular attention to platelet count, hemoglobin level, and coagulation profile. Appropriate inquiries should be made with regard to allergies and former tolerance of sedative medications. The clinician should ensure that the patient understands the procedure, including risks and benefits, and that proper informed consent is obtained and documented before proceeding.

VII. STEP-BY-STEP GUIDE TO THE EXAMINATION

A. The patient's **dentures** should be removed.

B. **An intravenous (IV) line** should be inserted to allow for administration of medications and saline contrast for study.

C. The American Heart Association association does not recommend **antibiotic prophylaxis** for patients undergoing endoscopic procedures. The reported incidence

TABLE 61.4 Preparation for Transesophageal Echocardiography

Patient must have had nothing by mouth (NPO) for at least 4 h prior to the procedure
Assess for possible contraindications:
History of odynophagia or dysphagia
History of mediastinal or cervical radiation that might have resulted in stricture formation
History of and workup for gastrointestinal bleeding
Allergies to and previous tolerance of sedative medications
Patient understanding of procedure and indications
Informed consent of patient

of transient bacteremia with endoscopy is no higher than the contamination rates reported with blood cultures.

D. A **blood pressure cuff** should be placed on the patient's arm.

E. **Electrocardiographic leads** should be applied and connected to the telemetry monitor.

F. A **pulse oximeter** should be applied to the patient's finger or ear.

G. A **nasal cannula** should be applied so that supplemental oxygen can be given as needed.

H. While sitting up, the patient should be asked to gargle **viscous 2% lidocaine** for one minute and then swallow it for topical anesthesia. **Cetacaine spray (10%) or xylocaine spray (4%)** is then sprayed on to the posterior tongue and upper pharynx. These procedures normally suppress the **gag reflex**, but if necessary, this can be verified using a tongue depressor or gloved finger; additional **topical anesthesia** is then applied until the reflex is dulled. By visualizing the area being sprayed, inadvertent spraying of the vocal cord and resultant laryngospasm can be avoided. Some operators advocate the use of drying agents to minimize oropharyngeal secretions (e.g., glycopyrrolate). We generally have not found a need for use of such agents, which can cause an increase in heart rate.

I. Have the patient lie down on the left side (left lateral decubitus position), facing the echo machine (alternatively, the patient can lie on the right side, with the machine on the right), with neck flexed. TEE can be performed with the patient sitting but is easier in the lateral position.

J. **Midazolam** is the preferred agent for sedation, having the benefit of a short half-life. It also produces an antegrade amnestic effect. Typically, give IV doses of 0.5 mg every 3 to 5 minutes until adequate sedation is achieved. The goal is to reduce anxiety without compromising respiratory drive and while maintaining the patient's ability to follow simple commands, such as swallowing when necessary. Check pulse oximetry and blood pressure before each dose. **Fentanyl**, a short-acting opioid analagesic, can be used for sedation (typically 25 mg IV per dose) in conjunction with midazolam, and may be better tolerated in patients with poor left ventricular function or renal impairment. An alternative sedative is **meperidine**, which is typically given in 12.5 to 25 mg IV doses. Meperidine possesses an analgesic effect and helps to suppress the gag reflex as well. Again, **check vital signs before and after each dose.** Additional doses of these sedatives and anxiolytics may be administered during the procedure if necessary.

K. With adequate sedation and topical anesthesia (diminution of gag reflex), **begin probe insertion.** There are two approaches that are generally used.

1. The first is the **digital technique,** which is especially useful with the larger multiplane probe. With this method, the bite guard is inserted onto the shaft of the probe such that after esophageal intubation the bite guard can be moved into place. The distal end of the probe is lubricated. The imaging surface of the transducer is placed toward the tongue. The tip of the transducer is placed under the index finger, and is slowly guided downward and posterior to the hypopharynx. At this point the patient is asked to swallow, and gentle pressure is applied with the other hand to guide the probe down. Swallowing results in relaxation of the upper esophageal sphincter. If resistance is met, stop, let the patient relax, and reattempt or redirect as needed. Using the finger as a guide will help center the probe in the region of the hypopharynx over the esophagus and avoid the lateral recesses.
2. An **alternative method is to use the rotary controls on the TEE probe** to guide the intubation. The bite guard is inserted first. The probe is inserted through the bite guard, and gentle anteflexion is applied as the probe is passed over the back of the tongue. The probe is then returned to the neutral position, or with slight retroflexion, as it is passed down into the esophagus. The patient is asked to swallow as the probe is advanced past the upper esophageal sphincter. The operator is still able to guide the probe if needed by insertion of a finger around the side of the bite guard.

Patients often gag as the probe enters the upper esophagus (even with adequate anesthesia); however, patients generally find it more comfortable once the probe has passed beyond this point (usually at 25 cm, past the level of the carina). The probe should be advanced to approximately 30 to 40 cm (midesophageal level).

In intubated patients, it is important to **secure the endotracheal tube firmly to one side of the mouth** to prevent dislodgment and inadvertent extubation. Direct visualization with a laryngoscope may be needed. **Sedation** is equally important in these patients, and given the tendency for partially sedated patients to bite on their tubes, a **paralyzing agent** is often required. Intubation in the supine position is not a problem because the airway is protected. Other catheters in the esophagus, such as feeding tubes or nasogastric tubes often have to be removed prior to the procedure; they may become interposed between the esophagus and the TEE probe, interfering with the images. If left in, these tubes may become dislodged by the TEE probe, and tube position should be reconfirmed after the echocardiographic examination.

For patients with tracheostomies, some operators will carefully and gently deflate the cuff to facilitate probe insertion.

VIII. IMAGING. TEE technology has undergone much evolution, from the initial monoplane views to the current multiplane probes. Monoplane TEE provides for images in the horizontal plane only, perpendicular to the shaft of the endoscope. Longitudinal relationships among cardiac structures are difficult to appreciate. With biplane TEE, the orthogonal longitudinal plane can also be obtained. Both monoplane and biplane systems required additional manipulation to obtain off-axis views, making the examination more difficult and more uncomfortable for the patient. With **multiplane TEE**, the transducer has a single array of crystals that can be rotated 180 degrees around the long axis, producing a continuum of transverse and longitudinal images from a single probe position. This minimizes the probe manipulation necessary to obtain intermediate and off-axis images. Consequently, multiplane TEE has increased sensitivity for detection of sometimes subtle abnormalities, including vegetations, periprosthetic leaks, left atrial appendage thrombi, and aortic dissection. The development of **real-time three-dimensional TEE** (see IIIC) offers the possibility of assessing cardiac structures volumetrically, although this technology is still in the process making its way into routine clinical practice.

A. Basic views. The TEE examination tends to be more goal directed than the transthoracic examination, as there may be time constraints imposed by how long the patient can tolerate the esophageal probe. Initial views should focus on the question at hand, but it is still important to perform a comprehensive and thorough examination. Most operators prefer to begin with upper esophageal views before proceeding to transgastric views. The order of views obtained is not important providing the operator develops a consistent and comprehensive approach.

The probe may inadvertently rotate during insertion and may require initial manipulation before starting the examination. The left atrium should be seen at the center of the screen. If the aorta is seen (which is posterior to the esophagus), then the probe must be rotated anteriorly. Slight retroflexion of the probe may be necessary to maintain adequate contact between the probe and esophagus. Air in the esophagus, which is interposed between the probe and the heart, may affect image quality. This generally lessens as the examination progresses (from ongoing peristaltic activity in the esophagus). Similarly, the presence of a hiatal hernia may compromise image quality.

Views obtained from multiplane TEE will be described first. These views are described in terms of degrees of rotation required to obtain particular images. At each transducer location, start array at 0 degrees and rotate to 180 degrees at 5- to 15-degree increments to obtain a complete sweep. The standard horizontal plane is designated as 0 degrees. At approximately 45 degrees, short-axis views are obtained. Ninety degrees is defined as the longitudinal plane, whereas at around 135 degrees, the true long-axis cardiac views are obtained. At 180 degrees a mirror image view of the standard horizontal plane is obtained. Given the variable anatomic relationships between structures, the degree of probe manipulation required to obtain the standard views will vary from patient to patient.

1. Upper esophagus (30 cm)—base of the heart (Fig. 61.2). With the array at 0 degrees, a five-chamber cross-sectional view of the left atrium, left ventricle, right atrium, right ventricle, and aortic valve is obtained. At 40 to 60 degrees, the

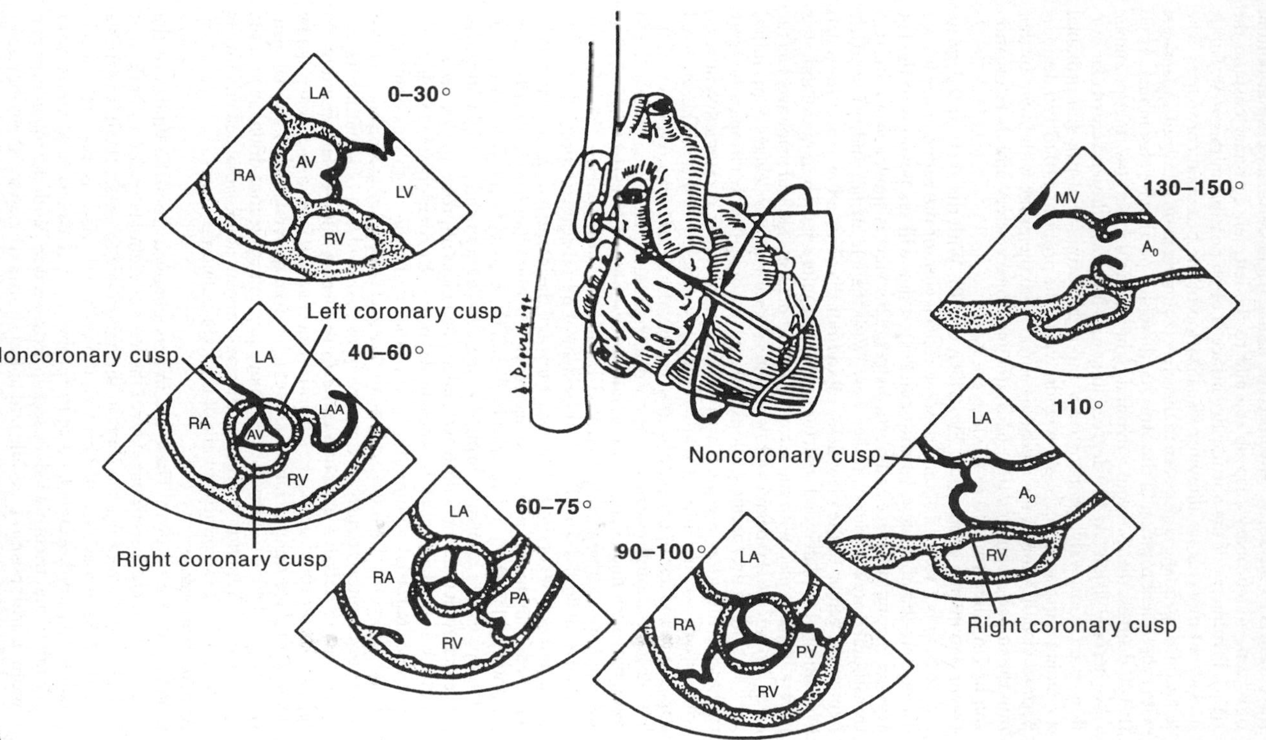

Figure 61.2. Schematic representation of selected multiplane transesophageal echocardiography views of the aorta and aortic valve from the upper esophagus. Ao, aorta; LA, left atrium; LV, left ventricle; RA, right atrium; RV, right ventricle; PA, pulmonary artery; PV, pulmonary valve; LAA, left atrial appendage; MV, mitral valve. (Modified from Roelandt JRTC, Pandian NG, eds. *Multiplane transesophageal echocardiography.* New York: Churchill Livingstone, 1996;15–68.)

three leaflets of the aortic valve become visible (right coronary cusp at bottom of screen, noncoronary cusp on top and to the left, left coronary cusp on the right). Planimetry of the aortic valve orifice is often possible in this view. Subtle in-and-out movements allow for visualization of the proximal coronaries. The left atrial appendage is also seen in this view (zooming in on the atrial appendage, with subsequent rotation of the array, facilitates inspection for thrombus). At 60 to 100 degrees, the tricuspid valve and right ventricular outflow tract/pulmonic valve become visible. At 120 degrees, long-axis images of the left ventricular outflow tract, aortic valve (noncoronary and right coronary cusps), and proximal ascending aorta are seen. Slight wighdrawal of the probe at 110 to 120 degreees permits visualization of the ascending aorta. With the probe withdrawn further into the upper esophagus (Fig. 61.3), the pulmonary artery and its bifurcation can be visualized (from 0 to 45 degrees).

2. **Lower and middle esophagus** (Fig. 61.4A and B). With the array at 0 degrees, a four-chamber view is obtained (some retroflexion of the probe is needed for a true four-chamber view, as with anteflexion one will see portions of the left ventricular outflow tract and aortic valve). This view is similar to an inverted transthoracic apical four-chamber view. With the left atrium and left ventricle kept in the center of the view field, rotation of the array allows for a thorough evaluation of the left-sided structures. Doppler interrogation of mitral inflow is generally performed with the array at 0 to 30 degrees. Skillful maneuvers as the array is rotated to 90 degrees allow for interrogation of both leaflets of the mitral valve, including the specific scallops of the posterior leaflet. Rotation of the array to 90 to 110 degrees reveals the two-chamber view (left atrium/left ventricle), with the anterior and inferior walls of the left ventricle visualized. The left atrial appendage and left upper pulmonary vein are also seen. Long-axis views of the left ventricular outflow tract, aortic valve (right and noncoronary cusps), and proximal ascending aorta are obtained by rotation to 120 to 140 degrees. The anterior mitral leaflet is particularly well visualized in these views. This complete sweep permits full delineation of the extent of mitral regurgitation.

   Similar views of right-sided structures and the interatrial septum can also be obtained from this position. At 0 degrees (in the four-chamber view as described previously), the septal and anterior leaflets of the tricuspid valve can be seen. The endoscope is then rotated to bring the interatrial septum and the right atrium to the center of view (some withdrawal or advancement of probe may be necessary to optimize visualization of the interatrial septum). By rotation of the multiplane array, the interatrial septum and fossa ovalis can be thoroughly examined for evidence of a patent foramen ovale or atrial septal defect. Agitated saline contrast can be given intravenously at this time to expose evidence of shunting; asking the patient to Valsalva or cough can help to identify right-to-left shunting. At approximately 100 degrees, the superior vena cava and inferior vena cava can be seen entering the right atrium, and the right atrial appendage can also be seen. This is a good view to identify anomalous pulmonary venous drainage into the right atrium or superior vena cava, or a sinus venosus atrial septal defect. Further rotation will allow for assessment of the right pulmonary veins.

3. **Transgastric views**

   a. **Proximal** (Fig. 61.5A). These are images obtained from the fundus of the stomach. A cross-sectional view of the left and right ventricles is obtained at 0 degrees. By rotating the shaft of the endoscope to center the left ventricle in the field of view, serial short-axis ("doughnut") views of the left ventricle can be obtained. Anteflexion of the probe will give rise to basal views, with the mitral and tricuspid valves seen in cross-section. With the transducer in a more neutral position, middle and apical short-axis views will be obtained.

      At 80 to 100 degrees, a two-chamber view of the left atrium (with appendage) and left ventricle (anterior and inferior walls of left ventricle, mitral leaflets, papillary muscles) will be obtained. At 120 degrees plus, a long-axis outflow tract view with aortic valve and ascending aorta will be visualized. The anteroseptal and posterior walls of the left ventricle are seen.

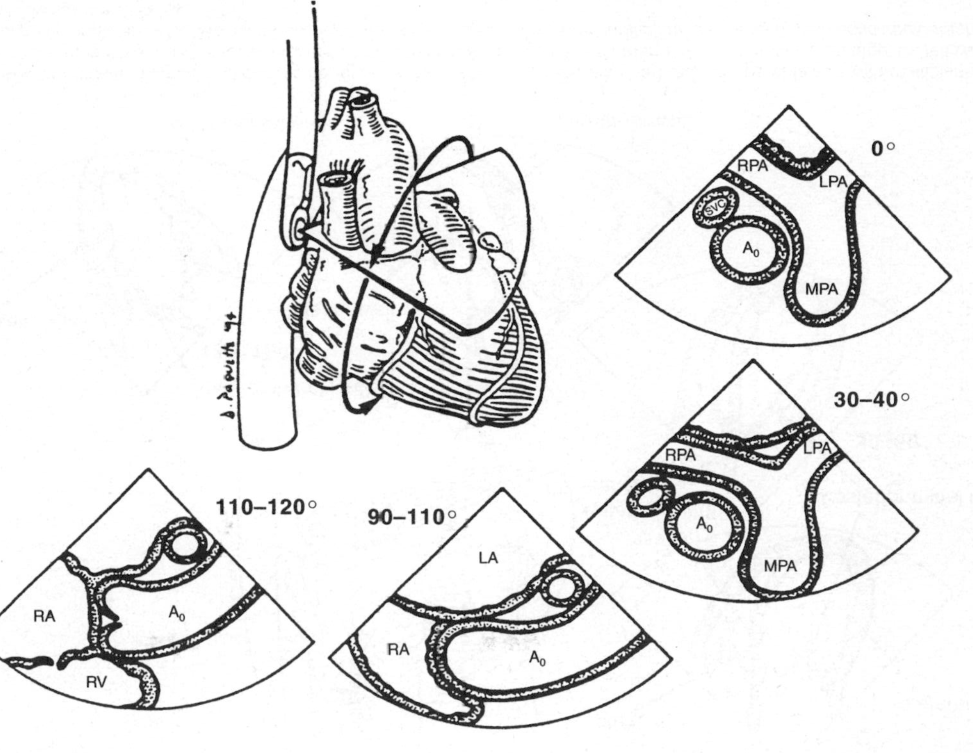

Figure 61.3. Schematic of some of the multiplane transesophageal echocardiography views of the aorta and pulmonary artery that can be obtained from the upper esophagus. Ao, aorta; LA, left atrium; LPA, left pulmonary artery; PA, main pulmonary artery; RA, right atrium; RPA, right pulmonary artery; RV, right ventricle; SVC, superior vena cava. (Modified from Roelandt JRTC, Pandian NG, eds. *Multiplane transesophageal echocardiography.* New York: Churchill Livingstone, 1996;15–68.)

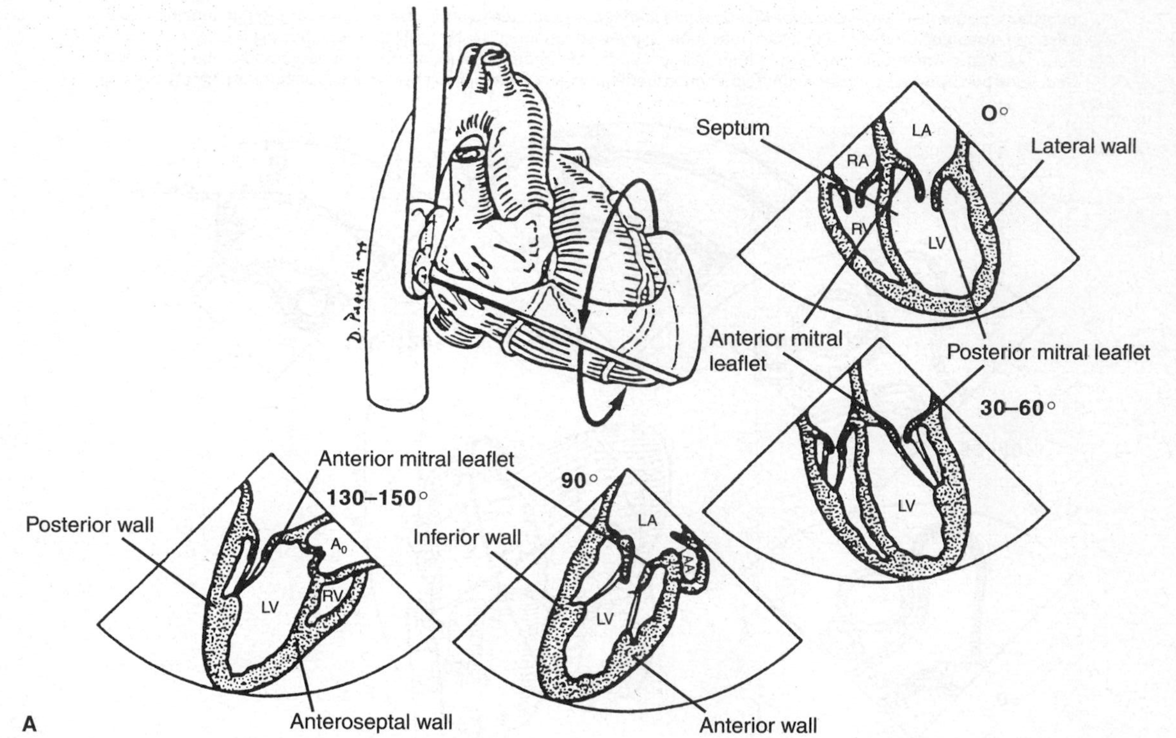

Figure 61.4A. Schematic diagram showing some representative sections of the left heart that can be obtained with multiplane transesophageal echocardiography from the lower and middle esophagus. Ao, aorta; LA, left atrium; LAA, left atrial appendage; LV, left ventricle; RA, right atrium; RV, right ventricle. (Modified from Roelandt JRTC, Pandian NG, eds. *Multiplane transesophageal echocardiography.* New York: Churchill Livingstone, 1996;15–68.)

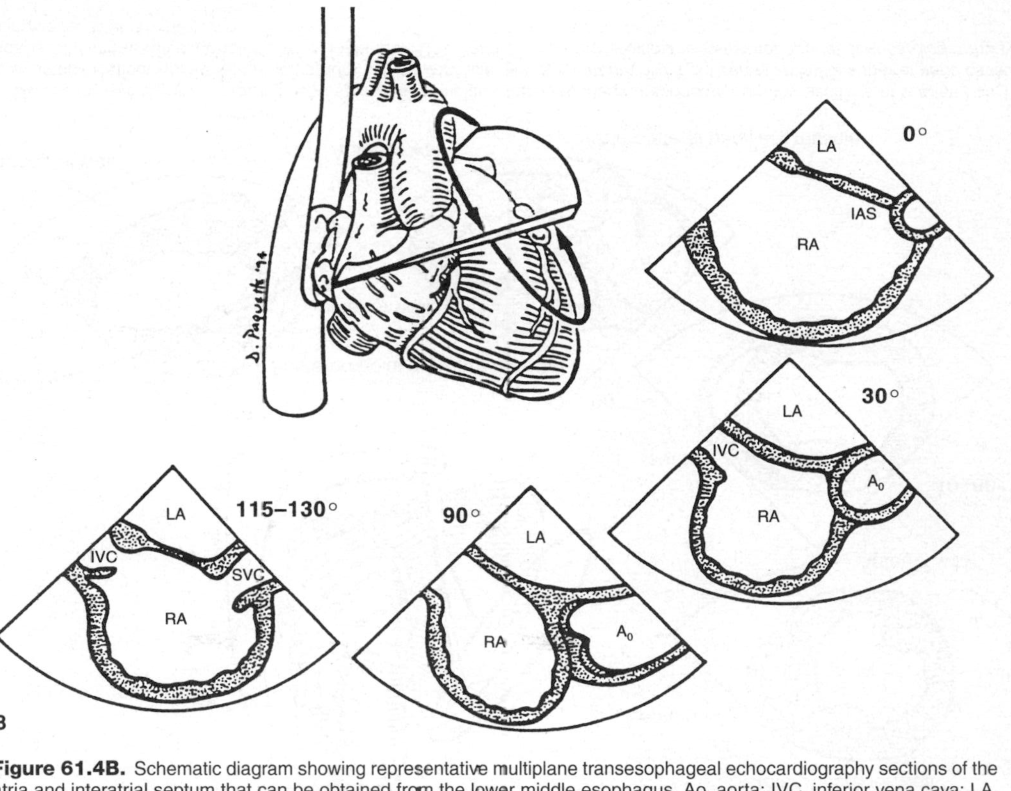

Figure 61.4B. Schematic diagram showing representative multiplane transesophageal echocardiography sections of the atria and interatrial septum that can be obtained from the lower middle esophagus. Ao, aorta; IVC, inferior vena cava; LA, left atrium; RA, right atrium; SVC, superior vena cava; IAS, interatrial septum. (Modified from Roelandt JRTC, Pandian NG, eds. *Multiplane transesophageal echocardiography.* New York: Churchill Livingstone, 1996;15–68.)

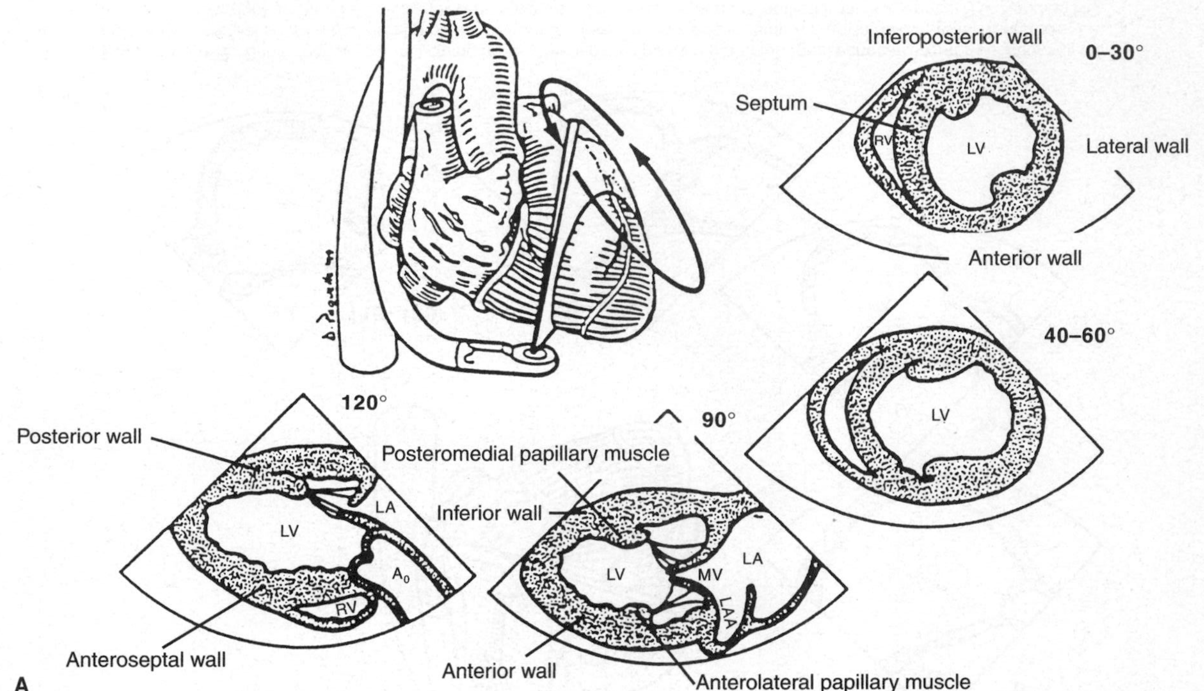

Figure 61.5A. Schematic diagram showing representative multiplane transesophageal echocardiography sections of the left heart from the proximal transgastric location. Ao, aorta; LA, left atrium; LV, left ventricle; RA, right atrium; RV, right ventricle; SVC, superior vena cava; LAA, left atrial appendage; MV, mitral valve. (Modified from Roelandt JRTC, Pandian NG, eds. *Multiplane transesophageal echocardiography.* New York: Churchill Livingstone, 1996:15–68.)

Depending on the alignment with the transducer, this view may be useful in obtaining velocities across the aortic valve.

Bringing the array back to 0 degrees and rotating the shaft of endoscope to center the right ventricle in view will allow for interrogation of the right-sided structures (Fig. 61.5B). At 30 to 60 degrees, the three leaflets of the tricuspid valve are visualized (anterior leaflet at bottom, posterior leaflet on top, and septal leaflet to the right). At around 70 to 80 degrees, the right ventricular inflow tract view (superior vena cava, tricuspid valve with anterior and posterior leaflets) is obtained. At 90 to 100 degrees, the right ventricular outflow and pulmonary valve become visible as well. At 110 to 130 degrees, the two-chamber view of the right ventricle and right atrium can be seen. By rotating to 130 to 150 degrees, the papillary muscles and chordae supporting the tricuspid valve are further delineated.

b. Deep transgastric. The probe is advanced further into the stomach with the tip anteflexed. At 0 degrees, a foreshortened five-chamber view is obtained. This view allows for Doppler interrogation of the aortic valve and left ventricular outflow tract. By rotating the multiplane array, different segments of the left ventricle apex can be visualized in the search for thrombus or aneurysm.

4. Aorta. Counterclockwise rotation of the endoscope brings the aorta into view. Typically the probe is advanced beyond the diaphragm and then slowly pulled back, following the aorta back to the arch. Rotation of the probe is required to keep the aorta in view in the center of the screen. At the level of the diaphragm, the aorta is posterior to the esophagus. In the midesophagus, the aorta is medial, whereas the ascending aorta and arch lie anterior to the esophagus. At 0 degrees, the aorta is seen as a circular structure. Long-axis images (at 100 to 130 degrees) provide additional information as needed at selected intervals. At the arch, the aorta is curved in front of the esophagus, presenting a sausage-shaped structure with the probe at 0 degrees. Gentle clockwise rotation will follow the arch back to the ascending aorta. The ascending aorta is visualized in the longitudinal planes as discussed with the other views. Multiplane TEE has reduced the so-called blind spot of the ascending aorta (where the trachea is interposed between the esophagus and aorta, an area that poses a problem during horizontal plane imaging).

B. Biplane probe. There are times at which a biplane probe may be used. This is a smaller probe, so it may be beneficial to use in certain cases when there might be difficulty in esophageal intubation with the multiplane probe. By manipulating the probe via rotation about the long axis and use of the rotary controls, intermediate and off-axis images in addition to the standard transverse and longitudinal views described earlier can be obtained. Through hands-on experience, the operator will come to be familiar with these maneuvers.

C. Three-dimensional (3D) probe. Three-dimensional probes use a two-dimensional array scanning along two axes simultaneously, allowing a pyramidal volume of data to be acquired. 3D TEE has been shown to be useful for assessing LV function and assessing valvular abnormalities. It can provide unique geometric insights into the mechanism of valvular function. However, its use is somewhat limited by relatively poor signal-to-noise ratio. Development of higher frequency probes and signal amplication technologies is expected to improve this exciting technology.

IX. PATIENT RECOVERY.

The patient's NPO status should be maintained until the gag reflex has returned. When the patient commences oral intake, he or she should initially take a small sip of ice water. If the water does not feel cold, then some topical anesthetic effect is still present. Until this has dissipated the patient should avoid any hot drinks so as to avoid scalding. Appropriate precautions should be followed if sedatives were used, as the effects persist for several hours. Patients may have dizziness and orthostatic symptoms for up to several hours, and should be instructed to sit or lie down if this occurs. Patients should not drive or operate heavy equipment until the next day.

X. PROBE CARE.

Following use, the probe should be cleaned with soap, water, and an enzymatic solution to remove saliva. The nonimmersible parts of the probe, such as

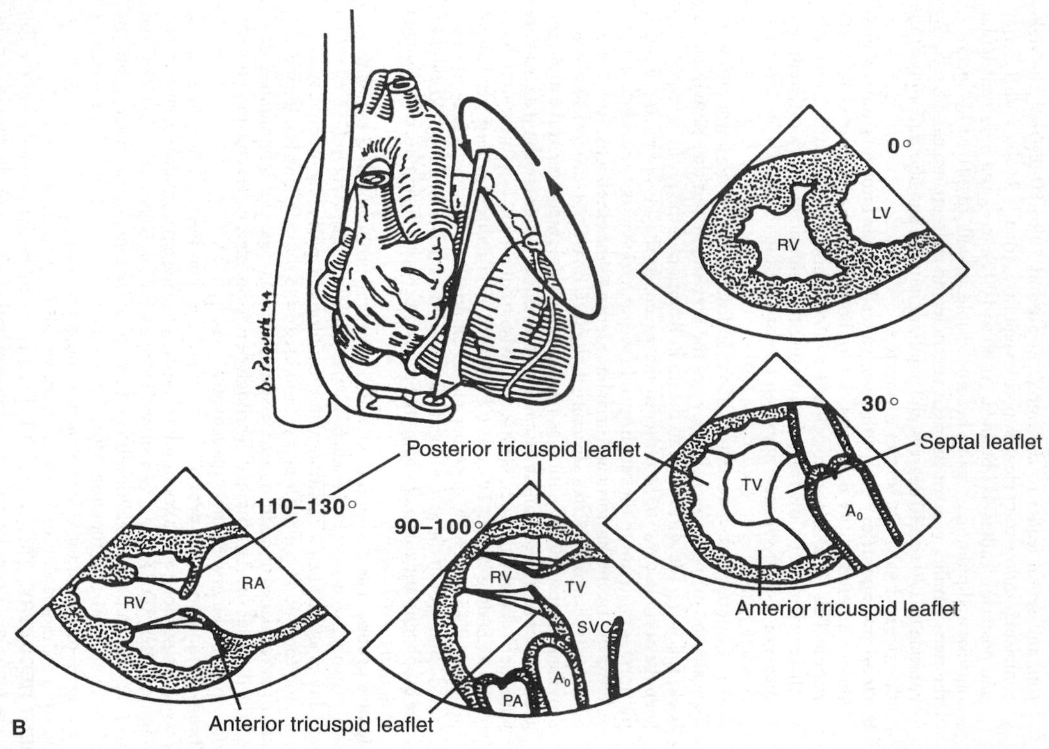

Figure 61.5B. Schematic of images from a transgastric, multiplane sweep through the right ventricle. LV, left ventricle; RA, right atrium; RV, right ventricle; TV, tricuspid valve; SVC, superior vena cava; PA, pulmonary artery; Ao, aorta. (Modified from Roelandt JRTC, Pandian NG, eds. *Multiplane transesophageal echocardiography.* New York: Churchill Livingstone, 1996: 15–68.)

the handle and rotary controls, should be cleaned with alcohol. Afterward the probe should be soaked in a glutaraldehyde solution for a minimum of 20 minutes and a maximum of several hours to eliminate bacteria. The probe should not soak in this solution overnight. It can then be rinsed with water and air dried. The probe should be inspected closely for any tears or perforations.

XI. COMPLICATIONS. In reported series, the incidence of major and minor complications is 2% to 3%, with most being minor complications. Major complications (death, esophageal perforation, significant arrhythmias, congestive heart failure, and aspiration) occur with a frequency of 0.3%, with a reported mortality of less than 0.01%. Reported minor complications include transient hypotension, hypertension (particularly with agitation), hypoxia, and arrhythmias (such as sustained ventricular tachycardia, nonsustained ventricular tachycardia, and transient atrioventricular block). Methemoglobinemia has been rarely reported due to the anesthetic spray and should be considered if cyanosis occurs. Other complications of intubation include tracheal intubation, laryngospasm, and vocal cord paralysis. Sore throat is not uncommon after the procedure and may persist for a day. Anaphylaxis and other allergic reactions can occur due to the medications used.

XII. PITFALLS. The improved resolution and anatomic detail provided by TEE, as compared with TTE, is what makes it such a powerful diagnostic tool. However, this can also lead to misinterpretation of normal structures. Trabeculations in the atrial appendage can be mistaken for thrombi, and lipomatous hypertrophy of the interatrial septum can be incorrectly labeled as a mass, as can the eustachian valve. The transverse and oblique sinuses can be mistaken for abscess cavities. Off-axis images may create the appearance of a mass on the aortic valve when one of the cusps is cut obliquely. The lungs can give rise to reverberation artifacts, which can erroneously be diagnosed as dissection flaps (presence in nonanatomic planes, lack of disruption of color Doppler of blood flow, and crossing of normal anatomy all favor diagnosis of artifact). Abnormal findings should be visualized and verified in several views to ensure that they do not represent imaging artifacts.

These pitfalls are best minimized by the experience of the operator, but variations in anatomy may provide diagnostic dilemmas for even the most skilled echocardiographer.

Suggested Readings

Cheitlin MD, et al. ACC/AHA/ASE 2003 Guideline Update for the Clinical Application of Echocardiography: summary article. A report of the American College of Cardiology/American Heart Association Task Force on Practice Guidelines. *J Am Coll Cardiol* 2003;42;954–970.

Douglas PS, et al. ACCF/ASE/ACEP/ASNC/SCAI/SCCT/SCMR 2007 appropriateness criteria for transthoracic and transesophageal echocardiography. *J Am Coll Cardiol* 2007;50;187–204.

Key Reviews

Khanderia BK, Seward JB, Tajik AJ. Critical appraisal of transesophageal echocardiography: limitations and pitfalls. *Crit Care Clin* 1996;12:235–251.

Khanderia BK, Tajik AJ, Seward JB. Multiplane transesophageal echocardiography: examinationtechnique, anatomic correlations and image orientation. *Crit Care Clin* 1996;12:203–233.

Peterson GE, Brickner ME, Reimold SC. Transesophageal echocardiography: clinical indications and applications. *Circulation* 2003;107:2398–2402.

Relevant Book Chapters

Griffin BP. Transesophageal echocardiography. In: Topol EJ, ed. *Textbook of cardiovascular medicine*, 3rd ed. Philadelphia: Lippincott Williams & Wilkins, 2006.

Oh JK, et al. Transesophageal and intracardiac echocardiography. In: Oh, JK, ed. *The echo manual*, 3rd ed. Philadelphia: Lippincott Williams & Wilkins, 2006.

XII Common Genetic Issues in Cardiovascular Disease

62 COMMON GENETIC ISSUES IN CARDIOVASCULAR DISEASE

Saif Anwaruddin and Eric J. Topol

Genetic abnormalities have been associated with all types of cardiovascular disease including coronary atherosclerosis, rhythm disorders, aortic disease, and structural heart disease. Since the initial descriptions of familial hypercholesterolemia (FH) and the mutations in the low-density-lipoprotein (LDL) receptor (LDL-R), genetic studies have fostered an improved understanding of the underlying pathophysiology of various cardiovascular disease states. Furthermore, the sequencing of the human genome has ushered in the era of cardiovascular genomics. The ability to efficiently scour through the massive amount of genomic information will ultimately result in an improved understanding of the contributions of genetics to cardiovascular disease.

This understanding would potentially lead to an improved ability to accurately diagnose disease, prevent progression, and risk-stratify at the individual level. Furthermore, this information will add to our understanding of the relationship between DNA variants and the response to drugs or other treatment modalities. The pharmacogenomic profiles developed may provide a refined approach to treatment with less toxicity. A more comprehensive assessment of future risk both for patient and potentially affected family members would also be feasible.

Although there are some examples within cardiovascular disease of simple monogenic disorders explained by principles of Mendelian inheritance, many of the entities, such as coronary atherosclerosis, acute myocardial infarction, and atrial fibrillation, are complex traits with multiple genes contributing to the phenotype. As opposed to Mendelian disorders, which are deterministic, complex traits are probabilistic.

Being able to define all the variations in all the genes that contribute to the susceptibility or protection from a complex trait will require extensive time and effort. Furthermore, the simple identification of genes involved does not address the issue of gene–gene and gene–environment interactions influencing complex traits. There have been extensive recent reports of genomic variants associated with risk of diseases. These variants are common, often accounting for 20% to 30% of the population attributable risk, but with an odds ratio of 1.2 or 1.3, for example, only 20% to 30% excess risk. These are common variants for common diseases. The hunt to find rare variants that induce susceptibility to common diseases with high risk (or protection) will be more challenging, but eminently feasible with sequencing technology and ultra-high throughput genotyping. At some point in the future, the major genomic underpinnings for most cardiovascular diseases will be known. Furthermore, the integration of all of the genomic variants for any cardiovascular disease has not been undertaken. What follows is a brief overview of what is known today about the genetic basis for a sampling of disease entities within cardiovascular medicine.

METHODOLOGY

The process of discovering relevant genetic underpinnings of generally complex traits requires an extensive analysis of genetic information in large populations. Complex traits without simple Mendelian patterns of inheritance are difficult to analyze given that there are often multiple genes involved, with many gene interactions being important. However, even before attempting this task, perhaps the single most significant goal is to accurately and concisely define the phenotype in question. In addition, many variations often exist within a single category of cardiovascular diseases such as hypertrophic cardiomyopathy and acute myocardial infarction. The ability to clearly define cases and controls is paramount to obtaining accurate and reproducible information.

There are three major methods of identifying DNA variants associated with cardiovascular disease. Of note, some of the single nucleotide polymorphism (SNP) variants that have been found are not in a gene, but actually in areas of the genome not associated with gene expression. It is not yet known how these variants exert their effect. Of note, the major variants for myocardial infarction (MI) (at 9p21) and atrial fibrillation (at 4q25) fall into this category of inter-gene (i.e., not in a gene).

GENOME WIDE ASSOCIATION STUDIES

Gene association studies utilize the concept that multiple SNPs, where a single nucleic acid substitution results in a different allele, can affect the risk of developing a disease in question. This is especially true in diseases of complex traits such as coronary artery disease and myocardial infarction. Using genes of interest in a particular disease phenotype, scans are conducted in areas of interest in both cases and controls in order to compare haplotype frequency to determine if a statistically significant difference between the two groups in the region of interest exists. One of the limitations of this technique is the inability to know whether the SNP of interest is involved in the pathogenesis or simply associated (in linkage disequilibrium) with another SNP that may actually be involved in the process. Utilizing this process of gene association across the entire genome is now possible with high throughput sequencing technology of up to 1 million SNPs assessed per individual and the term "genome wide" association has been coined. The SNPs assessed are tagging tiny bins of the genome, such that in a genome of an individual of European ancestry there are only about 250,000 bins, most of which are sampled by current high-throughput genotyping. Each bin is typically inherited as a block (haplotype). The breakdown of the genome into bins via the International Haplotype map was critical to making current genome wide association studies possible.

LINKAGE ANALYSIS

Linkage analysis is another tool used to identify genes possibly involved in the pathogenesis of complex traits. The use of linkage analysis begins without any assumptions as to the potential involvement of various genes. It is based on the idea that during the process of meiosis when recombination events occur, they tend to involve loci on a particular chromosome that are closer together than farther apart. By following the inheritance of certain known loci, assumptions can be made about the presence of alleles that cosegregate with them. Using linkage analysis, the potential exists to identify these known loci as markers and determine the transmission through a pedigree and its relationship to the phenotype in question. In doing so, it may be possible to suggest that an allele in proximity to known loci may be associated with a particular phenotype. The logarithm of odds ratio (LOD score) is used to estimate the (distance) relationship between the known locus of interest and an unknown locus thought to be associated with the disease phenotype. An LOD score of 3 is used to classify such a statistically meaningful linkage.

GENE EXPRESSION PROFILING

The identification of certain disease alleles or loci associated with disease-causing genes provides valuable information but remains limited in its scope. The statistical association of genes and disease **does not prove causation or even involvement** in disease. Gene expression profiling takes this concept one step forward in trying to delineate gene expression. The presence of transcription profiles may provide more useful information in terms of relevance of findings made in gene association studies or linkage analysis.

Technology now permits the evaluation of large genomes in a rapid fashion in order to derive expression profiles, which can then be compared between diseased and healthy individuals to draw conclusions about which genes are transcriptionally active in certain phenotypes.

I. CORONARY ATHEROSCLEROSIS AND ATHEROTHROMBOSIS. Coronary atherothrombosis and atherosclerosis remain significant causes of morbidity and mortality in the population as a whole. There is a great deal of variation in presentation in atherosclerosis and in acute MI. The presence of atherosclerosis is necessary but not sufficient for atherothrombosis. There are separate factors involved that predispose to plaque rupture and thrombosis. Even within the category of plaque rupture, the clinical phenotypes vary significantly, as reflected by the spectrum of diseases that constitute the acute coronary syndromes. These entities are complex traits and are influenced by multiple pathways. Inflammation, endothelial dysfunction, and dyslipidemias are only a few of the pathways influencing the development of atherothrombosis and atherosclerosis. Delineating the genetic basis, in most cases, is a work in progress, but may help to broaden our understanding of disease.

A. Dyslipidemia: familial hyperlipidemia and other genetic variants. Dyslipidemia is a known risk factor for the development of atherosclerosis. Familial hyperlipidemia (FH) is a well-characterized, albeit relatively uncommon, entity defined by elevated levels of serum LDL levels, which predispose to coronary atherosclerosis. Often these patients can develop atherosclerotic disease between 20 and 30 years of age. In FH, the dyslipidemia is often severe and not responsive to standard lifestyle and pharmacologic interventions.

1. **Autosomal dominant.** The underlying problem in this form of FH has to do with an abnormality in the clearance of the LDL-R, and, as a consequence, elevated levels of LDL persist. There are close to 900 known mutations of LDL-R and these appear to affect many aspects of LDL-R function. Alterations in the gene range from point mutations to gene rearrangements. Homozygotes and heterozygotes for FH vary in terms of the severity of lipid levels. Typically these patients and affected family members develop premature coronary atherosclerosis and myocardial infarction.
2. **Autosomal recessive.** Occurs as a result of a mutation in the LDL-R adaptor protein 1 (LDLRAP1) gene. The phenotype of this form of FH is milder than the autosomal dominant form of the disease and more amenable to treatment with lipid-lowering agents.
3. **Familial defective apolipoprotein B.** The cellular mechanisms involved in cholesterol metabolism are complex, and there are many potential targets where mutations can significantly affect phenotype. One such example is a point mutation in the apolipoprotein B (apoB) component of the LDL molecule. The Arg3500Gln substitution in the apoB (APOB) gene results in the inability of LDL to bind to its LDL-R. This mutant allele is more common in European populations as a cause of hyperlipidemia, but the phenotype appears to be less severe than in the LDL-R defective form of FH.
4. **PCSK-9.** A rare form of FH involves the proprotein convertase subtilisin/kexin type 9 gene. Although a few mutations have been identified, the consequence of these mutations are still not clearly defined, although it is believed to be involved in cholesterol metabolism and lipoprotein handling. Recently, specific mutations in PCSK-9 have been described, which result in lower LDL levels and confer a protection against coronary atherosclerosis.

In addition to the FH syndromes, there is a multitude of genes involved in more frequently occurring types of dyslipidemia. Phenotypically, these forms of dyslipidemia are less severe and more amenable to treatment than observed in the FH population. A recent study genotyping 93 SNPs in 13 genes identified a significant correlation between identified haplotypes and the phenotypic variance observed in LDL and high-density lipoprotein (HDL) cholesterol. Given the importance of dyslipidemia in cardiovascular disease, the potential exists to extrapolate this genetic data to assess cardiovascular risk.

B. Endothelial function. *MEF2a* is a transcription factor that localizes to the endothelial cell of coronary arteries and is believed to be important in the function of endothelial cells. Mutation in the *MEF2a* gene was described in a large family with autosomal dominant transmission of coronary atherothrombosis and has since been replicated. A 21 base-pair deletion in exon 11 was thought to result in loss of function. Other mutations in the same gene have been described in association with a similar phenotype. Given the putative role for *MEF2a* in the endothelium, it is likely that compromise of endothelial function and integrity as a result of the mutation may predispose to atherosclerosis and eventual atherothrombosis.

C. Inflammation. The case for inflammation as a significant participant in acute myocardial infarction has been made stronger recently by the discovery, through linkage analysis to a locus at 13q12-13, of a 4 SNP haplotype in the gene ALOX5AP. This variant was found to confer an increased risk of both stroke and myocardial infarction. The protein from this gene normally encodes a 5-lipoxygenase activating protein that is involved in the leukotriene pathway and those carriers of the variant had higher levels of leukotriene-B4. Another haplotype variant of the ALOX5AP gene was found to confer an increased risk of myocardial infarction in a British cohort. This same group also discovered a multiple SNP marker variant of the LTA4H gene also involved in the inflammation pathway.

The potential clinical relevance of this genetic information was noted in a trial in patients with previous myocardial infarction. Carriers of either the ALOX5AP variant or the LTA4H variant were randomized to a 5-lipoxygenase activating protein (FLAP) inhibitor (DG-031) versus placebo. Those receiving the FLAP blocker had a significant reduction in biomarkers of inflammation. Although clinical outcomes were not recorded, the potential exists as a viable target for preventing future myocardial infarction.

D. Thrombosis/Hypercoagulability. Tendency toward thrombosis appears to confer an additional risk toward development of MI and coronary atherosclerosis. Variants in the factor V gene (1691A) and prothrombin gene (20210A) were both found to confer an increased risk of coronary artery disease in a meta-analysis of more than 66,000 cases.

E. Novel SNPs without specified role. Recently, two separate groups of investigators identified variants conferring an increased risk of myocardial infarction and coronary artery disease on chromosome 9p21 (Fig. 62.1). There were multiple SNPs described in this region. However, the sequence variants do not appear to code a protein but rather appear to be in proximity to genes CDKN2A and CDKN2B, which code proteins vital to regulation of cellular proliferation and apoptosis. These findings were screened for and validated in multiple populations of a cumulative 40,000 individuals and have since been confirmed by many other groups. The 9p21 variants have a homozygote (two copies) risk of 1.64 and a population attributable risk of more than 20% in those of European ancestry. This means that if one could eliminate this gene variant there would be eradication of more than 20% of heart attacks among Europeans, indicating the importance of this finding. It is not yet known whether these variants carry risk in other ancestries. Although the functionality of this region is not yet known, there is mounting evidence to suggest the importance of noncoding regions in influencing gene expression.

There are many other variants of genes involved in various pathways discussed previously that are believed to confer an increased risk of myocardial infarction and coronary artery disease (Table 62.1).

II. CONNECTIVE TISSUE ABNORMALITIES AND DISEASE OF THE AORTA. Genetic mutations in affecting the connective tissue and extracellular matrix typically affect multiple organ systems, but often the most devastating and lethal effects arise from those upon the cardiovascular system. Aortic dissection and rupture are often the consequences of such abnormalities, and what follows is a brief description of three such disorders.

A. Marfan's syndrome. This disorder is inherited in an autosomal dominant fashion with variable penetrance, and it affects the connective tissue, leading to abnormalities of organs of the cardiovascular, skeletal, and ocular systems. The genetic defect

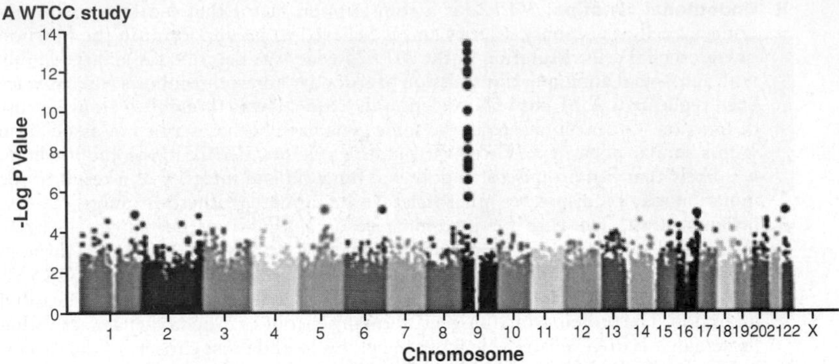

Figure 62.1. Signal-Intensity Plot of the Wellcome Trust Case Control Consortium (WTCCC) study displaying the relationship between the single nucleotide polymorphisms (SNPs) believed important in coronary artery disease and the distribution of p-values. As can be seen here, there is a significant association between the 9q21 locus and coronary artery disease (CAD). The rs1333049 SNP is the main SNP in 9q21 and 22% of the patients in the WTCCC study were homozygous for this allele and 50% of the remaining were carriers. (From Samani, et al. *N Engl J Med* 2007;357:447. Copyright 2007 *Massachusetts Medical Society. All rights reserved.* Reproduced with permission.)

TABLE 62.1 Gene Variants Associated with CAD and MI

Gene	SNP	Odds ratio	Potential gene function
VAMP8	3'UTR	1.75	Involved in platelet degranulation
HNRPUL1	Intron	1.92	Involved in mRNA processing
Connexin 37 gene (Japanese)	C1019T	1.4	Important in endothelial integrity
Plasminogen-activator inhibitor type I	4G-668/5G	1.6	Produced in endothelium and involved in thrombosis
Stromelysin-1 (Japanese women)	5A-1171/6A	4.7	Matrix metalloproteinase
TNFSF4	A/G (Intron 1)	1.4	Important in OX40 ligand pathway in T lymphocytes
LPA	I4399M	3.14	Component of lipoprotein(a), assoc. with severe CAD and elevated Lp(a) levels
MHC2A	A-168-G	1.39	Affects expression of MHC molecules involved in adaptive immunity
Lymphotoxin-alpha (LTA)	A-252-G	1.69	Proinflammatory, ?affecting adhesion molecule production
LGALS2	C-3279-T	1.57	Affects galectin-2 production, which in turn may affect LTA levels
Thrombospondin-4 (THBS4)	A-387-P	3.07	Affects endothelial cell function
Thrombospondin-1 (THBS1	N700S	8.16	Affects vWF size and important in thrombus stabilization
ApoE	G-219-T (m) T-3932-C (f)	1.5 2.0	Located in LDL receptor binding domain, determinant of ε4 allele

CAD, Coronary artery disease; MHC, major histocompatability complex; LDL, low-density lipoprotein; LTA, vWF, von Willebrand factor.

is in the fibrillin-1 (FBN1) gene on chromosome 15q21. Often the diagnosis is made on clinical grounds alone. The classic features of tall stature, arachnodactyly, dolichostenomelia, pectus excavatum, ectopia lentis, and a positive family history all support a diagnosis of Marfan's syndrome. The cardiovascular system is affected, and the most common cause of death in these patients is from aortic dissection. Other common related problems include aortic dilation, mitral valve prolapse, tricuspid valve prolapse, and arrhythmias. When patients with Marfan's syndrome present with dissection they are typically younger and do not have hypertension.

The FBN1 gene is responsible for producing a key constituent of microfibrils, which are important in the extracellular matrix. Microfibrils add to the elastic properties of extracellular tissue. There are multiple mutations in the FBN1 gene that have been recognized and appear to affect different aspects of cellular processing of fibrillin-1. There are no specific relationships between mutations and phenotypes as of yet. The diagnosis of Marfan's syndrome, however, generally is made on a clinical basis and genetic testing is rarely utilized for diagnosis alone.

B. Ehlers-Danlos syndrome. Ehlers-Danlos syndrome is a connective tissue disease that involves defects in proteins that are involved in the formation of collagen. There are multiple types of Ehlers-Danlos based on the collagen type affected; however, the cardiovascular system is involved prominently in type IV. The defect in this subtype is localized to chromosome 2q24.3-q31 and involves the gene for type III procollagen. Aortic dissections are the primary cause of death and often involve both the thoracic and abdominal aortas.

C. Loeys-Dietz syndrome. Loeys-Dietz syndrome is a disorder characterized by hypertelorism, cleft palate, and vascular disease in the form of arterial aneurysms and dissection. It is inherited in an autosomal dominant fashion. Clinically, these patients are at high risk of aortic dissection. The genetic defect identified in this group of patients involves the transforming growth factor beta (TGF-β) receptors 1 and 2 (TGFBR1 and TGFBR2). Phenotypically, these patients appear similar (with the exception of the craniofacial abnormalities) to Ehlers-Danlos patients with vascular involvement. The relevance of this distinction is that those with Loeys-Dietz appear to have much lower intraoperative mortality during corrective vascular surgery.

III. CARDIOMYOPATHIES. Primary disease of the myocardium affects both systolic and diastolic function and often results in heart failure or other adverse events over time. Many of the nonischemic cardiomyopathies have a strong genetic component to explain their phenotype. Perhaps the most clinically relevant entities include dilated cardiomyopathy and hypertrophic cardiomyopathy. Cardiomyopathies can also occur as a secondary process in response to a separate unrelated factor (i.e., hypertension) and it is unknown to what degree genetic susceptibility determines the myocardial response/remodeling over time. Until recently, the classification of cardiomyopathies has been based on phenotype and morphologic characteristics. However, with an improved knowledge of the genetics of these disorders, a new understanding and appreciation for the underlying mechanisms of disease in these disorders will undoubtedly influence how these entities are treated in the future.

A. Dilated cardiomyopathy. Dilated cardiomyopathy (DCM) is characterized by dilation of one or both of the ventricular chambers resulting in severe systolic dysfunction and characterized by congestive heart failure. Almost half of all DCM cases are thought to be genetic, and in many cases the pattern of inheritance is autosomal dominant. Many cases of DCM are secondary to other etiologies. There are many genes that have been associated with this phenotype and although the products of most of these genes are important structural proteins, there are others involved in the handling of calcium and regulation of energy within the myocytes. Again, however, there are often subtle differences in the various types of DCM such as age of onset and degree of clinical symptoms, all of which may suggest separate genetic abnormalities at play. Genetic screening for this disorder has been limited to research to this point and is not used to confirm or establish a diagnosis. Table 62.2 lists some of the genetic variants believed associated with various dilated cardiomyopathy phenotypes.

TABLE 62.2 Genetic Variants Associated with Dilated Cardiomyopathies

Gene	Location	Type of cardiomyopathy	Function of gene product
Lamin A/C (LMNA)	1p1–q21	Dilated	Affects structure of nucleus in myocytes
Thymopoietin (LAP2)	12q22	Dilated	Maintains functional integrity of nucleus
β-myosin heavy chain (MYH7)	14q11	Dilated	Part of sarcomere, and mutations may affect contractile mechanism
Actin (ACTC)	15q14	Dilated	Vital part of contractile apparatus of myocyte
Cardiac muscle LIM protein (CLP)	11p15	Dilated	Functions as a stretch sensor in myocyte
Phospholamban	6q22	Dilated	Controls muscle relaxation through calcium regulation via calcium-ATPase
Desmin (DES)	2q35	Dilated	Cytoskeletal protein involved in stabilization of sarcomere and mutation may affect contractile force
Dystrophin (DMD)	Xp21	Dilated—X linked	More commonly involved in Duchenne's and Becker's muscular. dystrophy, mutations can affect transduction of contractile force
Troponin T (TNNT2)	1q32	Dilated	Mutations affect contractile force
Presenilin Genes (PSEN1 and 2)		Dilated	

B. Hypertrophic cardiomyopathy. Hypertrophic cardiomyopathy (HCM) is a highly variable and heterogeneous disease process that affects the myocardium, with clinical manifestations varying from completely asymptomatic to severe (sudden cardiac death). The broad range of phenotypes and significant selection bias resulted in an overestimation of the mortality rate associated with this disease. The clinical spectrum of disease is wide, and being able to accurately predict outcomes remains challenging. The clinical variability of HCM is not limited to the presenting phenotype, but also related to age of presentation, clinical course, and eventual outcomes, making it very challenging to properly identify a phenotype of interest. The characteristic phenotype is an asymmetrically hypertrophied myocardium with a small ventricular chamber and occasionally an LV outflow tract (with systolic anterior motion of the mitral valve) and/or an intracavitary gradient.

Mutations in 11 separate genes have been identified and are thought to account for more than one-half of all types of HCM. The genes involved encode proteins of the cardiac sarcomere unit. The products of these genes involved include troponin T, troponin I, β-myosin heavy chain, myosin light chains, myosin-binding protein C, α-myosin light chain, α-tropomyosin, and actin, among others. Hundreds of mutations have been identified in these genes. The importance of properly characterizing a phenotype as heterogeneous as HCM has been illustrated by the example of glycogen storage diseases mimicking the appearance of hypertrophic cardiomyopathy. Mutations in the genes for AMP-activated protein kinase gamma2 (PRKAG2) and lysosome-associated membrane protein 2 (LAMP2) were found in phenotypes that closely resembled HCM but were differentiated based on serum protein levels and ventricular preexcitation.

TABLE 62.3 Genetic Variants of ARVC

ARVC Variant	Chromosome/Gene	Comments
ARVC1	14q23–24/TGFβ-3	
ARVC2	1q41.1–q43/RYR2	Autosomal dominant. Ryanodine receptor involved in Ca^{2+} release into cytosol
ARVC3	14q12–q22	Discovered in a study of three small families
ARVC4	2q32	Some family members from affected cohort had involvement of left ventricle
ARVC5	3p23/LAMR1	Mutant form of LAMR1 leads to alterations in cardiac myocyte gene expression
ARVC6	10p13-p14/PTPLA	Protein tyrosine phosphatases involved in cell growth and PTPLA is primarily found in cardiac tissue
ARVC7	10q.22.3 2q35/DES	
ARVC8	6p24/DSP	Desmoplakin is a constituent protein of desmosomes. In some this form is associated with keratoderma and wooly hair
ARVC9	12p11/PKP2	Plakophilins are part of desmosome and also found in the nucleus regulating transcription
ARVC10	18q12/DSG2	Codes for desmogleins involved in desmome cell adhesion. Occur in AD and AR (Naxos, Carvajal) forms
ARVC11	18q21/DSC2	Codes for desmocollin, a desmosomal cadherin protein

Adapted from Moric Janiszewska, et al. *Europace* 2007.

C. Arrhythmogenic right ventricular cardiomyopathy. Arrhythmogenic right ventricular cardiomyopathy (ARVC) is a primary abnormality resulting in fibrofatty infiltration into the myocardium, primarily the right ventricle. Clinical manifestations include right ventricular dysfunction and lethal ventricular arrhythmias. Diagnosis often includes a battery of tests, including an electrocardiogram demonstrating repolarization abnormalities and an epsilon wave, magnetic resonance imaging (MRI) or computed tomography (CT) demonstrating fibrofatty infiltration of the right ventricle, endomyocardial biopsy, and often a positive family history. ARVC can be inherited in both an autosomal dominant and autosomal recessive fashion. Mutations in genes encoding desmoplakin, desmoglein-2, cardiac ryanodine receptor, and plakophilin-2 have all been associated with the autosomal dominant form of the disease. Mutations in plakoglobin are associated with the autosomal recessive form, particularly Naxos disease, a variant associated with the triad of ARVC, wooly hair and palmoplantar keratoderma. There are 11 subtypes of ARVC, which are distinguished on the basis of the gene involved and are described further in Table 62.3.

D. Left ventricular noncompaction. Left ventricular (LV) noncompaction is a relatively uncommon disease of the myocardium resulting in a trabeculated appearance of the LV cavity. This disorder can occur in isolation or in association with other congenital anomalies. Over time, it is thought that noncompaction can proceed to dilated cardiomyopathy with severe systolic dysfunction. The Cypher/ZASP gene, and genes encoding NKX2.5 and α-dystrobrevin proteins are thought to be involved in the pathogenesis.

IV. ARRHYTHMOGENIC DISORDERS

A. Brugada syndrome. Disorders of conduction system of the heart lead to significant clinical manifestations, most notably ventricular arrhythmias and sudden cardiac death. Two entities, long QT syndrome and Brugada syndrome, have been well described, and their respective genetic abnormalities have been characterized. Brugada syndrome was initially described by Josep and Pedro Brugada in 1992. Clinically, ventricular arrhythmias and sudden cardiac death occur, particularly in middle-aged men. Characteristic electrocardiographic features can help to make the diagnosis, and, in some cases, certain drugs, including sodium channel blockers and tricyclic antidepressants can unmask the abnormality on a surface electrocardiogram. The genetic basis for this disorder has been traced to the gene for the alpha subunit of the cardiac sodium channel (*SCN5A*) on chromosome 3. The phenotype is typically inherited in an autosomal dominant fashion, and there are many mutations of the *SCN5A* gene that have been described. Genetic testing in this disease phenotype is used to confirm a clinical diagnosis; however, a negative screen of known mutations of the *SCN5A* gene does not necessarily exclude the diagnosis. There are many polymorphisms, including those in promoter regions for *SCN5A,* that are not part of genetic testing.

B. Long QT syndrome. Long QT Syndrome (LQTS) encompasses a range of disorders characterized clinically by syncope and sudden cardiac death, with electrocardiographic abnormalities in the QT interval and in the T wave morphology. LQTS can be inherited in a typical autosomal dominant or recessive fashion. Recent data suggest, however, that in type 1 and 2 LQTS, there may be transmission distortion resulting in increased carriers among children of affected females. There are nine different types of LQTS based on the type of gene involved. Studies have examined and confirmed a relationship between the gene involved and event-free survival stratified on the basis of gender and duration of QT_c prolongation. The various forms of LQTS are often distinguishable by clinical features and genetic abnormalities. One such distinguishing feature is that those with long QT syndrome 1 (LQT1) are typically at higher risk during periods of exercise, whereas those with the long QT syndrome 3 variant (LQT3) are at higher risk during sleep. The *KCNQ1* gene encodes the catecholamine sensitive portion of the potassium channel responsible for conducting the delayed rectifier current (I_{Ks}) in the LQT1 variant, whereas the *SCN5A* gene is affected in the LQT3 variant. The underlying defect involving the sodium channel results in a prolonged depolarization current, whereas defects involving the potassium channel result in a longer QT duration secondary to inability to re-establish repolarization within the myocyte. The autosomal recessive phenotypes (Jervell and Lange-Nielsen 1 and 2) are associated with bilateral sensorineural hearing loss.

Hundreds of mutations are believed to be responsible in LQTS. However, most of the prognostic information available is based on the gene involved and not the specific mutation. Having the genotypic information can help in prognosis and in determining response to therapy. The rates of ventricular arrhythmias and sudden cardiac death vary based on the gene involved, as does response to therapy. This information would be particularly helpful in trying to decide between medical therapy, ICD implantation, or both. Table 62.4 lists the nine variants of LQTS and the genes involved.

C. Atrial fibrillation. Atrial fibrillation (AF) is the most common of the arrhythmic disorders. It is increasing in prevalence. A major breakthrough has occurred in the genomics of AF with the finding that variants at 4q25 carry a risk of 1.6 and a population attributable risk of more than 30% in individuals of both European and Asian ancestry. The 4q25 variants are near a gene—PITX2—which is involved in left–right symmetry of the heart in development. But it has not yet been proven how the variants at 4q25 exert their effect. Other genes contribute to a much smaller degree to the risk of AF. Genes in the ACE gene, the gene encoding the cardiac potassium channel (KCNQ1, KCNJ2, KCNE2, KCNH2), and the connexin 40 gene (GJA5) have all been implicated as possible candidates.

V. VALVULAR HEART DISEASE

A. Mitral valve prolapse. Mitral valve prolapse is a common disorder that appears to have a strong genetic component, and the genetic form is likely inherited in an autosomal dominant fashion with variable penetrance. Although it occurs in an idiopathic form, it is also associated with other valvular syndromes such as bicuspid

TABLE 62.4 Genetic Variants Associated with Long QT Syndrome

LQT variant	Gene	Mode of inheritance	Function of gene product
LQT1	*KCNQ1*	Autosomal Dominant	Catecholamine sensitive portion of I_K channel
LQT2	*KCNH2*	Autosomal Dominant	Alpha subunit of I_{Kr} potassium channel
LQT3	*SCN5A*	Autosomal Dominant	Cardiac sodium channel
LQT4	*ANK2*	Autosomal Dominant	Ankyrin protein
LQT5	*KCNE1*	Autosomal Dominant	Beta subunit of I_{Ks} potassium channel
LQT6	*KCNE2*	Autosomal Dominant	Beta subunit of I_{Ks} potassium channel
LQT7	*KCJNE2*	Autosomal Dominant	Subunit of I_{Kr} potassium channel
Jervell and Lange-Nielsen Type 1	*KCNQ1*	Autosomal Recessive	Subunit I_K channel
Jervell and Lange-Nielsen Type 2	*KCNE1*	Autosomal Recessive	Beta subunit of I_{Ks} potassium channel

aortic valve and connective tissue diseases, which typically affect cardiovascular function such as Marfan's syndrome, osteogenesis imperfecta, and Ehlers Danlos syndrome. Prolapse of the mitral valve occurs primarily in the connective tissue matrix of the valve itself. Myxomatous degeneration of the valve tissue leads to redundant tissue and weakening of both the valve and subvalvular apparatus. Clinically this manifests as displacement of the mitral valve leaflets into the left atrium during systole and may progress to mitral regurgitation and eventual congestive heart failure with occasional rupture of the chordae. Although surgical repair and replacement has improved the long-term prognosis of this disorder, understanding the genetic basis of this disease may allow the earlier diagnosis and development of therapies to prevent progression. The genetic determinants of this phenotype are delineated further in Table 62.5.

B. Bicuspid aortic valve and aortic valve calcification. Aortic valve disease can be divided into two different types based on clinical characteristics: bicuspid aortic valve and calcific aortic valvular disease. Calcific aortic valvular disease is typically a disease of the elderly and appears to be affected by those risk factors predisposing toward coronary artery disease. Bicuspid aortic disease is believed to be a congenital abnormality that is typically discovered earlier on in life and is associated with disease of the aorta. What these two disorders have in common is the eventual progression to calcification of the aortic valve itself. With regards to

TABLE 62.5 Genetic Variants in Mitral Valve Prolapse

Gene	Location	Comments
MMVP1	Chromosome 16	
MMVP2	Chromosome 11p15.4 and 13q31.1-32.1	Autosomal dominant familial MVP
Gene for Filamin A	Chromosome Xq28	X-linked. Affects aortic and mitral valve

TABLE 62.6 Cardiovascular Manifestations of Systemic Metabolic Disease

Metabolic disorder	Gene/protein defect	Effect upon cardiovascular system	Comments
Anderson-Fabry	α-Galactosidase deficiency	Accumulation of globotriaosylce-ramide. Cardiomyopathy in form of LV hypertrophy, lethal arrhythmias, coronary ischemia.	X-linked
Hereditary Hemochromatosis	*HFE*, a MHC class I like protein, ferroportin??, hepcidin, hemojuvelin, and transferrin receptor-2	Iron deposition involves the heart and results in cardiomyopathy	Can be acquired via transfusion associated hemochromatosis
Niemann-Pick	Defect in sphingomyelinase	Accumulation of sphingomyelin in cardiac tissue leading to cardiomegaly	Affected children do not survive past first few years of life
Hurler's Syndrome (Type 1 Mucopolysaccha-ridosis)	Deficiency in α-L-iduronidase	Biventricular enlargement, endocardial fibrosis, valvular disease	Autosomal recessive
Hunter's Syndrome (Type 2 Mucopolysaccha-ridosis)	Deficiency in iduronate sulphatase	Cardiac involvement includes valvular disease	X linked
Danon Disease	Deficiency in lysosome associated protein type 2	Cardiac involvement includes LVH, CHF, and preexcitation	X-linked
Gaucher's Disease	Deficiency of glucocerebrosidase	Accumulation of glucocerebroside leading to cardiomyopathy, also calcification of aorta, aortic and mitral valves	
Pompe Disease	Defect in glycogen storage	Biventricular concentric hypertrophy	Autosomal recessive transmission
L-Carnitine deficiency	OCTN2 gene mutations affecting transport of carnitine	Cardiomegaly, dilated cardiomyopathy.	Carnitine transport is vital for mitochondrial function. Cardioprotective benefits may be derived from protection from free radical damage.

TABLE 62.7 Common Chromosomal Abnormalities and Associated Cardiovascular Disease

Syndrome	Chromosomal abnormality	Associated CV abnormality
Down Syndrome	Trisomy 21	Endocardial cushion defect, mitral valve prolapse, tetralogy of Fallot
Turner Syndrome	45X	Coarctation of the aorta, bicuspid AV, anomalous PV return
Patau Syndrome	Trisomy 13	Dextrocardia, ASD/VSD, bicuspid AV
Edward Syndrome	Trisomy 18	PDA, left SVC
Fragile X Syndrome	FMR1 gene (X chromosome) with trinucleotide repeats	Mitral valve disease

ASD, Atrial septal defect; AV, aortic valve; PV, pulmonary valve; PDA, patent ductus arteriosus; SVC, superior vena cava; VSD, ventricular septal defect.

bicuspid aortic valve, small studies suggested involvement of *NKX2.5* and *KCNJ2* genes in the pathogenesis. More compelling evidence for mutations in *NOTCH1* on chromosome 9 has suggested that this transmembrane protein with transcriptional regulatory activity is vital not only for aortic valve development but also for calcification. In families with bicuspid aortic valves and other congenital abnormalities mutations in this gene have been identified. It is thought that mutations in the *NOTCH1* gene may allow the normally repressed transcription factor Runx2 to facilitate the development of valvular endothelial cells into osteoblast-like cells and promote valvular calcification.

VI. INBORN ERRORS OF METABOLISM. Cardiovascular disease is often a manifestation of genetic abnormalities in separate pathways, which produce secondary effects upon the cardiovascular system. Many of these genetic mishaps occur in multiple pathways essential to metabolism, and their resultant phenotypes often impose upon the cardiovascular system. Table 62.6 lists some examples of metabolic abnormalities and the associated cardiac manifestations.

VII. CHROMOSOMAL ABNORMALITIES AND CARDIOVASCULAR DISEASE. Chromosomal abnormalities that occur at the time of development can have serious implications with regard to the proper growth and development of a child. Although neuropsychiatric development is often delayed, the cardiovascular system is also affected in many of these disorders and often survival may be limited due to the severity of congenital defects. Table 62.7 lists common syndromes associated with chromosomal structural abnormalities and the associated cardiovascular findings.

Suggested Readings

1. Wang L, Fan C, Topol SE, et al. Mutation of MEF2A in an inherited disorder with features of coronary artery disease. *Science* 2003;302:1578–1581.
2. Helgadottir A, Manolescu A, Helgason A, et al. A variant of the gene encoding leukotriene A4 hydrolase confers ethnicity-specific risk of myocardial infarction. *Nat Genet* 2006;38:68–74.
3. Hakonarson H, Thorvaldsson S, Helgadottir A, et al. Effects of a 5-lipoxygenase-activating protein inhibitor on biomarkers associated with risk of myocardial infarction: a randomized trial. *JAMA* 2005;293:2245–2256.
4. Cohen JC, Boerwinkle E, Mosley TH Jr, et al. Sequence variations in PCSK9, low LDL, and protection against coronary heart disease. *N Engl J Med* 2006;354:1264–1272.
5. Topol EJ, Smith J, Plow EF, et al. Genetic susceptibility to myocardial infarction and coronary artery disease. *Hum Mol Genet* 2006;15[Spec No 2]:R117–123.
6. Hirashiki A, Yamada Y, Murase Y, et al. Association of gene polymorphisms with coronary artery disease in low- or high-risk subjects defined by conventional risk factors. *J Am Coll Cardiol* 2003;42:1429–1437.
7. Ye Z, Liu EH, Higgins JP, et al. Seven haemostatic gene polymorphisms in coronary disease: meta-analysis of 66,155 cases and 91,307 controls. *Lancet* 2006;367:651–658.
8. Wang X, Ria M, Kelmenson PM, et al. Positional identification of TNFSF4, encoding OX40 ligand, as a gene that influences atherosclerosis susceptibility. *Nat Genet* 2005;37:365–372.
9. Swanberg M, Lidman O, Padyukov L, et al. MHC2TA is associated with differential MHC molecule expression and susceptibility to rheumatoid arthritis, multiple sclerosis and myocardial infarction. *Nat Genet* 2005;37:486–494.

10. Helgadottir A, Thorleifsson G, Manolescu A, et al. A common variant on chromosome 9p21 affects the risk of myocardial infarction. *Science* 2007;316:1491–1493.
11. McPherson R, Pertsemlidis A, Kavaslar N, et al. A common allele on chromosome 9 associated with coronary heart disease. *Science* 2007;316:1488–1491.
12. Topol EJ, McCarthy J, Gabriel S, et al. Single nucleotide polymorphisms in multiple novel thrombospondin genes may be associated with familial premature myocardial infarction. *Circulation* 2001;104:2641–2644.
13. Arnett DK, Baird AE, Barkley RA, et al. Relevance of genetics and genomics for prevention and treatment of cardiovascular disease: a scientific statement from the American Heart Association Council on Epidemiology and Prevention, the Stroke Council, and the Functional Genomics and Translational Biology Interdisciplinary Working Group. *Circulation* 2007;115:2878–2901.
14. Kamisago M, Sharma SD, DePalma SR, et al. Mutations in sarcomere protein genes as a cause of dilated cardiomyopathy. *N Engl J Med* 2000;343:1688–1696.
15. Chen Q, Kirsch GE, Zhang D, et al. Genetic basis and molecular mechanism for idiopathic ventricular fibrillation. *Nature* 1998;392:293–296.
16. Schulze-Bahr E, Eckardt L, Breithardt G, et al. Sodium channel gene (SCN5A) mutations in 44 index patients with Brugada syndrome: different incidences in familial and sporadic disease. *Hum Mutat* 2003;21:651–652.
17. Antzelevitch C. Brugada syndrome. *Pacing Clin Electrophysiol* 2006;29:1130–1159.
18. Moss AJ, Shimizu W, Wilde AA, et al. Clinical aspects of type-1 long-QT syndrome by location, coding type, and biophysical function of mutations involving the KCNQ1 gene. *Circulation* 2007;115:2481–2489.
19. Ashrafian H, Watkins H. Reviews of translational medicine and genomics in cardiovascular disease: new disease taxonomy and therapeutic implications cardiomyopathies: therapeutics based on molecular phenotype. *J Am Coll Cardiol* 2007;49:1251–1264.
20. Karkkainen S, Peuhkurinen K. Genetics of dilated cardiomyopathy. *Ann Med* 2007;39:91–107.
21. Schmitt JP, Kamisago M, Asahi M, et al. Dilated cardiomyopathy and heart failure caused by a mutation in phospholamban. *Science* 2003;299:1410–1413.
22. Disse S, Abergel E, Berrebi A, et al. Mapping of a first locus for autosomal dominant myxomatous mitral-valve prolapse to chromosome 16p11.2-p12.1. *Am J Hum Genet* 1999;65:1242–1251.
23. Freed LA, Acierno JS, Jr., Dai D, et al. A locus for autosomal dominant mitral valve prolapse on chromosome 11p15.4. *Am J Hum Genet* 2003;72:1551–1559.
24. Nesta F, Leyne M, Yosefy C, et al. New locus for autosomal dominant mitral valve prolapse on chromosome 13: clinical insights from genetic studies. *Circulation* 2005;112:2022–2030.
25. Kyndt F, Schott JJ, Trochu JN, et al. Mapping of X-linked myxomatous valvular dystrophy to chromosome Xq28. *Am J Hum Genet* 1998;62:627–632.
26. Samani NJ, Erdmann J, Hall AS, et al. Genomewide association analysis of coronary artery disease. *N Engl J Med* 2007;357:443–453.
27. Fox CS, Parise H, D'Agostino RB, Sr, et al. Parental atrial fibrillation as a risk factor for atrial fibrillation in offspring. *JAMA* 2004;291:2851–2855.
28. Gollob MH, Jones DL, Krahn AD, et al. Somatic mutations in the connexin 40 gene (GJA5) in atrial fibrillation. *N Engl J Med* 2006;354:2677–2688.
29. Gudbjartsson DF, Arnar DO, Helgadottir A, et al. Variants conferring risk of atrial fibrillation on chromosome 4q25. *Nature* 2007;448:353–357.
30. Moric-Janiszewska E, Markiewicz-Loskot G. Review on the genetics of arrhythmogenic right ventricular dysplasia. *Europace* 2007;9:259–266.
31. Garg V, Muth AN, Ransom JF, et al. Mutations in NOTCH1 cause aortic valve disease. *Nature* 2005;437:270–274.
32. Maron BJ, Towbin JA, Thiene G, et al. Contemporary definitions and classification of the cardiomyopathies: an American Heart Association Scientific Statement from the Council on Clinical Cardiology, Heart Failure and Transplantation Committee; Quality of Care and Outcomes Research and Functional Genomics and Translational Biology Interdisciplinary Working Groups; and Council on Epidemiology and Prevention. *Circulation* 2006;113:1807–1816.
33. Arad M, Maron BJ, Gorham JM, et al. Glycogen storage diseases presenting as hypertrophic cardiomyopathy. *N Engl J Med* 2005;352:362–372.
34. Roberts R. Genomics and cardiac arrhythmias. *J Am Coll Cardiol* 2006;47:9–21.
35. Robinson PN, Arteaga-Solis E, Baldock C, et al. The molecular genetics of Marfan syndrome and related disorders. *J Med Genet* 2006;43:769–787.
36. Guertl B, Noehammer C, Hoefler G. Metabolic cardiomyopathies. *Int J Exp Pathol* 2000;81:349–372.
37. Gelb BD. Genetic basis of congenital heart disease. *Curr Opin Cardiol* 2004;19:110–115.
38. Levine RA, Slaugenhaupt SA. Molecular genetics of mitral valve prolapse. *Curr Opin Cardiol* 2007;22:171–175.
39. Schwartz PJ, Spazzolini C, Crotti L, et al. The Jervell and Lange-Nielsen syndrome: natural history, molecular basis, and clinical outcome. *Circulation* 2006;113:783–790.

CARDIOVASCULAR DRUGS XIII

APPENDIX

Michael A. Militello

This appendix includes most of the available cardiovascular drugs used in clinical practice. The tables are arranged in two different schemes; they are alphabetical according to drug class and/or therapeutic class. Each table contains:

- brand and generic name of each drug
- usual starting doses and maximum doses where available
- mechanism of action
- indications, both labeled and unlabeled
- side effects that occur in more than 1% of the population, or if less than 1%, those that are considered potentially life-threatening
- comments

The tables include some drug interactions but are not exhaustive. Many of the medications, both cardiovascular and noncardiovascular, have significant drug interactions; one should be aware of these when prescribing any new medication.

Drug	Dose	Mechanism of action	Indications	Side effects	Comments
Adrenergic Antagonists—Peripheral					
Guanadrel (Hylorel)	Initial oral: 5 mg twice daily Maximum: 150 mg/d	Inhibits peripheral adrenergic neurons by initially decreasing the release of norepinephrine and then causing depletion of neuronal norepinephrine	Labeled: Hypertension	—Orthostatic hypotension —Edema (see Comments) —Depression —Diarrhea —Drowsiness/fatigue —Dry mouth —Angina —Sexual dysfunction	—Contraindicated in patients with pheochromocytoma, CHF, and patients on MAOIs —Significant sodium and water retention occurs —Use with caution in patients with PUD, renal dysfunction, and asthma —Discontinue 2–3 d before surgery because of risk of cardiovascular collapse during anesthesia induction —Exaggerated response to vasopressors
Guanethidine (Ismelin)	Initial oral: 10 mg/d Maximum: 300 mg/d		Labeled: Hypertension	—Orthostatic hypotension —Edema (see Comments) —Depression —Diarrhea (may be severe) —Drowsiness/fatigue —Dry mouth —Angina —Sexual dysfunction	—Contraindicated in patients with pheochromocytoma, CHF, and patients on MAOIs —Exaggerated response to exogenous administered vasopressors —May aggravate asthma —Significant sodium and water retention occurs —Do not increase doses more frequently than every 5–7 d

Reserpine (Various)	Initial oral: 0.1–0.5 mg/d Maximum: 0.25 mg/d (see Comments)	Binds to central and peripheral adrenergic neurons, destroying storage vesicles for norepinephrine and dopamine, thus decreasing sympathetic outflow	Labeled: Hypertension, psychotic states (decreases agitation of patients in psychotic states)	—Depression (see Comments) —Drowsiness —Nasal congestion —Nausea/vomiting/abdominal cramps —↑Gastric acid production —Edema (see Comments) —Sexual dysfunction	—High incidence of severe depression —Rarely used because of high incidence of side effects —Significant sodium and water retention occurs —Use cautiously in patients with depression, PUD, renal dysfunction, or gallstones
General information		Centrally acting α_2 agonist decreases sympathetic outflow		—Sedation —Dry mouth —Hypotension —Dizziness —Sexual dysfunction —Bradycardia —Nausea —Headache	—Abrupt withdrawal causes rebound hypertension —Rebound hypertension can be severe with concurrent administration of β-blockers
Clonidine (Catapres) (Catapres-TTS)	Initial oral: 0.1 mg twice daily Maximum: 2.4 mg/d Transdermal patch TTS 1–0.1 mg/24 h TTS-2–0.2 mg/24 h TTS-3–0.3 mg/24 h	See General Information for α-adrenergic antagonists	Labeled: Hypertension Unlabeled: Hypertensive urgencies, alcohol and opiate withdrawal, smoking cessation, Tourette's syndrome	—See General Information for α-adrenergic antagonists —Depression	—CrCl <10 mL/min reduce dose by 25%–50% —When initiating a patch in a patient on clonidine, full oral doses must be given the first day, then 1/2 dose the second day, and then 1/2 of the second day's dose on the third day, then discontinue PO —Patches are replaced weekly —15% of patients develop contact dermatitis with patches

(*continued*)

Drug	Dose	Mechanism of action	Indications	Side effects	Comments
Guanfacine (Tenex)	Initial oral: 1 mg/d Maximum: 2 mg/d	See General Information for α-adrenergic antagonists	Labeled: Hypertension Unlabeled: Opiate withdrawal, migraine headache prophylaxis	—See General Information for α-adrenergic antagonists —Constipation	—Risk of rebound hypertension usually less severe because of long half-life
Guanabenz (Wytensin)	Initial oral: 4 mg twice daily Maximum: 32 mg/d	See General Information for α-adrenergic antagonists	Labeled: Hypertension	—See General Information for α-adrenergic antagonists —Muscular weakness	
Methyldopa (Aldomet)	Initial oral: 250 mg 2–4 times daily Maximum: 2000 mg/d	See General Information for α-adrenergic antagonists	Labeled: Hypertension, hypertensive emergency (IV only)	—See General Information for α-adrenergic antagonists —Peripheral edema —Hemolytic anemia —Drug fever	—Positive Coombs test 10%–20% of patients within 6–12 mo —Hemolytic anemia <1% —SLE-like syndrome —Hepatitis is rare —Measure Coombs test at baseline, 6 and 12 mo
Methyldopate HCl	IV: 250 mg 3–4 times daily up to 1000 mg 4 times			—Depression —Nightmares —Hepatocellular injury —Anxiety	
α-Adrenergic Antagonists					
General information				—Orthostatic hypotension —Dizziness —Lightheadedness —Drowsiness —Headache —Dry mouth —Malaise	—Give first dose and increased doses at bedtime to limit orthostatic hypotension

Doxazosin (Cardura)	Initial oral: 1 mg/d Maximum: 16 mg/d	Peripherally acting α_1 receptor antagonist	Labeled: Hypertension	See General Information for α-adrenergic antagonists	—Doses $>$4 mg/d will increase risk of orthostatic hypotension —Recent data suggest that doxazosin provides worse outcomes as compared to chlorthalidone in the management of hypertension and that doxazosin should not be considered as first-line therapy for hypertension.
Phentolamine (Regitine)	Hypertensive crisis: 5–20 mg IV push every 1–2 h Pheochromocytoma diagnosis: 5 mg IV Extravasation: see Comments	Competitive nonselective α-adrenergic antagonist having similar affinities for α_1 andα_2 receptors	Labeled: Hypertensive crisis in patients with pheochromocytoma, diagnosis of pheochromocytoma, management of skin necrosis in patients with norepinephrine extravasation	—Hypotension —Tachycardia —Arrhythmias —Angina —Nausea/vomiting/diarrhea —Exacerbates PUD —Nasal congestion —Flushing —Exacerbates PUD —Nasal congestion —Flushing	—Very short duration with a half-life 19 min —May be used to treat extravasation of dopamine and epinephrine —Disulfiram reaction may occur —Has positive inotropic and chronotropic effects —Extravasation: 5–10 mg diluted in 10 mL of normal saline. Phentolamine is injected in multiple sites around the area of extravasation with 27- to 30-gauge needles changing the needle after each injection. This should be done within 12 h of extravasation. Skin color should return to normal within 1 h if treatment was effective

(*continued*)

Drug	Dose	Mechanism of action	Indications	Side effects	Comments
Prazosin (Minipress)	Initial oral: 1 mg 2–3 times daily Maximum: 20 mg/d	Peripherally acting α_1 receptor antagonist	Labeled: Hypertension Unlabeled: Raynaud's syndrome, benign prostatic hypertrophy, CHF	See General Information for α-adrenergic antagonists	—Few patients benefit from doses >40 mg/d
Terazosin	Initial oral: 1 mg/d Maximum: 20 mg/d	Peripherally acting α_1 receptor antagonist	Labeled: Hypertension, BPH	See General Information for α-adrenergic antagonists	—10 mg/d is the maximum dose for BPH
Angiotensin-Converting Enzyme Inhibitors					
General Information		Inhibits the conversion of angiotensin I to angiotensin II by blocking ACE		—Cough —Acute renal failure —Angioedema —Hyperkalemia —Proteinuria —Hypotension —Headache —Rash —Neutropenia/ agranulocytosis —Dizziness	—Angioedema occurs infrequently, usually with first dose; however, it may occur at any time during therapy. —Severe hypotension seen in patients who are volume depleted or elderly, consider lower initial doses —Contraindicated in pregnancy and bilateral renal artery stenosis or unilateral renal artery stenosis in patients with solitary kidney

					—Neutropenia and/or agranulocytosis has been reported with many ACE-I —Hematologic abnormalities usually associated with collagen vascular disorders, higher doses, and renal dysfunction
Benazepril (Lotensin)	Initial oral: 10 mg/d (see Comments) Maximum : 80 mg/d	See General Information for ACE-I	Labeled: Hypertension	—See General Information for ACE-I	—May need to use twice daily —Use lower doses with renal insufficiency
Captopril (Capoten)	Initial oral: 6.25–2.5 mg 2–3 times daily (see Comments) Maximum: 150–450 mg/d	See General Information for ACE-I	Labeled: Hypertension, HF, treatment of LV dysfunction post-MI, diabetic nephropathy	—See General Information for ACE-I —Neutropenia/ agranulocytosis —Abnormal taste	—Most patients do not have an increased response to doses greater than 100 mg three times daily —Not a prodrug —Reduce dose in patients with renal dysfunction —Food decreases extent of absorption —Target dosage for HF: 50 mg three times daily —Generics are available
Enalapril (Vasotec)	Initial oral: 2.5 mg 1–2 times daily (see Comments) Maximum: 40 mg/d divided doses IV: 0.625–1.25 mg every 6 h given over 5 min	See General Information for ACE-I	Labeled: Hypertension, HF (symptomatic and asymptomatic)	—See General Information for ACE-I —Neutropenia/ agranulocytosis —Abnormal taste	—Reduce dose in patients with renal dysfunction —Target dosage for HF: 10 mg twice daily —Generics are available

(*continued*)

Drug	Dose	Mechanism of action	Indications	Side effects	Comments
Fosinopril (Monopril)	Initial oral: 10 mg/d (see Comments) Maximum: 80 mg/d divided doses	See General Information for ACE-I	Labeled: Hypertension and HF	—See General Information for ACE-I —Neutropenia/ agranulocytosis	—Dual routes of elimination and may be useful in patients with significant renal dysfunction
Lisinopril (Zestril/ Prinivil)	Initial oral: 2.5 mg/d (see Comments) Maximum: 40 mg/d	See General Information for ACE-I	Labeled: Hypertension, HF, and post–MI	—See General Information for ACE-I —Abnormal taste —Neutropenia	—Not a prodrug —Reduce dose in patients with renal failure —Target dosage for HF: 20 mg/d —Generics are available
Moexipril (Univasc)	Initial oral: 7.5 mg/d (see Comments) Maximum: 30 mg/d divided doses	See General Information for ACE-I	Labeled: Hypertension	—See General Information for ACE-I —Abnormal taste —Neutropenia	—Food decreases extent of absorption —Reduce dose in patients with renal dysfunction
Perindopril (Aceon)	Initial oral: 4 mg/d (see Comments) Maximum: 16 mg/d	See General Information for ACE-I	Labeled: Essential hypertension	—See General Information for ACE-I	
Quinapril (Accupril)	Initial oral: 10 mg/d (see Comments) Maximum: 80 mg/d	See General Information for ACE-I	Labeled: Hypertension and HF agranulocytosis	—See General Information for ACE-I —Neutropenia/	—Reduce dose in patients with renal dysfunction —Target dosage for HF: 20 mg twice daily
Ramipril (Altace)	Initial oral: 2.5 mg/d (see Comments) Maximum: 10 mg/d divided doses	See General Information for ACE-I	Labeled: Hypertension, and symptomatic HF post-MI	—See General Information for ACE-I —Neutropenia/agranulocytosis	—Reduce dose in patients with renal dysfunction
Trandolapril (Mavik)	Initial oral: 1–2 mg/d (see Comments) Maximum: 8 mg/d divided doses	See General Information for ACE-I	Labeled: Hypertension	—See General Information for ACE-I	—Reduce dose in patients with hepatic and renal dysfunction

Angiotensin II Receptor Blockers					
General information		Selectively binds to the angiotensin II (AT1) receptor in vascular smooth muscle and in the adrenal cortex, thereby inhibiting the effects of angiotensin II		—Hypotension —Dizziness —Headache	—Use smaller initial doses in patients on diuretics or with suspected volume depletion —Contraindicated in pregnancy and bilateral renal artery stenosis or unilateral renal artery stenosis in patients with solitary kidney —Contraindicated in pregnancy
Candesartan (Atacand)	Initial oral: 16 mg/d Maximum: 32 mg /d	See General Information for angiotensin II receptor blockers	Labeled: Hypertension	—See General Information for angiotensin II receptor blockers	—See General Information for angiotensin II receptor blockers —Rare cases of angioedema have been reported with ARBs —Also available with hydrochlorothiazide
Eprosartan (Teveten)	Initial oral: 600 mg/d Maximum: 800 mg/d	See General Information for angiotensin II receptor blockers	Labeled: Hypertension	—See General Information for angiotensin II receptor blockers	—See General Information for angiotensin II receptor blockers —Rare cases of angioedema have been reported with ARBs —Also available with hydrochlorothiazide
Irbesartan (Avapro)	Initial oral: 150 mg/d	See General Information for angiotensin II receptor blockers	Labeled: Hypertension	See General Information for angiotensin II receptor blockers	—See General Information for angiotensin II receptor blockers —Adverse effects were greater with placebo in clinical trials than with irbesartan

(*continued*)

Drug	Dose	Mechanism of action	Indications	Side effects	Comments
	Maximum: 300 mg/d		Unlabeled: CHF in patients intolerant to ACE-I		—See General Information for angiotensin II receptor blockers —Rare cases of angioedema have been reported with ARBs —Also available with hydrochlorothiazide
Losartan (Cozaar)	Initial oral: 50 mg/d Maximum: 100 mg/d	See General Information for angiotensin II receptor blockers	Labeled: Hypertension Unlabeled: CHF in patients intolerant to ACE-I	—See General Information for angiotensin II receptor blockers —Hyperkalemia —Diarrhea —Dyspepsia —Insomnia	—Hepatotoxicity has been reported —Reduce dose in patients with hepatic dysfunction (25 mg/d) —Use lower initial doses in patients with suspected volume depletion or on diuretic therapy —E-3174 metabolite is 40 times as potent as losartan
Olmesartan (Benicar)	Initial oral: 20 mg/d Maximum: 40 mg/d	See General Information for angiotensin II receptor blockers	Labeled: Hypertension	—See General Information for angiotensin II receptor blockers	—See General Information for angiotensin II receptor blockers —Rare cases of angioedema have been reported with ARBs —Also available with hydrochlorothiazide
Telmisartan (Micardis)	Initial oral: 40 mg/d Maximum: 80 mg/d	See General Information for angiotensin II receptor blockers	Labeled: Hypertension	—See General Information for angiotensin II receptor blockers	—See General Information for angiotensin II receptor blockers —Rare cases of angioedema have been reported with ARBs —Also available with hydrochlorothiazide

Valsartan (Diovan)	Initial oral: 80 mg/d Maximum: 320 mg/d	See General Information for angiotensin II receptor blockers	Labeled: Hypertension and treatment of HF (NYHA class II–IV) in patients who cannot tolerate ACE inhibitors.	—See General Information for angiotensin II receptor blockers —Neutropenia has been reported	—See General Information for angiotensin II receptor blockers —Hepatotoxicity has been reported —Initiate therapy with lower doses in patients with hepatic dysfunction and in patients with CrCl <20–30 mL/min —Addition of valsartan to ACE-I has not been shown to improve outcomes —Rare cases of angioedema have been reported with ARBs —Also available with hydrochlorothiazide
Direct Renin Inhibitor					
Aliskiren (Tekturna)	Initial: 150 mg/d Maximum: 300 mg/d	Direct renin inhibitor preventing the conversion of angiotensinogen to angiotensin	Labeled: Hypertension	—Diarrhea —Angioedema —Hyperkalemia most common in diabetics on ACE-I	—Avoid in pregnancy —High-fat meals decrease absorption
Antiarrhythmics					
Class Ia General Information			Decrease phase 0 depolarization rate, slow intracardiac conduction, and prolong refractory period. Effects are associated with sodium and potassium channel blockade.	—Proarrhythmic —Torsade de pointes	—ECG effects: Prolongs QRS, QT, and (±) PR

(continued)

Drug	Dose	Mechanism of action	Indications	Side effects	Comments
Quinidine (Various)	Initial oral: 200–400 mg every 6–8 h	See General Information for class Ia antiarrhythmics	Labeled: Atrial fibrillation and flutter, ventricular arrhythmias	—Diarrhea	—May produce hypotension secondary to α-blocking activity
				—Nausea/vomiting/abdominal cramping —Rash —Hypotension —Fever —Cinchonism—tinnitus, blurred vision, headache, and/or delirium —Platelet-mediated thrombocytopenia —Lupus-like syndrome	—IV not recommended because of hypotension —Vagolytic effect may enhance AV nodal conduction —Each salt form has varying degrees of quinidine base: sulfate (83%), gluconate (62%), and polygalacturonate (60%) —Quinidine will increase digoxin levels and enhance warfarin's effect —Amiodarone will increase quinidine levels —Therapeutic range 2–6 mg/L

Procainamide (Pronestyl, Procan)	Initial oral: 50 mg/kg/d (normal renal function) *Immediate release:* give every 3–4 h *Sustained release:* give every 6–8 h Maximum: 9 g/d IV: Loading dose 14–17 mg/kg up to 1500 mg; infuse at 20 mg/min Maintenance: 2–4 mg/min	See General Information for class Ia antiarrhythmics	Labeled: Ventricular arrhythmias Unlabeled: Atrial arrhythmias	—Drug-induced SLE —GI symptoms —Hypotension (IV) —Rash —Insomnia/confusion —Chemical hepatitis (rare) —Myopathy —Agranulocytosis	—50%–85% of patients develop (+) ANA and 30%–50% will develop symptoms of SLE —Adjust dose in patients with renal dysfunction —50% eliminated renally —Hepatic elimination by acetylation: there are slow and fast acetylators —Slow acetylators are at higher risk for developing drug-induced SLE: fever, arthralgia, rash, pericarditis, and pleuritis —Heart block, bradycardia, and asystole may occur —Therapeutic range: procainamide 4–10 mg/L; NAPA <20 mg/L
Disopyramide (Norpace)	Initial oral Load: 300–400 mg	See General Information for class Ia antiarrhythmics	Labeled: Ventricular arrhythmias	—Dry mouth —Urinary retention —Constipation —Blurred vision	—Anticholinergic adverse effects limit its usefulness —Significant negative inotropic activity and may be useful in patients with hypertrophic obstructive cardiomyopathy

(*continued*)

Drug	Dose	Mechanism of action	Indications	Side effects	Comments
	Maintenance: Immediate release: 100–200 mg every 6 h Sustained release: 200–400 mg every 12 h Maximum: 1.6 g/d		Unlabeled: Atrial arrhythmias	—Hypotension —Nausea/vomiting —Heart block —Hypoglycemia —Nervousness	—Adjust dosage in patients with CHF, renal insufficiency, hepatic disease, and the elderly —May speed AV nodal conduction secondary to vagolytic effects —Therapeutic range 2–6 mg/L
Class Ib General Information		Decrease phase 0 depolarization rate and slow intracardiac conduction. Moderate sodium channel blocking activity. Shorten action potential duration and refractory period in ventricular tissue.		—Drowsiness —Slurred speech (perioral numbness) —Confusion/disorientation —Seizures —Paresthesias —Coma —Proarrhythmia —Tremor	—CNS side effects usually occur at levels >5mg/L: Seizures, coma, psychosis, tinnitus, tremor —ECG effects: no significant effects
Lidocaine (Xylocaine)	IV: Loading dose: 1–1.5 mg/kg given over 2 min; repeat every 5–10 min to a maximum of 3 mg/kg. Maintenance: 1–4 mg/min	See General Information for class Ib antiarrhythmics	Labeled: Acute treatment of ventricular arrhythmias	—See General Information for class Ib antiarrhythmics —Cardiac depression (with high levels) —Tinnitus —Bradycardia/asystole	—Metabolized in the liver and dependent on liver blood flow —Use lower maintenance doses in patients with HF and liver disease —Levels should be monitored with infusions lasting greater than 24 h and with signs and symptoms of toxicity

					—Acute phase reactant α-acid glycoprotein binds to lidocaine, and total lidocaine levels may be high with normal free lidocaine levels —Half-life may double after 24–48 h of continuous infusions —Therapeutic levels: 1.5–5 mg/L
Mexiletine (Mexitil)	Initial oral: 400 mg one time, then 200–300 mg every 8 h Maximum: 1200 mg/d	See General Information for class Ib antiarrhythmics	Labeled: Ventricular arrhythmias Unlabeled: Reducing pain associated with diabetic neuropathy	—See General Information for class Ib antiarrhythmics —Nausea/vomiting/anorexia —Thrombocytopenia (rare) —AV block	—CNS side effects similar to lidocaine. —Should be given with food to decrease GI side effects —40% of patients complain of minor CNS side effects —Commonly used with other antiarrhythmics —Reduce dose in patients with hepatic disease and CHF —Reduced dosages may be required in patients with CrCl $<$10 mL/min —Therapeutic levels: 0.5–2 mg/L
Class Ic General Information		Decrease phase 0 depolarization rate and slow intracardiac conduction. Velocity to the greatest degree. Most potent sodium channel blockers		—Bradycardia —Heart block —Proarrhythmia —Worsen HF —Dizziness	—ECG effects: Prolong PR interval and QRS complex; little to no effect on QT interval —Generally avoided in patients with structural heart disease because of increased mortality —May worsen HF

(*continued*)

Drug	Dose	Mechanism of action	Indications	Side effects	Comments
Flecainide (Tambocor)	Initial oral: 50 mg every 12 h Maximum: 300 mg/d Pill in Pocket: See comments	See General Information for class Ic antiarrhythmics	Labeled: Paroxysmal atrial fibrillation and flutter, paroxysmal supraventricular tachycardias (AVNRT), ventricular arrhythmias (see Comments)	—See General Information for class Ic antiarrhythmics —Significant (–) inotropy —Blurred vision —Headache —GI upset —Neutropenia	—Increases threshold for electrical defibrillation —Reduce dose in patients with HF, liver disease, or renal insufficiency —Therapeutic drug levels: 0.2–1 mg/L —Pill in Pocket: This dosing is for very select patients who convert to NSR after in-hospital dose testing. Patients may receive 300 mg if >70 kg or 200 mg if <70 kg once, if they revert to atrial fibrillation at home.
Propafenone (Rythmol)	Initial oral: 150 mg every 8 h Maximum: 1200 mg/d Initial SR dosing: 225 mg every 12 h Maximum SR dosing: 425 mg every 12 h	See General Information for class Ic antiarrhythmics	Labeled: Ventricular arrhythmias	—See General Information for class Ic antiarrhythmics —Metallic/bitter taste	—Exhibits β-blocking activity; therefore, may worsen asthma or obstructive lung disease

	Pill in Pocket See Comments		Unlabeled: Supraventricular arrhythmias	—Headache —GI upset —Cholestatic jaundice (rare)	—Reduce dose in patients with hepatic disease —Therapeutic drug levels not established] —Pill in Pocket: This dosing is for very select patients who convert to NSR after in-hospital dose testing. Patients may receive 600 mg if >70 kg or 450 mg if <70 kg once, if they revert to atrial fibrillation at home
Class II β-Blockers	See β-Blockers	See β-adrenergic antagonists	See β-Blockers	See β-Blockers	See β-Blockers
Class III Amiodarone (Cordarone)	Oral loading: 800–1600 mg/d for 1–3 wk, then 600–800 mg/d for 4 wk	Potassium channel blocker, sodium channel blocker, β-blocker activity, and calcium channel blocking activity	Labeled: Ventricular arrhythmias Unlabeled: Atrial arrhythmias	—Hyper/hypothyroidism —Chemical hepatitis —Pulmonary fibrosis —Bradycardia —Heart block	—ECG effect: Sinus bradycardia, prolong PR interval, QRS complex, and QT interval —IV administration may cause hypotension secondary to amiodarone's vasodilating effects as well as solubilizing agent Tween-80

(*continued*)

Drug	Dose	Mechanism of action	Indications	Side effects	Comments
	Oral maintenance: 100–400 mg/d IV: Initial 150 mg over 10 min, then 1 mg/min for 6 h, then 0.5 mg/min for 18 h			—Proarrhythmia —Torsade de pointes (rare) —Peripheral neuropathy —Tremor —Blue/gray skin discoloration —Photosensitivity —Corneal microdeposits —GI upset	—Long half-life range 25–100 d —Adverse effects may be prolonged after discontinuation because of long half-life —GI upset limits large oral doses —Desethylamiodarone active metabolite —Use lowest possible maintenance dose to limit toxicity —IV concentrations of >2 mg/mL may cause phlebitis Therapeutic drug levels: 1–2 mg/L
Dofetilide (Tikosyn)	Oral: Initial dose dependent on renal function:	Pure potassium channel blocker. Dofetilide blocks the inward K rectifier potassium channel, thereby prolonging refractory period of myocardial tissue.	Labeled:	—Proarrhythmia specifically torsade de pointes —Headache	—ECG effect: QTc prolongation

	Maintenance of normal sinus rhythm in patients with atrial fibrillation or flutter of more than 1 wk duration who have been converted to normal sinus rhythm. Because dofetilide can cause life-threatening ventricular arrhythmias, it should be reserved for patients in whom AF/AFL is highly symptomatic Dofetilide is indicated for the conversion of AF and AFL to NSR.	—Contraindicated medications include: cimetidine, hydrochlorothiazide, ketoconazole, itraconazole, megestrol, prochlorperazine, trimethoprim, and verapamil, as well as medications that prolong QT interval —Baseline QTC should be ≤440 msec in patients without ventricular conduction abnormalities or ≤500 msec in patients with ventricular conduction abnormalities.

(*continued*)

Drug	Dose	Mechanism of action	Indications	Side effects	Comments
	Calculated CrCl (mL/min) — *Dofetilide Dose* >60 — 500 μg twice daily 40–60 — 250 μg twice daily 20–39 — 125 μg twice daily <20 — CONTRAINDICATED Subsequent dosing will depend on the degree of QTc prolongation (see Comments)				—ECG should be obtained 2–3 h post dose (peak plasma concentrations) to determine effect on QTc interval. If QTc prolongs >15% of baseline or if QTc >500 msec (550 msec in patients with ventricular conduction abnormalities) after the first dose, then decrease the dose by half —Prolongations in QTc of >15% of baseline, or if QTc >500 msec (550 msec in patients with ventricular conduction abnormalities) after second and subsequent doses, the drug should be discontinued —Only facilities that have received adequate education and only physicians who have registered with the company can dispense or prescribe dofetilide —A 72-h admission for initiating therapy is required

Ibutilide (Corvert)	IV: For patients >60 kg, 1 mg infused over 10 min followed by another 1-mg infusion over 10 min, if patient did not convert to NSR infusion, separated by 10 min	—Increase sodium influx —May block potassium channels —Exact mechanism is controversial	Labeled: Conversion of atrial fibrillation or flutter	—Proarrhythmia —1.7% risk of inducing ventricular arrhythmias requiring cardioversion —Torsade de pointes	—ECG effect: Prolongs QT interval —Patients must be off all medications that prolong the QT interval for at least 5 half-lives before receiving ibutilide
	Patients <60 kg give: 0.01 mg/kg in the same fashion as above			—AV block	—Monitor patient for at least 4 h or until QT interval normalizes, whichever is longer —Correct serum magnesium and potassium levels before initiating therapy —Therapeutic drug levels not useful
Sotalol (Betapace)	Initial oral: 80 mg every 12 h (see Comments)	Potassium channel blocker and β-blocker	Labeled: Ventricular arrhythmias	—See General Information for β-blockers —Proarrhythmia	—ECG effect: Sinus bradycardia, prolongs QT and PR interval —See General Information for β-adrenergic antagonists
	Maximum: 320 mg/d in divided doses		Unlabeled: Atrial fibrillation	—Torsade de pointes	—Reduce dose in patients with renal dysfunction —High incidence of proarrhythmic effect —Limit QT-interval prolongation to <550 msec —Therapeutic drug levels: not clinically useful

(*continued*)

Drug	Dose	Mechanism of action	Indications	Side effects	Comments
Class IV General information		Prolong AV nodal refractory period			—ECG effects: Prolongs PR interval and sinus bradycardia —Avoid in patients with WPW and atrial fibrillation
Diltiazem (Cardizem)	IV: Loading dose: 0.25 mg/kg given over 2 min; if no response in 5–10 min then repeat loading dose with 0.35 mg/kg (see diltiazem under calcium channel blockers Maintenance: 5–15 mg/h	See General Information for class IV antiarrhythmics	See diltiazem under calcium channel blockers	See diltiazem under calcium channel blockers	See diltiazem under calcium channel blockers
Verapamil (Various)	IV: 2.5–10 mg given over 2 min may repeat 10-mg dose at 30 min Maximum: 20 mg Maintenance: 5–10 mg/h continuous infusion	See General Information for class IV antiarrhythmics	See verapamil under calcium channel blockers	See verapamil under calcium channel blockers	See verapamil under calcium channel blockers —Use lower doses in elderly patients

Others					
Adenosine (Adenocard)	IV: 6 mg rapid IV push; if no response, 12 mg rapid IV push; if no response, may repeat once	α_1 receptor agonist leading to depression of AV nodal conduction and SA node firing tachycardia	Labeled: Conversion of paroxysmal supraventricular	—Facial flushing —Shortness of breath —Chest pressure —Nausea —Arrhythmias —May provoke bronchospasm in asthmatic patients	—Doses should be given at most proximal point to the patient —Follow each dose with a 10–20 mL NS flush —May decrease dose if giving through a central catheter —Half-life about 9 s —Patients taking methylxanthine may not respond —May produce transient asystole
Digoxin (Lanoxin)	IV: Load: 10–15 μ/kg: 50% given initially, then 25% in 6 h and 25% 6 h after second dose (see Comments) Maintenance: 0.0625–0.5 mg/d depending on renal function and patient size	Increases AV nodal refractory period secondary to increase in vagal tone and sympathetic withdrawal	Labeled: HF slows ventricular response in patients with atrial fibrillation/flutter and paroxysmal atrial tachycardia	—Bradycardia —AV block —Anorexia —Nausea —Diarrhea —Abdominal pain —Blurred vision —Yellow/green halo around light —Confusion —Proarrhythmia	—ECG effects: Prolongs PR interval, depresses ST segment, and flattens T wave —Use lower loading doses in the elderly and in patients with uremia —Bioavailability of oral tablets is 70%; therefore, patients may require less if given IV digoxin —Many of the side effects are signs of digoxin toxicity

(*continued*)

Drug	Dose	Mechanism of action	Indications	Side effects	Comments
					—Effects are diminished with increased sympathetic tone —Therapeutic drug levels: 1–2 ng/mL —Toxicity may be seen in patients with therapeutic levels
Anticoagulants *direct thrombin inhibitor*					
Argatroban (Argatroban)	HIT/HITTs: Initial dose: 2 μg/kg/min infusion Maximum: 10 μg/kg/min PCI dosing: Initial bolus: 350 μg/kg given over 3–5 min Initial maintenance infusion: 25 μg/kg/min Check ACT in 5–10 min	Direct thrombin inhibitor. Directly and reversibly binds to the active site of thrombin	Labeled: An anticoagulant for prophylaxis or management of thrombosis in patients with heparin-induced thrombocytopenia and as an anticoagulant in patients with or at risk for heparin-induced thrombocytopenia undergoing PCI	—Bleeding —Hypotension —Nausea —Vomiting —Fever	—Patients with moderate to severe hepatic dysfunction require dosage adjustments, and an initial dose of 0.5 μg/kg/min should be used in patients with HIT/HITTs —No need to adjust for renal failure —Monitor with aPTT 2 h after initiation or infusion and 2 h after dosage adjustments. Goal aPTT is 1.5 to 3 times control

If ACT <300 s then rebolus with 150 μg/kg and increase rate by 5 μg/kg min If the ACT is >450 s, the infusion rate should be decreased to 15 μg/kg/min, and the ACT checked 5–10 min later ACT should be monitored throughout the procedure	—Argatroban will elevate INR. When initiating warfarin therapy discontinue argatroban when INR is >4 and recheck INR 4–6 h later. If subtherapeutic then restart argatroban —No reversal agent available —Consider using lower initial doses in patients with hepatic congestion

(*continued*)

Drug	Dose	Mechanism of action	Indications	Side effects	Comments
Bivalirudin (Angiomax)	PTCA without stenting Initial bolus: 1 mg/kg bolus given rapidly. Maintenance infusion: 2.5 mg/kg/h for 4 h If continued anticoagulation after 4 h is needed, then decrease the infusion dose to 0.2 mg/kg/h for 20 h (see Comments)	Direct thrombin inhibitor Directly and reversibly binds to thrombin's active site and exosite 2, thereby inactivating its activity.	Labeled: Anticoagulant in patients with unstable angina undergoing percutaneous transluminal coronary angioplasty	—Bleeding	—Renally clean and infusion doses should be adjusted with long-term administration —Half-life is about 25 min; however, increase to 3.5 h in patients with creatinine clearance <10 mL/min —As compared to glycoprotein IIb/IIIa inhibitors and heparin during PCI; Bivalirudin in patients with low to moderate risk had similar outcomes with fewer bleeding episodes; patients with low to moderate risk had similar outcomes with fewer bleeding episodes
	REPLACE 2 Initial bolus: 0.75 mg/kg given rapidly		Unlabeled: Anticoagulant in patients undergoing PCI with stent placement		—Current studies are evaluating the use of bivalirudin in patients with HIT and undergoing bypass surgery

	Maintenance infusion: 1.75 mg/kg/h for the duration of procedure (see Comments)				—No reversal agent available —Reduce maintenance infusion in patients with renal insufficiency
Lepirudin (rDNA) (Refludan)	IV Loading dose: 0.4 mg/kg over 15–20 s	Directly and irreversibly binds to thrombin, inactivating its activity	Labeled: Anticoagulation in patients with heparin-induced thrombocytopenia and associated thromboembolic disease	—Bleeding —Abnormal liver function	—Monitor aPTT to goal of 1.5–2.5 above control
	Maintenance infusion: 0.15 mg/kg/h (see Comments)			—Rash —Cough/bronchospasm/ dyspnea	—Reduce dose in patients with CrCl <60 mL/min or serum creatinine >1.5 mg/dL (refer to package insert); avoid when CrCl <10 mL/min —No reversal agent bleeding complications
	Dose is dependent on renal function and lower bolus, and initial infusion doses should be used.			—Anaphylaxis	—7 cases of anaphylaxis have been reported. In 6 cases patients had received lepirudin in the past. Of the 7 patients with anaphylaxis, 5 died. Routine readministration of lepirudin should be done cautiously, or use an alternative agent

(*continued*)

Drug	Dose	Mechanism of action	Indications	Side effects	Comments
	Continuous infusion should be avoided in patients with a creatinine clearance <10 mL/min				—Expensive ($500–700/d) —Limited data are available for subcutaneous administration for managing DVT
Heparin (Various)	Various dosing regimens	Binds to antithrombin III, increasing its ability to inactive thrombin, as well as activated factors IX, X, XI, XII	Labeled: Management and prophylaxis of venous and arterial thrombosis	—Bleeding —Thrombocytopenia (see Comments) —Elevated AST/ALT —Osteoporosis (long-term therapy) —Hyperkalemia	—Heparin-induced thrombocytopenia occurs in two forms: antibody mediated and non–antibody mediated —10%–15% of patients will have lower platelet levels —1%–3 % of those with heparin-associated thrombocytopenia will go on to develop antibody-mediated HIT
Fondaparinux (Arixtra)	2.5 mg subcutaneously every 24 h starting 6–8 h after surgery once hemostasis has occurred. Duration of therapy is generally 5–9 d	Binds antithrombin III, leading to selective inhibition of activated factor X (factor Xa). It has no effects on thrombin (factor IIa)	Labeled: DVT prophylaxis in patients undergoing hip fracture surgery, hip replacement surgery, and knee replacement surgery	—Bleeding —Rash and pruritus at injection site —Mild elevation in serum aminotransferases —Thrombocytopenia	—Avoid use in patients with impaired renal function (CrCl <30 mL/min) —Avoid use in patients with body weight <50 kg —Half-life between 17 and 21 h —No reversal agent available —Fondaparinux reaches maximum antifactor Xa activity 3 h after injection

Low–Molecular-Weight Heparin (LMWH)					
General information		Antifactor Xa activity greater than antithrombin activity; however, each LMWH has different degrees of antifactor Xa/IIa ratios		—Bleeding —Thrombocytopenia —Rash —Hematoma at injection site —Fever	—LMWH, have a different antifactor Xa/IIa ratio and are not considered interchangeable —LMWH, produce less HIT —Patients with heparin-induced thrombocytopenia secondary to unfractionated heparin have a high cross-reactivity to LMWH (up to 90%). Therefore, avoid use in patients with HIT or suspected HIT —LMWH are renally cleared and are either contraindicated in patients with severe renal insufficiency or used with extreme caution
Dalteparin (Fragmin)	DVT Prophylaxis: *Abdominal surgery:* 2500 IU subcutaneously starting 1–2 h before surgery, then give 2500 IU subcutaneously once daily ***or*** abdominal surgery associated with a high risk of thromboembolic	See General Information for LMWH	Labeled: —Prophylaxis against DVT in patients at high risk for thromboembolic complications undergoing abdominal surgery and those having hip replacement surgery —Prophylaxis of ischemic complications in patients with unstable angina non-Q-wave MI	See General Information for LMWH	—Renal elimination primary route of elimination

(*continued*)

Drug	Dose	Mechanism of action	Indications	Side effects	Comments
	complications: 5000 IU subcutaneously the evening before surgery, then daily postoperatively ***or*** 2500 IU 1–2 h before surgery, then 2500 IU 12 h later, then 5000 IU once daily **Hip replacement surgery dosing options:** ***Postoperative initiation:*** 2500 IU subcutaneously starting 4–8 h after surgery once hemostasis is achieved, then 5000 IU subcutaneously daily				

Preoperative initiation

Option 1:

Day of surgery give 2500 IU subcutaneously within 2 h before surgery, then give 2500 IU subcutaneously starting 4–8 h after surgery once hemostasis is achieved, then 5000 IU subcutaneously daily

Option 2:

Evening before surgery give 5000 IU subcutaneously (10–14 h before surgery), then give 5000 IU subcutaneously starting 4–8 h after surgery once hemostasis is achieved, then 5000 IU subcutaneously daily

(*continued*)

Drug	Dose	Mechanism of action	Indications	Side effects	Comments
	Unstable angina/Non-Q wave MI: 120 IU/kg (10,000 IU maximum) subcutaneously every 12 h for 5–8 d				
Enoxaparin (Lovenox)	**DVT Prophylaxis: *Hip or knee replacement surgery:*** 30 mg subcutaneously every 12 h beginning 12–24 h postoperatively once hemostasis has been achieved; may be given up to 14 d ***Hip replacement surgery Option 2:*** 40 mg subcutaneously 12 h before surgery, then 40 mg once daily for 3 wk	See General Information for LMWH	Labeled: DVT prophylaxis —Hip replacement surgery —Knee replacement surgery —Abdominal surgery —Medical patients due to severely restricted mobility during acute illness DVT treatment —Inpatient treatment of DVT with or without PE in conjunction with warfarin	See General Information for LMWH	—Highest antifactor Xa/IIa ratio —Contraindicated in patients with a creatinine clearance less than 30 mL/min —Little dosing data have been obtained in extremely obese patients; should be tried cautiously —Reduce dose in patients with creatinine clearance <30 mL/min

Abdominal surgery: 40 mg subcutaneously daily initial dose given 2 h before surgery	—Outpatient treatment of DVT in patients without PE in conjunction with warfarin Treatment of unstable angina/non-Q-wave MI (NSTEMI) when given with aspirin
Medical patients during acute illness: 40 mg subcutaneously once daily **DVT treatment:** ***Inpatient management of DVT with or without PE:*** 1 mg/kg subcutaneously every 12 h or 1.5 mg/kg subcutaneously once daily ***Outpatient management of DVT without PE:*** 1 mg/kg subcutaneously every 12 h	

(*continued*)

Drug	Dose	Mechanism of action	Indications	Side effects	Comments
	Unstable angina/non-Q-wave MI: 1 mg/kg subcutaneously every 12 h for 2–8 d				
Tinzaparin (Innohep)	DVT management dosing: 175 anti-Xa IU/kg given subcutaneously once daily for 6d or until patient is on warfarin	See General Information for LMWH	Labeled: In-hospital treatment of symptomatic DVT with or without PE in conjunction with warfarin	See General Information for LMWH	—Kidney is the major route of elimination and should be used cautiously in patients with moderate to severe renal dysfunction. Accumulation of the drug will occur in these patients and may increase the risk of bleeding
Oral Anticoagulants					
General information		Indirect-acting anticoagulants by altering the synthesis of coagulation factors II, VII, IX, X, by interfering with vitamin K utilization		—Bleeding —Skin necrosis —Purple-toe syndrome —Dermatitis —Cholesterol microembolization —Alopecia	—Avoid large initial doses to reduce risk of hemorrhage and necrosis secondary to the initial decrease in proteins C and S —Maintain INR between 2–3 for most indications except for mechanical heart valves where the range is 2.5–3.5 —Contraindications: Pregnancy, severe uncontrolled hypertension, unreliable patients, hemorrhage tendencies —In addition to PT/INR, monitor for evidence of bleeding or bruising and hemoglobin and hematocrit

Warfarin (Coumadin)	Initial oral: see Comments	See General Information for oral anticoagulants	Labeled: Provide management of and prophylaxis for DVT and PE, thromboembolic complications of AF, and cardiac valve replacement, and reduce the risk of death, recurrent MI, and thromboembolic events after MI	See General Information for oral anticoagulants	—Initiating warfarin therapy is variable; however, 5–10 mg/d is typical —Patients with malabsorption syndromes may require higher doses of warfarin —Numerous drug–drug and food–drug interactions
β-Adrenergic antagonists					
General information		β-Receptor blockade		—Bradycardia —Bronchospasm in predisposed patients —CHF exacerbation —Dizziness —Fatigue —Depression —Sleep disturbances —Hypotension —Sexual dysfunction —Dyslipidemia	—Contraindications: bradycardia, greater than first-degree heart block, cardiogenic shock, acute HF, asthma, or severe bronchospastic lung disease —β-Blockers possess a high degree of interpatient variability between dose and effect —β_1-Selective β-blockers lose selectivity with high doses —Abrupt withdrawal of β-blockers may cause rebound hypertension and may precipitate angina in patients with CAD —β-Blockers blunt hypoglycemic reactions —β-Blockers have produced profound hypertension in patients abruptly withdrawing from clonidine

(*continued*)

Drug	Dose	Mechanism of action	Indications	Side effects	Comments
Acebutolol (Sectral)	Initial oral: 200 mg 1–2 times daily Maximum: 1200 mg/d	β_1-Selective adrenergic blocker with intrinsic sympathomimetic and membrane-stabilizing activity	Labeled: Hypertension and ventricular premature complexes	—See General Information for β-adrenergic blockers	—Resting heart rate will be increased because of intrinsic sympathomimetic activity
Atenolol (Tenormin)	Initial oral: 25 mg/d (see Comments) Maximum: 200 mg/d	β_1-Selective adrenergic blocker Hypertension,	Labeled: information for angina pectoris and MI		—Adjust dose in patients with renal insufficiency —Lower incidence of CNS adverse effects because of low penetration into CNS
	IV (see Comments) Acute MI 5 mg IV over 5 min, then repeat in 10 min, then start oral therapy		Unlabeled: Supraventricular arrhythmias, ventricular arrhythmias, migraine headache prophylaxis, alcohol withdrawal, anxiety, esophageal varices rebleeding		
Betaxolol (Kerlone)	Initial oral: 10 mg/d	β_1-Selective adrenergic blocker with intrinsic sympathomimetic activity	Labeled: Hypertension	—See General Information for β-adrenergic blockers	—Usually seen as eye drops —Systemic effects may be seen with ophthalmic administration

Bisoprolol (Zebeta)	Maximum: 40 mg/d Initial oral: 2.5–5 mg/d Maximum: 20 mg/d	β_1-Selective adrenergic blocker	Labeled: Hypertension Unlabeled: Angina pectoris, supraventricular arrhythmias, ventricular premature complexes	—See General Information for β-adrenergic blockers	—Adjust dose in patients with renal dysfunction
Carteolol (Cartrol)	Initial oral: 2.5 mg/d Maximum: 10 mg/d	Nonselective β-adrenergic blocker with intrinsic sympathomimetic activity	Labeled: Hypertension Unlabeled: Angina pectoris	—See General Information for β-adrenergic blockers	—Adjust dose in patients with renal dysfunction
Esmolol (Brevibloc)	IV: Loading dose 500 μg/kg over 1 min Maintenance dose: 25–300 μg/kg/min Titrate by 25–50 μg/kg/min every 5–10 min. Some patients may need a second 500 μg/kg load during titration phase	β_1-Selective adrenergic blocker	Labeled: Supraventricular arrhythmias and sinus tachycardia Unlabeled: Angina pectoris and as adjunctive therapy for acute aortic dissection	—See General Information for β-adrenergic blockers —Nausea —Vomiting —Inflammation and induration at injection site commonly occurs —Extravasation may cause skin necrosis	—Half-life = 9 min —Metabolized in blood via red blood cell esterases to active and inactive metabolites —Active metabolites may accumulate in patients with significant renal impairment —IV concentrations should not exceed 10 mg/mL
Metoprolol (Lopressor)	Initial oral: 25–50 mg twice daily	β_1-Selective adrenergic blocker	Labeled: Hypertension, angina pectoris, and MI	—See General Information for β-adrenergic blockers	

(*continued*)

Drug	Dose	Mechanism of action	Indications	Side effects	Comments
	Maximum: 450 mg/d IV: Acute MI, 5 mg every 2 min for 3 doses		Unlabeled: Ventricular arrhythmias, supraventricular arrhythmias, migraine prophylaxis, essential tremor, aggressive behavior, antipsychotic-induced akathisia, stable CHF		
Nadolol (Corgard)	Initial oral: 40 mg/d Maximum: 320 mg/d	Nonselective β-adrenergic blocker	Labeled: Hypertension and angina pectoris Unlabeled: Ventricular arrhythmias, migraine prophylaxis, essential tremor, lithium-induced tremor, Parkinsonian tremor, aggressive behavior, antipsychotic-induced-akathisia, esophageal varices rebleeding, anxiety, decreased intraocular pressure	—See General Information for β-adrenergic blockers	—Adjust dose in patients with renal dysfunction

Penbutolol (Levatol)	Initial oral: 20 mg/d Maximum: 80 mg/d	Nonselective β-adrenergic blocker with intrinsic sympathomimetic activity	Labeled: Hypertension	—See General Information for β-adrenergic blockers	—High lipid solubility leads to increased CNS penetration and depression —Systemic effects may be seen with ophthalmic administration
Pindolol (Visken)	Initial oral: 5 mg twice daily Maximum: 60 mg/d	Nonselective β-adrenergic blocker with intrinsic sympathomimetic and membrane-stabilizing activity	Labeled: Hypertension Unlabeled: Ventricular arrhythmias, anxiety, antipsychotic-induced akathisia	—See General Information for β-adrenergic blockers	—Adjust dose in patients with severe renal and/or hepatic dysfunction
Propranolol (Inderal)	Initial oral: 10 mg 3–4 times daily Maximum: 480 mg/d	Nonselective β-adrenergic blocker with membrane-stabilizing activity	Labeled: Hypertension, angina pectoris, supraventricular and ventricular arrhythmias, digitalis-induced tachyarrhythmias, MI, pheochromocytoma, migraine prophylaxis, hypertrophic obstructive cardiomyopathy, essential tremor	—See General Information for β-adrenergic blockers	—IV dose is much smaller than oral dose because of high first-pass effect —Oral dosage form available as immediate-release, sustained-release formulation, and oral solution

(*continued*)

Drug	Dose	Mechanism of action	Indications	Side effects	Comments
	IV (see Comments): 1 mg slow IV push 2–10 min given every 5 min to a maximum of 0.15 mg/kg				—High lipid solubility leads to increased CNS penetration and depression —Adjust dosage downward in patients with liver dysfunction and in geriatric patients
			Unlabeled: Alcohol withdrawal, esophageal varices rebleeding, anxiety, acute panic disorders, thyrotoxicosis		
Timolol	Initial oral:	Nonselective β-adrenergic blocker	Labeled: Hypertension, ventricular arrhythmias, MI, glaucoma	—See General Information for β-adrenergic blockers	—Systemic effects may be seen with ophthalmic administration
(Blocadren)	10 mg twice daily Maximum: 60 mg/d				
			Unlabeled: Migraine prophylaxis, essential tremor, anxiety		

Beta/Alpha Antagonists					
Carvedilol (Coreg)	Initial oral: CHF: 3.125 mg twice daily (see Comments) HTN: 6.25 mg twice daily Maximum: CHF: 50 mg twice daily HTN: 50 mg/d	Nonselective β-adrenergic blocker and α_1-adenergic blocker	Labeled: Mild to moderate (NYHA class II-III) HF, essential hypertension	—See General Information for β-adrenergic blockers	—Patients with CHF should be started on carvedilol only after stabilization on ACE-I, diuretics, and/or digitalis —CHF: dose should be titrated no sooner than every 2 weeks to maximum tolerated doses. Patients weighing <85 kg maximum dose is 25 mg twice daily. —Carvedilol is available in controlled release formulation: Carvedilol CR Coreg to Coreg CR conversion: Coreg 3.125 mg every 12 h — Coreg CR 10 mg/d Coreg 6.25 mg every 12 h — Coreg CR 20 mg/d Coreg 12.5 mg every 12 h — Coreg CR 40 mg/d Coreg 25 mg every 12 h — Coreg CR 80 mg/d
Labetalol (Normodyne/ Trandate)	Initial oral: 100 mg twice daily Maximum: 2400 mg/d IV dosing: *Multiple injection method* 20 mg IV push over 2 min may repeat every 10 min to a cumulative dose of 300 mg	Nonselective β-adrenergic blocker and α_1-adrenergic blocker	Labeled: Hypertension Unlabeled: Hypertensive crisis, pheochromocytoma, acute aortic dissection, clonidine withdrawal hypertension	—See General Information for β-adrenergic blockers	—May be effective as a single agent in patients with acute aortic dissection —IV labetalol has 7:1 β-to-α activity, whereas oral labetalol has 3:1 β-to-α activity —Because of long half-life, labetalol is not recommended as a continuous infusion

(*continued*)

Drug	Dose	Mechanism of action	Indications	Side effects	Comments
	Intermittent infusion method Initiate dose at 2 mg/min until satisfactory response, then discontinue infusion to a maximum of 300 mg; may repeat when blood pressure begins to rise				
Calcium channel blockers					
Dihydropyridine					
General information		Blocks calcium channels in vascular smooth muscle-producing vasodilatation of peripheral and coronary arteries. Reflex increases in sympathetic tone negates the effects on SA and AV nodal conduction		—Peripheral edema —Flushing —Headache —Dizziness —Rash —Hypotension	—It is no longer recommended to use immediate-release dihydropyridine calcium channel blockers to acutely lower blood pressure because of potential for inducing stroke and MI. Also, large doses of short-acting calcium channel blockers *may* increase risk of MI —Calcium channel blockers have many drug interactions because of hepatic metabolism
Amlodipine (Norvasc)	Initial oral: 2.5 mg/d Maximum: 10 mg/d	See General Information for dihydropyridine calcium channel blockers	Labeled: Hypertension and stable and vasospastic angina	See General Information for dihydropyridine calcium channel blockers	—Reduce dose in patients with hepatic dysfunction

Felodipine (Plendil)	Initial oral: 5 mg/d Maximum: 40 mg/d	See General Information for dihydropyridine calcium channel blockers	Labeled: Hypertension	See General Information for dihydropyridine calcium channel blockers	—Reduce dose in patients with hepatic dysfunction —Grapefruit juice increases bioavailability and should be avoided
Isradipine (DynaCirc)	Initial oral: 2.5 mg twice daily Maximum: 20 mg/d	See General Information for dihydropyridine calcium channel blockers	Labeled: Hypertension	See General Information for dihydropyridine calcium channel blockers	—Doses greater than 10 mg/d add no benefit
Nicardipine (Cardene)	Initial oral: 20 mg twice daily Maximum: 120 mg/d	See General Information for dihydropyridine calcium channel blockers	Labeled: Hypertension (immediate and sustained release and IV) and stable angina (immediate release only)	See General Information for dihydropyridine calcium channel blockers	—Consider lower initial doses in patients with hepatic dysfunction
Nifedipine (Procardia, Adalat)	Initial oral: 10 mg three times daily Maximum: 180 mg/d (see Comments)	See General Information for dihydropyridine calcium channel blockers	Labeled: Hypertension and vasospastic angina (sustained release only) Unlabeled: Migraine headache prophylaxis, primary pulmonary hypertension, lower esophageal sphincter spasm	See General Information for dihydropyridine calcium channel blockers —Gingival hyperplasia (rare)	—Reduce dose in patients with cirrhosis —Grapefruit juice increases bioavailability and should be avoided
Nisoldipine (Sular)	Initial oral: 20 mg/d Maximum: 60 mg/d	See General Information for dihydropyridine calcium channel blockers	Labeled: Hypertension	See General Information for dihydropyridine calcium channel blockers	—Grapefruit and high-fat meals increase bioavailability and should be avoided —Reduce dose in patients with hepatic dysfunction

(*continued*)

Drug	Dose	Mechanism of action	Indications	Side effects	Comments
Benzothiazepine					
Diltiazem (Cardizem, Dilacor)	Initial oral: 30 mg three times daily Maximum: 360 mg/d (See diltiazem under antiarrhythmics for IV dosing)	Calcium channel blockade produces vasodilation of coronary and peripheral arteries as well as decreasing heart rate and prolonging AV nodal conduction	Labeled: Hypertension angina and supraventricular arrhythmias	—Negative inotropic —Headache —Flushing —Dizziness —Edema —Bradycardia —AV block —Hypotension	—Avoid patients with WPW and atrial fibrillation —Consider reduced doses in patients with hepatic dysfunction
Diphenyl alkylamine					
Verapamil (Calan, Isoptin)	Initial oral: 80 mg three times daily Maximum: 480 mg/d	Calcium channel blockade produces vasodilation of coronary and peripheral arteries as well as decreasing heart rate and prolonging AV nodal conduction	Labeled: Hypertension, angina, supraventricular arrhythmias Unlabeled: Migraine and cluster headache prophylaxis, exercise-induced asthma, hypertrophic obstructive cardiomyopathy; nocturnal leg cramps	—Negative inotropic —Constipation —Hypotension —Bradycardia —AV block	—Avoid in patients with WPW and atrial fibrillation —Consider reduced doses in patients with hepatic dysfunction

Miscellaneous					
Bepridil (Vascor)	Initial oral: 200 mg/d Maximum: 400 mg/d	Type 4 calcium channel blocker, has properties similar to typical calcium channel blockers, and may inhibit fast sodium channels	Labeled: Stable angina	—Dizziness —Headache —Nausea/dyspepsia/ abdominal pain/anorexia —Weakness —Bradycardia —Nervousness —Diarrhea —Torsade de pointes	—Causes QT prolongation —Many patients cannot tolerate side effects —Reserved for patients who are either intolerant or maximized to other antianginals —Data is lacking for dosage adjustments in patients with hepatic dysfunction
Diuretics					
Loop					
General Information		Block chloride reabsorption in the ascending loop of Henle, sodium, and water then follow	See individual agent	—Decreases serum electrolytes: K, Cl, Mg, Ca, phosphate, Na —Ototoxicity —Tinnitus —Hyperuricemia —Hyperglycemia —Rash —Azotemia —Dyslipidemia	—Loop diuretic gain access to the lumen of the nephron by organic acid pump and do not rely on glomerular filtration —Overdiuresis may cause a hypochloremic metabolic alkalosis —Additive ototoxic effects when loop diuretics are added to other ototoxic drugs
Bumetanide (Bumex)	Initial oral: 0.5 mg 1–2 times daily Maximum: 10 mg/d	See General Information for loop diuretics	Labeled: Edema	—See General Information for loop diuretics	—Onset 10–30 min —IV Furosemide: bumetanide ratio is 40:1 —IV PO conversion 1:1 —IV doses up to 0.5–1 mg should be given over 1–2 min

(*continued*)

Drug	Dose	Mechanism of action	Indications	Side effects	Comments
	IV: 0.5–1 mg to a maximum of 10 mg/d				—IV doses 3–5 mg should be given over 10 min —IV doses >5 mg should be infused at 0.25 mg/min to reduce risk of ototoxicity —Continuous infusions of bumetanide have been used —Contains a sulfhydryl group, and patients allergic to sulfonamides may have a cross-reaction
Ethacrynic acid (Edecrin)	Initial oral: 50 mg/d Maximum: 400 mg/d IV: 50 mg or 0.5–1 mg/kg to a maximum of 100 mg/d; infuse over several minutes	See General Information for loop diuretics	Labeled: Edema	—See General Information for loop diuretics	—Onset within 30 min —Safest alternative in patients allergic to bumetanide, furosemide, torsemide, or thiazides, because it contains no sulfhydryl group —50 mg of IV ethacrynic acid, approximately 35 mg furosemide, approximately 1 mg bumetanide —Give IV doses slowly to limit ototoxicity

Furosemide (Lasix)	Initial oral: 20 mg 1–3 times daily Maximum: 480 mg/d (see Comments) IV: Variable doses >120 mg should be infused at 4 mg/min	See General Information for loop diuretics	Labeled: Edema and hypertension Unlabeled: Hypercalcemia	—See General Information for loop diuretics	—To limit ototoxicity doses, >120 mg should be infused at 4 mg/min —IV PO conversion 1:2 —Bioavailability may be decreased in patients with CHF —IV Furosemide bumetanide ratio is 40:1 —IV continuous infusions may be beneficial in certain patients. Initiate infusion at 10 mg/h to a maximum dose of 40 mg/h —Contains a sulfhydryl group, and patients allergic to sulfonamides may have a cross-reaction
Torsemide (Demadex)	Initial oral: 5 mg/d Maximum: 200 mg/d IV: 10–20 mg but variable Give IV doses over 2 min	See General Information for loop diuretics	Labeled: Edema and hypertension	—See General Information for loop diuretics	—5–10 mg torsemide; approximately 20 mg IV furosemide —IV PO conversion 1:1 —Bioavailability similar in healthy individuals when compared to patients with CHF —Contains a sulfhydryl group, and patients allergic to sulfonamides may have a cross-reaction

(*continued*)

Drug	Dose	Mechanism of action	Indications	Side effects	Comments
Diuretics ***Thiazide and thiazide-like diuretics***					
General information		Interfere with sodium ion transport in the distal convoluted tubule with chloride and water excretion being enhanced	Labeled: Edema and hypertension Unlabeled: Diabetes insipidus, prophylaxis of renal calculus associated with hypercalcemia	—Decreases in serum electrolytes: K, Mg, Cl, Na —Decreases calcium and uric acid levels —Dehydration —Rash —Hypersensitivity reactions —Dyslipidemia —Hyperglycemia —Hematologic abnormalities (rare) —Photosensitivity	—Thiazides are not effective in patients with CrCl <30 mL/min —Patients allergic to sulfonamide-derived drugs may be allergic to thiazide diuretics —Recommended first-line therapy for hypertension —Synergistic diuresis when added to loop diuretics —Avoid use in patients with elevated serum calcium levels and in disease states that increase serum calcium levels
Chlorothiazide	Initial oral: 500 mg 1–2 times daily Maximum: 2000 mg/d IV: 250–1000 mg 1–2 times daily	See General Information for thiazide and thiazide-like diuretics	See General Information for thiazide and thiazide-like diuretics	See General Information for thiazide and thiazide-like diuretics	—Only thiazide available for intravenous administration

Chlorthalidone (Hygroton)	Initial oral: 25 mg/d Maximum: 100 mg/d	See General Information for thiazide and thiazide-like diuretics	See General Information for thiazide and thiazide-like diuretics	See General Information for thiazide and thiazide-like diuretics	—Thiazide-like diuretic —Doses >25 mg rarely improve diuresis —Recent data from the ALL-HAT trial determined that chlorthalidone should be considered as first-line therapy in patients with hypertension
Hydro-chlorothiazide (Hydro-Diuril)	Initial oral: 12.5–25 mg/d Maximum: 50 mg/d	See General Information for thiazide and thiazide-like diuretics	See General Information for thiazide and thiazide-like diuretics	See General Information for thiazide and thiazide-like diuretics	—See General Information under Comments for thiazides and like diuretics
Indapamide (Lozol)	Initial oral: 1.25–2.5 mg/d Maximum: 5 mg/d	See General Information for thiazide and thiazide-like diuretics	See General Information for thiazide and thiazide-like diuretics	See General Information for thiazide and thiazide-like diuretics	—Thiazide-like diuretic
Metolazone (Zaroxolyn)	Initial oral: 2.5–10 mg/d Maximum: 20 mg/d	See General Information for thiazide and thiazide-like diuretics	See General Information for thiazide and thiazide-like diuretics	See General Information for thiazide and thiazide-like diuretics	—Thiazide-like diuretics —May be useful in patients with CrCl <30 mL/min —Long half-life may cause prolonged diuresis —Hypokalemia may limit duration of therapy

(*continued*)

Drug	Dose	Mechanism of action	Indications	Side effects	Comments
Potassium sparing					
Amiloride (Midamor)	Initial oral: 5 mg/d Maximum: 20 mg/d	Acts directly on the distal convoluted tubule and collecting ducts to decrease active transport of sodium and potassium	Labeled: Adjunctive diuretic to thiazide and loop diuretics Unlabeled: Reduce lithium-associated polyuria, hyperaldosteronism	—Nausea/vomiting/diarrhea —Headache —Rash —Hyperkalemia —Hyperchloremic metabolic acidosis —Hyponatremia —Gynecomastia —Impotence	—Weak diuretic effect, and its use is to help prevent hypokalemia in patients on potassium-wasting diuretics —Use cautiously in patients with renal dysfunction secondary to potential for hyperkalemia —Avoid use in patients with serum potassium levels $>$5.5 mEq/L —Avoid use in diabetic patients with microalbuminuria
Eplerenone (Inspra)	Initial oral: 50 mg/d	Competitive inhibitor of aldosterone at the mineralocorticoid receptors	Labeled: Hypertension	—Diarrhea —Dizziness —Gynecomastia (less common than spironolactone)	—Do not use in males with a serum creatinine $>$2 mg/dL and in females with a serum creatinine $>$1.8 mg/dL
	Maximum: 50 mg twice daily		Unlabeled: Adjunctive treatment in patients post MI with LV dysfunction	—Abnormal vaginal bleeding —Hyperkalemia	—Avoid potassium supplements and potassium-sparing diuretics —Eplerenone is metabolized by the cytochrome P450 3A4 isoenzyme and should be avoided with potent inhibitors of this enzyme

Spironolactone (Aldactone)	Initial oral: 50 mg 1–2 times daily	Competitive inhibitor of aldosterone at the mineralocorticoid receptors	Labeled: Primary aldosteronism, edema, hypertension, and hypokalemia associated with loop or thiazide diuretics	—Hyperkalemia —Fatigue —Gynecomastia —Sexual dysfunction —Breast tenderness in women	—Long half-life of metabolites —Use cautiously in patients with renal dysfunction secondary to hyperkalemia
	Maximum: 400 mg/d		Unlabeled: Adjunctive therapy for patients with class III–IV HF	—Nausea/vomiting/ diarrhea —Confusion	—Reduces morbidity and mortality in severe HF when added to standard HF therapy. Patients in the randomized Aldactone evaluation study were enrolled if serum creatinine was less than 2.5 mg/dL and serum potassium level was less than 5 mmol/L —Gynecomastia occurred in about 10% of patients receiving spironolactone
Triamterene (Dyrenium)	Initial oral: 50 mg/d Maximum: 300 mg/d	Acts directly on the distal convoluted tubule and collecting ducts to decrease active transport of sodium and potassium	Labeled: Edema and hypokalemia associated with loop or thiazide diuretics	—Rash —Hyperkalemia —Nausea/vomiting/diarrhea —Hyponatremia —Megaloblastic anemia (see Comments)	—Use cautiously in patients with renal dysfunction secondary to hyperkalemia —May cause metabolic acidosis —Megaloblastic anemia may occur in alcoholic cirrhosis

(*continued*)

Drug	Dose	Mechanism of action	Indications	Side effects	Comments
Carbonic anhydrase inhibitors					
Acetazolamide (Diamox)	Initial oral: 250 mg 1–4 times daily	Carbonic anhydrase inhibitor	Labeled: Edema, centrencephalic epilepsies, glaucoma, acute mountain sickness	—Malaise —Anorexia —Diarrhea	—Not useful as a diuretic for long-term treatment; looses effectiveness within 24–48 h
	Maintenance: Varies			—Metallic taste —Depression —Rash —Black stools	—Causes a metabolic acidosis —Reduce dose in patients with renal dysfunction —Ineffective when CrCl <10 mL/min —May be used acutely for metabolic alkalosis
	IV: 250–500 mg once daily for edema				
Vasopressin Antagonists					
Conivaptan (Vaprisol)	Loading dose: 20 mg infused over 30 minutes Maintenance dose: 20 mg infused over 24 h. If adequate results not achieved, the infusion can be increased to 40 mg over 24 h. Infusion should not exceed 4 d	Dual $V_{1a\ and\ 2}$ receptor inhibitor. Predominate free water excretion occurs through the inhibition of V_2 receptors in the renal-collecting ducts	Labeled: indicated in the treatment of euvolemic and hypervolemic hyponatremia	—Infusion site reactions —Orthostatic hypotension —Gastrointestinal	Monitor for resolution of hyponatremia to prevent rapid changes in serum sodium levels and to monitor for efficacy

Inotropic Agents					
Inamrinone (Inocor)	Loading dose: 0.5 mg/kg given over 5 min (see Comments)	Myocardial cell phosphodiesterase inhibitor that results in an increase in intracellular CAMP, thereby increasing contractility. It is also a potent vasodilator by direct effects on vascular smooth muscle	Labeled: Short-term management of CHF	—Thrombocytopenia —Ventricular arrhythmias	—If hypotension occurs during loading dose, decrease the rate of administration and give over 15–20 min
	Maintenance dose: 5–5 μg/kg/min			—Hypotension —Nausea —Hepatotoxicity —Hypersensitivity reactions	—Half-life prolonged in patients with HF —Thrombocytopenia dose and duration dependent occurring within 48–72 h. Reversible upon discontinuation —Consider dosage adjustment in patients with renal failure and liver dysfunction —Long half-life (4–6 h) may cause prolonged hypotension in patients —**Note generic name change**

(*continued*)

Drug	Dose	Mechanism of action	Indications	Side effects	Comments
Dopamine (Intropin)	1–3 μg/kg/min primarily dopamine effects	Mixed α, β, and dopaminergic agonist	Labeled: Hypotension, shock secondary to cardiac origin septicemia, and trauma	—Tachycardia —Ventricular arrhythmias —Hypertension	—Dose-dependent effects; lower doses produce an increase in renal blood flow, in medium-range doses, β effects predominate; and in higher doses, α effects predominate
	5–10 μg/kg/min primarily β effects 10–20 μg/kg/min primarily α effects			—Headache —Nausea	—Central line is recommended —Skin necrosis may occur with extravasation —Short half-life <2 min —Central line required when given by continuous infusion
Dobutamine (Dobutrex)	2.5–20 μg/kg/min	Relatively selective β-receptor agonist	Labeled: Short-term inotropic support in patients with acute cardiac decompensation	—Tachycardia —Hypotension/hypertension —Ventricular arrhythmias —Nausea —Headache —Myocardial ischemia	—Dose-dependent tachycardia —Tachyphylaxis may occur with prolonged administration —Long-term home administration in dependent patients may have an increase in mortality, secondary to ventricular arrhythmias —May be used in combination with phosphodiesterase inhibitors

Epinephrine (Adrenalin)	0.01–0.05 μg/kg/min primarily β effects 0.05–1 μg/kg/min α and β effects	Mixed α and β agonist	Labeled: Ventricular stand-still, shock, anaphylaxis	—Tachycardia —Flushing —Hypertension —Restlessness —Exacerbation of narrow-angle glaucoma —Ventricular arrhythmias	—May decrease renal and splanchnic blood flow secondary to vasoconstriction —Increase myocardial oxygen demand —Central line required for continuous infusion —Extravasation may lead to skin necrosis —Short half-life, approximately 2 min —Central line required when given by continuous infusion
Isoproterenol (Isuprel)	2–20 μg/kg/min	Nonselective β-receptor agonist	Labeled: Shock, heart block, Adams-Stokes attacks, bronchospasm Unlabeled: Bradycardia until temporary pacing can be accomplished, torsade de pointes	—Tachycardia —Ventricular arrhythmias —Hypotension —Myocardial ischemia —Mild tremors —Nervousness —Flushing	—Short half-life <5 min —May worsen myocardial ischemia —More likely to induce arrhythmias than other inotropic agents —May be effective in patients with β-blocker overdose
Milrinone (Primacor)	Loading dose: 50 μg/kg Maintenance dose: 0.375–7.5 μg/kg/min	Myocardial cell phosphodiesterase inhibitor that results in an increase in intracellular cAMP thus Increased contractility. It is also a potent vasodilator by direct effects on vascular smooth muscle	Labeled: Short-term management of CHF	—Hypotension —Ventricular arrhythmias —Supra ventricular arrhythmias —Angina —Chest pain —Headache —Tremor —Thrombocytopenia (rare)	—Thrombocytopenia occurs in <1% of patients —Long-term therapy may increase mortality secondary to ventricular arrhythmias —May be used in combination with dobutamine because of different mechanism of action —May be useful in patients with β-blocker overdose to increase contractility

(*continued*)

Drug	Dose	Mechanism of action	Indications	Side effects	Comments
Lipid-lowering agents ***Bile Acid Resins***					
Cholestyramine (Questran (*Light*))	Initial oral: 4 g 1–2 times daily (anhydrous cholestyramine) Maximum: 24 g/d divided doses (anhydrous cholestyramine)	Bind intestinal bile acids preventing enterohepatic recycling leading to increased stool elimination of bile acid	Labeled: Hyper-cholesterolemia, and relief of partial biliary obstruction pruritus Unlabeled: *Clostridium difficile* toxin binder, adjunct to thyroid and digitalis overdose	—Constipation —Flatulence —Abdominal pain —Bloating —Heartburn —Steatorrhea —Diarrhea —Hypertriglyceridemia	—4 g of cholestyramine = 5 g of colestipol —Many drug interactions: digoxin, thyroid hormones, warfarin, fat-soluble vitamins, others —Separate from other medications —May raise triglycerides —High rate of noncompliance secondary to taste —No systemic effects
Colestipol (Colestid)	Initial oral: 5 g 1–2 times daily Maximum: Powder 30 g/d divided doses Tablets 16 g/d divided doses	See cholestyramine	Labeled: Hyper-cholesterolemia Unlabeled: Adjunct to digitalis overdose	See cholestyramine	

Colesevelam (WelChol)	Initial dose: 3 tablets (1875 mg) twice daily with food or 6 tablets once daily with a meal Maximum dose: 7 tablets daily in divided doses	See cholestyramine	Labeled: Hyper-cholesterolemia	See cholestyramine	—May interfere with other medications absorption. Take 2 h before to 4 h after other medications —More convenient for patients because of tablet formulation
Fibric Acids					
Clofibrate (Atromid-S)	Initial oral: 1 g twice daily	—Exact mechanism unknown; however, triglyceride and VLDL clearance is increased and decreases cholesterol synthesis	Labeled: Type III, IV, and V hyperlipidemia	—Nausea —Dyspepsia —Flatulence —Myalgia —Increases AST/ALT	—Rarely used because it increases risk of cholelithiasis and hepatic malignancy (animal studies) with no substantial cardiovascular benefits
				—Renal failure (rare)	—Monitor liver function tests and CBC
				—Anemia, agranulocytosis, leukopenia	—Contraindicated in patients with significant hepatic and renal dysfunction, primary biliary cirrhosis, and pregnancy —Reduce dose in patients with renal dysfunction —Enhance effects of warfarin, insulin, and sulfonylureas

(*continued*)

Drug	Dose	Mechanism of action	Indications	Side effects	Comments
Fenofibrate (Tricor)	Initial oral: 48–145 mg/d	—Exact mechanism unknown —Inhibits triglyceride synthesis and stimulates catabolism of VLDL	Labeled: Types IV and V hyperlipidemia	—Rash —Gastrointestinal disturbances	—Combination with a HMG-CoA reductase inhibitor may increase risk of rhabdomyolysis
	Maximum dose: 145 mg/d			—Increases AST/ALT —Arthralgia —Headache —Flulike symptoms —Dyspepsia	—Contraindicated in patients with severe hepatic and renal disease, and gall bladder disease —Monitor liver function tests —Reduce dose to 48 mg/d in the elderly and patients with renal dysfunction —May enhance effects of warfarin —Bile acid sequestrants decrease absorption
Gemfibrozil (Lopid)	Initial oral: 600 mg twice daily	—Exact mechanism unknown; however, there is inhibition of lipolysis, decreased VLDL levels, and increased HDL levels	Labeled: Types IV and V hyperlipidemia, and reduces risk of coronary heart disease in type IIb patients	—Dyspepsia —Abdominal pain —Cholelithiasis —Diarrhea —Fatigue —Mild to moderate hyperglycemia —Rash —Hepatotoxicity —Drowsiness/dizziness —Blurred vision	—Associated with rhabdomyolysis when given with statins —Occasional hematologic abnormalities —Monitor liver function tests —May enhance warfarin effects

HMG-CoA reductase inhibitors					
General information		Inhibit HMG-CoA, the rate-controlling enzyme for endogenous cholesterol production		—Heartburn/flatulation/nausea —Rash/pruritus —Increased creatine phosphokinase —Myalgia —Lenticula opacities —Gynecomastia —Hepatotoxicity	—Many statins are substrates for cytochrome P450 system 3A4 to different degrees, and inhibitors of this enzyme may increase statin levels, increasing risk for rhabdomyolysis —Pravastatin and fluvastatin are not metabolized by the CYP 3A4 system —Rhabdomyolysis is rare but increases with concomitant administration of cyclosporine, gemfibrozil, niacin, erythromycin, itraconazole, and ketoconazole —May enhance warfarin effects —Monitor liver function periodically —Statins produce a dose-dependent reduction in LDL
Atorvastatin (Lipitor)	Initial oral: 10 mg/d Maximum: 80 mg/d	See General Information for HMG-CoA reductase inhibitors	Labeled: Hyper-cholesterolemia and mixed lipidemia	See General Information for HMG-CoA reductase inhibitors	—Greatest effect on LDL cholesterol and triglycerides
Fluvastatin (Lescol)	Initial oral: 20–40 mg/d Maximum: 80 mg/d	See General Information for HMG-CoA reductase inhibitors	Labeled: Hyper-cholesterolemia	See General Information for HMG-CoA reductase inhibitors	—Weakest effect on LDL

(*continued*)

Drug	Dose	Mechanism of action	Indications	Side effects	Comments
Lovastatin (Mevacor)	Initial oral: 10–20 mg/d Maximum: 80 mg/d	See General Information for HMG-CoA reductase inhibitors	Labeled: Hypercholesterolemia, and slow the progression of atherosclerosis	See General Information for HMG-CoA reductase inhibitors	—Taking with evening meals increases absorption
Pravastatin (Pravachol)	Initial oral: 10–20 mg/d Maximum: 40 mg/d	See General Information for HMG-CoA reductase inhibitors	Labeled: Slow progression of atherosclerosis, primary prevention of coronary events, and hypercholesterolemia	See General Information for HMG-CoA reductase inhibitors	
Rosuvastatin (Crestor®)	Initial oral: 5–10 mg/d Maximum: 40 mg/day	See General Information for HMG-CoA reductase inhibitors	Labeled: Reduce elevated TC, LDL-C, ApoB, non–HDL-C, and triglyceride levels and increase HDL-C in patients with primary hypercholesterolemia and mixed dyslipidemia	—Proteinuria	—Low potential for drug interactions with the cytochrome P450 enzyme system

				—See General Information for HMG-CoA reductase inhibitors	—Dose can be taken with or without food and is independent of time of day —90% of drug is excreted in the feces —Higher doses may cause proteinuria. Clinical significance yet to be determined.
Simvastatin (Zocor)	Initial oral: 5–10 mg/d Maximum: 40 mg/d	See General Information for HMG-CoA reductase inhibitors	Labeled: Hyper-cholesterolemia and coronary heart disease	See General Information for HMG-CoA reductase inhibitors	
Others					
Niacin (nicotinic acid) (Various)	Initial oral: 100 mg 2–3 times daily titrated to 3 g/d Maximum: 8 g/d divided doses	—Exact mechanism unknown —Inhibition of lipolysis, reduced LDL and VLDL synthesis, and increased lipoprotein lipase activity may be involved	Labeled: Vitamin B_3 replacement Unlabeled: Hyper-cholesterolemia	—Facial flushing —Hyperuricemia —Flushing minimized with aspirin —Hyperglycemia	—Sustained release formulations are avoided because of greater risk for hepatotoxicity —Effective for decreased TC, LDL, and triglycerides, and increased HDL
				—Gastric irritation —Pruritus —Chemical hepatitis	—Food helps to decrease GI intolerance

(*continued*)

Drug	Dose	Mechanism of action	Indications	Side effects	Comments
Ezetimibe (Zetia)	Initial dose: 10 mg once daily Maximum dose: 10 mg/d	Ezetimibe acts at the brush-border cells and blocks intestinal absorption of meal-derived cholesterol and bile acids in the small intestine	Labeled: —Primary hyper-cholesterolemia (monotherapy and in combination with statins —Homozygous familial hyper-cholesterolemia —Homozygous sitosterolemia	—Abdominal pain and diarrhea —Headache —Sinusitis —Dizziness —Chest pain	—Avoid use in patients with moderate to severe hepatic dysfunction —This drug has little systemic effect —Take this medication 2 h before or 4 h after a bile acid sequestrant
Nitrates					
General information		Biotransformation of nitrates release nitric oxide, causing vasodilatation through cAMP. Venous dilation predominates.		—Headache —Hypotension (large doses) —Flushing —Dizziness —Rash —Nausea —Methemoglobinemia —Reflex tachycardia	—Long-term nitrate use without nitrate-free intervals leads to nitrate tolerance; with loss of hemodynamic and antianginal effects; mechanism is controversial —Tolerance can be limited by providing a nitrate-free interval of 10–12 h —Headache and postural hypotension usually decrease over several days of therapy —Causes coronary artery dilation and improves collateral blood flow

Isosorbide dinitrate (Isordil, Sorbitrate)	Initial oral: 10 mg three times daily allowing for a 12-h nitrate-free interval Maximum: 40 mg/dose	—See General Information for nitrates	Labeled: Prevention of anginal attacks Unlabeled: HF when used in combination with hydralazine	—See General Information for nitrates	—Used in combination with hydralazine in CHF
Isosorbide Mononitrate (Imdur, Ismo, Monoket)	Initial oral: Immediate release 10–20 mg two times daily separated by 7 h Sustained release: 15–30 mg/d	—See General Information for nitrates	Labeled: Prevention of anginal attacks	—See General Information for nitrates	—Longer half-life may lead to nitrate tolerance with frequent dosing
Nitroglycerin Paste (Nitrol)	Initial: $\frac{1}{2}$–4 inches every 6 h holding one dose to allow for a 1 h nitrate-free interval	—See General Information for nitrates	Labeled: Prevention of anginal attacks	—See General Information for nitrates	—Inconvenient for long-term therapy because of ointment being messy —Dose absorbed is related to skin surface area in which ointment is applied —Quick onset once applied to skin
Nitroglycerin Patch	0.2–0.8 mg/h patch on for 12 h and off for 12 h	—See General Information for nitrates	Labeled: Prevention of anginal attacks	—See General Information for nitrates —Contact dermatitis	—Some patients develop a contact dermatitis with certain patches —Inform patients to rotate patch sites

(*continued*)

Drug	Dose	Mechanism of action	Indications	Side effects	Comments
(Various) Nitroglycerin SL (Nitrostat, Nitrolingual spray)	Use as needed for chest pain 0.4 mg every 5 min three times per day	—See General Information for nitrates	Labeled: Acute for nitrates treatment or prophylaxis of anginal attacks	—See General Information for nitrates	—Each spray delivers 0.4 mg of nitroglycerin —Most common sublingual tablet is 0.4 mg (0.3–0.6 mg) —Effective for acute anginal attacks and prophylaxis of angina for known exertional activities —Tablets start degrading once bottle is opened and if stored correctly should be replaced every 3–6 mo
Nitroglycerin IV (Tridil)	IV: 5–10 μg/min initially then increase by 5–10 μg/min every 5–10 min for relief of chest pain	—See General Information for nitrates	Labeled: Perioperative hypertension, CHF with acute MI, angina Unlabeled: Hypertensive crisis; pulmonary hypertension	—See General Information for nitrates	—Methemoglobinemia may occur with high doses —May increase intracranial pressure —IV formulation is poorly soluble

Miscellaneous antianginal medication					
Ranolazine (Ranexa)	Initial dose: 500 mg every 12 h Maximum dose: 1000 mg every 12 h	Exact mechanism of action is unclear. May be related to changing myocardial energy production from free fatty acid to glucose, improving efficiency of ATP production, and also to sodium channel inhibition	Labeled: Treatment of chronic angina in combination with amlodipine, beta-blockers or nitrates	—Dizziness —Constipation — QT prolongation	—Monitor for QT prolongation —Monitor for drug interactions with the cytochrome P450 enzymes especially CYP 3A4 —Strong CYP 3A4 inhibitors increase the levels of ranolazine that may increase the risk of QT prolongation
Platelet inhibitors ***Cyclooxygenase inhibitor***					
Aspirin	Initial oral: 162–325 mg once d Maintenance: 81–325 mg/d	Irreversibly acetylate platelet cyclo-oxygenase decreasing the formation of thromboxane A_2 from arachidonic acid	Labeled: Analgesic, antipyretic, anti-inflammatory, MI, TIAs, CVA	—Bleeding —Gastric ulceration —Nausea/dyspepsia/ heartburn —Hemolytic anemia —Tinnitus (large doses or overdose)	—Food and enteric coating decreases gastric upset

(*continued*)

Drug	Dose	Mechanism of action	Indications	Side effects	Comments
Glycoprotein IIb/IIIa inhibitors					
Abciximab (ReoPro)	PCI: 0.25 mg/kg 10–60 min before intervention immediately followed by 0.125 μg/kg/min (maximum 10-μg/min) for 12 h Unstable angina with PCI: 0.25 mg/kg starting 18–24 h before PCI, immediately followed by 0.125 μg/kg/min (maximum 10 μg/min), infusion ending 1 h after intervention	Murine-derived monoclonal antibody Fab fragment to the human GP IIb/IIIa receptor on the platelet surface, inhibiting platelet aggregation	Labeled: Percutaneous coronary intervention and unstable angina when PCI is planned within 24 h	—Bleeding —Thrombocytopenia —Hypersensitivity reactions	—Platelet function returns to normal usually within 48 h; abciximab can be seen in the circulation bound to platelets for up to 10 d —Data is lacking for readministration of abciximab —Thrombocytopenia is rare and usually transient —Low immunogenicity —Full-dose abciximab with half-dose reteplase, should similar mortality result when compared to full-dose reteplase

Eptifibatide (Integrilin)	Acute coronary syndrome: Loading dose: 180 μg/kg bolus Maintenance dose: CrCl $\geq$50 mL/min 2 μg/kg/min for a maximum of 96 h CrCl $\leq$ 50 mL/min 1 μg/kg/min for a maximum of 96 h Contraindicated if dependent on renal dialysis (see Comments) PCI: Bolus dose: Double bolus of 180 μg/kg. Give first bolus of 180 μg/kg, then initiate the infusion and give second bolus 10 min after first dose. Maintenance infusion: CrCl $\geq$50 mL/min 2 μg/kg/min; infuse for 18 h after PCI	Heptapeptide antagonist that reversibly inhibits GP IIb/IIIa receptor on the platelet surface, inhibiting platelet aggregation	Labeled: —Acute coronary syndromes (unstable angina and non-Q-wave MI) with or without PCI —PCI with or without stent placement	—Bleeding —Thrombocytopenia	—Infusions should be continued for 18–24 h after PCI or atherectomy —All patients should receive aspirin —Most patients in clinical studies also received heparin before and during intervention —Use lower doses in patients with renal dysfunction —Data is emerging for use in ST-segment elevation MI in combination with half-dose thrombolytics

(continued)

Drug	Dose	Mechanism of action	Indications	Side effects	Comments
	CrCl $\leq$50 mL/min 1 μg/kg/min; infuse for 18 h after PCI Contraindicated if dependent on renal dialysis				
Tirofiban (Aggrastat)	Acute coronary syndrome: 0.4 μg/kg/min for 30 min, then 0.1 μg/kg/min for 96 h For patients with CrCl <30 mL/min, the dose should be cut in half	Nonpeptide antagonist that reversibly inhibits GP IIb/IIIa receptor on the platelet surface inhibiting platelet aggregation	Acute coronary syndrome in patients who are being treated medically and those undergoing PTCA or atherectomy	—Bleeding —Thrombocytopenia	—Infusions should continue for 12–24h after PTCA or atherectomy —Heparin and aspirin should be given concomitantly before and during PCI
Others					
Clopidogrel (Plavix)	Initial oral: 75 mg/d PCI: Initial oral: 300–600 mg once then maintenance Maintenance: 75 mg/d	Inhibition of adenosine diphosphate–induced platelet aggregation	Labeled: —Reduce the risk of MI, stroke, and/or peripheral arterial disease in patients with a completed MI, stroke, and/or peripheral arterial disease —Acute coronary syndromes	—Bleeding —Diarrhea —Headache —Dizziness —Abdominal pain/nausea/dyspepsia —Purpura —Rash	—Most side effects when compared to aspirin in clinical trials were less in the clopidogrel-treated group —Maximum effects are seen 3–7 d after initiating therapy —11 cases of TTP have been reported —Recent data suggest that clopidogrel be continued for at least 1 y after coronary artery stent placement

			Unlabeled: Adjunctive therapy after coronary artery stent placement with aspirin		
Ticlopidine (Ticlid)	Initial oral: 250 mg twice daily	See clopidogrel for mechanism of action information	Labeled: Reduce risk of thrombotic stroke in patients with completed thrombotic stroke or stroke precursors Unlabeled: Adjunctive therapy for coronary artery stent placement and alternative to aspirin in patients unable to take aspirin	—Bleeding —Diarrhea —Nausea/dyspepsia/vomiting/anorexia —Rash —Neutropenia —Purpura	—Severe neutropenia occurs in 0.8% of patients and has been associated with death —CBC with differential should be measured at baseline and every 2 wk for the first 3 mo of therapy —Patients should be monitored for fevers or other signs of infection —Case reports of TTP have been reported with ticlopidine —Maximum pharmacologic effects obtained 3–7 d after initiating therapy

(*continued*)

Drug	Dose	Mechanism of action	Indications	Side effects	Comments
Dipyridamole (Persantine)	Initial oral: 25–100 mg four times daily IV for stress test: 0.142 mg/kg/min over 4 min (0.57 mg/kg) to a maximum dose of 60 mg	Antiplatelet mechanism not established but related to inhibition of adenosine reuptake, phosphodiesterase inhibition, and inhibition of thromboxane A_2 formation Stress testing: Coronary vasodilation by preventing degradation of adenosine	Labeled: Adjunct to warfarin therapy to prevent postoperative thromboembolic events of cardiac valve and intravenously for stress test	—Exacerbation of angina —Dizziness —Hypotension —Tachycardia —Headache —Rash —GI distress —Dyspnea	—Methylxanthines antagonize the effects of dipyridamole and should be discontinued for 36–48 h before administration —Aminophylline 50–250 mg over 30–60 s may be given to reverse dipyridamole effects —Use with caution in patients with bronchospastic lung disease; may exacerbate asthma
Cilostazol (Pletal)	Initial oral dose: 100 mg twice daily	Selective phosphodiesterase inhibitor causing both vasodilation and antiplatelet effects	Labeled: Intermittent claudication to reduce symptoms Unlabeled: Adjunct to aspirin therapy in patients receiving coronary artery stent placement	—Headache —Palpitations —Diarrhea —Peripheral edema	—Take on an empty stomach —Do not use in patients with heart failure of any severity This is based on the historical trials of phosphodiesterase inhibitors in HF and potential for increasing mortality —Should not be used first-line in coronary artery stent placement because of mixed results from clinical trials

Alteplase, tPA (Activase)	*Acute MI accelerated (front loaded):* Patients >67 kg total dose = 100 mg 15 mg IV bolus, then 50 mg over 30 min, then 35 mg over 60 min Patients ≤67 kg total dose <100 mg 15 mg IV bolus, then 0.75 mg/kg (50 mg max) over 30 min, then 0.5 mg/kg (35 mg max) over 60 min *Acute ischemic stroke:* 0.9 mg/kg over 60 min with 10% of total dose given over the first min *Pulmonary embolism:* 100 mg given over 120 min	rTPA binds to clot-bound plasminogen to catalyze conversion to plasmin. The specificity for clot-bound plasminogen decreases systemic fibrinolysis	Labeled: Acute ST-segment elevation MI, pulmonary embolism, and acute ischemic stroke	—Bleeding —Intracranial hemorrhage (0.7%) —Hypotension —Nausea/vomiting —Epistaxis	—Acute MI patients should receive aspirin and heparin during TPA infusion —Pulmonary embolism heparin should be started at the end of the alteplase infusion —TPA is not specific for fresh clot and binds to any clot-bound plasminogen —No antigenicity; therefore may be used without risk of antibody formation —Short half-life of about 4 min —Considered superior to streptokinase —Risk of intracranial hemorrhage > streptokinase —Age >65 years old and weight <70 kg are independent risk factors for intracranial hemorrhage
Reteplase, rPA	Acute MI 10 units over 2 min followed by a second 10-U bolus in 30 min	Single stranded mutant of wild-type TPA with similar action to TPA with less high-affinity fibrin binding, but increased potency	Labeled: Acute ST segment elevation MI	—Bleeding	—Combination half-dose reteplase with full-dose Abciximab was evaluated in the GUSTO V trial and found not to be inferior to reteplase full dose. There was no mortality benefit at 1 year —Intracranial hemorrhage

(*continued*)

Drug	Dose	Mechanism of action	Indications	Side effects	Comments
Streptokinase, SK (Streptase)	Acute MI: Intravenous: 1.5 million IU over 60 min Intracoronary 20,000 IU followed by 2000 IU/min for 60 min (total dose = 140,000 IU) Pulmonary embolism: 250,000 IU given IV over 30 min, then 100,000 IU/h for 24 h. May continue for 72 h if DVT suspected DVT: 250,000 IU given IV over 30 min, then 100,000 IU/h for 72 h Arterial thrombosis or embolism: 250,000 IU given IV over 30 min, then 100,000 IU/h for 24–72 h	Binds to clot-bound and circulating plasminogen; this complex then catalyzes conversion of plasminogen to plasmin. Not specific for clot-bound plasminogen and therefore produces a systemic fibrinolytic state.	Labeled: Acute ST segment elevation MI, pulmonary embolism, DVT, arterial thrombosis or embolism, occlusion of cannulae	—Bleeding —Bronchospasm —Periorbital swelling —Angioedema edema —Anaphylaxis —Hypotension —Rash —Intracranial hemorrhage (0.2%) —Fever —Urticaria	—Patients should not receive streptokinase if within the last 1–4 y they have received APSAC or streptokinase —Intracranial hemorrhage occurs less often than with alteplase —Heparin usually not given with streptokinase; if needed, the heparin is initiated 4 h after streptokinase infusion without a bolus

	Arteriovenous cannulae occlusion: Instill 250,000 IU in 2 mL of solution into each occluded limb of cannula slowly. Clamp off cannula for 12 h. After treatment aspirate contents, flush with saline, and reconnect cannula.				
Tenecteplase (TNK-ase)	Acute MI: Single IV bolus given over 5 s	TNK-TPA binds to clot-bound plasminogen to catalyze conversion to plasmin. The point mutations increase fibrin specificity, decrease clearance, and decrease inhibition from plasminogen activator inhibitor 1	Labeled: Acute ST-segment elevation MI	—Bleeding —Intracranial hemorrhage —Hypotension may occur	—Bleeding and rates of intracranial hemorrhage are dose dependent. Dose greater than 0.5 mg/kg conferred a higher risk —Efficacy was no different than patients treated with alteplase. On subgroup analysis, patients presenting >4 h but <6 h had a lower mortality rate if treated with tenecteplase —Single IV bolus is more convenient than rate-adjusted infusions and double-bolus methods —Heparin infusions were continued for 48–72 h

(*continued*)

Drug	Dose	Mechanism of action	Indications	Side effects	Comments
	Weight (kg)	*Dose (mg)*			
	<60	30	—		—Enoxaparin has been used with tenecteplase
	≥ 60 to <70	35			—Half-dose tenecteplase and full-dose glycoprotein IIb/IIIa inhibitors are being evaluated for ST-segment elevation MI
	≥ 70 to <80	40			
	≥ 80 to <90	45			
	≥ 90	50			
Urokinase (Abbokinase)	Pulmonary embolism: 4400 IU/kg over 10 min, then 4400 IU/kg/h for 12 h Intracoronary infusion: 750,000 IU over 2 h; 6000 IU/min for 2 h Large-vessel thrombi: 4400 IU/kg over 10 min, then 4400 IU/kg/h for 24–72 h	Directly activates plasminogen; causes less systemic fibrinolysis than streptokinase	Labeled: Pulmonary embolism, intracoronary administration for coronary artery thrombosis, intravenous catheter clearance	—Bleeding —Allergic reactions —Fever/chills/rigors	—Less antigenic than streptokinase —Shorter half-life than streptokinase; therefore, it produces less systemic fibrinolysis

Vasodilators					
Diazoxide	IV bolus: 1–3 mg/kg (150 mg max) over 30 s (see Comments)	Direct relaxation of arteriolar smooth muscle	Labeled: Hypertensive emergencies (IV) and hypoglycemia (PO)	—Hypotension —Nausea/vomiting —Dizziness —Hyperglycemia —Edema	—Not used often because of unpredictable lowering of blood pressure —Causes hyperglycemia via inhibition of insulin release and decreasing peripheral utilization of glucose
	IV Infusion: 10–30 mg/min up to 5 mg/kg until blood pressure controlled; may repeat every 4–24 h as needed (see Comments)			—Thrombocytopenia —Hirsutism	—May induce cerebral or myocardial ischemia —Significant sodium and water reabsorption with repeated dosing —Oral therapy may be used for chronic hypoglycemia related to insulin-secreting tumors —IV therapy should not be used for more than 10 days
Hydralazine (Apresoline)	Initial oral: 10–25 mg 3–4 times daily Maximum: 600 mg/d (see Comments)	Direct relaxation of arteriolar smooth muscle	Labeled: Hypertension (PO), hypertensive emergencies (IV) Unlabeled: HF	—Palpitations —Flushing —Tachycardia —Myocardial ischemia —Headache —Nausea/vomiting/anorexia —Hypotension	—Hydralazine IV has unpredictable effects and is rarely used for hypertensive emergencies —Long-term use may lead to drug-induced SLE —Increases intracranial pressure —May increase myocardial oxygen demand and potentially causes myocardial ischemia

(*continued*)

Drug	Dose	Mechanism of action	Indications	Side effects	Comments
	IV: 10–20 mg 4–6 times daily up to 40 mg/dose			—Drug-induced SLE —Sodium and water retention	—Doses as high as 2 gm/d have been safely used
Fenoldopam (Corlopam)	IV: 0.025–0.3 μg/kg/min (see Comments)	Dopamine-1 receptor agonist causing smooth muscle relaxation, causing vasodilation and increased renal blood flow	Labeled: Short-term management of hypertensive emergencies and urgencies	—Hypotension —Headache —Flushing —Nausea —Tachycardia —Hypokalemia (rarely)	—Some clinical trials used doses of up to 1.6 μg/kg/min —Most patients respond to 0.1–0.8 μg/kg/min —Increased renal blood flow, increased CrCl in clinical trials —Short half-life of 5–10 min —Natriuresis and diuresis can be seen —Very expensive —Blood pressure-lowering effects equal to that of nitroprusside —Use with caution in patients with glaucoma —No toxic metabolites —Recently presented data suggest there is no role for fenoldopam in the prevention of contrast-induced nephropathy

Minoxidil (Loniten)	Initial oral: 2.5–5 mg/d Maximum: 100 mg/d in divided doses	Direct vasodilator with primary effect on arterial smooth muscle	Labeled: Hypertension Unlabeled: HF	—Significant reflex tachycardia —Sodium and water retention —Edema —Weight gain —Hypertrichosis —Breast tenderness —Gynecomastia —Headache	—Use with β-blockers to decrease reflex tachycardia —Sodium and water retention will occur, and patients commonly need diuretics
Nicardipine IV	Initial IV Dose: 5 mg/h increase by 2.5 mg/h every 15 minutes until a maximum of 15 mg/h; once blood pressure goal is achieved, decrease dose to 3 mg/h and titrate as needed	See calcium channel blockers	Hypertensive emergency	See calcium channel blockers	—Peripheral IV infusions need to be rotated every 12 h to minimize risk of phlebitis
Nitroprusside (sodium) (Nipride)	IV: 0.3–10 μg/kg/min Most patients require 3 μg/kg/min Doses should not exceed 10 μg/kg/min for more than 10 min (see Comments)	Direct vasodilation occurs secondary to the liberation of the nitroso group from the nitrosocyanide structure. It possesses a balanced effect on both veins and arteries.	Labeled: Hypertensive emergencies, and management of acute CHF	—Hypotension —Thiocyanate toxicity —Cyanide toxicity —Headache —Nausea —Confusion —Metabolic acidosis	—Doses of 10 μg/kg/min for greater than 10 min increases the risk of developing cyanide toxicity —Short half-life of about 3 min —Patients with hepatic failure are at an increased risk of developing cyanide toxicity: this is suspected in patients with a metabolic acidosis, venous hyperoxemia, increased lactate, air hunger, confusion, seizures, ataxia, and potentially stroke

(*continued*)

Drug	Dose	Mechanism of action	Indications	Side effects	Comments
					—Patients with suspected cyanide toxicity should receive inhaled amyl nitrite while administering 300 mg of IV sodium nitrite, then administer 12.5 mg of IV sodium thiosulfate. If symptoms reappear administer half the amount of sodium nitrite and sodium thiosulfate. These modalities shift cyanide conversion to thiocyanate. Cyanide levels are not helpful because it may take up to 5 d to receive results —Thiocyanate is a neurotoxin causing confusion psychosis, lethargy, tinnitus, convulsions, and hyperreflexia Hemodialysis removes thiocyanate from the blood. Levels are typically not monitored unless infusion of >3 d or when high doses are used in patients with renal failure

Ambrisentan (Letairis)	Initial dose: 5 mg/d Maximum dose: 10 mg/d	Endothelin receptor antagonist (types ET-A and ET-B)	Labeled: Management of patients with pulmonary hypertension with class II or III symptoms to improve exercise capacity and delay clinical worsening	—Hepatotoxicity —Peripheral edema —Nasal congestion —Teratogenic	—Patients tolerating 5 mg/d should have their dose increased to 10 mg/d —Contraindicated in pregnancy. Women of childbearing age should use 2 forms of birth control unless they have received a tubal ligation or have certain IUDs. —Women must have a negative pregnancy test before initiating therapy and monthly pregnancy tests to assure they are not pregnant —Monitor for drug interactions with the cytochrome P450 enzyme system —Liver function tests (LFT) need to be performed before initiating therapy and monthly to monitor for liver function abnormalities —If LFTs increase >3 times the upper limit of normal but <5 times the upper limit of normal, then reduce dose or discontinue therapy and monitor LFTs every two weeks until they decrease <3 times the upper limit of normal

(*continued*)

Drug	Dose	Mechanism of action	Indications	Side effects	Comments
					—If measured LFT >5 times the upper limit of normal but <8 times the upper limit of normal, then discontinue therapy and monitor levels frequently until levels drop to <3 times the upper limit of normal. At that time may reinitiate therapy with more frequent measurements of LFTs —If at any time the LFTs are >8 times the upper limit of normal, therapy should be discontinued and not reinitiated —Like bosentan, ambrisentan can only be obtained through a specialized distribution program called the Letairis Education and Access Program (LEAP)
Bosentan (Tracleer)	Initial oral dose: 62.5 mg twice daily for 4 wk	Endothelin receptor antagonist (types ET-A and ET-B)	Labeled: Management of pulmonary arterial hypertension in patients with WHO class III or IV symptoms	—Severe hepatocellular damage (11%) —Teratogenic —Headache —Flushing —Hypotension	—Initial dose is 62.5 mg twice daily; after 4 wk if this dose is tolerated, then increase dose to 125 mg twice daily. Monitor aminotransferase and bilirubin levels at baseline and then monthly

Maintenance oral dose: 125 mg twice daily (see Comments)	—Fatigue —Pruritus —Edema —Anemia	—Monitor liver function tests more frequently in patients who develop elevations of at least 3 times upper limit of normal —If ALT/AST levels are >3 but ≤5 times upper limit of normal, then repeat and confirm test; if still elevated, reduce dose or discontinue therapy and monitor levels every 2 wk. If ALT/AST levels return to normal, then continue or reintroduce therapy. —If ALT/AST levels are >5 but ≤8 times upper limit of normal, repeat test. If confirmed, stop therapy and monitor ALT/AST levels every 2 wk until they return to baseline. At this time may consider reintroduction of therapy —If ALT/AST levels are >8 times upper limit of normal, confirm with another test and if correct discontinue therapy and bosentan should not be reintroduced —After reintroduction of therapy, monitor ALT/AST levels at 3 d and then as above —Women of childbearing potential must have a negative baseline and monthly pregnancy test to be considered appropriate for therapy

(continued)

Drug	Dose	Mechanism of action	Indications	Side effects	Comments
					—Bosentan is only available as direct shipment from the company. Patients must be enrolled in the company's database for distribution. The cost is about $3500/mo —Bosentan is a potent inducer of the CYP 3A4 isoenzyme. This enzyme is the most ubiquitous of the CYP enzymes and is responsible for the metabolism of a number of medications. It is important to inform women of childbearing years that hormonal birth control methods may not be reliable methods and that other steps need to be used to assure adequate birth control —Bosentan is metabolized by the CYP 3A4 and 2C9 isoenzymes, and inhibitors of this enzyme may cause elevated levels of bosentan

Nesiritide (Natrecor)	Bolus dose: 2 μg/kg given over 1 min Maintenance infusion: 0.01 μg/kg/min for 48 h (see Comments for titration)	Recombinant human b type or brain natriuretic peptide. rhBNP binds to guanylate cyclase receptors in vascular smooth muscle and endothelial cells, increasing intracellular levels of cGMP causing venous and arterial dose-dependent reduction in PCWP and systemic blood pressure. Nesiritide causes a mild natriuresis as well.	Labeled: Intravenous management of acutely decompensated HF in patients who have rest or with minimal activity.	—Hypotension —Headache —Dizziness	—Avoid in patients with cardiogenic shock, aortic stenosis, and systolic blood pressures less than 90 mm Hg —Monitor urine output, blood pressure, and symptoms of HF —Infusions for more than 48 h have not been fully studied —Use lower intravenous diuretic doses when initiating nesiritide —Patients with baseline marginal blood pressures consider not giving initial bolus dose —About 70% of the peak blood pressure effect is seen within 15 min of initiation —Half-life approximately 18 min —Patients who develop hypotension may continue to be hypotensive for 2–2.5 h after drug discontinuation Reinitiating infusion can be done at a 30% reduction in dose —Dose titration can be done but is not encouraged secondary to increasing side effects (hypotension)

(*continued*)

Drug	Dose	Mechanism of action	Indications	Side effects	Comments
					—In clinical trials, dosage titrations were done in patients with pulmonary artery catheters and hemodynamic monitoring. Dosage increases were done by titrating the dose by 0.005 μg/kg/min every 3 h up to a maximum dose of 0.03 μg/kg/min —Elimination occurs by binding to cell surface receptors, internalization and lysosomal proteolysis, proteolytic cleavage by neutral endopeptidase, and renal filtration
Epoprostenol (Flolan)	Initial dose is 2 μg/kg/min, and increase every 15 min until dose-limiting pharmacologic or adverse effects are seen. Once this occurs, decrease dose by 2 μg/kg/min until symptoms are relieved. This will be the chronic dose	Prostaglandin I_2 is a vasodilator of the systemic as well as the pulmonary arteries. Also, it inhibits platelet aggregation	Labeled: Primary pulmonary hypertension and pulmonary hypertension related to scleroderma in patients failing conventional therapy	—Jaw pain —Hypotension —Headache —Rash —Diarrhea —Joint pain —Noncardiogenic pulmonary edema —Line-related infections	—During chronic infusions, doses may need to be adjusted upward or downward depending on the clinical response of the patient —The half-life is 3–5 min Therefore, abrupt discontinuation of medications will not be tolerated by most patients —All patients need a chronic indwelling central catheter, which may be a source of infection —Noncardiogenic pulmonary edema can be seen with epoprostenol

					—Most patients complain of jaw pain —Patients must be able to prepare infusion bags at home and understand how to use miniature infusion pumps
Vasopressors					
Dopamine (Intropin)	See dopamine under inotropic agents	Mixed α, β, and dopaminergic antagonists	See dopamine under inotropic agents	See dopamine under inotropic agents	—Initially may see initial vasodilatation then vasoconstriction —α effects are typically seen with doses greater than 10 μg/kg/min —Central line required when given by continuous infusion
Epinephrine (Adrenalin)	See epinephrine under inotropic agents	Mixed α and β antagonist	See epinephrine under inotropic agents	See epinephrine under inotropic agents	—See epinephrine under inotropic agents —With lower doses, β effects predominate, and with higher doses, α effects predominate —Vasopressor of choice in septic shock —Acidemia may blunt pressor effects —Endotracheal administration in cardiac arrest is 2–2.5 times that of IV —Central line required when given by continuous infusion

(*continued*)

Drug	Dose	Mechanism of action	Indications	Side effects	Comments
Norepinephrine (Levophed)	0.1–3.5 μg/kg/min	Mixed α and β antagonist	Hypotension	—Hypertension —Headache —Trembling —Ventricular arrhythmias	—Primary effect is vasoconstriction —Administer by central line —Extravasation may cause skin necrosis —Decreases renal splanchnic, hepatic, and peripheral blood flow due to vasoconstriction —β effects are usually off set by baroreceptor-mediated vagal stimulation —Central line required when given by continuous infusion
Phenylephedrine (Neo-Synephrine)	0.5–15 μg/kg/min	Pure α-antagonist	Hypotension	—Bradycardia —Hypertension —Myocardial ischemia	—No β effects —Useful in patients with tachycardia from mixed α/β antagonists —Administer by central line —Extravasation may cause skin necrosis —Central line required when given by continuous infusion
Miscellaneous agents					
Aminocaproic acid (Amicar)	IV: 4–5 g given over 1 h, then 1 g/h for 8 h or until bleeding stops	Inhibits activation of plasminogen to plasmin	Labeled: Enhance hemostasis when fibrinolysis contributes to bleeding	—Hypotension —Bradycardia —Rash —Headache —Myopathy —Tinnitus —GI irritation	—Reduce dose by 25% in patients with oliguria or ESRD: accumulates in this patient population —Decreased platelet function —Monitoring: fibrinogen, fibrin split products —Rapid infusions may cause hypotension, bradycardia, and arrhythmias —Randomized data lacking for counteracting thrombolytics

Digoxin Immune Fab (Digibind)	Dependent on total body stores of digoxin or digitoxin. If the amount of ingested or total body stores is unknown, then 20 vials should be administered. Infuse dose over 15–30 min through a 0.22-μm filter	Digoxin immune Fab binds to serum digoxin, decreasing free digoxin from binding to receptors	Labeled: Management of life-threatening digoxin or digitoxin toxicity	—Anaphylaxis —Serum sickness —Hypokalemia —Erythema at injection site	—Onset within 30 min —Many digoxin assays report inaccurate digoxin levels after Digibind therapy —Patients with known allergy to sheep proteins may have an anaphylactic reaction to Digibind —Patients with severe renal failure may have a delayed rebound toxicity with Digibind therapy —Each vial of digoxin immune Fab binds 0.6 mg of digoxin or digitoxin
Protamine sulfate	Variable: 1 mg binds about 100 U of heparin sodium; usual range 25–50 mg Maximum: 50 mg IV once	Protamine is a strong base that complexes with heparin (acid) and forms an inactive stable salt	Labeled: Heparin overdose	—Hypotension (see Comments) —Bradycardia (see Comments) —Dyspnea —Transient flushing —Hypersensitivity reactions (see Comments)	—Rapid onset of action and heparin neutralization occurs within 5 min —Hypotension, bradycardia, dyspnea, and flushing may occur with rapid administration —Hypersensitivity reactions, including anaphylaxis, occur in <1% of patients —Patients predisposed to hypersensitivity reactions include: patients allergic to fish, diabetics on insulin-containing protamine, and vasectomized males

(*continued*)

Drug	Dose	Mechanism of action	Indications	Side effects	Comments
Vitamin K—Phytonadione (Mephyton, AquaMephyton)	Variable: Range 0.5–10 mg subcutaneously, or IV 2.5–10 mg orally	Replete vit. K stores needed for the formation of blood coagulation factors II, VII, IX, and X in liver	Labeled: Hypoprothrombinemia secondary to: coumarin or indandione overdose, antibacterial therapy, malabsorption states and decreased synthesis, and prophylaxis and management of hemorrhage disease of newborns	—Rare hypersensitivity reactions	—Anaphylaxis has occurred in some patients

ACE, angiotensin-converting enzyme
AF, atrial fibrillation
AFL, atrial flutter
ALT, alanine aminotransferase
ANA, antinuclear antibody
APSAC, Anisoylated plasminogen streptokinase activator
aPTT, activated partial thromboplastin time
ARB, angiotensin II receptor blocker
AST, aspartate aminotransferase
AV, atrioventricular
AVNRT, atrioventricular node reentry tachycardia
BPH, benign prostatic hypertrophy
CBC, complete blood count
CHF, congestive heart failure
CNS, central nervous system
CrCl, creatine clearance
CVA, cardiovascular accident
DVT, deep venous thrombosis
ECG, electrocardiogram
ET, endothelin
GI, gastrointestinal
GP, glycoprotein
HDL, high-density lipoprotein
HIT, heparin-induced thrombocytopenia
HITT, heparin-induced thrombocytopenia and thrombosis
HMG-CoA, 3-hydroxy-3-methylglutaryl coenzyme A
HTN, hypertension
INR, international normalized ratio
LMWH, low–molecular-weight heparin
LV, left ventricular
MAOI, monoamine oxidase inhibitor
MI, myocardial infarction
NAPA, N-ACETV1-Procainamide
NS, normal saline
NSR, normal sinus rhythm
NYHA, New York Heart Association
PCI, percutaneous coronary intervention
PCWP, pulmonary capillary wedge pressure
PE, pulmonary embolism
PT, prothrombin
PTCA, percutaneous transluminal coronary angioplasty
PUD, peptic ulcer disease
rTPA, recombinant tissue plasminogen activator
SA, sinoatrial
SLE, systemic lupus erythematosus
TC, total cholesterol
TPA, tissue plasminogen activator
TTP, thrombotic thrombocytopenic purpura
TIA, transient ischemic attack
VLDL, very-low-density lipoprotein
WHO, World Health Organization
WPW, Wolff-Parkinson-White (syndrome)

INDEX

Page numbers followed by t indicate table; those in *italics* indicate figure.